ESSENTIALS OF Paramedic Care

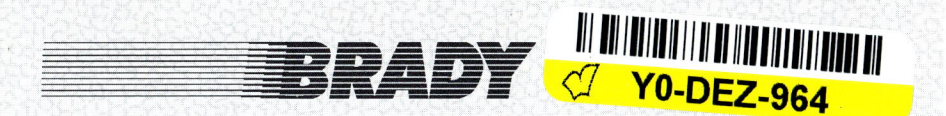

Instructor's Resource Manual

SECOND EDITION

Tony Crystal, ScD, EMT-P, RPhT

BRYAN E. BLEDSOE, DO, FACEP, EMT-P
Adjunct Associate Professor of Emergency Medicine
The George Washington University Medical Center
Washington, DC
and
Emergency Physician
Midlothian, Texas

ROBERT S. PORTER, MA, NREMT-P
Senior Advanced Life Support Educator
Madison County Emergency Medical Services
Canastota, New York
and
Flight Paramedic
AirOne, Onondaga County Sheriff's Department
Syracuse, New York

RICHARD A. CHERRY, MS, NREMT-P
Clinical Assistant Professor of Emergency Medicine
Technical Director for Medical Simulation
Upstate Medical University
Syracuse, New York

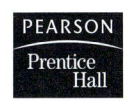

PEARSON
Prentice Hall

Upper Saddle River, New Jersey 07458

Dedication

This Instructor's Resource Manual is dedicated to all the hard-working EMS educators making a difference in the improvement of prehospital care.

Publisher: Julie Levin Alexander
Publisher's Assistant: Regina Bruno
Executive Editor: Marlene McHugh Pratt
Senior Managing Editor for Development: Lois Berlowitz
Project Development: Triple SSS Press Media Development
Assistant Editor: Matthew Sirinides
Director of Marketing: Karen Allman
Executive Marketing Manager: Katrin Beacom
Marketing Coordinator: Michael Sirinides
Director of Production and Manufacturing: Bruce Johnson
Managing Editor for Production: Patrick Walsh
Production Liaison: Faye Gemmellaro
Production Editor: Heather Willison/Carlisle Publishing Services
Manufacturing Manager: Ilene Sanford
Manufacturing Buyer: Pat Brown
Senior Design Coordinator: Cheryl Asherman
Cover Design: Blair Brown
Cover Photography: Eddie Sperling
Composition: Carlisle Publishing Services
Printing and Binding: Banta Harrisonburg
Cover Printer: Phoenix Color

Studentaid.ed.gov, the U.S. Department website on college planning assistance, is a valuable tool for anyone intending to pursue higher education. Designed to help students at all stages of schooling, including international students, returning students, and parents, it is a guide to the financial aid process. This website presents information on applying to and attending college as well as on funding your education and repaying loans. It also provides links to useful resources, such as state education agency contact information, assistance in filling out financial aid forms, and an introduction to various forms of student aid.

NOTICE ON CARE PROCEDURES

This Instructor's Resource Manual reflects current EMS practices based on the 1998 U.S. Department of Transportation's EMT-Paramedic National Standard Curriculum. It is the intent of the authors and publisher that this manual be used as part of a formal Emergency Medical Technician-Paramedic education program taught by qualified instructors and supervised by a licensed physician. The procedures described in this manual are based upon consultation with EMS and medical authorities. The authors and publisher have taken care to make certain that these procedures reflect currently accepted clinical practice; however, they cannot be considered absolute recommendations.

The material in this manual contains the most current information available at the time of publication. However, federal, state, and local guidelines concerning clinical practices, including, without limitation, those governing infection control and universal precautions, change rapidly. The reader should note, therefore, that the new regulations may require changes in some procedures.

It is the responsibility of the reader to familiarize himself or herself with the policies and procedures set by federal, state, and local agencies as well as the institution or agency where the reader is employed. The authors and the publisher of this manual disclaim any liability, loss, or risk resulting directly or indirectly from the suggested procedures and theory, from any undetected errors, or from the reader's misunderstanding of the text. It is the reader's responsibility to stay informed of any new changes or recommendations made by any federal, state, and local agency as well as by his or her employing institution or agency.

NOTICE ON CPR AND ECC

The national standards for Cardiopulmonary Resuscitation (CPR) and Emergency Cardiovascular Care (ECC) are reviewed and revised on a regular basis and may change slightly after this manual is printed. It is important that you know the most current procedures for CPR and ECC, both for the classroom and your patients. The most current information may be obtained from the appropriate credentialing agency.

Copyright © 2007 by Pearson Education, Inc., Upper Saddle River, New Jersey 07458. Pearson Prentice Hall. All rights reserved. Printed in the United States of America. This publication is protected by Copyright and permission should be obtained from the publisher prior to any prohibited reproduction, storage in a retrieval system, or transmission in any form or by any means, electronic, mechanical, photocopying, recording, or likewise. For information regarding permission(s), write to: Rights and Permissions Department.

Pearson Prentice Hall™ is a trademark of Pearson Education, Inc.
Pearson® is a registered trademark of Pearson plc.
Prentice Hall® is a registered trademark of Pearson Education, Inc.

Pearson Education Ltd.
Pearson Education Singapore, Pte. Ltd.
Pearson Education Canada, Ltd.
Pearson Education—Japan
Pearson Education Australia Pty., Limited

Pearson Education North Asia Ltd.
Pearson Educación de Mexico, S.A. de C.V.
Pearson Education Malaysia, Pte. Ltd.
Pearson Education, Upper Saddle River, New Jersey

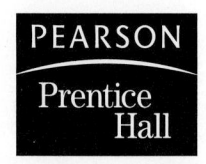

10 9 8 7 6 5 4 3 2 1
ISBN: 0-13-171167-9

CONTENTS
Instructor's Resource Manual

Acknowledgments vii
Letter to Instructor ix
How to Integrate This Manual with *Essentials of Paramedic Care*,
   2nd Edition Brady Learning Materials xi
   Using Your Student Text Features xi
   Using the Package xii
   Additional Resources xiii
Tips for Program/Classroom Success xv
   About the 1998 EMT-Paramedic Curriculum xv
   Instructor Responsibilities xvii
   About Learning xx
   Classroom Tools xxii
   Instructing Students with Learning Disablities xxv
   Websites and Other Resources xxvii
Test-Taking Hints and Guidelines for Your Students xxxi
Transition Guide 1 xxxiii
Transition Guide 2 xlvii

DIVISION 1: Introduction to Advanced Prehospital Care 1

CHAPTER 1
Introduction to Advanced Prehospital Care 3

CHAPTER 2
Medical/Legal Aspects of Advanced Prehospital Care 77

CHAPTER 3
Anatomy and Physiology 97

CHAPTER 4
General Principles of Pathophysiology 149

CHAPTER 5
Life-Span Development 173

CHAPTER 6
General Principles of Pharmacology 189

CHAPTER 7
Medication Administration 221

CHAPTER 8
Airway Management and Ventilation 265

CHAPTER 9
Therapeutic Communications 309

DIVISION 2: Patient Assessment ... 323

CHAPTER 10
History Taking ... 325

CHAPTER 11
Physical Exam Techniques ... 349

CHAPTER 12
Patient Assessment in the Field ... 383

CHAPTER 13
Clinical Decision Making ... 415

CHAPTER 14
Communications ... 431

CHAPTER 15
Documentation ... 451

DIVISION 3: Trauma Emergencies ... 469

CHAPTER 16
Trauma and Trauma Systems ... 471

CHAPTER 17
Blunt Trauma ... 483

CHAPTER 18
Penetrating Trauma ... 499

CHAPTER 19
Hemorrhage and Shock ... 513

CHAPTER 20
Soft-Tissue Trauma ... 533

CHAPTER 21
Burns ... 553

CHAPTER 22
Musculoskeletal Trauma ... 571

CHAPTER 23
Head, Facial, and Neck Trauma ... 591

CHAPTER 24
Spinal Trauma ... 609

CHAPTER 25
Thoracic Trauma ... 623

CHAPTER 26
Abdominal Trauma ... 643

DIVISION 4: Medical Emergencies ... 655

CHAPTER 27
Pulmonology ... 657

CHAPTER 28
Cardiology ... 671

CHAPTER 29
Neurology 721

CHAPTER 30
Endocrinology 739

CHAPTER 31
Allergies and Anaphylaxis 755

CHAPTER 32
Gastroenterology 773

CHAPTER 33
Urology and Nephrology 787

CHAPTER 34
Toxicology and Substance Abuse 801

CHAPTER 35
Hematology 823

CHAPTER 36
Environmental Emergencies 835

CHAPTER 37
Infectious Disease 861

CHAPTER 38
Psychiatric and Behavioral Disorders 885

CHAPTER 39
Gynecology 909

CHAPTER 40
Obstetrics 923

DIVISION 5: Special Considerations/Operations 943

CHAPTER 41
Neonatology 945

CHAPTER 42
Pediatrics 979

CHAPTER 43
Geriatric Emergencies 1031

CHAPTER 44
Abuse and Assault 1063

CHAPTER 45
The Challenged Patient 1083

CHAPTER 46
Acute Interventions for the Chronic-Care Patient 1105

CHAPTER 47
Assessment-Based Management 1127

CHAPTER 48
Operations 1195

CHAPTER 49
Responding to Terrorist Acts 1271

ACKNOWLEDGMENTS
Instructor's Resource Manual

With this second edition of *Essentials of Paramedic Care Instructor's Resource Manual*, exciting new ideas and approaches have been introduced to better equip instructors to educate and train EMT-Paramedics. Since the first edition, many individuals have provided a strong educational foundation on which the second edition was built. It is important to acknowledge those who have given so much of their talents and insight to this current edition and those who have contributed to the previous edition as well.

LESSON DEVELOPMENT SPECIALIST

David M. Habben, NREMT-P
EMS Instructor/Consultant
Boise, Idaho

Tony Crystal, Sc. D., EMT-P, RPhT
Director, Emergency Medical Services
Lake Land College
Mattoon, Illinois

TEACHING STRATEGIES SPECIALIST

Heather Davis, MS, NREMT-P
Clinical Coordinator
UCLA-DFH Paramedic Education
Inglewood, California

TEST ITEM SPECIALISTS

We also wish to thank the following individuals for coordination of test questions in the *Prentice Hall TestGen* that accompanies *Essentials of Prehospital Care*. The quality of work was excellent, and their assistance is appreciated.

Melissa Alexander, M.S., NREMT-P
Learning Solutions in EMS
Fairfax, Virginia

Tony Crystal ScD, EMT-P, RPhT
Director, Emergency Medical Services
Lake Land College
Mattoon, Illinois

LETTER TO INSTRUCTOR
Instructor's Resource Manual

As we enter the twenty-first century, dynamic changes will be taking place in EMS and health care in general. With shorter hospital stays, an increase in home care activities, and the general changes in society, the number and types of patients receiving prehospital care are increasing. We have come a long way from "The White Paper" of 1966 (*Accidental Death and Disability: The Neglected Disease of Modern Society*) to the present, and we still have a long way to go. The skills needed and types of treatment rendered by EMS personnel have changed in recent years and will continue to change. Skills and treatment modalities once reserved for physicians and other specialists are now being performed by EMT-Paramedics, EMT-Intermediates, and EMT-Basics.

The National Highway Traffic Safety Administration has developed a series of documents to help guide our path. The *EMS Agenda for the Future* serves as a guideline for EMS providers, health care organizations and institutions, governmental agencies, and policy makers committed to improving health care in their communities, and aims to ensure that EMS efficiently contributes to that goal. The *EMS Education Agenda for the Future* serves as a guideline that provides EMS educational outcomes designed to meet the needs of the public. This system also emphasizes the integration of EMS within the overall health care system. The *National EMS Research Agenda* serves as a guideline for EMS research and for elevating the science of EMS and prehospital care to the next level. The *Trauma System Agenda for the Future* documents the importance of full implementation of quality trauma systems across the United States to provide optimal care for injured patients and to enhance the country's readiness to respond to future acts of terrorism. The *National EMS Scope of Practice Model* project will help take the *EMS Agenda for the Future* into the streets.

This Instructor's Resource Manual has been developed to provide you with resources needed to effectively present the materials related to Paramedic Care. It not only covers the materials in the National Standard Curriculum, but incorporates numerous references to a variety of Brady/Prentice Hall Health products to enhance student education, evaluate student progress, and provide for remediation of materials, as needed. These materials have been developed by a team of EMS educators and production professionals to bring you state-of-the-art resources for today's EMS educational programs.

Tony Crystal, ScD, EMT-P, RPhT
Director, Emergency Medical Services
Lake Land College
Mattoon, Illinois

Preface

How to Integrate This Manual with *Essentials of Paramedic Care,* 2nd Edition Brady Learning Materials

USING YOUR STUDENT TEXT FEATURES

The key to keeping your students engaged is often knowing when and how to integrate their assigned chapter materials into your lectures and discussions. Following are tips on the key text features and how to use them.

- **DOT Objectives.** This feature references the appropriate curriculum objectives contained in each chapter. The list of objectives includes the DOT objective in addition to the page reference on which the objective is covered. Student understanding of the link between these objectives and ultimately their exams is a giant step toward understanding how to study for the exams.
- **Key Terms.** Tell your students that these key terms will be found in each chapter and to use the page references on which the terms first appear. It's often easier than sending them to the index.
- **Running Glossary.** This feature highlights terms and definitions directly next to the paragraph in which the terms are first presented. This is another quick reference for saving time and reinforcing difficult-to-remember medical terminology and EMS references.
- **Figures.** Updated illustrations and photos help to explain, enhance, and demonstrate key concepts.
- **Tables.** The tables summarize and condense difficult or complex subjects. Some contain photos to enhance and better explain content. Many EMT-Paramedic students are visual learners and may require a boost to their reading skills. As the saying goes, a picture is worth a thousand words, and students find that when they see information in a graphic manner, the material is better understood.
- **Content Review.** Lists, mnemonics, and summaries of key information for quick reference and review make the Content Review a concise feature.
- **Procedures.** Key information and step-by-step approaches are summarized and presented for easy reference in illustrated procedures. In presenting the materials to teach EMT-Paramedics, it is understood that it sometimes can take many words to thoroughly cover a topic. This may sometimes overwhelm students and hinder their ability to sort out the more important information they need. Students need to be able to integrate the didactic material so they can apply it to the psychomotor skills they are expected to perform. Procedures are resources that help to facilitate this educational process, and instructors should consider using them as part of their toolbox.
- **Summary.** Students need a concise review of important chapter information. The Summary is intended to briefly recap the topic of the chapter and flag important points. It is a quick review but certainly does not cover any specific point in depth. Students should find it helpful in bringing together the many pieces of information that a chapter covers. It is an excellent reinforcement tool. Encourage students to read the summaries and reflect back on the chapters to identify those areas that require more study in order for them to better understand the material.
- **Review Questions.** These ask students to recall certain information and to apply the principles they've just learned.

USING THE PACKAGE

This section offers examples and ideas on how to combine or mix and match the *Essentials of Paramedic Care, 2nd Edition* suite of products or "toolbox" into your classroom. The following list offers ideas on how to enhance your classroom with each product.

- **Student CD.** This all-new in-text CD contains multiple-choice quizzes, case studies with questions and rationales, interactive animations and exercises, virtual tours, a drug guide, EMS scenes, and an audio glossary. Assign its use during or after each chapter. The Student CD has been designed specifically for this text. It is a tool for those students who benefit from using a computer as part of their learning style. Those who take advantage of this CD will find that it is not only helpful with retention of the course material but is also fun to use. Encourage students to take advantage of this resource. Use this CD for those difficult-to-learn concepts; they are brought to life with video and animation. Also included on this CD are *Patho Pearls*, snapshots of pathological considerations students will encounter in the field; *Cultural Considerations*, which convey different experiences and issues to consider when providing care for patients from other cultures; and *Legal Notes*, instances in which legal or ethical considerations should be evaluated.

- **Workbook.** The Workbook contains matching exercises, multiple-choice questions, short-answer questions, street scenes questions, labeling exercises, case studies and questions, references to other resources, and skill performance checklists. Students should be strongly encouraged to use the workbook side-by-side with the text. Those students who need more direct mentoring may require specific assignments to complete in order for this resource to be most effective for them.

- **EMT Achieve: Paramedic Test Preparation.** This program enables students to practice test-taking on-line. Four 180-question tests contain questions across the major content areas found in national and state examinations. In addition, each content area has two 25-question tests. Once students take a test, they can see their results, targeting areas of improvement. Before going on to another test, they can take quizzes in each of the content areas. All test questions have rationales and are reinforced with text, photos, illustrations, and video clips. Visit *www.prenhall.com/emtachieve/*.

- **TestGen.** The former Test Manager has been thoroughly updated and reviewed. It contains more than 2,000 exam-style questions, including references to DOT objectives and the student text. The questions in the TestGen are well-designed multiple-choice questions that represent a complete cross-section of the course objectives. Consider composing tests of various lengths throughout the course at regular intervals so students can be evaluated on as much of the course material as possible. TestGen will allow students to become comfortable with the multiple-choice format and style of testing; it is the one most commonly used for state certification examinations and the National Registry.

- **Companion Website.** The accompanying website contains quizzes, labeling exercises, links, and state EMS office listings. This tool is another important resource for students who have access to the Internet. Visit *www.bradybooks.com/paramedic*. If students have not already discovered this site on their own, show them where it is located. Also, if students don't have access to the Internet, consider helping them "make the connection."

- **PowerPoint® Presentation.** Every chapter of this PowerPoint® Presentation has been updated. All chapters include additional illustrations and photos as well as a new Image Bank containing all artwork from the textbooks. PowerPoint® slides are a wonderful tool to help teach topics in an EMT-Paramedic course, and there are several advantages to using them. First, many are developed specifically for this particular textbook and work extremely well with the ancillary materials provided to assist students and support instructors. The slides flow with the topics of the textbook in order to provide continuity. Second, the slides have been designed from an educational perspective for an instructor by an instructor. Third, this presentation is also customizable. You can delete or add slides and even delete or add photographs or other resources. Personalize them for your classroom without starting from scratch. These slides are meant to give you a base to work from; changes to text and photographs and insertion or deletion of text can be done easily. Here are some tips for using the slides:
  - Use them sparingly.
  - Review well in advance.
  - Test equipment before class.
  - Have a backup plan in case of equipment failure.
  - Don't use a whiteboard or wall that will cause a glare when used as a screen.
  - Pay attention to the lighting level in the room.

- **OneKey.** This new distance-learning program for didactic portions of the course is offered on one of three platforms: Course Compass, Blackboard, or Web CT. OneKey includes the IRM, PowerPoints®, TestGen, and Companion Website for instruction. You can use this learning program for all your needs in one place. Features include:
  - Course outline
  - On-line grade book, which automatically keeps track of students' performance on quizzes, class participation, and attendance
  - Ability to upload questions authored off-line and to randomize question order for each student
  - Ability to add your own URLs and course links, set up discussion boards, and modify navigation features
  - A virtual classroom for real-time sessions and communication with students
  - Web links
  - Ability to include your teaching assistants into course creation/management
- **Advanced Life Support Skills.** This highly visual manual guides readers through 26 practical skills in detail. Step-by-step procedures are shown in full color and are accompanied by rationales. In addition, each skill includes Key Terms, Objectives, Introduction, Equipment, Assessment, Overview, Rationales, Problem Solving, Ongoing Assessment, Geriatric/Pediatric Notes, Case Studies, and Review Questions. This accessible, easy-to-follow format helps readers understand what, how, and why each skill is performed and is perfect for initial or refresher training.
- **Advanced Life Skills Review.** Over 150 minutes of video show 26 skills close-up, step-by-step for thorough review, so that students can see exactly how skills should be performed. A companion to the *Advanced Life Support Skills* text, this powerful package is all students need to study for their practical exams.
- **Brady Skills Series: Advanced Life Support.** Over 3 hours of video on four tapes/CDs; contains 26 skills in the following format:
  - *Introduction*—what you'll see; indications, contraindications, assessment, as appropriate; also to include video clips for actual scenes
  - *Equipment*—to include variations; photos/illustrations and text
  - *Overview*—quick run through the entire skill
  - *Skill Close-up*—step-by-step for each skill with commentary by authors, and problem-solving by the authors

ADDITIONAL RESOURCES

- **Review Manual for the EMT-Paramedic.** This is the text for helping students pass national and state examinations. All items are written and tested by educators and offer proven authoritative information. This text blends a collection of practice exam questions with helpful test-taking tips and student hints. All questions are keyed to *Paramedic Care: Principles & Practice, 2nd Edition* and *Essentials of Paramedic Care, 2nd Edition*. Rationales are also provided for all answers.
- **Paramedic National Standards Self-Test.** Based on the 1998 National Standard Curriculum and the AHA's *2000 Handbook of Emergency Cardiovascular Care for Healthcare Providers*, this self-test format enables students to target areas for further study. Includes multiple-choice and scenario-based questions to sharpen test-taking skills, and provides a section on preparing for practical exams. Answers are referenced to *Paramedic Care: Principles & Practice, 2nd Edition* and *Essentials of Paramedic Care, 2nd Edition*.

INTRODUCTION
Tips for Program/Classroom Success

ABOUT THE 1998 EMT-PARAMEDIC CURRICULUM

The Instructor's Resource Manual that accompanies *Essentials of Paramedic Care, 2nd Edition* builds upon the knowledge and skills gained by experienced instructors who have taught the EMT-Paramedic National Standard Curriculum. Their knowledge of the curriculum, coupled with extensive field and/or instructional experience, has shaped the many materials included in this manual.

This educational program is based on the 1998 U.S. Department of Transportation EMT-Paramedic National Standard Curriculum and is divided into five volumes. Division 1 is entitled *Introduction to Advanced Prehospital Care* and addresses the fundamentals of paramedic practice, including pathophysiology, pharmacology, medication administration, and advanced airway management. Division 2, *Patient Assessment*, builds on the assessment skills of the EMT-Basic with special emphasis on advanced patient assessment at the scene. Division 3, *Trauma Emergencies*, discusses advanced prehospital care from the mechanism of injury analysis to shock/trauma resuscitation. Division 4, *Medical Emergencies*, is the most extensive and addresses paramedic-level care of medical emergencies. Particular emphasis is placed on the most common medical problems as well as serious emergencies, such as respiratory and cardiovascular emergencies. Division 5, *Special Considerations/Operations*, includes neonatal, pediatric, geriatric, home health care, and specially challenged patients, as well as incident command, ambulance services, rescue, hazardous materials, crime scene operations, and responding to terrorist acts.

Length of Course

The emphasis of paramedic education should be competence of the graduate, not the amount of education that they receive. The time involved in educating a paramedic to an acceptable level of competence depends on many variables. Based on the experience in the pilot and field testing of the National Standard Curriculum, it is expected that the average program, with average students, will achieve average results in approximately 1,000–1,200 hours of instruction. This can be further broken down to 500–600 hours classroom and practical lab, 250–300 hours clinical, and 250–300 hours field internship. Be sure to consult with your state agency for specific minimum times for these areas.

The length of this course will vary according to a number of factors, including, but not limited to the following:

- Students' basic academic skills competence.
- Faculty-to-student ratio.
- Student motivation.
- Students' prior emergency/health care experience.
- Students' prior academic achievements.
- Clinical and academic resources available.
- Quality of the overall educational program.

EMT-Basic is a prerequisite for the paramedic course. It helps to form a foundation for the paramedic student and because the National Standard Curriculum module titles are the same, it will give the student a general overview on what topics to expect. In addition to the EMT-Basic prerequisite, the Paramedic curriculum has identified coursework in anatomy and physiology as either a pre- or co-requisite. A mastery of anatomy and physiology, beyond that covered in the anatomy and physiology review of each section of the program, is assumed throughout this curriculum. EMS educational programs have many opportunities to address anatomy and physiology in paramedic education. For programs that have access to formal anatomy and physiology classes, an appropriate-level course can be identified as a pre- or co-requisite to paramedic training. For other programs, anatomy and physiology can be "front loaded" in the paramedic course, or presented throughout the course.

As it has been six years since the U.S. DOT EMT-Paramedic National Standard Curriculum was revised, there have been a number of changes made by most of the authorities that approve EMT-Paramedic courses. EMT-Paramedic instructors must ensure that they stay current with curriculum changes that will affect their courses.

Educational Philosophy

Education standards are needed to guide program managers and instructors in making appropriate decisions about what material to cover in classroom instruction. Additionally, these standards are used as one component of program evaluation in the accreditation process and are used by publishers to develop instructional materials. In most allied health professions, education standards are developed by professional associations with broad community input. The complexity, interdisciplinary nature, and state government oversight of EMS necessitates a slightly different approach.

Where We Are

Currently the content of most EMS education programs is based on a national standard curriculum. The National Standard Curriculum (NSC) is funded, developed, and updated periodically by the U.S. Department of Transportation, National Highway Traffic Safety Administration (NHTSA). The National Standard Curriculum has been developed for all nationally recognized levels of EMS education and consists of detailed, highly prescriptive objectives and declarative material. Because these documents are closely tied to scope of practice and because their revision is the only national venue for the discussion of scope of practice, the NSC revision process is time consuming and expensive.

Many EMS education programs and faculty strictly follow the NSC in defining the content of their courses. A typical measure of quality for EMS programs has been their adherence to the current NSC. Although the use of the NSC has contributed to the standardization of EMS education, the quality and length of programs still vary nationally. The reliance on the NSC has decreased flexibility, limited creativity, and made the development of alternative delivery methods difficult. The strict focus on the NSC may result in the development of narrow technical and conceptual skills without consideration for the broad range of professional competencies expected of today's entry-level EMS providers.

Where We Want to Be in 2010

The National EMS Education Standards will be derived from the National EMS Scope of Practice Model. Each National EMS Education Standards document will provide the minimal terminal objectives necessary for successful program completion of a level of EMS provider identified in the National EMS Scope of Practice Model. All programs must adhere to these standards, but there will be significant flexibility in how to achieve the standards. The standards will be designed to encourage creativity in delivery methods such as problem-based learning, computer-aided instruction, distance learning, programmed self-instruction, and others. Without the constraint of an unduly prescriptive NSC, EMS educational institutions are held more accountable for the content and quality of their instruction. This would require institutions to, at a minimum, conduct evaluations of both educational process and outcome quality.

With less prescriptive curriculum standards, it will be much easier to modify curriculum content, both locally and nationally. Changes based on research, practice analysis, future direction of the profession, and experience are quickly reflected in education content, and these changes are communicated to programs through a variety of mechanisms. Although all programs must meet national standards, they will be encouraged to continually improve and excel.

There will be a variety of outstanding instructional materials including instructor lesson plans available from publishers, educational institutions, and other interested parties to support local EMS instruction. EMS instructors will utilize published materials or develop their own for classroom use.

The scope of practice for EMS providers will not be defined by education standards or curriculum. National EMS Education Standards will be designed to prepare EMS providers who are competent to perform within a specific scope of practice. Education will support, rather than define, scope of practice. The scope of practice for EMS providers will be based on the National EMS Scope of *Practice Model.*

Further information may be found in the U.S. Department of Transportation's *EMS Education Agenda for the Future: A Systems Approach.*

Interventions

The goal of EMS is to prevent or reduce morbidity and mortality from illness or injury. Toward that end result, the roles and responsibilities of the modern paramedic include:

- Having fulfilled prescribed requirements by a credentialing agency to practice the art and science of prehospital medicine in conjunction with medical direction.
- Possessing the knowledge, skills, and attitudes consistent with the expectations of the public and the profession.
- Recognizing that they are an essential component of the continuum of care and serve as linkages among health resources.
- Striving to maintain high-quality, reasonable-cost health care by delivering patients directly to appropriate facilities.
- Being a proactive patient advocate in affecting long-term health care by working in conjunction with other provider agencies, networks, and organizations.
- Participating in public education, health promotion, and participation in injury and illness prevention programs.
- Functioning as a facilitator of access to care, as well as an initial treatment provider.
- Being accountable to medical direction, the public, and peers.
- Recognizing the importance of research and actively participating in the design, development, evaluation, and publication of research.
- Seeking to take part in life-long professional development and peer evaluation, and assuming an active role in professional and community organizations.

INSTRUCTOR RESPONSIBILITIES

Many of us can remember a favorite teacher or instructor. Think back to what made that person special. Chances are the memorable instructor was a dynamic, knowledgeable person who took the job seriously yet was able to interject a sense of informality and fun that made learning the material easy and enjoyable.

Instructors who fit this description (and who probably became role models for many of their students) didn't get that way by accident. In addition to countless hours behind the desk or podium and in front of the keyboard learning about or presenting information on their chosen subjects, they also worked to develop a solid foundation of knowledge about the needs of student learners.

For the most part, students in paramedic programs are adult learners. This is significant, because adults learn differently than children do. They also have very different needs and motivational factors. Understanding these needs and motivations is the key to being a successful EMS instructor.

So what do adult learners require? Simply put, adult learners want to have a reason for being in the classroom. In other words, when adult learners sit down in the classroom, they expect to find out how the information being presented is pertinent to their needs.

Sometimes, the relevance of the learning is obvious and does not need to be clarified—for example, the idea that direct pressure stops most bleeding. The reasons for learning other information may take more explanation on the part of the instructor—for example, why learning and using correct terminology is important. The relevance of learning to student needs can sometimes be emphasized through textbook case studies or through the relation of personal experiences by the instructor.

This leads to another important aspect of adult learners. They have life experiences that are important to them. The life experiences that adult learners bring to the classroom can be a tremendous motivational tool for the student as well as the instructor. Perhaps a student is taking the EMT-Paramedic course because he or she was first on the scene of an accident and felt helpless at being unable to assist the victim. It is easy to see that this student will be highly motivated and will understand the reason for learning the material presented in class. For another example, a group of students might be in class because they plan to volunteer together with their local ambulance service. Their motivation will likely be quite high. Students such as the ones just described are some of the easiest for an instructor to teach.

Unfortunately, few paramedic classes will be so straightforward. Paramedic classes usually contain a mix of students with a wide variety of motivations and life experiences. Reaching out to and making the class meaningful for such a range of students is a real challenge for the instructor. In order to do so, the instructor must employ a variety of educational techniques. The following sections will be helpful to instructors in making the paramedic program a valuable experience.

Basic Course Coordination

The following section may be one of the most important for first-time instructors to read. Experienced instructors may also pick up some tips to help make teaching their paramedic courses a little easier.

Teaching a paramedic course involves much more than just preparing a lecture and presenting the material in class. Course coordination is the essential framework that holds the class together and can determine how successful the learning experience will be for students.

Depending on where the course is taught, much of the course coordination work may be done for the instructor. For example, an EMS instructor who teaches a program at a community college may have the schedule preset, books available at the campus bookstore, and access to audiovisual needs at a moment's notice. Other instructors may be asked to hold classes for a community agency and will be responsible for everything from site selection to equipment rental. Although the amount of work that goes into coordinating the course will vary, there are some basic components of course coordination that should be considered in any setting.

Regulations. The first area to look at when coordinating a paramedic program is the arena of state and local regulations. Many states have specific requirements that must be met before teaching of the course can begin. These requirements can range from applying for course approval to designating a physician sponsor for the course.

One of the easiest ways to get into serious trouble as an instructor is to ignore or not comply with applicable state and local regulations. Take the time to learn which regulations apply to teaching in your specific area.

Schedule. A great deal of time should be invested in developing a course schedule that works for the students as well as for the instructor. An EMT-Paramedic course contains a lot of information. Any course schedule should be paced to allow proper absorption and retention of the material. Generally, an 8-hour-a-day, 5-day-a-week course should not be considered. Exceptions can be made when a specific group of students being trained has a demonstrated history of EMS experience, but most adult learners have other obligations that would not permit them to take such a full-time course. Many instructors will schedule an EMT-Paramedic course for 3- to 4-hour blocks. These blocks for the most part work well in terms of teaching specific sections or chapters of the text. When scheduling the time for each class session, remember to build in enough time at the beginning of each class to give the quiz or to handle any administrative details.

The suggested amount of time it takes to teach a full EMT-Paramedic course is 1,000–1,200 hours. Given the amount of material to be covered, there is little to no extra time in the course. When setting the schedule, pay attention to the suggested teaching time listed in the front of each chapter of this manual.

Facility Selection. Forethought and planning in selecting the site where the course will be taught will save an instructor from hours of headache. A comfortable, complete facility can have a profound effect on the students' ability to learn and on the instructor's ability to present the material. When selecting a facility for the course, a number of factors need to be considered.

The site needs to be large enough to hold the number of students enrolled in the course comfortably. If the space available is limited, it can be maximized through proper arrangement of the tables and chairs or desks. Experiment with various setups to find the best placements for the size of the room. Keep in mind that the students need to be able to see the instructor and any audiovisual materials that are used.

The students need room to move around as well as adequate space to sit comfortably. There also needs to be room for the instructor to move around in the front of the class. Some instructors are roamers and need a lot of space, whereas others are more "home oriented" and tend to stay at the podium or front table. Evaluate your own style and factor that into the site selection.

Remember also that an EMT-Paramedic course is very much skills-oriented. There must be plenty of room to break the students up into small groups to practice skills. A facility with access to more than one classroom is ideal. An appropriate facility is one that is relatively free from distractions. Trying to hold an entire EMT-Paramedic course in the kitchen of the fire station will more than likely prove a frustrating experience for the instructor. Even more important, an environment with too many distractions detracts from the learning process for the students.

Make sure the heating ventilation and air-conditioning systems for the facility are appropriate and working. If the classroom temperature is too hot or too cold, the students will pay more attention to trying to get comfortable and less attention to the instructor. Also avoid sites where the HVAC system is too noisy.

Other site selection factors to be considered include availability of restrooms, water fountains, and adequate parking for the students.

Course Materials and Resources. Not having required course materials in place for the class reflects poorly on the instructor. Planning far enough in advance can prevent most of the problems related to course materials. Some materials such as textbooks or workbooks can be ordered well ahead of time. Remember that it never hurts to order a few more texts than you think you'll need. It's more expensive to have to order just one or two books at a time.

Access to a copy machine is an absolute necessity. Everything from handouts to quizzes to CPR cards must be copied. It's probably best to do the copying of materials for the course every few class sessions instead of trying to make all the copies for the entire course in one sitting. Sometimes schedules and topics change slightly, and smaller and more frequent copy jobs will prevent having to redo a quiz or handout. Leave yourself plenty of time to do the copying. It's inappropriate to take the first 30 minutes of the class time making copies.

Also, think about materials you'll need for skills demonstrations and practices and for role-playing scenarios. The lesson plans in this manual list the resources you'll need for such activities on the first page of each lesson.

If you are teaching in a dedicated classroom with equipment storage on site, equipment availability is generally not a problem. There may be times, however, when it is necessary to obtain extra pieces of equipment. Reserve such equipment far in advance to keep from being caught short when the equipment is actually needed.

Additional Instructors. There will be times at which another instructor may be invited to class, either to help with skills or to serve as guest lecturer. Guest lecturers can be valuable in several ways. They can give a new slant to required information and provide useful supplementary knowledge. They can spark student interest by providing a break in the routine. They can also give students the opportunity to observe different teaching styles and techniques, something that can be valuable for the regular instructor as well.

When a guest instructor is invited, he or she should be provided with both lesson objectives and a lesson plan. Plan on observing a first-time guest lecturer to get a sense of his or her instructional abilities and success in covering the objectives. Be alert for tendencies to deviate from the topic excessively. When additional instructors are used for skills practice sessions, a ratio of one instructor for every four to five students is probably most appropriate.

Final Considerations. In terms of coordinating a course, the instructor's best friend and worst enemy is time. If there is enough time, almost anything can be accomplished. If there isn't any time, nothing can be accomplished. The bottom line is that in order to make your course a truly successful one, take care of as many details as far in advance of the course as possible.

Preparation for State and/or National Certification

The successful end of an EMT-Paramedic course will be the completion by students of all requirements for state and/or national certification as EMT-Paramedics. Both students and instructors should have a very clear understanding of what those requirements are.

There are some other things that can be done to help increase students' chances of passing the written and practical examinations for certification.

Written Exams. Most of the state certification exams as well as the National Registry written exam use the multiple-choice format. There are definite keys to successfully passing multiple-choice examinations. One of the best ways to prepare students for taking certification exams is to make multiple-choice examinations a part of the course from the very beginning. Doing so will hone students' test-taking skills and will prepare them for the format they are most likely to see. Each chapter in this manual contains a multiple-choice quiz to build student familiarity with the format and the student workbook contains thousands of test questions. In addition, Prentice Hall TestGen for *Essentials of Paramedic, 2nd Edition*, allows you to easily prepare multiple-choice tests custom tailored to your students' needs. The new online product, *EMT Achieve: Paramedic Test Preparation* (*www.prenhall.com/emtachieve*), provides practice with immediate scoring and rationales and quizzes by module with immediate instructor access by students.

If multiple-choice testing reveals some deficiencies in student understanding of chapter material, you might assign some of the Reinforcement Handouts available with each lesson. The Chapter Review provides a fill-in-the-blank format, while other handouts offer a variety of approaches for reviewing chapter content. Additional reinforcement materials can be found on the Student CD and Companion Website provided by Prentice Hall at *www.prenhall.com/bledsoe*.

Practical Exams. Students fear practical examinations from the first day of the paramedic course right up through test day. Nothing an instructor can do will completely eliminate this apprehension. The fear is generally of performance, not ability.

One of the best techniques to help relieve some of their anxiety is to have the students practice their skills at every opportunity. This will build their confidence and provide an opportunity for the instructor to stress some of the finer points of the more detailed skills.

It will be helpful to discuss the state and national examination process with the students at the first class session. Allow them to ask questions and give them frank answers. *Provide each of your students with the test-taking hints provided in this Instructor's Resource Manual.*

ABOUT LEARNING

Psychomotor Development

The work that paramedics do is very much oriented to practical skills. These skills are based upon a sound foundation of cognitive knowledge and the understanding of when and how to apply that knowledge in appropriate settings. At least 50 percent of the paramedic course will be spent teaching, demonstrating, and performing skills. The time, effort, and energy you put into the teaching of skills in the classroom will directly affect the future success of your students as competent EMT-Paramedics.

There are many ways of teaching the necessary skills in a paramedic course. No single method is correct for all instructors at all times. The appropriateness of methods used will depend on factors such as the number of students in the class, their motivations for being in the class, and the individual differences in learning styles among students in a particular class.

To be most effective at teaching skills in an EMT class, instructors must be competent in and fully aware of the skills criteria used locally. Some states or localities use a packet of skill sheets containing separate skill sheets for each discrete skill. Other areas may use the skill sheets developed by the National Registry of EMTs. Still other areas use both. Take the time to review and study such materials prior to the start of the course and before each class session in which skills will be taught.

Skill Demonstrations

Demonstrating a skill for paramedic students can be one of the most difficult and challenging responsibilities for an instructor. The pressure to perform is enormous because so much is riding on the outcome. Even an instructor who is very comfortable with his or her skills may suffer from intimidation or performance anxiety.

The first time a skill is demonstrated for the students is critical to the students' performance of that skill in the future. The first time most students see a skill performed leaves a strong impression; if a part of the skill was demonstrated incorrectly, the students are likely to repeat the mistake. It is easy to see why this first demonstration of a skill is so crucial and why it can produce anxiety for the instructor.

There are things that you as an instructor can do to help alleviate this anxiety. First and foremost, have faith in your ability. Many instructors have been paramedics for years and have the background and experience to support their textbook knowledge. Also, EMS instructors have been through the class before and, in many cases, have helped with skills training even before becoming instructors themselves. Have the confidence to realize that you know the skills and are more than capable of presenting them to the class.

It may be helpful for the instructor to practice certain skills prior to the class session. Review the skill sheet and the materials found in the textbook as well as the instructor manual. It may also be helpful for the students to hear another instructor narrate the written steps of the skill as it is being demonstrated. Learning increases as the number of the students' senses are stimulated. You might also consider videotaping a demonstration of the skill before the class. This allows for greater control of any possible mistakes; the taped demonstration can also then be used with other classes.

The disadvantage to videotaping is that if the production quality is poor, it can distract students who will pay more attention to inadequacies of the lighting, script, or sound than the skill being demonstrated. Also, remember that the best way to become more comfortable with demonstrating skills in front of the class is by demonstrating skills repeatedly. As with public speaking, the only thing that makes it any easier is doing it often.

When demonstrating a skill to your students, remember that as adult learners they bring a multitude of life experiences with them. They may also have some experience with a particular skill and may offer comments, feedback, or suggestions. Do not discount such input. Instructors have a tendency to teach something the way they themselves were taught, and too often they fail to keep an open mind to other ways a skill might be performed or taught. The most important thing to remember is that a different technique is not necessarily wrong as long as the principles of the skill are correct. The best instructors are flexible and adapt to new information or circumstances and to the needs of their students.

Scenarios for Learning

One of the best ways for instructors to integrate cognitive knowledge with practical skills is through the use of scenarios.

Scenarios are beneficial to the students in a number of ways. They can add a sense of realism to the course. They also can give students a hint of the pressures they will face in the real world. Scenarios promote interaction among the students and can go far in terms of enhancing student bonding and camaraderie/team building. Student performance in the scenarios will provide instructors with an opportunity to evaluate how well the students have grasped both the skill and the ideas in the textbook that are behind it.

There are some basic points that instructors should keep in mind when running patient care scenarios in the classroom setting:

- The scenario has to be doable. Giving students impossible scenarios sets them up for failure and can destroy their confidence.
- The scenario has to be winnable. A winnable scenario is one in which students have the opportunity to see an improvement in patient outcome based on their care.
- Each scenario should be evaluated and feedback provided to the students. Providing feedback on student performance will help reinforce positive performances and eliminate mistakes.
- Keep the scenario simple. The "busload of hypochondriacs that goes off the cliff into a toxic waste dump" scenario may be fun, but it's complicated, uses up too much precious time, and probably involves so many considerations that students actually learn very little.
- Start using scenarios early in the course. Even on the first night of class an appropriate scenario can be run. Consider a simple CPR call or a call for choking.
- Use scenarios often. Many instructors will use a scenario in every class session.

Like most things, scenarios work most effectively and smoothly when you take the time to plan them out in advance. There are detailed instructions for scenarios in this manual that make such planning easier. There are also collections of ready-to-go scenarios available from publishers. Your own experiences as a paramedic, however, may make the best, most effective scenarios for your class. There are many benefits to using personal experiences as a basis for scenarios. Real calls that you have been on have a different flavor from generic scripts borrowed from books. This heightens the sense of their realism. In addition, after the students have played out the scenario, you can tell them what actually happened and compare notes. By objectively evaluating your responses to the call with the students, you can demonstrate to them that there is no such thing as a "perfect" call. This will help remind them that there is always room for improvement, even for the instructor.

One key to running successful scenarios is the use of an appropriate evaluation tool. A proper evaluation tool need not be fancy—in fact, the simpler the better. An evaluation tool can consist of nothing more than a sheet of paper containing appropriate information about the call and room to write notes and comments about student performance. The evaluation tool can even be incorporated into the scenario planning sheet.

When developing your own classroom scenarios, always use a scenario planning sheet. A well-prepared planning sheet should ensure similar learning outcomes for students even if other instructors use the sheet to run the scenario. The planning sheet should contain the following:

- Description of the call
- Environmental factors that might affect the call
- Pertinent findings in the scene size-up, initial assessment, focused history and physical exam, and baseline and follow-up vital signs
- An area for information about such things as interventions performed and time at which they were done
- A list of the objectives for the call—what you are trying to teach the students with this scenario
- A list of equipment needed to run the call
- Moulage instructions if pertinent
- Instructions to the "patient"
- A space for any additional comments in which you can evaluate student performance (Leaving enough space to write comments probably works better than trying to develop a complicated checklist of things the students should have done in the scenario.).

One of the easiest ways to incorporate scenarios into the classroom is to pair the students up into responder teams and place a different team on call for each class session. This gives the students both a feel for what it's like to be on duty and an opportunity to apply their skills in a fairly realistic setting. The on-call crew should check at the beginning of the class to ensure that the jump kits to be used are complete and operational. It's also a good idea to assign a second crew as backup in case the first crew needs additional help.

There are many ways to make scenarios an everyday part of the class. Evaluate the characteristics of your facility and your students to determine the best way to use scenarios in your classes.

Assisting Student Learning

The type and amount of information covered in paramedic courses can be overwhelming for students if they are not prepared to study effectively. Unfortunately, many adult learners lack the tools and background for efficient study. For a large percentage of your students, the paramedic course represents a first return to the classroom in many years. For some students the paramedic course may be their first formal experience as adult learners. Much has changed in the way of educational methodology and technology since they were in school, and tools and resources taken for granted today were often unavailable then and are thus unfamiliar to these students. Anything that you can do as an instructor to help such students study more effectively is an investment that will pay off handsomely for both the students, in terms of their future employment prospects, and for your EMS system, in terms of better-trained, more capable EMT-Paramedics.

As adult learners, paramedic students must take responsibility for their own learning. It would be extremely difficult for most paramedic students to make it through the course without studying for a substantial amount of time outside the classroom. It is not unusual for students to spend three to four hours studying for each hour spent in the classroom. To help students get the most from their study time, you might consider suggesting some of the following strategies for success that have worked for others in the past:

- Encourage the formation of study groups. A study group can help students put pieces of information together in ways that "click" as they hadn't when students were studying on their own. Often a member of the study group can explain a concept in a way that allows another student to understand something that wasn't grasped in class. Some students will feel more comfortable asking that "stupid" question in a small group setting rather than the classroom. One problem with study groups, however, is that if students misunderstand something, the misinformation will be more widely circulated and it may take some time for the instructor to become aware that this has occurred. If your students do form study groups, pay attention to what your evaluation tools reveal about student understanding of key concepts and ideas.
- Use the student workbooks that are available with the basic textbook. Workbooks include many different types of activities that will reinforce what students have read in the text.
- Make yourself available for questions before and after class as well as during breaks. Some students are shy about classroom participation and will hesitate to bring up what they may see as "silly" questions.
- Use computer resources if available. There are some excellent computer programs that can enhance student understanding of key ideas—test banks for reviewing course knowledge, and anatomy models for illustrating how the body works, for example. If a classroom computer is available, consider purchasing one or more of these programs and make it (them) available for student use at appropriate times. (See "High-Tech Options" later in the introductory material.)
- Pace yourself when delivering lectures. Give students enough time to write their notes. Monitor the students' nonverbal cues that indicate they are ready to continue. When pencils stop moving, then pick up the topic and carry on with the lecture.
- Consider giving students outlines of your lecture with plenty of spaces for them to write notes. Most of today's computer presentation software can generate such simplified outlines from the more detailed lecture preparations.
- Finally, encourage the students to seek to balance study, work, and play in their lives. Retention of course material will be enhanced if students are relatively relaxed and not overloading any one area of their lives. (The same will be true for their EMS careers.) This material should be covered during the "Well-Being of the EMT" section of the course.

CLASSROOM TOOLS

The instructional media an instructor will use in the classroom will vary with equipment and resource materials available. The instructor's comfort level with a particular medium also affects what resources are used in the classroom. Experimenting with different media is strongly encouraged; this will increase the instructor's familiarity with other media and enlarge the pool of resources he or she is likely to draw on.

Remember also that it is important to avoid saturating students with one type of audiovisual material. There may be an entire slide set for the course, but it may not be the soundest educational policy to use nothing but those slides as you teach the course. Students learn differently and different media will reach or interest different students.

Think of technology as critical to your classroom presentation. The following tips and techniques will guide you through the technology maze.

PowerPoint® Presentations

PowerPoint® presentations and slides are a wonderful tool to help teach topics in a paramedic course, and there are a number of advantages to using them. First, slides developed specifically for a particular textbook work extremely well with that text and other ancillary materials associated with it, such as the instructor's manual and the workbook. This Instructor's Resource Manual tells you specifically which slides to use for which part of a lecture. The material presented in the slides is consistent with what students learn in their reading. Additionally, use of such slide programs can decrease preparation time for the instructor. The *Essentials of Paramedic Care, 2nd Edition* PowerPoint® Presentation is customizable if an instructor doesn't wish to be tied to a program prepared by someone else.

Disadvantages in the use of slides are usually related to equipment problems and a tendency to overuse the medium. In order for the slide presentation to be successful, the projector has to be working, and your computer must be in good working order so that there is no danger of the presentation freezing. Also remember that lighting conditions in the room must be appropriate for the projection of the slides. If there are no shades for the windows and class is held during daylight hours, students may have trouble seeing the images. Keep in mind, if this is the case, that you can change the design colors on the presentation to make it easier to read.

Videotapes

The age of video has not left EMS instruction untouched. The sheer volume and range of subjects available in commercial training tapes today is tremendous. The many timely topics available in the format lend a state-of-the-art feel to the classroom. Also, students are extremely comfortable with the medium, probably more so than with any other.

Videotapes offer vivid, dynamic images and sounds that excite and stimulate most students and instructors. Real-life footage conveys the nature of EMS work in a way that other audiovisual aids cannot. Videos can be an excellent choice for dramatizing a specific point an instructor wants to make. Perhaps most important, difficult procedures can be shown on tape over and over until students understand the concept or skill.

The disadvantages of videotape use include heavy reliance on the equipment. The TV has to be operating correctly, as do the VCR and the videotape cassette. If any one component fails, the entire presentation fails. Initial outlay to purchase the equipment can be expensive. Also, in a large class setting it may be difficult to position the video monitor so that all students have a good view of it. Finally, the fact that so many topics are available on tape may tempt instructors to overuse this audiovisual aid in the classroom.

Tips for using videotapes include:

- Always preview the tape for quality and appropriateness of the material.
- Never put in a video and then leave the classroom. Videos should not be used to baby-sit the students.
- Have a backup plan in case of equipment failure.
- Preset the video for the appropriate starting point before class.
- Use short, pertinent video segments instead of always running entire tapes. The shorter segments can have a more profound impact.
- Be prepared to pause the tape and ask or answer pertinent questions.
- Set up the TV/VCR before class so that you can check to ensure sight and sound quality throughout the room.

Using videotapes in the classroom can add a dynamic boost to your lectures. Sprinkle them liberally throughout the course and watch the impact they have on students.

Whiteboards

This modern-day relative of the chalkboard can be found in nearly every classroom setting. Students expect to see a writing surface of one type or another in a classroom, and the simplicity, spontaneity, and versatility that whiteboards make possible can hardly be matched.

The major limit on the use of the whiteboard is the instructor's imagination. Even if a lesson plan calls for a class to be lecture based, a particular point that needs to be emphasized or explained can be written on the board. The variety of colors available for use on the whiteboard enlivens presentations. Complicated or detailed drawings or formulas can be written on the board before class, allowing more time for discussion during the lesson. Finally, with no bulbs to burn out or other electronics to fail, whiteboards are extremely reliable.

The disadvantages of whiteboards are relatively few and often instructor related. Poor penmanship on the part of the instructor can leave students frustrated. The dry-erase markers used on whiteboards can dry up, leaving the instructor with few options. In very large classroom settings, it may be difficult for all students to see the board. Finally, inadvertent use of a permanent marker may ruin a whiteboard.

Here are some tips for using whiteboards:

- Use blue or black for the main color, and use a bright color such as red or green to highlight key words or concepts.
- Never use the yellow marker, as yellow will be nearly invisible to most students sitting any distance away.
- Don't talk to the board while you are writing—your listeners are in the seats.
- Draw complex images before the class starts.
- Print legibly.
- Use letters large enough for all to see.
- Do not allow permanent markers in the classroom, especially in the marker tray.
- Watch for spelling and grammatical errors.
- Give students ample time to write material down in their notebooks before erasing it.

Whiteboards are a wonderful visual aid that when used appropriately can make the instructor's job easier, while providing students with a familiar and colorful visual stimulus.

Making It Real—Moulage Tips

Moulage is the application of materials to a volunteer "patient" to simulate injuries and other significant clinical signs. EMS instructors have used moulage techniques for years to enhance the realism of scenarios for their students. A well-done job of moulage creates an impressively real patient, whereas a poorly handled job detracts from the scenario and from student learning.

The application of makeup and other objects to simulate injuries has long been a staple in Hollywood films. However, EMS instructors do not need access to the movie industry's makeup artists to learn to create effects that are believable and accurate in "patients." Some great moulage techniques can be achieved with minimal amounts of material and training. Contrary to what some may think, applying good moulage does not have to be a time-consuming ordeal. The benefit of moulage is lost if it takes an hour to apply the makeup.

Basic Moulage Techniques. Injuries are not perfect, so it's difficult to make a "bad" injury. Here are some basic rules that will allow the instructor to create realistic injuries and signs easily:

- First and foremost, remember that "less is more." A light application of whites, blues, and grays will have a more profound impact than a heavily applied layer of clown white when simulating paleness or cyanosis.
- Simplicity is the key in creating realistic "injuries" in a short period of time. Most injuries can be simulated with a few commonly available items. A basic list of supplies for moulage can be found later in this section.
- Always apply a light application of cold cream under any injuries or skin signs that you apply. Cold cream helps the makeup stay on the skin and makes the removal of the makeup much easier for the "patient."
- Accuracy is important in creating believable injuries. Placing a giant bruise over the entire area of the chest to simulate a pneumothorax probably does more to detract from the scenario than illustrate it.
- To simulate cyanosis, try a light application of blue to the nail beds, ear lobes, and around the lips after applying a basic underlay of white or light gray.
- Use a mixture of water with a small amount of glycerin to simulate diaphoresis. Keep the mixture in a small spray bottle and apply immediately prior to the arrival of the "rescuers."

- To simulate burns, apply a layer of cold cream followed by a base coat of red to the entire area. Lay some tissue over the area and then apply some water-soluble lubricant such as K-Y® jelly over the tissue. Gently break the tissue by rolling it from the center of the "burned" area toward the edges. This will create a remarkably realistic looking second-degree burn.
- Use activated charcoal applied with a cotton swab around the edges of the nares and the mouth and tongue to simulate a respiratory burn.
- Place a small amount of effervescent tablet in a simulated chest wound. Just prior to "rescuer" arrival, place a few drops of water on the tablet to help simulate a sucking chest wound. The bubbling action is usually quite impressive.
- Whenever there is a chance that the "patient" may "bleed" or "ooze," be sure to place a tarp under the patient to avoid staining the carpet or flooring underneath the patient.

The best way to become comfortable with moulage is to use it often. Experiment with different materials and household items. Remember that because real injuries are not perfect, *it's difficult to go wrong if you keep it simple.*

Resources for Moulage. Putting together a useful moulage kit does not have to be expensive or complicated. One of the biggest decisions to make is whether to build your own kit or purchase one of the commercially available injury simulation kits. There are advantages and disadvantages to each approach. Commercially available kits usually contain a variety of fake injuries made from rubber or plastic that can be either strapped on or held in place by spirit gum. They also contain a variety of colored makeup. The advantage to this type of moulage kit is its completeness.

The biggest drawback to such kits is the price. Some of the more elaborate kits can cost hundreds of dollars. Also, many of the injuries included are not very realistic, and the time that it takes an instructor to develop a level of expertise using the kits may be unreasonable for most EMS instructors.

Another drawback is that using a single source for moulage materials and techniques limits the development of the instructor's skill in using moulage as a resource. An instructor forced by circumstances to use a kit other than his or her own may have difficulty moulaging patients.

An alternative to purchasing a ready-made kit is putting together a kit of your own. Most of the materials are inexpensive, and this will also give you the flexibility to be creative. Experiment with different items and find the things that work the best for you. Some items that such a kit might contain include the following:

- Cold cream—for applying under makeup.
- Plumber's putty—to use as a modeling clay when building injuries.
- Eye shadow—a variety of shades to simulate cyanosis and bruises.
- Dirt—a container of dirt is handy to help make realistic road rashes and other injuries.
- Halloween makeup—haunt the costume aisles of your local store in October. A wide variety of makeup colors and simulated injuries are available. Hint: Shop the day after Halloween to get bargain prices.
- Chicken bones—for use in the simulation of open fractures. Place them in a bag and lightly crush them to obtain realistic bone fragments. Be sure to sanitize the bones prior to use.
- Clear plastic cups—crushed, they provide pieces of very good looking "glass" for use in an injury
- Fake blood—one of those items that can be purchased commercially. Many instructors have also come up with their own recipes that work well. Try to avoid any red dyes that stain too easily.
- Knife handles—use just the handle of a knife and build putty around the knife end to simulate an impaled object.
- Effervescent tablets—to help simulate chest wounds.
- Condoms—filled with a little water or K-Y jelly for creating simulated evisceration.
- Brushes—variety of makeup brushes for applying colors for cyanosis and bruising.
- Activated charcoal—for burn moulage.

INSTRUCTING STUDENTS WITH LEARNING DISABILITIES

Each adult learner who enrolls in an EMS course possesses a unique personality and a unique ability to learn. Factors such as learning ability and style, preexisting knowledge, life experience, and motivation will contribute to the level of achievement of each student. Very few, if any, adult education classes will contain a truly homogeneous group of students. Competent educators realize this and use the strengths of each learner to achieve the desired educational outcomes. As a result, instructors have a responsibility to identify students who may be deficient in learning skills and to provide appropriate remediation and support.

Learning disabilities do not mean a lack of intelligence. Many famous people have overcome learning disabilities to contribute their talents to all walks of life—Albert Einstein, Winston Churchill, Cher, Walt Disney, Whoopi Goldberg, Bruce Jenner, and Woodrow Wilson, just to name a few. Although not all people with learning disabilities will achieve success, even in modest terms, many can complete training programs in a wide variety of fields such as EMS. The message is this: Students with learning disabilities of any age can learn.

In recent decades, state and federal governments have extended protection to students with learning disabilities through a wide variety of court decisions and laws, such as the Americans with Disabilities Act (ADA) of 1990. Today educational institutions must have operational plans aimed at identifying and assisting students with learning disabilities. Adult learners who have benefited from these programs in their primary and secondary educations are aware of these laws and are entering EMS programs in greater numbers than in the past. They will request—and rightly so—the educational accommodations and compensatory mechanisms that have helped them achieve prior learning success. EMS educators, therefore, will be asked to develop a wide variety of instructional strategies—diverse methods of presentation that will not only enrich the educational experience of students with learning disabilities, but of all the students in a class. Of the many types of learning disabilities, the ones that an EMS instructor can expect to encounter most frequently are "academic skills disorders." Of particular concern are developmental reading disorders, such as dyslexia. It may be necessary for a student with a reading impairment to go over a paragraph many times to reach an understanding. The assignment of a complex chapter on anatomy, for example, can seem like an impossible task.

If a student with a reading disorder (or any other learning disability) appears in a paramedic course, an instructor has a legal and/or ethical responsibility to seek appropriate remediation. For example, assistance for a dyslexic student may include referral to a reading skills program or to a service that provides "audiobooks." In most cases, however, moderate assistance on the part of the instructor can help adult learners deficient in one or more skills—especially if they have received remediation during their earlier education.

In deciding upon a course of action for students with a learning disabilities, an EMS educator must be careful not to confuse the educational process with certification. The educational component is designed to facilitate the acquisition of cognitive knowledge and psychomotor skills necessary to obtain a certificate or license to practice EMS. Although many EMS educational institutions work closely with the entities that certify and license EMS providers, the two processes—education and certification—must remain separate. The EMS educator's only concern should be that of preparing the student for the credentialing process. In the case of the students with learning disabilities, the educator should focus on strategies that will help each student accomplish the instructional objectives while providing "reasonable" remediation and compensation measures.

Point out this distinction to students with learning disabilities. It would not be ethical to have such students—or any other students for that matter—assume that completion of an EMS course assures success in the certification or licensure process. As a result, an EMS educator should urge students with learning disabilities to initiate early contact with the certifying or licensing agency to determine what accommodations will be accepted or made for them during the certification process.

All EMS instructors in the twenty-first century should investigate the programs, laws, and regulations related to learning disabilities specified by local, state, and federal governments. Some sources of information are listed in "Resources for Teaching Students with Learning Disabilities" at the end of the introductory material.

Most important, keep in mind that the majority of adults with learning disabilities function as normal, productive members of society. They aspire to the same educational goals as people without learning disabilities—and, in many cases, with a higher motivation. Far too often, however, they become frustrated by an inability to learn using the same method or at the same rate as other students.

An astute EMS educator must seek to create new opportunities for the students with learning disabilities. One of the best resources is a caring educator willing to take the time to recognize learning disabilities and then to provide the additional assistance—videos, audiotapes, and teamwork with other students—that can mean the difference between success and failure.

WEBSITES AND OTHER RESOURCES

Following are lists of various types of resources that instructors might find valuable. The lists are not all-inclusive, and instructors should add to them and create a file that suits their needs. Although all information has been checked and is current at time of publication, contact and website information may change.

Professional Organizations

(NOTE: Access to some areas of organizational website may be limited to members only)

American Ambulance Association
1255 Twenty-Third Street
Washington, D.C. 20037-1174
202-452-8888
www.the-aaa.org

American College of Emergency Physicians
P.O. Box 619911
Dallas, TX 75261-9911
800-798-1822
www.acep.org

American Heart Association
7272 Greenville Ave.
Dallas, TX 75231
800-242-8721
www.americanheart.org

Association of Air Medical Services
526 King Street, Suite 415
Alexandria, Virginia 22314-3143
703-836-8732
www.aams.org

Citizen CPR Foundation
P.O. Box 15945-314
Lenexa, KS 66285-5945
913-495-9816
www.citizencpr.com

Emergency Nurses Association
915 Lee Street
Des Plaines, IL 60016-6569
800-900-9659
www.ena.org

National Association of EMS Educators
Foster Plaza 6
681 Andersen Drive
Pittsburgh, PA 15220-2766
412-920-4775
www.naemse.org

National Association of EMS Physicians
P.O. Box 15945-281
Lenexa, KS 66285-5945
800-228-3677
www.naemsp.org

National Association of EMTs
P.O. Box 1400
Clinton, MS 39060-1400
800-34-NAEMT
www.naemt.org

National Association for Search and Rescue
4500 Southgate Place, Suite 100
Chantilly, VA 20151-1714
703-222-6277
www.nasar.org

National Association of State EMS Directors
111 Park Place
Falls Church, VA 22046-4513
703-538-1799
www.nasemsd.org

National Council of State EMS Training Coordinators
201 Park Washington Court
Falls Church, VA 22046-4513
703-538-1794
http://www.ncsemstc.org

National Emergency Medical Services Alliance
1947 Camino Vida Roble
Carlsbad, CA 92008
619-431-7054

National Registry of EMTs
6610 Busch Blvd.
P.O. Box 29233
Columbus, OH 43229
614-888-4484
www.nremt.org

Introduction **xxvii**

EMS Websites

One of the big advantages of owning a computer today is the availability of information through the Internet. To steer a course through this electronic maze, we've compiled a list of websites at which instructors can find information they can use in developing lectures or enhancing student knowledge of emergency medicine. These sites have the potential to provide access to a whole new realm of information and entertainment for you and your students.

Each of these EMS websites has been visited and reviewed for appropriateness and content. Remember to bookmark the sites for easy access to them the next time you are surfing.

News Groups

emsvillage.com
prehospitalperspective.net

These news groups are excellent places to learn about the latest trends in EMS. They also offer the opportunity to ask questions and gain insights into what other EMS providers across the country are doing.

In addition, many EMS organizations support list servers where members can ask questions and interact with other EMS professionals.

Web Sites

www.bennye.com
    Make up and kits for applying moulage

www.bradybooks.com
    The home page of the publisher of *Essential of Paramedic Care*.

www.cdc.gov
    The home page for the Centers for Disease Control and Prevention. An excellent source of information on infectious diseases.

www.cpem.org
    Teaching resource for instructors in prehospital pediatrics.

www.fire-ems.net
    The fire and EMS information network. A site that features everything from chat areas to website development for fire and EMS services.

www.jems.com/
    JEMS on-line. *The Journal of Emergency Medical Services* home page.

www.LessStress.com
    This site contains a prehospital care simulator.

www.lifeart.com
    A source for medical clip art that can be useful for overheads and handouts.

www.merck.com
    The famous Merck manual on-line.

www.ncemsf.org/
    The National EMS Collegiate Foundation. This home page contains information about EMS educational programs around the country.

www.nhtsa.dot.gov/portal/site/nhtsa/menuitem
    The home page for the National Highway Traffic Safety Administration. Download curricula for all of the EMT levels.

www.osha.gov
    The home page for the Occupational Safety and Health Administration. Information from ergonomics to OSHA documents.

www.pcrf.mednet.ucla.edu/
    The Prehospital Care Research Forum is dedicated to the promotion, education, and dissemination of prehospital research.

www.shrs.pitt.edu/emergency/index.html
    The Center for Emergency Medicine's site with information about the revision of the EMT-Intermediate and EMT-Paramedic Curricula.

www.ptialaska.net/~bearmt/
    Information on an inexpensive AED Trainer.

www.trauma.org/prehospital/ph-images.html
    Prehospital images of accident scenes and the like.

Books

Brown, C. *Square Pegs and Round Holes*. Lake Worth, FL: EES Publications, 1990.

An easy-to-use text designed specifically for EMS instructors. Not quite as meaty as the McClincy text listed below, but it still contains some good information.

Hoff, R. *I Can See You Naked*. Kansas City, MO: Andrews and McMeel, 1992.

Once you get past the title, you will find a text that contains pertinent information on public speaking.

Martini, F. H., Bartholomew, E. F., and Bledsoe, B. E., *Anatomy and Physiology for Emergency Care*. Upper Saddle River, NJ: Brady-Prentice Hall, 2002.

Anatomy and physiology text for students in emergency care and allied health programs requiring an overview of the human body's systems.

McClincy, W. *Instructional Methods in Emergency Services*. 2nd edition. Upper Saddle River, NJ: Brady-Prentice Hall, 2002.

This text is the most comprehensive manual to date on methods of instruction for EMS personnel. Experienced and new instructors alike will find this book to be a valuable source of information.

Nixon, R. G. *Communicable Diseases and Infection Control for EMS*. Upper Saddle River, NJ: Brady-Prentice Hall, 2000.

Oosterhof, A. *Classroom Applications of Educational Measurement*. Columbus, OH: Merrill, 2000.

This text is directed toward theory and makes a nice addition to the libraries of those instructors who want more information on evaluation tools.

Simmons, S. *How to Be the Life of the Podium*. New York: AMACOM, 1993.

This book contains quips, quotes, and stories that can be used to spice up almost any presentation.

U.S. Department of Transportation. *Paramedic and EMT-Intermediate National Standard Curricula*. Washington, DC: GPO, 1999.

Journals

ACLS Alert
3525 Piedmont Rd. NE
Six Piedmont Center
Suite 400
Atlanta, GA 30305

Annals of Emergency Medicine
P.O. Box 619911
Dallas, TX 75261

EMS Insider
Jems Communications
1947 Camino Vida Roble
Carlsbad, CA 92008
619-431-9797

Emergency
6200 Yarrow Drive
P.O. Box 159
Carlsbad, CA 92008
800-854-6449

Emergency Medical Services
Creative Age Publications
7628 Densmore Ave.
Van Nuys, CA 91406
818-782-7328

Emergency Training
Miller Landing
Building 200
150 N. Miller Road
Akron, OH 44333
216-836-0600

Journal of Emergency Medical Services
P.O. Box 370
Escondido, CA 92033
800-334-8152

Journal of Emergency Medicine
Pergamon Press
660 White Plains Road
Tarrytown, NY 10591

911 Magazine
18201 Weston Pl.
Tustin, CA 92680
714-544-7776

Prehospital Emergency Care
Hanley & Belfus, Inc., Medical Publishers
210 South 13th Street, Philadelphia, PA 19107
800-962-1892
215-546-7293
Fax 215-790-9330
www.hanleybelfus.com

Rescue
Jems Communications
P.O. Box 370
Escondido, CA 92033
800-334-8152

Topics in Emergency Medicine
200 Orchard Ridge Dr.
Gaithersburg, MD 2087
800-638-8437

Video Producers
Pulse/Emergency Medical Update
P.O. Box 11380
Winslow, WA 98110
800-327-3841

For Students with Learning Disabilities

This partial listing has been compiled from sources available at the time of the publication of the Instructor's Resource Manual. Changes in laws, regulations, and/or technology may have an affect on the resources available in the future.

Alliance for Technology Access (ATA)
2175 East Francisco Blvd., Suite L
San Rafael, CA 94901
415-455-4575
FAX: 415-455-0491
www.atacess.org
> Provides access to supportive technology for people with disabilities.

Association on Higher Education and Disability (AHEAD)
P.O. Box 21192
Columbus, OH 43221
614-488-4972
FAX: 614-488-1174
www.ahead.org
> Provides information about full participation in higher education for people with disabilities.

Council for Learning Disabilities (CLD)
P.O. Box 40303
Overland Park, KS 66204
913-492-8755
FAX: 913-942-2546
www.cldinternational.org
> Offers enhancement for the education and development of the learning disabled.

Division of Adult Education and Literacy Clearinghouse
U.S. Department of Education
Office of Vocational and Adult Education
400 Maryland Avenue, SW
Washington, DC 20202
202-205-9996
FAX: 202-205-8873
www.ed.gov
> Links the adult education community with existing resources in adult education available through the Adults in Education Act.

HEATH Resource Center
National Clearinghouse on Postsecondary Education for Individuals with Disabilities
American Council on Education
One Dupont Circle, NW, Suite 800
Washington, DC 20036
202-939-9320
FAX: 202-833-4760
www.ACENET.edu
> Collects and disseminates information about postsecondary education for individuals with disabilities.

National Association for Adults with Special Learning Needs (NAASLN)
P.O. Box 716
Bryn Mawr, PA 19010
610-525-8336
FAX: 610-525-8337
www.naasln.org/
> Provides information for helping adults with special learning needs.

National Center for Learning Disabilities (NCDL)
381 Park Avenue South, Suite 1420
New York, NY 10016
212-545-7510
FAX: 212-545-9665
www.ncld.org
> Provides programs and services to promote a better understanding and acceptance of learning disabilities.

Rebus Institute
1499 Bayshore Blvd., Suite 146
Burlingame, CA 94010
415-697-7424
FAX: 415-697-3734
> Disseminates information on adult issues related to specific learning disabilities and Adult Attention Deficit Disorders (AADD)

Recording for the Blind and Dyslexic (RFBD)
20 Roszel Road
Princeton, NY 20542
609-452-0606
800-221-4792
www.rfbd.org
> Offers free recordings and speech software versions of books for the blind and dyslexic.

U.S. Department of Education
National Library of Education
Office of Educational Resource and Improvement
Institute of Education Sciences
455 New Jersey Ave., NW
Washington, DC 20208
202-219-2221
www.ed.gov
> Houses the Educational Resources Information Center (ERIC)—the source of a wide variety of educational literature and resources.

Test-Taking Hints and Guidelines for Your Students

The following list of helpful hints is probably most appropriate for the end-of-course examination, state certification, or the National Registry written examination. Consider photocopying this section and giving it directly to your students.

- Study from your class notes and the workbook that accompanies the course text. Do not cram the night before, as cramming may hinder your efforts rather than help.
- Relax the evening before the examination and get a good night's sleep. You are usually in better mental shape if you are well rested. If you exercise regularly, consider doing your usual routine. A brisk walk before the exam can help you relax and it also reduces stress, especially if you worked during the day of the exam.
- Avoid anything that may overstimulate or tranquilize you. Too much coffee or caffeinated beverages will not be helpful.
- Eat a sensible meal about two hours prior to the exam. A large meal just before an examination may make you feel tired. Drink a small glass of water just prior to entering the exam room if you are thirsty. Too much to drink before a test may mean frequent restroom breaks. Most standardized tests do not give you extra time for breaks.
- Wear comfortable clothing that is appropriate for the climate and environment. It is a good idea to bring a light sweater or sweatshirt to the exam. Many exam rooms are large and it is sometimes difficult to control the temperature.
- Plan to arrive early for the exam. You do not want to feel rushed and you may need some extra time if you encounter unexpected delays en route.
- Make sure that you bring any exam supplies that you are responsible for. Make a list so you do not forget. It can be frustrating if you need to go home and get a photo ID card or ask to borrow a pencil.
- Carefully follow the instructions of the examination proctor. Do not begin the exam or make any entries on the answer form until you are instructed to do so. Ask questions if you do not understand any part of the instructions.
- Once the exam begins, pace yourself. Determine how many questions and how much time you are allowed (a 100-question exam given over three hours allows an average of three and one-half minutes per question). Note the time the test starts so you can keep track of how much time remains at any given time. If you spend too much time on one question, you may find yourself rushed in order to finish. (It may be a good idea to bring your own watch in case a clock is not available and so that you're not dependent on the proctors counting down the time. Calculator watches may not be allowed in the examination. The examination proctor can advise.)
- After carefully reading the question, read all the answer choices before making a final decision as to the correct answer and marking the answer sheet. You may be sure you have figured out the correct response after reading only the first or second choice, but reading all the answers gives you some additional reinforcement that you are correct. Many times there are a few answers that you can eliminate almost immediately, making your final decision easier.
- Read each question carefully. Make sure you understand what is being asked. Does the question say "**all the following _EXCEPT_**" or "which of the following is _NOT_"? If so, that means that they are looking for the one answer that doesn't fit. Take an extra few seconds to make sure you picked the correct answer.
- When presented with a scenario question with patient-specific or scenario-specific information, consider reading the scenario, then the question and all answer choices, then return to the question to extract the relevant information and decide on the answer.
- Occasionally you may have a question that is very difficult or confusing. Consider skipping this question and moving to the next. Mark the question clearly (do not write in the examination booklet if a separate answer sheet is provided), so you know you need to return and deal with it later. In addition, because most of these tests use a standardized testing sheet, make sure you skip to the next answer row. Obviously, misaligned answers will be read as wrong by a computer or answer key. This important detail needs the close attention of the test taker.

- If you have a question that you are struggling with you should move on. Remember there is a time limit and you don't want to feel rushed as time is running out. If you know one or more of the answers are definitely wrong, mark them (do not write in the examination booklet if a separate answer sheet is provided) as such so that when you return to the question you have fewer answers to consider. It is also possible to have your memory jogged by information in a later question.
- Once you make a decision and mark the answer sheet, be reluctant to change it. Unless you are sure the first answer marked is wrong, making a change may not be the right thing to do.
- If all else fails and you can't determine or remember what is the right answer, consider guessing. It is probably not to your advantage to leave any blank answers, as they will be scored as incorrect answers.
- Once you have answered all the questions go back and check your work to ensure completeness. Make sure you have marked an answer for every question. Don't second-guess yourself. This is the time to make sure you have filled in all the answers according to the instructions, and that there are no stray marks on the answer sheet. Remember to completely erase any answer you want to change.

Congratulations on your decision to make a difference in emergency medical services.

Transition Guide 1

From: Brady, *Essentials of Paramedic Care*, First Edition.
To: Brady, *Essentials of Paramedic Care*, Second Edition.

The following Transition Guide will help you coordinate course materials for Brady, *Essentials of Paramedic Care*, Second Edition if you previously used Brady, *Essentials of Paramedic Care*, First Edition for class instruction.

Transition Guide 1	Brady First Edition	Brady Second Edition
DIVISION ONE		
Introduction to Advanced Prehospital Care	Chap 1, pp. 2–71	Chap 1, pp. 2–63
Part 1: Introduction to Advanced Prehospital Care	Chap 1, pp. 6–8	Chap 1, pp. 6–8
Description of the Profession	Chap 1, pp. 6–7	Chap 1, pp. 6–7
Paramedic Characteristics	Chap 1, p. 7	Chap 1, p. 7
The Paramedic: A True Health Professional	Chap 1, pp. 7–8	Chap 1, p. 7
Expanded Scope of Practice	Chap 1, p. 8	Chap 1, p. 8
Part 2: EMS Systems	Chap 1, pp. 9–24	Chap 1, pp. 8–23
History of EMS	Chap 1, pp. 9–12	Chap 1, pp. 9–12
Today's EMS Systems	Chap 1, pp. 12–24	Chap 1, pp. 12–23
Part 3: Roles and Responsibilities of the Paramedic	Chap 1, pp. 24–32	Chap 1, pp. 23–31
Primary Responsibilities	Chap 1, pp. 25–27	Chap 1, pp. 23–26
Additional Responsibilities	Chap 1, pp. 27–28	Chap 1, pp. 26–27
Professionalism	Chap 1, pp. 28–32	Chap 1, pp. 27–31
Part 4: The Well-Being of the Paramedic	Chap 1, pp. 33–52	Chap 1, pp. 31–47
Basic Physical Fitness	Chap 1, pp. 33–37	Chap 1, pp. 31–34
Personal Protection from Disease	Chap 1, pp. 37–41	Chap 1, pp. 34–38
Death and Dying	Chap 1, pp. 41–45	Chap 1, pp. 38–41
Stress and Stress Management	Chap 1, pp. 45–50	Chap 1, pp. 41–45
General Safety Considerations	Chap 1, pp. 50–52	Chap 1, pp. 45–47
Part 5: Illness and Injury Prevention	Chap 1, pp. 52–59	Chap 1, pp. 47–53
Epidemiology	Chap 1, pp. 52–53	Chap 1, pp. 47–48
Prevention within EMS	Chap 1, pp. 53–56	Chap 1, pp. 48–50
Prevention in the Community	Chap 1, pp. 56–59	Chap 1, pp. 50–53
Part 6: Ethics in Advanced Prehospital Care	Chap 1, pp. 59–70	Chap 1, pp. 53–62
Overview of Ethics	Chap 1, pp. 60–63	Chap 1, pp. 53–56
Ethical Issues in Contemporary Paramedic Practice	Chap 1, pp. 64–70	Chap 1, pp. 56–62

Transition Guide 1	Brady First Edition	Brady Second Edition
Medical/Legal Aspects of Advanced Prehospital Care	Chap 2, pp. 72–93	Chap 2, pp. 64–83
Legal Duties and Ethical Responsibilities	Chap 2, pp. 74–78	Chap 2, pp. 66–69
Legal Accountability of the Paramedic	Chap 2, pp. 78–82	Chap 2, pp. 69–73
Paramedic-Patient Relationships	Chap 2, pp. 82–90	Chap 2, pp. 73–79
Resuscitation Issues	Chap 2, pp. 90–92	Chap 2, pp. 79–81
Crime and Accident Scenes	Chap 2, p. 92	Chap 2, p. 81
Documentation	Chap 2, pp. 92–93	Chap 2, pp. 81–82
Anatomy and Physiology	Chap 3, pp. 93–261	Chap 3, pp. 84–238
Part 1: The Cell and the Cellular Environment	Chap 3, pp. 96–116	Chap 3, pp. 88–104
The Normal Cell	Chap 3, pp. 96–104	Chap 3, pp. 88–94
The Cellular Environment: Fluids and Electrolytes	Chap 3, pp. 104–113	Chap 3, pp. 94–101
Acid-Base Balance	Chap 3, pp. 113–116	Chap 3, pp. 101–104
Part 2: Body Systems	Chap 3, pp. 116–261	Chap 3, pp. 104–235
The Integumentary System	Chap 3, pp. 116–119	Chap 3, pp. 105–107
The Blood	Chap 3, pp. 119–130	Chap 3, pp. 107–116
The Musculoskeletal System	Chap 3, pp. 130–152	Chap 3, pp. 117–138
The Head, Face, and Neck	Chap 3, pp. 153–166	Chap 3, pp. 138–151
The Spine and Thorax	Chap 3, pp. 166–177	Chap 3, pp. 151–160
The Nervous System	Chap 3, pp. 177–195	Chap 3, pp. 160–177
The Endocrine System	Chap 3, pp. 195–206	Chap 3, pp. 177–188
The Cardiovascular System	Chap 3, pp. 206–226	Chap 3, pp. 188–205
The Respiratory System	Chap 3, pp. 226–240	Chap 3, pp. 205–217
The Abdomen	Chap 3, pp. 240–243	Chap 3, pp. 217–220
The Digestive System	Chap 3, pp. 243–246	Chap 3, pp. 220–223
The Spleen	Chap 3, p. 246	Chap 3, p. 223
The Urinary System	Chap 3, pp. 246–252	Chap 3, pp. 223–228
The Reproductive System	Chap 3, pp. 252–260	Chap 3, pp. 228–235
General Principles of Pathophysiology	Chap 4, pp. 262–319	Chap 4, pp. 239–290
Part 1: How Normal Body Processes Are Altered by Disease and Injury	Chap 4, pp. 264–295	Chap 4, pp. 241–267
Pathophysiology	Chap 4, p. 264	Chap 4, p. 241
How Cells Respond to Change and Injury	Chap 4, pp. 265–271	Chap 4, pp. 241–246
Fluids and Fluid Imbalances	Chap 4, pp. 271–275	Chap 4, pp. 246–250
Acid-Base Derangements	Chap 4, pp. 275–277	Chap 4, pp. 250–252

Transition Guide 1	Brady First Edition	Brady Second Edition
Genetics and Other Causes of Disease	Chap 4, pp. 277–283	Chap 4, pp. 252–257
Hypoperfusion	Chap 4, pp. 283–295	Chap 4, pp. 257–267
Part 2: The Body's Defenses against Disease and Injury	Chap 4, pp. 295–319	Chap 4, pp. 268–288
Self-Defense Mechanisms	Chap 4, pp. 296–299	Chap 4, pp. 268–271
The Immune Response	Chap 4, pp. 299–302	Chap 4, pp. 271–273
Inflammation	Chap 4, pp. 302–307	Chap 4, pp. 273–279
Variances in Immunity and Inflammation	Chap 4, pp. 308–311	Chap 4, pp. 279–282
Stress and Disease	Chap 4, pp. 312–318	Chap 4, pp. 282–288
Life-Span Development	Chap 5, pp. 320–337	Chap 5, pp. 291–306
Infancy	Chap 5, pp. 321–326	Chap 5, pp. 292–296
Toddler and Preschool Age	Chap 5, pp. 326–329	Chap 5, pp. 296–298
School Age	Chap 5, pp. 329–330	Chap 5, pp. 298–299
Adolescence	Chap 5, pp. 330–331	Chap 5, pp. 299–300
Early Adulthood	Chap 5, p. 332	Chap 5, pp. 300–301
Middle Adulthood	Chap 5, p. 332	Chap 5, p. 301
Late Adulthood	Chap 5, pp. 332–337	Chap 5, pp. 301–305
General Principles of Pharmacology	Chap 6, pp. 338–411	Chap 6, pp. 307–372
Part 1: Basic Pharmacology	Chap 6, pp. 340–360	Chap 6, pp. 309–326
General Aspects		Chap 6, pp. 309–311
Names	Chap 6, pp. 340–341	Chap 6, pp. 309–310
Sources	Chap 6, p. 341	Chap 6, p. 310
Reference Materials	Chap 6, pp. 341–342	Chap 6, pp. 310–311
Components of a Drug Profile	Chap 6, p. 342	Chap 6, p. 311
Legal Aspects		Chap 6, pp. 311–313
Legal	Chap 6, pp. 343–344	
Patient Care: The Safe and Effective Administration of Medications	Chap 6, pp. 344–348	Chap 6, pp. 313–316
Pharmacology	Chap 6, pp. 348–360	Chap 6, pp. 316–326
Part 2: Drug Classifications	Chap 6, pp. 360–410	Chap 6, pp. 326–370
Classifying Drugs	Chap 6, pp. 360–361	Chap 6, p. 327
Drugs Used to Affect the Nervous System	Chap 6, pp. 361–378	Chap 6, pp. 327–342
Drugs Used to Affect the Cardiovascular System	Chap 6, pp. 378–390	Chap 6, pp. 343–353
Drugs Used to Affect the Respiratory System	Chap 6, pp. 390–394	Chap 6, pp. 353–356

Transition Guide 1	Brady First Edition	Brady Second Edition
Drugs Used to Affect the Gastrointestinal System	Chap 6, pp. 395–398	Chap 6, pp. 356–359
Drugs Used to Affect the Eyes	Chap 6, p. 398	Chap 6, pp. 359–360
Drugs Used to Affect the Ears	Chap 6, pp. 398–399	Chap 6, p. 360
Drugs Used to Affect the Endocrine System	Chap 6, pp. 399–405	Chap 6, pp. 360–366
Drugs Used to Treat Cancer	Chap 6, pp. 405–406	Chap 6, p. 366
Drugs Used to Treat Infectious Diseases and Inflammation	Chap 6, pp. 406–408	Chap 6, pp. 366–368
Drugs Used to Affect the Skin	Chap 6, p. 409	Chap 6, p. 368
Drugs Used to Supplement the Diet	Chap 6, p. 409	Chap 6, pp. 368–369
Drugs Used to Treat Poisoning and Overdoses	Chap 6, p. 410	Chap 6, p. 370
Medication Administration	Chap 7, pp. 412–495	
Intravenous Access and Medication Administration		Chap 7, pp. 373–453
Part 1: Principles and Routes of Medication Administration	Chap 7, pp. 414–448	Chap 7, pp. 375–405
General Principles		Chap 7, pp. 375–378
Medical Direction	Chap 7, pp. 414–415	Chap 7, p. 376
Body Substance Isolation	Chap 7, p. 415	Chap 7, p. 376
Medical Asepsis	Chap 7, pp. 415–416	Chap 7, pp. 376–377
Disposal of Contaminated Equipment and Sharps	Chap 7, p. 416	Chap 7, p. 377
Medication Administration and Documentation	Chap 7, p. 417	Chap 7, p. 378
Percutaneous Drug Administration	Chap 7, pp. 417–421	Chap 7, pp. 378–381
Pulmonary Drug Administration	Chap 7, pp. 421–425	Chap 7, pp. 381–385
Enteral Drug Administration	Chap 7, pp. 425–432	Chap 7, pp. 385–390
Parenteral Drug Administration	Chap 7, pp. 432–448	Chap 7, pp. 390–405
Part 2: Intravenous Access, Blood Sampling, and Intraosseous Infusion	Chap 7, pp. 448–487	Chap 7, pp. 405–442
Intravenous Access	Chap 7, pp. 448–480	Chap 7, pp. 405–435
Intraosseous Infusion	Chap 7, pp. 480–487	Chap 7, pp. 435–442
Part 3: Medical Mathematics	Chap 7, pp. 487–495	Chap 7, pp. 442–449
Metric System	Chap 7, pp. 487–490	Chap 7, pp. 442–444
Medical Calculations	Chap 7, pp. 490–495	Chap 7, pp. 444–449
Airway Management and Ventilation	Chap 8, pp. 496–573	Chap 8, pp. 454–531
Respiratory Problems	Chap 8, pp. 498–500	Chap 8, pp. 456–458
Respiratory System Assessment	Chap 8, pp. 500–508	Chap 8, pp. 458–468

Transition Guide 1	Brady First Edition	Brady Second Edition
Basic Airway Management	Chap 8, pp. 508–515	Chap 8, pp. 468–474
Advanced Airway Management	Chap 8, pp. 516–562	Chap 8, pp. 474–519
Managing Patients with Stoma Sites	Chap 8, pp. 562–563	Chap 8, pp. 520–521
Suctioning	Chap 8, pp. 563–565	Chap 8, pp. 521–522
Gastric Decompression	Chap 8, pp. 565–566	
Gastric Distension and Decompression		Chap 8, pp. 522–523
Oxygenation	Chap 8, pp. 566–567	Chap 8, pp. 523–525
Ventilation	Chap 8, pp. 567–572	Chap 8, pp. 525–529
Therapeutic Communications	Chap 9, pp. 574–587	Chap 9, pp. 532–544
Basic Elements of Communication	Chap 9, pp. 575–577	Chap 9, pp. 533–535
Communication Techniques	Chap 9, pp. 577–587	Chap 9, pp. 535–543
DIVISION 2		
History Taking	Chap 10, pp. 590–607	Chap 10, pp. 546–563
Establishing Patient Rapport	Chap 10, pp. 591–594	Chap 10, pp. 547–550
The Comprehensive Patient History	Chap 10, pp. 594–602	Chap 10, pp. 550–558
Special Challenges	Chap 10, pp. 602–606	Chap 10, pp. 558–561
Physical Exam Techniques	Chap 11, pp. 608–696	Chap 11, pp. 564–650
Physical Examination Approach and Overview	Chap 11, pp. 610–622	Chap 11, pp. 565–576
Overview of a Comprehensive Examination	Chap 11, pp. 622–629	Chap 11, pp. 576–584
Anatomical Regions	Chap 11, pp. 630–689	Chap 11, pp. 585–642
Physical Examination of Infants and Children	Chap 11, pp. 690–695	Chap 11, pp. 642–647
Recording Examination Findings	Chap 11, pp. 695–696	Chap 11, p. 647
Patient Assessment in the Field	Chap 12, pp. 698–754	Chap 12, pp. 651–703
Scene Size-Up	Chap 12, pp. 701–712	Chap 12, pp. 654–663
The Initial Assessment	Chap 12, pp. 712–722	Chap 12, pp. 663–673
The Focused History and Physical Exam	Chap 12, pp. 722–743	Chap 12, pp. 673–691
The Detailed Physical Exam	Chap 12, pp. 744–750	Chap 12, pp. 692–698
Ongoing Assessment	Chap 12, pp. 751–754	Chap 12, pp. 698–701
Clinical Decision Making	Chap 13, pp. 756–768	Chap 13, pp. 704–715
Clinical Judgment		Chap 13, p. 705
Paramedic Practice	Chap 13, pp. 757–759	Chap 13, pp. 705–708

Transition Guide 1	Brady First Edition	Brady Second Edition
Critical Thinking Skills	Chap 13, pp. 759–763	Chap 13, pp. 708–710
Thinking under Pressure	Chap 13, pp. 764–765	Chap 13, pp. 710–711
The Critical Decision Process	Chap 13, pp. 765–767	Chap 13, pp. 711–714
Communications	Chap 14, pp. 770–787	Chap 14, pp. 716–734
Verbal Communication	Chap 14, pp. 773–774	Chap 14, p. 718
Written Communication	Chap 14, p. 774	Chap 14, pp. 718–720
The EMS Response	Chap 14, pp. 775–778	Chap 14, pp. 720–726
Communication Technology	Chap 14, pp. 779–783	Chap 14, pp. 726–730
Reporting Procedures	Chap 14, pp. 783–786	Chap 14, pp. 730–732
Regulation	Chap 14, pp. 786–787	Chap 14, pp. 732–733
Documentation	Chap 15, pp. 788–812	Chap 15, pp. 735–758
Uses for Documentation	Chap 15, pp. 790–791	Chap 15, pp. 736–738
General Considerations	Chap 15, pp. 792–799	Chap 15, pp. 738–745
Elements of Good Documentation	Chap 15, pp. 799–802	Chap 15, pp. 745–748
Narrative Writing	Chap 15, pp. 802–808	Chap 15, pp. 748–753
Special Considerations	Chap 15, pp. 808–810	Chap 15, pp. 753–755
Consequences of Inappropriate Documentation	Chap 15, pp. 810–811	Chap 15, pp. 755–756
Closing	Chap 15, p. 811	Chap 15, p. 756
DIVISION 3		
Trauma and Trauma Systems	Chap 16, pp. 814–823	Chap 16, pp. 760–769
Trauma	Chap 16, pp. 815–816	Chap 16, pp. 761–762
The Trauma Care System	Chap 16, p. 816	Chap 16, p. 762
Trauma Center Designation	Chap 16, pp. 817–818	Chap 16, pp. 762–764
Your Role as an EMT-Paramedic	Chap 16, pp. 819–823	Chap 16, pp. 764–767
Blunt Trauma	Chap 17, pp. 824–857	Chap 17, pp. 770–801
Kinetics of Blunt Trauma	Chap 17, pp. 826–827	Chap 17, pp. 771–773
Types of Trauma	Chap 17, pp. 827–829	
Blunt Trauma	Chap 17, pp. 829–857	Chap 17, pp. 774–799
Penetrating Trauma	Chap 18, pp. 858–877	Chap 18, pp. 802–820
Physics of Penetrating Trauma	Chap 18, pp. 859–869	Chap 18, pp. 803–811
Specific Tissue/Organ Injuries	Chap 18, pp. 869–873	Chap 18, pp. 811–816
Special Concerns with Penetrating Trauma	Chap 18, pp. 874–877	Chap 18, pp. 816–818

Transition Guide 1	Brady First Edition	Brady Second Edition
Hemorrhage and Shock	Chap 19, pp. 878–909	Chap 19, pp. 821–851
Hemorrhage	Chap 19, pp. 880–896	Chap 19, pp. 822–837
Shock	Chap 19, pp. 896–908	Chap 19, pp. 837–849
Soft-Tissue Trauma	Chap 20, pp. 910–951	Chap 20, pp. 852–890
Pathophysiology of Soft-Tissue Injury	Chap 20, pp. 912–929	Chap 20, pp. 854–868
Dressing and Bandage Materials	Chap 20, pp. 929–931	Chap 20, pp. 869–871
Assessment of Soft-Tissue Injuries	Chap 20, pp. 932–936	Chap 20, pp. 871–875
Management of Soft-Tissue Injury	Chap 20, pp. 936–951	Chap 20, pp. 875–888
Burns	Chap 21, pp. 952–985	Chap 21, pp. 891–923
Pathophysiology of Burns	Chap 21, pp. 954–969	Chap 21, pp. 892–906
Assessment of Thermal Burns	Chap 21, pp. 969–975	Chap 21, pp. 906–912
Management of Thermal Burns	Chap 21, pp. 975–978	Chap 21, pp. 912–915
Assessment and Management of Electrical, Chemical, and Radiation Burns	Chap 21, pp. 978–985	Chap 21, pp. 915–921
Musculoskeletal Trauma	Chap 22, pp. 986–1022	Chap 22, pp. 924–957
Prevention Strategies	Chap 22, p. 988	Chap 22, p. 926
Pathophysiology of the Musculoskeletal System	Chap 22, pp. 988–996	Chap 22, pp. 926–933
Musculoskeletal Injury Assessment	Chap 22, pp. 996–1002	Chap 22, pp. 933–938
Musculoskeletal Injury Management	Chap 22, pp. 1002–1022	Chap 22, pp. 938–955
Head, Facial, and Neck Trauma	Chap 23, pp. 1024–1067	Chap 23, pp. 958–999
Pathophysiology of Head, Facial, and Neck Injury	Chap 23, pp. 1026–1045	Chap 23, pp. 960–978
Assessment of Head, Facial, and Neck Injuries	Chap 23, pp. 1045–1053	Chap 23, pp. 978–985
Head, Facial, and Neck Injury Management	Chap 23, pp. 1053–1067	Chap 23, pp. 985–997
Spinal Trauma	Chap 24, pp. 1068–1097	Chap 24, pp. 1000–1029
Pathophysiology of Spinal Injury	Chap 24, pp. 1070–1076	Chap 24, pp. 1001–1007
Assessment of the Spinal Injury Patient	Chap 24, pp. 1076–1083	Chap 24, pp. 1007–1014
Management of the Spinal Injury Patient	Chap 24, pp. 1083–1097	Chap 24, pp. 1014–1027
Thoracic Trauma	Chap 25, pp. 1098–1131	Chap 25, pp. 1030–1060
Pathophysiology of Thoracic Trauma	Chap 25, pp. 1101–1119	Chap 25, pp. 1032–1048
Assessment of the Thoracic Trauma Patient	Chap 25, pp. 1119–1125	
Assessment of the Chest Injury Patient		Chap 25, pp. 1048–1053

Transition Guide 1	Brady First Edition	Brady Second Edition
Management of the Chest Injury Patient	Chap 25, pp. 1125–1131	
Management of the Thoracic Trauma Patient		Chap 25, pp. 1053–1058
Abdominal Trauma	Chap 26, pp. 1132–1151	Chap 26, pp. 1061–1078
Pathophysiology of Abdominal Injury	Chap 26, pp. 1135–1143	Chap 26, pp. 1062–1069
Assessment of the Abdominal Injury Patient	Chap 26, pp. 1143–1149	Chap 26, pp. 1069–1074
Management of the Abdominal Injury Patient	Chap 26, pp. 1149–1151	Chap 26, pp. 1074–1077
DIVISION 4		
Pulmonology	Chap 27, pp. 1154–1195	Chap 27, pp. 1080–1084
Pathophysiology	Chap 27, pp. 1158–1161	Chap 27, pp. 1084–1086
Assessment of the Respiratory System	Chap 27, pp. 1162–1172	Chap 27, pp. 1086–1098
Management of Respiratory Disorders	Chap 27, pp. 1172–1173	Chap 27, p. 1098
Specific Respiratory Diseases	Chap 27, pp. 1173–1195	Chap 27, pp. 1098–1118
Cardiology	Chap 28, pp. 1196–1339	Chap 28, pp. 1121–1242
Part 1: Cardiovascular Anatomy and Physiology, ECG Monitoring and Dysrhythmia Analysis	Chap 28, pp. 1202–1279	Chap 28, pp. 1127–1185
Review of Cardiovascular Anatomy and Physiology	Chap 28, pp. 1202–1205	Chap 28, pp. 1127–1130
Electrocardiographic Monitoring	Chap 28, pp. 1206–1219	Chap 28, pp. 1130–1142
Dysrhythmias	Chap 28, pp. 1219–1279	Chap 28, pp. 1142–1185
Part 2: Assessment and Management of the Cardiovascular Patient	Chap 28, pp. 1280–1336	Chap 28, pp. 1186–1240
Assessment of the Cardiovascular Patient	Chap 28, pp. 1280–1290	Chap 28, pp. 1186–1194
Management of Cardiovascular Emergencies	Chap 28, pp. 1290–1306	Chap 28, pp. 1194–1211
Managing Specific Cardiovascular Emergencies	Chap 28, pp. 1307–1336	Chap 28, pp. 1211–1237
Prehospital ECG Monitoring	Chap 28, pp. 1336–1339	Chap 28, pp. 1237–1240
Neurology	Chap 29, pp. 1340–1377	Chap 29, pp. 1243–1279
Pathophysiology	Chap 29, pp. 1342–1344	Chap 29, pp. 1245–1247
General Assessment Findings	Chap 29, pp. 1344–1353	Chap 29, pp. 1247–1255
Management of Specific Nervous System Emergencies	Chap 29, pp. 1353–1377	Chap 29, pp. 1255–1277
Endocrinology	Chap 30, pp. 1378–1393	Chap 30, pp. 1280–1294
Endocrine Disorders and Emergencies	Chap 30, pp. 1380–1393	Chap 30, pp. 1282–1293

Transition Guide 1	Brady First Edition	Brady Second Edition
Allergies and Anaphylaxis	Chap 31, pp. 1394–1405	Chap 31, pp. 1295–1305
Pathophysiology	Chap 31, pp. 1396–1399	Chap 31, pp. 1296–1299
Assessment Findings in Anaphylaxis	Chap 31, pp. 1400–1401	Chap 31, pp. 1299–1301
Management of Anaphylaxis	Chap 31, pp. 1401–1403	Chap 31, pp. 1301–1303
Assessment Findings in Allergic Reaction	Chap 31, p. 1403	Chap 31, p. 1303
Management of Allergic Reactions	Chap 31, pp. 1403–1404	Chap 31, p. 1303
Gastroenterology	Chap 32, pp. 1406–1429	Chap 32, pp. 1306–1327
General Pathophysiology, Assessment, and Treatment	Chap 32, pp. 1407–1412	Chap 32, pp. 1307–1311
Specific Illnesses	Chap 32, pp. 1412–1429	Chap 32, pp. 1311–1325
Urology and Nephrology	Chap 33, pp. 1430–1453	Chap 33, pp. 1328–1348
General Mechanisms of Nontraumatic Tissue Problems	Chap 33, p. 1433	Chap 33, p. 1330
General Pathophysiology, Assessment, and Management	Chap 33, pp. 1433–1438	Chap 33, pp. 1331–1335
Renal and Urologic Emergencies	Chap 33, pp. 1439–1453	Chap 33, pp. 1335–1347
Toxicology and Substance Abuse	Chap 34, pp. 1454–1495	Chap 34, pp. 1349–1388
Epidemiology	Chap 34, p. 1456	Chap 34, p. 1351
Poison Control Centers	Chap 34, pp. 1456–1457	Chap 34, p. 1351
Routes of Toxic Exposure	Chap 34, pp. 1457–1458	Chap 34, pp. 1352–1353
General Principles of Toxicologic Assessment and Management	Chap 34, pp. 1458–1461	Chap 34, pp. 1353–1355
Ingested Toxins	Chap 34, pp. 1461–1463	Chap 34, pp. 1356–1357
Inhaled Toxins	Chap 34, p. 1464	Chap 34, pp. 1357–1358
Surface-Absorbed Toxins	Chap 34, pp. 1464–1465	Chap 34, pp. 1358–1359
Specific Toxins	Chap 34, pp. 1465–1480	Chap 34, pp. 1359–1372
Injected Toxins	Chap 34, pp. 1480–1488	Chap 34, pp. 1372–1380
Substance Abuse and Overdose	Chap 34, pp. 1488–1492	Chap 34, pp. 1380–1381
Alcohol Abuse	Chap 34, pp. 1492–1495	Chap 34, pp. 1381–1386
Hematology	Chap 35, pp. 1496–1513	Chap 35, pp. 1389–1404
General Assessment and Management	Chap 35, pp. 1500–1506	Chap 35, pp. 1392–1397
Managing Specific Patient Problems	Chap 35, pp. 1506–1513	Chap 35, pp. 1397–1403

Transition Guide 1	Brady First Edition	Brady Second Edition
Environmental Emergencies	Chap 36, pp. 1514–1553	Chap 36, pp. 1405–1438
Homeostasis	Chap 36, pp. 1516–1517	Chap 36, p. 1407
Pathophysiology of Heat and Cold Disorders	Chap 36, pp. 1517–1520	Chap 36, pp. 1407–1411
Heat Disorders	Chap 36, pp. 1521–1526	Chap 36, pp. 1411–1416
Cold Disorders	Chap 36, pp. 1526–1534	Chap 36, pp. 1416–1423
Near-Drowning and Drowning	Chap 36, pp. 1535–1538	Chap 36, pp. 1423–1426
Diving Emergencies	Chap 36, pp. 1538–1546	Chap 36, pp. 1426–1433
High Altitude Illness	Chap 36, pp. 1546–1549	Chap 36, pp. 1433–1436
Nuclear Radiation	Chap 36, pp. 1549–1553	
Infectious Disease	Chap 37, pp. 1554–1605	Chap 37, pp. 1439–1485
Public Health Principles	Chap 37, pp. 1556–1557	Chap 37, pp. 1441–1442
Public Health Agencies	Chap 37, p. 1557	Chap 37, p. 1442
Microorganisms	Chap 37, pp. 1557–1561	Chap 37, pp. 1443–1446
Contraction, Transmission, and Stages of Disease	Chap 37, pp. 1562–1564	Chap 37, pp. 1446–1449
Infection Control	Chap 37, pp. 1564–1570	Chap 37, pp. 1449–1454
Assessment of the Patient with Infectious Disease	Chap 37, pp. 1570–1572	Chap 37, pp. 1454–1455
Selected Infectious Diseases	Chap 37, pp. 1572–1603	Chap 37, pp. 1455–1483
Preventing Disease Transmission	Chap 37, pp. 1604–1605	Chap 37, pp. 1483–1484
Psychiatric and Behavioral Disorders	Chap 38, pp. 1606–1629	Chap 38, pp. 1486–1508
Behavioral Emergencies	Chap 38, pp. 1607–1608	Chap 38, pp. 1487–1488
Pathophysiology of Psychiatric Disorders	Chap 38, pp. 1608–1609	Chap 38, pp. 1488–1489
Assessment of Behavioral Emergency Patients	Chap 38, pp. 1609–1613	Chap 38, pp. 1489–1492
Specific Psychiatric Disorders	Chap 38, pp. 1613–1624	Chap 38, pp. 1492–1502
Management of Behavioral Emergencies	Chap 38, pp. 1624–1626	Chap 38, pp. 1502–1504
Violent Patients and Restraint	Chap 38, pp. 1626–1629	Chap 38, pp. 1504–1507
Gynecology	Chap 39, pp. 1630–1639	Chap 39, pp. 1509–1517
Assessment of the Gynecological Patient	Chap 39, pp. 1631–1633	Chap 39, pp. 1510–1511
Management of Gynecological Emergencies	Chap 39, pp. 1633–1634	Chap 39, p. 1512
Specific Gynecological Emergencies	Chap 39, pp. 1634–1639	Chap 39, pp. 1512–1516
Obstetrics	Chap 40, pp. 1640–1677	Chap 40, pp. 1518–1552
The Prenatal Period	Chap 40, pp. 1641–1647	Chap 40, pp. 1519–1525
General Assessment of the Obstetric Patient	Chap 40, pp. 1648–1651	Chap 40, pp. 1525–1527
General Management of the Obstetric Patient	Chap 40, p. 1651	Chap 40, p. 1527

Transition Guide 1	Brady First Edition	Brady Second Edition
Complications of Pregnancy	Chap 40, pp. 1652–1662	Chap 40, pp. 1527–1537
The Puerperium	Chap 40, pp. 1662–1670	Chap 40, pp. 1537–1544
Abnormal Delivery Situations	Chap 40, pp. 1670–1674	Chap 40, pp. 1544–1547
Other Delivery Complications	Chap 40, pp. 1674–1675	Chap 40, pp. 1548–1549
Maternal Complications of Labor and Delivery	Chap 40, pp. 1675–1677	Chap 40, pp. 1549–1550
DIVISION 5		
Neonatology	Chap 41, pp. 1680–1711	Chap 41, pp. 1554–1584
General Pathophysiology, Assessment, and Management	Chap 41, pp. 1682–1689	Chap 41, pp. 1556–1563
The Distressed Newborn	Chap 41, pp. 1689–1700	Chap 41, pp. 1563–1573
Specific Neonatal Situations	Chap 41, pp. 1701–1711	Chap 41, pp. 1574–1582
Pediatrics	Chap 42, pp. 1712–1797	Chap 42, pp. 1585–1666
Role of the Paramedics in Pediatric Care	Chap 42, pp. 1714–1716	Chap 42, pp. 1587–1589
General Approach to Pediatric Emergencies	Chap 42, pp. 1716–1725	Chap 42, pp. 1589–1597
General Approach to Pediatric Assessment	Chap 42, pp. 1726–1736	Chap 42, pp. 1597–1606
General Management of Pediatric Patients	Chap 42, pp. 1736–1753	Chap 42, pp. 1606–1623
Specific Medical Emergencies	Chap 42, pp. 1753–1780	Chap 42, pp. 1623–1648
Trauma Emergencies	Chap 42, pp. 1780–1789	Chap 42, pp. 1648–1656
Sudden Infant Death Syndrome (SIDS)	Chap 42, pp. 1789–1790	Chap 42, pp. 1656–1657
Child Abuse and Neglect	Chap 42, pp. 1790–1793	Chap 42, pp. 1657–1661
Infants and Children with Special Needs	Chap 42, pp. 1794–1797	Chap 42, pp. 1661–1664
Geriatric Emergencies	Chap 43, pp. 1798–1851	Chap 43, pp. 1667–1714
Epidemiology and Demographics	Chap 43, pp. 1800–1802	Chap 43, pp. 1669–1671
General Pathophysiology, Assessment, and Management	Chap 43, pp. 1802–1812	Chap 43, pp. 1671–1680
System Pathophysiology in the Elderly	Chap 43, pp. 1812–1818	Chap 43, pp. 1680–1685
Common Medical Problems in the Elderly	Chap 43, pp. 1819–1845	Chap 43, pp. 1685–1708
Trauma in the Elderly Patient	Chap 43, pp. 1845–1851	Chap 43, pp. 1708–1713
Abuse and Assault	Chap 44, pp. 1852–1865	Chap 44, pp. 1715–1728
Partner Abuse	Chap 44, pp. 1853–1856	Chap 44, pp. 1716–1718
Elder Abuse	Chap 44, p. 1856	Chap 44, pp. 1718–1720
Child Abuse	Chap 44, pp. 1858–1862	Chap 44, pp. 1720–1723
Sexual Assault	Chap 44, pp. 1862–1865	Chap 44, pp. 1724–1727

Transition Guide 1 **xliii**

Transition Guide 1	Brady First Edition	Brady Second Edition
The Challenged Patient	Chap 45, pp. 1866–1883	Chap 45, pp. 1729–1745
Physical Challenges	Chap 45, pp. 1867–1874	Chap 45, pp. 1730–1736
Mental Challenges and Emotional Impairments	Chap 45, p. 1874	Chap 45, p. 1736
Developmental Disabilities	Chap 45, pp. 1874–1876	Chap 45, pp. 1736–1738
Pathological Challenges	Chap 45, pp. 1876–1882	Chap 45, pp. 1738–1743
Other Challenges	Chap 45, pp. 1882–1883	Chap 45, pp. 1743–1744
Acute Interventions for the Chronic–Care Patient	Chap 46, pp. 1884–1919	Chap 46, pp. 1746–1777
Epidemiology of Home Care	Chap 46, pp. 1885–1891	Chap 46, pp. 1747–1753
General System Pathophysiology, Assessment, and Management	Chap 46, pp. 1892–1896	Chap 46, pp. 1753–1757
Specific Acute Home Health Situations	Chap 46, pp. 1897–1919	Chap 46, pp. 1757–1776
Assessment-Based Management	Chap 47, pp. 1920–1935	Chap 47, pp. 1778–1792
Effective Assessment	Chap 47, pp. 1922–1927	Chap 47, pp. 1779–1784
The Right Equipment	Chap 47, pp. 1927–1928	Chap 47, pp. 1784–1785
General Approach to the Patient	Chap 47, pp. 1928–1932	Chap 47, pp. 1785–1788
Presenting the Patient	Chap 47, pp. 1932–1934	Chap 47, pp. 1788–1790
Review of Common Complaints	Chap 47, p. 1934	Chap 47, pp. 1790–1791
Operations	Chap 48, pp. 1936–2034	Chap 48, pp. 1793–1889
Part 1: Ambulance Operations	Chap 48, pp. 1940–1953	Chap 48, pp. 1798–1809
Ambulance Standards	Chap 48, pp. 1940–1942	Chap 48, pp. 1798–1800
Checking Ambulances	Chap 48, pp. 1942–1943	
Checking and Maintaining Ambulances		Chap 48, pp. 1800–1801
Ambulance Deployment and Staffing	Chap 48, pp. 1943–1944	Chap 48, pp. 1801–1802
Safe Ambulance Operations	Chap 48, pp. 1944–1949	Chap 48, pp. 1802–1806
Utilizing Air Medical Transport	Chap 48, pp. 1949–1952	Chap 48, pp. 1806–1809
Part 2: Medical Incident Command	Chap 48, pp. 1953–1972	
Part 2: Medical Incident Management		Chap 48, pp. 1809–1830
Origins of the Incident Management System	Chap 48, pp. 1953–1954	
Origins of Emergency Incident Management		Chap 48, pp. 1810–1811
Command at Mass-Casualty Incidents	Chap 48, pp. 1954–1958	
Command		Chap 48, pp. 1811–1816
Support of Incident Command	Chap 48, pp. 1958–1960	Chap 48, pp. 1816–1819
Division of Functions	Chap 48, pp. 1960–1962	
Division of Operations Functions		Chap 48, pp. 1819–1820

xliv ESSENTIALS OF PARAMEDIC CARE

Transition Guide 1	Brady First Edition	Brady Second Edition
Functional Groups within an EMS Branch	Chap 48, pp. 1962–1969	
Functional Groups with an EMS Branch		Chap 48, pp. 1820–1827
Disaster Management	Chap 48, pp. 1969–1970	Chap 48, pp. 1827–1828
Meeting the Challenge of Mass Casualty Incidents	Chap 48, pp. 1970–1972	
Meeting the Challenge of Multiple-Casualty Incidents		Chap 48, pp. 1828–1830
Part 3: Rescue Awareness and Operations	Chap 48, pp. 1972–2001	Chap 48, pp. 1830–1857
Role of the Paramedic	Chap 48, pp. 1972–1973	Chap 48, pp. 1830–1831
Protective Equipment	Chap 48, pp. 1973–1975	Chap 48, pp. 1831–1833
Safety Procedures	Chap 48, pp. 1976–1977	Chap 48, pp. 1833–1834
Rescue Operations	Chap 48, pp. 1977–1980	Chap 48, pp. 1835–1838
Surface Water Rescues	Chap 48, pp. 1981–1987	Chap 48, pp. 1838–1845
Hazardous Atmosphere Rescues	Chap 48, pp. 1987–1990	Chap 48, pp. 1845–1847
Highway Operations and Vehicle Rescues	Chap 48, pp. 1990–1995	Chap 48, pp. 1847–1851
Hazardous Terrain Rescues	Chap 48, pp. 1995–2000	Chap 48, pp. 1851–1857
Part 4: Hazardous Materials Incidents	Chap 48, pp. 2001–2019	Chap 48, pp. 1857–1872
Role of the Paramedic	Chap 48, pp. 2001–2002	Chap 48, pp. 1857–1858
Incident Size-Up	Chap 48, pp. 2002–2009	Chap 48, pp. 1858–1863
Specialized Terminology	Chap 48, pp. 2009–2010	Chap 48, pp. 1863–1865
Contamination and Toxicology Review	Chap 48, pp. 2010–2014	Chap 48, pp. 1865–1868
Approaches to Decontamination	Chap 48, pp. 2014–2017	Chap 48, pp. 1868–1871
Hazmat Protection Equipment	Chap 48, pp. 2017–2018	Chap 48, p. 1871
Medical Monitoring and Rehabilitation	Chap 48, pp. 2018–2019	Chap 48, p. 1872
Importance of Practice	Chap 48, p. 2019	Chap 48, p. 1872
Part 5: Crime Scene Awareness	Chap 48, pp. 2019–2033	Chap 48, pp. 1872–1885
Approach to the Scene	Chap 48, pp. 2020–2022	Chap 48, pp. 1873–1875
Specific Dangerous Scenes	Chap 48, pp. 2023–2026	Chap 48, pp. 1875–1879
Tactical Considerations	Chap 48, pp. 2026–2031	Chap 48, pp. 1879–1883
EMS at Crime Scenes	Chap 48, pp. 2031–2033	Chap 48, pp. 1883–1885
Responding to Terrorist Acts	n/a	Chap 49, pp. 1890–1904
Explosive Agents	n/a	Chap 49, p. 1892
Nuclear Detonation	n/a	Chap 49, pp. 1893–1895
Chemical Agents	n/a	Chap 49, pp. 1895–1900
Biological Agents	n/a	Chap 49, pp. 1900–1902
General Considerations regarding Terrorist Attacks	n/a	Chap 49, pp. 1902–1903

Transition Guide 2

From: Mosby, *Paramedic Textbook*, Third Edition

To: Brady, *Essentials of Paramedic Care*, Second Edition

The following Transition Guide will help you coordinate course materials for Brady, *Essentials of Paramedic Care*, Second Edition if you previously used Mosby, *Paramedic Textbook*, Third Edition for class instruction.

Transition Guide 2	Mosby Third Edition	Brady Second Edition
PART ONE		
Emergency Medical Service Systems: Roles and Responsibilities	Chap 1, pp. 2–21	Chap 1, pp. 8–23
Emergency Medical Services System Development	Chap 1, pp. 3–7	Chap 1, pp. 9–12
Current Emergency Medical Services Systems	Chap 1, pp. 7–10	Chap 1, pp. 12–16
National Emergency Medical Services Group Involvement	Chap 1, p. 10	Chap 1, p. 7
Paramedic Education	Chap 1, p. 11	Chap 1, pp. 16–18
Licensure, Certification, and Registration	Chap 1, p. 11	Chap 1, pp. 16–18
Professionalism	Chap 1, pp. 11–13	Chap 1, pp. 27–31
Roles and Responsibilities of the Paramedic	Chap 1, pp. 13–15	Chap 1, pp. 23–31
Medical Direction for Emergency Medical Services	Chap 1, pp. 15–16	Chap 1, pp. 13–14
Improving System Quality	Chap 1, p. 16	Chap 1, pp. 20–21
Emergency Medical Services Research	Chap 1, pp. 16–20	Chap 1, p. 21–23
The Well-Being of the Paramedic	Chap 2, pp. 22–41	Chap 1, pp. 31–47
Wellness Components	Chap 2, pp. 23–32	Chap 1, pp. 31–34
Stress	Chap 2, pp. 32–37	Chap 1, pp. 41–45
Dealing with Death, Dying, Grief, and Loss	Chap 2, pp. 37–39	Chap 1, pp. 38–41
Prevention of Disease Transmission	Chap 2, pp. 39–40	Chap 1, pp. 34–38
Injury Prevention	Chap 3, pp. 42–53	Chap 1, pp. 47–53
Injury Epidemiology	Chap 3, p. 43	Chap 1, pp. 47–48
Overview of Injury Prevention	Chap 3, pp. 43–46	Chap 1, pp. 47–53
Feasibility of Emergency Medical Services Involvement	Chap 3, pp. 46–50	Chap 1, pp. 47–53
Participation in Prevention Programs	Chap 3, pp. 50–52	Chap 1, pp. 50–53

Transition Guide 2	Mosby Third Edition	Brady Second Edition
Medical/Legal Issues	Chap 4, pp. 54–71	Chap 2, pp. 64–83
Legal Duties and Ethical Responsibilities	Chap 4, p. 55	Chap 2, pp. 66–69
The Legal System	Chap 4, pp. 55–58	Chap 2, pp. 66–69
Legal Accountability of the Paramedic	Chap 4, pp. 58–61	Chap 2, pp. 70–73
Paramedic-Patient Relationships	Chap 4, pp. 61–65	Chap 2, pp. 73–79
Resuscitation Issues	Chap 4, pp. 65–69	Chap 2, pp. 79–81
Crime Scene Responsibilities	Chap 4, p. 69	Chap 2, p. 81
Documentation	Chap 4, pp. 69–70	Chap 2, pp. 81–82
Ethics	Chap 5, pp. 72–79	Chap 1, pp. 53–62
Ethics Overview	Chap 5, pp. 73–76	Chap 1, pp. 53–56
A Rapid Approach to Emergency Ethical Problems	Chap 5, p. 76	Chap 1, pp. 54–55
Ethical Tests in Health Care	Chap 5, p. 76	Chap 1, pp. 54–55
Resolving Ethical Dilemmas	Chap 5, pp. 76–77	Chap 1, pp. 55–56
Ethical Issues in Contemporary Paramedic Practice	Chap 5, pp. 77–79	Chap 1, pp. 56–62
PART TWO		
Review of Human Systems	Chap 6, pp. 82–149	
Anatomy and Physiology		Chap 3, pp. 84–238
Terminology	Chap 6, pp. 83–84	Chap 3, p. 87
Cell Structure	Chap 6, pp. 84–90	Chap 3, pp. 88–90
Tissues	Chap 6, pp. 90–92	Chap 3, pp. 90–91
Organ Systems	Chap 6, pp. 92–143	Chap 3, pp. 91–94
Special Senses	Chap 6, pp. 144–148	
General Principles of Pathophysiology	Chap 7, pp. 150–195	Chap 4, pp. 239–290
Section One—Cellular Physiology	Chap 7, pp. 152–171	Chap 3, pp. 94–104
Basic Cellular Review	Chap 7, p. 152	Chap 3, p. 94
Cellular Environment	Chap 7, pp. 152–171	Chap 3, pp. 94–104
Section Two—Cellular Injury and Disease	Chap 7, pp. 172–193	Chap 4, pp. 241–267
Alterations in Cells and Tissues	Chap 7, pp. 172–176	Chap 4, pp. 241–246
Hypoperfusion	Chap 7, pp. 176–181	Chap 4, pp. 257–267
Self-Defense Mechanisms	Chap 7, pp. 181–185	Chap 4, pp. 268–271
Variances in Immunity and Inflammation	Chap 7, pp. 185–187	Chap 4, pp. 279–282
Stress and Disease	Chap 7, pp. 187–189	Chap 4, pp. 282–288
Genetics and Familial Diseases	Chap 7, pp. 189–193	Chap 4, pp. 252–257

Transition Guide 2	Mosby Third Edition	Brady Second Edition
Life Span Development	Chap 8, pp. 196–211	Chap 5, pp. 291–306
Newborn	Chap 8, pp. 197–201	
Infancy		Chap 5, pp. 292–296
Toddler and Preschool Years	Chap 8, pp. 201–203	Chap 5, pp. 296–298
School-Age Years	Chap 8, pp. 203–204	Chap 5, pp. 298–299
Adolescence	Chap 8, pp. 204–206	Chap 5, pp. 299–300
Early Adulthood	Chap 8, p. 206	Chap 5, pp. 300–301
Middle Adulthood	Chap 8, pp. 206–207	Chap 5, p. 301
Late Adulthood	Chap 8, pp. 207–210	Chap 5, pp. 301–305
PART THREE		
Therapeutic Communications	Chap 9, pp. 214–225	Chap 9, pp. 532–544
Communication	Chap 9, pp. 215–216	Chap 9, pp. 533
Internal Factors in Effective Communication	Chap 9, pp. 216–217	Chap 9, pp. 533–540
External Factors in Effective Communication	Chap 9, pp. 217–218	Chap 9, pp. 533–540
Patient Interview	Chap 9, pp. 218–219	Chap 9, pp. 537–540
Strategies for Obtaining Information	Chap 9, pp. 219–220	Chap 9, pp. 537–540
Methods of Assessing Mental Status during the Interview	Chap 9, pp. 220–221	Chap 9, p. 537–540
Special Interview Situations	Chap 9, pp. 221–223	Chap 9, pp. 540–543
History Taking	Chap 10, pp. 226–233	Chap 10, pp. 546–563
Content of the Patient History	Chap 10, p. 227–228	Chap 10, pp. 547–558
Techniques of History Taking	Chap 10, pp. 228–231	Chap 10, pp. 551–558
Special Challenges	Chap 10, pp. 231–233	Chap 10, pp. 550–558
Techniques of Physical Examination	Chap 11, pp. 234–279	Chap 11, pp. 564–650
Physical Examination: Approach and Overview	Chap 11, pp. 235–238	Chap 11, pp. 565–576
Mental Status	Chap 11, pp. 238–240	Chap 11, pp. 576–578
General Survey	Chap 11, pp. 240–250	Chap 11, pp. 576–584
Anatomical Regions	Chap 11, pp. 250–274	Chap 11, pp. 585–642
Physical Examination of Infants and Children	Chap 11, pp. 274–277	Chap 11, pp. 642–647
Physical Examination of Older Adults	Chap 11, pp. 277–278	
Patient Assessment	Chap 12, pp. 280–289	Chap 12, pp. 651–703
Scene Size-Up and Assessment	Chap 12, pp. 281–282	Chap 12, pp. 654–663
Patient Assessment Priorities	Chap 12, p. 282	

Transition Guide 2	Mosby Third Edition	Brady Second Edition
Initial Assessment	Chap 12, pp. 282–286	Chap 12, pp. 663–673
Focused History and Physical Examination—Medical Patients	Chap 12, p. 286	Chap 12, pp. 683–691
Focused History and Physical Examination—Trauma Patients	Chap 12, pp. 286–287	Chap 12, pp. 673–691
Rapid Trauma Physical Examination	Chap 12, p. 287	
Detailed Physical Examination	Chap 12, p. 287	Chap 12, pp. 692–698
Ongoing Assessment	Chap 12, pp. 287–288	Chap 12, pp. 698–701
Care of Medical versus Trauma Patients	Chap 12, p. 288	
Clinical Decision Making	Chap 13, pp. 290–297	Chap 13, pp. 704–715
The Spectrum of Prehospital Care	Chap 13, p. 291	Chap 13, p. 705
Critical Thinking Process for Paramedics	Chap 13, pp. 291–293	Chap 13, pp. 708–710
Fundamental Elements of Critical Thinking for Paramedics	Chap 13, p. 293	Chap 13, pp. 708–711
Field Application of Assessment-Based Patient Management	Chap 13, p. 293–294	Chap 13, pp. 708–711
Putting It All Together—"The Six Rs"	Chap 13, pp. 294–295	Chap 13, p. 713–714
Assessment-Based Management	Chap 14, pp. 298–305	Chap 47, pp. 1778–1792
Effective Assessment	Chap 14, pp. 299–302	Chap 47, pp. 1779–1784
The Right Stuff	Chap 14, p. 302	Chap 47, pp. 1784–1785
Optional Take-In Equipment	Chap 14, p. 302	Chap 47, p. 1785
General Approach to the Patient	Chap 14, p. 303	Chap 47, pp. 1785–1788
Presenting the Patient	Chap 14, pp. 303–304	Chap 47, pp. 1788–1790
Communications	Chap 15, pp. 306–317	Chap 14, pp. 716–734
Phases of Communications during a Typical		
Emergency Medical Services Event	Chap 15, pp. 307–308	Chap 14, pp. 720–726
Role of Communications in Emergency		
Medical Services	Chap 15, pp. 308–310	Chap 14, pp. 720–726
Communications Systems	Chap 15, pp. 310–314	Chap 14, pp. 726–730
Components and Functions of Dispatch Communications Systems	Chap 15, pp. 314–315	Chap 14, pp. 726–730
Regulation	Chap 15, p. 315	Chap 14, pp. 732–733
Procedures for Emergency Medical Services Communications	Chap 15, pp. 315–316	Chap 14, pp. 730–732

l ESSENTIALS OF PARAMEDIC CARE

Transition Guide 2	Mosby Third Edition	Brady Second Edition
Documentation	Chap 16, pp. 318–329	Chap 15, pp. 735–758
Importance of Documentation	Chap 16, p. 319	Chap 15, pp. 736–738
General Considerations	Chap 16, p. 320	Chap 15, pp. 738–745
The Narrative	Chap 16, pp. 320–326	Chap 15, pp. 748–753
Elements of a Properly Written EMS Document	Chap 16, p. 326	Chap 15, pp. 745–748
Systems of Narrative Writing	Chap 16, p. 326–327	Chap 15, pp. 748–753
Special Considerations of Documentation	Chap 16, pp. 327–328	Chap 15, pp. 753–755
Document Revision/Correction	Chap 16, p. 328	Chap 15, p. 747
Consequences of Inappropriate Documentation	Chap 16, pp. 328	Chap 15, pp. 755–756
PART FOUR		
Pharmacology	Chap 17, pp. 332–387	
General Principles of Pharmacology		Chap 6, pp. 307–372
Section One—Drug Information	Chap 17, pp. 334–337	Chap 6, pp. 309–326
Historical Trends in Pharmacology	Chap 17, p. 334–337	Chap 6, p. 309
Section Two—Mechanisms of Drug Action	Chap 17, pp. 337–351	Chap 6, pp. 316–326
General Properties of Drugs	Chap 17, pp. 337–347	Chap 6, pp. 316–326
Drug Interactions	Chap 17, p. 347	Chap 6, pp. 316–317
Drug Forms, Preparations, and Storage	Chap 17, p. 348	Chap 6, pp. 321–322
Drug Profiles and Special Considerations in Drug Therapy	Chap 17, pp. 348–351	Chap 6, p. 314–316
Section Three—Drugs That Affect the Nervous System	Chap 17, pp. 351–364	Chap 6, pp. 327–342
Review of Anatomy and Physiology	Chap 17, pp. 351–364	Chap 6, pp. 327–342
Section Four—Drugs That Affect the Cardiovascular System	Chap 17, pp. 364–368	Chap 6, pp. 343–353
Review of Anatomy and Physiology	Chap 17, pp. 364–368	
Section Five—Drugs That Affect the Blood	Chap 17, pp. 368–369	Chap 6, pp. 350–353
Anticoagulants, Fibrinolytics, and Blood Components	Chap 17, pp. 368–369	Chap 6, pp. 350–353
Section Six—Drugs That Affect the Respiratory System	Chap 17, pp. 370–372	Chap 6, pp. 353–356
Review of Anatomy and Physiology	Chap 17, pp. 370–372	
Section Seven—Drugs That Affect the Gastrointestinal System	Chap 17, pp. 372–374	Chap 6, pp. 356–359
Review of Anatomy and Physiology	Chap 17, pp. 372–374	
Section Eight—Drugs That Affect the Eye and Ear	Chap 17, pp. 374–375	Chap 6, pp. 359–360
Treatment of Eye Disorders	Chap 17, pp. 374–375	

Transition Guide 2 **li**

Transition Guide 2	Mosby Third Edition	Brady Second Edition
Section Nine—Drugs That Affect the Endocrine System	Chap 17, pp. 375–376	Chap 6, pp. 360–366
Review of Anatomy and Physiology	Chap 17, pp. 375–376	Chap 6, pp. 360–366
Section Ten—Drugs That Affect the Reproductive System	Chap 17, pp. 376–377	
Treatment of Disorders of the Reproductive System	Chap 17, pp. 376–377	
Section Eleven—Drugs Used in Neoplastic Diseases	Chap 17, p. 377	Chap 6, pp. 366
Antineoplastic Agents	Chap 17, p. 377	Chap 6, pp. 366
Section Twelve—Drugs Used in Infectious Disease and Inflammation	Chap 17, pp. 378–381	Chap 6, pp. 366–368
Treatment of Infectious Disease and Inflammation	Chap 17, pp. 378–381	
Section Thirteen—Drugs That Affect the Immunological System	Chap 17, pp. 381–382	
Review of Anatomy and Physiology	Chap 17, pp. 381–382	
Venous Access and Medication Administration	Chap 18, pp. 388–427	Chap 7, pp. 373–453
Mathematical Equivalents Used in Pharmacology	Chap 18, pp. 389–391	Chap 7, pp. 442–449
Drug Calculations	Chap 18, pp. 391–396	Chap 7, pp. 444–449
Drug Administration	Chap 18, pp. 396–397	Chap 7, p. 378
Medical Asepsis	Chap 18, p. 397	Chap 7, pp. 376–377
Universal Precautions in Medication Administration	Chap 18, p. 397	Chap 7, p. 376
Enteral Administration of Medications	Chap 18, pp. 397–399	Chap 7, pp. 385–390
Parenteral Administration of Medications	Chap 18, pp. 399–420	Chap 7, pp. 390–405
Administration of Percutaneous Medications	Chap 18, pp. 420–423	Chap 7, pp. 378–381
Special Considerations for Pediatric Patients	Chap 18, p. 423	
Obtaining a Blood Sample	Chap 18, pp. 423–424	Chap 7, pp. 431–434
Disposal of Contaminated Items and Sharps	Chap 18, p. 425	Chap 7, p. 377
PART FIVE		
Airway Management and Ventilation	Chap 19, pp. 430–498	Chap 8, pp. 454–531
Section One—Respiratory Physiology	Chap 19, pp. 431–449	See Chapter 3
Mechanics of Respiration	Chap 19, pp. 431–437	See Chapter 3
Measurement of Gases	Chap 19, pp. 437–438	Chap 8, pp. 462–464
Pulmonary Circulation	Chap 19, pp. 438–449	Chap 8, pp. 462–464
Section Two—Respiratory Pathophysiology	Chap 19, pp. 449–453	Chap 8, pp. 458–468
Foreign Body Airway Obstruction	Chap 19, pp. 449–452	Chap 8, pp. 457–458

Transition Guide 2	Mosby Third Edition	Brady Second Edition
Aspiration by Inhalation	Chap 19, pp. 452–453	Chap 8, p. 458
Section Three—Airway Evaluation	Chap 19, pp. 453–497	Chap 8, pp. 458–468
Essential Parameters of Airway Evaluation	Chap 19, pp. 453–454	Chap 8, pp. 458–468
Supplemental Oxygen Therapy	Chap 19, pp. 455–459	Chap 8, pp. 523–525
Ventilation	Chap 19, pp. 459–464	Chap 8, pp. 525–529
Airway Management	Chap 19, pp. 464–466	Chap 8, pp. 468–519
Suction	Chap 19, pp. 466–469	Chap 8, pp. 521–522
Mechanical Adjuncts in Airway Management	Chap 19, pp. 469–472	Chap 8, pp. 471–474
Advanced Airway Procedures	Chap 19, pp. 472–490	Chap 8, pp. 474–519
Pharmacological Adjuncts to Airway Management and Ventilation	Chap 19, pp. 490–492	Chap 8, pp. 494–497
Translaryngeal Cannula Ventilation	Chap 19, pp. 492–494	
Cricothyrotomy	Chap 19, pp. 494–497	Chap 8, pp. 512–519
PART SIX		
Trauma Systems and Mechanism of Injury	Chap 20, pp. 500–519	
Trauma and Trauma Systems		Chap 16, pp. 760–769
Epidemiology of Trauma	Chap 20, pp. 501–503	Chap 16, pp. 761–769
Section One—Kinematics	Chap 20, pp. 503–504	Chap 17, pp. 771–774
Energy	Chap 20, pp. 503–504	Chap 17, pp. 772–773
Section Two—Blunt Trauma	Chap 20, pp. 504–513	Chap 17, pp. 774–801
Blunt Trauma	Chap 20, pp. 504–506	Chap 17, pp. 774–777, 779–785
Restraints	Chap 20, pp. 506–508	Chap 17, pp. 777–779
Organ Collision Injuries	Chap 20, pp. 508–510	Chap 17, p. 775
Other Motorized Vehicular Collisions	Chap 20, pp. 510–511	Chap 17, pp. 787–790
Pedestrian Injuries	Chap 20, p. 511	Chap 17, p. 788
Other Causes of Blunt Trauma	Chap 20, pp. 511–513	Chap 17, pp. 790–799
Section Three—Penetrating Trauma	Chap 20, pp. 513–517	Chap 18, pp. 802–820
Penetrating Trauma	Chap 20, pp. 513–517	Chap 18, pp. 802–820
Hemorrhage and Shock	Chap 21, pp. 520–537	Chap 19, pp. 821–851
Hemorrhage	Chap 21, pp. 521–522	Chap 19, pp. 822–837
Tissue Oxygenation	Chap 21, pp. 522–523	Chap 19, pp. 838–839
The Body as a Container	Chap 21, pp. 523–524	Chap 19, pp. 838–839
Capillary-Cellular Relationship in Shock	Chap 21, pp. 524–526	Chap 19, pp. 838–839
Classifications of Shock	Chap 21, pp. 526–527	
Stages of Shock	Chap 21, p. 527	Chap 19, pp. 839–841
Uncompensated Shock	Chap 21, pp. 527–529	

Transition Guide 2	Mosby Third Edition	Brady Second Edition
Management and Treatment Plan for the Patient in Shock	Chap 21, pp. 529–536	Chap 19, pp. 843–849
Integration of Patient Assessment and the Treatment Plan	Chap 21, p. 537	Chap 19, pp. 849
Soft Tissue Trauma	Chap 22, pp. 538–557	Chap 20, pp. 852–890
Anatomy and Physiology	Chap 22, pp. 539–540	See Chapter 3
Pathophysiology	Chap 22, pp. 540–542	Chap 20, pp. 854–868
Pathophysiology and Assessment of Soft Tissue Injuries	Chap 22, pp. 542–547	Chap 20, pp. 854–860
Management Principles for Soft Tissue Injuries	Chap 22, pp. 547–549	Chap 20, pp. 871–888
Hemorrhage and Control of Bleeding	Chap 22, pp. 549–551	Chap 20, pp. 861–863
Dressing Materials Used with Soft Tissue Trauma	Chap 22, pp. 551–552	Chap 20, pp. 869–871
Management of Specific Soft Tissue Injuries Not Requiring Closure	Chap 22, pp. 552–556	Chap 20, pp. 864–867
Special Considerations for Soft Tissue Injuries	Chap 22, pp. 556–557	Chap 20, pp. 867–869
Burns	Chap 23, pp. 558–579	Chap 21, pp. 891–923
Incidence and Patterns of Burn Injury	Chap 23, pp. 559–561	Chap 21, p. 892–902
Classifications of Burn Injury	Chap 23, pp. 561–565	Chap 21, pp. 902–906
Pathophysiology of Burn Shock	Chap 23, pp. 565–566	Chap 21, pp. 904–906
Assessment of the Burn Patient	Chap 23, pp. 566–567	Chap 21, pp. 906–912
General Principles in Burn Management	Chap 23, pp. 567–569	Chap 21, pp. 912–921
Inhalation Burn Injury	Chap 23, pp. 569–570	Chap 21, pp. 914–915
Chemical Burn Injury	Chap 23, pp. 570–573	Chap 21, pp. 917–919
Electrical Burn Injuries	Chap 23, pp. 573–576	Chap 21, pp. 915–917
Radiation Exposure	Chap 23, pp. 576–578	Chap 21, pp. 919–921
Head and Facial Trauma	Chap 24, pp. 580–605	
Head, Facial, and Neck Trauma		Chap 23, pp. 958–999
Maxillofacial Injury	Chap 24, pp. 581–584	Chap 23, pp. 972–977
Ear, Eye, and Dental Trauma	Chap 24, pp. 585–589	Chap 23, pp. 996–997
Anterior Neck Trauma	Chap 24, pp. 590–593	Chap 23, pp. 977–978
Head Trauma	Chap 24, pp. 593–596	Chap 23, pp. 961–966
Brain Trauma	Chap 24, pp. 596–603	Chap 23, pp. 966–972
Injury Rating Systems	Chap 24, pp. 603–605	Chap 23, pp. 982–984

Transition Guide 2	Mosby Third Edition	Brady Second Edition
Spinal Trauma	Chap 25, pp. 606–629	Chap 24, pp. 1000–1029
Spinal Trauma: Incidence, Morbidity, and Mortality	Chap 25, p. 607	Chap 24, p. 1001
Traditional Spinal Assessment Criteria	Chap 25, pp. 607–609	Chap 24, pp. 1001–1004
Review of Spinal Anatomy and Physiology	Chap 25, p. 609	See Chapter 3
General Assessment of Spinal Injury	Chap 25, pp. 609–611	Chap 24, pp. 1001–1004
Classifications of Spinal Injury	Chap 25, pp. 611–614	
Evaluation and Assessment of Spinal Cord Injury	Chap 25, pp. 614–615	Chap 24, pp. 1007–1014
General Management of Spinal Injuries	Chap 25, pp. 615–626	Chap 24, pp. 1014–1027
Cord Injury Presentations	Chap 25, pp. 626–627	Chap 24, pp. 1005–1007
Nontraumatic Spinal Conditions	Chap 25, pp. 627–628	
Assessment and Management of Nontraumatic Spinal Conditions	Chap 25, p. 628	
Thoracic Trauma	Chap 26, pp. 630–643	Chap 25, pp. 1030–1060
Skeletal Injury	Chap 26, pp. 631–633	Chap 25, pp. 1035–1038
Closed Pneumothorax	Chap 26, pp. 633–638	Chap 25, pp. 1038–1043
Heart and Great Vessel Injury	Chap 26, pp. 638–640	Chap 25, pp. 1043–1047
Other Thoracic Injuries	Chap 26, pp. 640–641	Chap 25, pp. 1047–1048
Abdominal Trauma	Chap 27, pp. 644–651	Chap 26, pp. 1061–1078
Mechanisms of Abdominal Injury	Chap 27, pp. 645–646	Chap 26, pp. 1062–1064
Specific Abdominal Injuries	Chap 27, pp. 646–649	Chap 26, pp. 1064–1066
Vascular Structure Injuries	Chap 27, p. 649	Chap 26, p. 1066
Assessment of Abdominal Trauma	Chap 27, p. 649	Chap 26, pp. 1069–1074
Management of Abdominal Trauma	Chap 27, pp. 649–650	Chap 26, pp. 1074–1077
Musculoskeletal Trauma	Chap 28, pp. 652–671	Chap 22, pp. 924–957
Classifications of Musculoskeletal Injuries	Chap 28, pp. 653–656	Chap 22, pp. 927–928
Inflammatory and Degenerative Conditions	Chap 28, pp. 656–658	Chap 22, pp. 932–933
Signs and Symptoms of Extremity Trauma	Chap 28, p. 658	Chap 22, pp. 935–937
Assessment of Musculoskeletal Injuries	Chap 28, pp. 658–660	Chap 22, pp. 933–938
Upper Extremity Injuries	Chap 28, pp. 660–664	Chap 22, pp. 947–948, 951–952
Lower Extremity Injuries	Chap 28, pp. 664–668	Chap 22, pp. 945–951
Open Fractures	Chap 28, pp. 668–669	Chap 22, p. 938

Transition Guide 2	Mosby Third Edition	Brady Second Edition
Straightening Angular Fractures and Reducing Dislocations	Chap 28, pp. 669–670	Chap 22, p. 939
Referral of Patients with Minor Musculoskeletal Injury	Chap 28, pp. 670–671	Chap 22, p. 955
PART SEVEN		
Cardiology	Chap 29, pp. 674–813	Chap 28, pp. 1121–1242
Risk Factors and Prevention Strategies	Chap 29, p. 676	Chap 28, p. 1126
Section One—Anatomy and Physiology of the Heart	Chap 29, pp. 676–681	Chap 28, pp. 1127–1185
Anatomy	Chap 29, pp. 676–677	Chap 28, pp. 1127–1130
Physiology	Chap 29, pp. 677–681	Chap 28, pp. 1127–1130
Section Two—Electrophysiology of the Heart	Chap 29, pp. 681–688	Chap 28, pp. 1129–1130
Electrical Activity of Cardiac Cells and Membrane Potentials	Chap 29, pp. 681–682	Chap 28, pp. 1129–1130
Cell Excitability	Chap 29, pp. 682–685	Chap 28, pp. 1129–1130
Electrical Conduction System of the Heart	Chap 29, pp. 685–688	Chap 28, p.
Section Three—Assessment of the Patient with Cardiac Disease	Chap 29, pp. 688–691	Chap 28, pp.
Assessment	Chap 29, pp. 688–691	Chap 28, pp.
Section Four—Electrocardiogram Monitoring	Chap 29, pp. 691–702	Chap 28, pp. 1130–1142
Basic Concepts of Electrocardiogram Monitoring	Chap 29, pp. 691–699	Chap 28, pp. 1130–1142
Relationship of the Electrocardiogram to Electrical Activity	Chap 29, pp. 699–702	Chap 28, pp. 1134–1141
Section Five—Electrocardiogram Interpretation	Chap 29, pp. 702–712	Chap 28, pp. 1141–1142
Steps in Rhythm Analysis	Chap 29, pp. 702–712	Chap 28, pp. 1141–1142
Section Six—Introduction to Dysrhythmias	Chap 29, pp. 713–777	Chap 28, pp. 1142–1185
Classification of Dysrhythmias	Chap 29, pp. 713–714	Chap 28, p. 1144
Dysrhythmias Originating in the Sinoatrial Node	Chap 29, pp. 714–722	Chap 28, pp. 1144–1149
Dysrhythmias Originating in the Atria	Chap 29, pp. 722–735	Chap 28, pp. 1150–1159
Dysrhythmias Sustained or Originating in the Atrioventricular Junction	Chap 29, pp. 735–738	Chap 28, pp. 1159–1170
Dysrhythmias Originating in the Ventricles	Chap 29, pp. 738–763	Chap 28, pp. 1171–1182
Dysrhythmias That Are Disorders of Conduction	Chap 29, pp. 763–777	Chap 28, pp. 1184–1185
Section Seven—Specific Cardiovascular Diseases	Chap 29, pp. 778–799	Chap 28, pp. 1211–1237
Pathophysiology and Management of Cardiovascular Disease	Chap 29, pp. 778–799	Chap 28, pp. 1211–1237

Transition Guide 2	Mosby Third Edition	Brady Second Edition
Section Eight—Techniques of Managing Cardiac Emergencies	Chap 29, pp. 799–809	Chap 28, pp. 1186–1240
Basic Cardiac Life Support	Chap 29, pp. 799–802	Chap 28, p. 1194
Defibrillation	Chap 29, pp. 802–804	Chap 28, pp. 1199–1204
Implantable Cardioverter Defibrillators	Chap 29, pp. 804–805	Chap 28, pp. 1179–1182
Synchronized Cardioversion	Chap 29, pp. 805–806	Chap 28, p. 1204
Transcutaneous Cardiac Pacing	Chap 29, pp. 806–807	Chap 28, p. 1206
Cardiac Arrest and Sudden Death	Chap 29, pp. 807–808	Chap 28, pp. 1229–1233
Termination of Resuscitation	Chap 29, pp. 808–809	Chap 28, pp. 1232–1233
PART EIGHT		
Pulmonary Emergencies	Chap 30, pp. 816–835	
Pulmonology		Chap 27, pp. 1080–1120
Pathophysiology	Chap 30, pp. 817–818	Chap 27, pp. 1084–1086
Scene Size-Up and Rescuer Safety	Chap 30, pp. 818–820	Chap 27, pp. 1086–1098
Obstructive Airway Disease	Chap 30, pp. 820–825	Chap 27, pp. 1101–1112
Pneumonia	Chap 30, pp. 825–828	Chap 27, pp. 1109–1110
Adult Respiratory Distress Syndrome	Chap 30, pp. 828–830	Chap 27, pp. 1100–1101
Pulmonary Thromboembolism	Chap 30, pp. 830–831	Chap 27, pp. 1114–1116
Upper Respiratory Infection	Chap 30, p. 831	Chap 27, pp. 1108–1109
Spontaneous Pneumothorax	Chap 30, pp. 831–832	Chap 27, p. 1116
Hyperventilation Syndrome	Chap 30, p. 832	Chap 27, pp. 1116–1117
Lung Cancer	Chap 30, pp. 832–833	Chap 27, pp. 1112–1113
Neurology	Chap 31, pp. 836–863	Chap 29, pp. 1243–1279
Anatomy and Physiology of the Nervous System	Chap 31, pp. 837–842	Chap 29, pp. 1245–1247
Neurological Pathophysiology	Chap 31, pp. 842–847	Chap 29, pp. 1247–1255
Pathophysiology and Management of Specific Central Nervous System Disorders	Chap 31, pp. 847–862	Chap 29, pp. 1255–1277
Endocrinology	Chap 32, pp. 864–881	Chap 30, pp. 1280–1294
Anatomy and Physiology of the Endocrine System	Chap 32, pp. 865–866	Chap 30, pp. 1281–1282
Specific Disorders of the Endocrine System	Chap 32, pp. 866–867	Chap 30, pp. 1282–1293
Disorders of the Pancreas: Diabetes Mellitus	Chap 32, pp. 867–876	Chap 30, pp. 1282–1288
Disorders of the Thyroid Gland	Chap 32, pp. 877–878	Chap 30, pp. 1289–1291
Disorders of the Adrenal Glands	Chap 32, pp. 878–880	Chap 30, pp. 1291–1293

Transition Guide 2	Mosby Third Edition	Brady Second Edition
Allergies and Anaphylaxis	Chap 33, pp. 882–891	Chap 31, pp. 1295–1305
Antigen-Antibody Reaction	Chap 33, p. 883	Chap 31, pp. 1296–1299
Allergic Reaction	Chap 33, p. 883	Chap 31, pp. 1298–1299
Localized Allergic Reaction	Chap 33, p. 884	Chap 31, p. 1303
Anaphylaxis	Chap 33, pp. 884–890	Chap 31, pp. 1299–1302
Gastroenterology	Chap 34, pp. 892–907	Chap 32, pp. 1306–1327
Gastrointestinal Anatomy	Chap 34, p. 893	See Chapter 3
Assessment of the Patient with Acute Abdominal Pain	Chap 34, pp. 893–897	Chap 32, pp. 1307–1311
Management of the Patient with an Abdominal Emergency	Chap 34, p. 897	Chap 32, pp. 1307–1311
Specific Abdominal Emergencies	Chap 34, pp. 897–903	Chap 32, pp. 1311–1325
Urology	Chap 35, pp. 908–919	
Urology and Nephrology		Chap 33, pp. 1328–1348
Anatomy and Physiology Review	Chap 35, pp. 909–911	See Chapter 3
Physical Examination for Patients with Genitourinary Disorders	Chap 35, p. 912	Chap 33, pp. 1331–1335
Management and Treatment Plan	Chap 35, pp. 912–917	Chap 33, pp. 1335–1345
Management	Chap 35, p. 917	Chap 33, p. 1347
Toxicology	Chap 36, pp. 920–969	
Toxicology and Substance Abuse		Chap 34, pp. 1349–1388
Section One—Poisonings	Chap 36, pp. 921–945	
Poison Control Centers	Chap 36, pp. 921–922	Chap 34, p. 1351
General Guidelines for Managing a Poisoned Patient	Chap 36, p. 922	Chap 34, pp. 1353–1355
Poisoning by Ingestion	Chap 36, pp. 922–931	Chap 34, pp. 1356–1357
Poisoning by Inhalation	Chap 36, pp. 932–935	Chap 34, pp. 1357–1358
Poisoning by Injection	Chap 36, pp. 935–944	Chap 34, pp. 1372–1380
Poisoning by Absorption	Chap 36, pp. 944–945	Chap 34, pp. 1358–1359
Section Two—Drug Abuse	Chap 36, pp. 945–955	Chap 34, pp. 1380–1381
Toxic Effects of Drugs	Chap 36, pp. 945–955	Chap 34, pp. 1380–1381
Section Three—Alcoholism	Chap 36, pp. 955–961	Chap 34, pp. 1381–1386
Alcohol Dependence	Chap 36, pp. 955–956	Chap 34, pp. 1381–1386
Ethanol	Chap 36, p. 956	Chap 34, pp. 1381–1384
Medical Consequences of Chronic Alcohol Ingestion	Chap 36, pp. 956–959	Chap 34, pp. 1384–1386

Transition Guide 2	Mosby Third Edition	Brady Second Edition
Alcohol Emergencies	Chap 36, pp. 959–961	Chap 34, pp. 1381–1386
Section Four—Management of Toxic Syndromes	Chap 36, pp. 961–962	
General Management Principles for Toxic Syndromes	Chap 36, pp. 961–962	Chap 34, pp. 1361, 1382–1383
Hematology	Chap 37, pp. 970–983	Chap 35, pp. 1389–1404
Blood and Blood Components	Chap 37, pp. 971–972	See Chapter 3
Specific Hematological Disorders	Chap 37, pp. 972–980	Chap 35, pp. 1397–1403
General Assessment and Management of Patients with Hematological Disorders	Chap 37, p. 980–982	Chap 35, pp. 1392–1397
Environmental Conditions	Chap 38, pp. 984–1003	
Environmental Emergencies		Chap 36, pp. 1405–1438
Thermoregulation	Chap 38, pp. 985–987	Chap 36, pp. 1407–1411
Hyperthermia	Chap 38, pp. 988–990	Chap 36, pp. 1411–1416
Hypothermia	Chap 38, pp. 990–993	Chap 36, pp. 1416–1422
Frostbite	Chap 38, pp. 993–995	Chap 36, pp. 1422–1423
Submersion	Chap 38, pp. 995–996	Chap 36, pp. 1423–1426
Diving Emergencies	Chap 38, pp. 997–1000	Chap 36, pp. 1426–1433
High-Altitude Illness	Chap 38, pp. 1000–1001	Chap 36, pp. 1433–1436
Infectious and Communicable Diseases	Chap 39, pp. 1004–1041	Chap 37, pp. 1439–1485
Public Health Principles Related to Infectious Diseases	Chap 39, pp. 1005–1009	Chap 37, pp. 1441–1442
Pathophysiology of Infectious Disease	Chap 39, pp. 1009–1011	Chap 37, pp. 1446–1449
Physiology of the Human Response to Infection	Chap 39, pp. 1011–1016	Chap 37, pp. 1443–1446
Stages of Infectious Disease	Chap 39, p. 1016	Chap 37, pp. 1448–1449
Human Immunodeficiency Virus	Chap 39, pp. 1016–1020	Chap 37, pp. 1456–1458
Hepatitis	Chap 39, pp. 1021–1023	Chap 37, pp. 1458–1461
Tuberculosis	Chap 39, pp. 1023–1025	Chap 37, pp. 1461–1463
Meningococcal Meningitis	Chap 39, pp. 1025–1026	Chap 37, pp. 1466–1468
Pneumonia	Chap 39, pp. 1026–1027	Chap 37, pp. 1463–1464
Tetanus	Chap 39, pp. 1027–1028	Chap 37, pp. 1476–1477
Rabies	Chap 39, p. 1028	Chap 37, pp. 1475–1476
Hantavirus	Chap 39, pp. 1028–1029	Chap 37, pp. 1473
Viral Diseases of Childhood	Chap 39, pp. 1029–1031	Chap 37, pp. 1465–66, 1469–71
Other Viral Diseases	Chap 39, pp. 1031–1032	Chap 37, pp. 1464–65, 1468–69

Transition Guide 2	Mosby Third Edition	Brady Second Edition
Sexually Transmitted Diseases	Chap 39, pp. 1032–1036	Chap 37, pp. 1478–1481
Lice and Scabies	Chap 39, pp. 1036–1038	Chap 37, pp. 1481–1482
Reporting an Exposure to an Infectious / Communicable Disease	Chap 39, pp. 1038–1039	Chap 37, pp. 1442
The Paramedic's Role in Preventing Disease Transmission	Chap 39, pp. 1039	Chap 37, pp. 1483–1484
Behavioral and Psychiatric Disorders	Chap 40, pp. 1042–1061	Chap 38, pp. 1486–1508
Understanding Behavioral Emergencies	Chap 40, pp. 1043–1044	Chap 38, pp. 1487–1488
Assessment and Management of Behavioral Emergencies	Chap 40, pp. 1045–1048	Chap 38, pp. 1489–92, 1502–04
Specific Behavioral and Psychiatric Disorders	Chap 40 pp. 1048–1057	Chap 38, pp. 1492–1502
Special Considerations for Patients with Behavioral Problems	Chap 40, pp. 1057–1060	Chap 38, pp.1502–1507
Gynecology	Chap 41, pp. 1062–1071	Chap 39, pp. 1509–1517
Organs of the Female Reproductive System	Chap 41, p. 1063	See Chapter 3
Menstruation and Ovulation	Chap 41, pp. 1063–1066	See Chapter 3
Specific Gynecological Emergencies	Chap 41, pp. 1066–1071	Chap 39, pp. 1512–1516
Obstetrics	Chap 42, pp. 1072–1097	Chap 40, pp. 1518–1552
Normal Events of Pregnancy	Chap 42, p. 1073	Chap 40, p. 1519
Specialized Structures of Pregnancy	Chap 42, pp. 1073–1074	Chap 40, pp. 1519–1522
Fetal Growth and Development	Chap 42, pp. 1074–1077	Chap 40, pp.1522–1525
Obstetrical Terminology	Chap 42, p. 1077	Chap 40, pp. 1524–1525
Patient Assessment	Chap 42, pp. 1077–1080	Chap 40, pp. 1525–1527
Complications of Pregnancy	Chap 42, pp. 1080–1091	Chap 40, pp.1527–1537
Delivery Complications	Chap 42, pp. 1091–1095	Chap 40, pp. 1544–1550
PART NINE		
Neonatology	Chap 43, pp. 1100–1115	Chap 41, pp. 1554–1584
Risk Factors Associated with the Need for Resuscitation	Chap 43, pp. 1101–1102	Chap 41, pp.1556–1559
Physiological Adaptations at Birth	Chap 43, pp. 1102–1103	Chap 41, p. 1557
Assessment and Management of the Neonate	Chap 43, pp. 1103–1106	Chap 41, pp. 1559–1563
Resuscitation of the Distressed Newborn	Chap 43, pp. 1106–1108	Chap 41, pp. 1563–1573
Postresuscitation Care	Chap 43, p. 1108	Chap 41, pp. 1566–1568
Neonatal Transport	Chap 43, pp. 1108–1109	Chap 41, p. 1573
Specific Situations	Chap 43, pp. 1109–1113	Chap 41, pp. 1574–1582
Psychological and Emotional Support	Chap 43, p. 1113	

Transition Guide 2	Mosby Third Edition	Brady Second Edition
Pediatrics	Chap 44, pp. 1116–1159	Chap 42, pp. 1585–1666
The Paramedic's Role in Caring for Pediatric Patients	Chap 44, p. 1117	Chap 42, pp. 1587–1589
Emergency Medical Services for Children	Chap 44, pp. 1117–1118	Chap 42, pp. 1588–1589
Growth and Development Review	Chap 44, pp. 1118–1120	Chap 42, pp. 1590–1593
Anatomy and Physiology Review	Chap 44, pp. 1120–1122	Chap 42, pp. 1593–1597
General Principles of Pediatric Assessment	Chap 44, pp. 1122–1124	Chap 42, pp. 1597–1606
General Principles of Patient Management	Chap 44, p. 1125	Chap 42, pp. 1606–1623
Specific Pathophysiology, Assessment, and Management	Chap 44, pp. 1125–1153	Chap 42, pp. 1623–1648
Infants and Children with Special Needs	Chap 44, pp. 1153–1157	Chap 42, pp. 1661–1664
Geriatrics	Chap 45, pp. 1160–1183	
Geriatric Emergencies		Chap 43, pp. 1667–1714
Demographics, Epidemiology, and Societal Issues	Chap 45, p. 1161	Chap 43, pp. 1669–1671
Living Environments and Referral Sources	Chap 45, p. 1161	Chap 43, pp. 1670–1671
Physiological Changes of Aging	Chap 45, pp. 1162–1165	Chap 43, pp. 1671–1680
General Principles in Assessment of the Geriatric Patient	Chap 45, p. 1166	Chap 43, pp. 1671–1680
System Pathophysiology, Assessment, and Management	Chap 45, pp. 1166–1180	Chap 43, pp. 1671–1685
Abuse and Neglect	Chap 46, pp. 1184–1195	
Abuse and Assault		Chap 44, pp. 1715–1728
Battering	Chap 46, pp. 1185–1188	Chap 44, pp. 1716–1718
Elder Abuse	Chap 46, pp. 1188–1189	Chap 44, pp. 1718–1720
Child Abuse	Chap 46, pp. 1189–1192	Chap 44, pp. 1720–1723
Sexual Assault	Chap 46, pp. 1192–1193	Chap 44, pp. 1724–1727
Patients with Special Challenges	Chap 47, pp. 1196–1209	
The Challenged Patient		Chap 45, pp. 1729–1745
Physical Challenges	Chap 47, pp. 1197–1199	Chap 45, pp. 1730–1736
Mental Challenges	Chap 47, pp. 1200–1201	Chap 45, pp. 1736–1738
Pathological Challenges	Chap 47, pp. 1201–1205	Chap 45, pp. 1738–1743
Culturally Diverse Patients	Chap 47, pp. 1205–1207	Chap 45, pp. 1743–1744
Terminally Ill Patients	Chap 47, p. 1207	Chap 45, p. 1744
Patients with Communicable Diseases	Chap 47, p. 1207	Chap 45, p. 1744
Financial Challenges	Chap 47, pp. 1207–1208	Chap 45, p. 1744

Transition Guide 2	Mosby Third Edition	Brady Second Edition
Acute Interventions for the Home Health Care Patient	Chap 48, pp. 1210–1228	
Acute Interventions for the Chronic-Care Patient		Chap 46, pp. 1746–1753
Overview of Home Health Care	Chap 48, pp. 1211–1213	Chap 46, pp. 1747–1753
General Principles and Assessment	Chap 48, pp. 1213–1214	Chap 46, pp. 1753–1757
Specific Acute Home Health Care Interventions	Chap 48, pp. 1214–1227	Chap 46, pp. 1757–1776
PART TEN		
Ambulance Operations	Chap 49, pp. 1230–1239	Chap 48, pp. 1798–1809
Ambulance Standards	Chap 49, p. 1231	Chap 48, pp. 1798–1800
Checking Ambulances	Chap 49, p. 1231	Chap 48, pp. 1800–1801
Ambulance Stationing	Chap 49, pp. 1231–1232	Chap 48, pp. 1801–1802
Safe Ambulance Operation	Chap 49, pp. 1232–1235	Chap 48, pp. 1802–1806
Aeromedical Transportation	Chap 49, pp. 1236–1238	Chap 48, pp. 1806–1809
Medical Incident Command	Chap 50, pp. 1240–1255	
Medical Incident Management (Part 2 of Chap 48)		Chap 48, pp. 1809–1830
Incident Command System	Chap 50, pp. 1241–1246	Chap 48, pp. 1810–1816
Mass Casualty Incidents	Chap 50, pp. 1246–1250	Chap 48, pp. 1811–1816
Principles and Technology of Triage	Chap 50, pp. 1250–1253	Chap 48, pp. 1820–1827
Critical Incident Stress Management	Chap 50, p. 1253	Chap 48, pp. 1829–1830
Rescue Awareness and Operations	Chap 51, pp. 1256–1275	Chap 48, pp. 1830–1857
Appropriate Training for Rescue Operations	Chap 51, pp. 1257–1258	Chap 48, pp. 1830–1834
Phases of a Rescue Operation	Chap 51, pp. 1258–1260	Chap 48, pp. 1835–1838
Rescuer Personal Protective Equipment	Chap 51, p. 1260	Chap 48, pp. 1831–1833
Surface Water Rescue	Chap 51, pp. 1260–1263	Chap 48, pp. 1838–1845
Hazardous Atmospheres	Chap 51, pp. 1263–1265	Chap 48, pp. 1845–1847
Highway Operations	Chap 51, pp. 1265–1270	Chap 48, pp. 1847–1851
Hazardous Terrain	Chap 51, pp. 1270–1273	Chap 48, pp. 1851–1856
Assessment Procedures During Rescue	Chap 51, pp. 1273–1274	Chap 48, pp. 1851–1856
Crime Scene Awareness	Chap 52, pp. 1276–1285	Chap 48, pp. 1872–1885
Approaching the Scene	Chap 52, pp. 1276–1278	Chap 48, pp. 1873–1875
The Dangerous Residence	Chap 52, p. 1278	Chap 48, pp. 1875–1876
Dangerous Highway Encounters	Chap 52, pp. 1278–1279	Chap 48, p. 1876–1877

Transition Guide 2	Mosby Third Edition	Brady Second Edition
Violent Street Incidents	Chap 52, p. 1279	Chap 48, pp. 1877–1878
Violent Groups and Situations	Chap 52, pp. 1279–1281	Chap 48, pp. 1878–1879
Safety Tactics	Chap 52, pp. 1281–1283	Chap 48, pp. 1880–1882
Tactical Patient Care	Chap 52, pp. 1283–1284	Chap 48, pp. 1882–1883
EMS at Crime Scenes	Chap 52, p. 1284	Chap 48, pp. 1883–1885
Hazardous Materials Incidents	Chap 53, pp. 1286–1305	Chap 48, pp. 1857–1872
Scope of Hazardous Materials	Chap 53, p. 1287	Chap 48, p. 1857
Laws and Regulations	Chap 53, pp. 1287–1288	Chap 48, p. 1857
Identification of Hazardous Materials	Chap 53, pp. 1288–1291	Chap 48, pp. 1860–1863
Personal Protective Clothing and Equipment	Chap 53, pp. 1291–1293	Chap 48, p. 1871
Health Hazards	Chap 53, pp. 1293–1295	Chap 48, pp. 1865–1868
Response to Hazardous Materials Emergencies	Chap 53, pp. 1295–1298	Chap 48, pp. 1858–1863
Medical Monitoring and Rehabilitation	Chap 53, pp. 1298–1299	Chap 48, p. 1872
Emergency Management of Contaminated Patients	Chap 53, pp. 1299–1301	Chap 48, pp. 1868–1871
Decontamination of Rescue Personnel and Equipment	Chap 53, p. 1301	Chap 48, pp. 1868–1871
Bioterrorism and Weapons of Mass Destruction	Chap 54, pp. 1306–1320	
Responding to Terrorist Acts		Chap 49, pp. 1890–1904
History of Biological Weapons	Chap 54, pp. 1307–1308	Chap 49, p. 1891
Critical Biological Agents	Chap 54, p. 1308	Chap 49, pp. 1900–1902
Methods of Dissemination	Chap 54, pp. 1308–1309	Chap 49, pp. 1900–1902
Specific Biological Threats	Chap 54, pp. 1309–1312	Chap 49, pp. 1900–1902
Nuclear and Radiological Threats	Chap 54, pp. 1312–1313	Chap 49, pp. 1893–1895
Incendiary Threats	Chap 54, p. 1313	Chap 49, p. 1892
Specific Chemical Threats	Chap 54, pp. 1313–1316	Chap 49, pp. 1895–1900
Explosive Threats	Chap 54, p. 1316	Chap 49, p. 1892
Department of Homeland Security	Chap 54, pp. 1316–1317	Chap 49, pp. 1902–1903

Essentials of Paramedic Care

Division 1

Introduction to Advanced Prehospital Care

Chapter 1

Introduction to Advanced Prehospital Care

INTRODUCTION

Before beginning on the long journey of paramedic education, your students should understand what the career of the EMT-Paramedic entails in the twenty-first century. This chapter outlines many of the basics that are involved in the paramedic profession.

The Emergency Medical Services (EMS) system, of which paramedics are a part, is a complex health care system made up of personnel, equipment, and resources established to deliver aid and emergency medical care to the community. It comprises both out-of-hospital and in-hospital care. The roles and responsibilities of the paramedic in this system have changed dramatically in the past 10 years. Advanced prehospital care is an enormous responsibility for which the paramedic must be mentally, physically, and emotionally prepared. Students must realize that they will be responsible for providing not only competent emergency care but also emotional support to patients and families. Students also need to realize that during their careers as paramedics they will be exposed to many kinds of physical and emotional stress. They will face situations involving infectious diseases, fear, physical danger, death, and dying. They must thus become familiar with the use of equipment and strategies that will help them remain physically and emotionally safe and healthy. By understanding safe practices, they will be better able to avoid harm from violent people, roadway hazards, and infectious diseases. They will be able to make appropriate choices about how they live rather than having a physical or emotional injury make that decision for them. They will also learn how they can take action to prevent illness and injury, not only in their own lives but in those of their co-workers and the patients they encounter.

Dealing, as they frequently do, with high-pressure, life-or-death situations, EMS providers frequently face ethical problems such as patients refusing care, conflicts regarding hospital destinations, and difficulties with advance directives. This chapter will also explore the fundamental principles and methods of ethics that apply to common prehospital situations.

PART 1: INTRODUCTION TO ADVANCED PREHOSPITAL CARE

TOTAL TEACHING TIME:
There is no specific time requirement for this topic in the National Standard Curriculum for Paramedic. Instructors should take into consideration such factors as the pace at which students learn, the size of the class, and breaks. The actual time devoted to teaching objectives is the responsibility of the instructor.

PART 2: EMS SYSTEMS

TOTAL TEACHING TIME:
There is no specific time requirement for this topic in the National Standard Curriculum for Paramedic. Instructors should take into consideration such factors as the pace at which students learn, the size of the class, and breaks. The actual time devoted to teaching objectives is the responsibility of the instructor.

PART 3: ROLES AND RESPONSIBILITIES OF THE PARAMEDIC

TOTAL TEACHING TIME: 3.81 HOURS
The total teaching time is only a guideline based on the didactic and practical lab averages in the National Standard Curriculum. Instructors should take into consideration such factors as the pace at which students learn, the size of the class, and breaks. The actual time devoted to teaching objectives is the responsibility of the instructor.

PART 4: THE WELL-BEING OF THE PARAMEDIC

TOTAL TEACHING TIME:
4.97 HOURS

The total teaching time is only a guideline based on the didactic and practical lab averages in the National Standard Curriculum. Instructors should take into consideration such factors as the pace at which students learn, the size of the class, and breaks. The actual time devoted to teaching objectives is the responsibility of the instructor.

PART 5: ILLNESS AND INJURY PREVENTION

TOTAL TEACHING TIME:
3.14 HOURS

The total teaching time is only a guideline based on the didactic and practical lab averages in the National Standard Curriculum. Instructors should take into consideration such factors as the pace at which students learn, the size of the class, and breaks. The actual time devoted to teaching objectives is the responsibility of the instructor.

PART 6: ETHICS IN ADVANCED PREHOSPITAL CARE

TOTAL TEACHING TIME:
2.44 HOURS

The total teaching time is only a guideline based on the didactic and practical lab averages in the National Standard Curriculum. Instructors should take into consideration such factors as: the pace at which students learn, the size of the class, and breaks. The actual time devoted to teaching objectives is the responsibility of the instructor.

CHAPTER OBJECTIVES

Part 1: Introduction to Advanced Prehospital Care (pp. 6–8)

After reading Part 1 of this chapter, you should be able to:

1. Describe the relationship between the paramedic and other members of the allied health professions. (pp. 6–7)
2. Identify the attributes and characteristics of the paramedic. (p. 7)
3. Explain the elements of paramedic education and practice that support its stature as a profession. (p. 7)
4. Define and give examples of the expanded scope of practice for the paramedic. (p. 8)

Part 2: EMS Systems (pp. 8–23)

After reading Part 2 of this chapter, you should be able to:

1. Describe key historical events that influenced the national development of Emergency Medical Services (EMS) systems. (pp. 9–12)
2. Define the following terms:
   - certification (p. 16)
   - EMS systems (p. 8)
   - ethics (p. 53)
   - health care professional (p. 17)
   - licensure (p. 16)
   - medical direction (pp. 13–14)
   - peer review (p. 21)
   - profession (p. 16)
   - professionalism (p. 21)
   - protocols (p. 14)
   - registration (p. 16)
3. Identify national groups important to the development, education, and implementation of EMS as well as the role of national associations, the National Registry of EMTs, and the roles of various EMS standard-setting agencies. (pp. 17–18)
4. Identify the standards (components) of an EMS system as defined by the National Highway Traffic Safety Administration. (p. 11)
5. Differentiate among EMS provider levels: First Responder, Emergency Medical Technician-Basic, Emergency Medical Technician-Intermediate, and Emergency Medical Technician-Paramedic. (p. 17)
6. Describe what is meant by "citizen involvement in the EMS system." (p. 14)
7. Discuss the role of the EMS physician in providing medical direction, prehospital and out-of-hospital care as an extension of the physician, the benefits of on-line and off-line medical direction, and the process for the development of local policies and protocols. (pp. 13–14)
8. Describe the relationship between a physician on the scene, the paramedic on the scene, and the EMS physician providing on-line medical direction. (p. 13)
9. Describe the components of continuous quality improvement and analyze its contribution to system improvement, continuing medical education, and research. (pp. 20–21)

10. Describe the importance, basic principles, process of evaluating and interpreting, and benefits of research. (pp. 21–23)

Part 3: Roles and Responsibilities of the Paramedic (pp. 23–31)

After reading Part 3 of this chapter, you should be able to:

1. Describe the attributes of a paramedic as a health care professional. (pp. 27–30)
2. Describe the benefits of paramedic continuing education and the importance of maintaining one's paramedic license/certification. (pp. 30–31)
3. List the primary and additional responsibilities of paramedics. (pp. 23–27)
4. Define the role of the paramedic relative to the safety of the crew, the patient, and bystanders. (p. 25)
5. Describe the role of the paramedic in health education activities related to illness and injury prevention. (p. 26)
6. Describe examples of professional behaviors in the following areas: integrity, empathy, self-motivation, appearance and personal hygiene, self-confidence, communications, time management, teamwork and diplomacy, respect, patient advocacy, and careful delivery of service. (pp. 28–30)
7. Identify the benefits of paramedics teaching in their community. (p. 26)
8. Analyze how the paramedic can benefit the health care system by supporting primary care for patients in the out-of-hospital setting. (p. 25)
9. Describe how professionalism applies to the paramedic while on and off duty. (p. 28)

Part 4: The Well-Being of the Paramedic (pp. 31–47)

After reading Part 4 of this chapter, you should be able to:

1. Discuss the concept of wellness and its benefits, components of wellness, and role of the paramedic in promoting wellness. (p. 31)
2. Discuss how cardiovascular endurance, weight control, muscle strength, and flexibility contribute to physical fitness. (pp. 31–34)
3. Describe the impact of shift work on circadian rhythms. (pp. 42–43)
4. Discuss the contributions that periodic risk assessments and warning sign recognition make to cancer and cardiovascular disease prevention. (pp. 32–33)
5. Differentiate proper from improper body mechanics for lifting and moving patients in emergency and nonemergency situations. (pp. 33–34)
6. Describe the problems that a paramedic might encounter in a hostile situation and the techniques used to manage the situation. (pp. 45–50)
7. Describe the considerations that should be given to using escorts, dealing with adverse environmental conditions, using lights and siren, proceeding through intersections, and parking at an emergency scene. (pp. 46–47)
8. Discuss the concept of "due regard for the safety of all others" while operating an emergency vehicle. (p. 47)
9. Describe the equipment available in a variety of adverse situations for self-protection, including body substance isolation steps for protection from airborne and bloodborne pathogens. (pp. 35–38, 45, 46–47)
10. Given a scenario where equipment and supplies have been exposed to body substances, plan for the proper cleaning, disinfection, and disposal of the items. (p. 37)
11. Describe the benefits and methods of smoking cessation. (p. 33)

12. Identify and describe the three phases of the stress response, factors that trigger the stress response, and causes of stress in EMS. (pp. 41–43)
13. Differentiate between normal/healthy and detrimental physiological and psychological reactions to anxiety and stress. (pp. 43–44)
14. Describe behavior that is a manifestation of stress in patients and those close to them, and describe how that behavior relates to paramedic stress. (pp. 44–45)
15. Identify and describe the defense mechanisms and management techniques commonly used to deal with stress, discuss research about possible problems with the use of critical incident stress management (CISM), and identify the appropriate mental health services that should be available to EMS personnel. (pp. 44–45)
16. Given a scenario involving a stressful situation, formulate a strategy to help adapt to the stress. (pp. 44–45)
17. Describe the stages of the grieving process (Kübler-Ross) and the unique challenges for paramedics in dealing with themselves, adults, children, and other special populations related to their understanding or experience of death and dying. (pp. 38–41)
18. Given photos of various motor-vehicle collisions, assess scene safety and propose ways to make the scene safer. (pp. 46–47)

Part 5: Illness and Injury Prevention (pp. 47–53)

After reading Part 5 of this chapter, you should be able to:

1. Describe the incidence, morbidity and mortality, and the human, environmental, and socioeconomic impact of unintentional and alleged unintentional injuries. (pp. 47–48)
2. Identify health hazards and potential crime areas within the community. (pp. 50–51)
3. Identify local municipal and community resources available for physical, socioeconomic crises. (pp. 48–49, 52–53)
4. List the general and specific environmental parameters that should be inspected to assess a patient's need for preventive information and direction. (pp. 50–53)
5. Identify the role of EMS in local municipal and community prevention programs. (pp. 47, 48–53)
6. Identify the injury and illness prevention programs that promote safety for all age populations. (pp. 50–53)
7. Identify patient situations where the paramedic can intervene in a preventive manner. (pp. 50–53)
8. Document primary and secondary injury prevention data. (pp. 50–53)

Part 6: Ethics in Advanced Prehospital Care (pp. 53–62)

After reading Part 6 of this chapter, you should be able to:

1. Define ethics and morals and distinguish between ethical and moral decisions in emergency medical service. (pp. 53–54)
2. Identify the premise that should underlie the paramedic's ethical decisions in out-of-hospital care. (pp. 54–55)
3. Analyze the relationship between the law and ethics in EMS. (p. 53)
4. Compare and contrast the criteria used in allocating scarce EMS resources. (pp. 59–60)
5. Identify issues surrounding advance directives in making a prehospital resuscitation decision and describe the criteria necessary to honor an advance directive in your state. (pp. 56–58)

FRAMING THE LESSON

Have students discuss what they think an EMS system is. How is the public involved? How are hospital staff members involved? Emphasize that the typical EMS system involves much more than just paramedics and ambulances. Give examples of how EMS systems in your general area are configured and how they respond to emergency calls.

Then have students list what they feel are the roles and responsibilities of a paramedic in the EMS system. The normal first responses will most likely relate to emergency patient care. Discuss the roles and responsibilities of the paramedic during a typical emergency call. Students may bring out the various aspects of patient assessment, treatment, and transportation. Also, encourage students to think about the many roles and responsibilities other than direct patient care. Prompt students to think about how paramedics can prepare themselves for their role, not only in learning the skills of a paramedic but in being ready to meet the physical demands of the career. Ask them also what emotional and moral challenges being a paramedic might present and how they think they can be ready for them. What leadership responsibilities do paramedics have at the scene of a call? What professional attitudes and attributes should paramedic have? How do students feel they can gain these during their education?

TEACHING STRATEGIES

People learn in a variety of ways. Some do better with the spoken word, whereas others prefer the written. Some prefer to work alone, whereas others profit from working in groups. Recognizing these different ways of acquiring knowledge, the authors of this *Instructor's Resource Manual* have provided a variety of teaching strategies for the different types of learners. These strategies are intended to foster higher-level cognitive skills and encourage creative learning and problem solving. For greatest effectiveness, incorporate these strategies into your class lecture. Symbols in the Lecture Outline indicate the points at which various exercises might be most appropriate. Other strategies can be used to preview the lesson or to summarize it.

The following strategies are keyed to specific sections of the lesson.

PART 1: INTRODUCTION TO ADVANCED PREHOSPITAL CARE

1. ***Breaking the Ice.*** Welcome students to the class and give them your name, title, and affiliation. Have students form a circle, while you stand in the center. Randomly beginning with any student, have that student give his or her name. Then, have the next student to the left say the name of the student to the right, and then introduce him- or herself. The third student in the circle will say the name of the first and second students, then his or her own, and so on. An alternative icebreaker is to divide the class in two. (If there is an odd number of students, you should join the smaller group.) Have students in each group count off and remember their numbers. Direct students to find the person in the other group who shares his or her number. Then have the pairs of students take several minutes to get acquainted, being sure to ask each other the following questions:

> What is your name?
> What makes you different from every other person?
> Why are you taking this course?

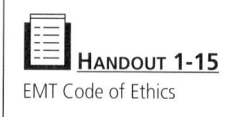

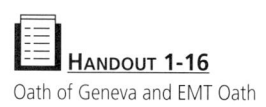

HANDOUT 1-15
EMT Code of Ethics

HANDOUT 1-16
Oath of Geneva and EMT Oath

After about 5 minutes for the interviews, let the students take turns introducing their partners to the class as a whole.

2. *Setting Ground Rules.* Take the time now to explain what you will expect of students during the course. Distribute a schedule of classes along with a listing of when readings and other written assignments should be completed. Explain your policy regarding missed classes or assignments. Outline the requirements for successful completion of the course, such as minimum exam scores, minimum percentage of courses attended, and clinical observation hours. Be sure students have or can get the textbooks and any other books or printed materials you will be using during the course. Briefly review the reading materials to give students a better understanding of the scope of the course. Note that at the beginning of each chapter you will distribute copies of an objectives checklist that outlines the knowledge and skills objectives that students must master. Explain your policy on tracking and testing and offering students access to your records on their performance. Also explain your policies on remediation and reexamination for students who do not master each chapter's content on their first attempt. Describe your requirements for student interaction with patients in either a hospital or field environment. Finally, describe your state's procedures and requirements for certification/licensure as an EMT-Paramedic.

3. *Highlighting the Need for Continuing Education.* Cover your state's continuing education policy. Identify resources for continuing education, such as other training centers, hospitals, colleges and universities, journals, videotapes, the Internet, and so on. Discuss the importance of lifelong learning. This activity empowers the student to locate challenging learning opportunities while still in the classroom. You can reinforce this positive behavior by asking about classes students have attended or by offering extra credit if they give a brief report on the subject matter to the class.

PART 2: EMS SYSTEMS

4. *Guest Lecturers.* Ask a representative from an area ambulance service to choose an emergency call to which more agencies than just his or hers responded. For example, the representative might cite a motor vehicle collision to which law enforcement, fire, and EMS were summoned. Then invite representatives from each involved agency, and from the emergency department to which the patient was transported, to discuss their agencies' roles at the scene and at the hospital. Try to have as many different agencies and departments as possible who would have been involved in the patient's care. For example, law enforcement, fire, and EMS for the on-scene aspect and an emergency department nurse, physician, X-ray technician, and others from the hospital. Students need to realize how far the scope of EMS systems can extend beyond the ambulance and crew.

5. *EMS Response Design.* Divide students into groups. Tell each group to design a community EMS response system and organizational chart. One example is a system in which the community has a BLS volunteer quick response team and a transporting paramedic ambulance response from a larger city 20 miles away. Another example is a system with a local fire department with EMT-Basics and a third-service paramedic ambulance. One more example is a small, rural community that relies on a volunteer BLS ambulance and a local clinic where patients can be transported. Have groups write examples of a typical response for their "community." Is air medical response available in their community? For what types of calls would it be requested? What level of hospital care is available locally? If patients are transported to the local community

hospital or clinic, where and how are they transferred to other facilities? Emphasize to students that many different types of EMS services and response configurations exist in the United States.

6. *Medical Direction Review.* Obtain a copy of the standing orders from an area paramedic service. Discuss with students which procedures are allowed by standing orders and which procedures require permission from on-line medical direction. Also discuss the importance of quality assurance, including peer review, to an EMS system. If possible, obtain copies of patient care reports from an area EMS agency and, after blacking out any information identifying the patient or crew, perform "peer reviews" on the reports. Have students review the reports for proper documentation, proper procedures, and so forth.

7. *Guest Speaker: Medical Director.* Have the medical director of the local EMS system visit the class. Let him or her explain to your students what it means to extend a medical license to someone. This will give your students a greater appreciation for the concept of medical direction. Ask the director to be ready to field any questions students might have about medical direction or EMS operations.

8. *Comparing Protocols.* Have students bring and share the protocol documents from their local agencies. Have them compare the presentations (manual v. pocket guide), formats (recipe or algorithm v. paragraphs), and the content (who has protocols for what) of the documents. The scope of practice may vary depending upon levels of providers, the history of EMS in the area, medical directors, continuing education requirements, and so on. Discuss who is ultimately responsible for the protocols, how to use them, and how to get them changed when needed. Encourage students to begin learning the protocols of the areas in which they plan to intern to make their transitions into those systems a little easier.

9. *Raising Public Awareness of EMS.* Let students design a public service announcement for radio, television, or newspapers about EMS system components. Topics could include proper use of 911, what information to give to a dispatcher, rendering first aid, warning signs of AMI or stroke, water safety, fire safety, and so forth. View the PSAs in class and consider submitting them to the proper media for use during EMS Week in May. This is a creative, kinesthetic activity that can be performed individually or in groups and tailored to the area in which students serve.

10. *EMS Provider-Level Survey.* Assign each student a different state in the United States. Have students write their state EMS offices requesting documents outlining the scope of practice and training course outline for various levels of EMS providers. When responses are received, compare scopes of practice and training for the same levels to determine how much they vary. States may have varying scopes of practice for the same level or may have levels in addition to the standard EMT-Basic, EMT-Intermediate, and EMT-Paramedic.

11. *EMS Research Investigation.* Divide students into several groups. Have each group discuss changes in prehospital care over the past several years and pick one specific change that has taken place. Then have the groups research their choices. Why was the procedure or skill initially added? What research into the procedure prompted the change? What is the current standard now? Students should use texts, EMS periodicals, and newsletters as sources. They will learn that until recently, most prehospital procedures were not based on sound scientific study. This activity will take time; give students several weeks to complete it.

PART 3: ROLES AND RESPONSIBILITIES OF THE PARAMEDIC

12. Defining Leadership Qualities. Divide students into groups and have them discuss good and bad leadership attitudes and attributes of supervisors and managers with whom they have had personal contact. Have the groups develop suggestions on how to improve bad attitudes and traits. What experiences have students had that would help them in leadership positions? Then have a spokesperson from each group present the results to the class.

13. Establishing a Dress Code. To promote professional appearance and good personal hygiene, set high standards in your classroom. If your teaching circumstances are appropriate, consider making a dress and hygiene code formal class policy, with penalties for not observing the standard. Consider requiring the internship uniform in class and hospital clinicals. Delineate what style pants, shirt, and shoes are acceptable. Make provisions for hair, facial hair, jewelry, undergarments, fingernails, makeup, and perfume. Be certain that any visitor could enter your classroom and be comfortable with your students. Also, you should be able to take your class anywhere (to the emergency department, dispatch, nursing home) and have them be received as professionals. This requirement will send a strong message about the seriousness of professionalism in EMS. These students will eventually be the managers and leaders of EMS in the future. Be sure they know how to represent all of us well.

PART 4: THE WELL-BEING OF THE PARAMEDIC

14. Gauging Basic Flexibility. Measure students' flexibility to give them an idea of their fitness levels. Many may be surprised at how stiff they have become over the years. Have students sit facing a wall, legs outstretched in front of them, heels against the wall. Shoes should be removed. Bend forward and sustain the maximum stretch possible for 5 seconds. Flexibility levels correspond to the following maximum stretches: fingertips only is poor, knuckles is good, and palms is excellent flexibility.

15. Healthy Diet Tracking. Have students go to *www.mypyramid.gov* and develop their customized food pyramid. Then have them keep track of the food they eat over a week's time. Discuss the results of their findings. Alternatively, bring in various snacks in single-serving containers, such as pretzels, popcorn, chips, crackers, candy, cookies, carrots, puddings applesauce, juice, pop, and so on. Have students categorize them by food group, then by nutritional value. Have them determine caloric content, calories from fat, and grams of fat, fiber, and protein. Reward students by allowing them to choose a snack to eat at break. This is a kinesthetic activity that has practical application in their work and personal lives. Teaching them to read a nutrition label is knowledge they can use the very next time they go to the grocery store.

16. Proper Lifting Technique Practice. Divide students into groups and distribute various types of patient-carrying devices, full jump kits, and other equipment commonly carried into a scene by paramedics. Under your supervision and/or the supervision of other clinical instructors, have the groups practice lifting patients on various devices, such as an ambulance gurney, scoop-stretcher, and stair-chair. If possible, have students practice lifting patients into an ambulance. Have groups practice good lifting and carrying techniques by carrying jump kits, airway kits, cardiac monitors, and other equipment for a set distance.

17. Personal Protective Equipment Practice. Provide each student with a pair of latex gloves, a pair of goggles or protective glasses, a surgical mask, and a surgical gown. Explain and demonstrate the correct technique for putting on each item. Emphasize each item's purpose and when it should be used. Then, have students put on each item themselves. Encourage students to help each other if necessary. Observe and correct errors.

18. *Proper Handwashing Techniques.* To demonstrate proper and thorough handwashing, try the following exercise. Have students dirty their hands with glitter. Send them to wash their hands with soap and water. Illustrate how much glitter has been left on their hands, and then on objects such as pens, desks, light switches, and so on. Most people do not employ proper handwashing techniques and so leave many germs on their hands to contaminate their surroundings. A variant on this activity is to coat items in the restroom with glitter. It becomes painfully obvious who does not properly wash his or her hands when glitter from the restrooms ends up all over the classroom. Reinforce this lesson by passing out travel-size bars of soap or waterless hand cleanser for each student to take home. For one more alternative exercise to stress good handwashing, bring a jar of creamy peanut butter to class and distribute a tongue depressor to each student. Have all students put a small amount of peanut butter onto a tongue depressor and then smear it all over their hands. (Students may want to remove jewelry before this exercise.) Then have them go to a sink or restroom and wash their hands with soap and water. If their handwashing is thorough, no odor of the peanut butter should remain on their hands. If any odor remains on their hands, have them rewash until they can no longer detect it.

PART 5: ILLNESS AND INJURY PREVENTION

19. *Injury Statistics.* Obtain a copy of the annual report of your state's statistics of deaths. The department of health and welfare or a similar state agency often will publish an annual report on the numbers of deaths caused by specific illnesses and traumatic incidents. Discuss with students the percentage of deaths that might have been prevented. Discuss risk factors, public education, community health, and other types of prevention programs.

20. *Designing a Safety or Prevention Program.* Divide the class into work teams and have them design a safety or prevention program for their agency. Be sure they address issues of researching the need, identifying the population to be served, financing the project, implementation, data collection and sharing, measuring the impact on the target population, benefits to EMS providers, and so on. These projects should be documented and presented to the class. This activity encourages critical thinking and creative problem solving. Communication skills are also exercised.

21. *Prevention Program Participation.* Contact local injury or illness prevention organizations or agencies, or law enforcement agencies, to locate an illness or injury prevention program that would benefit from student involvement. Such programs might include blood pressure clinics, car seat installation projects, CPR marathons, and so on. If several possibilities exist, allow each student to pick the program in which he or she is most interested. You may also discuss holding an open house at your school where students would perform blood pressure checks, medication listing, and so forth. Alternatively, have students chart the prevention resources available in the community by completing Handout 1-12, "Illness and Injury Prevention."

HANDOUT 1-12
Illness and Injury Prevention

22. *Class Safety Survey.* Pick busy intersections in your community and on a specified date and time have one or two students observe each of these intersections to count the number of vehicles in which drivers and passengers were or were not wearing seatbelts. At the end of the specified time, have students return to a central point and tabulate the results. Determine the percentage of vehicles in which the occupants were wearing seatbelts. Share that information with local law enforcement and public health agencies.

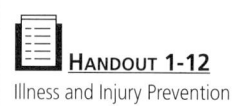

23. Documenting with Injury Prevention in Mind. Create a list of language and phrases that helps students to document injury prevention behaviors. Examples include such things as: "seatbelts used," "airbag deployed," "no helmet used," "knee and elbow pads intact," "many area rugs in the home," "no handrail available on stairs," "gloves and goggles worn." Many experienced paramedics may not be including this information on their run sheets because the commitment to prevention is relatively new to EMS. Therefore, students may not be able to learn this from their preceptors. Arm them with this positive habit when they enter the field.

24. Community Needs Assessment. As a class project, conduct a needs assessment of your community. Have students pick a lead person, then brainstorm what types of illness and injury prevention programs would be appropriate. Once the potential programs are identified, have each student pick one specific type of program. Have students determine if their programs are already in place in the community. If they are, have students contact the agencies or programs and gather information from them, such as number of citizens served, services offered, and similar facts. Then have students report their findings to the class.

PART 6: ETHICS IN ADVANCED PREHOSPITAL CARE

25. Identifying Moral/Ethical Issues. To help students identify moral versus ethical issues, use the newspaper or a videotape of the evening news. Select several stories and, for each, help students determine whether it demonstrates a legal, moral, or ethical violation or issue. Applying these concepts to actual events will help students learn the difference between the types of conflict. Adult learners need application to real life in order to "know" something rather than simply to "memorize" it. To expand on this activity, ask students to find newspaper or magazine articles from the lay press that discuss ethical issues. Between health care, politics, and violence, this should be no problem! Have students share their articles and identify the following: the issue, the affected parties, consequences of each possible action, and potential solutions. This exercise forces students to read, to stay current on events outside of EMS, and to conduct a literature search. Sharing their articles in class improves public speaking and oral communication skills.

26. Reinforcing Professional Ethics. Post an enlarged copy of the EMT Code of Ethics in your classroom. (See Handout 1-15 in this manual.) When issues arise or behavior dictates, ask students to read aloud from the posting. Remind students that paramedics have adopted this code as professionals, and those wishing to join their ranks as professional paramedics will have to align their behavior and decisions accordingly. Your classroom is the perfect place to instill values and professional behavior. Never feel bad about pushing your students in the classroom, for it is here that they are learning the profession of paramedicine. Employers, patients, and other professionals will appreciate these high standards when your students graduate.

27. Prehospital DNR Survey. Assign each student a state in the United States to contact. Have students request information, such as laws or polices, dealing with EMS providers' ability to honor or accept DNR orders in the prehospital setting. Are actual laws in place regarding this issue? Does the state have special programs, such as the Comfort One program, that allow EMS providers to honor DNR orders in the field? What agency administers the program? Does the state have any laws regarding unattended deaths? Once the students have obtained the information, have them present it to the class and compare the requirements of the different states.

The following strategy can be used at various points throughout the lesson or to help summarize and demonstrate what students have learned:

Cultural Considerations, Legal Notes, and Patho Pearls. The Student CD-ROM contains this series of informative features to enhance the student's understanding of the material covered in this chapter.

TEACHING OUTLINE

Chapter 1, "Introduction to Advanced Prehospital Care," is the first lesson in Division 1, *Introduction to Advanced Prehospital Care*. Distribute Handout 1-1 so that students can familiarize themselves with the learning goals for this chapter. If students have any questions about the objectives, answer them at this time.

Then present the chapter. One possible lecture outline follows. In the outline, the parenthetical references in regular type are references to text pages; those in bold type are references to figures or tables.

PART 1: INTRODUCTION TO ADVANCED PREHOSPITAL CARE (PP. 6–8)

I. Introduction. EMS has made significant advances. The paramedic of the twenty-first century is a highly trained health care professional. (p. 6) (**Fig. 1-1, p. 6**)

II. Description of the paramedic profession. The primary task of the paramedic is to provide emergency medical care in an out-of-hospital setting. (pp. 6–7) (**Fig. 1-1, p. 6**)

   A. Highest level of prehospital care provider (p. 6)
   1. Need for ability to make independent judgments in a timely manner
   2. Operates under the license of medical direction
   3. Requirements of licensing or credentialing

   B. Part of the continuum of patient care (p. 6)
   C. Responsibility to provide the best possible care regardless of the patient's ability to pay (p. 7)
   D. Emerging roles and responsibilities (p. 7)
   1. Education
   2. Health promotion
   3. Injury/illness prevention programs

   E. Responsibility to act in the best interest of the patient (p. 7)
   F. Responsibility and accountability (p. 7)
   1. System medical director
   2. Employer
   3. Public
   4. Peers

III. Paramedic characteristics. Regardless of the type of service provider you work for, your success as a paramedic will depend upon your having or developing certain professional characteristics. (p. 7)

   A. Must be flexible to meet the demands of the ever-changing emergency scene (p. 7)
   B. Must be a confident leader with the following qualities: (p. 7)
   1. Excellent judgment
   2. Ability to prioritize decisions
   3. Ability to develop rapport with a wide variety of patients
   4. Ability to function independently at an optimum level

HANDOUT 1-1
Chapter 1 Objectives Checklist

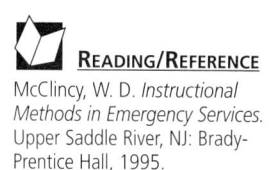

TEACHING STRATEGY 1
Breaking the Ice

TEACHING STRATEGY 2
Setting Ground Rules

READING/REFERENCE
McClincy, W. D. *Instructional Methods in Emergency Services.* Upper Saddle River, NJ: Brady-Prentice Hall, 1995.

POWERPOINT PRESENTATION
Chapter 1 PowerPoint slides 5–6

POWERPOINT PRESENTATION
Chapter 1 PowerPoint slides 7–12

TEACHING TIP
Offer an orientation to the new DOT curriculum to preceptors involved in your course. This will be a direct benefit to students during their field internships. Most preceptors were educated before adoption of the new curriculum and may not be familiar with the changes in terminology, the expanded pharmacology, or home-care therapies. Many people react to change by feeling threatened, which does not create a healthy learning environment. Be proactive by including preceptors in these changes for the future in EMS education. This will demonstrate to preceptors that you value them as part of the educational team.

POWERPOINT PRESENTATION
Chapter 1 PowerPoint slide 13

TEACHING STRATEGY 3
Highlighting the Need for Continuing Education

POWERPOINT PRESENTATION
Chapter 1 PowerPoint slides 14–18

TEACHING TIP
Invite your training center's medical director to the first day of class to address new students. Have him or her delineate the expectations he or she has of the students. Encourage the students to discuss their interest and commitment to prehospital care. Students need to know under whose license they perform. Familiarity with the medical director is often a question asked of students by accrediting bodies such as the JRC.

POWERPOINT PRESENTATION
Chapter 1 PowerPoint slides 19–23

POWERPOINT PRESENTATION
Chapter 1 PowerPoint slides 4–9

SLIDES/VIDEOS
Mention and periodically show the videotape magazine series 24-7 EMS or its predecessor *Pulse/Emergency Medical Update*, which offers continuing education credits.

TEACHING TIP
Distribute subscription order forms from various EMS periodicals and suggest students subscribe to one or more.

SLIDES/VIDEOS
"The History of Modern EMS: Making a Difference, 2E," JEMS/Mosby 2004.

TEACHING STRATEGY 4
Guest Lecturers

TEACHING TIP
Outline your local EMS service's organizational chart.

TEACHING STRATEGY 5
EMS Response Design

IV. The paramedic: A true health professional. Despite its relative youth as a profession, the field of emergency medicine is now recognized as an important part of the health care system. (p. 7)

  A. EMS is important part of health care system. (p. 7)
  B. The paramedic is a true health care professional. (p. 7)
  C. Professional development is a never-ending, career-long pursuit. (p. 7)
  D. EMT-Paramedic National Standard Curriculum sets standards for paramedic education. (p. 7)
  E. Participation in community organizations and research projects (p. 7)
  F. Paramedics must follow codes of professional ethics and etiquette. (p. 7)

V. Expanded scope of practice. Paramedics must be willing to step up to their expanding roles, or persons from other health care disciplines will fill them. (p. 8)

  A. Critical care transport (p. 8)
  B. Primary care (p. 8)
  C. Tactical EMS (p. 8)
  D. Industrial medicine (p. 8)
  E. Sports medicine (p. 8)

PART 2: EMS SYSTEMS (PP. 8–23)

I. Introduction. An Emergency Medical Services (EMS) system is a comprehensive network of personnel, equipment, and resources established to deliver aid and emergency medical care to the community. (pp. 8–9)

  A. Consists of out-of-hospital and in-hospital components (p. 8)
   1. Out-of-hospital components
      a. Members of the community trained in first aid and CPR
      b. Communications system
      c. EMS providers
         i. First responders, EMTs, and paramedics
      d. Fire/rescue and hazardous materials services
      e. Public utilities
         i. Power and gas companies, and so on
      f. Resource centers
         i. Poison control centers, and so on
   2. In-hospital components
      a. Emergency nurses
      b. Emergency physicians and specialty physicians
      c. Ancillary services
         i. Radiology, respiratory therapy, and so on
      d. Specialty physicians
         i. Trauma surgeons, cardiologists, and so on
      e. Rehabilitation services
  B. Citizen activation of the EMS system (p. 9)
  C. Dispatch center (p. 9)
   1. Collects information
   2. Sends appropriate response
   3. Provides prearrival instructions to caller
  D. First Responder (p. 9)
   1. Law enforcement
   2. Fire department
   3. Other community members

   E. Ambulance response (p. 9)
      1. Basic life support
      2. Advanced life support
      3. Tiered response
   F. Local hospital (p. 9)
   G. Specialty facilities (p. 9)
   H. Specialty physicians (p. 9)

II. History of EMS. (pp. 9–12)
   A. Ancient times (p. 9)
      1. Good Samaritan
      2. Sumerian and Mesopotamian protocols
      3. 1500 B.C.E.
         a. Edwin Smith scroll
         b. Book of Wounds
      4. Code of Hammurabi
         a. Law of the claw
         b. Medical fees and penalties
   B. Eighteenth and nineteenth centuries (p. 9)
      1. Napoleonic Wars
         a. Flying ambulance (ambulance volante)
         b. Triage
      2. U.S. Civil War
         a. Triage and transport of wounded soldiers
         b. Improvised hospitals in houses, barns, and churches
      3. First civilian ambulance service
         a. Cincinnati, Ohio (1865)
      4. New York City Health Department Ambulance Service (1869)
   C. Twentieth century (pp. 10–11)
      1. World War II
         a. Battlefield ambulances
         b. Transportation to appropriate facilities
      2. Korean and Vietnamese conflicts
         a. Soldiers treated in battlefield
         b. Evacuation by helicopter
      3. Post-1960s developments
         a. Mortician-operated ambulances withdrew due to costs and demand for additional services.
         b. Fire and police departments began providing EMS.
         c. Growth of volunteer and independent local EMS provider agencies
         d. Publication of *Accidental Death and Disability: The Neglected Disease of Modern Society* in 1966
            i. Highlighted deficiencies in prehospital emergency care
            ii. Set guidelines for development of EMS systems, training, ambulances, equipment
         e. National Highway Safety Act (1966)
            i. Matching grants for EMS services
            ii. Development of effective EMS systems
         f. First EMT-Ambulance program (1969)
         g. White House grants $9 million to EMS demonstration projects (1971)
         h. Department of Health, Education, and Welfare funds five-state initiative for development of regional EMS systems (1972)

POWERPOINT PRESENTATION
Chapter 1 PowerPoint slides 10–26

READING/REFERENCE
National Academy of Sciences, National Research Council. *Accidental Death and Disability: The Neglected Disease of Modern Society*. Washington, DC: U.S. Department of Health, Education, and Welfare, 1966.

>   >   i. Emergency Medical Services Systems Act (1973)
>   >   i. Listed 15 components of an EMS system
>   >   a. Manpower
>   >   b. Training
>   >   c. Communications
>   >   d. Transportation
>   >   e. Emergency facilities
>   >   f. Critical care units
>   >   g. Public safety agencies
>   >   h. Consumer participation
>   >   i. Access to care
>   >   j. Patient transfer
>   >   k. Standardized record keeping
>   >   l. Public information and education
>   >   m. System review and evaluation
>   >   n. Disaster management plans
>   >   o. Mutual aid
>   >   ii. System financing and medical direction omitted from legislation
>   >   iii. Amended in 1976 and 1979
>   >   j. First EMT-Paramedic curriculum (1977)
>   >   k. Congressional Omnibus Budget Reconciliation Act essentially wipes out federal funding for EMS (1981)
>   >   l. NHTSA initiates Statewide EMS Technical Assessment Program based on 10 key components of EMS system (1988)
>   >   i. Regulation and policy
>   >   ii. Resources management
>   >   iii. Human resources and training
>   >   iv. Transportation
>   >   v. Facilities
>   >   vi. Communications
>   >   vii. Trauma systems
>   >   viii. Public information and education
>   >   ix. Medical direction
>   >   x. Evaluation
>   D. *EMS Agenda for the Future* (pp. 11–12)
>   1. Published in 1996 as an opportunity to examine what has been learned during the prior three decades and to create a vision for the future for EMS in the United States
>   2. Continued development of 14 EMS attributes
>   a. Integration of health services
>   b. EMS research
>   c. Legislation and regulation
>   d. System finance
>   e. Human resources
>   f. Medical direction
>   g. Education systems
>   h. Public education
>   i. Prevention
>   j. Public access
>   k. Communication systems
>   l. Clinical care
>   m. Information systems
>   n. Evaluation

III. **Today's EMS systems.** Each community must develop an EMS system that best meets its needs. (pp. 12–23)

READING/REFERENCE

National Highway Traffic Safety Administration. *EMS Agenda for the Future*. Washington, DC: U.S. Department of Transportation, 1996. National Highway Traffic Safety Administration. *EMS Education Agenda for the Future: A System Approach*. Washington, DC: U.S. Department of Transportation, 2004.

POINT TO EMPHASIZE

Each community must develop an EMS system that best meets its needs.

POINT TO EMPHASIZE

A chain is only as strong as its weakest link. Designing an EMS system without involving the public may result in poor performance of that system.

POWERPOINT PRESENTATION

Chapter 1 PowerPoint slides 27–74

A. Local and state-level agencies (p. 12)
   1. Planning board
      a. Develops budget
      b. Selects qualified administrative staff
   2. Policies
   3. Quality assurance/improvement
   4. Allocation of funds to local systems
   5. Enacting legislation
      a. Prehospital practice
      b. Licensing/certification of field providers
      c. Enforcement of state EMS regulations
      d. Appointment of regional advisory councils
B. Medical direction (pp. 13–14)
   1. Medical director (**Fig. 1-2, p. 13**)
      a. Legally responsible for all clinical and patient-care aspects of system
      b. Extension of medical director's license
      c. Medical director's role in an EMS system
         i. Educate and train personnel
         ii. Participate in personnel and equipment selection
         iii. Develop clinical protocols in cooperation with expert EMS personnel
         iv. Participate in quality improvement and problem resolution
         v. Provide direct input into patient care
         vi. Interface between the EMS system and other health care agencies
         vii. Advocate within the medical community
         viii. Serve as the "medical conscience" of the EMS system, including advocating for quality patient care
   2. On-line medical direction
      a. Direct orders to prehospital care providers by radio or telephone
      b. May be delegated to MICN, PA, or paramedic
      c. Immediate access to medical consultation
      d. Telemetry
      e. Intervening physician
   3. Off-line medical direction
      a. Policies, procedures, and practices set up in advance of a call
      b. Protocols
      c. Standing orders
      d. Protocols and standing orders address the four "Ts" of emergency care
         i. Triage
         ii. Treatment
         iii. Transport
         iv. Transfer
C. Public information and education (p. 14)
   1. Recognition of an emergency
   2. System access
   3. Basic life support assistance
D. Communications (pp. 15–16)
   1. Communications network of regional EMS system plan
      a. Citizen access
      b. Single control center (**Fig. 1-3, p. 15**)
      c. Operational communications capabilities
      d. Medical communications capabilities
      e. Communications hardware
      f. Communications software

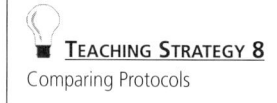

TEACHING STRATEGY 6
Medical Direction Review

TEACHING STRATEGY 7
Guest Speaker

TEACHING STRATEGY 8
Comparing Protocols

TEACHING TIP
Ask students to imagine they are driving through a strange town that does not have an E-911 system when a passenger in the car suddenly passes out. How would they access care? What number would they dial?

TEACHING STRATEGY 9
Raising Public Awareness of EMS

> **POINT TO EMPHASIZE**
> An effective EMS dispatching system places BLS care on scene within 4 minutes of onset and ALS care in less than 8 minutes.

> **READING/REFERENCE**
> Steele, S. *Emergency Dispatching: A Medical Communicator's Guide.* Upper Saddle River, NJ: Brady, 1993.

> **TEACHING STRATEGY 10**
> EMS Provider-Level Survey

> **TEACHING TIP**
> Explain the accreditation process for paramedic training programs in the United States. The Committee on Allied Health Education of the American Medical Association establishes standards for paramedic training programs. Those schools that meet the standard become accredited.

> **TEACHING TIP**
> List some emergency situations and their locations. Now have your students identify the proper mode of transportation of each patient to the appropriate facility. They will be amazed at the many factors that play into the correct decision.

> **TEACHING TIP**
> Have students list the specialty centers in your system.

    2. Emergency Medical Dispatcher (EMD)
       a. Basic telecommunications skills
       b. Medical interrogation
       c. Prearrival instructions
       d. Dispatch prioritization
    3. EMS dispatch
       a. EMS system status management
       b. Priority dispatching
       c. Prearrival instructions to callers
       d. Goal of dispatch:
          i. BLS in less than 4 minutes
          ii. ALS in less than 8 minutes
          iii. Goal met on at least 90 percent of calls
E. Education and certification (pp. 16–18)
    1. Initial education and continuing education
    2. Initial education
       a. Cognitive
       b. Affective
       c. Psychomotor
    3. Certification
    4. Licensure
    5. Registration
    6. Reciprocity
    7. Certification levels
       a. First Responder (FR)
       b. EMT-Basic (EMT-B)
       c. EMT-Intermediate (EMT-I)
       d. EMT-Paramedic (EMT-P)
    8. National Registry of EMTs
    9. Professional organizations
    10. Professional journals
F. Patient transportation (pp. 18–19)
    1. Ground transport
    2. Air transport
    3. Equipment standards
       a. American College of Surgeons Committee on Trauma
       b. American College of Emergency Physicians (ACEP)
    4. KKK-A-1822 federal specifications for ambulances
       a. Type I
       b. Type II
       c. Type III
G. Receiving facilities (pp. 19–20)
    1. Categorization
    2. Regionalized available services
       a. American College of Surgeons categories of trauma centers
          i. Level I
             a) Highest level of trauma care
          ii. Level II
             a) May not have specialty pediatrics or a neurosurgeon on site
          iii. Level III
             a) Generally does not have immediate surgical facilities available
    3. Emergency department with physician
    4. Commitment to participate in EMS system
    5. Receive emergency patients regardless of ability to pay
    6. Medical audit procedures
    7. Participate in multiple-casualty preparedness plans

H. Mutual aid and mass-casualty preparation (p. 20)
   1. Disaster plan
   2. Coordinated central management agency
   3. Integration of all EMS system components
   4. Flexible communications system
I. Quality assurance and improvement (pp. 20–21)
   1. A Leadership Guide to Quality Improvement for EMS Systems
      a. Leadership
      b. Information and analysis
      c. Strategic quality planning
      d. Human resources development and management
      e. EMS process management
      f. EMS system results
      g. Satisfaction of patients and other stakeholders
   2. Quality assurance (QA)
   3. Continuous quality improvement (CQI)
   4. "Take-it-for-granted" quality
      a. Highest level of professionalism
      b. Rules of evidence
         i. There must be a theoretical basis for the change
         ii. There must be ample research
         iii. It must be clinically important
         iv. It must be practical, affordable, and teachable
      c. Peer review
      d. Ethics
   5. Service quality
      a. Customer satisfaction
J. Research (pp. 21–23)
   1. Identify problem, reason for study, and hypothesis
   2. Identify published knowledge
   3. Select best study design
   4. Begin study and collect data
   5. Analyze and correlate data
   6. Assess and evaluate results against hypothesis
   7. Write and publish study
   8. Evidence-Based Medicine (EBM)
      a. Conscientious, explicit, and judicious use of the current best evidence in making decisions about the care of individual patients
      b. Combines clinical expertise with the best available clinical evidence from systematic research
K. System financing (p. 23)
   1. Fee-for-service (p. 23)
   2. Public utility model (p. 23)
   3. Failsafe franchise (p. 23)

PART 3: ROLES AND RESPONSIBILITIES OF THE PARAMEDIC (PP. 23–31)

I. Introduction. EMS and paramedic roles and responsibilities have changed dramatically in recent years. Modern paramedic needs a strong knowledge of pathophysiology and of the most current medical technology. (p. 23) (Fig. 1-4, p. 24)

II. Primary responsibilities. The paramedic's diverse responsibilities include emergency medical care for the patient and a variety of other responsibilities before, during, and after a call. (pp. 23–26)

TEACHING STRATEGY 11
EMS Research Investigation

POINT TO EMPHASIZE
Before responding to a call, a paramedic must be mentally, physically, and emotionally able to meet the demands of the job.

POWERPOINT PRESENTATION
Chapter 1 PowerPoint slides 4–15

A. Preparation (pp. 23–24)
   1. Protocols, policies, procedures
   2. Communications system
   3. Local geography
   4. Support agencies
B. Response (p. 24)
   1. Personal safety is the number-one priority.
   2. Always follow basic safety precautions while en route to call.
      a. Wear a seatbelt.
      b. Obey posted speed limits.
      c. Monitor the road for potential hazards.
   3. Know when to call for assistance.
      a. Multiple patients
      b. Motor vehicle collisions
      c. Hazardous materials
      d. Rescue situations
      e. Violent individuals (patients or bystanders)
      f. Use of a weapon
      g. Knowledge of previous violence
C. Patient assessment and management (p. 25)
   1. Scene size-up
   2. Patient assessment and management (**Fig. 1-25, p. 25**)
D. Appropriate disposition of patients (p. 25)
   1. Transportation to the appropriate facility
   2. Receiving facilities
   3. Other types of disposition
      a. Primary care
      b. "Treat and release"
E. Patient transfer (pp. 25–26)
   1. Questions concerning patient's best interests
   2. Verbal report and copy of patient's chart
   3. Transfer of care to contact person
F. Documentation (p. 26) (**Fig. 1-6, p. 26**)
G. Returning to service (p. 26)
   1. Prepare the unit.
   2. Review the call.

III. Additional responsibilities. In addition to emergency response, paramedics' duties involve taking an active role in promoting positive health practices in the community. (pp. 26–27)

A. Community involvement (p. 26)
   1. BLS instruction
   2. Injury prevention programs
   3. Benefits
      a. Enhances visibility of EMS
      b. Promotes positive image
      c. Puts forth EMS personnel as positive role models
      d. Integration with other agencies
B. Cost containment (p. 27)
   1. Promoting wellness
   2. Illness and injury prevention
C. Citizen involvement in EMS (p. 27)

IV. Professionalism. In addition to meeting requirements for initial and ongoing education, *professionalism* refers to the conduct or qualities that characterize a practitioner in a particular field or occupation. (pp. 27–31)

A. Professional ethics (p. 27)
   1. Oath of Geneva
   2. EMT Code of Ethics
B. Professional attitudes (pp. 27–28)
   1. Professionals place their patients first.
   2. Professionals set high standards.
   3. Professionals act responsibly on and off duty.
   4. Professionalism is an attitude, not a matter of pay.
C. Professional attributes (pp. 28–30)
   1. Leadership (**Fig. 1-7, p. 28**)
      a. Self-confidence
      b. Established credibility
      c. Inner strength
      d. Ability to remain in control
      e. Ability to communicate
      f. Willingness to make a decision
      g. Willingness to accept responsibility for the consequences of the team's actions
   2. Integrity
      a. Single most important behavior: honesty
   3. Empathy
      a. Being supportive and reassuring
      b. Demonstrating an understanding of the patient's and family's feelings
      c. Demonstrating respect for others
      d. Having a calm, compassionate, and helpful demeanor
   4. Self-motivation
      a. Completing assigned duties without being asked or told to do so
      b. Completing all duties and assignments without the need for direct supervision
      c. Correctly completing all paperwork in a timely manner
      d. Demonstrating a commitment to continuous quality improvement
      e. Accepting constructive feedback in a positive manner
      f. Taking advantage of learning opportunities
   5. Appearance and personal hygiene
   6. Self-confidence
   7. Communication
   8. Time management
   9. Teamwork and diplomacy
      a. Place the success of the team ahead of personal self-interest.
      b. Never undermine the role or opinion of another team member.
      c. Provide support for members of the team, both on and off duty.
      d. Remain open to suggestions from team members and be willing to change for the benefit of the patient.
      e. Openly communicate with everyone.
      f. Above all, respect the patient, other care providers, and the community you serve.
   10. Respect for others
   11. Patient advocacy
   12. Careful delivery of service
      a. Mastering and refreshing skills
      b. Performing complete equipment checks
      c. Careful and safe ambulance operations
   13. Following policies, procedures, and protocols
D. Continuing education and professional development (pp. 30–31)

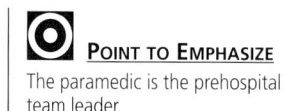

POINT TO EMPHASIZE
The paramedic is the prehospital team leader.

TEACHING STRATEGY 12
Defining Leadership Qualities

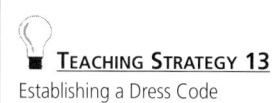

TEACHING STRATEGY 13
Establishing a Dress Code

POINT TO EMPHASIZE
The paramedic should always be an advocate for the patient.

READING/REFERENCE
Monosky, K. "2004 JEMS Salary & Workplace Survey." *JEMS*, Oct. 2004.

POWERPOINT PRESENTATION
Chapter 1 PowerPoint slide 4

POWERPOINT PRESENTATION
Chapter 1 PowerPoint slides 5–24

POINT TO EMPHASIZE
For strength and stamina on the job, and in life itself, eat well, stay physically fit, and avoid potentially addictive and harmful substances.

TEACHING TIP
If you have an employee fitness center at or near your location, negotiate a student rate. Encourage students to exercise before class or at lunch. Allow them to eat snacks or lunch foods during class or at breaks so that the lunch hour can be spent working out. Exercise will improve strength, flexibility, and cardiovascular and mental health. You will likely observe that students develop increased patience and improved dispositions, and have fewer sick days. Instilling these good habits can increase the length of service your students give to EMS.

TEACHING STRATEGY 14
Gauging Basic Flexibility

TEACHING STRATEGY 15
Healthy Diet Tracking

TEACHING TIP
Instead of a coffee fund, offer a bottled water service to encourage students to drink more water daily. You will find that for a dollar or two per month, students can purchase cold, great-tasting water to replace the coffee or pop they were drinking.

PART 4: THE WELL-BEING OF THE PARAMEDIC (PP. 31–47)

I. Introduction. Well-being is a fundamental aspect of top-notch performance in EMS. (p. 31)

   A. Physical well-being (p. 31)
   B. Mental well-being (p. 31)
   C. Emotional well-being (p. 31)

II. Basic physical fitness. For strength and stamina on the job, and in life itself, eat well, stay physically fit, and avoid potentially addictive and harmful substances. (pp. 31–34)

   A. Core elements (pp. 31–32)
      1. Muscular strength is achieved with regular exercise.
         a. Isometric exercise
            i. Active exercise performed against stable resistance
         b. Isotonic exercise
            i. Active exercise during which muscles are worked through their range of motion
      2. Cardiovascular endurance (aerobic capacity) (p. 32)
         a. Exercise at least three days a week to reach target heart rate (**Table 1-1, p. 32**)
         b. Brisk walk
         c. Stationary bike
      3. Flexibility (p. 32)
         a. Strengthen main muscle groups regularly.
         b. Stretching exercises
   B. Nutrition (p. 32)
      1. The most difficult part is altering established habits.
      2. Good nutrition is fundamental to well-being.
      3. Major food groups
         a. Grains/breads
         b. Vegetables
         c. Fruits
         d. Dairy products
         e. Meat/fish
      4. Avoid or minimize intake of
         a. Fat
         b. Salt
         c. Sugar
         d. Cholesterol
         e. Caffeine
      5. Target diet
         a. 40 percent carbohydrates
         b. 40 percent proteins
         c. 20 percent fat
      6. Eat properly sized portions.
      7. Learn to read and heed food labels. (**Fig. 1-8, p. 32**)
      8. Your body needs plenty of fluids; drink water instead of soft drinks.
   C. Preventing cancer and cardiovascular disease (pp. 32–33)
      1. Stress management
      2. Exercise
      3. Diet
      4. Risk-assessment screenings
      5. Self-examinations
   D. Habits and addictions (p. 33)
      1. Overuse or abuse of substances

2. Caffeine and nicotine
   3. Alcohol and smoking
   4. In overcoming habits and addictions, the first step has to be yours.
  E. Back safety (pp. 33–34)
   1. Correct posture (**Fig. 1-9, p. 34**)
   2. Proper lifting techniques
   3. Heed your own body signals.
   4. Do not reach, or lift, and twist at the same time.

III. Personal protection from disease. Take all necessary precautions to minimize your risk of catching a disease while caring for others. (pp. 34–38)
  A. Infectious diseases (p. 35)
   1. Any disease caused by the growth of pathogenic microorganisms (**Table 1-2, p. 35**)
   2. Bloodborne diseases
      a. HIV/AIDS
      b. Hepatitis B
   3. Airborne diseases
      a. Tuberculosis
      b. Influenza
      c. Pneumonia, bacterial and viral
   4. Incubation period
  B. Infection-control practices (pp. 35–38)
   1. Body substance isolation (BSI)
   2. Personal protective equipment
      a. Protective gloves (**Fig. 1-10, p. 36**)
      b. Masks and protective eyewear
      c. HEPA and N-95 respirators
      d. Gowns
      e. Resuscitation equipment
   3. Handwashing
      a. One of the most important infection control practices
      b. Soap and water
      c. Scrub at least 15 seconds.
   4. Vaccinations and screening tests
      a. Immunizations
         i. Rubella (German measles)
         ii. Measles
         iii. Mumps
         iv. Chicken pox
         v. Tetanus/diphtheria
         vi. Polio
         vii. Influenza
         viii. Hepatitis B
         ix. Lyme disease
      b. Screening tests
         i. Tuberculosis (PPD)
   5. Decontamination of equipment
      a. Properly dispose of single-use PPE in biohazard-labeled red bag. (**Fig. 1-11, p. 37**)
      b. Properly dispose of needles and sharp objects in puncture-proof containers.
      c. Proper cleaning of nondisposable equipment
         i. Cleaning
            a) Washing with soap and water

POINT TO EMPHASIZE
Pay particular attention to keeping your back fit and use proper lifting and moving techniques.

TEACHING STRATEGY 16
Proper Lifting Technique Practice

POWERPOINT PRESENTATION
Chapter 1 PowerPoint slides 25–42

READING/REFERENCE
West, K. "AIDS Update." *JEMS*, Dec. 2002.

READING/REFERENCE
EMS Safety: Techniques and Applications (FA-144). Washington, DC: Federal Emergency Management Agency (FEMA), 1994.

POINT TO EMPHASIZE
Body substance isolation precautions protect the patient as well as the paramedic.

TEACHING STRATEGY 17
Personal Protective Equipment Practice

POINT TO EMPHASIZE
The most important, easiest, and most overlooked infection control practice is thorough handwashing.

TEACHING STRATEGY 18
Proper Handwashing Techniques

POINT TO EMPHASIZE
Keep all vaccinations, boosters, and health screenings current.

> **TEACHING TIP**
>
> Teaching about death and dying can be tricky because you may resurrect latent feelings and emotions of your own. But emotion can be a very powerful teaching tool. If you feel comfortable doing it, relate a story of how you experienced each phase of the grief process following a personal loss.

> **POWERPOINT PRESENTATION**
>
> Chapter 1 PowerPoint slides 43–45

> **TEACHING TIP**
>
> Have a hospital chaplain come to your class and speak on how to communicate with a dying patient and his or her family.

> **POINT TO EMPHASIZE**
>
> Most people can withstand either high stress for short periods of time or low stress for long periods of time. No one can withstand high stress for long periods of time without suffering serious physical or psychological illness.

        ii. Disinfecting
           a) Kills many microorganisms
        iii. Sterilizing
           a) Kills all microorganisms
    6. Postexposure procedures (Fig. 1-12, p. 38)
        a. Immediately wash affected area with soap and water.
        b. Get a medical evaluation.
        c. Take appropriate immunization boosters.
        d. Notify agency's infection control liaison.
        e. Document circumstances surrounding the exposure.

IV. Death and dying. The smart paramedic recognizes and deals with death in a healthy manner through appropriate grief work and stress management. (pp. 38–41)

  A. The most personally uncomfortable and challenging of prehospital situations (p. 38)
  B. Paramedics encounter death more often than other people. (p. 38)
  C. Loss, grief, and mourning (pp. 38–39)
    1. Stages
        a. Denial, or "Not me"
        b. Anger, or "Why me?"
        c. Bargaining, or "Okay, but first let me . . ."
        d. Depression, or "Okay, but I haven't . . ."
        e. Acceptance, or "Okay, I'm not afraid."
    2. Mistaken belief that paramedics can handle death better
    3. Grief is a feeling.
    4. Mourning is a process.
    5. Needs and expectations of children regarding death (Table 1-3, p. 40)
        a. Newborn to 3 years
        b. Ages 3 to 6
        c. Ages 6 to 9
        d. Ages 9 to 12
        e. Ages 12 to 18
  D. What to say (pp. 39–41)
    1. You never know how people will respond.
    2. For safety reasons, position yourself between them and the door.
    3. Do not deliver news to a large group.
    4. Find out who is who among the survivors.
    5. Introduce yourself.
    6. Don't hesitate to use the words "dead" or "died."
    7. Use gentle eye contact, remember the power of touching an arm or holding a hand
        a. Loved one has died.
        b. There is nothing more anyone could have done.
        c. Your EMS service is available to assist survivors if needed.
        d. Information about local procedures for out-of-hospital death
    8. Do not include statements about God's will, relief from pain, or subjective assumptions.
  E. When it is someone you know (p. 41)
    1. In small communities, calls often involve people whom paramedics know.
    2. People may be greatly relieved to see a familiar, trusted face.
    3. Find a way to manage the stress if it is too much.
    4. The paramedic must grieve as well.

V. Stress and stress management. To manage stress, identify your personal stressors, the amount of stress you can take before it becomes a problem, and the specific stress-management techniques that work for you. (pp. 41–45)
   A. Stress (p. 41)
      1. Hardship or strain
      2. Physical or emotional response
   B. A stressor (p. 41)
      1. The stimulus that causes the stress.
   C. Adapting to stress is a dynamic, evolving process. (p. 41)
      1. Defensive strategies
      2. Coping
      3. Problem-solving skills
   D. EMS has abundant stressors. (p. 41)
      1. Administrative stressors
      2. Scene-related stressors
      3. Emotional and physical stressors
   E. Things to learn about job-related stress (p. 42)
      1. Your personal stressors
      2. Amount of stress you can take before it becomes a problem
      3. Stress-management strategies that work for you
   F. Three phases of stress response (p. 42)
      1. Stage I: Alarm
         a. "Fight-or-flight" phenomenon
      2. Stage II: Resistance
         a. When individual begins to cope with stress
      3. Stage III: Exhaustion
         a. Prolonged exposure to the same stressors
   G. Shift work (pp. 42–43)
      1. Disruption of biorhythms of the body known as circadian rhythms
         a. Cycles that occur approximately every 24 hours
         b. Hormonal and body temperature fluctuations
         c. Appetite and sleep cycles
         d. Other bodily processes
         e. Sleep deprivation for night workers
      2. How to minimize stress if you sleep in the daytime
         a. Sleep in a cool, dark place.
         b. Stick to sleeping at your anchor time; do not attempt to revert to a daytime schedule.
         c. Unwind appropriately after a shift in order to rest well.
         d. Post a "day sleeper" sign on your front door; turn off the phone.
   H. Signs of stress (p. 43) (Table 1-4, p. 43)
      1. Physical
         a. Nausea/vomiting
         b. Lack of coordination
         c. Fatigue
      2. Emotional
         a. Anxiety
         b. Depression
         c. Desire to hide
         d. Anger
      3. Cognitive
         a. Confusion
         b. Lowered attention span
         c. Poor concentration

POWERPOINT PRESENTATION
Chapter 1 PowerPoint slides 46–55

TEACHING TIP
Paramedics are human. Even paramedic instructors experience stress. Share with the class an emotionally critical incident that affected you. Your passion and sincerity are crucial to driving home this point. Teach by your example.

TEACHING TIP
Ask students if any of them would like to share how they felt experiencing a loss.

TEACHING TIP
At the end of one class session announce, "At the beginning of the next class, we will have an oral quiz. I will ask you questions on material from the beginning of the course through this week's assignment." When they arrive for that class, poll students to see which signs and symptoms of stress they experienced.

TEACHING TIP
Ask your students how they would approach a colleague to whom they were close if he or she began to exhibit signs of cumulative stress after years in the streets.

    4. Behavioral
        a. Withdrawal
        b. Unusual behavior
        c. Crying spells
    5. Burnout
  I. Common techniques for managing stress (p. 44)
    1. Detrimental (temporary sense of relief, but don't cure the problem)
        a. Substance abuse
        b. Overeating
        c. Chronic complaining
        d. Cutting off others and their support
        e. Avoidance behaviors
        f. Dishonesty about one's own health and well-being
    2. Beneficial (healthy techniques)
        a. Controlling breathing
        b. Reframe
        c. Attend to the medical needs of the patient
        d. Taking care of yourself
        e. Exercise regularly.
        f. Do something you enjoy and find relaxing.
        g. Pay close attention to your diet.
        h. Quit smoking.
        i. Create non-EMS circle of friends.
        j. Take a vacation or days off.
        k. Say "no" to offers of overtime shifts.
        l. Listen to music, meditate, learn positive thinking.
        m. Learn guided imagery and progressive relaxation techniques.

SLIDES/VIDEOS
"Critical Incident Stress," University of Maryland, Department of EMS, Department of Instructional Media.

  J. Specific EMS stress (pp. 44–45)
    1. Daily stress
    2. Small incidents
    3. Large incidents and disasters
  K. Mental health services (p. 45)
    1. Psychological first aid
        a. Not a treatment or intervention technique
            i. Practical palliative care
        b. Components
            i. Listening
            ii. Conveying compassion
            iii. Assessing needs
            iv. Ensuring that basic physical needs are met
            v. Not forcing personnel to talk
            vi. Providing or mobilizing family or significant others
            vii. Encouraging, but not forcing, social support
            viii. Protecting rescuers and victims from additional harm

POINT TO EMPHASIZE
An injured EMT becomes part of the problem, not part of the solution. Training and proper use of equipment beat out needless heroics every time.

  L. Disaster mental health services (p. 45)
    1. Emotional well-being of victims and rescuers
    2. New evidence on role of CISM and CISD
    3. Mental health professionals to provide psychological first aid

VI. General safety considerations. The topic of scene safety is vast and requires career-long attention. (pp. 45–47)

POWERPOINT PRESENTATION
Chapter 1 PowerPoint slides 56–58

  A. Interpersonal relations (pp. 45–46)
    1. Treat every person you meet with dignity and respect.
    2. Pay attention to cultural diversity.
  B. Roadway safety (pp. 46–47)
    1. One of the greatest hazards in EMS is the motor vehicle.
    2. Acquire training for rescue and safe use of rescue equipment.

3. Learn safety principles.
      a. Safely following an emergency vehicle escort
      b. Intersection management
      c. Noting hazardous conditions
      d. Evaluating the safest parking place
      e. Safely approaching a vehicle
      f. Patient compartment safety
      g. Safely using emergency lights and siren

PART 5: ILLNESS AND INJURY PREVENTION (PP. 47–53)

I. Introduction. How many injuries and deaths could be prevented? How many deaths due to chronic illnesses could have been prevented by better health education? Illness and injury prevention is a paramedic's duty and responsibility. (p. 47)

II. Epidemiology. Injury is one of our nation's most important health problems. (pp. 47–48)

  A. U.S. Department of Transportation facts (p. 47)
     1. Injuries have surpassed stroke as the third leading cause of death in the United States in people ages 1–44.
     2. Unintentional injuries cause 70,000 deaths and millions of nonfatal injuries each year.
     3. Leading causes are motor-vehicle collisions, fires, burns, falls, drowning, and poisons.
     4. Estimated lifetime cost of injuries will exceed $114 billion.
     5. For every death from injury, an estimated 19 hospitalizations and 254 ED visits also occur.
  B. Motor-vehicle "collisions," not accidents (p. 47)
  C. Epidemiology (p. 47)
     1. Study of the factors that influence the frequency, distribution, and causes of injury, disease, and other health-related events in the population
  D. Years of productive life (p. 47)
     1. Subtract the age at death from 65
  E. Injury risk (pp. 47–48)
     1. Real or potentially hazardous situation that puts people in danger
  F. Injury-surveillance program; injury risk and statistics (p. 48)
  G. Teachable moments shortly after an injury (p. 48)
  H. Primary prevention (p. 48)
  I. Secondary prevention (p. 48)
  J. Tertiary prevention (p. 48)

III. Prevention within EMS. Every day, paramedics witness the tragic effects of preventable injuries. (pp. 48–50)

  A. Perform CPR and life-saving procedures every day. (p. 48)
  B. Medical personnel are high-profile role models. (p. 48)
  C. EMS providers are often looked to for medical advice and direction. (p. 48)
  D. EMS providers comprise a "great arsenal" in the war to prevent disease and injury. (p. 48)
  E. Organizational commitment (pp. 48–49)
     1. Protection of EMS providers
     2. Education of EMS providers (**Fig. 1-13, p. 49**)
     3. Data collection

POINT TO EMPHASIZE
Injuries are among our nation's most important health problems. Paramedics and other EMS personnel see many more injuries than the average person, and are often looked to for advice and direction. EMS providers are an obvious choice to help prevent injury and illness.

POWERPOINT PRESENTATION
Chapter 1 PowerPoint slides 4–5

POWERPOINT PRESENTATION
Chapter 1 PowerPoint slides 6–9

TEACHING STRATEGY 19
Injury Statistics

POINT TO EMPHASIZE
Injuries result from interaction with potential hazards in the environment, which means that they may be predictable and preventable.

POINT TO EMPHASIZE
Emphasize to students throughout the course that personal safety is always their first priority.

POWERPOINT PRESENTATION
Chapter 1 PowerPoint slides 10–21

TEACHING TIP
Have students include injury prevention in any appropriate practice scenarios during the course. Take advantage of teachable moments.

TEACHING STRATEGY 20
Designing a Safety or Prevention Program

TEACHING TIP

To keep students conscious of safety and prevention throughout the course, periodically ask them at the beginning of class sessions what safety or prevention activities they have been involved in. This can be anything from always wearing their seatbelts to exercising regularly, or instructing CPR courses and so on.

POWERPOINT PRESENTATION
Chapter 1 PowerPoint slides 22–25

TEACHING STRATEGY 21
Prevention Program Participation

TEACHING STRATEGY 22
Class Safety Survey

TEACHING STRATEGY 23
Documenting with Injury Prevention in Mind

TEACHING STRATEGY 24
Community Needs Assessment

TEACHING TIP

Have students as a group write short safety and prevention messages, such as "Always Wear Seatbelts" or "Don't Drink and Drive." Once a list is compiled, have students contact businesses with large outdoor billboards. Ask the businesses to display one of the safety or prevention messages on their board for one week. This works especially well during designated prevention weeks such as a drinking-and-driving awareness week, when messages concentrate on one specific topic.

TEACHING STRATEGY 25
Identifying Moral/Ethical Issues

POWERPOINT PRESENTATION
Chapter 1 PowerPoint slides 4–5

POWERPOINT PRESENTATION
Chapter 1 PowerPoint slides 6–16

   4. Financial support
   5. Empowerment of EMS providers
F. EMS provider commitment (p. 49)
   1. Body substance isolation precautions
   2. Physical fitness
   3. Stress management
   4. Seeking professional care and counseling
   5. Drive safely.
G. Scene safety (pp. 49–50)
   1. Assess and maintain scene safety.

IV. Prevention in the community. EMS has a responsibility not only to prevent injury and illness among EMS workers but also to promote prevention among the public. (pp. 50–53)

A. Areas of need (pp. 50–51)
   1. Infants and children
      a. Low birth weight
      b. Unrestrained children in motor vehicles
      c. Bicycle-related injuries
      d. Household fire and burn injuries
      e. Violent acts
      f. Firearm injuries
   2. Geriatric patients
      a. Falls
         i. Largest number of preventable injuries for persons over 75
      b. The aging process
   3. Motor vehicle collisions
      a. Term "motor-vehicle accident" does not accurately reflect the causation of incidents; something, in fact, causes the "accident."
      b. About half of all MVC deaths are alcohol related.
   4. Work and recreation hazards
      a. 22 percent of work-related disabling injuries are to the back.
      b. Another 22 percent are injuries to eyes, hands, and fingers.
      c. Sports injuries
   5. Medications
      a. Take only medications that are prescribed to you.
      b. Medications improperly taken—too much, or too little, or not completely—cause problems.
   6. Early discharge
B. Implementation of prevention strategies (pp. 51–53)
   1. Preserve the safety of the response team.
   2. Recognize scene hazards.
   3. Document findings. (**Fig. 1-14, p. 52**)
   4. Engage in on-scene education.
   5. Know your community resources.
   6. Conduct a community needs assessment.

PART 6: ETHICS IN ADVANCED PREHOSPITAL CARE (PP. 53–62)

I. Introduction. Though most paramedics do not see ethics as a difficult part of their job, ethical questions frequently arise. These include refusal of care, hospital destinations, advance directives, confidentiality, consent, the obligation to provide care, and research. (p. 53)

II. Overview of ethics. Morals are defined as social, religious, or personal standards of right and wrong, whereas ethics are the rules or standards that

28 ESSENTIALS OF PARAMEDIC CARE

©2007 Pearson Education, Inc.
Essentials of Paramedic Care, 2nd ed.

govern the conduct of the members of a particular group or profession. (pp. 53–56)

A. Relationship of ethics to law and religion (p. 53)
B. Making ethical decisions (pp. 53–54)
   1. Ethical relativism
   2. Golden Rule
   3. Deontological method
   4. Consequentialism
C. Codes of ethics (p. 54)
   1. American Medical Association
   2. American College of Emergency Physicians
   3. American Nurses Association
   4. Emergency Nurses Association
   5. National Association of EMTs
D. Fundamental questions (p. 54)
   1. What is in the patient's best interest?
   2. Elements to help determine the answer
      a. Written statement describing the patient's desires
      b. Verbal statement of what the patient does and does not want
      c. Wishes of family members
E. Fundamental principles (pp. 54–55)
   1. Bioethics
   2. Beneficence
      a. Doing good for the patient
   3. Nonmaleficence
      a. Obligation not to harm the patient
   4. Autonomy
      a. Patient's right to determine what happens to him or her
   5. Justice
      a. Obligation to treat all patients fairly
F. Resolving ethical conflicts (pp. 55–56)
   1. State the action in a universal form.
   2. List the implications or consequences of the action.
   3. Compare them to relevant values.
   4. Quick ways to test ethics
      a. Impartiality test
         i. Would you be willing to have this done to you?
      b. Universalizability test
         ii. Would you want this action performed in all relevantly similar circumstances?
      c. Interpersonal justifiability test
         iii. Can the action be defended or justified to others?

III. **Ethical issues in contemporary paramedic practice.** A sound understanding of fundamental methods of ethical decision making will help you to make sound choices in the field. (pp. 56–62)

A. Resuscitation attempts (pp. 56–58)
   1. DNR orders
   2. Advance directives
B. Confidentiality (pp. 58–59)
C. Consent (p. 59)
D. Allocation of resources (pp. 59–60)
   1. Multiple-casualty incidents
   2. Triage

TEACHING STRATEGY 26
Reinforcing Professional Ethics

POINT TO EMPHASIZE
The single most important question a paramedic has to answer when faced with an ethical challenge is, "What is in the patient's best interest?"

POINT TO EMPHASIZE
The first rule of EMS is, "First, do no harm" (*Primum non nocere*).

TEACHING TIP
The EMS trade magazines are good sources of legal and ethical issues. Frequently a section is devoted to news, current events, or current cases in EMS. Use these resources when preparing case studies for discussion and application of ethical principles. Using references that are readily available to students encourages them to read the current literature relevant to our industry.

TEACHING STRATEGY 27
Prehospital DNR Survey

READING/REFERENCE
American College of Emergency Physicians. "Code of Ethics for Emergency Physicians." *Annals of Emergency Medicine*, 30 (1997).
Heilicser, B., C. Stocking, and M. Siegler. "Ethical Dilemmas in Emergency Medical Services: The Perspective of the Emergency Medical Technician." *Annals of Emergency Medicine*, 27 (1996).

Iserson, K. V., et al. *Ethics in Emergency Medicine*. 2nd ed. Tucson, AZ: Galen Press, 1995.

POWERPOINT PRESENTATION
Chapter 1 PowerPoint slides 17–27

TEACHING TIP
To discuss the topic of patient's rights versus family wishes in the case of sudden death, ask your class this question: "Does implied consent supersede a spouse's wish not to have resuscitative measures taken?"

E. Obligation to provide care (p. 60)
   1. Without regard for ability to pay
   2. HMOs
F. Teaching (p. 60)
   1. Patients advised students are working on them
   2. Number of attempts of a procedure made by students
G. Professional relations (pp. 60–61)
   1. Physician orders something paramedic believes is contraindicated.
   2. Physician orders something paramedic believes is medically acceptable but not in patient's best interest.
   3. Physician orders something paramedic believes is medically acceptable but morally wrong.
H. Research (pp. 61–62)
   1. Goal of patient care is to improve the patient's condition.
   2. Goal of research is to help future patients.

IV. Chapter Summary (p. 62). This is an exciting time for EMS and pre-hospital medicine. The paramedic of the twenty-first century is a true health care professional who can provide a significant impact on health care.

EMS has evolved over many years. Today, a comprehensive EMS system provides a continuum of care from First Responder to hospital and rehabilitative staff, from the mechanic who maintains the ambulance fleet to the emergency physician. It is a total team effort. The paramedic is the leader of the prehospital emergency medical team. You must undertake the responsibility of preparing yourself to do the job and of continually updating your knowledge and skills. The best paramedics are those who make a commitment to excellence.

As a paramedic, you must attend first to your own well-being in order to maintain the health and fitness to help others and to be a positive role model. Additionally, each member of EMS shares the responsibility of promoting wellness and preventing illness and injury among co-workers and in the community. As a paramedic, you also have the responsibility to behave ethically by acquiring a foundation in ethical values and having a system for making ethical decisions.

ASSIGNMENTS

Assign students to complete Chapter 1, "Introduction to Advanced Prehospital Care" of the workbook. Also assign them to read Chapter 2, "Medical/Legal Aspects of Advanced Prehospital Care," before the next class.

EVALUATION

Chapter Quiz and Scenario Distribute copies of the Chapter Quizzes provided in Handouts 1-2 through 1-7 to evaluate student understanding of this chapter. Make sure each student reads the scenarios to reinforce critical thinking on the scene. Remind students not to use their notes or textbooks while taking the quizzes.

Student CD Quizzes for every chapter are contained on the dynamic and highly visual in-text student CD.

Companion Website Additional quizzes for every chapter are contained in this exciting website.

WORKBOOK
Chapter 1 Activities

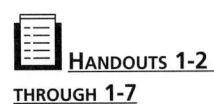

READING/REFERENCE
Textbook, pp. 64–83

HANDOUTS 1-2 THROUGH 1-7
Chapter 1 Quizzes

HANDOUTS 1-8 THROUGH 1-13
Chapter 1 Scenarios

PARAMEDIC STUDENT CD
Student Activities

COMPANION WEBSITE
http://www.prenhall.com/bledsoe

TestGen   You may wish to create a custom-tailored test using *Prentice Hall TestGen for Essentials of Paramedic Care,* 2nd Edition to evaluate student understanding of this chapter.

On-line Test Preparation (for students and instructors)   Additional test preparation is available through Brady's new on-line product, *EMT Achieve: Paramedic Test Preparation* at *http://www.prenhall.com/emtachieve/*. Instructors can also monitor student mastery on-line.

Review Manual for the EMT-Paramedic   This comprehensive exam review contains hundreds of test questions and rationales, including scenarios, along with two 180-question practice tests on CD.

REINFORCEMENT

Handouts   If classroom discussion or performance on the quiz indicates that some students have not fully mastered the chapter content, you may wish to assign some or all of the Reinforcement Handouts for this chapter.

Student CD (students)   A wide variety of material on this CD-ROM will reinforce and also expand student knowledge and skills.

PowerPoint Presentation (for instructors)   The PowerPoint material developed for this chapter offers useful reinforcement of chapter content.

Companion Website (for students)   Additional review quizzes and links to EMS resources will contribute to further reinforcement of the chapter.

OneKey   On-line support is offered for this course on one of three platforms: CourseCompass, Blackboard, or Web CT. Includes the IRM, PowerPoints, TestGen, and Companion Website for instruction. Ask your local sales representative for more information.

Brady Skills Series: Advanced Life Skills (Video or CD)   Have your students watch the skills come to life on VHS or CD-ROM, or they can purchase the highly visual, full-color text with step-by-step procedures and rationales.

TESTGEN
Chapter 1

EMT ACHIEVE: PARAMEDIC TEST PREPARATION
Mistovich & Beasley. *EMT Achieve: Paramedic Test Preparation*. http://www.prenhall.com/emtachieve/

REVIEW MANUAL FOR THE EMT-PARAMEDIC
Cherry & Mistovich. *Review Manual for the EMT-Paramedic,* 3rd edition.

HANDOUTS 1-14 THROUGH 1-26
Reinforcement Activities

PARAMEDIC STUDENT CD
Student Activities

POWERPOINT PRESENTATION
Chapter 1

COMPANION WEBSITE
http://www.prenhall.com/bledsoe

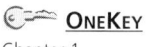

ONEKEY
Chapter 1

ADVANCED LIFE SUPPORT SKILLS
Larmon & Davis. *Advanced Life Support Skills.*

ADVANCED LIFE SKILLS REVIEW
Larmon & Davis. *Advanced Life Skills Review.*

BRADY SKILLS SERIES: ALS
Larmon & Davis. *Brady Skills Series: ALS.*

PARAMEDIC NATIONAL STANDARDS SELF-TEST
Miller. *Paramedic National Standards Self-Test,* 4th edition.

HANDOUT 1-1

Student's Name _____

CHAPTER 1 OBJECTIVES CHECKLIST

PART 1: INTRODUCTION TO ADVANCED PREHOSPITAL CARE

Knowledge	Date Mastered
1. Describe the relationship between the paramedic and other members of the allied health professions.	
2. Identify the attributes and characteristics of the paramedic.	
3. Explain the elements of paramedic education and practice that support its stature as a profession.	
4. Define and give examples of the expanded scope of practice for the paramedic.	

PART 2: EMS SYSTEMS

Knowledge	Date Mastered
1. Describe key historical events that influenced the national development of Emergency Medical Services (EMS) systems.	
2. Define the following terms: • certification • EMS systems • ethics • health care professional • licensure • medical direction • peer review • profession • professionalism • protocols • registration	
3. Identify national groups important to the development, education, and implementation of EMS as well as the role of national associations, the National Registry of EMTs, and the roles of various EMS standard-setting agencies.	
4. Identify the standards (components) of an EMS system as defined by the National Highway Traffic Safety Administration.	
5. Differentiate among EMS provider levels: First Responder, Emergency Medical Technician-Basic, Emergency Medical Technician-Intermediate, and Emergency Medical Technician-Paramedic.	
6. Describe what is meant by "citizen involvement in the EMS system."	

HANDOUT 1-1 Continued

Knowledge	Date Mastered
7. Discuss the role of the EMS physician in providing medical direction, prehospital and out-of-hospital care as an extension of the physician, the benefits of on-line and off-line medical direction, and the process for the development of local policies and protocols.	
8. Describe the relationship between a physician on the scene, the paramedic on the scene, and the EMS physician providing on-line medical direction.	
9. Describe the components of continuous quality improvement and analyze its contribution to system improvement, continuing medical education, and research.	
10. Describe the importance, basic principles, process of evaluating and interpreting, and benefits of research.	

PART 3: ROLES AND RESPONSIBILITIES OF THE PARAMEDIC

Knowledge	Date Mastered
1. Describe the attributes of a paramedic as a health care professional.	
2. Describe the benefits of paramedic continuing education and the importance of maintaining one's paramedic license/certification.	
3. List the primary and additional responsibilities of paramedics. Define the role of the paramedic relative to the safety of the crew, the patient, and bystanders.	
4. Describe the role of the paramedic in health education activities related to illness and injury prevention.	
5. Describe examples of professional behaviors in the following areas: integrity, empathy, self-motivation, appearance and personal hygiene, self-confidence, communications, time management, teamwork and diplomacy, respect, patient advocacy, and careful delivery of service.	
6. Identify the benefits of paramedics teaching in their community.	
7. Analyze how the paramedic can benefit the health care system by supporting primary care for patients in the out-of-hospital setting.	
8. Describe how professionalism applies to the paramedic while on and off duty.	

PART 4: THE WELL-BEING OF THE PARAMEDIC

Knowledge	Date Mastered
1. Discuss the concept of wellness and its benefits, components of wellness, and role of the paramedic in promoting wellness.	

HANDOUT 1-1 Continued

OBJECTIVES

Knowledge	Date Mastered
2. Discuss how cardiovascular endurance, weight control, muscle strength, and flexibility contribute to physical fitness.	
3. Describe the impact of shift work on circadian rhythms.	
4. Discuss the contributions that periodic risk assessments and warning sign recognition make to cancer and cardiovascular disease prevention.	
5. Differentiate proper from improper body mechanics for lifting and moving patients in emergency and nonemergency situations.	
6. Describe the problems that a paramedic might encounter in a hostile situation and the techniques used to manage the situation.	
7. Describe the considerations that should be given to using escorts, dealing with adverse environmental conditions, using lights and siren, proceeding through intersections, and parking at an emergency scene.	
8. Discuss the concept of "due regard for the safety of all others" while operating an emergency vehicle.	
9. Describe the equipment available in a variety of adverse situations for self-protection, including body substance isolation steps for protection from airborne and bloodborne pathogens.	
10. Given a scenario where equipment and supplies have been exposed to body substances, plan for the proper cleaning, disinfection, and disposal of the items.	
11. Describe the benefits and methods of smoking cessation.	
12. Identify and describe the three phases of the stress response, factors that trigger the stress response, and causes of stress in EMS.	
13. Differentiate between normal/healthy and detrimental physiological and psychological reactions to anxiety and stress.	
14. Describe behavior that is a manifestation of stress in patients and those close to them, and describe how that behavior relates to paramedic stress.	
15. Identify and describe the defense mechanisms and management techniques commonly used to deal with stress, discuss research about possible problems with the use of critical incident stress management (CISM), and identify the appropriate mental health services that should be available to EMS personnel.	
16. Given a scenario involving a stressful situation, formulate a strategy to help adapt to the stress.	

HANDOUT 1-1 Continued

Knowledge	Date Mastered
17. Describe the stages of the grieving process (Kübler-Ross) and the unique challenges for paramedics in dealing with themselves, adults, children, and other special populations related to their understanding or experience of death and dying.	
18. Given photos of various motor-vehicle collisions, assess scene safety and propose ways to make the scene safer.	

PART 5: ILLNESS AND INJURY PREVENTION

Knowledge	Date Mastered
1. Describe the incidence, morbidity and mortality, and the human, environmental, and socioeconomic impact of unintentional and alleged unintentional injuries.	
2. Identify health hazards and potential crime areas within the community.	
3. Identify local municipal and community resources available for physical, socioeconomic crises.	
4. List the general and specific environmental parameters that should be inspected to assess a patient's need for preventive information and direction.	
5. Identify the role of EMS in local municipal and community prevention programs.	
6. Identify the injury and illness prevention programs that promote safety for all age populations.	
7. Identify patient situations where the paramedic can intervene in a preventive manner.	
8. Document primary and secondary injury prevention data.	

PART 6: ETHICS IN ADVANCED PREHOSPITAL CARE

Knowledge	Date Mastered
1. Define ethics and morals and distinguish between ethical and moral decisions in emergency medical service.	
2. Identify the premise that should underlie the paramedic's ethical decisions in out-of-hospital care.	
3. Analyze the relationship between the law and ethics in EMS.	
4. Compare and contrast the criteria used in allocating scarce EMS resources.	
5. Identify issues surrounding advance directives in making a prehospital resuscitation decision and describe the criteria necessary to honor an advance directive in your state.	

HANDOUT 1-2

Student's Name _____

CHAPTER 1 QUIZ

PART 1: INTRODUCTION TO ADVANCED PREHOSPITAL CARE

Write the letter of the best answer in the space provided.

_____ 1. The National Standard Curriculum for paramedic training is published by the:
   A. National Registry of EMTs.
   B. U.S. Department of Transportation.
   C. National Association of State EMS Training Coordinators.
   D. U.S. Department of Health, Education, and Welfare.

_____ 2. As a rule, as a paramedic's use of a skill or procedure decreases:
   A. the more frequently he should review that skill or procedure.
   B. his retention of that skill or procedure remains the same.
   C. the less he needs to practice that skill or procedure.
   D. it is evidence that the skill or procedure may no longer be necessary.

_____ 3. Providing care at home without transport to a hospital is an example of the extended scope of:
   A. critical care.   C. primary care.
   B. industrial medicine.   D. advanced care.

_____ 4. The paramedic's emerging roles and responsibilities include:
   A. minor surgery.   C. industrial medicine.
   B. prescribing medications.   D. extended pediatric care.

_____ 5. Through research over the years, it has been found that:
   A. all EMS treatments used have been proven beneficial.
   B. little scientific evidence supports many prehospital practices.
   C. all current paramedic practices have been scientifically proven.
   D. treatments have been scientifically proven effective before they are used in the field.

_____ 6. According to the EMT-Paramedic: National Standard Curriculum Education Model, a pre- or co-requisite of the paramedic training course is:
   A. EMT-Intermediate.   C. First Responder.
   B. EMT-Basic.   D. advanced cardiac life support.

_____ 7. The EMT-Paramedic student should be competent in:
   A. chemistry.   C. mathematics.
   B. biology.   D. psychology.

_____ 8. Which of the following is TRUE regarding the 1998 EMT-Paramedic: National Standard Curriculum?
   A. It requires approximately the same number of hours as the previous curriculum.
   B. It requires a less extensive foundation of medical knowledge than the previous curriculum.
   C. A human anatomy and physiology course is a prerequisite.
   D. Content regarding the pathophysiology of illnesses and injuries is basically the same as in the previous curriculum.

_____ 9. Paramedics may function only under the direction of:
   A. the state EMS director.
   B. the system's medical director.
   C. the National Registry of EMTs.
   D. the emergency department charge nurse.

HANDOUT 1-2 Continued

_____ 10. A state or provincial agency typically provides a paramedic's:
   A. standing orders.
   B. medical control.
   C. license or registration.
   D. liability insurance.

CHAPTER 1 QUIZ

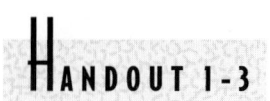

PART 2: EMS SYSTEMS

Write the letter of the best answer in the space provided.

_____ 1. One member of the in-hospital component of an EMS system is the:
  A. First Responder.
  B. EMT.
  C. paramedic.
  D. respiratory therapist.

_____ 2. A _____ emergency response system sends multiple levels of emergency care personnel to a single incident.
  A. basic
  B. public utility model
  C. tiered
  D. failsafe franchise

_____ 3. The _____ defined 10 elements necessary to all EMS systems.
  A. 1966 National Highway Safety Act
  B. 1973 Emergency Medical Services Systems Act
  C. 1981 Consolidated Omnibus Budget Reconciliation Act
  D. 1988 Statewide EMS Technical Assessment Program

_____ 4. State EMS agencies are responsible for all of the following EXCEPT:
  A. allocating funds to local systems.
  B. enforcing state EMS regulations.
  C. developing local quality assurance programs.
  D. certifying field providers.

_____ 5. The responsibility for all clinical and patient-care aspects of an EMS system rests with the:
  A. senior paramedic.
  B. system's medical director.
  C. EMS system director.
  D. quality assurance committee.

_____ 6. A well-designed communications plan for an EMS system should include:
  A. multiple control centers.
  B. operational communications capabilities.
  C. satellite uplinks.
  D. federally approved medical protocols.

_____ 7. The failsafe franchise represents an example of EMS:
  A. system financing.
  B. quality improvement.
  C. communications technology.
  D. research.

_____ 8. The evaluation of objective data such as response times, adherence to protocols, and patient survival is emphasized by:
  A. hospital categorization.
  B. QA programs.
  C. peer reviews.
  D. research programs.

_____ 9. An effective EMS dispatching system aims to place a BLS unit on the scene of an emergency in:
  A. the "golden hour."
  B. 14 minutes.
  C. 8 minutes.
  D. 4 minutes.

_____ 10. Training curricula for four levels of prehospital providers have been issued by the:
  A. American College of Emergency Physicians.
  B. American College of Surgeons Committee on Trauma.
  C. Department of Transportation.
  D. Department of Health, Education, and Welfare.

HANDOUT 1-3 Continued

_____ 11. The process by which a governmental agency grants permission to engage in a given occupation to an applicant who has attained the degree of competency required to ensure the public's protection is called:
   A. registration.
   B. licensure.
   C. certification.
   D. recognition.

_____ 12. In 1973, Congress passed an act that made EMS systems eligible for funding if they included 15 components. This act was called the:
   A. Ryan White Act.
   B. Emergency Medical Services System Act.
   C. National Highway Safety Act.
   D. Statewide EMS Technical Assessment Act.

_____ 13. One of the four Ts of emergency care is:
   A. trauma.
   B. triage.
   C. telemetry.
   D. tactical.

_____ 14. Guidelines for permitting a new medication, process, or procedure to be used in EMS are the:
   A. laws of medicine.
   B. rules of ethics.
   C. laws of research.
   D. rules of evidence.

_____ 15. Which is NOT an EMT-I skill?
   A. patient restraint
   B. advanced airway management
   C. advanced cardiac life support
   D. intravenous fluid therapy

CHAPTER 1 QUIZ

PART 3: ROLES AND RESPONSIBILITIES OF THE PARAMEDIC

Write the letter of the best answer in the space provided.

_____ 1. EMS has changed dramatically over the past 10 years. Today, paramedic emergency care emphasizes all of the following actions EXCEPT:
   A. providing competent emergency care.
   B. prescribing certain medications to patients who are not transported.
   C. providing emotional support to patients and their families.
   D. drawing on a strong knowledge of pathophysiology.

_____ 2. The paramedic's primary responsibilities include:
   A. community involvement.
   B. primary care.
   C. documentation.
   D. continuing education.

_____ 3. Identifying a patient's mechanism of injury is accomplished as part of which primary responsibility of a paramedic?
   A. patient assessment
   B. recognition of injury
   C. scene size-up
   D. appropriate disposition

_____ 4. The force or forces that cause(d) an injury are called the:
   A. kinematics of injury.
   B. chief complaint.
   C. nature of trauma.
   D. mechanism of injury.

_____ 5. The American College of Surgeons categorizes receiving facilities by the level of care they provide. A hospital that has surgery facilities available but no specialty physicians on site is classified as:
   A. Level I.
   B. Level II.
   C. Level III.
   D. Level IV.

_____ 6. A primary responsibility of the paramedic is returning to service after a call. Aspects of this include:
   A. reviewing the call with crew members.
   B. providing the ED staff a copy of your prehospital care report.
   C. turning the patient over to the hospital staff.
   D. calling your dispatch center for your run report times.

_____ 7. The term used to describe members of health care professions, apart from physicians and nurses, that includes paramedics, respiratory therapists, and laboratory technicians is:
   A. ancillary health professions.
   B. paramedical health professions.
   C. allied health professions.
   D. auxiliary health professions.

_____ 8. Leadership, integrity, and empathy are a few of the paramedic's professional:
   A. attitudes.
   B. attributes.
   C. duties.
   D. responsibilities.

_____ 9. Completing assigned duties without being asked or told is one example of the professional attribute of:
   A. self-confidence.
   B. time management skills.
   C. careful delivery of service.
   D. self-motivation.

HANDOUT 1-4 Continued

_____ 10. An example of the professional attribute of teamwork and diplomacy is:
   A. mastering and refreshing skills.
   B. being supportive and reassuring.
   C. placing the success of the team ahead of personal self-interest.
   D. accepting constructive feedback in a positive manner.

CHAPTER 1 QUIZ

PART 4: THE WELL-BEING OF THE PARAMEDIC

Write the letter of the best answer in the space provided.

_____ 1. An active exercise performed against stable resistance, in which muscles are exercised in a motionless manner, is called:
   A. isotonic.
   B. isometric.
   C. anaerobic.
   D. aerobic.

_____ 2. Exercising vigorously enough to raise your pulse to its target heart rate will increase:
   A. flexibility.
   B. muscle strength.
   C. cardiovascular endurance.
   D. respiratory endurance.

_____ 3. Which of the following is NOT one of the major food groups?
   A. grains/breads
   B. fruits
   C. dairy products
   D. carbohydrates

_____ 4. Foods from one food group contain vitamins A and C, potassium, and fiber. You should eat 2 to 4 servings a day of this food group, which is:
   A. vegetables.
   B. fruits.
   C. grains/breads.
   D. carbohydrates.

_____ 5. In general, you should avoid or minimize your intake of which of the following?
   A. complex carbohydrates
   B. oils
   C. caffeine
   D. protein

_____ 6. Your body needs plenty of fluids to flush food through your system and eliminate toxins. The drink that is more thirst quenching and better for you is:
   A. diet sodas.
   B. milk.
   C. coffee.
   D. water.

_____ 7. Which of the following is TRUE regarding back fitness?
   A. One of the best exercises for the back is the old-fashioned sit-up.
   B. While important for appearance, posture has little to do with the risk of back injury.
   C. Abdominal muscles are crucial to overall spinal-column strength and safe lifting.
   D. Smoking has not been shown to contribute to intervertebral disc deterioration.

_____ 8. Important principles of lifting include:
   A. positioning the load as far from your body as comfortably possible.
   B. keeping your palms down whenever possible.
   C. pulling rather than pushing, when given a choice.
   D. exhaling during the lift.

_____ 9. Microorganisms capable of producing disease, such as bacteria and viruses, are called:
   A. pathogens.
   B. infections.
   C. germs.
   D. microbes.

_____ 10. An example of a disease transmitted by airborne droplets is:
   A. hepatitis B.
   B. chicken pox.
   C. AIDS.
   D. staphylococcal skin infections.

_____ 11. Acquired Immune Deficiency Syndrome (AIDS) has an incubation period of:
   A. several months or years.
   B. 1 to 3 days.
   C. 2 to 6 weeks.
   D. 10 to 12 days.

HANDOUT 1-5 Continued

_____ 12. The time between contact with a disease organism and the appearance of the first symptoms is called the:
   A. contagious period.
   B. asymptomatic period.
   C. incubation period.
   D. developmental period.

_____ 13. Body substance isolation (BSI) is a strict form of infection control that:
   A. outlines procedures to use if you believe the patient may have an infectious disease.
   B. assumes that all blood and other body fluids are infectious.
   C. requires the use of protective gloves, mask, and gown for every patient contact.
   D. dictates minimal physical contact with a patient.

_____ 14. Equipment used by EMS personnel to protect against injury and the spread of infectious disease is called:
   A. biohazard protective equipment (BPE).
   B. infection protective equipment (IPE).
   C. patient protective equipment (PPE)
   D. personal protective equipment (PPE)

_____ 15. In cases where you suspect your patient is infected with tuberculosis, use a(n):
   A. HEPA respirator.
   B. plastic respirator.
   C. cotton mask.
   D. surgical mask.

_____ 16. A situation that would usually call for the use of a gown as protection would be:
   A. any patient contact.
   B. childbirth.
   C. venous bleeding.
   D. tuberculosis.

_____ 17. HIV/AIDS, hepatitis B, and tuberculosis are diseases of great concern because they are:
   A. contagious.
   B. untreatable.
   C. transmitted by airborne pathogens.
   D. life-threatening.

_____ 18. The most important infection-control practice is:
   A. wearing protective gloves when in contact with every patient.
   B. placing a mask on both yourself and the patient.
   C. proper handwashing.
   D. being up-to-date on all vaccinations and immunizations.

_____ 19. Contaminated wastes such as bloody dressings and bandages should be disposed of:
   A. only at the hospital emergency department.
   B. in a red bag with a biohazard seal.
   C. in a cardboard box and sealed with tape.
   D. in any normal garbage container.

_____ 20. In most areas, an EMS provider who has had an exposure should do all of the following EXCEPT:
   A. immediately wash the infected area with a disinfecting agent.
   B. get a medical evaluation.
   C. take the proper immunization boosters.
   D. notify the agency's infection-control liaison.

_____ 21. The use of a chemical or a physical method to kill all microorganisms on an object is called:
   A. cleaning.
   B. washing.
   C. disinfecting.
   D. sterilizing.

_____ 22. According to Elisabeth Kübler-Ross, there are five predictable stages of loss. They include:
   A. denial.
   B. elation.
   C. fear.
   D. confusion.

HANDOUT 1-5 Continued

_____ 23. The dying patient who is sad, mourning things not accomplished and dreams that will not come true, is in which stage of loss?
   A. denial
   B. anger
   C. depression
   D. acceptance

_____ 24. How people of different ages cope with death varies. When dealing with children from age 3 to 6 years, you should:
   A. encourage sharing of memories to facilitate the grief response.
   B. encourage the child to talk about and/or draw pictures of his feelings.
   C. locate a support group for the child.
   D. see if a trusted friend can provide appropriate support.

_____ 25. When telling a survivor that a loved one has died, your message should include the:
   A. use of encouraging statements, such as the person is "no longer in pain."
   B. use of terms such as *passed on* instead of the harsh word *dead*.
   C. statement that it was "God's will" (if the survivor is religious).
   D. statement that "There was nothing more anyone could have done."

_____ 26. Though stress is usually understood to be harmful, some stress is beneficial. It is called:
   A. positive stress.
   B. antistress.
   C. eustress.
   D. distress.

_____ 27. As a person adapts to stress, he or she develops:
   A. defensive strategies.
   B. resistance.
   C. illusions.
   D. desensitization.

_____ 28. To manage stress, you must:
   A. learn to become detached.
   B. think of patients only as signs and symptoms, not as people.
   C. know the amount of stress you can take before it becomes a problem.
   D. immerse yourself in work.

_____ 29. The three phases of a stress response include:
   A. excitement.
   B. exhaustion.
   C. fear.
   D. desensitization.

_____ 30. The physiological phenomena that occur over intervals of approximately 24 hours are:
   A. anchor time events.
   B. second-wind responses.
   C. hormonal rhythms.
   D. circadian rhythms.

_____ 31. In situations where your stress response threatens your ability to handle the moment, you should:
   A. concentrate on the medical needs of the patient.
   B. "retreat" and get away from the stressor.
   C. take medication to help you temporarily deal with the situation.
   D. increase your breathing rate and the amount of oxygen in your system.

_____ 32. All of the following are clearly defined types of EMS stress EXCEPT:
   A. small incident.
   B. cumulative.
   C. daily.
   D. large incident or disaster.

_____ 33. Psychological first aid includes:
   A. assessing needs.
   B. conveying compassion.
   C. not forcing personnel to talk.
   D. all of these

_____ 34. An emotional warning sign of excessive stress is:
   A. fatigue.
   B. difficulty in making decisions.
   C. withdrawal.
   D. depression.

HANDOUT 1-5 Continued

_____ **35.** Because one of the greatest hazards in EMS is motor vehicles, you should learn:
    A. basic engine repair.
    B. how to safely approach a vehicle in which someone is slumped over the wheel.
    C. high-speed pursuit driving.
    D. to closely follow escort vehicles, such as police cars.

CHAPTER 1 QUIZ

PART 5: ILLNESS AND INJURY PREVENTION

Write the letter of the best answer in the space provided.

_____ 1. _____ recently surpassed stroke as the third leading cause of death in the United States.
   A. AIDS
   B. Alzheimer's disease
   C. Injuries
   D. Hepatitis B

_____ 2. _____ are among the leading causes of death from unintentional injuries.
   A. Firearms
   B. Environnemental exposures
   C. Industrial machinery
   D. Falls

_____ 3. Years of productive life is calculated based on the age of death being:
   A. 60.
   B. 65.
   C. 70.
   D. 75.

_____ 4. For every one death caused by injury, there are _____ emergency department visits.
   A. 254
   B. 358
   C. 419
   D. 523

_____ 5. Instead of motor-vehicle "accident," we now use the term motor vehicle:
   A. incident.
   B. collision.
   C. mishap.
   D. casualty.

_____ 6. The study of factors that influence the frequency, distribution, and causes of injury, disease, and other health-related events in a population is:
   A. anthropology.
   B. sociology.
   C. epidemiology.
   D. pathology.

_____ 7. Keeping an injury from occurring is _____ prevention.
   A. primary
   B. secondary
   C. tertiary
   D. initial

_____ 8. EMS organizational commitment is vital to the development of any prevention activities. Organizational commitment includes:
   A. body substance isolation precautions.
   B. safe driving.
   C. data collection.
   D. stress management.

_____ 9. The first priority of EMS providers is to:
   A. care for the patient.
   B. protect themselves from harm.
   C. provide public education.
   D. fulfill their obligation to their employer.

_____ 10. The most frequent cause of injury to children younger than 6 years old is:
   A. firearms.
   B. vehicle/bicycle collisions.
   C. physical abuse.
   D. falls.

_____ 11. _____ are responsible for over half of all deaths from unintentional injuries.
   A. Motor vehicle collisions
   B. Firearms
   C. Falls
   D. Burns

HANDOUT 1-6 Continued

_____ 12. About half of all motor-vehicle fatalities involve:
   A. pedestrians.
   B. elderly patients.
   C. alcohol.
   D. drivers falling asleep.

_____ 13. Twenty-two percent of all disabling injuries in the workplace are to the patient's:
   A. back.
   B. hips.
   C. legs.
   D. arms.

_____ 14. The largest number of preventable injuries for persons over 75 years of age are:
   A. motor vehicle collisions.
   B. firearms related.
   C. burns.
   D. falls.

_____ 15. Patient documentation forms should include _____, which is (are) the best on-scene determinant of patient care
   A. statements from bystanders
   B. patient health insurance verifications
   C. mechanisms of injury
   D. patients' consents

CHAPTER 1 QUIZ

PART 6: ETHICS IN ADVANCED PREHOSPITAL CARE

Write the letter of the best answer in the space provided.

_____ 1. The rules or standards that govern the conduct of members of a particular group or profession are known as:
   A. guidelines.
   B. morals.
   C. ethics.
   D. laws.

_____ 2. Social, religious, or personal standards of right and wrong are:
   A. ethics.
   B. morals.
   C. mores.
   D. beliefs.

_____ 3. Allowing a person to decide how to behave and accepting whatever decision that person makes is called:
   A. consequentialism.
   B. the deontological method.
   C. ethical relativism.
   D. the nonmaleficence method.

_____ 4. Utilitarians who believe that the purpose of an action should be to bring the greatest happiness to the greatest number of people believe in:
   A. consequentialism.
   B. the deontological method.
   C. ethical relativism.
   D. the nonmaleficence method.

_____ 5. The single most important question a paramedic has to answer when faced with an ethical challenge is:
   A. "What are my protocols?"
   B. "What are the patient's family's wishes?"
   C. "What is in the patient's best interest?"
   D. "Does the patient have a valid DNR?"

_____ 6. The principle of doing good for the patient is:
   A. autonomy.
   B. justice.
   C. beneficence.
   D. nonmaleficence.

_____ 7. The obligation to treat all patients fairly is:
   A. autonomy.
   B. justice.
   C. beneficence.
   D. nonmaleficence.

_____ 8. A competent adult patient's right to determine what happens to his own body is:
   A. autonomy.
   B. justice.
   C. beneficence.
   D. nonmaleficence.

_____ 9. The Latin phrase *primum non nocere*, or "First, do no harm," sums up the principle of:
   A. autonomy.
   B. justice.
   C. beneficence.
   D. nonmaleficence.

_____ 10. One of the three basic steps in solving an ethical problem is:
   A. stating the action in a situation-specific form.
   B. listing the implications or consequences of the action.
   C. comparing implications or consequences to current protocols.
   D. applying the impartiality test.

HANDOUT 1-7 Continued

_____ 11. Asking whether you can justify or defend your actions to others is called the:
   A. interpersonal justifiability test.
   B. universalizability test.
   C. autonomizability test.
   D. relevantability test.

_____ 12. A general principle for paramedics to follow regarding advance directives is:
   A. always follow the family's wishes.
   B. accept verbal DNR orders from other health care providers.
   C. when in doubt, resuscitate.
   D. do not accept any DNR order under any circumstance in the prehospital setting.

_____ 13. A competent patient of legal age has the right to decide what health care he or she does not wish to receive. To exercise this right, a patient must have:
   A. an attorney present to witness the patient's decision.
   B. an advance directive document physically with him or her.
   C. the mental faculties to weigh the risks and benefits.
   D. a consultation with his personal physician.

_____ 14. An ethical issue raised by the role of a paramedic as a preceptor is whether:
   A. the paramedic may function in the hospital setting.
   B. patients should be informed that a student is caring for them.
   C. the paramedic can allow the student to perform advanced skills under his supervision.
   D. the paramedic should allow the student to drive the EMS vehicle.

_____ 15. One of the three most common sources of conflict between physicians and paramedics is a situation in which:
   A. the physician refuses to allow the paramedic to perform a procedure.
   B. the physician orders something that the paramedic believes is medically acceptable but morally wrong.
   C. the physician allows the paramedic to perform a procedure that is detrimental to the patient.
   D. the physician requires the paramedic to obtain on-line direction for all advanced procedures.

HANDOUT 1-8

Student's Name _____

CHAPTER 1 SCENARIO

PART 1: INTRODUCTION TO ADVANCED PREHOSPITAL CARE

Review the following real-life situation. Then follow the directions at the end of the scenario.

You and your EMT-Basic partner are assigned to Medic-5 one morning. At 10:40 you are dispatched to a motor vehicle crash on Clear Creek Road. A bystander has called 911 on his cell phone to report that a car ahead of him has swerved off the road, plunged into a ditch, and hit a tree. The crash has occurred in a rural portion of the county some distance from your quarters, so you have an extended response time. A local First Responder team has also been dispatched, with an ETA of 10 minutes.

Your unit arrives some 20 minutes after being dispatched, and you find the First Responder team already on scene. One of the First Responders is holding manual C-spine stabilization on a male in his 30s lying on the ground next to the crushed vehicle. Other First Responders are readying a cervical collar and oxygen. As you approach the patient, you can easily see that his shirt and pants are soaked with blood. Another First Responder is applying direct pressure to the patient's right upper leg.

The lead First Responder has completed the initial assessment and tells you that the patient is conscious, alert, and breathing; he has bruising to the chest and a large open wound, possibly a fracture, to the right thigh. He apparently got out of the vehicle on his own and collapsed due to the leg injury before responders arrived. You advise the First Responders to apply the cervical collar and high concentration oxygen. You examine the patient's chest and note the bruising as well as some breathing difficulty. As you quickly examine the leg wound, you note an open femur fracture. The patient appears to have lost a large amount of blood. Your assessment shows he has a rapid and thready pulse, an increased respiratory rate, and cool, moist skin.

Based on your initial assessment, you have your partner radio for a helicopter response to the scene for transport to the area trauma center. You continue your patient assessment and find no other serious injuries. While waiting for the helicopter, you and your partner apply the cardiac monitor, noting no abnormalities, and assist the First Responders in applying a traction splint to the injured leg and immobilizing the patient on a long spine board. You contact medical control at the trauma center and have time to start two large-bore IVs before the helicopter arrives.

A deputy sheriff who is also on scene assists in setting up a landing zone, and the helicopter arrives. The helicopter crew's critical care paramedic quickly reassesses the patient. The patient is loaded into the helicopter within 5 minutes of its landing. He is taken to St. Luke's Medical Center, the designated trauma facility for the area.

1. Describe the characteristics displayed by the paramedic at the scene.

2. What aspects of patient care exhibited during this call might not have been available 30 years ago?

HANDOUT 1-9

Student's Name _____

CHAPTER 1 SCENARIO

PART 2: EMS SYSTEMS

Review the following real-life situation. Then answer the questions that follow.

A call comes in to the 911 dispatch center from Damon, a resident on Hohman Avenue, who reports that a motor vehicle collision involving a car with two elderly occupants has just taken place. The dispatcher sends police, fire department, and EMS vehicles to the scene.

Damon, who phoned in the call and is also a local volunteer firefighter and First Responder, runs out to see if he can help. He finds that the car has run head-on into a large tree. In the car, a woman in the passenger seat is holding a man who is slumped into her lap. Damon determines that the scene is safe and moves to check the woman. As he does, she tells him that her husband, who is a diabetic, appeared to have a seizure while they were driving that caused him to lose control of the car and hit the tree.

As Damon is checking the woman, a fire truck arrives. Another firefighter/First Responder helps maintain stabilization of the woman's head while Damon checks her husband. He is breathing but still unconscious, and his legs appear to be wedged in place by crumpled metal. Meanwhile, the police and EMS units have arrived. The police officer directs traffic around the accident scene while the EMS crew assumes control of the patients and, with the aid of the firefighters, begins the process of removing the victims from the car. The senior paramedic, having had a chance to study the scene, now radios dispatch requesting a second ambulance.

The response team members remove the woman fairly easily. The EMTs immobilize her, treat a gash on her head, and transport her to the hospital in the first EMS unit. Extricating her husband takes longer. EMS personnel remain with him in the vehicle, stabilizing him and protecting him from debris. Once the team has freed the patient's legs, they immobilize him and remove him from the car. ALS procedures are initiated and he is transported rapidly to the hospital in the second ambulance, which has arrived during the extrication process.

The emergency department has already been alerted to the collision by the dispatcher, and crews of both ambulances give radio reports as they begin transporting the patients. Thus, the ED physicians and nurses are prepared to treat both patients on their arrival.

1. What components of the EMS system were involved in this scenario?

2. What are the dispatcher's primary roles?

3. What responsibilities did Damon, the First Responder, assume?

4. Why is teamwork so important to the functioning of the EMS system in this scenario?

HANDOUT 1-10 Student's Name _____

CHAPTER 1 SCENARIO

PART 3: ROLES AND RESPONSIBILITIES OF THE PARAMEDIC

Review the following real-life situation. Then answer the questions that follow.

Medic 3 from the Springfield substation has been dispatched to assist an elderly woman who has fallen down a flight of stairs. While checking in on her, a neighbor found her and called 911. The crew had just finished cleaning and restocking the ambulance after a run when they received the dispatch.

Medic 3 reaches the patient's house about 6 minutes after receiving the call. A quick scene size-up assures the crew that the scene is safe. The neighbor lets them into the house and leads them to the patient. As she does, she tells them that the woman, Mrs. Gombert, apparently tripped sometime yesterday, fell down the stairs, hurt her leg, and has been unable to move since then.

The crew finds Mrs. Gombert lying at the foot of the stairs. They note that she is highly anxious and somewhat confused. The neighbor states that Mrs. Gombert often appears confused and fears that she is growing senile.

The senior paramedic, Jo, takes charge of the call. She directs the other members of the crew as they carefully provide spinal immobilization, perform an initial assessment and physical exam, immobilize Mrs. Gombert's right hip and leg, and carefully move her to a long spine board. Following protocol, the crew administers oxygen, starts an IV, attaches and monitors an ECG machine, and prepares the patient for transport. While doing these tasks, the crew speaks gently to Mrs. Gombert, telling her what they are doing and seeking to calm and reassure her.

En route to the hospital, Jo radios a report of Mrs. Gombert's condition and the expected time of arrival to the emergency department. Despite an apparent fractured hip and dehydration, reassessment indicates that the patient is stable, and she is transported without incident. Upon arrival at the hospital, Jo turns Mrs. Gombert over to the ED personnel with an oral update on her condition. Jo prepares a written run report describing the circumstances under which the patient was found, a brief history related by the patient and the neighbor, vital signs taken at the scene and during transport, and care given by the EMS crew. As Jo writes the report, the other crew members once again clean and restock the ambulance. When all personnel are through with their tasks, Jo informs the dispatcher that Medic 3 is back in service and ready for another call.

1. How does this scenario illustrate the overall purpose of paramedic emergency care?

2. What primary responsibilities of the paramedic are demonstrated in this scenario?

Handout 1-11

Student's Name _____

CHAPTER 1 SCENARIO

PART 4: THE WELL-BEING OF THE PARAMEDIC

Review the following real-life situation. Then answer the questions that follow.

Lately you have noticed that your partner seems to have changed. He used to get to work at least a half hour before your shift started; now he's just barely on time. Wearing his uniform, he used to look like an ad in a catalog; now it just barely meets the standards of your service. He used to be easy-going and consistently good-natured; now everything and everyone seems to make him angry.

Today presented a good example of the changes you've observed. This morning at change of shift, you were told that a mandatory training session for a new piece of equipment had been scheduled for your next day off. He's been grousing about the training session and the "damn administration who think they own us every minute of every day." The irony is that he had been on the committee that had recommended the purchase of the equipment. Then about mid-morning, when you transported Mrs. Jonas (one of your "regulars") for her radiation treatment, he was very short-tempered and rude to her. You were particularly surprised by that, because he had told you once that she reminded him of his grandmother. You've also heard rumors that he's having some troubles at home, but he's said nothing about them to you.

1. What do you think is going on with your partner?

2. What should you do?

HANDOUT 1-12

Student's Name _____

CHAPTER 1 SCENARIO

PART 5: ILLNESS AND INJURY PREVENTION

Review the following real-life situation. Then answer the questions that follow.

You have a well-deserved day off and are taking advantage of it by driving to a nearby resort town for some fishing. It's a weekday and traffic is light on the county road with a speed limit of 45 mph. Suddenly, about a quarter-mile ahead, a 1972 Pontiac traveling in the opposite direction weaves, then crosses into opposing traffic. Predictably, the car crashes nearly head-on into another car on your side of the road.

You quickly use your cell phone to call for emergency assistance as you pull up to the scene. You park your vehicle safely on the side of the road, then proceed with a quick scene assessment. You decide the scene is safe to approach, so you begin assessing the patients. One adult male was in the car that crossed the median, and two adults and two children are in the other car. The driver of the first car was not restrained by a seat belt and so was thrown from the vehicle. You note several empty beer cans in the car. The driver is lying on the ground, approximately 15 feet from the crash site. Your initial assessment shows him to be pulseless and apneic. His neck is angulated.

The adults in the second vehicle were wearing seat belts, both airbags deployed, and the young children in the back seat are in car seats. The children are frightened and crying but appear uninjured. Both adults are conscious and breathing, talking, and appear stable. The local fire department and volunteer ambulance arrives within a few minutes and takes over assessment and treatment of the patients. You give the lead EMT a report of your assessment. The lead EMT calls for a second ambulance. Law enforcement arrives shortly, and you give your report to the officer, also.

When you go back to work the next day, a message from the lead EMT of the ambulance service is waiting for you. You return his call and receive an update on the incident. The first driver was dead at the scene. An autopsy revealed a blood-alcohol level of .18, over twice the legal limit. The family in the other car was doing well and had only received some minor abrasions and contusions. They all spent one night in the hospital for observation, but were released the next morning.

1. In what areas of this scenario would injury prevention programs have been useful?

2. What "teachable moments" exist in this scenario?

HANDOUT 1-13

Student's Name _____

CHAPTER 1 SCENARIO

PART 6: ETHICS IN ADVANCED PREHOSPITAL CARE

Review the following real-life situation. Then answer the questions that follow.

At 2 A.M., Medic 6 is dispatched to assist EMT-Basics on the scene of an attempted suicide. On arrival they find the scene in the kitchen under control, with one EMT getting a history of the patient, a 24-year-old female, from her distraught husband. The other EMT is rechecking blood pressure, which is only 78 palpated, down from 84/60. The patient's cut wrists are bandaged, and the EMTs, who have been there less than 5 minutes, are preparing to apply a PASG. Meanwhile, the husband states that he woke up and found his wife unconscious on the kitchen floor with blood everywhere. He explains that she has been troubled over a recent miscarriage. While setting up the IV and preparing to intubate per protocols, the paramedics quickly explain the need for these treatments to the husband, who nods affirmatively while watching.

As the paramedics prepare to transport, the husband tells them that he wants his wife to go to Doctor's Hospital, where her physician has privileges. The medics explain that, per protocol, she must go to County Hospital because it is the closest hospital with a psychiatric ward and works with the county health department on social service and mental health referrals. The husband continues to insist on transport to Doctor's Hospital and refuses to allow further treatment until the paramedics agree. The paramedics finally agree and transport the patient to Doctor's Hospital, where her physical wounds are treated and she is released.

Three days later, the paramedic crew learns that another duty crew later transported the same woman to County Hospital, suffering from a sedative overdose. The husband was at work and the call came in from a neighbor. These medics started an IV per protocol and gave naloxone per medical direction, but the woman was pronounced dead after 40 minutes of resuscitation efforts at the hospital.

1. Discuss how this scenario illustrates the conflict of implied consent versus the wishes of the husband.

2. How could the paramedics have resolved this ethical dilemma in the patient's best interest?

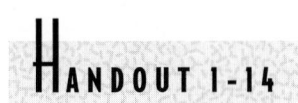

CHAPTER 1 REVIEW

PART 1: INTRODUCTION TO ADVANCED PREHOSPITAL CARE

Write the word or words that best complete each sentence in the space provided.

1. The paramedic is the _____ level of prehospital care.
2. The ability to make _____ judgments in a(n) _____ manner can mean the difference between life and death for the patient.
3. Paramedics may only function under the direction and license of the EMS system's _____ _____.
4. Licensing or credentialing is typically provided by a(n) _____ or _____ agency.
5. As a paramedic, you must realize that you are an essential component in the _____ of care.
6. Emerging roles and responsibilities of the paramedic include public _____, health _____, and participation in injury and illness _____, _____.
7. If you always act in the best interest of the _____, you will seldom have problems.
8. Paramedic students should be competent in _____, _____, and _____ before training begins.
9. The 1998 EMT-Paramedic: National Standard Curriculum provides for a much improved understanding of the _____ of various illnesses and injury processes.
10. Professional development should be a _____, _____ pursuit.

HANDOUT 1-15 Student's Name _____

PART 1: INTRODUCTION TO ADVANCED PREHOSPITAL CARE

EMT CODE OF ETHICS

Professional status as an Emergency Medical Technician-Paramedic is maintained and enriched by the willingness of the individual practitioner to accept and fulfill obligations to society, other medical professionals, and the profession of Emergency Medical Technician. As an Emergency Medical Technician at the basic level or an Emergency Medical Technician-Paramedic, I solemnly pledge myself to the following code of professional ethics.

A fundamental responsibility to the Emergency Medical Technician is to conserve life, to alleviate suffering, to promote health, to do no harm, and to encourage the quality and equal availability of emergency medical care.

The Emergency Medical Technician provides services based on human need, with respect for human dignity, unrestricted by consideration of nationality, race, creed, color, or status.

The Emergency Medical Technician does not use professional knowledge and skills in any enterprise detrimental to the public well-being.

The Emergency Medical Technician respects and holds in confidence all information of a confidential nature obtained in the course of professional work unless required by law to divulge such information.

The Emergency Medical Technician, as a citizen, understands and upholds the law and performs the duties of citizenship; as a professional, the Emergency Medical Technician has the never-ending responsibility to work with concerned citizens and other health care professionals in promoting a high standard of emergency medical care to all people.

The Emergency Medical Technician shall maintain professional competence and demonstrate concern for the competence of other members of the Emergency Medical Services health care team.

The Emergency Medical Technician assumes responsibility in defining and upholding standards of professional practice and education.

The Emergency Medical Technician assumes responsibility for individual professional actions and judgment, both in dependent and independent emergency functions, and knows and upholds the laws that affect the practice of the Emergency Medical Technician.

The Emergency Medical Technician has the responsibility to be aware of and participate in matters of legislation affecting the Emergency Medical Technician and the Emergency Medical Services System.

The Emergency Medical Technician adheres to standards of personal ethics that reflect credit upon the profession.

Emergency Medical Technicians, or groups of Emergency Medical Technicians, who advertise professional services, do so in conformity with the dignity of the profession.

The Emergency Medical Technician has an obligation to protect the public by not delegating to a person less qualified, any service that requires the professional competence of an Emergency Medical Technician.

The Emergency Medical Technician will work harmoniously with and sustain confidence in Emergency Medical Technician associates, the nurse, the physician, and other members of the Emergency Medical Services health care team.

HANDOUT 1-15 Continued

The Emergency Medical Technician refuses to participate in unethical procedures, and assumes the responsibility to expose incompetence or unethical conduct of others to the appropriate authority in a proper and professional manner.

The National Association of Emergency Medical Technicians

HANDOUT 1-16 Student's Name _____

PART 1: INTRODUCTION TO ADVANCED PREHOSPITAL CARE

OATH OF GENEVA

I solemnly pledge myself to consecrate my life to the service of humanity; I will give to my teachers the respect and gratitude which is their due; I will practice my profession with conscience and dignity; the health of my patient will be my first consideration; I will respect the secrets which are confided in me; I will maintain by all the means in my power the honor and noble traditions of the medical profession; my colleagues will be my brothers; I will not permit considerations of religion, nationality, race, party, politics, or social standing to intervene between my duty and my patient; I will maintain the utmost respect for human life from the time of conception; even under threat, I will not make use of my medical knowledge contrary to the laws of humanity. I make these promises solemnly, freely, and upon my honor.

The EMT Oath

Be it pledged as an Emergency Medical Technician, I will honor the physical and judicial laws of God and man. I will follow that regimen which, according to my ability and judgment, I consider for the benefit of patients and abstain from whatever is deleterious and mischievous, nor shall I suggest any such counsel. Into whatever homes I enter, I will go into them for the benefit of only the sick and injured, never revealing what I see or hear in the lives of men unless required by law.

I shall also share my medical knowledge with those who may benefit from what I have learned. I will serve unselfishly and continuously in order to help make a better world for mankind.

While I continue to keep this oath unviolated, may it be granted to me to enjoy life and the practice of the art, respected by all men, in all times. Should I trespass or violate this oath, may the reverse be my lot. So help me God.

Adopted by the National Association of Emergency Medical Technicians, 1978

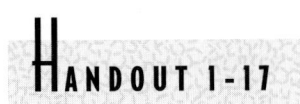

CHAPTER 1 REVIEW

PART 2: EMS SYSTEMS

Write the word or words that best complete each sentence in the space provided.

1. In the eighteenth century, Jean Larrey developed a method of sorting patients by severity of their injuries that is called _____.

2. In 1966, Congress passed the National _____ _____ _____, which established the U.S. Department of Transportation.

3. Medical policies, procedures, and practices that are available to providers either on-line or off-line are called _____ _____.

4. An evaluation program that emphasizes service and uses customer satisfaction as the ultimate indicator of system performance is called _____ _____ _____.

5. The Statewide _____ _____ _____ Program defined 10 elements necessary to all EMS systems.

6. The _____ _____ is the physician who is legally responsible for all of the clinical and patient-care aspects of an EMS system.

7. _____ medical direction occurs when a qualified physician gives direct orders to a prehospital care provider by either radio or telephone.

8. _____ medical direction refers to medical policies, procedures, and practices that medical direction has established in advance of the call.

9. A licensed physician who attempts to assist EMS providers with patient care at a scene is called a(n) _____ _____.

10. The four Ts of Emergency Care are _____, _____, _____, and _____.

11. The EMS person responsible for assignment of emergency medical resources to a medical emergency is the _____ _____ _____.

12. A job or trade that involves mastery of a specialized body of knowledge or skills is a(n) _____.

13. The process by which an agency or association grants recognition to an individual who has met its qualifications is _____.

14. The process by which a governmental agency grants permission to engage in a given occupation to an applicant who has attained the degree of competency required to ensure the public's protection is _____.

15. The process of entering your name and essential information within a particular record is called _____.

16. The four nationally recognized curricula for EMS providers are _____, _____, _____, and _____.

17. Paramedics accompanying specially trained law enforcement officers on operations such as hostage rescues and drug raids are practicing in the expanded role of _____ _____.

18. The General Services Administration developed standards for three types of ambulance vehicle design. A conventional cab and chassis on which a module ambulance body is mounted, with no passageway between the driver's and patient compartments, is called a Type _____.

HANDOUT 1-17 Continued

19. The conduct and qualities that characterize a practitioner in a particular field or occupation are called _____.

20. The rules or standards that govern the conduct of members of a particular group or profession are called _____.

Handout 1-18

Student's Name _____

PART 2: EMS SYSTEMS

EMS TRUE OR FALSE

Indicate if the following statements are true or false by writing T or F in the space provided.

_____ 1. The First Responder's role is to stabilize the patient until the EMT or paramedic arrives.

_____ 2. Most EMS systems today receive the largest part of their operating expenses directly from the federal government.

_____ 3. The 15 components of an EMS system were laid out in the "White Paper" of 1966.

_____ 4. The director or manager of an EMS system is legally responsible for all of the clinical and patient-care aspects of the system.

_____ 5. Medical direction communications may be delegated to a mobile intensive care nurse or a physician assistant.

_____ 6. If an intervener physician is present at an emergency scene and direct medical control does exist, the on-line physician has ultimate responsibility.

_____ 7. The four Ts of emergency medical care are triage, treatment, transport, and transfer.

_____ 8. Standing orders take precedence over on-line communications.

_____ 9. In priority dispatching, medical dispatchers interrogate callers, prioritize symptoms, select appropriate responses, and give prearrival instructions.

_____ 10. The goal of emergency response is for BLS care to arrive in less than 4 minutes and ALS care to arrive in less than 8 minutes.

_____ 11. Ambulances that display the "Star of Life" symbol must meet the standards set by the NAEMT.

_____ 12. The U.S. Department of Transportation has developed curricula for four levels of prehospital care providers.

_____ 13. EMT-Intermediates should successfully complete an ACLS and PALS course.

_____ 14. Ethics refers to the moral conduct or qualities that characterize a practitioner in a particular field or occupation.

_____ 15. "Failsafe franchise" refers to an advanced form of EMS communications.

Handout 1-19

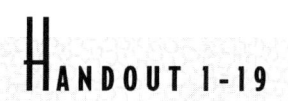

Student's Name _____

CHAPTER 1 REVIEW

PART 3: ROLES AND RESPONSIBILITIES OF THE PARAMEDIC

Write the word or words that best complete each sentence in the space provided.

1. The primary responsibility of the paramedic that includes familiarity with all local EMS protocols, policies, and procedures is _____.
2. During an emergency response, _____ _____ is a paramedic's number-one priority.
3. The force or forces that cause(d) an injury are called the _____ _____ _____.
4. A patient's general medical condition or complaint is called the _____ _____ _____.
5. Potential hazards at an emergency scene are assessed during the _____ _____.
6. You should look for and immediately treat life-threatening conditions during the _____ _____.
7. Most commonly, patient priority is based on the _____ _____ _____.
8. Proper record keeping helps to ensure _____ _____ _____ _____ _____ from the emergency scene to the hospital setting.
9. The highest level of trauma care is delivered at a Level _____ facility.
10. Basic health care provided at the patient's first contact with the health care system is called _____ _____.
11. Additional responsibilities of the paramedic may include teaching CPR to the public or other demonstrations. These are aspects of _____ _____.
12. The term used to describe the ancillary health care professions, apart from physicians and nurses, is _____ _____ _____.
13. Self-confidence, establishing credibility, and inner strength are characteristics of _____.
14. The paramedic should always be a(n) _____ for the patient, acting in his or her best interests.
15. The best paramedics are those who make a commitment to _____.

HANDOUT 1-20

Student's Name _____

PART 3: ROLES AND RESPONSIBILITIES OF THE PARAMEDIC

ROLES AND RESPONSIBILITIES LISTING

Complete each of the following lists.

1. List the eight primary responsibilities of a paramedic.

   _____   _____
   _____   _____
   _____   _____
   _____   _____

2. List four additional responsibilities of a paramedic.

   _____
   _____
   _____
   _____

3. List the 12 professional attributes of a paramedic.

   _____
   _____
   _____
   _____
   _____
   _____
   _____
   _____
   _____
   _____
   _____
   _____

4. List four ways in which a paramedic can show empathy with a patient.

   _____
   _____
   _____
   _____

Handout 1-21

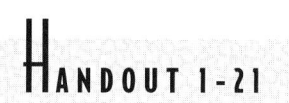

Student's Name _____

CHAPTER 1 REVIEW

PART 4: THE WELL-BEING OF THE PARAMEDIC

Write the word or words that best complete each sentence in the space provided.

1. Core elements of physical fitness are _____ _____, _____ _____, and _____.

2. Active exercise performed against stable resistance, where muscles are exercised in a motionless manner, is called _____ exercise.

3. Active exercise during which muscles are worked through their range of motion is called _____ exercise.

4. The five major food groups are _____, _____, _____, _____, and _____.

5. For a healthy diet you should avoid or minimize intake of _____, _____, _____, _____, and _____.

6. If given a choice when lifting, _____, do not _____.

7. Always avoid _____ and _____ when lifting.

8. Any disease caused by the growth of microorganisms, which may spread from person to person, is called a(n) _____ _____.

9. Microorganisms capable of producing disease, such as bacteria and viruses, are called _____.

10. While hepatitis B is a(n) _____ borne disease, tuberculosis is a(n) _____ borne disease.

11. The time between contact with a disease organism and the appearance of the first symptoms is called the _____ period.

12. A strict form of infection control that is based on the assumption that all blood and other body fluids are infectious is _____ _____ _____.

13. Equipment used by EMS personnel to protect against injury and the spread of infectious disease is called _____ _____ _____.

14. In addition to protective gloves, the paramedic should wear a _____ and _____ _____ whenever blood spatter is likely to occur, as with arterial bleeding or oral suctioning.

15. Whenever caring for a patient with tuberculosis, you should wear a _____ _____ _____ _____ respirator.

16. Perhaps the most important infection-control practice is _____.

17. Washing an object with cleaners such as soap and water is called _____.

18. Cleaning with an agent that can kill some microorganisms on the surface of an object is called _____.

19. The use of a chemical or physical method such as pressurized steam to kill all microorganisms on an object is called _____.

20. Any occurrence of blood or body fluids coming in contact with nonintact skin, mucous membranes, or delivered by parenteral contact is called a(n) _____.

HANDOUT 1-21 Continued

21. There are five predictable stages of loss. The inability to believe the reality of the event is called the _____ stage.

22. The patient is in the _____ stage of loss when he mourns things not accomplished and dreams that will not come true.

23. Generally, children ranging in age from _____ to _____ believe death is a temporary state, and may ask continually when the dead person will return.

24. When a patient of yours has died, a basic element of your message to survivors should include a statement that the loved one has _____.

25. Adaptation to stress involves the development of _____ strategies, _____, and _____ skills.

26. Your job in managing stress is to learn your personal _____.

27. The three phases of a stress response are: Stage I, or _____; Stage II, or _____; and Stage III, or _____.

28. Physiological phenomena that occur at approximately 24-hour intervals are _____ _____.

29. A set of hours when a night-shift worker can reliably expect to rest without interruption is called _____ _____.

30. _____ occurs when coping mechanisms no longer buffer job stressors.

31. Warning signs of excessive stress fall into four categories. These categories include _____, _____, _____, and _____.

32. For long-term well-being, the best stress-management technique is to take care of _____.

33. _____ _____ _____ can provide the information and education needed for rescuers to understand trauma, what to expect, and where to get help if needed.

34. Mental health professionals should be available during the 2 months following a critical incident to screen and assist anyone who may be developing _____ _____ _____.

35. Principles of roadway safety include evaluating the safest _____ _____ when arriving at a roadway incident.

Handout 1-22

Student's Name _____

PART 4: THE WELL-BEING OF THE PARAMEDIC

WELL-BEING BASICS LISTING

Complete the following lists.

1. List the five basics of physical fitness.

   _____
   _____
   _____
   _____
   _____

2. List the five major food groups.

   _____
   _____

3. List the five minimum pieces of recommended PPE.

   _____
   _____
   _____
   _____
   _____

4. List at least five warning signs of excessive stress.

   _____
   _____
   _____
   _____
   _____

5. List the five stages of loss, as defined by Elisabeth Kübler-Ross.

   _____
   _____

HANDOUT 1-22 Continued

6. List at least five types of calls that have a higher-than-normal potential for causing stress in EMS personnel.

   _____

   _____

   _____

   _____

   _____

Handout 1-23

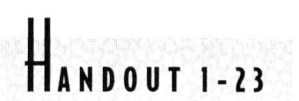

Student's Name _____

CHAPTER 1 REVIEW

PART 5: ILLNESS AND INJURY PREVENTION

Write the word or words that best complete each sentence in the space provided.

1. _____ is the study of factors that influence the frequency, distribution, and causes of injury, disease, and other health-related events in a population.

2. The calculation made by subtracting the age at death from 65 produces what is called _____ _____ _____ _____.

3. _____ is the intentional or unintentional damage to a person resulting from acute exposure to thermal, mechanical, electrical, or chemical energy or from the absence of such essentials as heat and oxygen.

4. A real or potentially hazardous situation that puts people in danger of sustaining injury is called a(n) _____ _____.

5. A(n) _____ _____ _____ is the ongoing and systematic collection, analysis, and interpretation of injury data essential to planning, implementing, and evaluating public health practice.

6. _____ _____ occur shortly after an injury, when the patient and observers remain acutely aware of what has happened and may be more receptive to teaching about how similar injury or illness could be prevented in the future.

7. Keeping an injury from ever occurring is called _____ prevention.

8. Medical care after an injury or illness that helps to prevent further problems from occurring is called _____ prevention.

9. Rehabilitation after an injury or illness that helps to prevent further problems from occurring is called _____ prevention.

10. An aspect of organizational commitment to illness and injury prevention is to assure the _____ of EMS providers.

11. An aspect of EMS provider commitment is managing _____ in personal, family, and work life.

12. The first priority of a paramedic is always _____ _____.

13. Areas in need of prevention activities include _____ _____ _____ in newborns, _____ firearm-related deaths, and _____ in the elderly.

14. Alcohol is a factor in about _____ of all motor-vehicle fatalities.

15. One prevention strategy is conducting a community _____ _____.

Handout 1-24

Student's Name _____

PART 5: ILLNESS AND INJURY PREVENTION

PREVENTION MATCHING

Write the letter of the term in the space next to the appropriate description.

A. epidemiology
B. years of productive life
C. injury
D. injury risk
E. primary prevention
F. secondary prevention
G. tertiary prevention
H. unintentional
I. teachable moments
J. EMS provider commitment
K. organizational commitment
L. safety
M. falls
N. alcohol
O. back

_____ 1. Collecting and distributing illness and injury data.

_____ 2. Keeping an injury from occurring.

_____ 3. The study of factors that influence the frequency, distribution, and causes of injury, disease, and other health-related events in a population.

_____ 4. A factor in about half of all motor-vehicle fatalities.

_____ 5. A real or potentially hazardous situation that puts people in danger of sustained injury.

_____ 6. Taking body substance isolation precautions.

_____ 7. Intentional or unintentional damage to a person resulting from acute exposure to thermal, mechanical, electrical, or chemical energy or from the absence of such essentials as heat and oxygen.

_____ 8. Medical care after an injury or illness that helps to prevent further problems from occurring.

_____ 9. Accounts for 22 percent of all disabling injuries in the workplace.

_____ 10. Always the paramedic's first priority.

_____ 11. The most frequent cause of injury to children under 6 years of age.

_____ 12. These occur shortly after an injury, when the patient and observers remain acutely aware of what has happened.

_____ 13. Rehabilitation after an injury or illness that helps to prevent further problems from occurring.

_____ 14. Type of injury that causes 70,000 deaths each year.

_____ 15. A calculation made by subtracting the age at death from 65.

HANDOUT 1-25

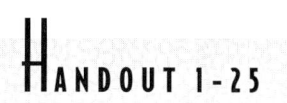

Student's Name _____

CHAPTER 1 REVIEW

PART 6: ETHICS IN ADVANCED PREHOSPITAL CARE

Write the word or words that best complete each sentence in the space provided.

1. The social, religious, or personal standards of right and wrong are called _____.
2. The rules or standards that govern the conduct of members of a particular group or profession are called _____.
3. Allowing each person to decide how to behave and accepting whatever decision that person makes is called _____ _____.
4. Saying people should just fulfill their duties is known as the _____ method.
5. Believing that actions can be judged as good or bad only after we know the consequences of those actions is called _____.
6. The single most important question a paramedic has to answer when faced with an ethical challenge is, "_____?"
7. The principle of doing good for the patient is called _____.
8. The obligation not to harm the patient is called _____.
9. A competent adult patient's right to determine what happens to his own body is called _____.
10. The obligation to treat all patients fairly is called _____.
11. *Primum non nocere* is Latin for "_____"
12. The first element in solving an ethical problem is, "State the action in a(n) _____ form."
13. The second element in solving an ethical problem is, "List the _____ or _____ of the action."
14. The third element in solving an ethical problem is, "Compare the results to _____ values."
15. One of the quick ways to test ethics is by asking whether you would be willing to undergo this procedure or action if you were in the patient's place. This is called the _____ test.
16. Asking whether you can defend or justify your actions to others is called the _____ _____ test.
17. The _____ test asks whether you would want this action performed in all relevantly similar circumstances.
18. The general principle for paramedics to follow regarding DNRs is, "When in doubt, _____."
19. Providing the most care to the most seriously injured patients is the _____ method of triage.
20. Military triage has traditionally concentrated on helping the _____ _____ _____.

Handout 1-26

Student's Name _____

PART 6: ETHICS IN ADVANCED PREHOSPITAL CARE

ETHICS LIST COMPLETION

Complete the following lists regarding ethics in advanced prehospital care.

1. List three different approaches for determining how a medical professional should behave under different circumstances.
   _____
   _____
   _____

2. List the four fundamental principles used in solving bioethics problems.
   _____
   _____
   _____
   _____

3. List the three steps in solving an ethical problem.
   _____
   _____
   _____

4. List the three quick ways to test ethics.
   _____
   _____
   _____

Chapter 1 Answer Key

Handout 1-2: PART 1: Introduction to Advanced Prehospital Care—Quiz

1. B	6. B		
2. A	7. C		
3. C	8. C		
4. C	9. B		
5. B	10. C		

Handout 1-3: PART 2: EMS Systems—Quiz

1. D	6. B	11. B
2. C	7. A	12. B
3. D	8. B	13. B
4. C	9. D	14. D
5. B	10. C	15. C

Handout 1-4: PART 3: Roles and Responsibilities of the Paramedic—Quiz

1. B	6. A
2. C	7. C
3. C	8. B
4. D	9. D
5. B	10. C

Handout 1-5: PART 4: The Well-Being of the Paramedic—Quiz

1. B	11. A	21. D	31. A
2. C	12. C	22. A	32. B
3. D	13. B	23. C	33. D
4. C	14. D	24. B	34. D
5. C	15. A	25. D	35. B
6. D	16. B	26. C	
7. C	17. D	27. A	
8. D	18. C	28. C	
9. A	19. B	29. B	
10. B	20. A	30. D	

Handout 1-6: PART 5: Illness and Injury Prevention—Quiz

1. C	6. C	11. A
2. D	7. A	12. C
3. B	8. C	13. A
4. A	9. B	14. D
5. B	10. D	15. C

Handout 1-7: PART 6: Ethics in Advanced Prehospital Care—Quiz

1. C	6. C	11. A
2. B	7. B	12. C
3. C	8. A	13. C
4. A	9. D	14. B
5. C	10. B	15. B

Handout 1-8: PART 1: Introduction to Advanced Prehospital Care—Scenario

1. The paramedic took control of the scene as a confident leader, interacting with First Responders and law enforcement. He functioned independently in ensuring that the correct prehospital care was initiated for the patient, and he prioritized treatment and transport of the patient, making the decision to transport by helicopter to the trauma center.
2. Advanced life support and paramedic-level care was not readily available. Prehospital care was provided primarily by basic life support personnel. EMS services were still using soft cervical collars, and cardiac monitoring and IVs would not have been used. The availability of a helicopter transport to a trauma center was also unlikely. This patient would most likely have been transported to the closest hospital by ground.

Handout 1-9: PART 2: EMS Systems—Scenario

1. First Responders, EMTs, and paramedics. Hospital personnel: emergency nurses and physicians. Support personnel: emergency medical dispatchers, firefighters, law enforcement.
2. The dispatcher serves as the primary point of contact with the public and assigns and directs appropriate medical care to the victim.
3. He alerted the EMS system by calling 911. He also performed a rapid triage of both patients and directed another First Responder in stabilizing one of the patients.
4. Teamwork is a vital component of EMS because many individuals with different types of training and skills must work together to see the incident through to completion. The individuals in the scenario recognize one another's talents and put aside individual egos in the best interests of the patients.

Handout 1-10: PART 3: Roles ad Responsibilities of the Paramedic—Scenario

1. The overall purpose of paramedic emergency care is to provide competent emergency medical care and emotional support for the patient and family members. In this case, through their professional support and care with Mrs. Gombert, the crew of Medic 3 provided the patient with both.
2. Among the responsibilities illustrated are response to the emergency; scene size-up and safety; patient assessment, treatment, and management; determination of the patient's disposition and transport; documentation of the call; and preparation of the ambulance for the next call, and finally, resuming in-service posture.

Handout 1-11: PART 4: The Well-Being of the Paramedic—Scenario

1. Your partner is showing classic signs and symptoms of excess stress. His coping mechanisms are no longer working. He is showing up to work later and is directing his anger toward patients and administrators. He is showing a change in his interaction with others. The common term for his condition is *burnout*.
2. Encourage your partner to talk to you. Discuss things that may be bothering him. Perhaps one particular situation is getting to him, or it could be an accumulation of unresolved problems over the years.

Encourage him to take some time off and increase time with his family and friends. If he continues to feel excessive anger, he may need professional counseling. Emphasize that his feelings are normal and seeking help does not make him any less of a professional.

Handout 1-12: PART 5: Illness and Injury Prevention—Scenario

1. The first and most obvious would be prevention of driving under the influence of alcohol. Other aspects of prevention illustrated here are seat belt usage and child car seat usage. The deployment of the airbags in the newer vehicle points to the growing number of safer vehicles.
2. DUI prevention, seat belt, and car seat usage can be discussed with the survivors and observers.

Handout 1-13: PART 6: Ethics in Advanced Prehospital Care—Scenario

1. Because the patient is unconscious, EMS providers, using implied consent, assume the patient would wish to be treated appropriately. This includes being transported to the most appropriate medical facility. The closest facility may not always be the most appropriate. In this case, the patient's husband wanted transport to a particular hospital because the patient's physician had privileges there. However, the hospital was not equipped to handle the psychiatric component of the patient's condition. The conflict involved the paramedics' wanting to do what was in the best interest of the patient and the husband's wanting transport to a less appropriate facility.
2. The paramedics should have explained why one hospital was more appropriate than the other. Proper patient care should have outweighed where the patient's physician had privileges. If time permitted, the paramedics could also have had medical control talk with the husband briefly by telephone. As a last resort, law enforcement could have been summoned if the husband became out of control, continuing to refuse proper care for his wife.

Handout 1-14: PART 1: Introduction to Advanced Prehospital Care—Review

1. highest
2. independent, timely
3. medical director
4. state, provincial
5. continuum
6. education, promotion, prevention programs
7. patient
8. mathematics, reading, writing
9. pathophysiology
10. never-ending, career-long

Handout 1-17: PART 2: EMS Systems—Review

1. triage
2. Highway Safety Act
3. medical direction (or control)
4. continuous quality improvement
5. EMS Technical Assessment
6. medical director
7. On-line
8. Off-line
9. intervener physician
10. triage, treatment, transport, transfer
11. emergency medical dispatcher
12. profession
13. certification
14. licensure
15. registration
16. First Responder, EMT-Basic, EMT-Intermediate, EMT-Paramedic
17. tactical EMS
18. I
19. professionalism
20. ethics

Handout 1-18: PART 2: EMS Systems—EMS True or False

1. T
2. F
3. F
4. F
5. T
6. T
7. T
8. F
9. T
10. T
11. F
12. T
13. F
14. F
15. F

Handout 1-19: PART 3: Roles and Responsibilities of the Paramedic—Review

1. preparation
2. personal safety
3. mechanism of injury
4. nature of illness
5. scene size-up
6. initial assessment
7. urgency of transport
8. continuity of patient care
9. I
10. primary care
11. community involvement
12. allied health professions
13. leadership
14. advocate
15. excellence

Handout 1-20: PART 3: Roles and Responsibilities of the Paramedic—Roles and Responsibilities Listing

1. Preparation
   Response
   Scene size-up
   Patient assessment
   Treatment and management
   Disposition and transfer
   Documentation
   Clean-up, maintenance, and review
2. Community involvement
   Support for primary care
   Citizen involvement
   Personal and professional development
3. Leadership
   Integrity
   Empathy
   Self-motivation
   Professional appearance and hygiene
   Self-confidence
   Communication skills
   Time management skills
   Diplomacy in teamwork

Respect
Patient advocacy
Careful delivery of service
4. Being supportive and reassuring
Demonstrating an understanding of the patient's feelings and the feelings of the family
Demonstrating respect for others
Having a calm, compassionate, and helpful demeanor.

Handout 1-21: PART 4: The Well-Being of the Paramedic—Review

1. muscular strength, cardiovascular endurance, flexibility
2. isometric
3. isotonic
4. grains/breads, vegetables, fruits, dairy products, meat/fish
5. fat, salt, sugar, cholesterol, caffeine
6. push, pull
7. twisting, turning
8. infectious disease
9. pathogens
10. blood, air
11. incubation
12. body substance isolation
13. personal protective equipment (PPE)
14. mask, protective eyewear
15. high efficiency particulate air (HEPA)
16. handwashing
17. cleaning
18. disinfection
19. sterilization
20. exposure
21. denial
22. depression
23. 3, 6
24. died
25. defensive, coping, problem-solving
26. stressors
27. alarm, resistance, exhaustion
28. circadian rhythms
29. anchor time
30. Burnout
31. physical, emotional, cognitive, behavioral
32. yourself
33. Mental health professionals
34. stress-related symptoms
35. parking place

Handout 1-22: PART 4: The Well-Being of the Paramedic—Well-Being Basics Listing

1. Cardiovascular endurance
Strength and flexibility
Nutrition and weight control
Freedom from addictions
Back safety
2. Grains/breads
Vegetables
Fruits
Dairy products
Meats/fish
3. Protective gloves
Masks and eyewear
HEPA and N-85 respirators
Gowns
Resuscitation equipment

4. Any five from Table 2-4, 37
5. Denial
Anger
Bargaining
Depression
Acceptance
6. Injury or death of an infant or child
Injury or death of someone known to EMS
Injury, death, or suicide of EMS worker
Extreme threat to EMS worker
Disaster or mass-casualty incident
Injury or death of civilian caused by EMS operations
Incidents that draw unusual media attention
Prolonged incident
Other significant events

Handout 1-23: PART 5: Illness and Injury Prevention—Review

1. Epidemiology
2. years of productive life
3. Injury
4. injury risk
5. injury surveillance program
6. Teachable moments
7. primary
8. secondary
9. tertiary
10. protection
11. stress
12. personal safety
13. low birth weight, unintentional, falls
14. half
15. needs assessment

Handout 1-24: PART 5: Illness and Injury Prevention—Prevention Matching

1. K
2. E
3. A
4. N
5. D
6. J
7. C
8. F
9. O
10. L
11. M
12. I
13. G
14. H
15. B

Handout 1-25: PART 6: Ethics in Advanced Prehospital Care—Review

1. morals
2. ethics
3. ethical relativism
4. deontological
5. consequentialism
6. What is in the patient's best interest?
7. beneficence
8. nonmaleficence
9. autonomy
10. justice
11. First, do no harm.
12. universal
13. implications, consequences
14. relevant
15. impartiality
16. interpersonal justifiability
17. universalizability
18. resuscitate
19. civilian
20. least seriously injured

Handout 1-26: PART 6: Ethics in Advanced Prehospital Care—Ethics List Completion

1. Ethical relativism
   Deontological method
   Consequentialism
2. Beneficence
   Nonmaleficence
   Autonomy
   Justice
3. State the action in a universal form.
   List the implications or consequences of the action.
   Compare them to relevant values.
4. Impartiality test
   Universalizability test
   Interpersonal justifiability test

Chapter 2

Medical/Legal Aspects of Advanced Prehospital Care

INTRODUCTION

Legal issues are an important concern of the paramedic. Paramedics must be familiar with the laws that affect EMS as well as the potential areas of liability they may encounter in the field. Paramedics must be prepared to make the best medical decisions and the most appropriate legal decisions. This chapter addresses general legal principles in addition to specific laws and legal concepts that affect the paramedic's daily practice.

TOTAL TEACHING TIME:
4.72 HOURS
The total teaching time is only a guideline based on the didactic and practical lab averages in the National Standard Curriculum. Instructors should take into consideration such factors as the pace at which students learn, the size of the class, and breaks. The actual time devoted to teaching objectives is the responsibility of the instructor.

CHAPTER OBJECTIVES

After reading this chapter, you should be able to:

1. Differentiate among legal, ethical, and moral responsibilities. (p. 66)
2. Describe the basic structure of the legal system and differentiate civil and criminal law. (pp. 66–67)
3. Differentiate licensure and certification. (p. 68)
4. List reportable problems or conditions and to whom the reports are to be made. (p. 69)
5. Define:

    - abandonment (p. 78)
    - advance directives (p. 80)
    - assault (p. 78)
    - battery (p. 78)
    - breach of duty (p. 70)
    - confidentiality (p. 73)
    - consent (expressed, implied, informed, involuntary) (p. 75)
    - Do Not Resuscitate orders (p. 80)
    - duty to act (p. 70)
    - emancipated minor (p. 76)
    - false imprisonment (p. 78)
    - immunity (p. 69)
    - liability (p. 66)

©2007 Pearson Education, Inc.
Essentials of Paramedic Care, 2nd ed.

- libel (p. 74)
- minor (p. 76)
- negligence (p. 70)
- proximate cause (p. 71)
- scope of practice (p. 68)
- slander (p. 74)
- standard of care (p. 70)
- tort (p. 67)

6. Discuss the legal implications of medical direction. (pp. 68, 72)
7. Describe the four elements necessary to prove negligence. (pp. 70–71)
8. Explain liability as it applies to emergency medical services. (pp. 66, 70–73)
9. Discuss immunity, including Good Samaritan statutes, as it applies to the paramedic. (pp. 69, 72)
10. Explain necessity and the standards for maintaining patient confidentiality that apply to the paramedic. (pp. 73–74)
11. Differentiate expressed, informed, implied, and involuntary consent and describe the process used to obtain informed or implied consent. (pp. 75–76)
12. Discuss appropriate patient interaction and documentation techniques regarding refusal of care. (pp. 76–77)
13. Identify legal issues involved in the decision not to transport a patient, or to reduce the level of care. (pp. 77, 79)
14. Describe the criteria and the role of the paramedic in selecting hospitals to receive patients. (p. 79)
15. Differentiate assault and battery. (p. 78)
16. Describe the conditions under which the use of force, including restraint, is acceptable. (pp. 78–79)
17. Explain advance directives and how they impact patient care. (pp. 80–81)
18. Discuss the paramedic's responsibilities relative to resuscitation efforts for patients who are potential organ donors. (pp. 80–81)
19. Describe how a paramedic may preserve evidence at a crime or accident scene. (p. 81)
20. Describe the importance of providing accurate documentation of an EMS response. (pp. 81–82)
21. Describe what is required to make a patient care report an effective legal document. (pp. 81–82)

FRAMING THE LESSON

Begin the class by reviewing the important points from Chapter 1, "Introduction to Advanced Prehospital Care." Discuss any aspects of the chapter not understood by students. Then go on to Chapter 2. Review the description of the profession, paramedic characteristics, the paramedic as a health care professional, and the expanded scope of practice. Begin a discussion on what physical attributes a paramedic would need to do his or her job successfully. Ask each student to state a healthy living habit and a bad living habit. These would include habits of diet, exercise, hygiene, attitude, and safety. Have them include activities of daily life as well as those related to EMS. Ask students to offer ideas as to what consequences the bad habits might have.

TEACHING STRATEGIES

People learn in a variety of ways. Some do better with the spoken word, whereas others prefer the written. Some prefer to work alone, whereas others profit from working in groups. Recognizing these different ways of acquiring knowledge, the authors of this *Instructor's Resource Manual* have provided a variety of teaching strategies for the different types of learners. These strategies are intended to foster higher-level cognitive skills and encourage creative learning and problem solving. For greatest effectiveness, incorporate these strategies into your class lecture. Symbols in the Lecture Outline indicate the points at which various exercises might be most appropriate. Other strategies can be used to preview the lesson or to summarize it.

The following strategies are keyed to specific sections of the lesson:

1. ***Reviewing Legal Basics.*** Show video clips that demonstrate each type of law discussed in class. With so many lawyer, police, and investigator shows on television these days, it is easy to find examples of constitutional, common, legislative, administrative, criminal, and civil law being either prosecuted, defended, or investigated. This is a visual activity.

2. ***Field Trip to Court.*** Arrange a field trip for students to attend a civil trial in your community. In preparation for the trial attendance, ask a local attorney to come to class to discuss and answer student questions regarding civil law, especially related to the medical profession.

3. ***Understanding Scope of Practice.*** Distribute your state's scope-of-practice document to students. If your county has additional limitations, distribute them as well. This is especially important because students learn a national curriculum in class but will work in a county or state with its own laws. This activity will help students to understand that just because they learned something in class does not mean they can necessarily perform a procedure or give a medication in the field.

4. ***Reviewing Licensing and Certification Requirements.*** This is a good time to discuss the certification and licensing requirements in your area. Distribute the necessary forms here, instead of at the end of the program. Perhaps create a timeline of certification steps, requirements, and fees. For example, in California, students must take a County Accreditation Exam before starting their field internship. Then, they must pass the National Registry exam, which is given in place of the state licensing exam. Then they make application to the state for a license, but need to have a course completion certificate, be issued a National Registry card, and pay a $180 fee. Explaining the process and empowering students to handle certification or licensure themselves promotes responsibility. Students and employers dislike surprises and mistakes when waiting for licensure at the end of a long program of education.

5. ***Understanding Breach of Duty.*** Create a list of negative behaviors by the paramedic and have students categorize them by mal/mis/nonfeasance. For situations that are not clear, facilitate a discussion about the injurious behavior. Whenever possible, have the case or example available to show students how the behavior was viewed by the courts in a previous, similar situation. This activity relates to the broader concept of negligence, which is extremely important to medical providers. By using real examples and case law, you help bridge the gap between classroom concepts and reality.

6. ***Stressing Confidentiality.*** Observe the principles of confidentiality in your classroom. Be sure ECGs, X-rays, CTs, and lab reports that you use as illustrations for students always have the patient's name blackened out or

removed. Do not allow identifying information to be relayed when discussing calls or clinical cases. Further reinforce the program's commitment to confidentiality by creating a statement to that effect, which students must sign before entering the clinical setting. A real and observable commitment to confidentiality will strengthen relationships with clinical partners and be appreciated by future employers and colleagues of your students.

The following strategies can be used at various points throughout the lesson or to help summarize and demonstrate what students have learned:

Role-Playing Legal Issues. Break students into groups of three or four. Give each group 15 to 20 minutes to develop a scenario in which a paramedic crew responds to a medical or trauma call that involves managing one to three patients. Have each group fill out a sample prehospital care report for each patient. Randomly draw a scenario, read it aloud, and let the class as a whole think about the situation. Then ask for individuals to play the parts of the paramedics, bystanders, and patient(s) in the scenario and take a 10- to 15-minute break while the "actors" prepare for their parts. Assign other students the roles of attorneys, jury members, doctors, and a judge in a lawsuit that has developed out of the scenario. Tell them to think about possible legal issues that might be raised by the scenario. After the break, explain that the patient has filed a negligence lawsuit based on a paramedic's alleged actions or failure to act. Emphasize the importance of including or considering all legal issues covered in the chapter, particularly the need for a complete and well-written prehospital care report. Let the courtroom scene play for about 30 to 45 minutes. Then review and discuss the case and other legal issues raised in this chapter. No other activity will better illustrate each component of a lawsuit for students than their having to research and act out the roles. This is a kinesthetic, visual, and auditory activity that is both fun and educational. It requires research, oral communication skills, and the ability to consider another's viewpoint.

Cultural Considerations, Legal Notes, and Patho Pearls. The Student CD-ROM contains this series of informative features to enhance the student's understanding of the material covered in this chapter.

TEACHING OUTLINE

Chapter 2, "Medical/Legal Aspects of Advanced Prehospital Care," is the second lesson in Division 1, *Introduction to Advanced Prehospital Care*. Distribute Handout 2-1 so that students can familiarize themselves with the learning goals for this chapter. If students have any questions about the objectives, answer them at this time.

Then present the chapter material. One possible lecture outline follows. In the outline, the parenthetical references in regular type are references to text pages; those in bold type are references to figures or tables.

I. Introduction. A paramedic must be prepared to make the best medical decisions and the most appropriate legal decisions. (p. 65)

A. Paramedics must be familiar with the legal issues they are likely to encounter in the field.

B. When faced with a specific legal question, rely on the advice of an attorney.

II. Legal duties and ethical responsibilities. Paramedics have specific legal duties to their patients, crews, medical directors, and the public. (pp. 66–69)

A. Liability/legal responsibilities (p. 66)
  1. Perform systematic patient assessment.
  2. Provide appropriate medical care.
  3. Maintain accurate and complete documentation of all incidents.

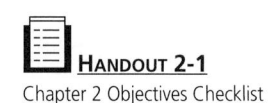

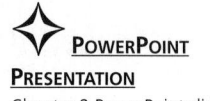

B. Ethical standards, not laws (p. 66)
  1. Promptly respond to both the physical and emotional needs of every patient.
  2. Treat all patients and their families with courtesy and respect.
  3. Maintain mastery of your skills and medical knowledge.
  4. Participate in continuing education programs, seminars, and refresher training.
  5. Critically review your performance and constantly seek improvement.
  6. Report honestly and in a manner respectful of patient confidentiality.
  7. Work cooperatively, showing respect for other emergency professionals.

C. The legal system (pp. 66–67)
  1. Sources of law
     a. Constitutional law
     b. Common law
     c. Legislative law
     d. Administrative law
  2. Categories of law
     a. Criminal law
     b. Civil law

D. Anatomy of a civil lawsuit (pp. 67–68)
  1. Incident
  2. Investigation
  3. Filing of the complaint
  4. Answering the complaint
  5. Discovery
     a. An examination before trial (deposition)
     b. An interrogatory
     c. Requests for document production
  6. Trial
  7. Decision
  8. Appeal
  9. Settlement

E. Laws affecting EMS and the paramedic (pp. 68–69)
  1. Scope of practice
  2. Licensure and certification
  3. Motor-vehicle laws
  4. Mandatory reporting requirements
     a. Spousal abuse
     b. Child abuse and neglect
     c. Elder abuse
     d. Sexual assault
     e. Gunshot and stab wounds
     f. Animal bites
     g. Communicable diseases
  5. Legal protections for the paramedic
     a. Immunity
     b. Good Samaritan laws
     c. Ryan White CARE Act

III. Legal accountability of the paramedic. Any deviation from the expected standard of care may expose a paramedic to allegations of negligence and liability for any resulting damages. (pp. 70–73)

A. Negligence and medical liability (pp. 70–72)
  1. Components of a negligence claim
     a. Duty to act

TEACHING STRATEGY 2
Field Trip to Court

TEACHING TIP
To show students what giving testimony is like, have them watch Court TV, if it is available. They will see the justice system in action. If possible, record a segment in which an EMT or paramedic is testifying and show it to your class. This will be a real eye-opener.

TEACHING TIP
Find the medical practice act that defines the scope and role of EMS workers in your state and bring copies to class to discuss with students.

TEACHING STRATEGY 3
Understanding Scope of Practice

TEACHING STRATEGY 4
Reviewing Licensing and Certification Requirements

TEACHING TIP
Present the following scenario to the class: you are a paramedic student and have just learned how to administer drugs during last week's class. You are on an emergency call where there are no paramedics. Now ask the class, "Do you perform the skill you know you are physically able to perform?"

POWERPOINT PRESENTATION
Chapter 2 PowerPoint slides 21–35

TEACHING STRATEGY 5
Understanding Breach of Duty

      b. Breach of duty
         i. Violation of standard of care
           a) Malfeasance
           b) Misfeasance
           c) Nonfeasance
         ii. *Res ipsa loquitur*
           a) "The thing speaks for itself."
         iii. Negligence per se
           a) Automatic negligence
      c. Actual damages
      d. Proximate cause
    2. Defenses to charges of negligence
      a. Good Samaritan laws
      b. Governmental immunity
      c. Statute of limitations
      d. Contributory or comparative negligence
B. Special liability concerns (pp. 72–73)
    1. Medical direction
    2. Borrowed servant doctrine
    3. Civil rights
    4. Off-duty paramedics

POWERPOINT PRESENTATION
Chapter 2 PowerPoint Slides 36–68

IV. Paramedic-patient relationships. Paramedics have legal and ethical duties to protect their patients' privacy and treat them with honesty, respect, and compassion. (pp. 73–79)

A. Confidentiality (pp. 73–74)
    1. Situations allowing release of patient information
      a. Patient consent for release of records
      b. Other medical care providers' need to know
      c. Legal requirement to release a patient's medical records
      d. Third-party billing requirements
    2. Health Insurance Portability and Accountability Act (HIPAA)
      a. Mandatory HIPAA training
      b. Patient privacy protections
      c. Patient inspection of their health records
    3. Defamation
      a. Libel
         i. False written communication
      b. Slander
         i. False oral communication
    4. Invasion of privacy

TEACHING STRATEGY 6
Stressing Confidentiality

B. Consent (pp. 75–78)
    1. Informed consent
      a. Needed from all competent adults
    2. Expressed consent
    3. Implied consent
    4. Involuntary consent
    5. Special consent situations
      a. Minor
         i. Usually under age 18
      b. Emancipated minor
         i. Person under 18 who, because of circumstances, is considered an adult
    6. Withdrawal of consent
    7. Refusal of service
      a. Be sure patient is competent adult.

b. Make multiple and sincere attempts to convince patient to accept care.
   c. Enlist help of others such as family and friends to convince patient to accept care.
   d. Be certain the patient is fully informed about the implications of decision and risks of refusing care.
   e. Consult with on-line medical direction.
   f. Have patient and witnesses sign release-from-liability form. (Fig. 2-1, p. 76)
   g. Advise patient that he may call again for help if needed.
   h. Attempt to get patient's family or friends to stay with him.
   i. Document the entire situation thoroughly on patient care report.
   8. Problem patients
      a. Violent, intoxicated, drug overdose victim, minor with no adult available to give consent
      b. Try to develop trust and rapport with patient.
      c. Involve law enforcement as necessary.
      d. Document in detail.
C. Legal complications related to consent (p. 78)
   1. Abandonment
   2. Assault and battery
   3. False imprisonment
D. Reasonable force (pp. 78–79)
   1. Minimal force necessary to ensure that an unruly or violent person does no harm to anyone
E. Patient transportation (p. 79)

V. Resuscitation issues. Generally, you are under obligation to begin resuscitative efforts when summoned to the scene of a patient who is unresponsive, pulseless, and apneic. Sometimes, however, you will determine that resuscitation is not indicated. (pp. 79–81)

A. Advance directives (pp. 80–81)
   1. Living wills
      a. Specification of the kind of medical treatment a person is willing to accept
   2. Durable Power of Attorney for Healthcare
   3. Do Not Resuscitate orders
      a. Indication by patient of what types of life-sustaining measures will be permitted if heart and respiratory functions cease
   4. Potential organ donation
B. Death in the field (p. 81)

VI. Crime and accident scenes. You should be familiar with crime-scene preservation issues, but you must not sacrifice patient care to preserve evidence or to become involved in detective work. (p. 81)

A. Contact law enforcement. (p. 81)
B. Protect yourself and the safety of other EMS personnel. (p. 81)
C. Initiate patient contact only when a crime scene has been deemed safe. (p. 81)
D. Do not move or touch anything unless it is necessary for patient care; protect evidence. (p. 81)
E. If you need to remove items from the scene, document your actions and notify police. (p. 81)

POINT TO EMPHASIZE
Abandonment is the number-one reason for legal suits against emergency services personnel. Make sure you document evidence of the mental capacity of the patient, his or her reason for refusing, and the fact that he or she understands your impression of the problem and the possible consequences of refusal.

READING/REFERENCE
Criss, E. "Prehospital Resuscitation Practices," *JEMS*. May 2003.

POWERPOINT PRESENTATION
Chapter 2 PowerPoint slides 69–74

TEACHING TIP
Consider in class the patient's rights versus family wishes in the case of sudden death. To generate discussion, ask if implied consent supersedes a spouse's wish not to have resuscitative measures taken.

POINT TO EMPHASIZE
Whether the paramedic can assess the validity of a living will or a DNR order in the patient's home is doubtful. State laws and local protocol should clearly define what constitutes a death pronouncement.

POWERPOINT PRESENTATION
Chapter 2 PowerPoint slides 75–77

POWERPOINT PRESENTATION
Chapter 2 PowerPoint slides 78–79

POINT TO EMPHASIZE
Sloppy/incomplete recording will imply sloppy/incomplete care. Assume you will have to review your prehospital care report 5 years from now; write it so that it will be legible at that time. Remember, lawyers love to discover disagreement and discrepancies in medical records.

WORKBOOK
Chapter 2 Activities

READING/REFERENCE
Textbook, pp. 84–238

HANDOUT 2-2
Chapter 2 Quiz

HANDOUT 2-3
Chapter 2 Scenario

PARAMEDIC STUDENT CD
Student Activities

COMPANION WEBSITE
http://www.prenhall.com/bledsoe

TESTGEN
Chapter 2

EMT ACHIEVE: PARAMEDIC TEST PREPARATION
Mistovich & Beasley. *EMT Achieve: Paramedic Test Preparation.*
www.prenhall.com/emtachieve/

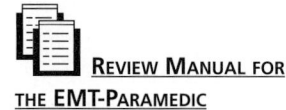

REVIEW MANUAL FOR THE EMT-PARAMEDIC
Cherry & Mistovich. *Review Manual for the EMT-Paramedic*, 3rd edition

VII. Documentation. The treatment of your patient does not end until you have properly documented the entire incident from initial response to transfer of patient care to the hospital emergency department staff. (pp. 81–82)

  A. Characteristics of good documentation (pp. 81–82)
      1. It is completed promptly after patient contact.
      2. It is thorough.
      3. It is objective.
      4. It is accurate.
      5. It maintains patient confidentiality.
  B. Written amendments (p. 82)
  C. Maintenance of records per state law (p. 82)

VIII. Chapter Summary (p. 82). It is in your best interest to learn and follow all state laws and local protocols related to your practice as a paramedic. Also be sure to receive good training and keep current by pursuing continuing education, reading industry journals, and obtaining recertification or relicensure as required by state law. Always act in good faith and use your common sense. High-quality patient care and high-quality documentation are always your best protection from liability.

ASSIGNMENTS

Assign students to complete Chapter 2, "Medical/Legal Aspects of Advanced Prehospital Care," of the workbook. Also assign them to read Chapter 3, "Anatomy and Physiology," before the next class.

EVALUATION

Chapter Quiz and Scenario Distribute copies of the Chapter Quiz provided in Handouts 2-2 and 2-3 to evaluate student understanding of this chapter. Make sure each student reads the scenario to reinforce critical thinking on the scene. Remind students not to use their notes or textbooks while taking the quiz.

Student CD Quizzes for every chapter are contained on the dynamic and highly visual in-text student CD.

Companion Website Additional quizzes for every chapter are contained on this exciting website.

TestGen You may wish to create a custom-tailored test using *Prentice Hall TestGen for Essentials of Paramedic Care,* 2nd Edition to evaluate student understanding of this chapter.

On-line Test Preparation (for students and instructors) Additional test preparation is available through Brady's new on-line product, *EMT Achieve: Paramedic Test Preparation* at h*ttp://www.prenhall.com/emtachieve/*. Instructors can also monitor student mastery on-line.

Review Manual for the EMT-Paramedic This comprehensive exam review contains hundreds of test questions and rationales, including scenarios, along with two 180-question practice tests on CD.

REINFORCEMENT

Handouts If classroom discussion or performance on the quiz indicates that some students have not fully mastered the chapter content, you may wish to assign some or all of the Reinforcement Handouts for this chapter.

Student CD (for students) A wide variety of material on this CD-ROM will reinforce and also expand student knowledge and skills.

PowerPoint Presentation (for instructors) The PowerPoint material developed for this chapter offers useful reinforcement of chapter content.

Companion Website (for students) Additional review quizzes and links to EMS resources will contribute to further reinforcement of the chapter.

OneKey On-line support is offered for this course on one of three platforms: CourseCompass, Blackboard, or Web CT. Includes the IRM, PowerPoints, TestGen, and Companion Website for instruction. Ask your local sales representative for more information.

Brady Skills Series: Advanced Life Skills (Video or CD) Have your students watch the skills come to life on VHS or CD-ROM, or they can purchase the highly visual, full-color text with step-by-step procedures and rationales.

HANDOUTS 2-4 AND 2-5
Reinforcement Activities

PARAMEDIC STUDENT CD
Student Activities

POWERPOINT PRESENTATION
Chapter 2

COMPANION WEBSITE
http://www.prenhall.com/bledsoe

ONEKEY
Chapter 2

ADVANCED LIFE SUPPORT SKILLS
Larmon & Davis. *Advanced Life Support Skills.*

ADVANCED LIFE SKILLS REVIEW
Larmon & Davis. *Advanced Life Skills Review.*

BRADY SKILLS SERIES: ALS
Larmon & Davis. *Brady Skills Series: ALS.*

PARAMEDIC NATIONAL STANDARDS SELF-TEST
Miller. *Paramedic National Standards Self-Test,* 4th edition.

HANDOUT 2-1

Student's Name _____

CHAPTER 2 OBJECTIVES CHECKLIST

Knowledge	Date Mastered
1. Differentiate among legal, ethical, and moral responsibilities.	
2. Describe the basic structure of the legal system and differentiate civil and criminal law.	
3. Differentiate licensure and certification.	
4. List reportable problems or conditions and to whom the reports are to be made.	
5. Define: • abandonment • advance directives • assault • battery • breach of duty • confidentiality • consent (expressed, implied, informed, involuntary) • Do Not Resuscitate orders • duty to act • emancipated minor • false imprisonment • immunity • liability • libel • minor • negligence • proximate cause • scope of practice • slander • standard of care • tort	
6. Discuss the legal implications of medical direction.	
7. Describe the four elements necessary to prove negligence.	
8. Explain liability as it applies to EMS.	
9. Discuss immunity, including Good Samaritan statutes, as it applies to the paramedic.	
10. Explain necessity and the standards for maintaining patient confidentiality that apply to the paramedic.	
11. Differentiate expressed, informed, implied, and involuntary consent and describe the process used to obtain informed or implied consent.	

HANDOUT 2-1 Continued

Knowledge	Date Mastered
12. Discuss appropriate patient interaction and documentation techniques regarding refusal of care.	
13. Identify legal issues involved in the decision not to transport a patient, or to reduce the level of care.	
14. Describe the criteria and the role of the paramedic in selecting hospitals to receive patients.	
15. Differentiate assault and battery.	
16. Describe the conditions under which the use of force, including restraint, is acceptable.	
17. Explain advance directives and how they impact patient care.	
18. Discuss the paramedic's responsibilities relative to resuscitation efforts for patients who are potential organ donors.	
19. Describe how a paramedic may preserve evidence at a crime or accident scene.	
20. Describe the importance of providing accurate documentation of an EMS response.	
21. Describe what is required to make a patient care report an effective legal document.	

Handout 2-2

Student's Name _____

CHAPTER 2 QUIZ

Write the letter of the best answer in the space provided.

_____ 1. As a paramedic, one of your ethical responsibilities is:
   A. transporting patients to whatever facility they request.
   B. attempting resuscitation on every patient in cardiac/respiratory arrest.
   C. treating all patients and their families with courtesy and respect.
   D. performing a skill or procedure that you have been trained to do, even if not within your scope of practice.

_____ 2. Your best protection from liability is to:
   A. provide as little advanced-level treatment as possible.
   B. always transport to the closest hospital.
   C. always be kind to patients, as "nice people" don't get sued.
   D. perform systematic assessments.

_____ 3. The area of law in which the federal, state, or local government will prosecute an individual on behalf of society for violating laws meant to protect society is:
   A. civil law.   C. law of torts.
   B. criminal law.   D. common law.

_____ 4. The filing of complaint, answering complaint, and settlement are three components of a:
   A. civil lawsuit.   C. legislative lawsuit.
   B. criminal lawsuit.   D. constitutional lawsuit.

_____ 5. If a paramedic intubates the esophagus of a patient instead of the trachea, does not confirm tube placement, and leaves the tube in place, he has breached his duty by:
   A. malfeasance.   C. nonfeasance.
   B. misfeasance.   D. cofeasance.

_____ 6. Elements of negligence include proof that the paramedic:
   A. committed the act on purpose.
   B. committed the act during the commission of a crime.
   C. was the proximate cause of actual damages to the patient.
   D. exceeded his scope of practice.

_____ 7. To show the existence of proximate cause, the plaintiff needs to prove that the damage to the patient was:
   A. reasonably foreseeable.
   B. willfully caused by the paramedic.
   C. caused by the paramedic's violation of a criminal law.
   D. the result of the paramedic's misdiagnosing the patient's condition.

_____ 8. A patient may sue you for violating his civil rights if you:
   A. exceed your scope of practice.
   B. fail to render care for a discriminatory reason.
   C. breach patient confidentiality.
   D. commit libel.

_____ 9. The act of injuring a person's character, name, or reputation by false or malicious statements spoken with malicious intent or reckless disregard for the falsity of those statements is called:
   A. libel.   C. assault.
   B. battery.   D. slander.

88 ESSENTIALS OF PARAMEDIC CARE

HANDOUT 2-2 Continued

_____ 10. If you respond to a 7-year-old child with a life-threatening injury and no parent or guardian is available, you may still treat the child because of:
   A. expressed consent.
   B. implied consent.
   C. involuntary consent.
   D. special consent.

_____ 11. If a competent adult refuses care, you should:
   A. have the patient placed in police custody.
   B. restrain the patient and transport.
   C. document the situation thoroughly.
   D. not argue with him and notify dispatch that you are back in service.

_____ 12. The termination of the paramedic-patient relationship without assurance that an equal or greater level of care will continue is:
   A. assault.
   B. abandonment.
   C. battery.
   D. false imprisonment.

_____ 13. A paramedic who starts an IV on a patient who does not consent to such treatment may be sued for:
   A. *res ipsa loquitur.*
   B. false imprisonment.
   C. nonfeasance.
   D. assault.

_____ 14. During transport of a patient to a health care facility, the level of care the patient receives must (may):
   A. be greater than the level of care received at the scene.
   B. be at least the same level of care received at the scene.
   C. be a lesser level of care than received at the scene if the patient agrees to it.
   D. be at least at the EMT-Basic level.

_____ 15. A document created to ensure that certain treatment choices are honored when a patient is unconscious or otherwise unable to express his choice of treatment is called a(n):
   A. DNR order.
   B. living will.
   C. advance directive.
   D. durable power of attorney.

_____ 16. If you have any doubt about whether a DNR order is valid, you should:
   A. withhold CPR.
   B. contact the patient's personal physician before beginning CPR.
   C. contact medical direction before beginning CPR.
   D. initiate resuscitation efforts.

_____ 17. Which type of instruction on a DNR order is legal?
   A. "Chemical code only"
   B. "Slow code"
   C. "Withhold CPR"
   D. all of these

_____ 18. When you are treating a patient at a crime scene, your responsibilities include:
   A. picking up weapons and other evidence and handing them to law enforcement so no one gets injured.
   B. cleaning up blood and body fluids on carpets, furniture, and so forth before leaving the scene to avoid further contamination.
   C. trying not to touch the body at all if the patient has an obvious mortal wound such as decapitation.
   D. entering the scene to treat the patient before law enforcement personnel arrive if necessary, as the patient is your primary concern.

_____ 19. Which of the following statements regarding documentation is true?
   A. Patient refusals do not need to be documented except for the release-from-liability form signed by the patient.
   B. Subjective statements such as "the patient was drunk" are appropriate.
   C. Altering a patient care report is permissible if both you and your partner agree on the changes.
   D. The patient report should be completed promptly after patient contact.

HANDOUT 2-2 Continued

_____ **20.** A legal document that allows a person to specify the kinds of medical treatment he wishes to receive should the need arise is called:
   A. a living will.
   B. a DNR order.
   C. medical proxy.
   D. durable power of attorney.

HANDOUT 2-3

Student's Name _____

CHAPTER 2 SCENARIO

Review the following real-life situation. Then answer the questions that follow.

A paramedic trainee is training on the job with a paramedic crew dispatched to the scene of a multivehicle collision. Air transport is unavailable due to inclement weather. Six patients require three BLS ambulances, each with two EMTs, and the paramedic ALS unit with its two paramedics and trainee. One ambulance transports two conscious patients with minor fractures and cuts that were stabilized on the scene. The second ambulance transports two more patients with similar stabilized injuries. The paramedic ALS unit will have to transport the most critical multitrauma patient, who is unconscious and will require both paramedics to monitor the IV, intubation, and bleeding control interventions they have already started. An EMT from the third ambulance will drive the paramedics' ALS vehicle.

This leaves one EMT and the paramedic trainee to transport the last patient in the third ambulance. Before the paramedics leave, they oversee the immobilization of this patient in an orthopedic frame with the PASG in place but not yet inflated and supervise the initiation of an IV of Ringer's. Oxygen is given by nonrebreather mask at 15 L/min per protocols. The EMT will drive, while the paramedic candidate rides with the patient, who is conscious, with a possible fractured pelvis, a blood pressure of 86/68, and a pulse rate of 120.

Before starting for the trauma center, the paramedic trainee rechecks the blood pressure and gets a systolic reading of 80. The PASG is inflated and the IV flow checked. A second blood pressure reading after inflation is 82/64; the pulse is 112. The 24-year-old male patient is diaphoretic, ashen, and complaining of pain. Pain-relieving and muscle-relaxing drugs are in the medications kit, but the candidate explains that the patient will get pain medication at the hospital when they arrive in about 4 minutes. The candidate continues to monitor the interventions and vital signs and ignores the patient's continued requests for pain medication. He is, however, concerned by the patient's threats to sue and wishes one of the paramedic crew members had been on board.

1. Could the paramedics be held negligent or be charged under *res ipsa loquitur*? Explain.

2. Describe the types of consent that could apply to this case. How is each used?

3. Did the paramedics adhere to the proper standard of care? Is abandonment an issue?

4. Did the paramedics act appropriately in leaving the trainee to act alone? Explain.

5. Write an example of how you would cover the medication issue on your prehospital report.

HANDOUT 2-4

Student's Name _____

CHAPTER 2 REVIEW

Write the word or words that best complete the following sentences in the space provided.

1. The best protection from liability is to perform _____ _____, provide appropriate _____ _____, and maintain accurate and complete _____.

2. The paramedic must treat patients and their families with _____ and _____.

3. A civil wrong committed by one individual against another is called a(n) _____.

4. The law that is derived from society's acceptance of customs and norms over time is called _____ law.

5. _____ is a process used to regulate occupations.

6. _____ refers to the recognition granted to an individual who has met predetermined qualifications to participate in a certain activity.

7. The range of duties and skills paramedics are allowed and expected to perform is their _____ _____ _____.

8. You may function as a paramedic only under the _____ _____ of a licensed physician through a delegation of authority.

9. The duties expected of the paramedic include operating an emergency vehicle _____ and _____.

10. An example of _____ is a paramedic breaching his duty by failing to immobilize a patient from a rollover motor-vehicle collision.

11. The maximum time period during which certain actions can be brought in court is called the _____ _____ _____.

12. _____ _____ is the action or inaction of the paramedic that immediately causes or worsens the damage suffered by a patient.

13. _____ is the act of injuring a person's character, name, or reputation by false or malicious statements written with malicious intent or reckless disregard for the falsity of those statements.

14. If your patient is able to make an informed decision about medical care, he is considered _____.

15. Consent for treatment granted by the authority of a court order is called _____ consent.

16. A person under the age of 18 years who is married, pregnant, a parent, a member of the armed forces, or financially independent and living away from home is considered a(n) _____ _____.

17. The unlawful touching of another individual without his consent is _____.

18. Intentional and unjustifiable detention of a person without his consent or other legal authority is called _____ _____.

19. Preserve _____ at a crime scene whenever possible.

20. A well-documented patient report is completed promptly after _____ _____.

92   ESSENTIALS OF PARAMEDIC CARE

MEDICAL/LEGAL MATCHING

Write the letter of the term in the space next to the appropriate description.

- **A.** liability
- **B.** criminal law
- **C.** civil law
- **D.** tort
- **E.** scope of practice
- **F.** immunity
- **G.** Good Samaritan law
- **H.** negligence
- **I.** duty to act
- **J.** battery
- **K.** standard of care
- **L.** malfeasance
- **M.** misfeasance
- **N.** nonfeasance
- **O.** proximate cause
- **P.** confidentiality
- **Q.** defamation
- **R.** implied consent
- **S.** abandonment
- **T.** assault

_____ 1. Termination of the paramedic-patient relationship without assurance that an equal or greater level of care will continue.

_____ 2. Consent for treatment that is presumed for a patient who is mentally, physically, or emotionally unable to grant consent.

_____ 3. Range of duties and skills paramedics are allowed and expected to perform.

_____ 4. Legal responsibility.

_____ 5. A breach of duty by failure to perform a required act or duty.

_____ 6. Exemption from legal liability.

_____ 7. An intentional false communication that injures another person's reputation or good name.

_____ 8. A formal contractual or informal legal obligation to provide care.

_____ 9. The unlawful touching of another individual without his consent.

_____ 10. A civil wrong committed by one individual against another.

_____ 11. A breach of duty by performance of a wrongful or unlawful act.

_____ 12. Provision that gives immunity to certain people who assist at the scene of a medical emergency.

_____ 13. Division of the legal system that deals with wrongs committed against society or its members.

_____ 14. Action or inaction of the paramedic that immediately causes or worsens the damage suffered by the patient.

_____ 15. The division of the legal system that deals with noncriminal issues and conflicts between two or more parties.

HANDOUT 2-5 Continued

_____ 16. Deviation from accepted standards of care recognized by law for the protection of others against the unreasonable risk of harm.

_____ 17. The degree of care, skill, and judgment that would be expected under similar circumstances by a similarly trained, reasonable paramedic in the same community.

_____ 18. A breach of duty by performance of a legal act in a manner that is harmful or injurious.

_____ 19. The principle of law that prohibits the release of medical or other personal information about a patient without the patient's consent.

_____ 20. An act that unlawfully places a person in apprehension of immediate bodily harm without his consent.

Chapter 2 Answer Key

Handout 2-2: Chapter 2 Quiz

1. C	6. C	11. C	16. D
2. D	7. A	12. B	17. C
3. B	8. B	13. D	18. C
4. A	9. D	14. B	19. D
5. B	10. B	15. C	20. A

Handout 2-3: Chapter 2 Scenario

1. Probably not; because the case meets neither the four elements of negligence nor the three areas of *res ipsa loquitur*, and the paramedics performed an accepted standard of care.
2. *Expressed*, by all patients who permitted care by arriving provider crews; probably *informed*, as provider crews likely explained treatment before they began any intervention; *implied*, for the unconscious patient being treated by the paramedic crew; possibly *expressed*, for the unconscious patient if related to one of the other conscious patients.
3. Crews provided standard care for the situation and followed medical direction; no.
4. They left a paramedic trainee, who should be capable of EMT field provider skills and be able to provide standard prehospital care for a BLS-level patient.
5. Discussion with patient should be along these lines: "Assured Mr. X that vital signs were improving, recognized he was in pain but assured him we would arrive at the hospital shortly; directed him to take slow, deep breaths to distract him from the pain."

Handout 2-4: Chapter 2 Review

1. systematic assessments, medical care, documentation
2. courtesy, respect
3. tort
4. common
5. Licensure
6. Certification
7. scope of practice
8. direct supervision
9. reasonably, prudently
10. nonfeasance
11. statute of limitations
12. Proximate cause
13. Libel
14. competent
15. involuntary
16. emancipated minor
17. battery
18. false imprisonment
19. evidence
20. patient contact

Handout 2-5: Medical/Legal Matching

1. S	6. F	11. L	16. H
2. R	7. Q	12. G	17. K
3. E	8. I	13. B	18. M
4. A	9. J	14. O	19. P
5. N	10. D	15. C	20. T

Chapter 3

Anatomy and Physiology

INTRODUCTION

In the study of emergency medical care, students must have a thorough understanding of human anatomy (the structures of the body) and human physiology (how the body functions under normal conditions) to aid in the assessment and management of patients. This chapter will discuss the anatomy and physiology of the human body.

CHAPTER OBJECTIVES

Part 1: The Cell and the Cellular Environment (p. 88)

After reading Part 1 of this chapter, you should be able to:

1. Describe the structure and function of the normal cell. (pp. 88–90)
2. List types of tissue. (pp. 90–91)
3. Define organs, organ systems, the organism, and system integration. (pp. 91–94)
4. Discuss the cellular environment (fluids and electrolytes), including osmosis and diffusion. (pp. 94–101)
5. Discuss acid–base balance and pH. (pp. 101–104)

Part 2: Body Systems (p. 105)

After reading Part 2 of this chapter, you should be able to:

1. Describe the anatomy and physiology of the integumentary system, including the skin, hair, and nails. (pp. 105–107)
2. Describe the anatomy and physiology of the hematopoietic system, including the components of the blood, and discuss hemostasis, the hematocrit, and hemoglobin. (pp. 107–116)
3. Describe the anatomy and physiology of the musculoskeletal system, including bones, joints, skeletal organization, and muscular tissue and structure. (pp. 117–138)
4. Describe the anatomy and physiology of the head, face, and neck and their relation to the physiology of the central nervous system. (pp. 138–151)

TOTAL TEACHING TIME
There is no specific time requirement for this topic in the National Standard Curriculum for Paramedic. Instructors should take into consideration such factors as the pace at which students learn, the size of the class, and breaks. The actual time devoted to teaching objectives is the responsibility of the instructor.

5. Describe the anatomy and physiology of the spine, including the cervical, thoracic, lumbar, and sacral spine and the coccyx. (pp. 151–155)
6. Describe the anatomy and physiology of the thorax, including its skeletal and muscular structure and the organs and vessels contained within it. (pp. 155–160)
7. Describe the anatomy and physiology of the nervous system, including the neuron, the central nervous system (brain and spine), and the peripheral nervous system (somatic, autonomic, sympathetic, and parasympathetic divisions). (pp. 160–178)
8. Describe the anatomy and physiology of the endocrine system, including the glands and other organs with endocrine activity. (pp. 177–188)
9. Describe the anatomy and physiology of the cardiovascular system, including the heart and the circulatory system. (pp. 188–200)
10. Describe the physiology of perfusion. (pp. 200–205)
11. Describe the anatomy of the respiratory system (upper and lower airway and pediatric airway) and the physiology of the respiratory system (respiration and ventilation and measures of respiratory function). (pp. 205–217)
12. Describe the anatomy and physiology of the abdomen, including its divisions and the organs and vessels contained within it. (pp. 217–220)
13. Describe the anatomy and physiology of the digestive system, including the digestive tract and the accessory organs of digestion, and also the spleen. (pp. 220–223)
14. Describe the anatomy and physiology of the urinary system, including the kidneys, ureters, urinary bladder, and urethra. (pp. 223–228)
15. Describe the anatomy and physiology of the female reproductive system, the menstrual cycle, and the pregnant uterus. (pp. 228–234)
16. Describe the anatomy and physiology of the male reproductive system. (pp. 234–235)

FRAMING THE LESSON

Begin the class by reviewing the important points from Chapter 2, "Medical/Legal Aspects of Advanced Prehospital Care." Discuss any aspects of the chapter not understood by students. Then go on to Chapter 3. Begin by displaying a skeleton or a diagram of the human body's internal organs. Ask the class to identify as many bones or organs as possible. Use this discussion to point out to students that as paramedics they will have to be familiar with these structures and organs, and not only where they lie but how they function. This chapter will highlight the areas they should know about.

TEACHING STRATEGIES

People learn in a variety of ways. Some do better with the spoken word, whereas others prefer the written. Some prefer to work alone, whereas others profit from working in groups. Recognizing these different ways of acquiring knowledge, the authors of this *Instructor's Resource Manual* have provided a variety of teaching strategies for the different types of learners. These strategies are intended to foster higher-level cognitive skills and encourage creative learning and problem solving. For greatest effectiveness, incorporate these strategies into your class lecture. Symbols in the Lecture Outline indicate the points at which various exercises might be most appropriate. Other strategies can be used to preview the lesson or to summarize it.

The strategies below are keyed to specific sections of the lesson:

1. ***Understanding Organ Systems.*** Have students create a "job description" for each organ system. Have them work in groups to list the function, location, benefits, and drawbacks of each "job." Let them share their descriptions in class. This activity encourages use of the right brain and improves oral communication skills.

2. ***Total Body Fluid Demonstration.*** Use a juicing machine (juice extractor) to graphically demonstrate the amount of fluid contained in the human body, as well as other forms of life. During the class session before the one covering Chapter 3, assign students to bring in various fruits and vegetables. Use the juicing machine to extract the fluid content, or juice, from each of the fruits and vegetables. Allow students to compare the amounts of fluids and amounts of solids that result. Correlate the fluid content of these items and the 65-percent water content of the average adult human.

3. ***Chemistry Panels.*** Add realism to your discussion of electrolytes by drawing a chemistry panel on students the week before this lesson. Have the hospital print reports on each for you. Students will enjoy this lesson if they can apply their new knowledge to themselves instantly. You can usually get your hospital laboratory to do this at minimal charge for the educational value it provides. Alternatives to this activity include having the panels drawn at a health fair or using generic lab reports from random patients.

4. ***Chemistry Experiments.*** Three simple experiments can introduce students to some of the concepts in this chapter. Divide students into three groups and have each group perform one of the following experiments for the class.

   - **Osmosis.** Fill a lambskin condom with a salt-water solution and place the filled condom in a clear glass container filled with tap water. Ask students to explain what happens.
   - **Diffusion.** Fill a container with water in which you have mixed various substances—salts or sugars, finely ground spices, grains of rice, and so on. Pour the mixture through sieves of varying degrees of fineness and coffee filters to demonstrate how some substances can pour easily through membranes while the membranes filter out others. Alternatively, demonstrate the concept of diffusion by making Kool-Aid in class. Students will be able to see an isotonic solution become hypertonic when the sugar is added and then become isotonic again when the sugar and food coloring dissolve to make the entire pitcher evenly concentrated in color and flavor. Of course, serve the Kool-Aid when you are finished. This activity is fun and visually appealing because Kool-Aid colors are usually quite bright.
   - **Buffer system.** Demonstrate the processes of the body's buffer system in dramatic fashion. Pour a couple of inches of vinegar into a clear wine bottle (with cork). Then pour a quarter of a cup or so of baking soda into the bottle and quickly place the cork in the top of the bottle. What happens? Ask students why this happened and how it relates to processes in the body. You can also demonstrate the effectiveness of the bicarbonate buffer system by using Alka-Seltzer to reduce the acidity of soda pop. Drop the tablet in and watch as it makes the pop flat in just seconds. You could further illustrate this by measuring the pH of the soda before and after the administration of the Alka-Seltzer.

5. ***Guest Speaker.*** Consider inviting a dermatologist to class to discuss the various layers of skin and care of the skin.

6. Understanding Blood Components. To illustrate the components of blood, draw a tube of blood from each student. Either have the lab spin down the tubes or wait several hours. Either way, the components of blood will separate out, and the plasma will be clearly visible from the formed elements. This kinesthetic activity personalizes the lesson because each student uses his or her own blood to examine and compare.

7. Working with Lab Reports. During discussion of the white blood cells, bring in several laboratory reports of CBCs with differentials. After taking precautions to ensure patient confidentiality, have students look for reports from patients with various disorders, such as a bacterial infection, viral infection, anemia, or leukemia. Having the report to look at, as well as a clinical presentation, will lend validity to the discussion.

8. Using a Skeleton to Identify Bones. Use the skeleton you have sitting in the corner of the classroom to label types of bones. Make strips of Post-it-type paper labeled with the words *flat*, *long*, *short*, and *irregular*. Students can take turns approaching the skeleton and labeling a bone with their strip of paper. Within a couple of trips to the skeleton, it will become obvious which types of bones are which. This activity will appeal to your visual learners as well as your kinesthetic learners.

9. Model Making. Have students use large and small rubber bands to construct a system of "muscles" that will allow a skeleton to move its various bones (e.g., bending its arm). Having them design the system reinforces the origin/insertion concept. Remember the old Chinese proverb: "Tell me and I will forget. Show me and I will remember. Let me do and I will understand."

10. Naming and Labeling Bones. Determine a list of bones that you want your students to know to mastery level. Practice naming and labeling those bones on your classroom skeleton. Next, encourage students to work toward the fastest times in labeling the skeleton. On an announced date, hold a "Speedy Skeleton" contest. Students will be timed while naming and identifying all of the bones on your predetermined list. Award prizes for fastest times and best accuracy if you like. Memorization with identification helps students to learn the information to mastery level, avoiding future memory degradation.

11. Coloring Book. A great source of anatomical drawings is *The Anatomy Coloring Book* (Wynn Kapit and Lawrence Elson. 2nd Edition. Addison-Wesley). Choose various illustrations of muscle groups and bones for students to color. Assign different areas of the body to students, and then combine the separate illustrations into one large body.

12. Representing the Meninges. Use a hard-boiled egg to demonstrate the layers of the meninges. The shell acts as the dura mater, the weblike lining that you can peel off the shell represents the arachnoid layer, and the egg white is the pia mater, which all protect the yolk, or the brain itself. Give students their own eggs to explore, and allow them to eat them afterwards.

13. Morgue Brains to Teach Anatomy. Ask your morgue assistant to borrow preserved brains. Frequently, from autopsies or cadavers, there will be a bucket of brains for students to hold and examine. The layers of meninges and the brain tissue itself will be visible to students. The topographical anatomy of the brain, such as fissures and gyri, will be available for identification, as well. Anatomy and physiology are difficult areas of the curriculum for students. Every visual and kinesthetic activity you create will improve retention and understanding of the material.

14. Anatomy Brain Puzzles. Create puzzles using parts of the brain. The anatomy of the brain is complex, and understanding the functions of the parts of the brain begins with knowing their location. Mount color copies of the brain on light cardboard. Using a utility knife, cut out visible structures. Then, place all of your puzzle pieces in an envelope for students. Students can practice reciting the function of each brain structure or area while they put their brain puzzles together. This activity enhances memory using right- and left-brain techniques while appealing to the visual and kinesthetic learner.

15. *Illustrating the Anatomy of the Spinal Cord.* Make a model of the spinal cord by using lengths of wire inside a cardboard tube from a roll of paper towels. The diameter allows for many individual pieces of wire, simulating the nerves housed within the spinal cord. The tube illustrates how the cord houses the nerves and protects them yet is vulnerable to compression, swelling, and lacerations. The cardboard, like the spinal cord, is strong, yet it can be bent and cut when enough force is applied.

16. *Creating Memory Aids.* Students are much more likely to remember the functions of each of the hormones if they create mnemonics or songs to help them. Assign to students a group of hormones, such as male or female reproductive, anterior pituitary, or those that promote homeostasis. Then allow them to work together in small groups to create jingles or songs about the hormones. Have them share their jingles in class so that all students are more likely to remember the seemingly endless list of endocrine system hormones.

17. *Dissecting a Heart.* Visit your butcher for beef hearts. They are usually readily available and will provide the best possible anatomy lesson for the heart itself. The thickness of the chamber walls, the size of the aorta, and the pericardium will all be "larger than life" when the student holds a heart in his or her hand. Additionally, beef hearts are quite large, so a group of four to eight students can easily share one heart. Allow dissection of the heart and labeling of the important structures. A photocopy from this text or a lab manual illustrating a cross-section would likely be useful as well.

18. *Inspecting Diseased Human Hearts.* Human hearts can be borrowed from your hospital pathology lab or medical school cadaver laboratory. Hearts affected by left ventricular hypertrophy, atrial fibrillation, mitral valve prolapse, and other pathologies will be collected there. Sometimes, they are preserved in jars, but frequently they are kept in buckets so that students can actually hold and examine the heart. You might also invite the pathologist to discuss the specimens. This activity illustrates both normal and abnormal anatomy as well as pathology.

19. *Airway Familiarization.* Ask your local butcher for a pig pluck, which is the trachea, esophagus, lungs, and heart of a pig. These can be kept without smelling for up to a week in the refrigerator. Let students intubate the trachea and ventilate the lungs. You will marvel at the wonderful demonstration of the alveoli, lung parenchyma, and even atelectasis. Because this specimen is fresh, it is even better than a human cadaver, which will lack the elasticity of the pig pluck. This activity is fun for your visual and kinesthetic learners but can be messy. Have lots of plastic bags, premoistened towelettes, and gloves on hand.

20. *Airway Anatomy Bowl.* Obtain diagrams of the upper and lower airway. You might either use large poster-size diagrams or use the airway diagrams on pages 206, 207, and 209 in the student text. Or you can duplicate the diagrams and distribute them for students to complete. In either case, cover any labels identifying the airway structures. Divide the class into a suitable number of teams. Equip each team with a buzzer, horn, or some noise-making device. Then use a pointer to indicate airway structures to be identified. The first team to signal gets first crack at naming the structure. If the team identifies the structure correctly, it gets 3 points. If the team fails to identify it correctly, it loses 2 points and the other teams signal again for the chance to name the structure. Identification at this level is worth 2 points, and misidentification costs 1 point. If the structure is still unidentified, go to a third round and award 1 point for a correct answer, with 0 points deducted for a wrong answer. Continue with the game until all structures have been identified. Award members of the team with the highest point total simple prizes such as key chains or pens.

21. Abdominal/Pelvic "Want Ads." To review the numerous organs of the abdominal and pelvic cavities, have students create abdominal/pelvic "personal ads." In these ads, each student will describe the appearance, job, and interests of an assigned organ. Students can guess which organ has placed the ad. This fun activity will help remind students of the appearance, function, and importance of each abdominal/pelvic organ or structure.

22. Organ Examination. If you have not already done so, obtain cow or pig abdominal organs from a local butcher for students to examine. Have them pay special attention to the difference in hollow and solid organs. Examination and dissection of these organs graphically demonstrate how injury and damage to solid organs may result in extensive bleeding. Stress to students that bleeding from internal organs generally has nowhere to go and remains in the abdominal cavity. Because of this, bleeding may not be immediately obvious in the prehospital setting.

23. Autopsy Observation. If possible, arrange through the coroner's office to have students observe an autopsy, paying particular attention to the abdomen. If this is not possible, the coroner's office or law enforcement training facility may have films or videos of autopsies for you to borrow. If you have a choice, attempt to obtain a film or video of an autopsy performed on someone with an abdominal injury.

24. Kidney Anatomy Puzzle. The anatomy of the kidney and its parts can be maddening for a student to try to learn. Color copy a photograph of the kidney, or several in different views—such as lateral or cross-sectional views—onto heavy cardstock. Then cut the cardstock into puzzle-shaped pieces. Have students learn the anatomy by putting together the puzzle pieces. This is a kinesthetic, right-brain activity that also requires concentration.

25. Kidney Organ Lab. Divide students into several small groups. Obtain several kidneys from a local grocery store or butcher and compare them to the structures labeled on a diagram of the kidney. Have enough kidneys available so that all students have a chance to inspect one.

The following strategy can be used at various points throughout the lesson or to help summarize and demonstrate what students have learned:

Cultural Considerations, Legal Notes, and Patho Pearls. The Student CD-ROM contains this series of informative features to enhance the student's understanding of the material covered in this chapter.

TEACHING OUTLINE

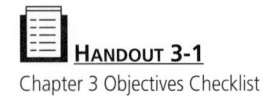

Chapter 3, "Anatomy and Physiology," is the third lesson in Division 1, *Introduction to Advanced Prehospital Care*. Distribute Handout 3-1 so that students can familiarize themselves with the learning goals for this chapter. If students have any questions about the objectives, answer them at this time.

HANDOUT 3-1
Chapter 3 Objectives Checklist

Then present the chapter. One possible lecture outline follows. In the outline, the parenthetical references in regular type are references to text pages; those in bold type are references to figures or tables.

PART 1: THE CELL AND THE CELLULAR ENVIRONMENT

I. The normal cell. The fundamental unit of the human body is the cell. (pp. 88–94) (**Fig. 3-1, p. 88**)

A. Cell structure (pp. 88–90)
  1. Cell membrane
     a. Outer covering that encircles and protects cells
  2. Cytoplasm
     a. Thick, viscous fluid that fills and gives shape to the cell
  3. Organelles
     a. Structures that perform specific functions within the cell
     b. Nucleus
     c. Endoplasmic reticulum
     d. Golgi apparatus
     e. Mitochondria
     f. Lysomes
     g. Peroxisomes

B. Cell function (p. 90)
  1. Movement
  2. Conductivity
  3. Metabolic absorption
  4. Secretion
  5. Excretion
  6. Respiration
  7. Reproduction

C. Tissues—groups of cells that perform a similar function (pp. 90–91)
  1. Epithelial tissue
  2. Muscle tissue
     a. Cardiac
     b. Smooth
     c. Skeletal
  3. Connective tissue
  4. Nerve tissue

D. Organs, organ systems, and the organism—important organ systems (pp. 91–92)
  1. Cardiovascular
  2. Respiratory
  3. Gastrointestinal
  4. Genitourinary
  5. Reproductive
  6. Nervous
  7. Endocrine
  8. Lymphatic
  9. Muscular
  10. Skeletal

E. System integration (pp. 92–94)
  1. Homeostasis
     a. Body's natural tendency to maintain a steady internal environment
     b. Significant amount of energy needed to maintain homeostasis
  2. Metabolism
     a. Building up and breaking down of substances by the body to produce energy
     b. Communication among cells is vital to metabolic processes

---

POWERPOINT PRESENTATION
Chapter 3 PowerPoint slides 4–29

TEACHING TIP
A fun way to illustrate the cell, cytoplasm, and organelles is to create "edible cells" using pudding as the cytoplasm and different candies as the organelles. Different small candies can represent different organelles, such as a gummy bear for the nucleus or licorice whips for flagella. This fun activity aids memorization of the function of the organelles by relating them to objects in the student's everyday life.

TEACHING TIP
Encourage students to role-play the various tissue types. They might do the wave for smooth muscle, play tag or telephone for nerve tissue, and form a ring of hands for connective tissue. This kinesthetic activity gets students out of their chairs and makes a lasting impression sure to stick in their memory.

TEACHING STRATEGY 1
Understanding Organ Systems

3. Endocrine signaling
   a. Paracrine signaling
   b. Autocrine signaling
   c. Synaptic signaling
4. Chemoreceptors
   a. Baroreceptors
   b. Alpha receptors
   c. Beta receptors
5. Negative feedback loop
6. Positive feedback loop

II. The cellular environment: fluids and electrolytes. Many pathological conditions, both medical and traumatic, adversely affect the fluid and electrolyte balance of the body. (pp. 94–101)

A. Water (pp. 94–98)
   1. Total body water (**Fig. 3-2, p. 94**) (**Table 3-1, p. 95**)
   2. Intracellular fluid
   3. Extracellular fluid
      a. Intravascular fluid
      b. Interstitial fluid
   4. Hydration
      a. Water is universal solvent
      b. Body requires a proper balance of intake and output to function properly
      c. Dehydration
         i. Abnormal decrease in body fluid caused by various mechanisms
            a) Gastrointestinal losses
            b) Increased insensible loss
            c) Increased sweating
            d) Internal losses
            e) Plasma losses
      d. Overhydration
         i. Edema
B. Electrolytes (pp. 98–99)
   1. Substances that dissociate into electrically charged particles when placed into water
   2. Chemical notation
   3. Ion
      a. Charged particle: atom or group of atoms whose electrical charge has changed from neutral to either positive or negative
      b. Cation
         i. Ion with a positive charge
         ii. Sodium (Na^+)
         iii. Potassium (K^+)
         iv. Calcium (Ca^{++})
         v. Magnesium (Mg^{++})
      c. Anion-ion with a negative charge
         i. Chloride (Cl^-)
         ii. Bicarbonate (HCO_3^-)
         iii. Phosphate (HPO_4^-)
C. Osmosis and diffusion (pp. 99–101)
   1. Solutions
      a. Isotonic
      b. Hypertonic

        c. Hypotonic
        d. Osmotic gradient
    2. Diffusion
        a. Movement of molecules through a membrane from an area of greater concentration to one of lesser concentration (**Fig. 3-3, p. 99**)
    3. Osmosis
        a. Movement of a solvent through a membrane (**Fig. 3-4, p. 100**)
    4. Active transport
        a. Movement of a substance through a cell wall from an area of lesser concentration to one of greater concentration
    5. Facilitated diffusion
        a. Movement of a substance through a cell membrane with the assistance of a carrier protein
    6. Water movement between intracellular and extracellular compartments (pp. 100–101)
        a. Osmolality
        b. Osmolarity
    7. Water movement between intravascular and interstitial compartments (p. 101)
        a. Osmotic pressure
        b. Oncotic force
        c. Hydrostatic pressure
        d. Filtration

III. Acid-base balance. Acid-base balance is a dynamic relationship that reflects the relative concentration of hydrogen ions in the body. (pp. 101–104)

A. The pH scale (pp. 101–102) (**Table 3-2, p. 102**)
    1. Acidosis
        a. High concentration of hydrogen ions
    2. Alkalosis
        a. Low concentration of hydrogen ions
B. Bodily regulation of acid-base balance (pp. 102–104) (**Fig. 3-5, p. 103; Fig. 3-6, p. 104**)
    1. Buffer (bicarbonate buffer) system
    2. Carbonic anhydrase
    3. Le Chatelier's principle

PART 2: BODY SYSTEMS

I. The integumentary system (pp. 105–107)

A. The skin (pp. 105–106) (**Fig. 3-7, p. 105**)
    1. Epidermis
    2. Dermis
    3. Subcutaneous tissue
B. The hair (pp. 106–107)
C. The nails (p. 107)(**Fig. 3-8, p. 107**)

II. The blood (pp. 107–116)

A. Hematopoietic system (pp. 107–108)
    1. Blood
    2. Bone marrow
    3. Liver
    4. Spleen
    5. Kidneys

POWERPOINT PRESENTATION
Chapter 3 PowerPoint slides 56–67

TEACHING STRATEGY 5
Guest Speaker: Dermatologist

READING/REFERENCE
Martini, F. *Fundamentals of Anatomy and Physiology.* Englewood Cliffs, NJ: Prentice Hall, 2001.

POWERPOINT PRESENTATION
Chapter 3 PowerPoint slides 5–8

TEACHING STRATEGY 6
Understanding Blood Components

POWERPOINT PRESENTATION
Chapter 3 PowerPoint slides 9–19

TEACHING STRATEGY 7
Working with Lab Reports

POINT OF INTEREST
About 2.5 million red blood cells die every second, but they are replaced just as quickly.

TEACHING TIP
Liken the process of clot formation to a beaver building a dam.

TEACHING TIP
Have a lean, muscular student or model display and demonstrate the anatomy and physiology of the musculoskeletal system. This is much more interesting than showing slides or transparencies. If possible, use body paint to highlight certain muscles or areas.

POWERPOINT PRESENTATION
Chapter 3 PowerPoint slides 20–50

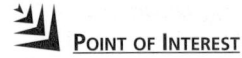

POINT OF INTEREST
The smallest bone in the body is the stirrup, which is located inside the ear. It is only 0.12 inch long and weighs about 0.0001 ounce. The largest bone is the femur.

TEACHING TIP
To show the wide range of motion of the upper extremities, demonstrate what a baseball pitcher does to throw a curveball. Break down each twist and turn of the shoulder, elbow, and wrist required to throw the pitch.

B. Components of blood (pp. 108–114)
  1. Plasma
  2. Red blood cells (erythrocytes) (**Fig. 3-9, p. 108**)
     a. Oxygen transport (**Fig. 3-10, p. 109; Fig. 3-11, p. 109**)
     b. Erythropoiesis
     c. Laboratory evaluation
        i. Hemoglobin (**Fig. 3-12, p. 110**)
        ii. hematocrit
  3. White blood cells (leukocytes)
     a. White blood cell processes
        i. Chemotaxis
        ii. Phagocytosis (**Fig. 3-13, p. 111**)
        iii. Leukopoiesis
     b. White blood cell categories
        i. Granulocytes (**Fig. 3-14, p. 111; Fig. 3-15, p. 112**)
           a) Basophils
           b) Eosinophils
           c) Neutrophils
        ii. Monocytes
        iii. Lymphocytes
     c. Immunity
        i. T cells
        ii. B cell
        iii. Autoimmune disease
        iv. Alterations in immune response
     d. Inflammatory process
        i. Platelets
C. Hemostasis (pp. 114–116) (**Fig. 3-16, p. 115**)
  1. Coagulation cascade (**Fig. 3-17, p. 116**)
     a. Intrinsic pathway
     b. Extrinsic pathway
     c. Common pathway
     d. Thrombin
  2. Thrombosis

III. The musculoskeletal system (pp. 117–138)

A. Skeletal tissue and structure (pp. 117–120)
  1. Protects vital organs
  2. Allows for efficient movement
  3. Stores salts and other materials for metabolism
  4. Produces red blood cells
  5. Bone structure (**Fig. 3-18, p. 118**)
     a. Haversian canals
     b. Osteocytes
        i. Osteoblast
        ii. Osteoclast
     c. Perforating canals
     d. Devascularization
     e. Diaphysis
     f. Epiphysis
     g. Metaphysis
     h. Medullary canal
     i. Periosteum
     j. Cartilage
  6. Joint structure
     a. Synarthroses
     b. Amphiarthroses

   c. Diarthroses, or synovial joints (**Fig. 3-19, p. 120**)
    i. Monaxial joints
    ii. Biaxial joints
    iii. Triaxial joints
   d. Ligaments
   e. Joint capsule (**Fig. 3-20, p. 121**)
   f. Synovial fluid
B. Skeletal organization (pp. 120–132) (**Fig. 3-21, p. 121**)
 1. Axial
 2. Appendicular
 3. The extremities
  a. Wrists and hands (**Fig. 3-22, p. 122; Fig. 3-23, p. 123**)
  b. Elbows (**Figs. 3-24 and 3-25, p. 124**)
  c. Shoulders (**Fig. 3-26, p. 125; Fig. 3-27, p. 126; Figs. 3-28 and 3-29, p. 127; Fig. 3-30, p. 128**)
  d. Ankles and feet (**Fig. 3-31, p. 129; Fig. 3-32, p. 130**)
  e. Knees (**Figs. 3-33 and 3-34, p. 130; Figs. 3-35, 3-36, and 3-37, p. 131**)
  f. Hips and pelvis (**Fig. 3-38, p. 132; Figs. 3-39 and 3-40, p. 133**)
C. Bone aging (pp. 132–134)
D. Muscular tissue and structure (pp. 134–138) (**Fig. 3-41, pp. 135–136; Fig. 3-42, p. 137; Fig. 3-43, p. 138**)
 1. Cardiac
  a. Automaticity
  b. Excitability
  c. Conductivity
 2. Smooth (involuntary)
 3. Skeletal (voluntary or striated)

IV. The head, face, and neck (pp. 138–151)

A. The head (pp. 138–143)
 1. The scalp
 2. The cranium (**Fig. 3-44, p. 139**)
 3. The meninges (**Fig. 3-45, p. 140**)
  a. Dura mater
  b. Pia mater
  c. Arachnoid membrane
 4. Cerebrospinal fluid
 5. The brain (**Fig. 3-46, p. 141**)
  a. Cerebrum
  b. Cerebellum
  c. Brainstem
  d. Midbrain
  e. Hypothalamus
  f. Thalamus
  g. Ascending reticular activating system
  h. Pons
  i. Medulla oblongata
  j. CNS circulation
  k. Blood-brain barrier
  l. Cerebral perfusion pressure
  m. Cranial nerves
  n. Ascending reticular activating system
B. The face (pp. 143–148)(**Fig. 3-47, p. 144**)

TEACHING STRATEGY 8
Using a Skeleton to Identify Bones

TEACHING STRATEGY 9
Model Making

TEACHING STRATEGY 10
Naming and Labeling Bones

TEACHING STRATEGY 11
Coloring Book

POWERPOINT PRESENTATION
Chapter 3 PowerPoint slides 51–65

TEACHING TIP
The skull is thick except in the temporal region. Bring in a skull and emphasize that the index of suspicion for blows to the side of the head should be high.

TEACHING STRATEGY 12
Representing the Meninges

TEACHING STRATEGY 13
Morgue Brains to Teach Anatomy

TEACHING STRATEGY 14
Anatomy Brain Puzzles

POINT OF INTEREST

The eye sees upside down, but the brain corrects the image. Rod cells in the retina help us to see in the dark but can only detect shades of gray. Cone cells allow us to see color when the light is bright. The human eye is so sensitive that under the best conditions, it is able to detect 10 million different color shades.

POWERPOINT PRESENTATION

Chapter 3 PowerPoint slides 66–73

TEACHING TIP

As in a geography class, have the students label a large drawing of the contents of the thorax.

POWERPOINT PRESENTATION

Chapter 3 PowerPoint slides 74–96

1. Bones of the face
   a. Zygoma
   b. Maxilla
   c. Mandible
   d. Nasal
2. The ear (**Fig. 3-48, p. 146**)
   a. Pinna
   b. Semicircular canals
3. The eye (**Fig. 3-49, p. 147**)
   a. Orbit
   b. Vitreous humor
   c. Retina
   d. Aqueous humor
   e. Iris
   f. Pupil
   g. Sclera
   h. Cornea
   i. Conjunctiva
   j. Lacrimal fluid
4. The mouth (**Figs. 3-50 and 3-51, p. 148**)

C. The neck (pp. 149–151) (**Fig. 3-52, p. 149**)
   1. Vasculature of the neck
   2. Airway structures
   3. Other structures of the neck (**Fig. 3-53, p. 150**)

V. The spine and thorax (pp. 151–160)

A. The spine (pp. 151–155)
   1. The vertebral column (**Fig. 3-54, p. 152**)
   2. Vertebra
      a. Vertebral body
      b. Spinal canal
      c. Pedicles
      d. Laminae
      e. Transverse process
      f. Spinous process
      g. Intervertebral disk
   3. Divisions of the vertebral column (**Fig. 3-55, p. 153**)
      a. Cervical spine
      b. Thoracic spine
      c. Lumbar spine
      d. Sacral spine
      e. Coccygeal spine
   4. The spinal meninges (**Fig. 3-56, p. 155**)

B. The thorax (pp. 155–160)
   1. Thoracic skeleton (**Fig. 3-57, p. 156**)
   2. Diaphragm
   3. Associated musculature (**Fig. 3-58, p. 157**)
   4. Trachea, bronchi, and lungs
   5. Mediastinum (**Fig. 3-59, p. 159**)
   6. Heart
   7. Great vessels—ligamentum arteriosum
   8. Esophagus

VI. The nervous system (pp. 160–177)

A. Organization of the nervous system (p. 160) (**Figs. 3-60 and 3-61, p. 161; Fig. 3-62, p. 162**)

1. Central nervous system (CNS)
2. Peripheral nervous system (PNS)
   a. Somatic nervous system
   b. Autonomic nervous system
      i. Sympathetic nervous system
      ii. Parasympathetic nervous system
B. Neuron as fundamental unit (pp. 160–162)
C. Central nervous system (pp. 162–171)
   1. Protective structures
      a. Bones (**Fig. 3-63, p. 163**)
      b. Meninges (**Fig. 3-64, p. 163**)
      c. Cerebrospinal fluid
   2. Brain (**Fig. 3-65, p. 164**)
      a. Divisions
         i. Cerebrum
         ii. Diencephalon
         iii. Mesencephalon or midbrain
         iv. Pons
         v. Medulla oblongata
         vi. Cerebellum
   3. Areas of specialization (**Fig. 3-66, p. 166**)
      a. Speech
      b. Vision
      c. Personality
      d. Balance and coordination
      e. Sensory
      f. Motor
      g. Reticular activating system (RAS) (**Fig. 3-67, p. 166**)
   4. Vascular supply (**Fig. 3-68, p. 167**)
      a. Carotid system
      b. Vertebrobasilar system
      c. Circle of Willis
   5. Spinal cord
      a. Gray matter
      b. White matter
   6. Spinal nerves (**Fig. 3-69, p. 168; Fig. 3-70, p. 170; Fig. 3-71, p. 170**) (**Table 3-3, p. 169**)
      a. Dermatomes
      b. Myotiomes
D. Peripheral nervous system (pp. 171–177) (**Fig. 3-72, p. 172**)
   1. Categories of peripheral nerves
      a. Somatic sensory nerves
      b. Somatic motor nerves
      c. Visceral (autonomic) sensory nerves
      d. Visceral (autonomic) motor nerves
   2. The somatic (voluntary) nervous system
   3. The autonomic (involuntary) nervous system (**Fig. 3-73, p. 173**)
      a. Sympathetic nervous system (**Fig. 3-74, p. 174; Fig. 3-75, p. 175; Fig. 3-76, p. 176**)
      b. Parasympathetic nervous system (**Fig. 3-77, p. 177; Figs. 3-78 and 3-79, p. 178**) (**Table 3-4, p. 179**)

VII. The endocrine system (pp. 177–178)

A. Organization of the endocrine system (pp. 177–179) (**Fig. 3-80, p. 180**) (**Table 3-5, pp. 181–182**)
B. Hypothalamus (pp. 179–180)

POINT OF INTEREST
One beer permanently destroys 10,000 brain cells. Unfortunately, brain cells do not regenerate.

POINT OF INTEREST
The brain is a greedy 3-pound organ, demanding 17 percent of cardiac output and 20 percent of all available oxygen.

POINT OF INTEREST
The spinal cord is about 17 inches long and weighs less than an ounce. It is a column of nervous tissue that acts like a relay station that connects the brain with all the other parts of the body.

TEACHING STRATEGY 15
Illustrating the Anatomy of the Spinal Cord

TEACHING STRATEGY 16
Creating Memory Aids

TEACHING TIP
Use the analogy of an elaborate system of thermostats to explain how the glands work.

POWERPOINT PRESENTATION
Chapter 3 PowerPoint slides 97–99

1. Located deep within cerebrum
2. Junction, or connection, between the CNS and endocrine system
3. Releases hormones that promote homeostasis (**Fig. 3-81, p. 183**)
    a. Growth hormone releasing hormone (GHRH)
    b. Growth hormone inhibiting hormone (GHIH)
    c. Corticotropin releasing hormone (CRH)
    d. Thyrotropin releasing hormone (TRH)
    e. Gonadotropin releasing hormone (GnRH)
    f. Prolactin releasing hormone (PRH)
    g. Prolactin inhibiting hormone (PIH)

C. Pituitary gland (pp. 180–184)
  1. Located below the hypothalamus
  2. Posterior pituitary
      a. Antidiuretic hormone (ADH)
          i. Causes retention of body water
      b. Oxytocin
          i. Causes uterine contraction and lactation
  3. Anterior pituitary
      a. Adrenocorticotropic hormone (ACTH)
          i. Targets adrenal cortexes
      b. Thyroid-stimulating hormone (TSH)
          i. Targets thyroid
      c. Follicle-stimulating hormone (FSH)
          i. Targets gonads
      d. Luteinizing hormone (LH)
          i. Targets gonads
      e. Prolactin (PRL)
          i. Targets mammary glands
      f. Growth hormone (GH)
          i. Targets almost all body cells

D. Thyroid gland (p. 184)
  1. Located in the neck
  2. Thyroxine (T_4)
      a. Stimulates cell metabolism
  3. Triiodothyronine (T_3)
      a. Stimulates cell metabolism
  4. Calcitonin
      a. Lowers blood calcium levels

E. Parathyroid glands (pp. 184–185)
  1. Located in the neck
  2. Parathyroid hormone (PTH)
      a. Increases blood calcium levels

F. Thymus gland (p. 185)
  1. Located in mediastinum just behind sternum
  2. Thymosin
      a. Promotes maturation of T lymphocytes

G. Pancreas (pp. 185–186) (**Fig. 3-82, p. 185**)
  1. Located in the upper retroperitoneum behind stomach and between duodenum and spleen
  2. Glucagon
      a. Increases blood glucose
  3. Insulin
      a. Decreases blood glucose

H. Adrenal glands (p. 186)
  1. Located on superior surface of kidneys
  2. Glucocorticoids
      a. Cortisol, the most important
      b. Increase blood glucose level

  3. Mineralocorticoids
   a. Aldosterone, the most important
   b. Contribute to salt and fluid balance
  4. Androgenic hormones
   a. Involved with sexual maturation
 I. Gonads (p. 187)
  1. Ovaries
   a. Estrogen
    i. Promotes and maintains secondary female sexual characteristics
   b. Progesterone
    i. Hormone of pregnancy
  2. Testes
   a. Testosterone
    i. Promotes and maintains secondary male sexual characteristics
 J. Pineal gland (p. 187)
  1. Located on roof of thalamus
  2. Melatonin
   a. Biological clock
 K. Other organs with endocrine activity (pp. 187–188)
  1. Placenta
   a. Human chorionic gonadotropin (hCG)
  2. Heart
   a. Atrial natriuretic hormone (ANH)

VIII. The cardiovascular system (pp. 188–205)

A. Anatomy of the heart (pp. 188–192) (**Fig. 3-83,** p. 188)
 1. Tissue layers (**Fig. 3-84,** p. 189)
  a. Endocardium
  b. Myocardium
  c. Pericardium
 2. Chambers (**Fig. 3-85,** p. 189)
  a. Atria
  b. Ventricles
  c. Interventricular septum
 3. Valves (**Fig. 3-86,** p. 190)
  a. Tricuspid valve
  b. Pulmonary valve
  c. Mitral valve
  d. Aortic valve
 4. Blood flow (**Fig. 3-87,** p. 191)
  a. Superior and inferior vena cava
  b. Right atrium
  c. Right ventricle
  d. Pulmonary arteries
  e. Pulmonary veins
  f. Left atrium
  g. Left ventricle
 5. Coronary circulation (**Fig. 3-88,** p. 192)
  a. Left coronary artery
   i. Anterior descending artery
   ii. Circumflex artery
  b. Right coronary artery
   i. Posterior descending artery
   ii. Marginal artery

POWERPOINT PRESENTATION
Chapter 3 PowerPoint slides 100–152

TEACHING STRATEGY 17
Dissecting a Heart

TEACHING STRATEGY 18
Inspecting Diseased Human Hearts

TEACHING TIP
Compare the pericardium with the pleura; both have visceral and parietal layers with a lubricating middle layer.

POINT OF INTEREST
Blood leaves the left heart at a rate of 3 feet per second. It takes about 1 minute for this blood to return from the toes to the right heart.

        c. Anterior great cardiac vein
        d. Lateral marginal veins
  B. Cardiac physiology (pp. 192–198)
      1. Cardiac cycle (Fig. 3-89, p. 193)
        a. Diastole
        b. Systole
      2. Nervous control of the heart (Fig. 3-90, p. 194)
        a. Chronotropy
        b. Inotropy
        c. Dromotropy
      3. Role of electrolytes
      4. Electrophysiology (Fig. 3-91, p. 195)
      5. Cardiac depolarization (Fig. 3-92, p. 196)
        a. Resting potential
        b. Action potential
        c. Depolarization
        d. Repolarization
      6. Cardiac conductive system (Fig. 3-93, p. 198)
        a. Excitability
        b. Conductivity
        c. Automaticity
        d. Contractility
  C. Anatomy of the peripheral circulation (pp. 198–200) (Fig. 3-94, p. 199)
      1. The arterial system (Fig. 3-95, p. 200)
      2. The venous system
      3. The lymphatic system (Fig. 3-96, p. 201)
  D. The physiology of perfusion (pp. 200–205)
      1. Components of the circulatory system (Fig. 3-97, p. 202)
        a. The pump (heart)
          i. Ejection fraction
          ii. Stroke volume
          iii. Preload
          iv. Cardiac contractile force
          v. Catecholamines
          vi. Afterload
          vii. Cardiac output
          viii. Peripheral vascular resistance
          ix. Compensatory mechanisms
        b. The fluid (blood)
          i. Plasma
          ii. Formed elements
        c. The container (blood vessels)
          i. Arteries
          ii. Veins
          iii. Capillaries
          iv. Sphincters
      2. Oxygen transport
        a. Respiration
        b. Fick principle
          i. Movement and utilization of oxygen by the body depend on:
            a) Adequate concentration of inspired oxygen
            b) Appropriate movement of oxygen across the alveolarlcapillary membrane into the arterial bloodstream
            c) Adequate number of red blood cells to carry the oxygen
            d) Proper tissue perfusion
            e) Efficient off-loading of oxygen at the tissue level
      3. Waste removal

TEACHING TIP

Bring in a very large rubber band to class and demonstrate the Frank-Starling mechanism with a student. This technique is also useful in evoking the sympathetic nervous system response.

IX. The respiratory system (pp. 205–217)

A. Upper airway anatomy (pp. 205–208) (Fig. 3-98, p. 206; Fig. 3-99. p. 207)
   1. The nasal cavity
   2. The oral cavity
   3. The pharynx
   4. The larynx
B. Lower airway anatomy (pp. 208–210) (Fig. 3-100, p. 209)
   1. The trachea
   2. The bronchi
   3. The alveoli (Fig. 3-101, p. 210)
   4. The lung parenchyma
   5. The pleura
C. The pediatric airway (p. 210) (Fig. 3-102, p. 211)
D. Physiology of the respiratory system: Knowledge of normal respiratory physiology will lay the groundwork for comprehension of important pathophysiology and will help to determine which actions will ensure optimum patient care. (pp. 210–217)
   1. Respiration and ventilation (Fig. 3-103, p. 212)
      a. The respiratory cycle
      b. Pulmonary circulation (Fig. 3-104, p. 213)
   2. Measuring oxygen and carbon dioxide levels (Table 3-6, p. 214)
      a. Partial pressure
      b. Oxygen concentration in the blood
      c. Carbon dioxide concentration in the blood
   3. Regulation of respiration
      a. Respiratory rate
      b. Nervous impulses from the respiratory center
      c. Stretch receptors
      d. Chemoreceptors
      e. Hypoxic drive
   4. Measures of respiratory function
      a. Total lung capacity (TLC)
      b. Tidal volume (V_T)
      c. Dead space volume (V_D)
      d. Alveolar volume (V_A)
      e. Minute volume (V_{min})
      f. Aveolar minute volume (V_{A-min})
      g. Inspiratory reserve volume (IRV)
      h. Expiratory reserve volume (ERV)
      i. Residual volume (RV)
      j. Functional residual capacity (FRC)
      k. Forced expiratory volume (FEV)

X. The abdomen (pp. 217–220)

A. Abdominal anatomy and physiology (pp. 217–218) (Fig. 3-105, p. 218)
   1. Peritoneal space
   2. Retroperitoneal space
   3. Pelvic space
   4. Abdominal quadrants
      a. Right upper
      b. Left upper
      c. Right lower
      d. Left lower
B. Abdominal vasculature (Fig. 3-106, p. 219)
   1. Abdominal aorta
   2. Iliac arteries
   3. Inferior vena cava

POWERPOINT PRESENTATION
Chapter 3 PowerPoint slides 153–196

TEACHING STRATEGY 19
Airway Familiarization

TEACHING TIP
Flypaper or insect traps illustrate the protective function of mucus in the respiratory tract. Bring in a full one for this lecture.

POINT OF INTEREST
Ask students why the tracheal rings are C-shaped. What would happen when they attempted to swallow huge bites of food if the rings were O-shaped?

TEACHING TIP
Bring in some clear plastic wrap and cooking oil to demonstrate the frictionless movement of the pleura.

TEACHING STRATEGY 20
Airway Anatomy Bowl

TEACHING TIP
Bring in a fireplace bellows or accordion to demonstrate inspiration and expiration.

TEACHING TIP
Start jogging in place and let students watch how your respiratory rate increases. Ask them to describe this process in biochemical terms.

TEACHING STRATEGY 21
Abdominal/Pelvic "Want Ads"

TEACHING STRATEGY 22
Organ Examination

TEACHING STRATEGY 23
Autopsy Observation

POWERPOINT PRESENTATION
Chapter 3 PowerPoint slides 197–204

PowerPoint Presentation
Chapter 3 PowerPoint slides 205–209
	C. Peritoneum
	    1. Peritoneum
	    2. Mesentery (**Fig. 3-107, p. 220**)

XI. The digestive system (pp. 220–223) (**Fig. 3-108, p. 221**)

  A. The digestive tract (pp. 220–222)
      1. Chyme
      2. Peristalsis
  B. Accessory organs (pp. 222–223)
      1. Liver
      2. Gallbladder
      3. Pancreas

Teaching Tip: Display a large drawing of the contents of the abdomen at the front of the class. Have students label the contents shown. Then have them trace the path of a bit of food from the mouth to the rectum.

PowerPoint Presentation: Chapter 3 PowerPoint slide 210

XII. The spleen (p. 223)

  A. Immunological functions (p. 223)
  B. Stores a large volume of blood (p. 223)

XIII. The urinary system (pp. 223–228) (**Fig. 3-109, p. 223**)

  A. The kidneys (pp. 224–228)
      1. Anatomy and physiology of the kidney (**Fig. 3-110, p. 224; 3-111, p. 225**)
      2. Overview of nephron physiology
          a. Glomerular
          b. Filtration
          c. Reabsorption
          d. Glomerular filtration rate
          e. Simple diffusion
          f. Osmosis
          g. Hyperosmolar
          h. Hypoosmolar
          i. Facilitated diffusion
          j. Active transport
      3. Tubular handling of water and electrolytes (**Table 3-7, p. 227**)
          a. Diuresis
          b. Antidiuresis
      4. Tubular handling of glucose and urea
      5. Control of arterial blood pressure
      6. Control of erythrocyte development
  B. The ureters (p. 228)
  C. The urinary bladder (p. 228)
  D. The urethra (p. 228)

PowerPoint Presentation: Chapter 3 PowerPoint slides 211–220

Teaching Strategy 24: Kidney Anatomy Puzzle

Teaching Strategy 25: Kidney Organ Lab

Point of Interest: The kidney has the highest blood supply per gram of any tissue in the body.

Teaching Tip: Compare the kidneys to a coffee filter. As a graphic demonstration, mix some sand in water. Then pour the water through the coffee filter and note the water after it is filtered.

XIV. The reproductive system (pp. 228–235)

  A. The female reproductive system (pp. 228–234)
      1. The external genitalia (**Fig. 3-112, p. 229**)
          a. Perineum
          b. Mons pubis
          c. Labia
          d. Clitoris
      2. The internal genitalia (**Fig. 3-113, p. 230; Fig. 3-114, p. 231**)
          a. Vagina
          b. Uterus
              i. Endometrium
              ii. Myometrium
              iii. Perimetrium

PowerPoint Presentation: Chapter 3 PowerPoint slides 220–234

Point of Interest: The uterus is normally the size of a small pear, but it stretches during pregnancy to about 12 inches.

            c. Fallopian tubes
            d. Ovaries
        3. The menstrual cycle
            a. The proliferative phase
            b. The secretory phase
            c. The ischemic phase
            d. The menstrual phase
            e. Menopause
        4. The pregnant uterus (**Fig. 3-115, p. 223**)
    B. The male reproductive system (pp. 234–235) (**Fig. 3-116, p. 235**)
        1. The testes
        2. The epididymis
        3. The vas deferens
        4. The prostate gland
        5. The penis

XV. Chapter summary (pp. 235–236). An understanding of human anatomy and physiology is basic to paramedic practice. This begins with an understanding of the basic organization of the human body, beginning with the cell and moving on to more complex structures: the tissues, organs, organ systems, and system integration within the organism itself.

Also critical is an understanding of the important body systems including the integumentary system; the blood; the musculoskeletal system; the head, face, and neck; the spine and thorax; the nervous, endocrine, cardiovascular, and respiratory systems; the abdomen, digestive system, and spleen; and the urinary and reproductive systems.

POINT OF INTEREST
Most women release one ripe egg every month for about 35 years. That adds up to more than 400 eggs. A woman's ovaries contain thousands of unripe eggs that never develop.

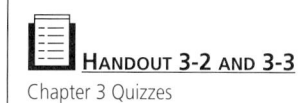

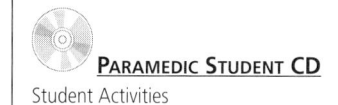

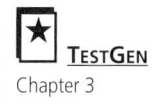

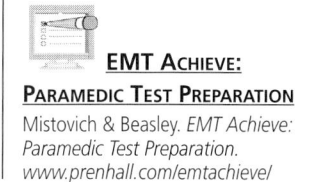

ASSIGNMENTS

Assign students to complete Chapter 3, "Anatomy and Physiology," of the workbook. Also assign them to read Chapter 4, "General Principles of Pathophysiology," before the next class.

EVALUATION

Chapter Quizzes Distribute copies of the Chapter Quiz provided in Handouts 3-2 and 3-3 to evaluate student understanding of this chapter. Make sure each student reads the scenario to reinforce critical thinking on the scene. Remind students not to use their notes or textbooks while taking the quiz.

Student CD Quizzes for every chapter are contained on the dynamic and highly visual in-text student CD.

Companion Website Additional quizzes for every chapter are contained on this exciting website.

TestGen You may wish to create a custom-tailored test using *Prentice Hall TestGen for Essentials of Paramedic Care*, 2nd Edition to evaluate student understanding of this chapter.

On-line Test Preparation (for students and instructors) Additional test preparation is available through Brady's new on-line product, *EMT Achieve: Paramedic Test Preparation* at *http://www.prenhall.com/emtachieve/*. Instructors can also monitor student mastery on-line.

WORKBOOK
Chapter 3 Activities

READING/REFERENCE
Textbook, pp. 239–290

HANDOUT 3-2 AND 3-3
Chapter 3 Quizzes

PARAMEDIC STUDENT CD
Student Activities

COMPANION WEBSITE
http://www.prenhall.com/bledsoe

TESTGEN
Chapter 3

EMT ACHIEVE: PARAMEDIC TEST PREPARATION
Mistovich & Beasley. *EMT Achieve: Paramedic Test Preparation.*
www.prenhall.com/emtachieve/

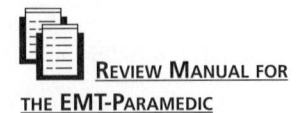

REVIEW MANUAL FOR THE EMT-PARAMEDIC
Cherry & Mistovich. *Review Manual for the EMT-Paramedic,* 3rd edition.

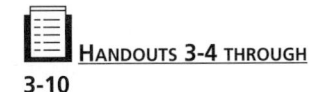

HANDOUTS 3-4 THROUGH 3-10
Reinforcement Activities

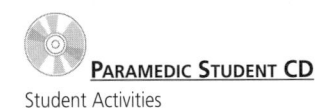

PARAMEDIC STUDENT CD
Student Activities

POWERPOINT PRESENTATION
Chapter 3

COMPANION WEBSITE
http://www.prenhall.com/bledsoe

ONEKEY
Chapter 3

ADVANCED LIFE SUPPORT SKILLS
Larmon & Davis. *Advanced Life Support Skills.*

ADVANCED LIFE SKILLS REVIEW
Larmon & Davis. *Advanced Life Skills Review.*

BRADY SKILLS SERIES: ALS
Larmon & Davis. *Brady Skills Series: ALS.*

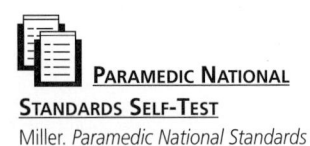

PARAMEDIC NATIONAL STANDARDS SELF-TEST
Miller. *Paramedic National Standards Self-Test,* 4th edition.

Review Manual for the EMT-Paramedic This comprehensive exam review contains hundreds of test questions and rationales, including scenarios, along with two 180-question practice tests on CD.

REINFORCEMENT

Handouts If classroom discussion or performance on the quiz indicates that some students have not fully mastered the chapter content, you may wish to assign some or all of the Reinforcement Handouts for this chapter.

Student CD (for students) A wide variety of material on this CD-ROM will reinforce and also expand student knowledge and skills.

PowerPoint Presentation (for instructors). The PowerPoint material developed for this chapter offers useful reinforcement of chapter content.

Companion Website (for students) Additional review quizzes and links to EMS resources will contribute to further reinforcement of the chapter.

OneKey On-line support is offered for this course on one of three platforms: CourseCompass, Blackboard, or Web CT. Includes the IRM, PowerPoints, TestGen, and Companion Website for instruction. Ask your local sales representative for more information.

Brady Skills Series: Advanced Life Skills (Video or CD) Have your students watch the skills come to life on VHS or CD-ROM, or they can purchase the highly visual, full-color text with step-by-step procedures and rationales.

HANDOUT 3-1

Student's Name _____

CHAPTER 3 OBJECTIVES CHECKLIST

PART 1: THE CELL AND THE CELLULAR ENVIRONMENT

After reading Part 1 of this chapter, you should be able to:

Knowledge	Date Mastered
1. Describe the structure and function of the normal cell.	
2. List types of tissue.	
3. Define organs, organ systems, the organism, and system integration.	
4. Discuss the cellular environment (fluids and electrolytes), including osmosis and diffusion.	
5. Discuss acid–base balance and pH.	

PART 2: BODY SYSTEMS

After reading Part 2 of this chapter, you should be able to:

Knowledge	Date Mastered
1. Describe the anatomy and physiology of the integumentary system, including the skin, hair, and nails.	
2. Describe the anatomy and physiology of the hematopoietic system, including the components of the blood, and discuss hemostasis, the hematocrit, and hemoglobin.	
3. Describe the anatomy and physiology of the musculoskeletal system, including bones, joints, skeletal organization, and muscular tissue and structure.	
4. Describe the anatomy and physiology of the head, face, and neck and their relation to the physiology of the central nervous system.	
5. Describe the anatomy and physiology of the spine, including the cervical, thoracic, lumbar, and sacral spine and the coccyx.	
6. Describe the anatomy and physiology of the thorax, including its skeletal and muscular structure and the organs and vessels contained within it.	
7. Describe the anatomy and physiology of the nervous system, including the neuron, the central nervous system (brain and spine), and the peripheral nervous system (somatic, autonomic, sympathetic, and parasympathetic divisions).	

HANDOUT 3-1 Continued

OBJECTIVES

Knowledge	Date Mastered
8. Describe the anatomy and physiology of the endocrine system, including the glands and other organs with endocrine activity.	
9. Describe the anatomy and physiology of the cardiovascular system, including the heart and the circulatory system.	
10. Describe the physiology of perfusion.	
11. Describe the anatomy of the respiratory system (upper and lower airway and pediatric airway) and the physiology of the respiratory system (respiration and ventilation and measures of respiratory function).	
12. Describe the anatomy and physiology of the abdomen, including its divisions and the organs and vessels contained within it.	
13. Describe the anatomy and physiology of the digestive system, including the digestive tract and the accessory organs of digestion, and also the spleen.	
14. Describe the anatomy and physiology of the urinary system, including the kidneys, ureters, urinary bladder, and urethra.	
15. Describe the anatomy and physiology of the female reproductive system, the menstrual cycle, and the pregnant uterus.	
16. Describe the anatomy and physiology of the male reproductive system.	

Handout 3-2

Student's Name _____

CHAPTER 3 QUIZ

PART 1: THE CELL AND THE CELLULAR ENVIRONMENT

Write the letter of the best answer in the space provided.

_____ 1. The main elements of the cell include:
   A. cytoplasm.
   B. eukaryotes.
   C. prokaryotes.
   D. granulocytes.

_____ 2. The basic structural unit of all plants and animals is the:
   A. DNA.
   B. cell.
   C. organelle.
   D. tissue.

_____ 3. The membrane of a cell allows certain substances to pass from one side to another but does not allow others to pass. This means the cell membrane is:
   A. dissociate.
   B. anaerobic.
   C. semipermeable.
   D. filterizable.

_____ 4. The thick fluid that fills a cell is called the:
   A. nucleus.
   B. endoplasm.
   C. ectoplasm.
   D. cytoplasm.

_____ 5. The organelle that contains the genetic material, DNA, and enzymes is the:
   A. nucleus.
   B. Golgi apparatus.
   C. endoplasmic reticulum.
   D. mitochondria.

_____ 6. A high-energy compound present in all cells is:
   A. cytoplasm.
   B. adenosine triphosphate.
   C. lysosome.
   D. deoxyribonucleic acid.

_____ 7. The seven major functions of cells include all of the following EXCEPT:
   A. metabolic absorption.
   B. conductivity.
   C. maintenance of homeostasis.
   D. secretion.

_____ 8. The tissue that lines internal and external body surfaces and protects the body is called:
   A. connective tissue.
   B. epithelial tissue.
   C. smooth tissue.
   D. muscle tissue.

_____ 9. A group of tissues functioning together is called a(n):
   A. organ.
   B. organ system.
   C. multifunction tissue.
   D. tissue group.

_____ 10. The type of muscle tissue found encircling blood vessels is:
   A. skeletal muscle.
   B. smooth muscle.
   C. connective muscle.
   D. cardiac muscle.

_____ 11. The lymphatic system includes the:
   A. heart.
   B. kidneys.
   C. spleen.
   D. pituitary gland.

_____ 12. The sum of all the cells, tissues, organs, and organ systems of a living being is called a(n):
   A. body.
   B. organism.
   C. structure.
   D. animal.

HANDOUT 3-2 Continued

_____ 13. Building up and breaking down of biochemical substances to produce energy is called:
   A. homeostasis.
   B. physiology.
   C. metabolism.
   D. endocrine signaling.

_____ 14. The body mechanisms working to reverse, or to compensate for, a pathophysiological process are known as a:
   A. negative feedback loop.
   B. positive feedback loop.
   C. pathological alteration.
   D. baroreceptor reflex mechanism.

_____ 15. What percentage of an average adult's body is water?
   A. 80 percent
   B. 75 percent
   C. 70 percent
   D. 65 percent

_____ 16. The fluid outside the body cells is called:
   A. intravascular fluid.
   B. interstitial fluid.
   C. extracellular fluid.
   D. intracellular fluid.

_____ 17. Approximately 75 percent of all body water is:
   A. intracellular.
   B. interstitial.
   C. extracellular.
   D. intravascular.

_____ 18. The normal tension in a cell, or the resistance of the skin to deformation, is called:
   A. overhydration.
   B. turgor.
   C. peritonitis.
   D. hydration.

_____ 19. Dehydration may be caused by internal losses such as:
   A. burns, surgical drains, or open wounds.
   B. diaphoresis.
   C. bowel obstruction.
   D. hyperventilation.

_____ 20. The chemical notation for sodium chloride is:
   A. HCO_3.
   B. Na^+.
   C. Ca^{++}.
   D. NaCl.

_____ 21. A major element of the body's atoms is:
   A. calcium.
   B. nitrogen.
   C. potassium.
   D. sodium.

_____ 22. Any charged atomic particle is called a(n):
   A. cation.
   B. ion.
   C. anion.
   D. electrolyte.

_____ 23. An ion with a negative charge is called a(n):
   A. anion.
   B. cation.
   C. electrolyte.
   D. dissociate.

_____ 24. The principal buffer of the body is:
   A. chloride.
   B. phosphate.
   C. bicarbonate.
   D. sodium.

_____ 25. The difference in concentration between solutions on opposite sides of a semipermeable membrane is called:
   A. the osmotic gradient.
   B. diffusion.
   C. osmosis.
   D. the facilitated balance.

HANDOUT 3-3

Student's Name _____

CHAPTER 3 QUIZ

PART 2: BODY SYSTEMS

Write the letter of the best answer in the space provided.

_____ 1. The skin is known collectively as the:
  A. integumentary system.
  B. inanition system.
  C. indagation system.
  D. inductotherm system.

_____ 2. The outermost layer of skin is the:
  A. epidermis.
  B. dermis.
  C. subcutaneous tissue.
  D. sebum.

_____ 3. The glands within the dermis that secrete a lubricant are called the:
  A. lymph glands.
  B. subcutaneous glands.
  C. sebaceous glands.
  D. soporiferous glands.

_____ 4. The cell from which the various types of blood cells can form is called a(n):
  A. erythropoietin.
  B. pluripotent stem cell.
  C. multipotent stem cell.
  D. unipotent progenitor.

_____ 5. A formed element of blood is:
  A. plasma.
  B. platelets.
  C. white blood cells.
  D. both B and C

_____ 6. Plasma is made up of 90 to 92 percent:
  A. proteins.
  B. carbohydrates.
  C. water.
  D. gases.

_____ 7. Each complete hemoglobin molecule can carry:
  A. one platelet.
  B. one red blood cell.
  C. four oxygen molecules.
  D. two white blood cells.

_____ 8. The effectiveness of oxygen transport depends on:
  A. red blood cell mass.
  B. pH.
  C. exercise.
  D. all of these

_____ 9. The packed cell volume of red blood cells per unit of blood is known as:
  A. hematocrit.
  B. hemolysis.
  C. sequestration.
  D. erythropoiesis.

_____ 10. Providing protection from foreign invasion is the job of the:
  A. leukocytes.
  B. erythrocytes.
  C. platelets.
  D. red blood cells.

_____ 11. The highly specialized member of the granulocytic series that can inactivate the chemical mediators of acute allergic reactions is the:
  A. neutrophil.
  B. monophil.
  C. basophil.
  D. eosinophil.

_____ 12. The "garbage collectors" of the immune system are the:
  A. macrophages.
  B. lymphocytes.
  C. monocytes.
  D. granulocytes.

©2007 Pearson Education, Inc.
Essentials of Paramedic Care, 2nd ed.

HANDOUT 3-3 Continued

_____ 13. The two basic subpopulations of lymphocytes are T cells and B cells. Which of the following is TRUE regarding T cells?
   A. T cells engulf foreign invaders and dead neutrophils.
   B. T cells produce antibodies to combat infections.
   C. T cells migrate to peripheral lymphatic tissues from the bone marrow.
   D. T cells are responsible for developing cell-mediated immunity.

_____ 14. After a local tissue injury occurs, the damaged tissues release chemical messengers that:
   A. decrease capillary permeability.
   B. attract white blood cells.
   C. cause vasoconstriction.
   D. reduce swelling.

_____ 15. The combined three mechanisms that work to prevent or control blood loss include all of the following EXCEPT:
   A. vascular spasms.
   B. inflammation.
   C. platelet plugs.
   D. stable fibrin blood clots.

_____ 16. The term for the process of three mechanisms that work to control blood loss is:
   A. homeostasis.
   B. sequestration.
   C. erythropoiesis.
   D. hemostasis.

_____ 17. One element of the coagulation cascade is the common pathway during which:
   A. tissue damage causes platelet aggregation and the formation of prothrombin activator.
   B. the prothrombin activator, in the presence of calcium, converts prothrombin to thrombin.
   C. platelets release substances that lead to the formation of prothrombin activator.
   D. thrombin, in the presence of calcium, converts fibrinogen to stable fibrin, which then traps blood cells and more platelets to form a clot.

_____ 18. Which of the following enhances blood clotting?
   A. vitamin D
   B. aspirin
   C. smoking
   D. low red blood cell count

_____ 19. Functions of the skeleton include:
   A. temperature regulation.
   B. storage of salts and other materials for metabolism.
   C. production of white blood cells.
   D. protection from pathogens and debris.

_____ 20. Small perforations of the long bones through which the blood vessels and nerves travel into the bone itself are called:
   A. perforating canals.
   B. diaphysis.
   C. haversian canals.
   D. osteoclasts.

_____ 21. The end of a long bone, including the growth plate and supporting structures underlying the joint, is called the:
   A. cancellous.
   B. epiphyseal.
   C. metaphysis.
   D. epiphysis.

_____ 22. The cavity within a bone that contains the marrow is called the:
   A. periosteum.
   B. haversian canal.
   C. epiphyseal.
   D. medullary canal.

_____ 23. Cartilage is the tissue that:
   A. provides the articular surfaces of the skeletal system.
   B. is responsible for the production of erythrocytes.
   C. stores fat in semiliquid form within the internal cavities of a bone.
   D. forms in a tendon.

_____ 24. Joints that do not permit movement are called:
   A. synovials.
   B. amphiarthroses.
   C. synarthroses.
   D. diarthroses.

HANDOUT 3-3 Continued

____ 25. Examples of a triaxial joint include:
   A. the hip and shoulder.
   B. the bases of the thumbs.
   C. the carpal bones of the wrist.
   D. the knees and elbows.

____ 26. The joint that allows articulation between the atlas and the axis of the spine is called a(n):
   A. pivot joint.
   B. hinge joint.
   C. condyloid joint.
   D. ellipsoidal joint.

____ 27. The hip and shoulder are examples of:
   A. pivot joints.
   B. hinge joints.
   C. ball-and-socket joints.
   D. saddle joints.

____ 28. Connective tissue that connects bone to bone and holds joints together is called a:
   A. tendon.
   B. ligament.
   C. joint.
   D. bursa.

____ 29. Bones of the head, thorax, and spine are known as the:
   A. appendicular skeleton.
   B. peripheral skeleton.
   C. axial skeleton.
   D. central skeleton.

____ 30. The single bone of the proximal upper extremity is the:
   A. femur.
   B. humerus.
   C. ulna.
   D. radius.

____ 31. The phalanges are found in the:
   A. foot.
   B. hand.
   C. skull.
   D. both A and B

____ 32. The bone on the thumb side of the forearm is called the:
   A. humerus.
   B. ulna.
   C. radius.
   D. olecranon.

____ 33. You would find the innominates and the ischial tuberosities in the:
   A. foot.
   B. hand.
   C. pelvis.
   D. skull.

____ 34. The attachment of a muscle to a bone that moves when the muscle contracts is called the:
   A. opposition.
   B. insertion.
   C. origin.
   D. fasciculus.

____ 35. Three membranes that protect the central nervous system are the dura mater, pia mater, and:
   A. cerebrospinal fluid.
   B. arachnoid.
   C. odontoid.
   D. medulla.

____ 36. The meninges and cerebrospinal fluid protect the:
   A. cerebrum.
   B. cerebellum.
   C. pons.
   D. all of these

____ 37. An expanding lesion within the cranium results in:
   A. a decrease in ICP.
   B. increased cerebral perfusion.
   C. damage to delicate brain tissue.
   D. all of these

____ 38. The portion of the brain that is the largest element of the nervous system and occupies most of the cranial cavity is the:
   A. cerebrum.
   B. cerebellum.
   C. pons.
   D. brainstem.

____ 39. The portion of the brain that controls much of endocrine function, the vomiting reflex, body temperature, and emotions is the:
   A. thalamus.
   B. pons.
   C. hypothalamus.
   D. medulla oblongata.

HANDOUT 3-3 Continued

_____ 40. Cerebral perfusion is exceptionally critical and depends on many factors. Which of the following is TRUE regarding cerebral perfusion?
  A. The pressure within the cranium resists blood flow and good perfusion to the central nervous system tissue.
  B. Mean arterial blood pressure must be at least 50 mmHg to perfuse the brain efficiently.
  C. Any edema or expanding mass within the cranium will displace CSF or blood.
  D. All of these are true.

_____ 41. Vitreous humor is a clear, watery fluid found in the:
  A. inner ear.
  B. posterior chamber of the eye.
  C. nose and mouth.
  D. outer layer of the meninges.

_____ 42. The short column of bone that forms the weight-bearing portion of a vertebra is called the:
  A. spinal canal.
  B. pedicles.
  C. laminae.
  D. vertebral body.

_____ 43. The posterior portions of the vertebra that help make up the foramen, or opening, of the spinal canal are the:
  A. pedicles.
  B. laminae.
  C. transverse processes.
  D. spinous processes.

_____ 44. Two vertebrae that differ from most vertebrae in not having discernable vertebral bodies are:
  A. C1 and C2.
  B. C1 and T1.
  C. T1 and T2.
  D. L1 and L2.

_____ 45. The divisions of the vertebral column include all of the following EXCEPT:
  A. cervical.
  B. transverse.
  C. lumbar.
  D. sacral.

_____ 46. The covering that protects the entire spinal cord and peripheral nerve roots is called the:
  A. spinous process.
  B. intervertebral disk.
  C. spinal meninges.
  D. white matter.

_____ 47. The thoracic skeleton consists of:
  A. 12 pairs of C-shaped ribs.
  B. the sternum.
  C. the clavicles.
  D. all of these

_____ 48. The 11th and 12th ribs are often termed "floating ribs" because they:
  A. have no posterior attachment.
  B. have no anterior attachment.
  C. have neither anterior nor posterior attachment and are attached only to other ribs.
  D. form the xiphoid process and are attached only to the sternum.

_____ 49. The union between the xiphoid process and the body of the sternum is called the:
  A. pulmonary hilum.
  B. carina.
  C. xiphisternal joint.
  D. sternal fusion.

_____ 50. The central medial region of the lung where the bronchi and pulmonary vasculature enter the lung is called the:
  A. carina.
  B. pulmonary hilum.
  C. alveolar junction.
  D. tracheobronchial branch.

_____ 51. The fibrous sac that surrounds the heart is called the:
  A. myocardium.
  B. epicardium.
  C. pericardium.
  D. pleuracardium.

_____ 52. The part of the nervous system that extends throughout the body is called the _____ nervous system.
  A. peripheral
  B. ventral
  C. somatic
  D. afferent

HANDOUT 3-3 Continued

_____ 53. The sympathetic nervous system is also known as the _____ division.
   A. feed or breed
   B. fight or flight
   C. slow or go
   D. stand or draw

_____ 54. The division of the autonomic nervous system that is responsible for controlling vegetative functions is the _____ nervous system.
   A. somatic
   B. afferent
   C. sympathetic
   D. parasympathetic

_____ 55. The fundamental unit of the nervous system is the:
   A. axion.
   B. soma.
   C. synaptic terminals.
   D. nerve cell, or neuron.

_____ 56. The axon is the portion of a nerve cell that:
   A. comes in physical contact with another nerve cell.
   B. is stimulated by environmental changes.
   C. conducts nerve impulses away from the soma.
   D. contains most of the metabolic machinery.

_____ 57. The membranes covering the brain and spinal cord are collectively called the:
   A. dura mater.
   B. meninges.
   C. pia mater.
   D. arachnoid membranes.

_____ 58. The portion of the brain that is the seat of consciousness and the center of higher mental functions is the:
   A. cerebellum.
   B. medulla oblongata.
   C. cerebrum.
   D. pons.

_____ 59. You will find the thalamus, the hypothalamus, and the limbic system inside the:
   A. cerebellum.
   B. midbrain.
   C. corpus callosum.
   D. diencephalon.

_____ 60. Involuntary actions such as temperature regulation, sleep, water balance, stress response, and emotions are the responsibility of the:
   A. cerebellum.
   B. midbrain.
   C. corpus callosum.
   D. diencephalon.

_____ 61. A portion of the brain that is NOT considered part of the brainstem is the:
   A. mesencephalon.
   B. pons.
   C. medulla oblongata.
   D. cerebellum.

_____ 62. The reticular activating system is responsible for:
   A. consciousness and the ability to respond to stimuli.
   B. posture, equilibrium, and muscle tone.
   C. respiratory, cardiac, and vasomotor activity.
   D. motor coordination and eye movement.

_____ 63. One of the two systems that join at the circle of Willis is the _____ system.
   A. venous sinuses
   B. internal jugular
   C. vertebrobasilar
   D. reticular activating

_____ 64. The _____ fibers transmit impulses to the central nervous system from the body.
   A. afferent
   B. efferent
   C. dermerent
   D. reflexerent

_____ 65. The 12 pairs of _____ nerves originate in the brain and supply nervous control to the head, neck, and certain thoracic and abdominal organs.
   A. cranial
   B. arachnoid
   C. anterolateral
   D. hexaxial

HANDOUT 3-3 Continued

_____ 66. When stimulated, the sympathetic nervous system:
   A. causes a rise in blood sugar.
   B. causes an increase in digestive activity.
   C. is mediated by the neurotransmitter acetylcholine.
   D. is responsible for controlling vegetative functions.

_____ 67. The topographical region of the body surface innervated by one nerve root is called a(n):
   A. myotome.   C. extensor.
   B. dermatome.   D. flexor.

_____ 68. There are eight major glands in the endocrine system. These include the:
   A. pseudothyroid.   C. pons.
   B. pancreas.   D. parietal.

_____ 69. The junction between the central nervous system and the endocrine system is the:
   A. hypothalamus.   C. thyroid.
   B. pituitary.   D. thymus.

_____ 70. The pancreas secretes two major hormones, including:
   A. prolactin.   C. aldosterone.
   B. calcitonin.   D. glucagon.

_____ 71. Epinephrine and norepinephrine are hormones released by the:
   A. gonads.   C. pituitary.
   B. thymus.   D. adrenal medulla.

_____ 72. The microscopic clusters of endocrine tissue found within the pancreas are known as:
   A. thymosins.   C. islets of Langerhans.
   B. circle of Willis.   D. Cushing's triad.

_____ 73. The pineal gland, located in the roof of the thalamus in the brain, releases the hormone:
   A. melatonin.   C. parathyroid hormone.
   B. cortisol.   D. human chorionic gonadotropin.

_____ 74. The cardiovascular system's two major components are the heart and:
   A. veins.   C. peripheral blood vessels.
   B. central blood vessels. D. arteries.

_____ 75. The heart consists of three tissue layers, including the:
   A. epithelium.   C. subcardium.
   B. endocardium.   D. parathelium.

_____ 76. The _____ consists of the visceral and parietal layers.
   A. epicardium   C. pericardium
   B. endocardium   D. intracardium

_____ 77. Which one of the following statements about the four chambers of the heart is correct?
   A. Atria are the inferior chambers of the heart.
   B. Ventricles are separated by the interventricular septum.
   C. Atria are the two largest chambers of the heart.
   D. Ventricles receive incoming blood from the body.

_____ 78. The heart contains the _____ valves.
   A. atrioventricular and semilunar   C. chordae and papillary
   B. epicardial and pericardial   D. arterial and ventricular

_____ 79. After blood circulates through the lungs and becomes oxygenated, it returns to the heart by way of the:
   A. pulmonary arteries.   C. pulmonary veins.
   B. myocardial arteries.   D. superior and inferior vena cava.

HANDOUT 3-3 Continued

_____ 80. Which one of the following statements about the circulation of blood is TRUE?
  A. Intracardiac pressures are higher on the left side of the heart.
  B. The left atrium sends oxygenated blood into the left ventricle.
  C. Pulmonary arteries are the only arteries that carry oxygenated blood.
  D. The right myocardium is thicker than the left myocardium.

_____ 81. The heart receives its nutrients from the:
  A. anterior great cardiac vein.   C. coronary arteries.
  B. blood within its chambers.   D. aorta.

_____ 82. The term "collateral circulation" refers to:
  A. both sides of the heart receiving blood at the same time.
  B. blood being sent from the atria into the ventricles.
  C. an alternate path for blood flow in case of blockage.
  D. blood flow to the lungs and heart at the same time.

_____ 83. Two or more blood vessels communicating to ensure circulation is called:
  A. anastomosis.   C. symbiosis.
  B. circumflexion.   D. ostiosis.

_____ 84. The connection points between the arterial and venous systems are called:
  A. lumens.   C. venules.
  B. capillaries.   D. tunica.

_____ 85. Which one of the following statements about arteries is TRUE?
  A. They carry oxygenated blood.
  B. They carry blood away from the heart.
  C. They carry blood under low pressure.
  D. They cannot change the size of their lumen.

_____ 86. The period of time from the end of one cardiac contraction to the end of the next is called the cardiac:
  A. fraction.   C. systole.
  B. diastole.   D. cycle.

_____ 87. Pressure in the filled ventricle at the end of diastole is called:
  A. afterload.   C. cardiac output.
  B. preload.   D. stroke volume.

_____ 88. The equation used to determine cardiac output is:
  A. stroke volume × heart rate.   C. preload × stroke volume.
  B. systolic pressure × heart rate.   D. preload × afterload.

_____ 89. Which one of the following statements about the nervous system's control of the heart is TRUE?
  A. In the heart's normal state, the sympathetic system is dominant.
  B. During sleep, the parasympathetic and sympathetic systems balance.
  C. In stressful situations, the sympathetic system becomes dominant.
  D. In the heart's normal state, the parasympathetic system is dominant.

_____ 90. A positive chronotropic agent will:
  A. increase heart rate.   C. strengthen cardiac contraction.
  B. increase respiratory rate.   D. speed impulse conduction.

_____ 91. Cardiac depolarization may be defined as:
  A. a negative charge on the outside of a cell.
  B. similar to the resting potential of cardiac cells.
  C. the opposite of the cell's resting state.
  D. the release of sodium and calcium from a cell.

HANDOUT 3-3 Continued

_____ 92. The return of a cardiac muscle cell to its pre-excitation resting state is called:
   A. resting potential.
   B. depolarization.
   C. action potential.
   D. repolarization.

_____ 93. The term "automaticity" refers to a cell's capability of:
   A. responding to electrical stimuli.
   B. propagating an electrical impulse from one cell to another.
   C. self-depolarizing.
   D. contracting or shortening.

_____ 94. The supplying of oxygen and nutrients to the body tissues is called:
   A. circulation.
   B. hydration.
   C. perfusion.
   D. output.

_____ 95. Cardiac output is the:
   A. amount of blood pumped by the heart with each contraction of the ventricles.
   B. force of the blood pumped by the heart with each contraction of the ventricles.
   C. resistance a contraction of the heart must overcome in order to eject blood.
   D. amount of blood pumped by the heart in 1 minute.

_____ 96. The resistance of the vessels to the flow of blood is called:
   A. afterload.
   B. preload.
   C. peripheral vascular resistance.
   D. cardiac contractile force.

_____ 97. Which of the following is NOT one of the three components of the circulatory system?
   A. siphon
   B. fluid
   C. container
   D. pump

_____ 98. The dependence on a set of conditions for oxygen movement and utilization is known as:
   A. the Fick principle.
   B. Cushing's triad.
   C. the Frank-Starling principle.
   D. the principle of Willis.

_____ 99. Which of the following represents the correct order of the airway structures from the mouth to the lungs?
   A. trachea, bronchi, larynx, pharynx
   B. pharynx, larynx, trachea, bronchi
   C. bronchi, trachea, pharynx, larynx
   D. larynx, pharynx, trachea, bronchi

_____ 100. The narrowest part of the airway in children is the _____ cartilage.
   A. thyroid
   B. cricoid
   C. hyoid
   D. erthymoid

_____ 101. Stimulation of laryngeal mucous membrane can cause all of the following EXCEPT:
   A. bradycardia.
   B. hypotension.
   C. cough.
   D. increased respiratory rate.

_____ 102. The trachea is maintained in an open position by:
   A. the Adam's apple.
   B. the carina.
   C. surfactant.
   D. cartilaginous C-rings.

_____ 103. The lungs are covered by the:
   A. visceral pleura.
   B. parenchyma.
   C. parietal pleura.
   D. none of these

_____ 104. The lung tissue receives most of its blood supply from:
   A. bronchial arteries.
   B. pulmonary arteries.
   C. bronchial veins.
   D. pulmonary veins.

_____ 105. In normal respiration, the size of the thoracic cavity can be increased by contracting the diaphragm and the:
   A. strap muscles.
   B. abdominal muscles.
   C. deltoid muscles.
   D. intercostal muscles.

HANDOUT 3-3 Continued

_____ **106.** Increases in carbon dioxide production can be caused by:
  A. fever.
  B. muscle exertion/shivering.
  C. metabolic processes (diabetic ketoacidosis).
  D. all of these

_____ **107.** During inspiration, the lungs become distended, activating the:
  A. stretch receptors.
  B. chemoreceptors.
  C. beta receptors.
  D. alpha receptors.

_____ **108.** In patients with chronic lung disease, the primary stimulus to breathe is:
  A. increased pH.
  B. increased carbon dioxide.
  C. decreased oxygen.
  D. none of these

_____ **109.** The average volume of gas inhaled in one respiratory cycle is called the:
  A. tidal volume.
  B. alveolar volume.
  C. minute volume.
  D. functional reserve capacity.

_____ **110.** The abdominal cavity is bound superiorly by the:
  A. ribs.
  B. pelvis.
  C. diaphragm.
  D. back muscles.

_____ **111.** The division of the abdominal cavity containing organs or portions of organs covered by the peritoneum is called the:
  A. peritoneal space.
  B. retroperitoneal space.
  C. pelvic space.
  D. abdoperitoneal space.

_____ **112.** Chyme is:
  A. fluid released by the liver and gallbladder that increases blood glucose.
  B. a mixture of ingested food and digestive secretions.
  C. a digestive enzyme produced in the pancreas.
  D. waste products of digestion eliminated through the anus.

_____ **113.** The wavelike muscular motion of the esophagus and bowel that moves food through the digestive system is called:
  A. peristalsis.
  B. peritonalsis.
  C. colycystalsis.
  D. duodenalsis.

_____ **114.** Accessory organs in the digestive system include the:
  A. stomach.
  B. pancreas.
  C. small bowel.
  D. rectum.

_____ **115.** The organ responsible for detoxifying the blood, removing damaged erythrocytes, and storing glycogen is the:
  A. liver.
  B. gallbladder.
  C. pancreas.
  D. spleen.

_____ **116.** An abdominal organ that is not an accessory organ of digestion but is part of the immune system is the:
  A. gallbladder.
  B. liver.
  C. pancreas.
  D. spleen.

_____ **117.** The microscopic structure in the kidney that produces urine is called a:
  A. Bowman's capsule.
  B. distal tubule.
  C. glomerulus.
  D. nephron.

_____ **118.** Which of the following is NOT true regarding the kidneys?
  A. Each kidney contains about 1 million nephrons.
  B. The left kidney lies behind the liver, and the right kidney lies behind the spleen.
  C. The kidneys are located in the left and right areas of the small of the back, or flanks.
  D. A healthy kidney in a young adult is about the size of a fist.

HANDOUT 3-3 Continued

_____119. Which of the following is one of the three general processes involved in formation of urine?
  A. glomerular osmosis
  B. secretion
  C. diffusion
  D. refiltration

_____120. The formation and passage of a dilute urine, which decreases blood volume, is called:
  A. hypoosmolarity.
  B. active transport.
  C. facilitated diffusion.
  D. diuresis.

_____121. Which of the following is TRUE regarding glucose and the kidneys?
  A. Glucose is prevented from entering Bowman's capsule and is not filtered.
  B. Glucose begins to be lost in urine when the blood glucose level exceeds about 180 mg/dL.
  C. Normally, glucose is not completely reabsorbed by the time filtrate leaves the proximal tubule.
  D. In uncontrolled diabetes mellitus type I, the body retains glucose and large amounts of water in the osmotic diuresis process.

_____122. A direct indicator of GFR is:
  A. blood urea nitrogen concentration.
  B. blood concentration of renin.
  C. blood concentration of creatinine.
  D. erythropoietin.

_____123. The kidneys regulate systemic arterial blood pressure by the release of:
  A. renin.
  B. creatinine.
  C. urea.
  D. erythropoietin.

_____124. The female external genitalia are known collectively as the:
  A. vagina.
  B. vulva.
  C. perineum.
  D. labia.

_____125. The _____ drains the urinary bladder.
  A. vagina
  B. mons pubis
  C. prepuce
  D. urethra

_____126. The part of the female internal genitalia that provides an outlet for menstrual blood and tissue leaving the body is called the:
  A. vagina.
  B. uterus.
  C. fallopian tube.
  D. urethra.

_____127. The normal site for fetal development is the:
  A. ovaries.
  B. uterus.
  C. urethra.
  D. fallopian tubes.

_____128. The fundus is the:
  A. uppermost portion of the uterus, above where the fallopian tubes connect.
  B. lower portion of the uterus, also called the cervix.
  C. upper two-thirds of the uterus, composed of smooth muscle.
  D. body, or corpus of the uterus.

_____129. The sloughing of the uterine lining is referred to as:
  A. endometriosis.
  B. pelvic inflammatory disease.
  C. the menstrual cycle.
  D. menopause.

_____130. Fertilization of the egg takes place during the:
  A. proliferative phase.
  B. secretory phase.
  C. ischemic phase.
  D. menstrual phase.

HANDOUT 3-4

Student's Name _____

CHAPTER 3 REVIEW

PART 1: THE CELL AND THE CELLULAR ENVIRONMENT

Write the word or words that best complete each sentence in the space(s) provided.

1. The basic structural unit of all plants and animals is the _____.
2. _____ means that a cell membrane allows certain substances, but not all, to pass through.
3. The thick fluid that fills a cell is the _____.
4. Structures that perform specific functions within a cell are called _____.
5. The organelle within a cell that contains the DNA is the _____.
6. _____ _____ is a high-energy compound present in all cells, especially muscle cells.
7. A group of cells that performs a similar function is called _____.
8. _____ tissue is the protective tissue that lines internal and external body surfaces.
9. The most abundant body tissue, providing support, connection, and insulation, is _____ tissue.
10. A group of tissues functioning together is a(n) _____.
11. A group of organs that works together is called a(n) _____ _____.
12. The sum of all the cells, tissues, organs, and organ systems of a living being is called a(n) _____.
13. _____ is the natural tendency of the body to maintain a steady and normal internal environment.
14. The total changes that take place during physiological processes are called _____.
15. A substance that, in water, separates into electrically charged particles is called a(n) _____.
16. Movement of a substance through a cell membrane against the osmotic gradient is called _____ _____.
17. Diffusion of a substance such as glucose through a cell membrane that requires the assistance of a "helper" is called _____ _____.
18. A substance that can crystallize and can diffuse through a membrane is called a(n) _____.
19. The pH is a measure of relative _____ _____ _____ acidity or alkalinity.
20. A pH below 7.35 is referred to as _____.

Handout 3-5

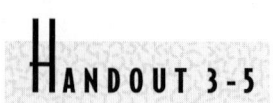

Student's Name _____

CHAPTER 3 REVIEW

PART 2: BODY SYSTEMS

Write the word or words that best complete each sentence in the space(s) provided.

1. The three layers of the skin, beginning with the outermost, are the _____, the _____, and the _____ layers.
2. Collectively, the skin is known as the _____ system.
3. The fatty secretion that helps keep the skin pliable and waterproof is called _____.
4. The organs included in the hematopoietic system are the _____, the _____, and the _____.
5. The cell from which the various types of blood cells can form is called a(n) _____ _____ _____.
6. _____ is the process through which pluripotent stem cells differentiate into various types of blood cells.
7. The hormone responsible for red blood cell production is the _____.
8. Components of blood include _____, which is the liquid part, and the formed elements, _____ _____ _____, _____ _____ _____, and _____.
9. _____ are red blood cells, and _____ are white blood cells.
10. _____ is the oxygen-bearing molecule in the red blood cells.
11. Each complete hemoglobin molecule can carry up to _____ oxygen molecules.
12. 2,3-Diphosphoglycerate is the chemical in red blood cells that affects _____ affinity for _____.
13. _____ is the process of producing red blood cells.
14. _____ is the destruction of red blood cells.
15. The trapping of red blood cells by an organ such as the spleen is called _____.
16. Placing a blood sample in a centrifuge and spinning it at high speed so that the cellular elements separate from the plasma will give you the blood's _____.
17. The process by which white blood cells follow chemical signals to an infection site is called _____.
18. The process in which white blood cells engulf and destroy an invader is called _____.
19. White blood cells are differentiated into three main immature forms known as _____, _____, and _____.
20. White blood cells are categorized as _____, _____, and _____.
21. The three mature forms of granulocytes are _____, _____, and _____.
22. The primary cells involved in the body's immune response are the _____.
23. _____ _____ is the condition in which the body makes antibodies against its own tissue.
24. A nonspecific defense mechanism that wards off damage from microorganisms or trauma is the _____ process.

HANDOUT 3-5 Continued

25. The combined three mechanisms that work to prevent or control blood loss are _____ spasms, _____ plugs, and _____ _____ blood clots.
26. The term for the process in which the body works to prevent or control blood loss is _____.
27. Plasmin dismantles a blood clot by a process known as _____.
28. Clot formation, which is extremely dangerous when it occurs in coronary arteries or cerebral vasculature, is called _____.
29. Functions of the skeleton include giving the body _____ form, protecting _____ _____, allowing for efficient _____, storage of _____ and other materials for metabolism, and producing _____ blood cells.
30. The small perforations of the long bones through which the blood vessels and nerves travel into the bone itself are called _____ canals.
31. A(n) _____ is a cell that helps in the creation of new bone during growth and bone repair.
32. The _____ is the central portion or shaft of a long bone.
33. The _____ is the growth zone of a bone.
34. The tissue within the internal cavity of a bone responsible for manufacture of erythrocytes is the _____ _____ _____.
35. _____ are immovable joints; _____ are joints that allow some very limited movement; and _____, or _____ joints, permit relatively free movement.
36. The three types of diarthroses are the _____, _____, and _____.
37. Movement of a body part toward the midline is called _____. Movement of a body part away from the midline is called _____.
38. The connective tissue that connects bone to bone is a(n) _____.
39. Joints are lubricated by _____ fluid.
40. The axial skeleton consists of the _____, _____, and _____. The appendicular skeleton consists of the bones of the _____, _____ _____, and pelvis (excepting the sacrum).
41. The bone of the proximal upper extremity is the _____, and the bones of the forearm are the _____ and _____.
42. The bones of the wrist are the _____ bones, the bones of the palm are the _____, and the bones of the fingers and toes are the _____.
43. The large bone of the proximal lower extremity is the _____.
44. The pairing of muscles that permits extension and flexion of limbs is called _____.
45. The _____ are the three membranes that surround and protect the brain and spinal cord. They include the _____ mater, the _____ mater, and the _____ membrane.
46. The _____ mater is the tough layer firmly attached to the interior of the skull. The _____ mater is the inner layer covering the convolutions of the brain and spinal cord. The _____ membrane is the middle layer.
47. The part of the brain that is the seat of consciousness and the center of the higher mental functions is the _____.
48. The portion of the brain that plays an important role in the fine control of voluntary muscular movements is the _____.
49. The cerebral hemispheres connect to the spinal cord at the _____.

HANDOUT 3-5 Continued

50. Although the brain accounts for only _____ percent of the body's total weight, it consumes about _____ percent of the body's oxygen.

51. The _____ _____ in the ear sense the motion of the head and provide positional sense for the body.

52. The fluid filling the posterior chamber of the eye is called _____ humor, and the fluid filling the anterior chamber of the eye is called _____ humor.

53. The fluid that lubricates the eye is called _____ fluid.

54. The major blood vessels traversing the neck are the _____ arteries and the _____ veins.

55. The vertebral column is made up of _____ bones.

56. The short column of bone that forms the weight-bearing portion of a vertebra is called the _____ _____.

57. The opening in the vertebrae that accommodates the spinal cord is called the _____ _____.

58. The thick, bony struts that connect the vertebral bodies with the spinous and transverse processes are called _____.

59. _____ are the posterior bones of the vertebra that help make up the foramen of the spinal canal.

60. The bony outgrowth of the vertebral pedicle that serves as a site for muscle attachment and articulation with the ribs is called the _____ process.

61. The prominence at the posterior part of a vertebra is the _____ process.

62. The cartilaginous pad between vertebrae that serves as a shock absorber is called the _____ _____.

63. The divisions of the vertebral column are the _____, _____, _____, _____, and _____ spines.

64. The _____ _____ are similar to those covering and protecting the structures within the cranium.

65. The greatest spacing between the spinal cord and the interior of the vertebral column is found in the _____ _____ and _____ _____ regions.

66. The thoracic skeleton is defined by _____ pairs of C-shaped ribs.

67. The union between the xiphoid process and the body of the sternum is called the _____ _____.

68. The muscular, dome-like structure that separates the abdominal cavity from the thoracic cavity is the _____.

69. The _____ _____ is the central medial region of the lung where the bronchi and pulmonary vasculature enter the lung.

70. The lungs are covered by the _____ _____, a smooth membrane that lines the exterior of the lungs.

71. The central nervous system is made up of the _____ and _____ _____.

72. The _____ nervous system extends throughout the body.

73. Voluntary bodily functions are controlled by the _____ nervous system.

74. The _____ nervous system controls involuntary bodily functions.

75. The _____ nervous system is the division of the autonomic nervous system that prepares the body for stressful situations.

HANDOUT 3-5 Continued

76. The _____ nervous system is the division of the autonomic nervous system that controls vegetative functions.
77. A(n) _____ is a substance that is released from the axon terminal of a presynaptic neuron upon excitation.
78. The membranes covering and protecting the brain and spinal cord are called the _____.
79. The portion of the brain lying beneath the cerebrum and above the brainstem is called the _____.
80. The _____ _____ is the lower portion of the brainstem, connecting the pons and the spinal cord. It contains major centers for control of _____, _____, and _____ activity.
81. The system responsible for consciousness is the _____ _____ system.
82. There are 12 pairs of _____ nerves that extend from the lower surface of the brain.
83. The _____ nervous system is often referred to as the "fight-or-flight" system, and the _____ nervous system is referred to as the "feed-and-breed" system.
84. Oxytocin, which stimulates uterine contractions and milk release, is produced by the _____ gland.
85. The _____ gland controls blood calcium levels.
86. Located in the neck, the _____ gland stimulates cell metabolism.
87. The adrenal gland produces the hormones _____ and _____.
88. Located in the upper retroperitoneum, the _____ produces insulin.
89. The _____ gland stimulates increased reabsorption of water into blood volume.
90. The _____ gland stimulates body growth in childhood.
91. Glucagon is a hormone produced by the _____.
92. The _____ in the male and the _____ in the female stimulate development of secondary sexual characteristics.
93. The "fight-or-flight" response to stress is stimulated by the _____ _____.
94. The _____ gland is in the mediastinum just behind the sternum.
95. The paired _____ glands are located on the superior surface of the kidneys.
96. The heart consists of three tissue layers: the _____, _____, and _____.
97. The two superior chambers of the heart are the _____. The larger, inferior chambers are the _____.
98. The heart contains two pairs of valves, the _____ valves and the _____ valves.
99. The _____ _____ _____ receives deoxygenated blood from the head and upper extremities. The _____ _____ _____ receives blood from the areas below the heart.
100. The only veins in the body that carry oxygenated blood are the _____ veins.
101. The term _____ refers to communication between two or more blood vessels.
102. The period of time from the end of one cardiac contraction to the end of the next is called the _____ _____.
103. The period of time when the myocardium is relaxed and cardiac filling and coronary perfusion occur is called _____.

HANDOUT 3-5 Continued

104. _____ is the period of the cardiac cycle when the myocardium is contracting.
105. The ratio of blood pumped from the ventricle to the amount of blood remaining at end of diastole is called the _____ _____.
106. The term _____ refers to the pressure within the ventricles at the end of diastole.
107. The term _____ refers to the resistance against which the heart must pump.
108. The amount of blood pumped by the heart in one minute is called the _____ _____.
109. The term _____ _____ refers to the amount of blood ejected by the heart in one cardiac contraction.
110. The term "chronotropy" pertains to heart _____.
111. The term "inotropy" pertains to cardiac _____ _____.
112. The term _____ pertains to the speed of impulse transmission.
113. A reversal of charges at a cell membrane so that the inside of the cell becomes positive in relation to the outside is called cardiac _____.
114. The normal electrical state of cells is called _____ _____.
115. The stimulation of myocardial cells that subsequently spreads across the myocardium is called the _____ _____.
116. The return of a muscle cell to its pre-excitation resting state is called _____.
117. The term _____ pertains to cells being able to respond to an electrical stimulus.
118. The term _____ pertains to cells being able to propagate the electrical impulse from one cell to another.
119. The pacemaker cells' capability of self-depolarization is called _____.
120. The supplying of oxygen and nutrients to the body tissues as a result of the constant passage of blood through the capillaries is called _____.
121. Inadequate perfusion of the body tissues is known as _____ or _____.
122. The circulatory system consists of three components: the _____ (_____), the _____ (_____), and the _____ (_____ _____).
123. The amount of blood delivered to the heart during diastole is called _____.
124. The strength of a contraction of the heart is called _____ _____ _____.
125. Epinephrine and norepinephrine are _____.
126. The upper airway extends from the mouth and nose to the _____.
127. The exchange of gases between a living organism and its environment is referred to as _____.
128. The lining in body cavities that handles air transport, usually containing small mucus-secreting cells, is called _____ _____.
129. _____ maneuver is pressure applied in a posterior direction to the anterior cricoid cartilage, occluding the esophagus.
130. _____ are the microscopic air sacs where most oxygen and carbon dioxide gas exchanges take place.
131. The term _____ means alveolar collapse.
132. The pressure exerted by each component of a gas mixture is called _____ _____.
133. The abbreviation for alveolar partial pressure is _____.

HANDOUT 3-5 Continued

134. The abbreviation for arterial partial pressure is _____.
135. FiO$_2$ is the FiO$_2$ concentration of _____ in inspired air.
136. Fever, muscle exertion, shivering, and metabolic processes may cause increased _____ production.
137. The mechanism that increases respiratory stimulation when PaO$_2$ falls is called _____ _____.
138. The abdominal cavity is divided into three spaces. The division containing those organs or portions of organs covered by the peritoneum is called the _____ space.
139. The division containing those organs posterior to the peritoneal lining is called the _____ space.
140. The division containing those organs located within the pelvis is the _____ space.
141. The abdomen is divided into four subregions by vertical and horizontal lines. The gallbladder, most of the liver, and a small portion of the pancreas are located in the _____ _____ quadrant.
142. The stomach, spleen, most of the pancreas, and transverse and descending colon are located in _____ _____ the quadrant.
143. The appendix and portions of the ascending colon, rectum, and female genitalia are located in _____ _____ the quadrant.
144. The sigmoid colon and portions of the urinary bladder, small bowel, descending colon, and rectum are located in the _____ _____ quadrant.
145. The _____ _____ is the internal passageway that begins at the mouth and ends at the anus.
146. _____ is the semifluid mixture of ingested food and digestive secretions found in the stomach and small intestine.
147. The wavelike muscular motion of the esophagus and bowel that moves food through the digestive system is called _____.
148. The three accessory organs to the digestive system are the _____, the _____, and the _____.
149. The abdominal aorta bifurcates into two large _____ arteries.
150. Fine fibrous tissue surrounding the interior of most of the abdominal cavity and covering most of the small bowel and some of the abdominal organs is called the _____.
151. The double fold of peritoneum that supports the major portion of the small bowel, suspending it from the posterior abdominal wall, is called the _____.
152. The microscopic structure within the kidney that produces urine is the _____.
153. The removal from blood of water and other elements, which enter the nephron tubule, is called _____ _____; the movement of a substance from a tubule back into the blood is called _____.
154. _____ _____ is the random motion of molecules from an area of high concentration to an area of lower concentration, while _____ _____ is a molecule-specific carrier in a cell membrane speeding the molecule's movement from a region of higher concentration to one of lower concentration.
155. _____ is the formation and passage of dilute urine, decreasing blood volume, while _____ is the formation and passage of a concentrated urine, preserving blood volume.

HANDOUT 3-5 Continued

156. The female external genitalia are known collectively as the _____, or the _____.

157. The _____ is a roughly diamond-shaped, skin-covered muscular tissue that separates the vagina from the anus.

158. The structures that protect the vagina and the urethra are the _____.

159. Although not truly a part of the female reproductive system, the _____ drains the urinary bladder.

160. The _____ is the female organ of copulation, forms the final passageway for the infant during childbirth, and provides an outlet for menstrual blood to leave the body.

161. The primary function of the _____ is to provide a site for fetal development.

162. The _____ is the uppermost portion of the uterus.

163. The fundal _____, measured in centimeters, is generally comparable to the _____ of gestation.

164. The inner layer of the uterine wall where the fertilized egg implants is called the _____.

165. The term _____ refers to the onset of menses, usually occurring between ages 10 and 14 years.

166. The _____ are the primary female gonads, or sex organs.

167. The function of the _____ _____ is to conduct the egg from the space around the ovaries into the uterine cavity.

168. The female sex hormones _____ and _____ control the ovarian-menstrual cycle, pregnancy, and lactation.

169. During the _____ phase of the menstrual cycle, the uterine lining thickens and becomes engorged with blood.

170. During the _____ phase, the ischemic endometrium is shed, along with a discharge of blood, mucus, and cellular debris.

171. The cessation of menses and ovarian function due to decreased secretion of estrogen is called _____.

172. The _____ is the small sac in which sperm cells are stored.

173. The _____ _____ is the duct that carries sperm cells to the urethra for ejaculation.

174. The _____ _____ is the gland that surrounds the male urinary bladder neck and is a major source of the fluid that combines with sperm to form semen.

175. The _____ are the primary male reproductive organs.

HANDOUT 3-6

Student's Name _____

COMPLETION

THE ROOT *CYT*

Fill in each blank with the appropriate word that includes the root "cyt," or cell.

1. _____ thick fluid that fills a cell
2. _____ clear liquid portion of the thick fluid that fills a cell
3. _____ structure of protein filaments that supports the internal structure of a cell
4. _____ red blood cell
5. _____ white blood cell
6. _____ blood cell responsible for clotting; also called a platelet
7. _____ a type of white blood cell that attacks foreign substances as part of the body's immune system
8. _____ a cell that has the ability to ingest other cells and substances such as bacteria and cell debris
9. _____ ingestion and digestion of bacteria and other substances by certain cells
10. _____ white blood cell with a single nucleus; the largest normal blood cell
11. _____ white blood cell with multiple nuclei that has the appearance of a bag of granules
12. _____ protein produced by a white blood cell that instructs neighboring cells to respond in a genetically preprogrammed fashion
13. _____ substance that is poisonous to cells
14. _____ poisonous (toxic) to cells

Handout 3-7

Student's Name _____

CHEMICAL NOTATION

Write the appropriate name of the element next to each chemical notation below.

1. H _____
2. O _____
3. C _____
4. N _____
5. Ca _____
6. Cl _____
7. Na _____
8. NaCl _____
9. H_2O _____
10. H_2CO_3 _____
11. Na^+ _____
12. K^+ _____
13. Ca^{++} _____
14. Mg^{++} _____
15. Cl^- _____
16. HCO_3^- _____
17. HPO_4^- _____

HANDOUT 3-8

Student's Name _____

ABDOMINAL MATCHING

Write the letter of the term in the space provided next to the appropriate description.

A. peritoneal space
B. retroperitoneal space
C. pelvic space
D. digestive tract
E. chyme
F. peristalsis
G. liver
H. pancreas
I. spleen
J. gallbladder
K. right upper quadrant
L. inferior vena cava
M. peritoneum
N. mesentery
O. left upper quadrant
P. right lower quadrant

_____ 1. Wavelike muscular motion of the esophagus and bowel that moves food through the digestive system.

_____ 2. The fine fibrous tissue surrounding the interior of most of the abdominal cavity and covering most of the small bowel and some of the abdominal organs.

_____ 3. Division of the abdominal cavity containing those organs posterior to the peritoneal lining.

_____ 4. Semifluid mixture of ingested food and digestive secretions found in the stomach and small intestine.

_____ 5. Double fold of peritoneum that supports the major portion of the small bowel, suspending it from the posterior abdominal wall.

_____ 6. A part of the immune system; the organ that performs some immunological functions and stores a large volume of blood.

_____ 7. Division of the abdominal cavity containing those organs located within the pelvis.

_____ 8. Internal passageway that begins at the mouth and ends at the anus.

_____ 9. The abdominal quadrant that contains the gallbladder, right kidney, most of the liver, some small bowel, a portion of the ascending and transverse colon, and a small portion of the pancreas.

_____ 10. The division of the abdominal cavity containing those organs or portions of organs covered by the peritoneum.

_____ 11. The small, hollow organ that receives bile from the liver and stores it until it is needed.

_____ 12. The abdominal quadrant that contains the stomach, spleen, left kidney, most of the pancreas, and a portion of the liver, small bowel, and transverse and descending colon.

_____ 13. The accessory organ of the digestive system responsible for detoxifying the blood, removing damaged or aged erythrocytes, and storing glycogen.

HANDOUT 3-8 Continued

_____ 14. The accessory organ of the digestive system responsible for the production of glucagon and insulin.

_____ 15. Located along the spinal column, it collects venous blood from the lower extremities and the abdomen, returning it to the heart.

_____ 16. The abdominal quadrant that contains the appendix and portions of the urinary bladder, small bowel, ascending colon, rectum, and female genitalia.

HANDOUT 3-9

Student's Name _____

ANATOMY OF THE KIDNEY

Write the letter of the term in the space provided next to the appropriate description.

A. hilum
B. cortex
C. medulla
D. pyramid
E. renal pelvis
F. glomerulus
G. papilla
H. Bowman's capsule
I. proximal tubule
J. descending loop of Henle
K. ascending loop of Henle
L. distal tubule
M. collecting tubule
N. collecting duct

_____ 1. The part of the tubule beyond Bowman's capsule.

_____ 2. The visible tissue structures within medulla of kidney.

_____ 3. The part of the tubule beyond the ascending loop of Henle.

_____ 4. The notched part of the kidney where the ureter and other structures join kidney tissue.

_____ 5. A part of the tubule beyond the distal tubule.

_____ 6. The part of the tubule beyond the proximal tubule.

_____ 7. The hollow, cup-shaped first part of the nephron tubule.

_____ 8. The outer tissue of the kidney.

_____ 9. The tip of the pyramid that juts into the hollow space of the kidney.

_____ 10. The part of the tubule beyond the descending loop of Henle.

_____ 11. A tuft of capillaries from which blood is filtered into a nephron.

_____ 12. The inner tissue of the kidney.

_____ 13. The hollow space of the kidney that junctions with a ureter.

_____ 14. The larger structure beyond a collecting tubule into which urine drips.

HANDOUT 3-10

Student's Name _____

UNDERSTANDING FEMALE REPRODUCTIVE ANATOMY

Write the name of each part of the female reproductive system indicated on the illustration below in the spaces provided.

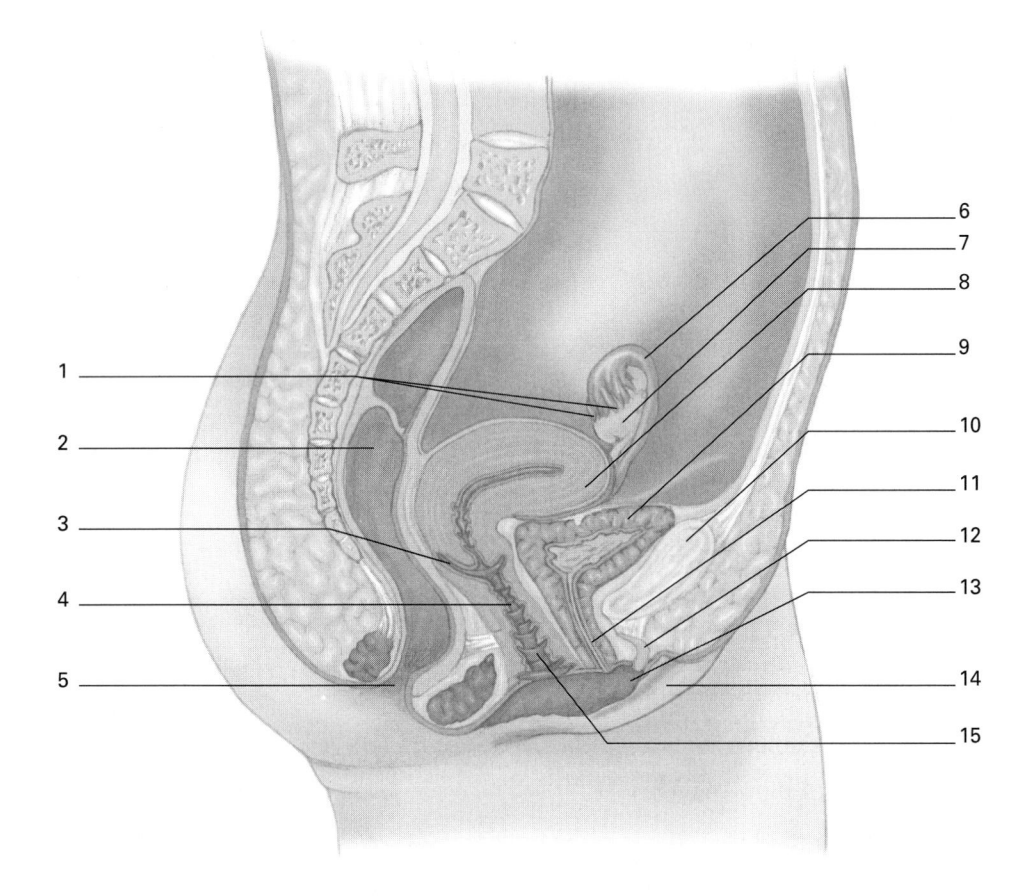

1. _____
2. _____
3. _____
4. _____
5. _____
6. _____
7. _____
8. _____
9. _____
10. _____
11. _____
12. _____
13. _____
14. _____
15. _____

144 ESSENTIALS OF PARAMEDIC CARE

Chapter 3 Answer Key

Handout 3-2: Part 1: The Cell and the Cellular Environment—Quiz

1. A
2. B
3. C
4. D
5. A
6. B
7. C
8. B
9. A
10. B
11. C
12. B
13. B
14. A
15. D
16. C
17. A
18. B
19. C
20. D
21. B
22. B
23. A
24. C
25. A

Handout 3-3: PART 2: Body Systems—Quiz

1. A
2. A
3. C
4. B
5. D
6. C
7. C
8. D
9. A
10. A
11. D
12. A
13. D
14. B
15. B
16. D
17. B
18. C
19. B
20. C
21. D
22. B
23. A
24. C
25. A
26. A
27. C
28. B
29. C
30. D
31. B
32. C
33. C
34. B
35. B
36. D
37. C
38. A
39. C
40. D
41. B
42. D
43. A
44. A
45. B
46. C
47. B
48. B
49. C
50. B
51. C
52. A
53. B
54. D
55. D
56. C
57. B
58. C
59. D
60. D
61. D
62. A
63. C
64. A
65. A
66. A
67. B
68. B
69. A
70. D
71. D
72. C
73. A
74. C
75. B
76. C
77. B
78. A
79. C
80. B
81. C
82. C
83. A
84. B
85. B
86. D
87. B
88. A
89. C
90. A
91. C
92. D
93. C
94. C
95. D
96. C
97. A
98. A
99. B
100. B
101. C
102. D
103. A
104. A
105. D
106. D
107. A
108. C
109. A
110. C
111. A
112. B
113. A
114. B
115. A
116. D
117. D
118. B
119. B
120. D
121. B
122. C
123. A
124. B
125. D
126. A
127. B
128. A
129. C
130. A

Handout 3-4: Part 1: The Cell and the Cellular Environment—Review

1. cell
2. Semipermeable
3. cytoplasm
4. organelles
5. nucleus
6. Adenosine triphosphate
7. tissue
8. Epithelial
9. connective
10. organ
11. organ system
12. organism
13. Homeostasis
14. metabolism
15. electrolyte
16. active transport
17. facilitated diffusion
18. crystalloid
19. potential of hydrogen
20. acidosis

Handout 3-5: Part 2: Body Systems—Review

1. epidermis, dermis, subcutaneous
2. integumentary
3. sebum
4. liver, spleen, kidneys
5. pluripotent stem cell
6. Hematopoesis
7. erythropoietin
8. plasma, red blood cells, white blood cells, platelets
9. Erythrocytes, leukocytes
10. Hemoglobin
11. four
12. hemoglobin's, oxygen
13. Erythropoiesis
14. Hemolysis
15. sequestration
16. hematocrit
17. chemotaxis
18. phagocytosis
19. myeloblasts, monoblasts, lymphoblasts
20. granulocytes, monocytes, lymphocytes
21. basophils, eosinophils, neutrophils
22. lymphocytes
23. Autoimmune disease
24. inflammatory
25. vascular, platelet, stable fibrin
26. hemostasis
27. fibrinolysis
28. thrombosis
29. structural, vital organs, movement, salts, red
30. haversian
31. osteoblast
32. diaphysis
33. metaphysis
34. red bone marrow
35. Synarthroses, amphiarthroses, diathroses, synovial
36. monaxial, biaxial, triaxial
37. adduction, abduction
38. ligament
39. synovial
40. head, thorax, spine, extremities, shoulder girdle
41. humerus, radius, ulna
42. carpal, metacarpals, phalanges
43. femur
44. opposition
45. meninges, dura, pia, arachnoid
46. dura, pia, arachnoid
47. cerebrum
48. cerebellum
49. brainstem
50. 2, 20
51. semicircular canals
52. vitreous, aqueous
53. lacrimal

54. carotid, jugular
55. 33
56. vertebral body
57. spinal canal
58. pedicles
59. Laminae
60. transverse
61. spinous
62. intervertebral disk
63. cervical, thoracic, lumbar, sacral, coccygeal
64. spinal meninges
65. upper lumbar, upper cervical
66. 12
67. xiphisternal joint
68. diaphragm
69. pulmonary hilum
70. visceral pleura
71. brain, spinal cord
72. peripheral
73. somatic
74. autonomic
75. sympathetic
76. parasympathetic
77. neurotransmitter
78. meninges
79. diencephalon
80. medulla oblongata, respiratory, cardiac, vasomotor
81. reticular activating
82. cranial
83. sympathetic, parasympathetic
84. pituitary
85. parathyroid
86. thyroid
87. epinephrine, norepinephrine
88. pancreas
89. pituitary
90. pituitary
91. pancreas
92. testes, ovaries
93. adrenal medulla
94. thymus
95. adrenal
96. endocardium, myocardium, pericardium
97. atria, ventricles
98. atrioventricular, semilunar
99. superior vena cava, inferior vena cava
100. pulmonary
101. anastomosis
102. cardiac cycle
103. diastole
104. Systole
105. ejection fraction
106. preload
107. afterload
108. cardiac output
109. stroke volume
110. rate
111. contractile force
112. dromotropy
113. depolarization
114. resting potential
115. action potential
116. repolarization
117. excitability
118. conductivity
119. automaticity
120. perfusion
121. hypoperfusion, shock
122. pump (heart), fluid (blood), container (blood vessels)
123. preload
124. cardiac contractile force
125. catecholamines
126. larynx
127. respiration
128. mucous membrane
129. Sellick's
130. Alveoli
131. atelectasis
132. partial pressure
133. PA
134. Pa
135. oxygen
136. CO_2
137. hypoxic drive
138. peritoneal
139. retroperitoneal
140. pelvic
141. right upper
142. left upper
143. right lower
144. left lower
145. digestive tract
146. Chyme
147. peristalsis
148. liver, gallbladder, pancrease
149. iliac
150. peritoneum
151. mesentery
152. nephron
153. glomerular filtration, reabsorption
154. Simple diffusion, facilitated diffusion
155. Diuresis, antidiuresis
156. vulva, pudendum
157. perineum
158. labia
159. urethra
160. vagina
161. uterus
162. fundus
163. height, weeks
164. endometrium
165. menarche
166. ovaries
167. fallopian tubes
168. estrogen, progesterone
169. proliferative
170. menstrual
171. menopause
172. epididymis
173. vas deferens
174. prostate gland
175. testes

Handout 3-6: Completion

1. cytoplasm
2. cytosol
3. cytoskeleton
4. erythrocyte
5. leukocyte
6. thrombocyte
7. lymphocyte
8. phagocyte
9. phagocytosis
10. monocyte
11. granulocyte

12. cytokine
13. cytotoxin
14. cytotoxic

Handout 3-7: Chemical Notation

1. hydrogen
2. oxygen
3. carbon
4. nitrogen
5. calcium
6. chlorine
7. sodium
8. sodium chloride
9. water
10. carbonic acid
11. sodium cation
12. potassium cation
13. calcium cation
14. magnesium cation
15. chloride anion
16. bicarbonate
17. phosphate

Handout 3-8: Abdominal Matching

1. F	5. N	9. K	13. G
2. M	6. I	10. A	14. H
3. B	7. C	11. J	15. L
4. E	8. D	12. O	16. P

Handout 3-9: Anatomy of the Kidney

1. I	5. M	9. G	13. E
2. D	6. J	10. K	14. N
3. L	7. H	11. F	
4. A	8. B	12. C	

Handout 3-10: Understanding Female Reproductive Anatomy

1. fimbriae of fallopian tube
2. rectum
3. cervix of uterus
4. vagina
5. anus
6. fallopian tube
7. ovary
8. uterus
9. urinary bladder
10. symphysis pubis
11. urethra
12. clitoris
13. labium major
14. labium minor
15. vaginal orifice

Chapter 4

General Principles of Pathophysiology

INTRODUCTION

In the study of all aspects of emergency medical care, students must learn what is normal before they can detect abnormalities. They must also understand basic human physiology (how the body functions under normal conditions) to aid them in the assessment of patients. This knowledge will enable them to distinguish changes in the body's functions in the presence of pathophysiology (disease or injury). When the ongoing activity that supports life is disturbed, the body seeks to compensate for it. If the body is unable to compensate, a variety of medical problems and emergencies can ensue. This chapter will discuss the probable causes of common assessment findings and help you choose effective treatments.

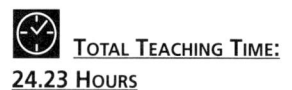

TOTAL TEACHING TIME: 24.23 HOURS

The total teaching time is only a guideline based on the didactic and practical lab averages in the National Standard Curriculum. Instructors should take into consideration such factors as the pace at which students learn, the size of the class, and breaks. The actual time devoted to teaching objectives is the responsibility of the instructor.

CHAPTER OBJECTIVES

Part 1: How Normal Body Processes Are Altered by Disease and Injury (p. 241)

After reading Part 1 of this chapter, you should be able to:

1. Discuss cellular adaptation, injury, and death. (pp. 241–246)
2. Discuss factors that precipitate disease in the human body. (pp. 246–251)
3. Analyze disease risk. (pp. 252–257)
4. Describe environmental risk factors and combined effects and interaction among risk factors. (pp. 252–257)
5. Discuss familial diseases and associated risk factors. (pp. 254–257)
6. Discuss hypoperfusion. (pp. 257–261)
7. Define cardiogenic, hypovolemic, neurogenic, anaphylactic, and septic shock. (pp. 261–265)
8. Describe multiple organ dysfunction syndrome. (pp. 265–267)

Part 2: The Body's Defenses Against Disease and Injury (pp. 268–290)

After reading Part 2 of this chapter, you should be able to:

1. Define the characteristics of the immune response. (pp. 271–273)
2. Discuss induction of the immune system. (pp. 272–273)
3. Describe the inflammation response and its systemic manifestations. (pp. 273–279)
4. Discuss the role of mast cells, the plasma protein system, and cellular components plus resolution and repair as part of the inflammation response. (pp. 274–279)
5. Discuss hypersensitivity. (pp. 279–280)
6. Describe deficiencies in immunity and inflammation. (pp. 280–282)
7. Describe homeostasis as a dynamic steady state. (p. 283)
8. Describe neuroendocrine regulation. (pp. 284–286)
9. Discuss the interrelationships between stress, coping, and illness. (pp. 286–288)

FRAMING THE LESSON

Begin the class by reviewing the important points from Chapter 3, "Anatomy and Physiology." Discuss any aspects of the chapter not understood by students. Then go on to Chapter 4. Before class, obtain copies of a standard personal and family history form for patient admissions used by local physicians, PAs, clinics, or hospitals. At the beginning of class, distribute the history forms and have students pair up. In each group, have students perform a history on their partner and the partner's family, as accurately as possible. List history of illnesses, including childhood diseases, immunizations, and vaccines. Also include the presence of any risk factors such as smoking or hazardous occupations. Have students refer to these completed histories during the discussion of family history and associated risk factors.

TEACHING STRATEGIES

People learn in a variety of ways. Some do better with the spoken word, whereas others prefer the written. Some prefer to work alone, whereas others profit from working in groups. Recognizing these different ways of acquiring knowledge, the authors of this *Instructor's Resource Manual* have provided a variety of teaching strategies for the different types of learners. These strategies are intended to foster higher-level cognitive skills and encourage creative learning and problem solving. For greatest effectiveness, incorporate these strategies into your class lecture. Symbols in the Lecture Outline indicate the points at which various exercises might be most appropriate. Other strategies can be used to preview the lesson or to summarize it.

The following strategies are keyed to specific sections of the lesson.

1. ***Total Body Fluid Demonstration.*** Use a juicing machine (juice extractor) to graphically demonstrate the amount of fluid contained in the human body, as well as other forms of life. During the class session before the one covering Chapter 4, assign students to bring in various fruits and vegetables. Use the juicing machine to extract the fluid content, or juice, from each of the fruits and vegetables. Allow students to compare the amounts of fluids and amounts of solids

that result. Correlate the fluid content of these items and the 65-percent water content of the average adult human.

2. Blood Bank Guest Speaker. Arrange to have a representative from a local blood bank or the American Red Cross visit the class to speak about blood typing and blood products.

3. Allergy Round Robin. Have each student write a list of 10 things that can cause an allergic/anaphylactic reaction. For each item on their lists, students should indicate the antigen's most probable route to enter the body. They should also indicate what they think would be the speed and severity of reaction. Finally, they might also list each item's most likely initial signs and symptoms (for example, drug reactions usually initially present as a rash, bee stings as redness and swelling around the sting site). After the students have completed their lists, call on class members in random order and have each present one item. As the presentations are made, reinforce the pathophysiology of an allergic reaction, the effects on various body systems, and the management of anaphylaxis. Listing items presented by students on the board might help to prevent duplication. Continue to call on students until they have no new items for the list.

4. Stress and Disease Guest Speaker. Invite a psychiatrist or other mental health professional to discuss the connection between stress and disease. This would also be a good time to bring in a representative from your local, regional, or state critical incident stress management team, if you did not already do so during the discussion of Chapter 1.

The following strategy can be used at various points throughout the lesson or to help summarize and demonstrate what students have learned.

Cultural considerations, legal notes, and patho pearls. The Student CD-ROM contains this series of informative features to enhance the student's understanding of the material covered in this chapter.

TEACHING OUTLINE

HANDOUT 4-1
Chapter 4 Objectives Checklist

Chapter 4, "General Principles of Pathophysiology," is the fourth lesson in Division 1, *Introduction to Advanced Prehospital Care*. Distribute Handout 4-1 so that students can familiarize themselves with the learning goals for this chapter. If students have any questions about the objectives, answer them at this time.

Then present the chapter. One possible lecture outline follows. In the outline, the parenthetical references in regular type are references to text pages; those in bold type are references to figures or tables.

I. Introduction. Paramedics who have a basic understanding of human physiology (how the body functions under normal conditions) and pathophysiology (how the body functions in the presence of disease or injury) will have a better understanding of the probable causes of common assessment findings and, consequently, will be better able to choose appropriate and effective treatments. (p. 240)

PART 1: HOW NORMAL BODY PROCESSES ARE ALTERED BY DISEASE AND INJURY

I. Pathophysiology (p. 241)

A. Pathology(p. 241)
    1. Study of disease and its causes

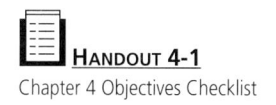

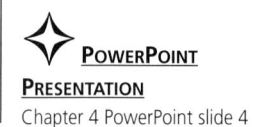

POWERPOINT
PRESENTATION
Chapter 4 PowerPoint slide 4

POWERPOINT PRESENTATION
Chapter 4 PowerPoint slides 5–16

B. Pathophysiology (p. 241)
  1. Study of how diseases alter normal physiology

II. How cells respond to change and injury. The body tends to maintain a constantly balanced environment and to adapt (i.e., correct or compensate) for any change that upsets the balance. (pp. 241–246)

  A. Cellular adaptation (pp. 241–243)
   1. Atrophy
      a. Decrease in cell size and increase in efficiency
   2. Hypertrophy
      a. Increase in cell size resulting from increased workload
   3. Hyperplasia
      a. Increase in number of cells resulting from increased workload
   4. Metaplasia
      a. Replacement of one type of cell by another type that is not normal for a particular tissue
   5. Dysplasia
      a. Change in cell size, shape, or appearance caused by external stressor
  B. Cellular injury (pp. 243–246)
   1. Hypoxic injury
      a. Due to oxygen deficiency
   2. Chemical injury
   3. Infectious injury
      a. Pathogens
      b. Possible outcomes
         i. Pathogen wins.
         ii. Pathogen and body battle to a draw.
         iii. Body defeats pathogen.
   4. Immunologic/inflammatory injury
   5. Injurious physical agents
   6. Injurious nutritional imbalances
   7. Injurious genetic factors
   8. Manifestations of cellular injury
      a. Anabolism
      b. Catabolism
      c. Cellular swelling
      d. Fatty change
  C. Cellular death: apoptosis and necrosis (p. 246)
   1. Apoptosis ("falling apart")
   2. Necrosis ("cell death")
      a. Coagulative
      b. Liquefactive
      c. Caseous
      d. Fatty
   3. Gangrenous necrosis
      a. Dry gangrene
      b. Wet gangrene
      c. Gas gangrene

POINT OF INTEREST
An adult needs about 1.5 to 2.0 quarts of water each day. The average person in an industrialized Western country eats about 30 tons of food in a lifetime.

TEACHING STRATEGY 1
Total Body Fluid Demonstration

TEACHING STRATEGY 2
Blood Bank Guest Speaker

POWERPOINT PRESENTATION
Chapter 4 PowerPoint slides 17–37

III. Fluids and fluid imbalances. Many pathological conditions, both medical and traumatic, adversely affect the fluid and electrolyte balance of the body. (pp. 246–250)

  A. Water (p. 246)
   1. Total body water (TBW)

2. Body fluid compartments
　　　a. Intracellular fluid
　　　　i. Fluid within body cells
　　　　ii. 75 percent of all body water
　　　b. Extracellular fluid
　　　　i. All fluid outside the body cells
　　　　ii. Intravascular fluid
　　　　iii. Interstitial fluid
B. Edema (p. 247)
　1. Accumulation of water in the interstitial space
　　a. Decrease in plasma oncotic force
　　b. Increased hypostatic pressure
　　c. Increased capillary permeability
　　d. Lymphatic channel obstruction
C. Intravenous therapy (pp. 247–250)
　1. Blood and blood components (**Fig. 4-1, p. 247**)
　　a. Plasma
　　　i. Liquid portion of blood
　　b. Formed elements
　　　i. Cellular portion of blood
　　　ii. Erythrocytes
　　　　a) Hemoglogin
　　　　b) Hematocrit
　　　　　1. Percentage of blood occupied by erythrocytes (**Fig. 4-2, p. 248**)
　　　iii. Leukocytes
　　　iv. Thrombocytes
　2. Fluid replacement (**Table 4-1, p. 249**)
　3. Transfusion reaction
　　a. Blood types
　　b. Rh types
　4. Intravenous fluids
　　a. Hemoglobin-Based Oxygen-Carrying Solutions (HBOCs)
　　　i. Compatible with all blood types
　　　ii. Do not require blood typing, testing, or cross-matching
　　　iii. PolyHeme
　　　iv. Hemopur
　　b. Colloids
　　　i. Substances consisting of large molecules or molecule aggregates that disperse evenly within a liquid without forming a true solution
　　　ii. Plasma protein fraction (albumin)
　　　iii. Salt poor albumin
　　　iv. Dextran
　　　v. Hetastarch
　　c. Crystalloids
　　　i. Substances capable of crystallization; in solution, can diffuse through a membrane (**Fig. 4-3, p. 250**)
　　　ii. Isotonic solutions
　　　　a) Normal saline
　　　　b) Lactated Ringers
　　　iii. Hypertonic solutions
　　　　a) Plasmanate
　　　　b) Dextran
　　　iv. Hypotonic solutions
　　　　a) D_5W (5 percent dextrose in water)

POINT TO EMPHASIZE
IVs started in the field cause more complications than those started in the hospital. Pay attention to aseptic technique.

TEACHING TIP
If possible, bring in a tube of blood from the emergency department and allow the red cells to settle. Nothing illustrates hematocrit better.

POINT OF INTEREST
About 2.5 million red blood cells die every second, but they are replaced just as quickly.

POINT TO EMPHASIZE
Blood products are only good for 21 days, while fresh frozen plasma is good for 6 months.

POINT TO EMPHASIZE
D_5W rapidly diffuses into the tissues; up to two thirds of normal saline and lactated Ringer's are lost to interstitial space within the first hour.

POWERPOINT PRESENTATION
Chapter 4 PowerPoint slides 38–43

POINT TO EMPHASIZE
As acid increases, bodily function decreases.

POWERPOINT PRESENTATION
Chapter 4 PowerPoint slides 44–61

IV. Acid-base derangements. Acid-base balance is a dynamic relationship that reflects the relative concentration of hydrogen ions (H^+) in the body. (pp. 250–252)

A. Acidosis and alkalosis (pp. 250–252)
　1. Respiratory acidosis
　　a. Caused by retention of CO_2
　2. Respiratory alkalosis
　　a. Caused by increased respiration and excessive elimination of CO_2
　3. Metabolic alkalosis
　　a. Alkalinity resulting from diuresis, vomiting, or overconsumption of sodium bicarbonate
　4. Metabolic acidosis
　　a. Acidity resulting from vomiting, diarrhea, diabetes, or medication (Fig. 4-4, p. 252)

V. Genetics and other causes of disease. Many diseases result from genetic causes, which are far more difficult to identify and treat than diseases that result from infections. (pp. 252–257)

A. Genetics, environment, lifestyle, age, and gender as causes of disease (pp. 252–253)
　1. DNA
　2. Multifactorial disorders
　　a. Genetics and environment
　3. Clinical factors
　　a. Effects on individuals
　　b. Effects on populations
　4. Epidemiological factors
　　a. Incidence
　　b. Prevalence
　　c. Mortality
B. Family history and associated risk factors (pp. 254–257)
　1. Immunologic disorders
　　a. Rheumatic fever
　　b. Allergies
　　c. Asthma
　2. Cancer
　3. Endocrine disorders
　　a. Type I diabetes
　　b. Type II diabetes
　4. Hematologic disorders
　　a. Hemophilia
　　b. Hemochromatosis
　　c. Anemia
　5. Cardiovascular disorders
　　a. Coronary artery disease
　　b. Hypertension
　6. Renal disorders
　7. Rheumatic disorders
　8. Gastrointestinal disorders
　　a. Crohn's disease
　　b. Peptic ulcers
　　c. Cholecystitis
　　d. Obesity

9. Neuromuscular disorders
    a. Multiple sclerosis
    b. Alzheimer's disease
10. Psychiatric disorders

VI. Hypoperfusion. Hypoperfusion is progressive and fatal if not corrected. (pp. 257–267)
  A. The pathophysiology of hypoperfusion (pp. 257–261)
    1. Causes of hypoperfusion
        a. Inadequate pump
            i. Inadequate preload
            ii. Inadequate cardiac contractile strength
            iii. Inadequate heart rate
            iv. Excessive afterload
        b. Inadequate fluid
            i. Hypovolemia
        c. Inadequate container
            i. Vasodilation with adequate fluid volume
            ii. Leak in vessel
    2. Shock at the cellular level
        a. Impaired use of oxygen (**Fig. 4-5, p. 259**)
            i. Aerobic metablolism
            ii. Anaerobic metabolism
        b. Impaired use of glucose
    3. Compensation and decompensation
        a. Compensated shock
            i. Body's mechanisms can maintain normal perfusion.
        b. Decompensated (progressive shock)
            i. Body's mechanisms may not be able to restore normal function.
            ii. Medical intervention may be able to correct problem.
        c. Irreversible shock
            i. Body's mechanisms unable to restore normal function.
            ii. Medical intervention ineffective
            iii. Death is inevitable.
  B. Types of shock (pp. 261–265)
    1. Cardiogenic
        a. Caused by insufficient cardiac output
        b. Evaluation and treatment
    2. Hypovolemic
        a. Caused by loss of intravascular fluid volume
        b. Evaluation and treatment
    3. Neurogenic
        a. Caused by brain or spinal injury
        b. Evaluation and treatment
    4. Anaphylactic
        a. Caused by allergic reaction
        b. Evaluation and treatment
    5. Septic
        a. Caused by infection
        b. Evaluation and treatment

POWERPOINT PRESENTATION
Chapter 4 PowerPoint slides 62–104

POINT TO EMPHASIZE
Shock, or hypoperfusion, has been described as a "momentary pause in the act of death."

READING/REFERENCE
Phrampus, P. "Concepts in Shock," *JEMS*, Mar. 2004.

SLIDES/VIDEOS
24-7 EMS: "Shock," Summer 2004.

TEACHING TIP
Bring in a very large rubber band to class and demonstrate the Frank-Starling mechanism with a student. This technique is also useful in evoking the sympathetic nervous system response.

C. Multiple organ dysfunction syndrome (pp. 265–267)
   1. Pathophysiology of MODS
      a. Infection
      b. Sepsis
      c. Septic shock
      d. MODS
      e. Death
   2. Clinical presentation of MODS
      a. 24 hours after resuscitation
         i. Low-grade fever
         ii. Tachycardia
         iii. Dyspnea
         iv. Altered mental status
         v. General hypermetabolic, hyperdynamic state
      b. Within 24 to 72 hours
         i. Pulmonary failure begins.
      c. Within 7 to 10 days
         i. Hepatic failure begins.
         ii. Intestinal failure begins.
         iii. Renal failure begins.
      d. Within 14 to 21 days
         i. Renal and hepatic failure intensifies.
         ii. Gastrointestinal collapse
         iii. Immune system collapse
      e. After 21 days
         i. Hematologic failure begins.
         ii. Myocardial failure begins.
         iii. Altered mental status resulting from encephalopathy
         iv. Death

PART 2: THE BODY'S DEFENSES AGAINST DISEASE AND INJURY

I. **Self-defense mechanisms.** The body has powerful ways of defending and healing itself, and medical intervention is needed only on occasion, when these natural defense mechanisms are unequal to the task and become overwhelmed. (pp. 268–271)

A. Infectious agents (pp. 268–270)
   1. Bacteria
      a. Antibiotics
      b. Exotoxins
      c. Endotoxins
      d. Septicemia
   2. Viruses
   3. Fungi
   4. Parasites
   5. Prions
B. Three lines of defense (pp. 270–271) (Table 4-2, p. 270)
   1. Anatomic barriers
      a. External
      b. Nonspecific
   2. Inflammatory response
      a. Internal
      b. Nonspecific
   3. Immune response
      a. Internal
      b. Specific

II. The immune response. The immune response is the body's detection of antigens and its production of substances to control or destroy them. (pp. 271–273)

A. How the immune response works (p. 271)
  1. Antigens
  2. Antibodies
  3. Immune response
  4. Immunity
B. Characteristics of the immune response and immunity (pp. 271–272) (**Table 4-3, p. 271**)
  1. Natural immunity versus acquired immunity
     a. Natural immunity
     b. Acquired immunity
  2. Humoral versus cell-mediated immunity
     a. Lymphocytes
     b. B lymphocytes
     c. Humoral immunity
     d. T lymphocytes
     e. Cell-mediated immunity
     f. Lymphocytes and the lymph system
C. Induction of the immune response (pp. 272–273)
  1. Antigens and immunogens
     a. Immunogens
     b. Antigenic immunogenicity
     c. Haptens
  2. Blood group antigens
     a. HLA antigens
     b. The Rh system
     c. The ABO system

POWERPOINT PRESENTATION
Chapter 4 PowerPoint slides 21–31

III. Inflammation. Also called inflammatory response, inflammation is the body's response to cellular injury. (pp. 273–279)

A. Inflammation contrasted to immune response (pp. 273–274)
  1. Inflammation response develops slowly; inflammation develops swiftly.
  2. Immune response is specific; inflammation is nonspecific.
  3. Immune response is long-lasting; inflammation is temporary.
  4. Immune response involves one type of white blood cell; inflammation involves platelets and many types of white cells.
  5. Immune response involves one type of plasma protein; inflammation involves several plasma protein systems.
B. How inflammation works (p. 274)
  1. Phases of inflammation; healing may take place after any phase.
     a. Phase 1: Acute inflammation
     b. Phase 2: Chronic inflammation
     c. Phase 3: Granuloma formation
     d. Phase 4: Healing
  2. Functions of inflammation
     a. Destroy and remove unwanted substances
     b. Wall off the infected and inflamed area
     c. Stimulate the immune response
     d. Promote healing
C. Acute inflammatory response (p. 274) (**Fig. 4-6, p. 275; Fig. 4-7, p. 276**)
D. Mast cells (pp. 274–277)
  1. Chief activators of inflammatory response
  2. Degranulation is stimulated by (**Fig. 4-28, p. 276**)
     a. Physical injury

POWERPOINT PRESENTATION
Chapter 4 PowerPoint slides 32–46

©2007 Pearson Education, Inc.
Essentials of Paramedic Care, 2nd ed.

CHAPTER 4 *General Principles of Pathophysiology* 157

    b. Chemical agents
    c. Immunologic and direct processes
  3. Vasoactive amines released during degranulation
    a. Histamine
    b. Serotonin
  4. Chemotactic factors released during degranulation
  5. Synthesis
    a. Leukotrienes
    b. Prostaglandins
E. Systemic responses of acute inflammation (p. 277)
  1. Endogenous pyrogen
  2. Acute phase reactants
F. Chronic inflammatory responses (pp. 277–278)
  1. Fibroblasts
  2. Pus
  3. Granuloma
G. Local inflammatory responses (p. 278)
  1. Vascular changes
  2. Exudation
    a. Dilutes toxins released by bacteria and the toxic products of tying cells
    b. Brings plasma proteins and leukocytes to the site to attack the invaders
    c. Carries away the products of inflammation, e.g., toxins, dead cells, pus
H. Resolution and repair (pp. 278–279)
  1. Outcomes of healing
    a. Resolution
    b. Regeneration
    c. Repair
  2. Debridement
  3. Extent of wounds and types of healing
    a. Minor wounds, primary intention
    b. More extensive wounds, secondary intention

IV. Variances in immunity and inflammation. Hypersensitivity is an example of the body's working "too well"; inflammation is an example of its not working well enough. (pp. 279–282)

A. Hypersensitivity (pp. 279–280)
  1. Types of hypersensitivity
    a. Allergy
    b. Autoimmunity
    c. Isoimmunity
  2. Types of reactions
    a. Immediate hypersensitivity reaction
    b. Delayed hypersensitivity reaction
  3. Mechanisms of hypersensitivity
    a. Type I
      i. IgE-mediated allergen reactions
    b. Type II
      i. Tissue-specific reactions
    c. Type III
      i. Immune complex–mediated reactions
    d. Type IV
      i. Cell-mediated reactions

POWERPOINT PRESENTATION
Chapter 4 PowerPoint slides 47–61

TEACHING STRATEGY 3
Allergy Round Robin

- **B.** Deficiencies in immunity and inflammation (pp. 280–282)
    1. Congenital immune deficiencies
    2. Acquired immune deficiencies
        a. Nutritional deficiencies
        b. Iatrogenic deficiencies
        c. Deficiencies caused by trauma
        d. Deficiencies caused by stress
        e. AIDS
    3. Replacement therapies for immune deficiencies
        a. Gamma globulin therapy
        b. Transplantation and transfusion
        c. Gene therapy

V. Stress and disease: The mind and body interact with a cause-and-effect relationship between stress and disease. (pp. 272–288)

- **A.** Concepts of stress (pp. 282–283)
    1. Stress
        a. Response to any noxious stimulus
    2. Stressor
        a. Stimulus or cause of stress
    3. General adaptation syndrome (GAS)
        a. Physiological effects
            i. Enlargement of the cortex of the adrenal gland
            ii. Atrophy of the thymus gland and other lymphatic structures
            iii. Development of bleeding ulcers of the stomach and duodenum
        b. Stages of GAS
            i. Stage I: Alarm
            ii. Stage II: Resistance or adaptation
            iii. Stage III: Exhaustion
        c. Physiological stress
    4. Psychological mediators and specificity
    5. Homeostasis as a dynamic steady state
        a. Dynamic steady state
        b. Turnover
- **B.** Stress responses:
    1. Psychoneuroimmunological regulation (pp. 284–287) (**Fig. 4-9, p. 284**)
    2. Neuroendocrine regulation
        a. Catecholamines (**Table 4-4, p. 285**)
        b. Cortisol
    3. Role of the immune system (**Table 4-5, p. 287**)
        a. Pathway 1
            i. Central nervous system to immune system
        b. Pathway 2
            i. Immune system to central nervous system
- **C.** Stress, coping, and illness interrelationships (pp. 287–288)
    1. Categories of stress
        a. Physiological
        b. Psychological
    2. Potential effects of stress based on effectiveness of coping
        a. In a healthy person
        b. In a symptomatic person
        c. In a person undergoing medical treatment

VI. Chapter Summary (p. 288). Pathophysiology is the study of how disease and injury alter normal physiology (body processes). The cell is the

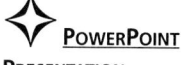

POWERPOINT PRESENTATION
Chapter 4 PowerPoint slides 62–71

TEACHING STRATEGY 4
Stress and Disease Guest Speaker

basic unit of life. The cells exist in an environment of fluids and electrolytes. When something interferes with normal cell function or the normal cell environment or normal cell intercommunication, disease can begin or advance.

Cells can be injured in a variety of ways, including hypoxia, chemicals, infectious agents, immunological/inflammatory injuries, and others. Diseases can be caused by genetic factors, environmental factors, or a combination of factors (multifactorial diseases).

The body responds to cellular injury in a variety of ways to restore homeostasis, the body's normal dynamic steady state. Cells can adapt through atrophy, hypertrophy, hyperplasia, metaplasia, and dysplasia. Negative feedback mechanisms work to correct, or compensate for, shock—if shock has not progressed too far.

Perfusion of the tissues is necessary to provide essential nutrients to the cells (especially oxygen and glucose) and to remove wastes. Inadequate perfusion, called hypoperfusion or shock, can be caused by a problem in any of the three parts of the cardiovascular system (the heart, the blood vessels, or the blood), sometimes abetted by problems with the respiratory or gastrointestinal system in which the normal intake and transfer of oxygen and glucose may be interrupted. If not corrected, shock continues in a downward spiral toward irreversible shock, possible multiple organ dysfunction syndrome (MODS), and death.

The body's chief means of self-defense is the immune system and the immune and inflammatory responses, which work to attack and destroy infectious agents and other unwanted invaders. Occasionally, the immune response system works "too well," as in hypersensitivity reactions, or not well enough, as in immune deficiency disorders. Stress can also contribute to disease through the interactions of the nerve, endocrine, and immune systems.

WORKBOOK
Chapter 4 Activities

READING/REFERENCE
Textbook, pp. 291–306

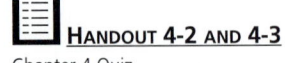

HANDOUT 4-2 AND 4-3
Chapter 4 Quiz

HANDOUT 4-4
Chapter 4 Scenario

PARAMEDIC STUDENT CD
Student Activities

COMPANION WEBSITE
http://www.prenhall.com/bledsoe

TESTGEN
Chapter 4

EMT ACHIEVE:
PARAMEDIC TEST PREPARATION
Mistovich & Beasley. EMT Achieve: Paramedic Test Preparation.
www.prenhall.com/emtachieve/

ASSIGNMENTS

Assign students to complete Chapter 4, "General Principles of Pathophysiology," of the workbook. Also assign them to read Chapter 5, "Life-Span Development," before the next class.

EVALUATION

Chapter Quiz and Scenario Distribute copies of the Chapter Quiz provided in Handouts 4-2, 4-3, and 4-4 to evaluate student understanding of this chapter. Make sure each student reads the scenario to reinforce critical thinking on the scene. Remind students not to use their notes or textbooks while taking the quiz.

Student CD Quizzes for every chapter are contained on the dynamic and highly visual in-text student CD.

Companion Website Additional quizzes for every chapter are contained on this exciting website.

TestGen You may wish to create a custom-tailored test using *Prentice Hall TestGen for Essentials of Paramedic Care*, 2nd Edition to evaluate student understanding of this chapter.

On-line Test Preparation (for students and instructors) Additional test preparation is available through Brady's new on-line product, *EMT Achieve: Paramedic Test*

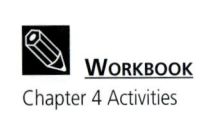

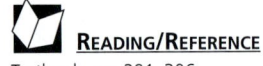

Preparation at *http://www.prenhall.com/emtachieve/*. Instructors can also monitor student mastery on-line.

Review Manual for the EMT-Paramedic This comprehensive exam review contains hundreds of test questions and rationales, including scenarios, along with two 180-question practice tests on CD.

REINFORCEMENT

Handouts If classroom discussion or performance on the quiz indicates that some students have not fully mastered the chapter content, you may wish to assign some or all of the Reinforcement Handouts for this chapter.

Student CD (for students) A wide variety of material on this CD-ROM will reinforce and also expand student knowledge and skills.

PowerPoint Presentation (for instructors) The PowerPoint material developed for this chapter offers useful reinforcement of chapter content.

Companion Website (for students) Additional review quizzes and links to EMS resources will contribute to further reinforcement of the chapter.

OneKey On-line support is offered for this course on one of three platforms: CourseCompass, Blackboard, or Web CT. Includes the IRM, PowerPoints, TestGen, and Companion Website for instruction. Ask your local sales representative for more information.

Brady Skills Series: Advanced Life Skills (Video or CD) Have your students watch the skills come to life on VHS or CD-ROM, or they can purchase the highly visual, full-color text with step-by-step procedures with rationales.

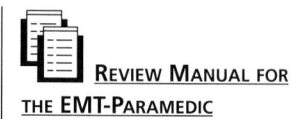

REVIEW MANUAL FOR THE EMT-PARAMEDIC
Cherry & Mistovich. *Review Manual for the EMT-Paramedic,* 3rd edition.

HANDOUTS 4-5 TO 4-7
Reinforcement Activities

PARAMEDIC STUDENT CD
Student Activities

POWERPOINT PRESENTATION
Chapter 4

COMPANION WEBSITE
http://www.prenhall.com/bledsoe

ONEKEY
Chapter 4

ADVANCED LIFE SUPPORT SKILLS
Larmon & Davis. *Advanced Life Support Skills.*

ADVANCED LIFE SKILLS REVIEW
Larmon & Davis. *Advanced Life Skills Review.*

BRADY SKILLS SERIES: ALS
Larmon & Davis. *Brady Skills Series: ALS.*

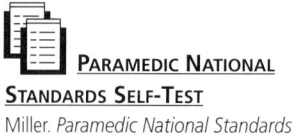

PARAMEDIC NATIONAL STANDARDS SELF-TEST
Miller. *Paramedic National Standards Self-Test,* 4th edition.

HANDOUT 4-1

Student's Name _____

CHAPTER 4 OBJECTIVES CHECKLIST

PART 1: HOW NORMAL BODY PROCESSES ARE ALTERED BY DISEASE AND INJURY

Knowledge	Date Mastered
1. Discuss cellular adaptation, injury, and death.	
2. Discuss factors that precipitate disease in the human body.	
3. Analyze disease risk.	
4. Describe environmental risk factors and combined effects and interaction among risk factors.	
5. Discuss familial diseases and associated risk factors.	
6. Discuss hypoperfusion.	
7. Define cardiogenic, hypovolemic, neurogenic, anaphylactic, and septic shock.	
8. Describe multiple organ dysfunction syndrome.	

PART 2: THE BODY'S DEFENSES AGAINST DISEASE AND INJURY

Knowledge	Date Mastered
1. Define the characteristics of the immune response.	
2. Discuss induction of the immune system.	
3. Describe the inflammation response and its systemic manifestations.	
4. Discuss the role of mast cells, the plasma protein system, and cellular components plus resolution and repair as part of the inflammation response.	
5. Discuss hypersensitivity.	
6. Describe deficiencies in immunity and inflammation.	
7. Describe homeostasis as a dynamic steady state.	
8. Describe neuroendocrine regulation.	
9. Discuss the interrelationships between stress, coping, and illness.	

HANDOUT 4-2

Student's Name _____

CHAPTER 4 QUIZ

PART 1: HOW NORMAL BODY PROCESSES ARE ALTERED BY DISEASE AND INJURY

Write the letter of the best answer in the space provided.

_____ 1. A decrease in cell size resulting from a decreased workload is called:
   A. hyperplasia.
   B. mitosis.
   C. atrophy.
   D. dysplasia.

_____ 2. An increase in the number of cells resulting from an increased workload is known as:
   A. hyperplasia.
   B. hypertrophy.
   C. atrophy.
   D. dysplasia.

_____ 3. Aerobic exercise gradually causes _____ of the myocardium.
   A. dilation
   B. atrophy
   C. hypertrophy
   D. hyperplasia

_____ 4. The most common cause of cellular injury is oxygen deficiency, or:
   A. ischemia.
   B. hypoxia.
   C. infarction.
   D. inflammation.

_____ 5. A microorganism capable of producing infection or disease is called a:
   A. parasite.
   B. lysosome.
   C. pathogen.
   D. fungus.

_____ 6. The constructive phase of metabolism in which cells convert nonliving substances into living cytoplasm is called:
   A. anabolism.
   B. catabolism.
   C. apoptosis.
   D. necrosis.

_____ 7. Necrosis means:
   A. an injured cell destroying itself.
   B. cell death.
   C. oxygen deficiency.
   D. a buildup of cell waste products.

_____ 8. Edema is excess fluid in the:
   A. interstitial space.
   B. extracellular space.
   C. intracellular space.
   D. intravascular space.

_____ 9. The component of blood that contains hemoglobin and transports oxygen is the:
   A. erythrocyte.
   B. leukocyte.
   C. thrombocyte.
   D. plasma.

_____ 10. Plasma is made up of approximately what percentage of water?
   A. 98 percent
   B. 92 percent
   C. 86 percent
   D. 82 percent

_____ 11. Intravenous fluids that contain proteins are called:
   A. colloids.
   B. crystalloids.
   C. plasma.
   D. albumins.

_____ 12. Lactated Ringer's solution is an example of a(n) _____ solution.
   A. isotonic
   B. hypertonic
   C. hypotonic
   D. normotonic

©2007 Pearson Education, Inc.
Essentials of Paramedic Care, 2nd ed.

HANDOUT 4-2 Continued

_____ 13. An electrolyte solution of sodium chloride in water is:
   A. D$_5$W.
   B. lactated Ringer's.
   C. normal saline.
   D. Hartman's solution.

_____ 14. A high concentration of hydrogen ions is known as:
   A. alkalosis.
   B. acidosis.
   C. carbonosis.
   D. base.

_____ 15. Impaired ventilation is the cause of:
   A. respiratory alkalosis.
   B. metabolic alkalosis.
   C. respiratory acidosis.
   D. metabolic acidosis.

_____ 16. Vomiting, diarrhea, or diabetes can cause:
   A. respiratory alkalosis.
   B. metabolic alkalosis.
   C. respiratory acidosis.
   D. metabolic acidosis.

_____ 17. Every human somatic cell contains how many pairs of chromosomes?
   A. 45
   B. 37
   C. 23
   D. 12

_____ 18. Diseases caused by a combination of genetic and environmental factors are called:
   A. multisystem failure.
   B. multifactorial disorders.
   C. multiple defect.
   D. geno-environmental disorders.

_____ 19. All of the following are immunologic disorders EXCEPT:
   A. diabetes.
   B. rheumatic fever.
   C. allergies.
   D. asthma.

_____ 20. The most common endocrine disorder is:
   A. pancreatitis.
   B. hemophilia.
   C. hypertension.
   D. diabetes mellitus.

_____ 21. The disease caused by a genetic clotting factor deficiency is:
   A. hemochromatosis.
   B. anemia.
   C. hemophilia.
   D. encephalitis.

_____ 22. A neuromuscular disorder known to be caused by a genetic defect is:
   A. cholecystitis.
   B. Huntington's disease.
   C. Crohn's disease.
   D. schizophrenia.

_____ 23. The supplying of oxygen and nutrients to the body tissues is called:
   A. circulation.
   B. hydration.
   C. perfusion.
   D. output.

_____ 24. Characteristics of impaired cellular metabolism in shock include impaired use of:
   A. sodium.
   B. glucose.
   C. hemoglobin.
   D. bicarbonate.

_____ 25. Your patient has received a large traumatic injury. Blood pressure is normal, but the heart rate and respiratory rate are increased, and the skin is cool and clammy. Your patient is in:
   A. homeostasis.
   B. compensated shock.
   C. decompensated shock.
   D. irreversible shock.

_____ 26. A drop in blood pressure in the patient described in Question 25 means the patient is in:
   A. homeostasis.
   B. compensated shock.
   C. decompensated shock.
   D. irreversible shock.

HANDOUT 4-2 Continued

_____ 27. Treatment for cardiogenic shock should include:
   A. placing the patient in the Trendelenburg position.
   B. rapid fluid replacement with a crystalloid solution.
   C. elevating the patient's head and shoulders.
   D. the application and inflation of the PASG.

_____ 28. The type of shock resulting from arteries' losing tone and dilating is known as:
   A. hypovolemic.   C. hemorrhagic.
   B. cardiogenic.   D. neurogenic.

_____ 29. The progressive impairment of two or more organ systems resulting from an uncontrolled inflammatory response to a severe illness or injury is called:
   A. multiple organ system failure.
   B. multiple organ dysfunction syndrome.
   C. multiple system failure.
   D. multiple sepsis syndrome.

_____ 30. The most common presentation of MODS within the first 24 hours after resuscitation includes:
   A. pulmonary failure.   C. general hypermetabolic state.
   B. immune system collapse.   D. hematologic failure.

HANDOUT 4-3

Student's Name _____

CHAPTER 4 QUIZ

PART 2: THE BODY'S DEFENSES AGAINST DISEASE AND INJURY

Write the letter of the best answer in the space provided.

_____ 1. The systemic spread of toxins through the bloodstream is called:
   A. infection.
   B. septicemia.
   C. pathogenia.
   D. toxemia.

_____ 2. Which of the following is NOT one of the three lines of defense for infection?
   A. anatomic barriers
   B. inflammatory response
   C. immune response
   D. febrile response

_____ 3. Which of the following begins within seconds of injury or invasion by a pathogen?
   A. immune response
   B. febrile response
   C. inflammatory response
   D. leukocyte response

_____ 4. Protection from infection or disease that is developed by the body after exposure to an antigen is called:
   A. acquired immunity.
   B. natural immunity.
   C. primary immune response.
   D. synthetic immunity.

_____ 5. The special type of leukocyte that is responsible for recognizing foreign antigens, producing antibodies, and developing memory is the:
   A. lymphocyte.
   B. cytoplast.
   C. thrombocyte.
   D. erythrocyte.

_____ 6. The type of white blood cell that does not produce antibodies but instead attacks antigens directly is the:
   A. T lymphocyte.
   B. B lymphocyte.
   C. IgM lymphocyte.
   D. IgD lymphocyte.

_____ 7. Someone is considered a universal donor if he has blood type:
   A. O.
   B. A.
   C. B.
   D. AB.

_____ 8. Which of the following statements is TRUE regarding the difference between the immune response and the inflammatory response?
   A. The immune response develops swiftly; inflammation develops slowly.
   B. The immune response is specific; inflammation is nonspecific.
   C. The immune response is temporary; inflammation is long-lasting.
   D. The immune response involves many types of white cells; inflammation involves one type of white blood cell.

_____ 9. One of the four functions of inflammation is:
   A. walling off the infected and inflamed area.
   B. attacking foreign substances.
   C. developing a memory for antigens.
   D. production of white blood cells.

_____ 10. The type of cells responsible for activating the inflammatory response are the:
   A. T cells.
   B. B cells.
   C. mast cells.
   D. plasma cells.

HANDOUT 4-3 Continued

_____ 11. The substance released by platelets that, through constriction and dilation of blood vessels, affects blood flow to an injured or affected site is called:
   A. histamine.
   B. serotonin.
   C. granules.
   D. pus.

_____ 12. A tumor or growth that forms when foreign bodies cannot be destroyed and is surrounded and walled off is called a:
   A. fibroblast.
   B. granuloma.
   C. melanoma.
   D. cyst.

_____ 13. Exudate has three functions at an inflammation site, one of which is:
   A. destruction of toxins released by bacteria.
   B. removal of plasma proteins and leukocytes from the site.
   C. carrying away the products of inflammation, e.g., toxins, dead cells, pus.
   D. all of these.

_____ 14. The complete healing of a wound and return of tissues to their normal structure and function is called:
   A. regeneration.
   B. repair.
   C. debridement.
   D. resolution.

_____ 15. The term autoimmunity refers to:
   A. an exaggerated immune response to an environmental antigen.
   B. an immune reaction between members of the same species, commonly of one person against the antigens of another person.
   C. a disturbance in the body's normal tolerance for self-antigens, such as hyperthyroidism or rheumatic fever.
   D. a severe allergic response that usually develops within minutes of reexposure.

_____ 16. Acquired immune deficiencies include:
   A. nutritional deficiencies.
   B. deficiencies caused by trauma.
   C. AIDS.
   D. all of these

_____ 17. In Stage I of the general adaptation syndrome, a person:
   A. experiences "burnout."
   B. begins to cope with the situation.
   C. experiences arousal of the sympathetic nervous system, mobilizing the "fight-or-flight" response.
   D. experiences an ensuing physical illness.

_____ 18. The dynamic steady state is also known as:
   A. turnover.
   B. homeostasis.
   C. stress.
   D. adaptation.

_____ 19. The physiological effects of catecholamines include:
   A. decreased glucose metabolism in the brain.
   B. bronchoconstriction.
   C. increased blood flow to the skin.
   D. increased glucose production in the liver.

_____ 20. The adrenal cortex releases a steroid hormone that regulates the metabolism of fats, carbohydrates, sodium, potassium, and proteins. That hormone is:
   A. cortisol.
   B. testosterone.
   C. growth hormone.
   D. beta-endorphines.

HANDOUT 4-4

Student's Name _____

CHAPTER 4 SCENARIO

Review the following real-life situation. Then answer the questions that follow.

You receive a call in the afternoon to proceed to a residential community of older citizens on a report that a patient has fallen. A postal worker noted the mail hadn't been picked up, so he checked the back of the house and heard someone moaning for help. When you arrive on scene, you find a 72-year-old female patient lying on the kitchen floor and complaining of right hip pain. As a precaution you immobilize her for possible spinal injuries. The patient tells you her name and states that she fell yesterday morning after her foot caught on the rug. During the fall, she heard a "crack" and afterwards could not get up because of the pain.

The patient's respiratory rate is 24 and slightly shallow; pulse is 120, weak and regular at the radial site; B/P is 90/60. Lungs are clear, neck veins are flat, and no edema is present. Determining skin turgor is difficult because, like many older people, the patient has lost underlying fat tissue. However, she complains of thirst and has dry mucous membranes. The skin is pale and cool. Capillary refill time is 3 seconds. The right lower extremity is shortened and rotated outward. There is a distal pulse, but it is weak. The patient can feel you touching her foot and can wiggle her toes. There is pain and discoloration (bruising) near the right greater trochanter. The ECG shows a sinus tachycardia at 120 beats per minute. There is no other pertinent past history, no use of medications, and no allergies. The patient weighs 110 pounds.

1. What do you think this patient's problems are?

2. What physical findings support your belief?

3. Develop a prehospital treatment plan for this patient.

168   ESSENTIALS OF PARAMEDIC CARE

Handout 4-5

Student's Name _____

CHAPTER 4 REVIEW

PART 1: HOW NORMAL BODY PROCESSES ARE ALTERED BY DISEASE AND INJURY

Write the word or words that best complete the following sentences in the space provided.

1. _____ is the natural tendency of the body to maintain a steady and normal internal environment.
2. An increase in cell size resulting from an increased workload is called _____.
3. An increase in the number of cells resulting from an increased workload is called _____.
4. A blockage in the delivery of oxygenated blood to the cells is called _____.
5. The destructive phase of metabolism in which cells break down complex substances into simpler substances to release energy is called _____.
6. A substance that can crystalloid and can diffuse through a membrane is called a(n) _____.
7. An increase in plasma bicarbonate due to diuresis, vomiting, or ingestion of too much sodium bicarbonate is called _____ _____.
8. Every human somatic cell contains _____ chromosomes.
9. The supplying of oxygen and nutrients to the body tissues as a result of the constant passage of blood through the capillaries is called _____.
10. In adequate perfusion of the body tissues is known as _____ or _____.
11. Characteristics of impaired cellular metabolism in shock include the impaired use of _____ and _____.
12. _____ metabolism is the second stage of metabolism and requires oxygen.
13. _____ metabolism is the first stage of metabolism and does not require oxygen.
14. The early stage of shock during which the body's compensatory mechanisms are able to maintain normal perfusion is called _____ shock.
15. _____ shock has progressed so far that no medical intervention can reverse the condition and death is inevitable.
16. _____ shock is caused by a loss of intravascular fluid volume.
17. _____ shock is the result of a brain or spinal cord injury.
18. The shock that develops as the result of infection carried by the bloodstream is called _____ shock.
19. The progressive impairment of two or more organ systems resulting from an uncontrolled inflammatory response is called _____ _____ _____ _____.
20. Patients in _____ shock should have their head and shoulders elevated, with fluid administration kept to a minimum.

HANDOUT 4-6

Student's Name _____

CHAPTER 4 REVIEW

PART 2: THE BODY'S DEFENSES AGAINST DISEASE AND INJURY

Write the word or words that best complete the following sentences in the space provided.

1. A single-cell organism with a cell membrane and cytoplasm, but having no organized nucleus, is a _____.

2. Toxic substances secreted by bacterial cells during their growth are called _____.

3. Molecules in the walls of certain gram-negative bacteria that are released when the bacterium dies or is destroyed, causing toxic effects on the host body, are called _____.

4. The systemic spread of toxins through the bloodstream is called _____.

5. An organism visible only under an electron microscope and that can grow only with the assistance of another organism is a(n) _____.

6. A marker on the surface of a cell that identifies it as "self" or "non-self" is a(n) _____.

7. A(n) _____ is a substance produced by B lymphocytes in response to the presence of a foreign antigen.

8. _____ is a long-term condition of protection from infection or disease.

9. The body's response to cellular injury is _____.

10. The substance released during the degranulation of mast cells is _____.

11. _____ are substances synthesized by mast cells during inflammatory response that cause vasoconstriction, vascular permeability, and chemotaxis and may also cause pain.

12. _____ is a liquid mixture of dead cells, bits of dead tissue, and tissue fluid that may accumulate in inflamed tissues.

13. Healing of a wound with a scar formation is called _____.

14. The cleaning up or removal of debris, dead cells, and scabs from a wound, principally through phagocytosis, is called _____.

15. _____ is an exaggerated or harmful immune response.

Handout 4-7

Student's Name _____

CHAPTER 4 COMPLETION

Complete each of the following lists.

PATHOGEN VERSUS THE BODY: THREE POSSIBLE OUTCOMES

1. _____
2. _____
3. _____

CAUSES OF CELLULAR INJURY

1. _____
2. _____
3. _____
4. _____
5. _____
6. _____
7. _____

TYPES OF SHOCK

1. _____
2. _____
3. _____
4. _____
5. _____

Chapter 4 Answer Key

Handout 4-2: Chapter 4 Quiz, Part 1

1. C	9. A	17. C	25. B
2. A	10. B	18. B	26. C
3. C	11. A	19. A	27. C
4. B	12. A	20. D	28. D
5. C	13. C	21. C	29. B
6. A	14. B	22. B	30. C
7. B	15. C	23. C	
8. A	16. D	24. B	

Handout 4-3: Chapter 4 Quiz, Part 2

1. B	8. B	15. C
2. D	9. A	16. D
3. C	10. C	17. C
4. A	11. B	18. B
5. A	12. B	19. D
6. A	13. C	20. A
7. A	14. D	

Handout 4-4: Chapter 4 Scenario

1. The patient appears to have a right hip fracture and is showing signs of hypovolemic shock.
2. The hip fracture is indicated by the shortened and rotated right lower extremity. The signs and symptoms of shock include an increased respiratory and pulse rate, with the pulse being weak. Blood pressure may be normal for her but could be slightly low. The patient is complaining of thirst and has dry mucous membranes. Her skin is pale and cool. Capillary refill time is increased. Due to the major blood vessels present in the hip and upper thigh area, internal bleeding could be causing the state of hypoperfusion.
3. The patient has already been immobilized due to the potential for spinal injuries. Airway and breathing are the first concerns. Her airway is obviously patent, so you should apply high-concentration oxygen with a nonrebreather mask. Depending on local protocols, the PASG may also be applied to stabilize the hip and treat the hypoperfusion. An IV line should be started, and a fluid bolus administered. However, be careful when administering fluids to elderly patients. Check frequently for any signs of pulmonary edema. As the patient has no allergies, administration of IV medication for pain, such as Demerol, would be appropriate before moving her. Continue to monitor the ABCs and a distal pulse in the injured extremity en route.

Handout 4-5: Chapter 4 Review, Part 1

1. Homeostasis
2. hypertrophy
3. hyperplasia
4. ischemia
5. catabolism
6. crystalloid
7. metabolic alkalosis
8. 46
9. perfusion
10. hypoperfusion, shock
11. oxygen, glucose
12. Aerobic
13. Anaerobic
14. compensated
15. Irreversible
16. Hypovolemic
17. Neurogenic
18. septic
19. multiple organ dysfunction syndrome
20. cardiogenic

Handout 4-6: Chapter 4 Review, Part 2

1. bacterium
2. exotoxins
3. endotoxins
4. septicemia
5. virus
6. antigen
7. antibody
8. Immunity
9. inflammation
10. histamine
11. Leukotrienes
12. Pus
13. repair
14. debridement
15. Hypersensitivity

Handout 4-7: Chapter 4 Completion

Pathogen versus the Body: Three Possible Outcomes

1. Pathogen wins.
2. Pathogen and body battle to a draw.
3. Body defeats pathogen.

Causes of Cellular Injury

1. Hypoxia
2. Chemicals
3. Infectious agents
4. Inflammatory reactions
5. Physical agents
6. Nutritional factors
7. Genetic factors

Types of Shock

1. Cardiogenic
2. Hypovolemic
3. Neurogenic
4. Anaphylactic
5. Septic

Chapter 5

Life-Span Development

INTRODUCTION

Although human anatomy and physiology remain basically the same throughout life, people do change over their life span. Besides the visible physical changes, we undergo changes in vital signs, body systems, and psychosocial development. Many of these changes will affect your assessment and care of patients. This chapter discusses changes and developmental stages.

CHAPTER OBJECTIVES

After reading this chapter, you should be able to:

1. Compare and contrast the physiological and psychosocial characteristics of the following life-span development stages:
   - Infant (pp. 292–296)
   - Toddler (pp. 296–298)
   - Preschooler (pp. 296–298)
   - School-aged (pp. 298–299)
   - Adolescent (pp. 299–300)
   - Early adult (pp. 300–301)
   - Middle-aged adult (p. 301)
   - Late-aged adult (pp. 301–305)

FRAMING THE LESSON

Begin the class by reviewing the important points from Chapter 4, "General Principles of Pathophysiology." Discuss any aspects of the chapter not understood by students. Then go on to Chapter 5. Ask students to think about their last family reunion, or large family gathering such as on a holiday. Ask them to think about the differences in the behavior and interactions of the various age groups represented—their own children, nieces and nephews, aunts and uncles, parents and grandparents. How did members of each of these age groups spend the day? How did they act and react to certain situations? How did they interact with each other?

TOTAL TEACHING TIME:
4.75 HOURS
The total teaching time is only a guideline based on the didactic and practical lab averages in the National Standard Curriculum. Instructors should take into consideration such factors as the pace at which students learn, the size of the class, and breaks. The actual time devoted to teaching objectives is the responsibility of the instructor.

TEACHING STRATEGIES

People learn in a variety of ways. Some do better with the spoken word, whereas others prefer the written. Some prefer to work alone, whereas others profit from working in groups. Recognizing these different ways of acquiring knowledge, the authors of this *Instructor's Resource Manual* have provided a variety of teaching strategies for the different types of learners. These strategies are intended to foster higher-level cognitive skills and encourage creative learning and problem solving. For greatest effectiveness, incorporate these strategies into your class lecture. Symbols in the Lecture Outline indicate the points at which various exercises might be most appropriate. Other strategies can be used to preview the lesson or to summarize it.

The following strategies are keyed to specific sections of the lesson.

1. Learning Vital Signs. Make laminated pocket cards with normal vital signs for students. There are getting to be so many developmental stages, it can be difficult to memorize vital signs for them all. Not only will your students use and appreciate the cards, but you will also be surprised at how often they end up in an ambulance or on the clipboard of a preceptor. Add your program's logo to them, and they can be a discrete marketing tool, too! As the instructor, you will have to decide which things you want students to know by heart and which you will allow them to use references for. For example, in pediatrics you might allow use of the Broselow tape because pediatric cases tend to be frightening for paramedics and are common sources of errors.

2. Getting to Know Them—Small Children. Not all of your students feel comfortable around small children. Arrange for those who have no children to spend time at a local child-care center, just to be around children of all ages. Another way of accomplishing this is to have children of all age groups come to the lab, where students can take their vital signs. Such measures are remarkably effective in decreasing anxiety for students and in improving their future care of pediatric patients.

3. Empathy Exercise. This exercise allows students to experience some of the specific physical limitations that the elderly face on a daily basis. For example, hearing loss in the elderly might be mimicked through the use of disposable wax ear plugs. Deteriorating eyesight might be simulated by placing a thin coat of petroleum jelly on the lenses of students' glasses or by having students who don't need glasses wear pairs of prescription glasses. Arthritis in the hands may be simulated by taping fingers into a static position. This exercise is only limited by the imagination of the instructor. Having students cope with these difficulties for all or part of the class should help heighten their sensitivity and awareness when they contact elderly patients in the field.

4. Learning about Aging. Have a "life-span panel" of guests varying in age from 30 to 80. Invite guests to share observations about noticeable changes in their bodies, feelings, concerns, and desires. Many will share stories about memory loss or not being able to enjoy the same foods they once did. Some will talk about developing new hobbies in retirement or losing close friends. A discussion like this is often enlightening to students and adds a human aspect to the issues discussed in this chapter.

5. Investigating Housing for the Elderly. Have students visit a variety of homes for aging adults. Create a list of questions for them to ask residents and staff. Information gathered might include: average age of resident, number of rooms or full apartments or houses, level of nursing care (if any), meals provided, social activities planned, most interesting resident, pets allowed, and so on. Have them bring brochures and information to share with the class.

This activity requires students to get acquainted with the facilities in their neighborhood or response district, exercise interviewing skills, and practice oral communication skills in the classroom report.

The following strategies can be used at various points throughout the lesson or to help summarize and demonstrate what students have learned.

Guest Speakers. Consider having guest speakers in each of your development groups as subject matter experts. Examples might include child-care workers, doctors and nurses, teachers, counselors, community organization leaders, nursing home workers, and so on. These people will frequently have excellent real-life examples that clearly illustrate the physiological and psychological needs and changes of people in the age groups with whom they work. Invite them to share their experiences at the beginning of class because you will only need them for 30 to 60 minutes, and it will likely be most convenient for them to drop by your class on their way to or from work. Not only are guest speakers fun and informative, by using them you can increase your network of community resources and exposure to the program.

Cultural Considerations, Legal Notes, and Patho Pearls. The Student CD-ROM contains this series of informative features to enhance the student's understanding of the material covered in this chapter.

TEACHING OUTLINE

Chapter 5, "Life-Span Development," is the fifth lesson in Division 1, *Introduction to Advanced Prehospital Care*. Distribute Handout 5-1 so that students can familiarize themselves with the learning goals for this chapter. If students have any questions about the objectives, answer them at this time.

Then present the chapter. One possible lecture outline follows. In the outline, the parenthetical references in regular type are references to text pages; those in bold type are references to figures or tables.

I. Introduction. Humans change over their lifetimes, not only physically but mentally as well. Some of the changes will require the paramedic to alter assessment and care procedures. This chapter discusses the developmental stages that occur over a lifetime and the physical and mental changes that accompany them. (p. 292)

A. Infancy (birth to 12 months) (p. 292)
B. Toddlerhood (12 to 36 months) (p. 292)
C. Preschool age (3 to 5 years) (p. 292)
D. School age (6 to 12 years) (p. 292)
E. Adolescence (13 to 18 years) (p. 292)
F. Early adulthood (20 to 40 years) (p. 292)
G. Middle adulthood (41 to 60 years) (p. 292)
H. Late adulthood (60 years and older) (p. 292)

II. Infancy. Infancy lasts from birth until about 12 months of age. (pp. 292–296)(**Fig. 5-2, p. 293**)

A. Physiological development (pp. 292–295)
  1. Vital signs (**Table 5-1, p. 292**)
  2. Weight
     a. 3 to 3.5 kg at birth
     b. Doubled in 4 to 6 months
     c. Tripled at 9 to 12 months

HANDOUT 5-1
Chapter 5 Objectives Checklist

SLIDES/VIDEOS
24-7 EMS: "Pediatric Assessment," Summer 2004.

POWERPOINT PRESENTATION
Chapter 5 PowerPoint slides 4–5

TEACHING STRATEGY 1
Learning Vital Signs

POWERPOINT PRESENTATION
Chapter 5 PowerPoint slides 6–27

POINT TO EMPHASIZE
Pediatric vital signs are age-related. Introduce the Broselow tape as an effective way to determine vital sign norms for each age group.

POINT TO EMPHASIZE

An infant's airway is shorter, narrower, less stable, and more easily obstructed than at any other stage in life.

SLIDES/VIDEOS

24-7 EMS: "Pediatric Respiratory Emergencies," Fall 2004.

TEACHING TIP

Encourage parents in your class to give real-life examples of the changes you discuss in class. Some might even have home videos of the very behaviors you are describing. This encourages participation by students and increases their interest in the subject matter. It is also both an auditory and visual experience.

TEACHING TIP

Using the popular cartoon strip Calvin and Hobbes is a fun way to illustrate the fear of monsters common to preschool-age children.

POWERPOINT PRESENTATION

Chapter 5 PowerPoint slides 28–38

TEACHING TIP

The Discovery Store at the Discovery Channel website (www.discovery.com) has numerous videos about life-span development—for example, "Body Story" and "Intimate Universe." Some are very current and short, so you can show several in this segment rather than just lecturing about development.

   3. Cardiovascular system
      a. Ductus venosus
         i. Ligamentum venosum
      b. Foramen ovale
         i. Fossa ovalis
      c. Ductus arteriosus
         i. Ligamentum arteriosum
   4. Pulmonary system
      a. Surfactant
      b. Nose breather
   5. Renal system
   6. Immune system
   7. Nervous system
      a. Reflexes
         i. Moro reflex—"startle reflex"
         ii. Palmar grasp
         iii. Rooting reflex
         iv. Sucking reflex
      b. Fontanelles
         i. Posterior close in 2 to 3 months
         ii. Anterior close in 9 to 18 months
      c. Sleep
         i. Newborns sleep 16 to 18 hours per day, which gradually decreases with age
   8. Musculoskeletal system
   9. Other developmental characteristics
B. Psychosocial development (pp. 295–296)
   1. Family process and reciprocal socialization
      a. Crying
         i. Only means of communication
      b. Attachment
         i. Secure attachment
         ii. Anxious resistant attachment
         iii. Anxious avoidant attachment
      c. Trust vs. mistrust
   2. Scaffolding
      a. Infants build on what they know
   3. Temperament
      a. Easy child
      b. Difficult child
C. Situational crisis and reactions to parental separation (p. 296)

III. Toddler and preschool age. In general, toddlers range in age from 12 months to 36 months; preschoolers from 3 years to 5 years. (pp. 296–298) (Fig. 5-2, p. 296; Fig. 5-3, p. 297) (Table 5-1, p. 292)

A. Physiological development (pp. 296–297)
   1. Cardiovascular system
   2. Pulmonary system
   3. Renal system
   4. Immune system
   5. Nervous system
   6. Musculoskeletal system
   7. Dental system
   8. Senses

B. Psychosocial development (pp. 297–298)
  1. Cognition
     a. Use of words at 10 months; understanding at 1 year
     b. Understanding of cause and effect at 18 to 24 months
     c. Separation anxiety between 18 and 24 months
     d. Development of "magical thinking" between 24 and 36 months
  2. Play
  3. Sibling relationships
  4. Peer group functions
  5. Parenting styles and their effects
     a. Authoritarian
     b. Authoritative
     c. Permissive
  6. Divorce and child development
  7. Television
  8. Modeling

IV. School age. School-aged children generally range from 6 to 12 years old. (pp. 298–299) (Fig. 5-4, p. 299) (Table 5-1, p. 292)

A. Physiological development (pp. 298–299)
B. Psychosocial development—levels of moral development (p. 299)
  1. Preconventional reasoning
  2. Conventional reasoning
  3. Postconventional reasoning

V. Adolescence. The age range of adolescence is roughly from 12 to 18 years. (pp. 299–300) (Fig. 5-5, p. 300) (Table 5-1, p. 292)

A. Physiological development (pp. 299–300)
  1. Girls usually finish growing by age 16.
  2. Boys usually finish growing by age 18.
  3. Reproductive maturity
B. Psychosocial development (p. 300)
  1. Family
  2. Development of identity
  3. Ethical development

VI. Early adulthood. Early adulthood lasts about from age 20 to age 40. (pp. 300–301) (Table 5-1, p. 292)

A. Physiological development (p. 301)
  1. Peak physical condition occurs from 19 years to 26 years, then the body begins its slowing process.
B. Psychosocial development (p. 301)
  1. Despite the stress of starting careers and families, this period is not associated with psychological problems related to well-being.

VII. Middle adulthood. Ranges between the ages of 41 and 60 years. (p. 301) (Table 5-1, p. 292)

A. Physiological development (p. 301)
  1. The body still functions at a high level with varying degrees of degradation based on the individual.
B. Psychosocial development (p. 301)
  1. Individuals in this age group become more task oriented as they see the time for accomplishing their lifetime goals recede.

TEACHING STRATEGY 2
Getting to Know Them—Small Children

POWERPOINT PRESENTATION
Chapter 5 PowerPoint slides 39–42

POINT TO EMPHASIZE
Adolescents want to be treated like adults.

POWERPOINT PRESENTATION
Chapter 5 PowerPoint slides 43–47

TEACHING STRATEGY 3
Empathy Exercise

POWERPOINT PRESENTATION
Chapter 5 PowerPoint slides 48–51

POINT TO EMPHASIZE
Cardiovascular health becomes a concern during middle adulthood.

POWERPOINT PRESENTATION
Chapter 5 PowerPoint slides 52–55

TEACHING STRATEGY 4
Learning about Aging

POINT TO EMPHASIZE
By the year 2030, patients 65 or older will represent 70 percent of all ambulance transports.

POWERPOINT PRESENTATION
Chapter 5 PowerPoint slides 56–68

TEACHING STRATEGY 5
Investigating Housing for the Elderly

SLIDES/VIDEOS
24-7EMS: "Geriatrics," Third Quarter 2005.

READING/REFERENCE
Criss, E. "The Elderly and Drug Interactions." *JEMS*, March 2002.

WORKBOOK
Chapter 5 Activities

READING/REFERENCE
Textbook, pp. 307–372

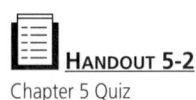

HANDOUT 5-2
Chapter 5 Quiz

HANDOUT 5-3
Chapter 5 Scenario

PARAMEDIC STUDENT CD
Student Activities

COMPANION WEBSITE
http://www.prenhall.com/bledsoe

TESTGEN
Chapter 5

EMT ACHIEVE: PARAMEDIC TEST PREPARATION
Mistovich & Beasley. *EMT Achieve: Paramedic Test Preparation.* www.prenhall.com/emtachieve/

VIII. Late adulthood. Late adulthood is the final developmental stage, beginning at about 60 years of age. (pp. 301–305) **(Fig. 5-6, p. 303) (Table 5-1, p. 292)**

  A. Physiological development (pp. 301–303)
  1. Vital signs
  2. Cardiovascular system
  3. Respiratory system
  4. Endocrine system
  5. Gastrointestinal system
  6. Renal system
  7. The senses
  8. Nervous system

  B. Psychosocial development (pp. 303–305)
  1. Housing
  2. Challenges
  3. Financial burdens
  4. Dying companions or death

IX. Chapter Summary (p. 305). The changes that take place during the span of a lifetime are innumerable. At some stages, the changes seem to occur almost daily. It is only through experience with patients at all of the various stages of life that you will come to feel comfortable dealing with each of them.

Remember that no matter what the stage of development, patience and a sincere desire to help a patient will help you to make the right decisions about emergency care.

ASSIGNMENTS

Assign students to complete Chapter 5, "Life-Span Development," of the workbook. Also assign them to read Chapter 6, "General Principles of Pharmacology," before the next class.

EVALUATION

Chapter Quiz and Scenario Distribute copies of the Chapter Quiz provided in Handouts 5-2 and 5-3 to evaluate student understanding of this chapter. Make sure each student reads the scenario to reinforce critical thinking on the scene. Remind students not to use their notes or textbooks while taking the quiz.

Student CD Quizzes for every chapter are contained on the dynamic and highly visual in-text student CD.

Companion Website Additional quizzes for every chapter are contained on this exciting website.

TestGen You may wish to create a custom-tailored test using *Prentice Hall TestGen for Essentials of Paramedic Care*, 2nd Edition to evaluate student understanding of this chapter.

On-line Test Preparation (for students and instructors) Additional test preparation is available through Brady's new on-line product, *EMT Achieve: Paramedic Test Preparation* at *http://www.prenhall.com/emtachieve/*. Instructors can also monitor student mastery on-line.

Review Manual for the EMT-Paramedic This comprehensive exam review contains hundreds of test questions and rationales, including scenarios, along with two 180-question practice tests on CD.

REINFORCEMENT

Handouts If classroom discussion or performance on the quiz indicates that some students have not fully mastered the chapter content, you may wish to assign some or all of the Reinforcement Handouts for this chapter.

Student CD (for students) A wide variety of material on this CD-ROM will reinforce and also expand student knowledge and skills.

PowerPoint Presentation (for instructors) The PowerPoint material developed for this chapter offers useful reinforcement of chapter content.

Companion Website (for students) Additional review quizzes and links to EMS resources will contribute to further reinforcement of the chapter material.

OneKey On-line support is offered for this course on one of three platforms: CourseCompass, Blackboard, or Web CT. Includes the IRM, PowerPoints, TestGen, and Companion Website for instruction. Ask your local sales representative for more information.

Brady Skills Series: Advanced Life Skills (Video or CD) Have your students watch the skills come to life on VHS or CD-ROM, or they can purchase the highly visual, full-color text with step-by-step procedures and rationales.

REVIEW MANUAL FOR THE EMT-PARAMEDIC
Cherry & Mistovich. *Review Manual for the EMT-Paramedic,* 3rd edition.

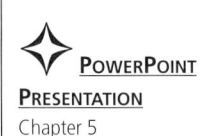

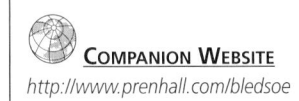

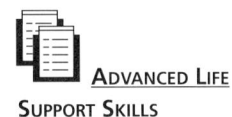

HANDOUTS 5-4 AND 5-5
Reinforcement Activities

PARAMEDIC STUDENT CD
Student Activities

POWERPOINT PRESENTATION
Chapter 5

COMPANION WEBSITE
http://www.prenhall.com/bledsoe

ONEKEY
Chapter 5

ADVANCED LIFE SUPPORT SKILLS
Larmon & Davis. *Advanced Life Support Skills.*

ADVANCED LIFE SKILLS REVIEW
Larmon & Davis. *Advanced Life Skills Review.*

BRADY SKILLS SERIES: ALS
Larmon & Davis. *Brady Skills Series: ALS*

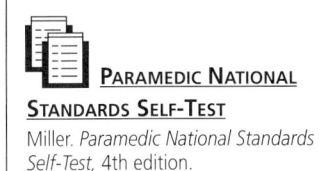

PARAMEDIC NATIONAL STANDARDS SELF-TEST
Miller. *Paramedic National Standards Self-Test,* 4th edition.

HANDOUT 5-1

Student's Name _____

OBJECTIVES

CHAPTER 5 OBJECTIVES CHECKLIST

Knowledge	Date Mastered
1. Compare and contrast the physiological and psychosocial characteristics of the following life-span development stages: • Infant • Toddler • Preschooler • School-aged • Adolescent • Early adult • Middle-aged adult • Late-aged adult	

HANDOUT 5-2

Student's Name _____

CHAPTER 5 QUIZ

Write the letter of the best answer in the space provided.

_____ 1. The greatest changes in the range of vital signs are in:
   A. pediatric patients.
   B. early adulthood patients.
   C. middle adulthood patients.
   D. late adulthood patients.

_____ 2. An infant's head is equal to what percentage of the total body weight?
   A. 10 percent
   B. 15 percent
   C. 20 percent
   D. 25 percent

_____ 3. After birth, an infant's cardiovascular system changes by constricting the ductus arteriosus. Once this closes:
   A. there is an immediate decrease in systemic vascular resistance.
   B. blood can bypass the lungs by moving from the pulmonary trunk directly into the aorta.
   C. there is a decrease in pulmonary vascular resistance.
   D. it becomes a fibrous cord embedded in the wall of the heart.

_____ 4. Lungs of a full-term fetus continually secrete surfactant whose purpose is to:
   A. hold the moist membranes of the lungs together.
   B. reduce the surface tension so lungs expand more easily.
   C. increase the efficiency of the oxygen–carbon dioxide exchange.
   D. regulate blood flow from the pulmonary arteries to the lungs.

_____ 5. Which of the following is true regarding an infant's pulmonary system?
   A. The infant is primarily a "mouth breather" until at least 4 weeks of age.
   B. An infant's lung tissue is prone to barotrauma.
   C. Breathing becomes ineffective at rates higher than 30 breaths per minute.
   D. Slow respiratory rates lead to rapid heat and fluid loss.

_____ 6. An infant can easily become dehydrated and develop water and electrolyte imbalance because:
   A. infants tend to perspire a great deal.
   B. urine is highly concentrated until the kidneys mature.
   C. their stool has a large amount of water in it.
   D. urine is a relatively dilute fluid with a specific gravity that rarely exceeds 1.0.

_____ 7. A reflex that occurs when a newborn is startled, causing the arms to throw wide and the fingers to spread, followed by a grabbing motion, is called the:
   A. palmar reflex.
   B. Moro reflex.
   C. rooting reflex.
   D. sucking reflex.

_____ 8. The purpose of the fontanelles is to allow for:
   A. growth of the heart and lungs.
   B. the growth of long bones.
   C. compression of the head during childbirth.
   D. intracranial pressure changes when the infant sucks.

_____ 9. The formation of a close personal relationship, especially through frequent or constant association, is called:
   A. bonding.
   B. secure attachment.
   C. scaffolding.
   D. anxious resistant attachment.

_____ 10. A stage of psychosocial development that lasts from birth to about 1½ years of age is:
   A. passive-aggressive.
   B. secure attachment.
   C. trust vs. mistrust.
   D. scaffolding.

HANDOUT 5-2 Continued

_____ 11. A child characterized by regularity in body functions, low or moderate intensity of reactions, and acceptance of new situations is called a(n):
   A. difficult child.
   B. easy child.
   C. quick-to-warm child.
   D. slow-to-warm child.

_____ 12. Which of the following is true regarding the physiological development of the toddler to school-aged child?
   A. The brain is now at 60 percent of adult weight.
   B. Chest muscles mature and can sustain excessively rapid respiratory rates.
   C. Passive immunity born with the infant will continue to function for a few more years.
   D. The kidneys are well developed by the toddler years.

_____ 13. The parenting style in which parents are demanding and desire instant obedience from a child is called:
   A. permissive.
   B. authoritarian.
   C. prescriptive.
   D. militaristic.

_____ 14. Which of the following statements best describes the psychosocial development of school-aged children?
   A. The development of a self-concept occurs at this age.
   B. The school-aged child strives for autonomy, and the parents strive for control.
   C. Capacity for logical, analytical, and abstract thinking is developed at this age.
   D. Separation anxiety is developed, and the child begins clinging and crying when a parent leaves.

_____ 15. School-aged children experience three levels of moral development. The punishment and obedience stage takes place at which level?
   A. postadaptive reasoning
   B. communicative reasoning
   C. preconventional reasoning
   D. cognitive reasoning

_____ 16. Depression and suicide are most common in which age group?
   A. adolescence
   B. early adulthood
   C. middle adulthood
   D. late adulthood

_____ 17. Cardiovascular health becomes a major concern, with cardiac output decreasing and cholesterol levels increasing, for which age group?
   A. adolescence
   B. early adulthood
   C. middle adulthood
   D. late adulthood

_____ 18. At 61 years of age and older, which of the following physiological changes takes place?
   A. Cortisol from the adrenal cortex is diminished by 50 percent.
   B. There is a 25 to 30 percent decrease in kidney mass.
   C. An increase in neurotransmitters in the nervous system results in a decrease in coordination.
   D. The ear canal atrophies and the eardrum thins.

_____ 19. A hearing loss of pure tones that increases with age is called:
   A. tone-deafness.
   B. presbycusis.
   C. audioporosis.
   D. cochlearitis.

_____ 20. The major cause of death for adults 40 years of age and older is:
   A. suicide.
   B. ill health.
   C. falls.
   D. motor vehicle crashes.

HANDOUT 5-3

Student's Name _____

CHAPTER 5 SCENARIO

Review the following real-life situation. Then answer the questions that follow.

"Hammond Medic 5, respond priority one to 1324 170th Street for a 7-year-old child who has been vomiting and has a fever. Cross street is Chestnut Ave. Time out is 1750." When you arrive on scene, the child's mother meets you at the door. She appears anxious and concerned. She leads you to the child's bedroom, where he is lying on the bed, obviously not feeling well, tightly holding a stuffed bear. His mother tells you he has been sick for a couple of days and came home from school sick today. He began to vomit frequently this afternoon and can't "keep anything down." The child looks at the paramedics and begins to whimper.

1. How would you approach this patient?

2. How would you conduct your physical exam of this patient?

3. What are the normal vital signs for a child this age?

Handout 5-4

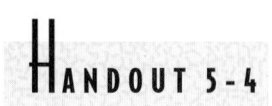

Student's Name _____

CHAPTER 5 REVIEW

Write the word or words that best complete the following sentences in the space provided.

1. The younger the child, the more _____ the pulse and respiratory rate.
2. The infant's head is equal to _____ percent of total body weight.
3. An infant's airway is _____, _____, less _____, and more _____ _____ than that of an adult.
4. The _____ _____ occurs when a newborn is startled, and its arms are thrown wide, fingers spread, and a grabbing motion follows.
5. The _____ _____ is a reflex in the newborn that is elicited by placing a finger firmly in the infant's palm.
6. The _____ _____ occurs when an infant's cheek is touched by a hand or cloth, and the hungry infant turns his head to the right or left.
7. The _____ _____ occurs when an infant's lips are stroked.
8. Diamond-shaped soft spots of fibrous tissue at the top of an infant's skull are called _____.
9. The formation of a close personal relationship, especially through frequent or constant association, is called _____.
10. _____ _____ _____ is a type of bonding that occurs when an infant learns to be uncertain about whether or not his caregivers will be responsive or helpful when needed.
11. A type of bonding that occurs when an infant learns that his caregivers will be responsive and helpful when needed is called _____ _____.
12. _____ _____ _____ is a type of bonding that occurs when an infant learns that his caregivers will not be responsive or helpful when needed.
13. _____ _____ _____ refers to a stage of psychosocial development that lasts from birth to about 1½ years of age.
14. _____ is a teaching/learning technique in which one builds on what has already been learned.
15. An infant who can be characterized by regularity of body functions, low or moderate intensity of reactions, and acceptance of new situations is called a(n) _____ _____.
16. An infant who can be characterized by a low intensity of reactions and a somewhat negative mood is called a(n) _____-_____-_____-_____ _____.
17. Children develop separation anxiety between the ages of _____ and _____ months.
18. A(n) _____ parenting style demands absolute obedience without regard to a child's individual freedom.
19. _____ parenting takes a tolerant, accepting view of a child's behavior.
20. The stage of moral development during which children desire approval from individuals and society is called _____ _____.
21. Because of _____, the adolescent prefers that parents not be present during physical examinations.
22. During middle adulthood, the body still functions at a high level with varying degrees of degradation based on the _____.

184 ESSENTIALS OF PARAMEDIC CARE

HANDOUT 5-4 Continued

23. The theoretical, species-specific, longest duration of life, excluding premature or "unnatural" death, is called _____ _____ _____.

24. The ability to learn and adjust _____ throughout life.

25. A theory that death is preceded by a 5-year period of decreasing cognitive functioning is called the _____-_____ _____.

Handout 5-5

Student's Name _____

NORMAL VITAL SIGNS

Complete the chart below, filling in pulse, respiration, and blood pressure for each of the developmental stages of life.

Life Stage	Pulse	Respirations	Blood Pressure
Infancy (at birth)			
Infancy (at one year)			
Toddler (12 to 36 months)			
Preschool age (3 to 5 years)			
School aged (6 to 12 years)			
Adolescence (13 to 18 years)			
Early adulthood (19 to 40 years)			
Middle adulthood (41 to 60 years)			
Late adulthood (61+ years)			

Chapter 5 Answer Key

Handout 5-2: Chapter 5 Quiz

1. A	6. D	11. B	16. A
2. D	7. B	12. D	17. C
3. C	8. C	13. C	18. B
4. B	9. A	14. A	19. B
5. B	10. C	15. C	20. B

Handout 5-3: Chapter 5 Scenario

1. Remember that patients in this age-group have developed decision-making skills and are allowed more self-regulation. It is important to talk to the child and not just the parent. Introduce yourself to this patient as you would any patient, and, even though it is not necessary with the parent there, ask permission to treat him or to take a look at him. While you can gain much of your medical history information from the mother, ask the patient questions also. A child this age can be a good source of information, especially about his current medical problem. Since this age-group begins to develop self-esteem, your inclusion of the patient in the process will help him psychologically, as well.
2. As above, be sure to involve the patient in the process. Do not ignore him and just talk with the parent. Explain what you are doing and why. Ask permission to perform vital signs and any portion of the physical exam you feel is necessary. The child will respond well to you if you treat him with respect, but do not forget he is a child. He is holding on to his stuffed bear. Allow him to continue to hold it if possible. You may even perform some portions of the physical exam on the bear first, to show the child what will happen. Be sure to get down to the patient's eye level or below when talking with him. You are an authority figure, especially in your uniform, so do whatever you can to allay his fears.
3. School-aged children have a pulse rate of 65 to 110 beats per minute, a respiratory rate of 18 to 30 breaths per minute, blood pressure of 97 to 112 systolic, and an average body temperature of 98.6°F.

Handout 5-4: Chapter 5 Review

1. rapid
2. 25
3. shorter, narrower, stable, easily obstructed
4. Moro reflex
5. palmar grasp
6. rooting reflex
7. sucking reflex
8. fontanelles
9. bonding
10. Anxious resistant attachment
11. secure attachment
12. Anxious avoidant attachment
13. Trust vs. mistrust
14. Scaffolding
15. easy child
16. slow-to-warm-up child
17. 18, 24
18. authoritarian
19. Permissive
20. conventional reasoning
21. modesty
22. individual
23. maximum life span
24. continues
25. terminal-drop hypothesis

Handout 5-5: Normal Vital Signs

Life Stage	Pulse	Respirations	Blood Pressure
Infancy (at birth)	100 to 180	30 to 69	60 to 90 systolic
Infancy (at one year)	100 to 160	30 to 60	87 to 105 systolic
Toddler (12 to 36 months)	80 to 110	24 to 40	95 to 105 systolic
Preschool age (3 to 5 years)	70 to 110	22 to 34	95 to 110 systolic
School aged (6 to 12 years)	65 to 110	18 to 30	97 to 112 systolic
Adolescence (13 to 18 years)	60 to 90	12 to 26	112 to 128 systolic
Early adulthood (19 to 40 years)	60 to 100	12 to 20	120/80
Middle adulthood (41 to 60 years)	60 to 100	12 to 20	120/80
Late adulthood (61+ years)	Depends on individual health status	Depends on individual health status	Depends on individual health status

Chapter 6: General Principles of Pharmacology

INTRODUCTION

The use of herbs and minerals to treat the ill has been documented for centuries, beginning with the ancient Egyptians, Arabs, and Greeks. Paramedics must have a fundamental knowledge of the medications they deliver to patients in prehospital emergency medicine. This chapter deals with general pharmacological principles and the classifications of drugs. It also serves as a reference text for drugs referred to in other chapters in this book.

CHAPTER OBJECTIVES

Part 1: Basic Pharmacology (p. 309)

After reading Part 1 of this chapter, you should be able to:

1. Describe important historical trends in pharmacology. (p. 309)
2. Differentiate among the chemical, generic (nonproprietary), official (USP), and trade (proprietary) names of a drug. (pp. 309–310)
3. List the four main sources of drug products. (p. 310)
4. List the authoritative sources for drug information. (pp. 310–311)
5. List legislative acts controlling drug use and abuse in the United States. (pp. 311–313)
6. Differentiate among Schedule I, II, III, IV, and V substances and list examples of substances in each schedule. (p. 312)
7. Discuss standardization of drugs. (p. 313)
8. Discuss special considerations in drug treatment with regard to pregnant, pediatric, and geriatric patients. (pp. 314–316)
9. Discuss the paramedic's responsibilities and scope of management pertinent to the administration of medications. (pp. 313–314)
10. Review the specific anatomy and physiology pertinent to pharmacology. (pp. 316–326)

> **TOTAL TEACHING TIME: 36.58 HOURS**
> The total teaching time is only a guideline based on the didactic and practical lab averages in the National Standard Curriculum. Instructors should take into consideration such factors as the pace at which students learn, the size of the class, and breaks. The actual time devoted to teaching objectives is the responsibility of the instructor.

11. List and describe general properties of drugs. (pp. 322–324)
12. List and describe liquid and solid drug forms. (pp. 321–322)
13. List and differentiate routes of drug administration. (pp. 320–321)
14. Differentiate between enteral and parenteral routes of drug administration. (pp. 320–321)
15. Describe mechanisms of drug action. (pp. 322–324)
16. List and differentiate the phases of drug activity, including the pharmaceutical, pharmacokinetic, and pharmacodynamic phases. (pp. 316–326)
17. Describe the processes called pharmacokinetics and pharmocodynamics, including theories of drug action, drug-response relationship, factors altering drug responses, predictable drug responses, iatrogenic drug responses, and unpredictable adverse drug responses. (pp. 316–326)
18. Differentiate among drug interactions. (p. 326)
19. Discuss considerations for storing and securing medications. (p. 322)
20. List the components of a drug profile by classification. (p. 311)

Part 2: Drug Classifications (p. 326)

After reading Part 2 of this chapter, you should be able to:

1. Describe how drugs are classified. (pp. 326–327)
2. Review the specific anatomy and physiology pertinent to pharmacology with additional attention to autonomic pharmacology. (pp. 327–370)
3. List and describe common prehospital medications, including indications, contraindications, side effects, routes of administration, and dosages. (pp. 327–370)
4. Given several patient scenarios, identify medications likely to be prescribed and those that are likely a part of the prehospital treatment regimen. (pp. 327–370)
5. Given various patient medications, assess the pathophysiology of a patient's condition by identifying classifications of drugs. (pp. 326–370)

FRAMING THE LESSON

Begin the class by reviewing the important points from Chapter 5, "Life-Span Development." Discuss any aspects of the chapter not understood by students. Then go on to Chapter 6. Ask students to name as many categories of drugs, both prescription and over-the-counter (OTC), as they can think of. These will most likely include medications to treat pain, coughs, flu, diabetes, poisonings, heart problems, gastrointestinal problems, psychological disorders, and so on. Vitamin supplements and herbal medications should also be mentioned. Stress the vast number of medications available, not only by prescription but OTC medications as well. If possible, invite a pharmacist or pharmacy technician to discuss the various types of medication that are now available over-the-counter that were available only by prescription in the past. Next, narrow the discussion to the types of medications that paramedics are likely to give in the prehospital setting. Stress the vital importance of accuracy in medication administration, not only in this chapter but in future chapters, as well. You may also suggest that students obtain a separate text on drug calculations and practice scenarios. Also have students obtain a package of index cards and make flash cards for their study of medications.

TEACHING STRATEGIES

People learn in a variety of ways. Some do better with the spoken word, whereas others prefer the written. Some prefer to work alone, whereas others profit from working in groups. Recognizing these different ways of acquiring knowledge, the authors of this *Instructor's Resource Manual* have provided a variety of teaching strategies for the different types of learners. These strategies are intended to foster higher-level cognitive skills and encourage creative learning and problem solving. For greatest effectiveness, incorporate these strategies into your class lecture. Symbols in the Lecture Outline indicate the points at which various exercises might be most appropriate. Other strategies can be used to preview the lesson or to summarize it.

The following strategies are keyed to specific sections of the lesson.

1. Recognizing Drug Reference Materials. Be sure to have copies of each of the drug reference materials listed in the text. Help students learn to use these references by having them look up drug information using each type of reference. It will quickly be obvious to them which references are easiest to use, most comprehensive, most accurate, and so on. Because many of these books are very expensive, ask your physician, hospital, or clinic contacts for past issues. Most offices replace their *Physician's Desk Reference (PDR)* every year.

2. Analyzing Drug Information. Help students learn the terms associated with pharmacology by locating the term or its meaning on drug advertisements. Pull the ads from magazines or photocopy them. Have students highlight the generic name, trade name, dose, supply options, side effects, indications, contraindications, and so on. Students are usually surprised about the number of side effects of most medications and by the sheer volume and variety of medications available today.

3. Guest Speaker. Arrange to have a pharmacist from the regional hospital visit the class and discuss some of the problems arising from the improper administration of medications. Ask the speaker, if possible, to bring samples of some outdated medications or medications that have developed discolorations or sediments so that students can actually see what they should check for before administering medications. If time permits, ask the pharmacist to discuss problems seen with interactions between OTC and prescribed medications in patients.

4. Recognizing Drug Forms and Routes. Create your own drug arsenal for use during this lecture. Find examples of every type of drug preparation, even those not given in the prehospital setting. Paramedics do encounter most medications at a patient's home or in the hospital. For instance, get nitroglycerin patches to illustrate transdermal administration, a decongestant spray for nasal administration, suppositories for rectal administration, and so on. You will likely find everything you need at your local drug store. Place the items in a display case so that students can see each type and understand their use. This lesson is important to prevent students from thinking narrowly about only the drugs they may administer in the prehospital setting. Additionally, it is visual, which helps them to remember the long list of terms associated with drug forms.

The following strategies can be used at various points throughout the lesson or to help summarize and demonstrate what students have learned.

Flash Cards. This is an excellent chapter for using flash cards, both in Part 1 and in Part 2. Students can prepare cards using pharmacological terminology, drug forms, and classifications of addictive medications, for starters. They can also make cards for prehospital medications, indications, contraindications, and dosage calculations. The medication or term should be on one side of the card and the description on the other.

Students can use the cards for individual study and review or to quiz each other. As an alternative method of presenting the material covered in this chapter, you may wish to consider incorporating discussion of the various classes of drugs into the appropriate medical/trauma lectures. For example, when covering neurological emergencies such as seizure and stroke, introduce the neurological medications. In this way, students receive a few drugs at a time related to the material associated with the drug. Helping students associate a medication with the indications for use prevents rote memorization and promotes actual learning of the medications. These associations can be drawn with nearly every lecture in your medical unit. Additional examples include diabetes medications with renal and endocrine emergencies, psych medications with behavioral emergencies, and breathing medications with respiratory emergencies.

Medications Familiarization Workshop. Divide the class into groups. Distribute a variety of medications and drug references to each group. Tell the groups they are to discover as much information as possible about each assigned medication. At the end of the time period, let the groups take turns presenting what they have discovered about each medication.

Cultural Considerations, Legal Notes, and Patho Pearls. The Student CD-ROM contains this series of informative features to enhance the student's understanding of the material covered in this chapter.

TEACHING OUTLINE

Chapter 6, "General Principles of Pharmacology," is the sixth lesson in Division 1, *Introduction to Advanced Prehospital Care*. Distribute Handout 6-1 so that students can familiarize themselves with the learning goals for this chapter. If students have any questions about the objectives, answer them at this time.

Then present the chapter. One possible lecture outline follows. In the outline, the parenthetical references in regular type are references to text pages; those in bold type are references to figures or tables.

Introduction. Pharmacology, beginning with the use of herbs and minerals to treat the sick and injured, has been documented as long ago as 2000 B.C. (p. 309)

PART 1: BASIC PHARMACOLOGY

I. **General aspects** (pp. 309–311)

A. Names. To study and converse about pharmacology, health care professionals must have a systematic method for naming drugs. (pp. 309–310)
 1. Chemical name
 2. Generic name
 3. Official name
 4. Brand name
B. Sources of drugs (p. 310)
 1. Plants
 2. Animals
 3. Minerals
 4. Laboratory (synthetic)

HANDOUT 6-1
Chapter 6 Objectives Checklist

POINT TO EMPHASIZE
Drugs are not magical. They cannot alter the body systems qualitatively, only quantitatively.

READING/REFERENCE
Bledsoe, B. E., and Clayden, D., *Prehospital Emergency Pharmacology*, 6th ed. Upper Saddle River, NJ: Brady, 2005.

TEACHING TIP
Provide drug packages, both over-the-counter and prescription, for visual aids in this section. Have students identify the generic and brand names. If the package inserts are available, they may even be able to find the chemical names of the drugs. This visual and kinesthetic activity will help students to recognize these medications when they later see them in the field.

POWERPOINT PRESENTATION
Chapter 6 PowerPoint slides 4–5

POWERPOINT PRESENTATION
Chapter 6 PowerPoint slides 6–19

TEACHING STRATEGY 1
Recognizing Drug Reference Materials

C. Reference materials. Using multiple sources and comparing the authors' statements about a drug may lead to the best available information about it. (pp. 310–311)
   1. *United States Pharmacopeia*
   2. *Physicians' Desk Reference*
   3. *Drug Information*
   4. *Monthly Prescribing Reference*
   5. *AMA Drug Evaluation*

D. Components of a drug profile. Paramedic students must become familiar with drug profiles—descriptions of their various properties—as they study specific medications. (p. 311)
   1. Names
   2. Classification
   3. Mechanism of action
   4. Indications
   5. Pharmacokinetics
   6. Side effects/adverse reactions
   7. Routes of administration
   8. Contraindications
   9. Dosage
   10. How supplied
   11. Special considerations

II. Legal aspects. Knowing and obeying the laws and regulations governing medications and their administration is an important part of the paramedic's career. (pp. 311–313)

A. Federal law (pp. 311–312)
   1. Pure Food and Drug Act of 1906
   2. Harrison Narcotic Act of 1914
   3. The Federal Food, Drug, and Cosmetic Act of 1938
   4. Durham-Humphrey Amendments
   5. Comprehensive Drug Abuse Prevention and Control Act of 1970 (**Table 6-1, p. 312**)
   6. Over-the-counter (OTC) medications

B. State laws and regulations (p. 312)

C. Local (p. 313)

D. Standards (p. 313)
   1. USP as official standard
   2. Assay
   3. Bioequivalence
   4. Bioassay

III. Patient care: the safe and effective administration of medications. Paramedics are responsible—legally, morally, and ethically—for the safe and effective administration of medications. (pp. 313–316)

A. Basic guidelines (p. 313)
   1. Know the precautions and contraindications.
   2. Practice proper technique.
   3. Know how to observe and document drug effects.
   4. Maintain a current knowledge of pharmacology.
   5. Establish and maintain professional relationships with other health care providers.
   6. Understand pharmacokinetics and pharmacodynamics.
   7. Have current medication references available.

TEACHING STRATEGY 2
Analyzing Drug Information

POWERPOINT PRESENTATION
Chapter 6 PowerPoint slides 20–23

POINT TO EMPHASIZE
The goal of drug dosing is to achieve the minimum therapeutic effect by the lowest dose possible and avoid toxic effects of higher doses. That is why we always start with lower doses of most emergency drugs. We can always give more.

TEACHING STRATEGY 3
Guest Speaker

POWERPOINT PRESENTATION
Chapter 6 PowerPoint slides 24–32

POINT TO EMPHASIZE
The fetus does not have a functioning blood-brain barrier, so the volume of distribution is different. All medications will enter the baby's brain.

> **TEACHING TIP**
> Your students may be wondering why they need to know this information. Point out to them, for example, that because lidocaine is metabolized in the liver, you must give lower doses to people with liver disease (alcoholics, hepatitis). Because insulin is eliminated by the kidneys, diabetics with renal failure may have higher levels of insulin and become hypoglycemic faster. This type of information is crucial and relates directly to street medicine.

> **POWERPOINT PRESENTATION**
> Chapter 6 PowerPoint slides 33–54

> **TEACHING STRATEGY 4**
> Recognizing Drug Forms and Routes

> **TEACHING TIP**
> Try a little "show and tell." Bring in samples of the different types of drug preparations and establish a reputation for being an interesting instructor.

8. Take careful drug histories including:
   a. Name, strength, and daily dose of prescribed drugs
   b. Over-the-counter drugs
   c. Vitamins
   d. Herbal medications
   e. Folk medicine or folk remedies
   f. Allergies
9. Evaluate the compliance, dosage, and adverse reactions.
10. Consult with medical direction when appropriate.

B. Six rights of medication administration (pp. 313–314)
   1. Right medication
   2. Right dose
   3. Right time
   4. Right route
   5. Right patient
   6. Right documentation

C. Special considerations (pp. 314–316)
   1. Pregnant patients
      a. Free drug availability
      b. FDA pregnancy categories (**Table 6-2, p. 315**)
   2. Pediatric patients (**Fig. 6-1, p. 316**)
   3. Geriatric patients

IV. **Pharmacology.** Pharmacology is the study of drugs and their interactions with the body. (pp. 314–326)

A. Pharmacokinetics (pp. 317–322)
   1. Review of physiology of transport
   2. Absorption
   3. Distribution
   4. Biotransformation
   5. Elimination
   6. Drug routes
      a. Enteral routes
         i. Absorption through the gastrointestinal tract
         ii. Oral (PO)
         iii. Orogastric/nasogastric tube (OG/NG)
         iv. Sublingual (SL)
         v. Buccal
         vi. Rectal (PR)
      b. Parenteral routes
         i. Delivery through any route outside the gastrointestinal tract
         ii. Intravenous (IV)
         iii. Endotracheal (ET)
         iv. Intraosseous (IO)
         v. Umbilical
         vi. Intramuscular (IM)
         vii. Subcutaneous (SC, SQ, SubQ)
         viii. Inhalation/nebulized
         ix. Topical
         x. Transdermal
         xi. Nasal
         xii. Instillation
         xiii. Intradermal
   7. Drug forms
      a. Solids
         i. Pills

                ii. Powders
               iii. Tablets
                iv. Suppositories
                 v. Capsules
             b. Liquids
                 i. Solutions
                ii. Tinctures
               iii. Suspensions
                iv. Emulsions
                 v. Spirits
                vi. Elixirs
               vii. Syrups
        8. Drug storage
    B. Pharmacodynamics (pp. 322–326)
        1. Actions of drugs
             a. Binding to a receptor site
                 i. Agonists
                ii. Antagonists
             b. Changing physical properties
             c. Chemically combining with other substances
             d. Altering a normal metabolic pathway
        2. Responses to drug administration
             a. Allergic reaction
             b. Idiosyncrasy
             c. Tolerance
             d. Cross tolerance
             e. Tachyphylaxis
             f. Cumulative effect
             g. Drug dependence
             h. Drug interaction
             i. Drug antagonism
             j. Summation
             k. Synergism
             l. Potentiation
             m. Interference
        3. Drug-response relationship
        4. Factors altering drug response
             a. Age
             b. Body mass
             c. Sex
             d. Environmental milieu
             e. Time of administration
             f. Pathologic state
             g. Genetic factors
             h. Psychological factors
        5. Drug interaction

TEACHING TIP
When discussing drug receptors, use the analogy of the "lock and key."

PART 2: DRUG CLASSIFICATIONS

I. Classifying drugs. Drugs can be classified in many ways. Grouping them according to their uses, as in this chapter, is a very practical way of classifying them. (p. 327)

II. Drugs used to affect the nervous system. The two major groupings of medications used to affect the nervous system are those that affect the central nervous system and those that affect the autonomic nervous system. (pp. 327–342)

POWERPOINT PRESENTATION
Chapter 6 PowerPoint slides 4–13

TEACHING TIP
Motivate students to learn this basic information because the vast majority of emergency drugs affect the autonomic nervous system.

POWERPOINT PRESENTATION
Chapter 6 PowerPoint slides 14–25

A. Central nervous system medications (pp. 327–336) (**Fig. 6-2, p. 328**)
   1. Analgesics and antagonists
      a. Opioid agonists
      b. Nonopioid analgesics
      c. Opioid antagonists
      d. Adjunct medications
      e. Opioid agonist-antagonists
   2. Anesthetics
   3. Antianxiety and sedative-hypnotic drugs
   4. Antiseizure or antiepileptic drugs (**Table 6-3, p. 332**)
   5. Central nervous system stimulants
   6. Psychotherapeutic medications (**Fig. 6-3, p. 334**)
   7. Drugs used to treat Parkinson's disease
B. Autonomic nervous system medications (pp. 336–342)
   1. Basic anatomy and physiology
   2. Drugs used to affect the parasympathetic nervous system (**Table 6-4, p. 340**)
      a. Cholinergics
      b. Anticholinergics
      c. Ganglionic blocking agents
      d. Neuromuscular blocking agents
      e. Ganglionic stimulating agents
   3. Drugs used to affect the sympathetic nervous system.
      a. Adrenergic receptors (**Table 6-5, p. 342**)
      b. Adrenergic agonists
      c. Adrenergic antagonists
      d. Skeletal muscle relaxants

III. Drugs used to affect the cardiovascular system. Cardiovascular care—and with it, understanding of cardiovascular drugs—remains an important and integral part of a paramedic's knowledge base. (pp. 343–353)

A. Cardiovascular physiology review (p. 343)
   1. Impulse generation and conduction
   2. Dysrhythmia generation
B. Classes of cardiovascular drugs (pp. 343–353)
   1. Antidysrhythmics (**Table 6-6, p. 343**)
      a. Sodium channel blockers (Class I)
      b. Beta-blockers (Class II)
      c. Potassium channel blockers (Class III)
      d. Calcium channel blockers (Class IV)
      e. Miscellaneous antidysrhythmics
   2. Antihypertensives
      a. Diuretics
      b. Adrenergic inhibiting agents
      c. Angiotensin converting enzyme (ACE) inhibitors
      d. Angiotensin II receptor antagonists
      e. Calcium channel blocking agents
      f. Direct vasodilators
   3. Hemostatic agents
      a. Antiplatelets
      b. Anticoagulants
      c. Fibrinolytics
   4. Antihyperlipidemic agents

IV. Drugs used to affect the respiratory system. Drugs that affect the respiratory system are useful in treating asthma and as cough suppressants, nasal decongestants, and antihistamines. (pp. 353–356)

  A. Antiasthmatic medications (pp. 353–355) (**Table 6-7, p. 354**)
     1. Beta$_2$ specific agents
     2. Nonselective sympathomimetics
     3. Methylxanthines
     4. Anticholinergics
     5. Glucocorticoids
     6. Leukotriene antagonists
  B. Drugs used for rhinitis and cough (pp. 355–356)
     1. Nasal decongestants
     2. Antihistamines
     3. Cough suppressants

V. Drugs used to affect the gastrointestinal system. The main purposes of drug therapy in the gastrointestinal system are to treat peptic ulcers, constipation, diarrhea, and emesis and to aid digestion. (pp. 356–359)

  A. Drugs used to treat peptic ulcer disease (pp. 356–358)
     1. H$_2$ receptor antagonists
     2. Proton pump inhibitors
     3. Antacids
     4. Anticholinergics
  B. Drugs used to treat constipation—laxatives (p. 358)
     1. Bulk-forming
     2. Surfactant
     3. Stimulant
     4. Osmotic
  C. Drugs used to treat diarrhea (p. 358)
  D. Drugs used to treat emesis (pp. 358–359)
     1. Antiemetics
     2. Serotonin antagonists
     3. Dopamine antagonists
     4. Cannabinoids
  E. Drugs used to aid digestion (p. 359)

VI. Drugs used to affect the eyes. Ophthalmic drugs are used to treat conditions involving the eyes, primarily glaucoma and trauma; others are used in diagnosing and examining the eyes. (pp. 359–360)

VII. Drugs used to affect the ears. Most drugs used to treat conditions involving the ear are aimed at eliminating underlying bacterial or fungal infections or at breaking up impacted ear wax. (p. 360)

VIII. Drugs used to affect the endocrine system. The endocrine system works in conjunction with the nervous system to regulate and maintain homeostasis. (pp. 360–366) (**Table 6-8, p. 363**)

  A. Drugs affecting the pituitary gland (p. 360)
     1. Anterior pituitary drugs
     2. Posterior pituitary drugs
  B. Drugs affecting the parathyroid and thyroid glands (pp. 360–361)
  C. Drugs affecting the adrenal cortex (p. 361)

D. Drugs affecting the pancreas (pp. 361–364)
   1. Insulin preparations
   2. Oral hypoglycemic agents
   3. Hyperglycemic agents
E. Drugs affecting the female reproductive system (pp. 364–365)
   1. Estrogens and progestins
   2. Oral contraceptives
   3. Uterine stimulants and relaxants
   4. Infertility agents
F. Drugs affecting the male reproductive system (p. 365)
G. Drugs affecting sexual behavior (pp. 365–366)

IX. Drugs used to treat cancer. Of the many known types of cancer, only a few are successfully treated with chemotherapy. (p. 366)

X. Drugs used to treat infectious diseases and inflammation. Infectious diseases may be treated with antimicrobial drugs developed to fight the bacteria, viruses, or "fungi" that cause them. (pp. 366–368)

A. Antibiotics (pp. 366–367)
B. Antifungal and antiviral agents (p. 367)
C. Other antimicrobial and antiparasitic agents (p. 367)
D. Nonsteroidal antiinflammatory drugs (NSAIDs) (p. 367)
E. Uricosuric drugs (p. 367)
F. Serums, vaccines, and other immunizing agents (p. 368)
G. Immune suppressing and enhancing agents (p. 368)

XI. Drugs used to affect the skin. Dermatologic drugs are common over-the-counter medications used to treat skin irritations. (p. 368)

XII. Drugs used to supplement the diet. Dietary supplements can help to maintain needed levels of essential nutrients and fluids. (pp. 368–369)

A. Vitamins and minerals (p. 369) (**Table 6-9, p. 369**)
B. Fluids and electrolytes (p. 369)

XIII. Drugs used to treat poisoning and overdoses. In general, treatment for poisoning and overdose aims at eliminating the substance. (p. 370)

A. Eliminating the substance (p. 370)
   1. Emptying the gastric contents
   2. Increasing gastric motility
   3. Alkalinizing the urine
   4. Filtering the substance from the blood
B. Actual antidotes are few. (p. 370)
   1. Receptor site antagonism
   2. Chelation

XIV. Chapter summary (p. 370). Pharmacology is a cornerstone of paramedic practice. Paramedics must have a solid understanding of its foundations (legal issues, terminology, drug forms, and routes), pharmacokinetics, and pharmacodynamics if they are to practice their profession safely. Additionally, paramedics must understand not only the medications they personally administer, but also the medications that their patients are taking on an ongoing basis. Though you are not likely to remember everything in this chapter after your first reading, with diligent study and practice you can master this information. This chapter has barely broken the surface of pharmacology. To continue your education, you should take the time to understand the mechanisms and interactions of the medications your patients are taking. If you do not already know them (you will not in the majority of cases as you begin your career), look them up. Many very useful drug references are available today. Most are small and can be easily carried with you on your unit or in your station.

Finally, pharmacology is a dynamic field with new discoveries being made every day. If you take your responsibilities as a paramedic seriously and remain current on the latest changes in this field, you can be sure that you can give your patients the care they deserve.

ASSIGNMENTS

Assign students to complete Chapter 6, "General Principles of Pharmacology," of the workbook. Also assign them to read Chapter 7, "Medication Administration," before the next class.

WORKBOOK
Chapter 6 Activities

READING/REFERENCE
Textbook, pp. 373–453

EVALUATION

Chapter Quiz and Scenario   Distribute copies of the Chapter Quizzes provided in Handouts 6-2 and 6-3 to evaluate student understanding of this chapter. Make sure each student reads the Scenario to reinforce critical thinking on the scene. Remind students not to use their notes or textbooks while taking the quiz.

Student CD   Quizzes for every chapter are contained on the dynamic and highly visual in-text student CD.

Companion Website   Additional quizzes for every chapter are contained on this exciting website.

TestGen   You may wish to create a custom-tailored test using *Prentice Hall TestGen for Essentials of Paramedic Care*, 2nd Edition to evaluate student understanding of this chapter.

On-line Test Preparation (for students and instructors)   Additional test preparation is available through Brady's new on-line product, *EMT Achieve: Paramedic Test Preparation* at *http://www.prenhall.com/emtachieve/*. Instructors can also monitor student mastery on-line.

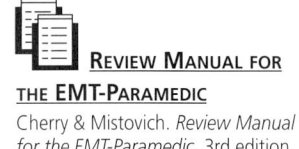

Review Manual for the EMT-Paramedic   This comprehensive exam review contains hundreds of test questions and rationales, including scenarios, along with two 180-question practice tests on CD.

HANDOUTS 6-2 AND 6-3
Chapter 6 Quizzes

HANDOUT 6-4
Chapter 6 Scenario

PARAMEDIC STUDENT CD
Student Activities

COMPANION WEBSITE
http://www.prenhall.com/bledsoe

TESTGEN
Chapter 6

EMT ACHIEVE: PARAMEDIC TEST PREPARATION
Mistovich & Beasley. *EMT Achieve: Paramedic Test Preparation.*
www.prenhall.com/emtachieve/

REVIEW MANUAL FOR THE EMT-PARAMEDIC
Cherry & Mistovich. *Review Manual for the EMT-Paramedic*, 3rd edition.

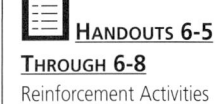

REINFORCEMENT

Handouts   If classroom discussion or performance on the quiz indicates that some students have not fully mastered the chapter content, you may wish to assign some or all of the Reinforcement Handouts for this chapter.

Student CD (for students)   A wide variety of material on this CD-ROM will reinforce and also expand student knowledge and skills.

PowerPoint Presentation (for instructors)   The PowerPoint material developed for this chapter offers useful reinforcement of chapter content.

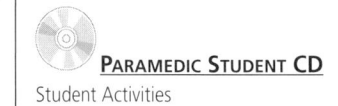

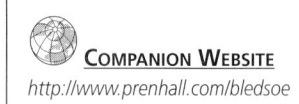

HANDOUTS 6-5 THROUGH 6-8
Reinforcement Activities

PARAMEDIC STUDENT CD
Student Activities

POWERPOINT PRESENTATION
Chapter 6

COMPANION WEBSITE
http://www.prenhall.com/bledsoe

ONEKEY
Chapter 6

ADVANCED LIFE SUPPORT SKILLS
Larmon & Davis. *Advanced Life Support Skills.*

ADVANCED LIFE SKILLS REVIEW.
Larmon & Davis. *Advanced Life Skills Review.*

BRADY SKILLS SERIES: ALS
Larmon & Davis. *Brady Skills Series: ALS.*

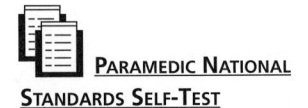

PARAMEDIC NATIONAL STANDARDS SELF-TEST
Miller. *Paramedic National Standards Self-Test,* 4th edition.

Companion Website (for students)   Additional review quizzes and links to EMS resources will contribute to further reinforcement of the chapter.

OneKey   On-line support is offered for this course on one of three platforms: Course Compass, Blackboard, or Web CT. Includes the IRM, PowerPoints, TestGen, and Companion Website for instruction. Ask your local sales representative for more information.

Brady Skills Series: Advanced Life Skills (Video or CD)   Have your students watch the skills come to life on VHS or CD-ROM, or they can purchase the highly visual, full-color text with step-by-step procedures and rationales.

Handout 6-1

Student's Name _____

CHAPTER 6 OBJECTIVES CHECKLIST

PART 1: BASIC PHARMACOLOGY

Knowledge	Date Mastered
1. Describe important historical trends in pharmacology.	
2. Differentiate among the chemical, generic (nonproprietary), official (USP), and trade (proprietary) names of a drug.	
3. List the four main sources of drug products.	
4. List the authoritative sources for drug information.	
5. List legislative acts controlling drug use and abuse in the United States.	
6. Differentiate among Schedule I, II, III, IV, and V substances and list examples of substances in each schedule.	
7. Discuss standardization of drugs.	
8. Discuss special considerations in drug treatment with regard to pregnant, pediatric, and geriatric patients.	
9. Discuss the paramedic's responsibilities and scope of management pertinent to the administration of medications.	
10. Review the specific anatomy and physiology pertinent to pharmacology.	
11. List and describe general properties of drugs.	
12. List and describe liquid and solid drug forms.	
13. List and differentiate routes of drug administration.	
14. Differentiate between enteral and parenteral routes of drug administration.	
15. Describe mechanisms of drug action.	
16. List and differentiate the phases of drug activity, including the pharmaceutical, pharmacokinetic, and pharmacodynamic phases.	
17. Describe the processes called pharmacokinetics and pharmacodynamics, including theories of drug action, drug-response relationship, factors altering drug responses, predictable drug responses, iatrogenic drug responses, and unpredictable adverse drug responses.	
18. Differentiate among drug interactions.	

©2007 Pearson Education, Inc.
Essentials of Paramedic Care, 2nd ed.

HANDOUT 6-1 Continued

OBJECTIVES

Knowledge	Date Mastered
19. Discuss considerations for storing and securing medications.	
20. List the components of a drug profile by classification.	

PART 2: DRUG CLASSIFICATIONS

Knowledge	Date Mastered
1. Describe how drugs are classified.	
2. Review the specific anatomy and physiology pertinent to pharmacology with additional attention to autonomic pharmacology.	
3. List and describe common prehospital medications, including indications, contraindications, side effects, routes of administration, and dosages.	
4. Given several patient scenarios, identify medications likely to be prescribed and those that are likely a part of the prehospital treatment regimen.	
5. Given various patient medications, assess the pathophysiology of a patient's condition by identifying classifications of drugs.	

Handout 6-2

Student's Name _____

CHAPTER 6 QUIZ

PART 1: BASIC PHARMACOLOGY

Write the letter of the best answer in the space provided.

_____ 1. Which of the following is one of the four drug names?
  A. biological name
  B. proper name
  C. official name
  D. sales name

_____ 2. The four main sources for drugs include:
  A. animals.
  B. plants.
  C. minerals.
  D. all of the these

_____ 3. For many years the primary source of insulin for treating diabetes mellitus was the extract of:
  A. primate pancreas.
  B. porcine pancreas.
  C. equine pancreas.
  D. bovine pancreas.

_____ 4. A compilation of drug inserts, the printed fact sheets that drug manufacturers supply with most medications, is found in the:
  A. *United States Pharmacopeia.*
  B. *Monthly Prescribing Reference.*
  C. *AMA Drug Evaluation.*
  D. *Physicians' Desk Reference.*

_____ 5. Name, classification, mechanism of action, indications, and so forth, are information contained in a drug's:
  A. profile.
  B. overview.
  C. synopsis.
  D. review.

_____ 6. According to the Controlled Substances Act of 1970, heroin is a Schedule 1 drug, meaning it:
  A. has a low abuse potential.
  B. has no accepted medical indications.
  C. may lead to limited psychological and/or physical dependence.
  D. has a low physical, but high psychological, dependence potential.

_____ 7. Drug legislation passed in the United States in 1906 to protect the public from adulterated or mislabeled drugs was the:
  A. Harrison Narcotic Act.
  B. Federal Food, Drug, and Cosmetic Act.
  C. Pure Food and Drug Act.
  D. Comprehensive Drug Abuse Prevention and Control Act.

_____ 8. According to the Controlled Substances Act of 1970, Valium, lorazepam, and phenobarbital are:
  A. Schedule V drugs.
  B. Schedule IV drugs.
  C. Schedule III drugs.
  D. Schedule II drugs.

_____ 9. The _____ test determines the amount and purity of a given chemical in a preparation.
  A. assay
  B. bioequivalence
  C. bioassay
  D. pharmacokinetics

_____ 10. How a drug is absorbed, distributed, metabolized, and excreted is called:
  A. bioequivalence.
  B. pharmacokinetics.
  C. pharmacodynamics.
  D. pharmacology.

©2007 Pearson Education, Inc.
Essentials of Paramedic Care, 2nd ed.

CHAPTER 6 *General Principles of Pharmacology*

HANDOUT 6-2 Continued

_____ 11. Which of the following is one of the six "rights" of medication administration?
   A. the right container
   B. the right doctor
   C. the right route
   D. the right pharmacy

_____ 12. Medication packages containing a single dose for a single patient are called:
   A. one-time-use packaging.
   B. dose packaging.
   C. single-patient packaging.
   D. unit packaging.

_____ 13. A medication that may deform or kill a fetus is called a(n):
   A. Category A drug.
   B. teratogenic drug.
   C. fetal risk drug.
   D. fundalgenic drug.

_____ 14. The _____ gives a good approximation of a child's weight based on his height.
   A. Roberts test
   B. Stanislav meter
   C. Weinstein ratio
   D. Broselow tape

_____ 15. How a drug interacts with the body to cause its effects is called:
   A. bioequivalence.
   B. pharmacokinetics.
   C. pharmacodynamics.
   D. pharmacology.

_____ 16. Facilitated diffusion is:
   A. the process in which carrier proteins transport large molecules across the cell membrane.
   B. movement of a substance without the use of energy.
   C. movement of solute in a solution from an area of higher concentration to an area of lower concentration.
   D. movement of molecules across a membrane from an area of higher pressure to an area of lower pressure.

_____ 17. Movement of solvent in a solution from an area of lower solute concentration to an area of higher solute concentration is called:
   A. filtration.
   B. passive transport.
   C. osmosis.
   D. diffusion.

_____ 18. The liver's partial or complete inactivation of a drug before it reaches the systemic circulation is the _____ effect.
   A. hepatic filtration
   B. first-pass
   C. liver-blood barrier
   D. antidrug

_____ 19. Which of the following is true regarding absorption?
   A. The body absorbs most drugs faster through intramuscular injection than through subcutaneous injection.
   B. Time-released medications may have an enteric coating that dissolves more readily in an acidic environment than in a more alkaline environment.
   C. The higher a drug's concentration, the slower the body will absorb it.
   D. No absorption needs to occur if a drug is injected intramuscularly, as it is already in the tissue.

_____ 20. Certain organs exclude some drugs from distribution. An example of this is the:
   A. arterial-venous barrier.
   B. endothelial barrier.
   C. blood-brain barrier.
   D. uterine-fetal barrier.

_____ 21. An example of the enteral route of drug administration is:
   A. sublingual.
   B. intravenous.
   C. subcutaneous.
   D. topical.

_____ 22. Drugs administered by the parenteral route are delivered:
   A. through the gastrointestinal tract.
   B. outside of the gastrointestinal tract.
   C. through an endotracheal or nasogastric tube.
   D. directly on the skin.

HANDOUT 6-2 Continued

_____ 23. Buccal administration of a drug is accomplished:
  A. by nasal spray.
  B. through a newborn's umbilical vein or artery.
  C. between the cheek and the gum.
  D. through an intraosseous needle.

_____ 24. A liquid form of a drug prepared using an alcohol extraction process is called a(n):
  A. solution.
  B. tincture.
  C. emulsion.
  D. spirit.

_____ 25. The force of attraction between a drug and a receptor is called:
  A. efficacy.
  B. binding.
  C. combining.
  D. affinity.

_____ 26. A drug's ability to cause the expected response is its:
  A. concentration.
  B. affinity.
  C. viability.
  D. efficacy.

_____ 27. An agonist is a drug that binds to a receptor:
  A. but does not cause it to initiate the expected response.
  B. and causes it to initiate the expected response.
  C. and stimulates some of its effects but blocks others.
  D. and causes a deformity on the binding site.

_____ 28. By developing a tolerance for morphine sulfate, a patient may develop a tolerance for other opioid agents. This is known as:
  A. tachyphylaxis.
  B. idiosyncrasy.
  C. cross tolerance.
  D. addiction.

_____ 29. An antagonist drug binds to a receptor:
  A. but does not cause it to initiate the expected response.
  B. and causes it to initiate the expected response.
  C. and stimulates some of its effects but blocks others.
  D. and causes a deformity on the binding site.

_____ 30. We use the analogy of a "lock and key" to describe drugs that:
  A. stimulate a receptor site.
  B. cause the body to increase the production of a substance.
  C. escort substances through cell membranes.
  D. reduce or eliminate an allergic reaction.

_____ 31. The period from the time that a drug's level drops below its minimum effective concentration until it is eliminated from the body is called:
  A. duration of action.
  B. therapeutic index.
  C. termination of action.
  D. biologic half-life.

_____ 32. Age affects the drug-response relationship because:
  A. infants and the elderly have less body fat.
  B. the digestive process in infants and the elderly is not as efficient.
  C. medication noncompliance occurs frequently in the elderly.
  D. the liver and kidney functions of the elderly have begun to deteriorate.

_____ 33. Factors affecting the standard drug-response relationship include:
  A. the gravity of the medication.
  B. the consistency of the medication.
  C. time of administration.
  D. brand name vs. generic medications.

HANDOUT 6-2 Continued

_____ **34.** The unintended adverse response known as summation is due to:
  A. unintentionally taking too much of one drug.
  B. one drug's enhancing the effect of another drug.
  C. a direct biochemical interaction between two drugs.
  D. two drugs that both have the same effect being given together.

_____ **35.** If a patient believes that a drug will have a given effect, then he is much more likely to perceive that the effect has occurred. This is known as the:
  A. substitution agent.   **C.** self-defense mechanism.
  B. phantom factor.   **D.** placebo effect.

HANDOUT 6-3

Student's Name _____

CHAPTER 6 QUIZ

PART 2: DRUG CLASSIFICATIONS

Write the letter of the best answer in the space provided.

_____ 1. Components of the central nervous system include:
   A. the autonomic nervous system.
   B. the brain and spinal cord.
   C. the "feed or breed" system.
   D. sensory nerves in the skin.

_____ 2. A drug that best demonstrates a class's common properties is called a(n):
   A. prototype.
   B. beta.
   C. omega.
   D. production.

_____ 3. The drug that best demonstrates the common properties of opioid agonists and illustrates their particular characteristics is:
   A. chloroform.
   B. morphine.
   C. heroin.
   D. codeine.

_____ 4. An agent that enhances the effects of other drugs is a(n):
   A. secondary medication.
   B. peripheral medication.
   C. booster medication.
   D. adjunct medication.

_____ 5. The prototype opioid antagonist is:
   A. opium.
   B. Versed.
   C. Narcan.
   D. ibuprofen.

_____ 6. Which of the following statements regarding opioid agonist-antagonist drugs is true?
   A. Respiratory depression is a common side effect in therapeutic doses.
   B. This class of drug is given in conjunction with other drugs to enhance their effects.
   C. This class of drug combines decreased sensation of pain with amnesia.
   D. This class of drug decreases pain response and has few respiratory depressant or addictive side effects.

_____ 7. The major difference between anesthetic and neuroleptanesthetic drugs is that the neuroleptanesthetic drugs:
   A. decrease pain sensation and produce amnesia while the patient remains conscious.
   B. induce a loss of all sensation, often impairing consciousness.
   C. are neuromuscular blocking agents that produce paralysis.
   D. include halothane, which is the prototype for this class of drug.

_____ 8. Benzodiazepines and barbiturates are the two main pharmacologic classes in the functional class of:
   A. antiseizure or antiepileptic drugs.
   B. analgesics and antagonists.
   C. antianxiety and sedative-hypnotic drugs.
   D. anesthetics.

_____ 9. The drug used primarily to treat absence seizures is:
   A. phenytoin.
   B. ethosuximide.
   C. phenobarbitol.
   D. carbamazepine.

_____ 10. The central nervous system stimulants known as the methylxanthines include:
   A. Ritalin.
   B. Dexedrine.
   C. theophylline
   D. amphetamine sulfate.

HANDOUT 6-3 Continued

_____ 11. Methylphenidate is the most commonly prescribed drug for:
   A. asthma.
   B. congestive heart failure.
   C. attention deficit hyperactivity disorder.
   D. motion sickness.

_____ 12. Muscle tremors and parkinsonism-like effects are common side effects of antipsychotic medications. These are known as:
   A. extrapyramidal symptoms.
   B. neuroleptic symptoms.
   C. psychotherapeutic symptoms.
   D. partial seizures.

_____ 13. The prototype phenothiazine drug is:
   A. Haldol.
   B. Thorazine.
   C. Benadryl.
   D. Ritalin.

_____ 14. Which of the following is true regarding phenothiazines and butyrophenones?
   A. Both have been the mainstays of psychiatry since the mid-1960s.
   B. These medications' therapeutic effects appear to come from blocking the alpha$_1$ adrenergic receptors in the peripheral nervous system.
   C. Medications in this group block dopamine receptors.
   D. Both are used to treat allergies by blocking histamine receptors.

_____ 15. Acute dystonic reactions are treated with:
   A. atropine.
   B. epinephrine.
   C. Dilantin.
   D. diphenhydramine.

_____ 16. SSRIs are used primarily as:
   A. antiseizure medications.
   B. Parkinson's disease medications.
   C. antidepressant medications.
   D. bipolar disorder medications.

_____ 17. Which of the following is an MAO inhibitor?
   A. Nardil
   B. Paxil
   C. Zoloft
   D. Prozac

_____ 18. The part of the nervous system that controls involuntary actions is the:
   A. central nervous system.
   B. peripheral nervous system.
   C. somatic nervous system.
   D. autonomic nervous system.

_____ 19. Stimulation of the parasympathetic nervous system results in:
   A. pupillary dilation.
   B. secretion by digestive glands.
   C. increase in heart rate and cardiac contractile force.
   D. bronchodilation.

_____ 20. The two main types of acetylcholine receptors are:
   A. nicotinic and muscarinic.
   B. alpha$_1$ and alpha$_2$.
   C. beta$_1$ and beta$_2$.
   D. parasympathomimetic and parasympatholytic.

_____ 21. The acronym SLUDGE is helpful in remembering the effects of cholinergic medication. The effects include:
   A. sedation.
   B. lactation.
   C. urination.
   D. dilation.

_____ 22. The effects of an atropine overdose include the description:
   A. "cold as ice."
   B. "blind as a bat."
   C. "sane as a saint."
   D. "wet as water."

_____ 23. Drugs that produce a state of paralysis without affecting consciousness are:
   A. ganglionic stimulating agents.
   B. ganglionic blocking agents.
   C. neuromuscular blocking agents.
   D. anticholinergics.

HANDOUT 6-3 Continued

_____ 24. Stimulation of the nerves leaving the collateral ganglia in the abdominal cavity causes:
  A. increased blood flow to the abdominal organs.
  B. increased digestive activity.
  C. relaxation of smooth muscle in the wall of the urinary bladder.
  D. retention of glucose stores in the liver.

_____ 25. Dopaminergic receptors, although not fully understood, are believed to cause:
  A. dilation of the renal, coronary, and cerebral arteries.
  B. constriction of peripheral arteries.
  C. an increase in respirations and blood flow to the respiratory system.
  D. constriction of the hepatic arteries.

_____ 26. Stimulation of the alpha$_1$ receptors results in:
  A. increased heart rate.   C. bronchodilation.
  B. renin release.   D. arteriole and venous constriction.

_____ 27. Stimulation of beta$_2$ receptors results in:
  A. increased heart rate.
  B. inhibition of contractions of the uterus.
  C. increased cardiac contractility.
  D. mydriasis.

_____ 28. Terbutaline specifically targets:
  A. alpha$_1$ receptors.   C. beta$_1$ receptors.
  B. alpha$_2$ receptors.   D. beta$_2$ receptors.

_____ 29. Lidocaine and phenytoin belong to the class of:
  A. calcium channel blockers.   C. sodium channel blockers.
  B. potassium channel blockers.   D. beta blockers.

_____ 30. Procainamide is indicated in the treatment of:
  A. atrial fibrillation with a rapid ventricular response.
  B. torsade de pointes.
  C. hypertension.
  D. congestive heart failure.

_____ 31. An endogenous nucleoside with a very short half-life (about 10 seconds), with alarming side effects such as shortness of breath and chest pain, is:
  A. Lanoxin.   C. Adenocard.
  B. magnesium.   D. verapamil.

_____ 32. Which class of drugs is used to decrease blood pressure by decreasing the amount of circulating angiotensin II and decreasing peripheral vascular resistance?
  A. calcium channel blockers   C. direct vasodilators
  B. ACE inhibitors   D. adrenergic inhibiting agents

_____ 33. Drugs used to treat high blood cholesterol are called:
  A. vasculotensives.   C. LDLs.
  B. ACE inhibitors.   D. antihyperlipidemics.

_____ 34. Activase is used to:
  A. break down thrombi.
  B. dilate blood vessels to reduce blood pressure.
  C. decrease the formation of platelet plugs.
  D. interrupt the clotting cascade.

_____ 35. Beta$_2$ specific agents used to treat asthma-induced shortness of breath include:
  A. Proventil.   C. Flovent.
  B. theophylline.   D. Deltasone.

HANDOUT 6-3 Continued

_____ 36. Medications that suppress the stimulus to cough in the central nervous system are called:
  A. antihistamines.
  B. expectorants.
  C. antitussives.
  D. mucolytics.

_____ 37. The hormone oxytocin causes uterine contraction and milk ejection. It is released by the:
  A. thyroid.
  B. pancreas.
  C. adrenal.
  D. posterior pituitary.

_____ 38. The substance that is secreted from the pancreatic islets by alpha cells and that increases blood glucose level is:
  A. insulin.
  B. glucagon.
  C. prolactin.
  D. luteinizing hormone.

_____ 39. A solution containing a modified pathogen that does not actually cause disease but still stimulates the development of antibodies specific to it is a(n):
  A. serum.
  B. vaccine.
  C. immunoglobulin.
  D. antibiotic.

_____ 40. The antidote for organophosphate poisoning is:
  A. epinephrine.
  B. lidocaine.
  C. Benadryl.
  D. atropine.

HANDOUT 6-4

Student's Name _____

CHAPTER 6 SCENARIO

Review the following real-life situation. Then answer the questions that follow.

You receive a call for a patient with chest pain. When you arrive on scene you find a 52-year-old male patient complaining of retrosternal chest pain radiating to the left arm. The patient describes his pain as a "squeezing" type and rates it as an 8 on a 1-to-10 scale. The pain began approximately 30 minutes earlier and has been getting steadily worse. The patient says he has never experienced a pain like this before. His respiratory rate is 16, normal depth; pulse is 90, strong and regular at the radial site; B/P is 130/82. His lungs are clear, JVD is normal, and no edema is present. The ECG shows a regular sinus rhythm. There is no other past pertinent history, no use of medications, and no complaint of allergies. The patient weighs 176 pounds. You explain your intended treatment to the patient, and he consents to your treatment and transport to the hospital. You begin your treatment by applying oxygen via a face mask, then start an IV.

Following your service's chest pain protocols, you prepare to administer nitroglycerin via sublingual spray.

1. Name the six "rights" of medication administration that you should follow with this and every patient.

2. What actions of nitroglycerin decrease chest pain?

3. What are the side effects of nitroglycerin? Which is of primary concern?

The nitroglycerin is given. The patient experiences a headache and tells you the pain is relieved a little, but he still rates it at about a 4 on the 1-to-10 scale. An additional dose of nitroglycerin brings no further improvement in the chest pain. Your protocols now allow you to administer morphine sulfate for the pain.

4. In therapeutic doses, what effects do you want from the morphine in this patient?

5. What side effects should you watch for when giving the morphine sulfate?

©2007 Pearson Education, Inc.
Essentials of Paramedic Care, 2nd ed.

HANDOUT 6-5

Student's Name _____

CHAPTER 6 REVIEW

PART 1: BASIC PHARMACOLOGY

Write the word or words that best complete the following sentences in the space provided.

1. A chemical used to diagnose, treat, or prevent disease is called a(n) _____.
2. The study of drugs and their interactions with the body is called _____.
3. Valium is the _____ name for the drug diazepam.
4. Diazepam is the _____ name for the drug Valium.
5. The four main sources of drugs are _____, _____, _____, and _____.
6. How a drug is absorbed, distributed, and eliminated is called _____.
7. The test that determines the amount and purity of a given chemical in a preparation in the laboratory is called the _____.
8. Phase _____ of new drug development involves testing a new drug on a limited population of patients who have the disease the drug is intended to treat.
9. Medication packages containing a single dose for a single patient are called _____ _____.
10. Movement of a molecule across a membrane from an area of higher pressure to an area of lower pressure is known as _____.
11. _____ _____ requires the use of energy to move a substance.
12. _____ is the measure of the amount of a drug that is still active after it reaches its target tissue.
13. The _____ _____ can prevent drugs from reaching a fetus.
14. The specific name given to the metabolism of drugs is _____.
15. A medication that is not active when administered but whose biotransformation converts it into active metabolites is called a(n) _____.
16. The tight junctions of the capillary endothelial cells in the central nervous system vasculature through which only non-protein-bound, highly lipid-soluble drugs can pass is known as the _____ _____ _____.
17. Oral, buccal, rectal, and sublingual are all _____ routes of drug administration.
18. IV, ET, IO, and IM are all _____ routes of drug administration.
19. Pills, tablets, and suppositories are all _____ forms of drugs.
20. Solutions, tinctures, and emulsions are all _____ forms of drugs.
21. Most drugs operate by binding to a(n) _____.
22. The process of binding of a drug or hormone to a target cell receptor and thus decreasing the number of receptors is _____ - _____.
23. A drug that binds to a receptor and causes it to initiate the expected response is a(n) _____.
24. A competitive antagonist's permanently binding with a receptor site is called _____.
25. An unintended response to a drug is called a(n) _____ _____.

212 ESSENTIALS OF PARAMEDIC CARE

HANDOUT 6-5 Continued

26. A drug effect that is unique to an individual, different than that seen or expected in the population in general, is called a(n) _____.

27. _____ is a rapidly occurring tolerance to a drug.

28. The _____ _____ is the ratio of a drug's lethal dose for 50 percent of the population to its effective dose for 50 percent of the population.

29. The time the body takes to clear one half of a drug is its _____ _____ - _____.

30. A drug's _____ _____ _____ describes the lengths of onset, duration, and termination of action, as well as the drug's minimum effective concentration and toxic level.

HANDOUT 6-6

Student's Name _____

CHAPTER 6 REVIEW

PART 2: DRUG CLASSIFICATIONS

Write the word or words that best complete the following sentences in the space provided.

1. The two major divisions of the nervous system are the _____ _____ _____ and the _____ _____ _____.
2. The drug that best demonstrates a class's common properties and illustrates its particular characteristics is called the _____.
3. A(n) _____ is a medication that relieves the sensation of pain.
4. _____ _____ are given concurrently with other drugs to enhance their effects.
5. A(n) _____ causes the absence of all sensations.
6. Opium is similar to natural pain-reducing peptides called _____.
7. Naloxone is the prototype _____ _____.
8. The state of decreased anxiety and inhibitions is called _____.
9. _____ is the instigation of sleep.
10. Grand mal seizures are treated with _____, _____, and _____.
11. The psychiatric disorder schizophrenia appears to be related to an increased release of _____.
12. _____ _____ are common side effects of antipsychotic medications, including muscle tremors and parkinsonism-like effects.
13. _____ _____ act by blocking the reuptake of norepinephrine and serotonin.
14. Nardil is the prototype drug for the pharmacologic class of drugs known as _____ _____.
15. _____ is the drug of choice for the management of bipolar disorder.
16. The two functional divisions of the autonomic nervous system are the _____ and the _____ nervous systems.
17. The space between nerve cells is the _____.
18. The chemical messenger that conducts a nervous impulse across a synapse is the _____.
19. The _____ _____ _____ controls involuntary actions.
20. The acronym SLUDGE stands for _____, _____, _____, _____, _____, and _____.
21. The two known types of sympathetic receptors are the _____ receptors and the _____ receptors.
22. Bronchodilation is the result of stimulation to the _____ (adrenergic) receptors.
23. $Beta_1$ stimulation results primarily in actions on the _____.
24. Norepinephrine, epinephrine, and dopamine are all _____.
25. The _____ _____ is the heart's dominant pacemaker.
26. The ability of all myocardial tissue to self-generate electrical impulses is called _____.

HANDOUT 6-6 Continued

27. Administration of _____ _____ _____ such as procainamide results in a widened QRS and prolonged QT.
28. The prototype beta-blocker drug is _____.
29. Beta blockers are indicated in the treatment of _____ resulting from excessive sympathetic stimulation.
30. The only two calcium channel blockers that affect the heart are _____ and _____.
31. _____ _____ _____ decrease conductivity through the AV node.
32. Side effects of the endogenous nucleoside _____ include shortness of breath and chest pain.
33. Antihypertensive drugs affect blood volume and control hypertension by manipulating _____.
34. In addition to their role in the treatment of hypertension, _____ _____ play an important role in the treatment of CHF by decreasing afterload.
35. _____ is used to increase cardiac output in CHF and to control the rate of ventricular response in atrial fibrillation.
36. Aspirin is given to patients suspected of having an MI because it decreases the formulation of _____ _____.
37. A drug that acts directly on thrombi to break them down is called a(n) _____.
38. Beta$_2$ specific agents are used in the treatment of asthma. _____ is the prototype.
39. A medication that is intended to increase the productivity of cough is called a(n) _____.
40. A(n) _____ is a medication used to prevent vomiting.
41. Hypersecretion of adrenocorticotropic hormone is called _____ disease.
42. _____ is a substance that decreases blood glucose levels.
43. _____ is contraindicated in a patient who has taken sildenafil recently.
44. Antibiotic agents are used to treat diseases caused by _____.
45. A solution containing whole antibodies for a specific pathogen is a(n) _____.

HANDOUT 6-7

Student's Name _____

MEDICATION CLASSIFICATION

Write the letter of the drug classification in the space provided next to the drug to which it applies. You may use the same letter more than once.

A. Antihistamines
B. Adrenergic agonists
C. Nonopioid analgesics
D. Adrenergic antagonists
E. Opioid agonists
F. Antiseizure drugs
G. Anticoagulants
H. Neuromuscular blocking agents
I. Fibrinolytics
J. Calcium channel blockers
K. Beta blockers
L. Direct vasodilators
M. Skeletal muscle relaxants
N. Sodium channel blockers
O. Anticholinergics

_____ 1. Aspirin

_____ 2. Ibuprofen

_____ 3. Morphine sulfate

_____ 4. Phenytoin

_____ 5. Atropine

_____ 6. Succinylcholine

_____ 7. Cardizem

_____ 8. Minipress

_____ 9. Scopolamine

_____ 10. Flexeril

_____ 11. Dibenzyline

_____ 12. Procainamide

_____ 13. Verapamil

_____ 14. Nitroglycerin

_____ 15. Xylocaine

_____ 16. Heparin

_____ 17. Apresoline

_____ 18. Propranolol

_____ 19. Activase

_____ 20. Benadryl

_____ 21. Dopamine

HANDOUT 6-8   Student's Name _____

AUTONOMIC NERVOUS SYSTEM REVIEW

Write the word or words that best complete the following sentences in the space provided.

1. The autonomic nervous system is responsible for control of _____ actions in the body.
2. The _____ nervous system is the subdivision of the autonomic nervous system that allows the body to function under stress and is sometimes referred to as the "fight-or-flight" system.
3. The subdivision of the autonomic nervous system that primarily controls basic, vegetative functions such as the digestion of food is the _____ nervous system.
4. The nerves of the autonomic nervous system exit the central nervous system and enter specialized structures called _____ _____.
5. Nerve fibers that exit the central nervous system and terminate in the autonomic ganglia are called _____ _____, while the fibers that exit the ganglia and terminate in the target tissues are called _____ _____.
6. The space between two nerve cells is called a(n) _____.
7. Specialized chemicals that conduct electrical impulses between nerve cells or between a nerve cell and its target tissue are called _____.
8. The neurotransmitter _____ is utilized in the preganglionic nerves of both the sympathetic and parasympathetic nervous systems.
9. _____ is the postganglionic neurotransmitter for the parasympathetic nervous system.
10. _____ is the postganglionic neurotransmitter for the sympathetic nervous system.
11. Synapses that use acetylcholine as the neurotransmitter are called _____ synapses.
12. Synapses that use norepinephrine as the neurotransmitter are called _____ synapses.
13. Nerves from the _____ _____ _____ stimulate secretion by sweat glands, constriction of vessels in the skin, increase in blood flow to skeletal muscles, and energy production.
14. Stimulating nerves from the _____ _____ results in reduced blood flow to the abdominal organs, decreased digestive activity, and release of glucose stored in the liver.
15. When the sympathetic nervous system is stimulated, the _____ _____ also releases the hormones _____ and _____.
16. The two known types of sympathetic receptors are the _____ and the _____ receptors.
17. _____ receptors cause peripheral vasoconstriction, mild bronchoconstriction, and stimulation of metabolism.
18. _____ receptors cause an increase in heart rate, cardiac contractile force, and cardiac automaticity and conductivity.
19. _____ receptors cause vasodilation and bronchodilation.
20. _____ receptors are believed to cause dilation of the renal, coronary, and cerebral arteries.
21. Drugs that stimulate the sympathetic nervous system are sometimes called _____ because they cause effects that "mimic" sympathetic stimulation.
22. Drugs that inhibit or block the sympathetic nervous system are sometimes called _____.

HANDOUT 6-8 Continued

23. When nerves from the _____ _____ _____ are stimulated, among the effects are pupillary constriction, secretion by digestive and salivary glands, increased smooth muscle activity along the digestive tract, bronchoconstriction, and reduced heart rate and cardiac contractile force.

24. The medications known as parasympatholytics are sometimes referred to as _____.

25. One example of a drug that blocks the actions of the parasympathetic nervous system is _____.

Chapter 6 Answer Key

Handout 6-2: Chapter 6 Quiz, Part 1

1. C
2. D
3. B
4. D
5. A
6. B
7. C
8. B
9. A
10. B
11. C
12. B
13. B
14. D
15. C
16. A
17. C
18. B
19. A
20. C
21. A
22. B
23. C
24. B
25. D
26. D
27. B
28. C
29. A
30. A
31. C
32. D
33. C
34. D
35. D

Handout 6-3: Chapter 6 Quiz, Part 2

1. B
2. A
3. B
4. D
5. C
6. D
7. A
8. C
9. B
10. C
11. C
12. A
13. B
14. C
15. D
16. C
17. A
18. D
19. B
20. A
21. C
22. B
23. C
24. C
25. A
26. D
27. B
28. D
29. C
30. A
31. C
32. B
33. D
34. A
35. A
36. C
37. D
38. B
39. B
40. D

Handout 6-4: Chapter 6 Scenario

1. Right medication, right dose, right time, right route, right patient, right documentation.
2. Nitroglycerin primarily dilates veins. This decreases preload and thus decreases myocardial workload.
3. The primary concern with nitroglycerin is orthostatic hypotension. Other side effects include headache and reflex tachycardia.
4. Morphine causes analgesia, euphoria, and sedation. It also decreases cardiac preload and afterload. It is useful in treating myocardial infarction and pulmonary edema.
5. Side effects at higher doses include respiratory depression and hypotension.

Handout 6-5: Chapter 6 Review, Part 1

1. drug
2. pharmacology
3. brand
4. generic
5. plants, animals, minerals, laboratory
6. pharmacokinetics
7. assay
8. 2
9. dose packaging
10. filtration
11. Active transport
12. Bioavailability
13. placental barrier
14. biotransformation
15. prodrug
16. blood-brain barrier
17. enteral
18. parenteral
19. solid
20. liquid
21. receptor
22. down-regulation
23. agonist
24. irreversible antagonism
25. side effect
26. idiosyncrasy
27. Tachyphylaxis
28. therapeutic index
29. biological half-life
30. plasma level profile

Handout 6-6: Chapter 6 Review, Part 2

1. central nervous system, peripheral nervous system
2. prototype
3. analgesic
4. Adjunct medications
5. anesthesia
6. endorphins
7. opioid antagonist
8. sedation
9. Hypnosis
10. carbamazepine, phenytoin, phenobarbitol
11. dopamine
12. Extrapyramidal symptoms
13. Tricyclic antidepressants
14. MAO inhibitors
15. Lithium
16. sympathetic, parasympathetic
17. synapse
18. neurotransmitter
19. autonomic nervous system
20. salivation, lacrimation, urination, defecation, gastric motility, emesis
21. adrenergic, dopaminergic
22. beta$_2$
23. heart
24. catecholamines
25. SA node
26. automaticity
27. sodium channel blockers
28. propranolol
29. tachycardias
30. verapamil, diltiazem
31. Calcium channel blockers
32. adenosine
33. preload
34. ACE inhibitors
35. Digoxin
36. platelet plugs
37. fibrinolytic
38. Albuterol
39. expectorant
40. antiemetic
41. Cushing's
42. Insulin
43. Nitroglycerin
44. bacteria
45. serum

Handout 6-7: Medication Classification

1. C
2. C
3. E
4. N or F
5. O
6. H
7. J
8. D
9. O
10. M
11. D
12. N
13. J
14. L
15. N
16. G
17. L
18. K
19. I
20. A
21. B

Handout 6-8: Autonomic Nervous System Review

1. involuntary
2. sympathetic
3. parasympathetic
4. autonomic ganglia
5. preganglionic nerves, postganglionic nerves
6. synapse
7. neurotransmitters
8. acetylcholine
9. Acetylcholine
10. Norepinephrine
11. cholinergic
12. adrenergic
13. sympathetic chain ganglia
14. collateral ganglia
15. adrenal medulla, epinephrine, norepinephrine
16. adrenergic, dopaminergic
17. Alpha$_1$
18. Beta$_1$
19. Beta$_2$
20. Dopaminergic
21. sympathomimetics
22. sympatholytics
23. parasympathetic nervous system
24. anticholinergics
25. atropine

Chapter 7

Medication Administration

INTRODUCTION

Medications or drugs are foreign substances placed into the human body to control or cure specific diseases. Paramedics may use medications to correct or prevent life-threatening situations and to stabilize and comfort patients in distress. Medication effectiveness depends on the correct medication, route, and technique of administration. Incorrect medication administration can have legal implications, as well as cause harm to the patient. This chapter discusses the routes and techniques used to deliver medications correctly to patients.

TOTAL TEACHING TIME:
19.49 HOURS
The total teaching time is only a guideline based on the didactic and practical lab averages in the National Standard Curriculum. Instructors should take into consideration such factors as the pace at which students learn, the size of the class, and breaks. The actual time devoted to teaching objectives is the responsibility of the instructor.

CHAPTER OBJECTIVES

Part 1: Principles and Routes of Medication Administration (p. 375)

After reading Part 1 of this chapter, you should be able to:

1. Review the specific anatomy and physiology pertinent to medication administration. (pp. 378–405)
2. Describe the indications, equipment needed, technique used, precautions, and general principles for the following:
   - inhalation routes of medication administration. (pp. 381–395)
   - parenteral routes of medication administration. (pp. 390–405)
   - percutaneous routes of medication administration. (pp. 378–381)
   - enteral routes of medication administration, including gastric tube administration and rectal administration. (pp. 385–390)
3. Describe the indications, contraindications, side effects, dosages, and routes of administration for medications commonly administered by paramedics. (pp. 378–405)
4. Discuss legal aspects affecting medication administration. (pp. 376, 377)

©2007 Pearson Education, Inc.
Essentials of Paramedic Care, 2nd ed.

5. Discuss the "six rights" of drug administration and correlate them with the principles of medication administration. (pp. 375–376)
6. Differentiate among the percutaneous routes of medication administration. (pp. 378–381)
7. Discuss medical asepsis and the differences between clean and sterile techniques. (pp. 376–377)
8. Describe uses of antiseptics and disinfectants. (p. 377)
9. Describe the use of body substance isolation (BSI) procedures when administering a medication. (p. 376)
10. Describe disposal of contaminated items and sharps. (p. 377)
11. Synthesize a pharmacologic management plan including medication administration. (pp. 375–405)

Part 2: Intravenous Access, Blood Sampling, and Intraosseous Infusion (p. 405)

After reading Part 2 of this chapter, you should be able to:

1. Review the specific anatomy and physiology pertinent to medication administration. (pp. 405–442)
2. Describe the indications, equipment needed, technique used, precautions, and general principles for the following:
   - peripheral venous or external jugular cannulation. (pp. 405–431)
   - intraosseous needle placement and infusion. (pp. 435–442)
   - obtaining a blood sample. (pp. 431–434)

Part 3: Medical Mathematics (p. 442)

After reading Part 3 of this chapter, you should be able to:

1. Review mathematical equivalents. (pp. 442–444)
2. Differentiate temperature readings between the centigrade and Fahrenheit scales. (p. 444)
3. Discuss formulas as a basis for performing drug calculations. (pp. 444–449)
4. Describe how to perform mathematical conversions from the household system to the metric system. (pp. 442–444)

FRAMING THE LESSON

Begin the class by reviewing the important points from Chapter 6, "General Principles of Pharmacology." Discuss any aspects of the chapter not understood by students. Then go on to Chapter 7. Ask students to name the various routes for administering medication. Write the names of the routes of administration on the board or flip chart. Then have students name various medications and identify the routes of administration for each, listing the medications under the routes on the board or flip chart. A review of aseptic techniques and body substance isolation precautions would also be appropriate for this chapter, as would a discussion on local EMS agencies' policies regarding possible exposure to a blood- or airborne pathogen. If needed, a brief overview of basic math principles would be appropriate. Consider having students obtain a separate text on pharmacological computations.

TEACHING STRATEGIES

People learn in a variety of ways. Some do better with the spoken word, whereas others prefer the written. Some prefer to work alone, whereas others profit from working in groups. Recognizing these different ways of acquiring knowledge, the authors of this *Instructor's Resource Manual* have provided a variety of teaching strategies for the different types of learners. These strategies are intended to foster higher-level cognitive skills and encourage creative learning and problem solving. For greatest effectiveness, incorporate these strategies into your class lecture. Symbols in the Lecture Outline indicate the points at which various exercises might be most appropriate. Other strategies can be used to preview the lesson or to summarize it.

The following strategies are keyed to specific sections of the lesson.

1. ***Medication Safety Measures.*** Administration of medications is serious business. Incorrect medication administration can be fatal for the patient. But improper handling of medications and the instruments for their administration can be harmful for the paramedic as well. Take time to stress the following safety measures before students begin skills lab or clinical rotation practice on the various techniques for administering medications.
   a. Remind students always to practice body substance isolation precautions, even in lab training. Good, safe behavior must be repeatedly reinforced.
   b. When administering drugs or starting IVs, always have a sharps container available. Used needles should not be recapped; they should be dropped directly into a sharps container.
   c. Teach students how to safely remove a protective cap from a needle. The correct method is the "two-hands loosen, one-hand drop" technique. One hand grasps the barrel of the syringe, while the other hand overlaps slightly and grasps the base of the protective cap. The second hand pushes against the first by lifting the cap straight up to loosen (but not remove) the cap. The hands should never come apart, and neither hand should ever pass beyond the tip of the needle. Once the cap is loosened, the second hand is released and moved away. The first hand now tips the syringe/needle down, and the loosened cap falls freely off. Have students practice this technique on straight writing pens with caps before they try it with syringes. Remind students never to use their mouths or an open-hands approach to remove the cap. If the hands are touching, they are more stable, even in the back of a moving ambulance. An open-hands approach increases the likelihood of one hand's passing over the needle end or pulling backward if the cap suddenly releases. Both of these techniques are unsafe and should be avoided.
   d. Although some IV needles and needles on syringes now have a protective guard that slips up over the needle after use, many still do not. Although sharps containers should always be available, occasionally EMS personnel encounter situations in which one is not on hand. Although recapping is *highly discouraged,* there is one reasonably safe method of recapping a needle. Stress to students that this should be used *only if absolutely necessary.* This technique reverses the two-hands loosen, one-hand drop method of uncapping with a "one-hand pick-up, two-hands secure" method. With the first hand holding the syringe/needle sharp, the paramedic uses the tip of the sharp to align the protective cap with the open end facing him. The second hand is kept away. With the first hand, the paramedic scoops up the protective cap to loosely cover the sharp's end. The second hand is now wrapped around the first, and its fingers grasp the base of the protective cap to secure it firmly to the syringe. This method maintains the closed-hand approach. The hand and fingers should never be placed over the end of the protective cap to press the cap on. Some protective caps have open ends, and if during the confusion of a run a paramedic picks up a discarded cap that is

shorter than the needle, he can easily stick himself with a dirty needle. Ultimately, each system should strive to have a sharps container available whenever sharps are used.

e. Protective caps for prefilled syringes come off fairly easily; however, caps for needles attached to syringes or IV lines (for medication drips) are more challenging. Inspection of such needles and caps usually reveals fins at the base of the needle and grooves along the inside of the protective cap. Such caps must be removed by lifting straight up using the two-hands loosen, one-hand drop technique. When the needle is attached to the syringe or IV line, it is usually given a quarter turn. If students try to twist the cap off the needle, they'll probably remove the needle they just attached. They will also encounter resistance because the fins and grooves are engaged. A student may become frustrated and use more force in attempting to remove the cap. This risks the cap and needle's suddenly jerking apart so that the needle sticks the student. Teach students to think problems through and use finesse, not force.

2. ***Learning Aseptic Techniques.*** The best place to learn aseptic technique is the operating room. Take a field trip as a class or in small groups on a lab day surgery. Have the experts there describe the sterile field and demonstrate sterile technique. This will also prepare students for clinical time for intubations with anesthesia services. Of all the people your students will encounter, OR nurses may be the most serious about asepsis! This activity gets your students out of the classroom, exposes them to a new learning environment, and gives you a chance to do some public relations with your clinical faculty.

3. ***MDI Familiarization.*** Order MDI placebos from your local pharmacy or MDI supplier. They are filled with air but give students a realistic sensation of the inhaler. Students should be better able to educate patients on proper use of the MDI once they experience the inhaler for themselves. While this activity certainly helps students understand the mechanics of the inhaler, it also serves as an empathy exercise, helping students to know how their patients feel when using an MDI.

4. ***Practicing ET Tube Administration.*** Allow students time to practice actually giving medications down the ET tube. Though administration through the ET tube seems like an easy skill, it does have several steps and requires some motor coordination to ensure that the ET tube is not displaced and continues to provide proper ventilation. Most intubation training mannequins have detachable lungs, so you can actually empty the fluid into the sink, allow the lung to air dry, and replace it the next day. You might even measure (in cc's) the volume of medication that actually gets into the lung, as much of it tends to stick in the ET tube itself. This will help students to realize the importance of a 5- to 10-mL saline flush following ET medication administration.

5. ***Working with Glass Ampules.*** Be sure you have enough ampules for everyone to break open at least one. Ampules of epinephrine are around 50 cents each. Not only can ampules be dangerous to open, but withdrawal of medication from them can also be difficult. Students commonly cause the medication to spill. Because many controlled substances such as morphine come in ampules, proper withdrawal is critical for narcotic inventory control.

6. ***Vein Location Labeling.*** Obtain or make a life-size outline of the human body in the anatomical position. This can be made from wrapping or butcher paper or drawn on a chalk or white board. Write the names of major veins used for peripheral IV access on small strips of paper. Put the strips of paper into a container and have each student pick out one strip. Then, using a marker or chalk, have students draw the vein in the proper location on the body diagram. An alternative to having a body outline on paper would be to use a student as

a model. Have the student model wear shorts or a swimsuit. Then, using a washable marker, have students draw their assigned veins on the model's body.

7. *Experimenting with Flow Rates.* Conduct a "flow rate experiment" in class to demonstrate the principles of volume replacement related to catheter and tubing size. Break your students into groups and assign varying combinations of catheter sizes and tubing to 1,000-mL bags of IV fluid. Of course, macrodrip tubing and a 1-gauge catheter will deliver greater volumes in less time than the other extreme of a 20-gauge catheter with microtubing. Let the students time how long it takes to administer all 1,000 mL of fluid and compare times and volumes. This is a kinesthetic activity that introduces the concept of research in your classroom. It also provides a very visual example of flow rates, rather than just talking about them.

8. *Medication Math Practice.* Have each student write on 3 × 5 cards a scenario involving the calculation of a correct drug dosage for a patient. Scenarios should include the chief complaint, the age and weight of the patient, and the drug to be given. Have students trade cards, calculate the drug dosage, and then present the scenario and the calculation to the class.

The following strategies below can be used at various points throughout the lesson or to help summarize and demonstrate what students have learned.

Practicing Medication Dosages. As students learn actual dosages of medications to administer, play "Simon Says on Drugs" to enhance their retention of the correct dosages. In the game, the student will either echo back (if it is correct) your description of the dosage or correct you (if it was the wrong dose) in order to take a step forward. The first student to reach the front of the classroom gets to be Simon. Here's an example: You say, "Give 6 mg atropine rapid IV push." The student says, "Give 6 mg adenosine rapid IV push." The student steps forward. If he had echoed you back verbatim, he would have been wrong and would have had to take a step back. This activity encourages healthy competition, is fun, and promotes rapid recognition of the material.

Mannequin Practice. Obtain mannequins for students to practice intravenous access, intramuscular injections, subcutaneous injections, and intraosseous access. Chicken legs may also be used for intraosseous drug administration practice. Clinical rotations: Have students schedule time with the regional hospital either in the emergency department or, if the hospital has one, with an IV team. If permitted by the hospital, have students perform IVs, subcutaneous and IM injections, and intraosseous access.

Cultural Considerations, Legal Notes, and Patho Pearls. The Student CD-ROM contains this series of informative features to enhance the student's understanding of the material covered in this chapter.

TEACHING OUTLINE

HANDOUT 7-1
Chapter 7 Objectives Checklist

Chapter 7, "Medication Administration," is the seventh lesson in Division 1, *Introduction to Advanced Prehospital Care*. Distribute Handout 7-1 so that students can familiarize themselves with the learning goals for this chapter. If students have any questions about the objectives, answer them at this time.

Then present the chapter. One possible lecture outline follows. In the outline, the parenthetical references in regular type are references to text pages; those in bold type are references to figures or tables.

PowerPoint Presentation
Chapter 7 PowerPoint slides 4–11

Teaching Tip
Stress the six rights of medication administration: right patient, right drug, right dose, right route, right time, right documentation.

Point to Emphasize
If you ever doubt the use or dosage of a medication, contact medical direction immediately.

Teaching Strategy 1
Medication Safety Measures

Point to Emphasize
Always take appropriate body substance isolation measures to decrease your risk of exposure to infectious material.

Teaching Strategy 2
Learning Aseptic Techniques

Point to Emphasize
Treat all blood and body fluids as potentially infectious.

PowerPoint Presentation
Chapter 7 PowerPoint slides 12–19

PART 1: PRINCIPLES AND ROUTES OF MEDICATION ADMINISTRATION

I. **General principles** (pp. 375–378)

   A. The six rights of drug administration. You can provide effective pharmacologic therapy and eliminate medication errors by following the six rights of drug administration; another good practice is to echo all drug orders from medical control. (pp. 375–376)
   1. Right person
   2. Right drug
   3. Right dose
   4. Right time
   5. Right route
   6. Right documentation

   B. Medical direction. Paramedics operate under the license of a medical director who is responsible for all of their actions. (p. 376)
   1. The medical director determines which medications paramedics deliver.
   2. Know all drug protocols in your system.

   C. Body substance isolation. Establishing routes for drug delivery presents the constant potential for exposure to blood and other body fluids. (p. 376)
   1. Always wear gloves.
   2. Goggles and mask
   3. Hand washing

   D. Medical asepsis. Many paramedic procedures, especially those related to drug administration, place the patient at increased risk for infection. (pp. 376–377)
   1. Sterilization
      a. Sterilize
      b. Medically clean techniques
         i. Careful handling of sterilized equipment
   2. Disinfectants and antiseptics

   E. Disposal of contaminated equipment and sharps. Properly handling needles and other sharps before and after patient use can prevent many accidental needle sticks. (p. 377)
   1. Minimize tasks performed in a moving ambulance.
   2. Immediately dispose of used sharps in sharps containers.
   3. Recap needles only as a last resort.

   F. Medication administration and documentation. Proper and thorough documentation of medication administration is extremely important. (p. 378)
   1. Indication for drug administration
   2. Dosage and route delivered
   3. Patient response to the medication
      a. Positive
      b. Negative
   4. Patient's condition and vital signs before and after medication administration

II. **Percutaneous drug administration.** Percutaneous medications are applied to and absorbed through the skin or mucous membranes. (pp. 378–381)

A. Transdermal administration (p. 378)
  1. Use BSI.
  2. Clean and dry patient's skin.
  3. Confirm indication, medication, dose, route, and expiration date.
  4. Apply medication to the site as specified by the manufacturer.
  5. Leave the medication in place for the required time.
B. Mucous membranes (pp. 378–381)
  1. Sublingual
      a. Through mucous membranes beneath the tongue
      b. Use appropriate BSI.
      c. Confirm indication, medication, dose, route, and expiration date.
      d. Have patient lift his tongue toward the top and back of oral cavity.
      e. Place the pill or direct spray between the underside of the tongue and the floor of the oral cavity. Have patient relax his tongue and mouth, let pill dissolve, and be careful not to swallow.
      f. Monitor patient for desirable or adverse effects.
  2. Buccal
      a. Through tissues between the cheek and gum
      b. Use appropriate BSI.
      c. Confirm indication, medication, dose, route, and expiration date.
      d. Place medication between patient's cheek and gum.
          i. Instruct patient to allow pill or preparation to dissolve and not to swallow it.
      e. Monitor patient for desirable or adverse effects.
  3. Ocular
      a. Through mucous membranes of the eyes (**Fig. 7-1, p. 380**)
      b. Use gloves and appropriate BSI.
      c. Confirm indication, medication, dose, route, and expiration date.
      d. Have patient lie supine or lay his head back and look toward ceiling.
      e. Pull the lower eyelid downward to expose the conjunctival sac. Never touch the eye.
      f. Use a medicine dropper to place prescribed dosage on the conjunctival sac, not directly on the eye unless instructed.
      g. Instruct patient to hold his eye(s) shut for 1 to 2 minutes.
  4. Nasal
      a. Through mucous membranes of nose (**Fig. 7-2, p. 380**)
      b. Use gloves and appropriate BSI.
      c. Confirm indication, medication, dose, route, and expiration date.
      d. Have patient blow his nose and tilt head backwards.
      e. Use medicine dropper or squeezable nebulizer to administer medication into the appropriate nare(s).
      f. Hold the nare(s) shut and/or tilt the head forward to distribute the medication.
      g. Monitor the patient for desirable and undesirable effects.
  5. Aural
      a. Through mucous membranes of ear and ear canal (**Fig. 7-3, p. 381**)
      b. Use gloves and appropriate BSI.
      c. Confirm indication, medication, route, dose, and expiration date.
      d. Determine the correct ear for administration.
      e. Have patient lie in lateral recumbent position with the affected ear upward.
      f. Manually open the ear canal: for adults, pull the ear up and back; for pediatric patients, pull it down and back.
      g. Administer appropriate dose of medication with medicine dropper.

POWERPOINT PRESENTATION
Chapter 7 PowerPoint slides 20–24

  h. Have patient continue to lie with ear up for 10 minutes.
  i. Monitor patient for desirable and undesirable effects.

III. Pulmonary drug administration. Special medications can be administered into the pulmonary system via inhalation or injection. (pp. 381–385)

  A. Nebulizer (pp. 381–382)
   1. Device that uses pressurized oxygen to disperse liquid as fine spray or mist (**Fig. 7-4, p. 382; Fig. 7-5, p. 383**)
   2. Confirm indication, medication, dose, route, and expiration date.
   3. Put medication in medication reservoir. Dilute with 3–5 cc sterile saline solution if not diluted.
   4. Assemble the nebulizer.
   5. Attach oxygen tubing to the oxygen port and oxygen source.
   6. Set regulator for 5–8 liters/minute.
   7. Place nebulizer in patient's mouth.
   8. For patients with inadequate tidal volume, attach nebulizer to BVM or ET tube, and have patient inhale slowly and deeply, holding in medication for 1 or 2 seconds before exhaling.

TEACHING STRATEGY 3
MDI Familiarization

  B. Metered dose inhaler (pp. 382–384) (**Fig. 7-6, p. 384**)
   1. Confirm indication, medication, dose, route, and expiration date.
   2. Insert medication canister into the plastic shell.
   3. Remove the cap from mouthpiece.
   4. Gently shake the MDI for 2–5 seconds.
   5. Instruct the patient to maximally exhale.
   6. Place mouthpiece in patient's mouth and have him form a seal with his lips.
   7. As patient inhales, press the canister's top downward to release medication.
   8. Have patient hold his breath for several seconds.
   9. Remove inhaler from patient's mouth and instruct him to breathe slowly.
   10. If a second dose is necessary, wait according to manufacturer's instructions. Then repeat.
   11. In acute respiratory emergency, use a nebulizer instead of MDI.

TEACHING STRATEGY 4
Practicing ET Tube Administration

  C. Endotracheal tube (pp. 384–385)
   1. Use if IV not yet started.
   2. Pulmonary absorption may be as fast as IV.
   3. Increase conventional doses from two to two and one-half times.
   4. Dilute medication with normal saline to create 10 mL of solution.
   5. Quickly inject down ET tube.
   6. If doing CPR, stop compression during administration.

POWERPOINT PRESENTATION
Chapter 7 PowerPoint slides 25–40

IV. Enteral drug administration. Enteral drug administration is the delivery of any medication that is absorbed through the gastrointestinal tract. (pp. 385–390) (**Fig. 7-7, p. 385**)

  A. Oral administration (pp. 386–387)
   1. Capsules
   2. Tablets
   3. Pills
   4. Enteric coated
     a. Time-release capsules and tablets
   5. Elixirs
   6. Emulsions
   7. Lozenges
   8. Suspensions
   9. Syrups

POINT TO EMPHASIZE
Never use household teaspoons to measure medications, as they vary significantly in volume.

228 ESSENTIALS OF PARAMEDIC CARE

©2007 Pearson Education, Inc.
Essentials of Paramedic Care, 2nd ed.

2. Equipment for oral administration
    a. Soufflé cup
    b. Medicine cup
    c. Medicine dropper
    d. Teaspoon
    e. Oral syringe
    f. Nipple
3. Principles of oral administration
    a. Use appropriate BSI.
    b. Note whether to administer with food or on an empty stomach.
    c. Gather equipment, mix liquids or suspensions, and prepare medications as needed.
    d. Confirm indication, medication, dose, route, and expiration date.
    e. Have patient sit upright (when not contraindicated).
    f. Place medication in patient's mouth. Allow self-administration when possible; assist when needed.
    g. Follow administration with 4–8 ounces of water or other liquid.
    h. Ensure patient has swallowed the medication.
B. Gastric tube administration (pp. 387–389) (**Proc. 7-1, p. 388**)
    1. Confirm proper tube placement.
    2. Irrigate gastric tube.
    3. Confirm indication, medication, dose, route, and expiration date.
    4. Prepare medication for delivery.
    5. Draw medication into 30- to 50-mL cone-tipped syringe and place the tip into open gastric tube. Administer medication into the tube.
    6. Draw 50–100 mL of warm normal saline into a cone-tipped syringe and attach to open end of tube. Gently inject the saline.
    7. Clamp off distal tube.
C. Rectal administration (pp. 389–390)
    1. Administration of liquid medication in the emergent setting
        a. Confirm indication and dose, and draw correct quantity of medication into a needleless syringe.
        b. Place hub of 14-gauge Teflon catheter (or endotracheal tube) on the end of the syringe. (**Fig. 7-8, p. 389; Fig. 7-9, p. 389**)
        c. Insert Teflon catheter in patient's rectum and inject medication.
        d. Withdraw the catheter and hold patient's buttocks together.
    2. Suppositories
    3. Small volume enema technique (**Fig. 7-10, p. 390**)
        a. Apply appropriate BSI and confirm need for enema.
        b. Confirm indication, medication, dose, route, and expiration date.
        c. Place patient on his left side, flex right leg to expose anus.
        d. Insert prelubricated rectal tip into the anus and advance 3 to 4 inches.
        e. Gently squeeze the medicated solution of the bottle into the rectum and colon.
        f. Hold buttocks together to enhance absorption.

V. Parenteral drug administration. *Parenteral* denotes any drug administration outside of the gastrointestinal tract; typically it involves the use of needles to inject medications into the circulatory system or tissues. (pp. 390–405)

A. Syringes and needles (pp. 390–391)
    1. Syringe (**Fig. 7-11, p. 391**)
    2. Hypodermic needle (**Fig. 7-12, p. 391**)
B. Medication packaging (pp. 391–397)
    1. Glass ampules (**Fig. 7-13, p. 392**) (**Proc. 7-2, p. 393**)
        a. Confirm medication indications and patient allergies.

POINT TO EMPHASIZE
Do not administer rectal medications in the presence of diarrhea, rectal bleeding, hemorrhoids, or any other situation involving severe anal irritation.

POWERPOINT PRESENTATION
Chapter 7 PowerPoint slides 41–95

TEACHING STRATEGY 5
Working with Glass Ampules

POINT TO EMPHASIZE
Always use the label printed directly on the container to confirm the correct medication.

  b. Confirm ampule label (name, dose, expiration).
  c. Hold ampule upright and tap its top to dislodge any trapped solution.
  d. Place gauze around the thin neck and snap it off with your thumb.
  e. Place the tip of the hypodermic needle inside the ampule and withdraw the medication into the syringe.
  f. Reconfirm the indication, drug, dose, and route.
  g. Administer medication appropriately via the indicated route.
  h. Properly dispose of the needle, syringe, and broken glass ampule.
 2. Single and multidose vials (**Fig. 7-14, p. 392**) (**Proc. 7-3, p. 394**)
  a. Confirm medication indications and patient allergies.
  b. Confirm the vial label (name, dose, expiration).
  c. Determine the volume of medication to be administered.
  d. Prepare syringe and hypodermic needle.
  e. Cleanse the vial's rubber top with an antiseptic alcohol preparation.
  f. Insert hypodermic needle into the rubber top and inject appropriate amount of air into the vial. Then withdraw the appropriate amount of medication.
  g. Reconfirm indication, drug, dose, and route.
  h. Administer appropriately via indicated route.
  i. Properly dispose of needle, syringe, and vial.
 3. Nonconstituted drug vial (**Fig. 7-15, p. 395**) (**Proc. 7-4, p. 396**)
  a. Confirm medication indications and patient allergies.
  b. Confirm vial's label (name, dose, expiration date).
  c. Remove all solution from the vial containing the mixing solution.
  d. With an alcohol preparation, cleanse the top of the vial containing the powdered drug and inject the mixing solution.
  e. Gently agitate or shake the vial to ensure complete mixture.
  f. Determine the volume of newly constituted medication to be administered.
  g. Prepare the syringe and hypodermic needle.
  h. Cleanse the medication vial's rubber stopper with an antiseptic alcohol preparation.
  i. Insert hypodermic needle into the rubber stopper and withdraw appropriate volume of medication.
  j. Reconfirm indication, drug, dose, and route.
  k. Administer appropriately via indicated route.
  l. Monitor patient for desired effects.
  m. Properly dispose of the needle, syringe, and vials.
 4. Prefilled or preloaded syringes (**Fig. 7-16, p. 397**)
  a. Confirm medication indications and patient allergies.
  b. Confirm prefilled syringe label (name, dose, expiration date).
  c. Assemble prefilled syringe; remove pop-off caps and screw together.
  d. Reconfirm indication, drug, dose, and route.
  e. Administer appropriately via the indicated route.
  f. Properly dispose of the needle and syringe.
 5. Intravenous medication solutions
C. Parenteral routes (pp. 397–405)
 1. Intradermal injections (**Fig. 7-17, p. 398**)
  a. Equipment
   i. BSI
   ii. Alcohol or betadine antiseptic preparation
   iii. Packaged medication
   iv. Tuberculin syringe
   v. 25- to 27-gauge needle, 3/8″–1″ long
   vi. Sterile gauze and adhesive bandage
  b. Intradermal injection steps
   i. Assemble and prepare equipment.

  ii. Apply BSI, confirm drug, indication, dosage, and need for intradermal injection.
  iii. Draw up medication as appropriate.
  iv. Prepare the site with alcohol or betadine.
  v. Pull patient's skin taut with nondominant hand.
  vi. Insert needle, bevel up, just under the skin, at a 10° to 15° angle.
  vii. Slowly inject the medication, look for a small bump, or wheal.
  viii. Remove the needle and dispose of it in the sharps container.
  ix. Place adhesive bandage over the site; use gauze for hemorrhage control as needed.
  x. Do not rub or massage the site.
2. Subcutaneous injection (**Fig. 7-18, p. 399**; **Fig. 7-19, p. 400**)
 a. Equipment needed
  i. BSI (gloves, goggles)
  ii. Alcohol or betadine antiseptic preparations
  iii. Packaged medication
  iv. Syringe (1 to 3 cc)
  v. 24- to 26-gauge hypodermic needle, 3/8"–1" long
  vi. Sterile gauze and adhesive bandage
 b. Administration technique (**Proc. 7-5, p. 401**)
  i. Assemble and prepare equipment.
  ii. Apply BSI, confirm drug, indication, dosage, and need for subcutaneous injection.
  iii. Draw up medication.
  iv. Prepare the site with alcohol or betadine.
  v. Gently pinch a 1-inch fold of skin.
  vi. Insert needle just into the skin at 45° angle with bevel up.
  vii. Pull the plunger back to aspirate tissue fluid.
  viii. If blood appears, needle is in blood vessel. Start procedure over again with new syringe.
  ix. If no blood appears, proceed to next step.
  x. Slowly inject the medication.
  xi. Remove needle and dispose of it in sharps container.
  xii. Place adhesive bandage over the site; use gauze for hemorrhage control if needed.
  xiii. Monitor patient.
  xiv. Gently rub or massage site.
3. Intramuscular injection (**Fig. 7-20, p. 402**)
 a. Sites and correlating volumes of medication (**Fig. 7-21, p. 403**)
  i. Deltoid, 2.0 mL
  ii. Dorsal gluteal, 5.0 mL or more
  iii. Vastus lateralis, 5.0 mL or more
  iv. Rectus femoris, up to 5.0 mL
 b. Equipment needed
  i. BSI (gloves and goggles)
  ii. Alcohol or betadine antiseptic preparation
  iii. Packaged medication
  iv. Syringe (1–5 mL)
  v. 21- to 23-gauge hypodermic needle, 3/8"–1" long
  vi. Sterile gauze and adhesive bandage
 c. Administration steps (**Proc. 7-6, p. 404**)
  i. Assemble and prepare needed equipment.
  ii. Apply BSI, confirm drug, indication, dosage, and need for IM injection.
  iii. Draw up medication as appropriate.
  iv. Prepare the site with alcohol or betadine.
  v. Stretch skin taut over the injection site with nondominant hand.

  vi. Insert needle just into skin at 90° angle, bevel up.
  vii. Pull back plunger to aspirate tissue fluid.
  viii. Slowly inject medication.
  ix. Remove needle and dispose of in sharps container.
  x. Place adhesive bandage over site; use gauze for hemorrhage control if needed.
  xi. Monitor patient.
  xii. Gently rub or massage site unless anticoagulant administered.

PART 2: INTRAVENOUS ACCESS, BLOOD SAMPLING, AND INTRAOSSEOUS INFUSION

I. Intravenous access. Venous circulation can deliver medications and fluids into the body and provides an invaluable tool for treating the sick and injured. (pp. 405–435)

 A. Indications for intravenous (IV) access (p. 405)
  1. Fluid and blood replacement
  2. Drug administration
  3. Obtaining venous blood specimens for lab analysis
 B. Types of intravenous access (pp. 406–407)
  1. Peripheral venous access
   a. Easy to master
   b. Arms, legs, neck (**Fig. 7-22, p. 406**)
   c. Start at distal end of extremity.
   d. Larger veins for fluid resuscitation
   e. Visualization and access usually easy
   f. Access while doing CPR or endotracheal intubation.
   g. Collapse in hypovolemia or circulatory failure
   h. Geriatric or pediatric patients' fragile veins
   i. Veins may roll and elude IV placement.
  2. Central venous access
   a. Deep veins: internal jugular, subclavian, femoral
   b. Near the heart for long-term use
   c. Transvenous pacing or monitoring central venous pressure
   d. Peripherally inserted central catheter (PICC)
   e. Typically restricted to the hospital setting
   f. Cannot be assessed during CPR, often require X-ray to confirm
 C. Equipment and supplies for venous access (pp. 407–414)
  1. Intravenous fluids
   a. Colloids
    i. Plasma protein fraction
    ii. Salt poor albumin
    iii. Dextran
    iv. Hetastarch
   b. Crystalloids
    i. Isotonic solutions
    ii. Hypertonic solutions
    iii. Hypotonic solutions
   c. Most common prehospital IV fluids
    i. Lactated Ringer's
    ii. Normal saline
    iii. Dextrose in water (D_5W) at 5 percent
   d. Blood
   e. Oxygen-carrying solutions
    i. Perfluorocarbons

POWERPOINT PRESENTATION
Chapter 7 PowerPoint slides 4–82

TEACHING STRATEGY 6
Vein Location Labeling

   ii. Hemoglobin-based oxygen-carrying solutions (HBOCs)
    a) PolyHeme
    b) Hemopure
  f. Packaging for intravenous fluids (**Fig. 7-23, p. 409**)
  g. Label
  h. Medication administration port
  i. Administration set port
2. Administration tubing (**Fig. 7-24, p. 410**)
  a. Microdrip (60 gtts/mL)
  b. Macrodrip (10 gtts/mL)
  c. Components of tubing
   i. Spike
   ii. Drip chamber
   iii. Drop former
   iv. Tubing
   v. Clamp
   vi. Flow regulator
   vii. Medication injection ports
   viii. Needle adapter
  d. IV extension tubing
  e. Electromechanical pump tubing
  f. Measured volume administration set
   i. Flanged spike
   ii. Clamp
   iii. Airway handle
   iv. Medication injection port
   v. Burette chamber
   vi. Float valve
   vii. Drip chamber
   viii. Flow regulator
   ix. Medication injection port
   x. Needle adapter
  g. Blood tubing
  h. Miscellaneous administration sets
3. In-line intravenous fluid heaters
4. Intravenous cannulas
  a. Over-the-needle catheter (**Fig. 7-25, p. 412**)
   i. Metal stylet
   ii. Flashback chamber
   iii. Telfon catheter
   iv. Hub
  b. Hollow-needle catheter (**Fig. 7-26, p. 413**)
  c. Catheter inserted through the needle (**Fig. 7-27, p. 413**)
  d. Cannula sizes
   i. 22-gauge
    a) Fragile veins such as in elderly or pediatric
   ii. 20-gauge
    a) Average adult who doesn't need fluid replacement
   iii. 18-gauge, 16-gauge, or 14-gauge
    a) Increase volume
    b) Viscous medications
5. Miscellaneous equipment
  a. Venous constricting band
  b. Alcohol and betadine
  c. Medical tape and adhesive bandage
  d. Clear membranes over the site

POINT TO EMPHASIZE
Do not use any IV fluids after their expiration date; any fluids that appear cloudy, discolored, or laced with particulate; or any fluid whose sealed packaging has been opened or tampered with.

TEACHING STRATEGY 7
Experimenting with Flow Rates

POINT TO EMPHASIZE
Intravenous access is painful and causes discomfort not only to those receiving it but also to family members watching a loved one in distress.

POINT TO EMPHASIZE
Never leave the constricting band in place for more than 2 minutes.

    D. Intravenous access in the hand, arm, and leg (pp. 414–416) (Proc. 7-7, p. 415)
      1. Most commonly used sites for IV access by paramedics
        a. Easily accessed
        b. Less likelihood of complications
      2. Technique
        a. Confirm indication, type of IV setup needed. Gather and arrange supplies and equipment beforehand.
          i. IV fluid
          ii. Administration set
          iii. Intravenous cannula
          iv. Tape or commercial securing device
          v. Venous blood drawing equipment
          vi. Venous constricting band
          vii. Antiseptic swab
        b. Prepare all needed equipment.
        c. Select venipuncture site.
        d. Place constricting band proximal to the site.
        e. Cleanse venipuncture site.
        f. Insert intravenous cannula into vein.
        g. Holding metal stylet stationary, slide Teflon catheter over needle into vein. Remove metal stylet and dispose of properly. Remove venous constricting band.
        h. Obtain venous blood samples as directed.
        i. Attach administration tubing to cannula.
        j. Apply antibiotic ointment to site and cover with adhesive bandage or commercial device. Loop distal tubing and secure in place.
        k. Label intravenous solution bag with date, time initiated, person initiating IV access.
        l. Continually monitor patient and flow rate.
    E. Intravenous access in the external jugular vein (pp. 416–418) (Proc. 7-8, p. 417)
      1. Offers many of the benefits afforded by central venous access
      2. Indications
        a. Consider only after all means of peripheral access are exhausted.
        b. Extremely painful; usually reserved for patients with decreased or total loss of consciousness.
      3. Technique
        a. Prepare all equipment as for peripheral IV access.
        b. Fill a 10-mL syringe with 3- to 5-mL of sterile saline.
        c. Attach distal part of syringe to flashback chamber of large-bore, over-the-needle catheter.
        d. Apply proper BSI—gloves and goggles.
        e. Place patient supine and/or in Trendelenburg position.
        f. Turn patient's head to the side opposite of access.
        g. Cleanse site with antiseptics.
        h. Occlude venous return by placing finger on external jugular just above clavicle.
        i. Position intravenous cannula parallel with the vein, midway between the angle of the jaw and the clavicle. Point the catheter at the medial third of the clavicle and insert it, bevel up, at a 10°–30° angle.
        j. Enter external jugular while withdrawing on the plunger of the attached syringe. See blood in the syringe or feel a pop as cannula enters the vein.

POINT TO EMPHASIZE
Consider accessing the external jugular only after you have exhausted other means of peripheral access or when a patient requires immediate fluid administration.

      k. Once inside vein, advance angiocatheter another 0.5 cm so tip of Teflon catheter lies within the lumen of the vein. Slide Teflon catheter into vein and remove metal stylet.
      l. Dispose of metal stylet appropriately.
      m. Obtain venous blood samples.
      n. Attach administration tubing to IV catheter. Allow fluid to flow freely for several seconds. Then set flow rate and secure in position.
      o. Monitor patient for complications.
F. Intravenous access with a measured volume administration set (p. 418) (**Proc. 7-9, p. 419**)
  1. Prepare tubing by closing all clamps, and insert flanged spike into IV solution bag's spike port.
  2. Open airway handle. Open uppermost clamp and fill burette chamber with approximately 20 mL of fluid.
  3. Squeeze drip chamber until fluid reaches the full line.
  4. Open bottom flow regulator to purge air through tubing.
  5. When all air is purged, close the bottom flow regulator.
  6. Continue to fill burette chamber with the designated amount of solution.
  7. Close uppermost clamp and open flow regulator to desired drip rate. Leave airway handle open.
G. Intravenous access with blood tubing (pp. 418–420)
  1. Prepare tubing by closing all clamps, and insert flanged spike into spike port of blood and/or normal saline solution (Y-configured tubing).
  2. Squeeze drip chamber until it is one-third full and blood covers the filter. Repeat for the normal saline if using Y-tubing.
  3. For straight tubing, piggyback secondary line of normal saline into blood tubing.
  4. Flush all tubing to the IV cannula or into a previously established IV line.
  5. Attach blood tubing to IV cannula or into previously established IV line.
  6. Ensure patency by infusing small amount of normal saline. Shut down when patency confirmed.
  7. Open clamp(s) and/or flow regulator(s) that allow blood to move from the bag to the patient.
  8. Adjust flow rate accordingly.
  9. When blood therapy is complete or must be discontinued, shut down flow regulator from blood supply and open regulator from normal saline solution.
H. Factors affecting intravenous flow rates (p. 420)
  1. Constricting band
  2. Edema at the puncture site
  3. Cannula abutting the vein wall or valve
  4. Administration set control valves
  5. IV bag height
  6. Completely filled drip chamber
  7. Catheter patency
I. Complications of peripheral intravenous access (pp. 421–422)
  1. Pain
  2. Local infection
  3. Pyrogenic reaction
  4. Allergic reaction
  5. Catheter shear

      6. Inadvertent arterial puncture
      7. Circulatory overload
      8. Thrombophlebitis
      9. Thrombus formation
    10. Air embolism
    11. Necrosis
    12. Anticoagulants
  J. Changing an IV bag or bottle (p. 422)
      1. Prepare new IV solution bag or bottle.
      2. Occlude the flow of solution from depleted bag or bottle.
      3. Remove the spike from the depleted bag or bottle.
      4. Insert spike into the new IV bag or bottle, ensuring drip chamber is filled appropriately.
      5. Open roller clamp to appropriate flow rate.
  K. Intravenous drug administration (pp. 423–431)
      1. Intravenous bolus administration (**Proc. 7-10, p. 424**)
        a. Equipment
          i. BSI
          ii. Alcohol antiseptic preparation
          iii. Packaged medication
          iv. Syringe
          v. 18- to 20-gauge hypodermic needle, 1″–1½″ long
          vi. Existing intravenous line with medication port
        b. Technique
          i. Assure primary IV is patent.
          ii. Confirm drug, indication, dose, and need for IV bolus.
          iii. Draw up medication or prepare a prefilled syringe.
          iv. Cleanse medication port nearest IV site with alcohol.
          v. Insert hypodermic needle through port membrane.
          vi. Pinch the IV line above the medication port.
          vii. Inject the medication.
          viii. Remove the hypodermic needle and syringe and release tubing.
          ix. Open flow regulator to allow a 20-cc fluid flush.
          x. Dispose of hypodermic needle and syringe appropriately.
          xi. Monitor patient for desired or undesired effects.
      2. Intravenous drug infusion (**Proc. 7-11, p. 426**)
        a. Information
          i. Name of medication
          ii. Total dosage in weight mixed in bag
          iii. Concentration (weight per single cc)
          iv. Expiration date
        b. Technique
          i. Establish primary IV line and assure patency.
          ii. Confirm administration indications and patient allergies.
          iii. Prepare infusion bag or bottle. (**Fig. 7-28, p. 425**)
          iv. Connect administration tubing to medication bag or bottle and fill drip chamber to fluid line.
          v. Place hypodermic needle on administration tubing's needle adapter and flush tubing with solution.
          vi. Cleanse medication administration port on primary line with alcohol and insert secondary line's hypodermic needle. Secure needle and line with tape.
          vii. Reconfirm indication, drug, dose, and route.
          viii. Shut down primary line so that no fluid will flow from primary solution bag.

POINT TO EMPHASIZE
Never administer intravenous infusions as a primary IV line.

   ix. Adjust secondary line to desired drip rate.
   x. Properly dispose of needle and syringe.
 3. Heparin lock and saline lock (**Fig.** 7-29, p. 427)
  a. Equipment
   i. IV cannula
   ii. Heparin lock
   iii. Syringe with 3–5 cc sterile saline
   iv. Tape or commercial securing device
   v. Venous blood drawing equipment
   vi. Venous constricting band
   vii. Antiseptic swab
  b. Steps
   i. Select venipuncture site.
   ii. Place constricting band proximal to puncture site.
   iii. Cleanse site with alcohol or betadine antiseptic.
   iv. Insert IV cannula into the vein.
   v. Slide Teflon catheter into vein.
   vi. Remove metal stylet and dispose of appropriately. Remove venous constricting band.
   vii. Obtain venous blood samples.
   viii. Attach heparin lock tubing to angiocatheter hub.
   ix. Cleanse medication port and inject 3–5 mL of sterile saline into the lock.
   x. Apply antibiotic ointment to site and cover with adhesive bandage. Secure tubing to patient.
  c. Equipment needed to administer IV medication bolus through heparin lock
   i. BSI
   ii. Alcohol antiseptic preparation
   iii. Packaged medication
   iv. Syringe
   v. 18- to 20-gauge hypodermic needle, 1″–1½″ long
  d. Technique
   i. Confirm drug, indication, dose, and need for IV bolus.
   ii. Draw up medication or prepare prefilled syringe.
   iii. Cleanse medication port nearest the IV site with alcohol.
   iv. Ensure that plastic clamp is open.
   v. Insert hypodermic needle through port membrane.
   vi. Inject medication as appropriate.
   vii. Remove hypodermic needle and dispose of appropriately.
   viii. Follow medication administration with 10 to 20 mL saline flush from another syringe.
   ix. Properly dispose of hypodermic needle and syringe.
   x. Monitor patient for desired or undesired effects.
 4. Venous access device
  a. Technique to prepare site
   i. Use BSI.
   ii. Fill 10-mL syringe with 7 mL of normal saline.
   iii. Place 21- or 22-gauge Huber needle on end of syringe.
   iv. Cleanse skin over injection port with povidone-iodine or alcohol preparation.
   v. Stabilize the site with one hand while inserting Huber needle at a 90° angle. Gently advance it until it meets resistance.
   vi. Pull back on plunger and observe for blood return, which confirms placement.
   vii. Slowly inject normal saline to assure patency.

      b. Medication administration technique
- **i.** Prepare medication, fluid, or blood for administration.
- **ii.** Attach a 21- or 22-gauge Huber needle to end of the syringe.
- **iii.** Cleanse skin over injection port with povidone-iodine or alcohol.
- **iv.** Insert needle into injection port at 90° angle until needle cannot be advanced further. Pull back plunger to observe for return of blood, confirming proper placement.
- **v.** Inject medication as appropriate.
- **vi.** Remove and dispose of syringe appropriately.
- **vii.** With another syringe and attached special needle, administer a bolus of heparinized saline to clear the catheter of any blood clots or obstructions.

      c. Fluid administration technique
- **i.** Prepare a primary IV line.
- **ii.** Attach Huber needle to primary IV administration tubing. Insert 10-mL syringe and hypodermic needle filled with 7 mL of normal saline solution into the tubing medication delivery port nearest the venous access device.
- **iii.** Cleanse skin over injection port with povidone-iodine or alcohol preparations.
- **iv.** Insert needle into injection port at 90° angle until it encounters resistance.
- **v.** Pinch administration tubing above medication administration port and pull back on syringe plunger. Observe for blood return, confirming proper placement.
- **vi.** Gently inject the 7 mL of normal saline solution.
- **vii.** Set primary line to appropriate flow rate.

      d. Administering secondary medicated infusion
- **i.** Prepare secondary line containing fluid, blood, or medicated solution for infusion.
- **ii.** Attach hypodermic needle to needle adapter of secondary line. Insert secondary line into a medication administration port on primary tubing.
- **iii.** Shut down primary line and infuse medicated solution.
- **iv.** When infusion is complete, administer bolus of heparinized saline to clear catheter of blood clots or obstructions.

5. Electromechanical infusion devices
   a. Infusion controllers
   b. Infusion pumps (**Fig. 7-30, p. 430; Fig. 7-31, p. 431**)

L. Venous blood sampling (pp. 431–434)
   1. Situations for obtaining venous blood
      a. During peripheral access
      b. Before drug administration
      c. When drug administration may be needed
   2. Equipment for drawing blood
      a. Blood tubes (**Fig. 7-32, p. 432**) (**Table 7-1, p. 432**)
         i. Red (no anticoagulant)
         ii. Blue (citrate)
         iii. Green (heparin)
         iv. Purple (EDTA)
         v. Gray (Fluoride)
      b. Miscellaneous equipment
   3. Obtaining venous blood
      a. Obtaining venous blood from IV angiocatheter
         i. Assemble and prepare all equipment. (**Fig. 7-33, p. 433**)
         ii. Establish IV access with angiocatheter.

> **POINT TO EMPHASIZE**
> Never stop to draw blood if it will delay critical measures.

iii. Attach end of leur adapter to hub of cannula or use a 20-mL syringe. (**Fig. 7-34, p. 433; Fig. 7-35, p. 434**)
   iv. In correct order, insert blood tubes so that rubber-covered needle punctures the self-sealing rubber top.
   v. Fill all blood tubes completely, and agitate tubes.
   vi. Tamponade vein and remove vacutainer and leur lock; attach IV line and assure patency.
   vii. Properly dispose of all sharps.
   viii. Label all blood tubes.
  b. Obtaining blood directly from a vein
   i. Assemble and prepare all equipment.
   ii. Apply constricting band and select appropriate puncture site.
   iii. Cleanse site with alcohol or betadine.
   iv. Insert end of leur sampling needle into vein and remove constricting band.
   v. In correct order, insert each blood tube so rubber-covered needle punctures self-sealing rubber top.
   vi. Gently agitate the tube to evenly mix anticoagulant with blood.
   vii. Place sterile gauze over site and remove sampling needle. Properly dispose of sharps.
   viii. Cover puncture site with gauze and tape or adhesive bandage.
   ix. Label all blood tubes.
  c. Complications from drawing blood
   i. Damage to vein wall
   ii. Hemoconcentration
   iii. Hemolysis
M. Removing a peripheral IV (pp. 434–435)

II. Intraosseous infusion. Intraosseous infusions involve inserting a rigid needle into the cavity of a long bone; any solution or drug that can be administered intravenously can be administered by the intraosseous route. (pp. 435–442)

A. Access site (p. 435)
  1. Most commonly the tibia (**Fig. 7-36, p. 436; Fig. 7-37, p. 437**)
    a. Pediatric
      i. Proximal tibia
    b. Adult
      i. Distal tibia
B. Equipment for intraosseous access (pp. 435–438) (**Fig. 7-38, p. 437**)
  1. Bone Injection Gun (B.I.G.) (**Fig. 7-39, p. 437**)
  2. F.A.S.T.1 (**Fig. 7-40, p. 438**)
  3. EZ-IO (**Fig. 7-41, p. 438**)
C. Placing an intraosseous infusion (pp. 438–441) (**Proc. 7-12, pp. 439–440**)
  1. Technique
    a. Determine the indication for intraosseous access.
    b. Assemble and check all equipment.
    c. Position the patient.
    d. Locate access site.
    e. Cleanse site with alcohol or betadine.
    f. Perform puncture.
    g. Remove trocar and attach saline-filled syringe.
    h. Slowly pull back plunger to attempt aspiration into syringe, confirming placement.
    i. Rotate plastic disk toward skin to secure needle.
    j. Remove the syringe and attach the administration tubing.
    k. Secure the needle.
    l. Periodically flush the needle to keep it patent.

POINT TO EMPHASIZE
Remove any IV that will not flow or has fulfilled its purpose.

POWERPOINT PRESENTATION
Chapter 7 PowerPoint slides 83–99

POINT TO EMPHASIZE
Initiate intraosseous lines only after 90 seconds or three unsuccessful attempts to establish peripheral IV access.

POINT TO EMPHASIZE
You must continually refresh your intraosseous access skills so that you can perform this technique properly when needed.

D. Intraosseous access complications and precautions (p. 441)
   1. Fracture
   2. Infiltration
   3. Growth plate damage
   4. Complete insertion
   5. Pulmonary embolism
E. Contraindications to intraosseous placement (p. 442)
   1. Fracture of tibia or femur on side of access
   2. Osteogenesis imperfecta
   3. Osteoporosis
   4. Establishment of a peripheral IV line

PART 3: MEDICAL MATHEMATICS

I. **Introduction.** Proper drug administration requires basic mathematical proficiency. (p. 442)

II. **Metric system** (pp. 442–444)

A. Conversion between prefixes (pp. 442–443) (**Example 1, p. 442; Example 2, p. 443; Example 3, p. 443; Example 4, p. 443**) (**Table 7-2, p. 442**)
B. Household and apothecary systems of measure (p. 443) (**Table 7-3, p. 443**)
C. Weight conversion (pp. 443–444) (**Example 5, p. 444**)
D. Temperature (p. 444) (**Example 6, p. 444; Example 7, p. 444**)
   1. Fahrenheit
   2. Celsius
E. Units (p. 444)

III. **Medication calculations** (pp. 444–449)

A. Introduction (p. 444)
   1. Oral medications
   2. Liquid parenteral medications
   3. Intravenous fluid administration
   4. Intravenous medication infusions
   5. Three facts
      a. Desired dose
      b. Dosage on hand
      c. volume on hand
B. Desired dose (p. 445)
C. Dosage on hand (p. 445)
D. Calculating dosages for oral medications (p. 445) (**Example 1, p. 445**)
E. Converting prefixes (p. 446) (**Example 2, p. 446**)
F. Calculating dosages for parenteral medications (pp. 446–447) (**Example 3, pp. 446–447**)
G. Calculating weight-dependent dosages (p. 447) (**Example 4, p. 447**)
H. Calculating infusion rates (pp. 447–449) (**Example 5, p. 448**)
I. Fluid volume over time (pp. 448–449) (**Example 6, pp. 448–449; Example 7, p. 449**)
J. Calculating dosages and infusion rates for infants and children (p. 449)

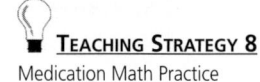

IV. **Chapter summary** (p. 449). Drug administration is a fundamental skill used in the treatment of the sick and injured. For medications to be effective, they must be *safely* delivered into the body by the *appropriate* route. Many different routes for drug delivery are available to the paramedic; however, specific drugs require specific routes for administration.

It is your responsibility to be familiar with all routes of drug delivery and the techniques for establishing and utilizing them. You will use some routes of medication administration infrequently, and they will quickly fade from memory. Nonetheless, someone's well-being may depend on your ability to utilize such a route in an emergency. Therefore, periodic review of all routes used in medication administration is highly recommended. In addition, you must accurately calculate many drug dosages. Dosage errors and inappropriate medication administration harm patient care and cast serious doubt on your ability.

ASSIGNMENTS

Assign students to complete Chapter 7, "Medication Administration," of the workbook. Also assign them to read Chapter 8, "Airway Management and Ventilation," before the next class.

EVALUATION

Chapter Quiz and Scenario Distribute copies of the Chapter Quiz provided in Handouts 7-3 to 7-5 to evaluate student understanding of this chapter. Make sure each student reads the scenario to reinforce critical thinking on the scene. Remind students not to use their notes or textbooks while taking the quiz.

Student CD Quizzes for every chapter are contained on the dynamic and highly visual in-text student CD.

Companion Website Additional quizzes for every chapter are contained on this exciting website.

TestGen You may wish to create a custom-tailored test using *Prentice Hall TestGen for Essentials of Paramedic Care*, 2nd Edition to evaluate student understanding of this chapter.

On-line Test Preparation (for students and instructors) Additional test preparation is available through Brady's new on-line product, *EMT Achieve: Paramedic Test Preparation* at *http://www.prenhall.com/emtachieve/*. Instructors can also monitor student mastery on-line.

Review Manual for the EMT-Paramedic This comprehensive exam review contains hundreds of test questions and rationales, including scenarios, along with two 180-question practice tests on CD.

REINFORCEMENT

Handouts If classroom discussion or performance on the quiz indicates that some students have not fully mastered the chapter content, you may wish to assign some or all of the Reinforcement Handouts for this chapter.

Student CD (for students) A wide variety of material on this CD-ROM will reinforce and also expand student knowledge and skills.

PowerPoint Presentation (for instructors) The PowerPoint material developed for this chapter offers useful reinforcement of chapter content.

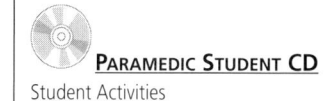

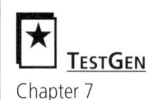

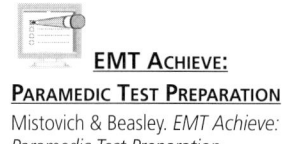

WORKBOOK
Chapter 7 Activities

READING/REFERENCE
Textbook, pp. 454–531

HANDOUTS 7-3 TO 7-5
Chapter 7 Quizzes

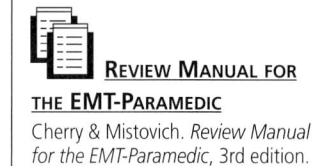

HANDOUT 7-6
Chapter 7 Scenario

PARAMEDIC STUDENT CD
Student Activities

COMPANION WEBSITE
http://www.prenhall.com/bledsoe

TESTGEN
Chapter 7

**EMT ACHIEVE:
PARAMEDIC TEST PREPARATION**
Mistovich & Beasley. *EMT Achieve: Paramedic Test Preparation*, www.prenhall.com/emtachieve/

REVIEW MANUAL FOR THE EMT-PARAMEDIC
Cherry & Mistovich. *Review Manual for the EMT-Paramedic*, 3rd edition.

HANDOUTS 7-7 THROUGH 7-10
Reinforcement Activities

PARAMEDIC STUDENT CD
Student Activities

POWERPOINT PRESENTATION
Chapter 7

COMPANION WEBSITE
http://www.prenhall.com/bledsoe

ONEKEY
Chapter 7

ADVANCED LIFE SUPPORT SKILLS
Larmon & Davis. *Advanced Life Support Skills*.

ADVANCED LIFE SKILLS REVIEW
Larmon & Davis. *Advanced Life Skills Review*.

BRADY SKILLS SERIES: ALS
Larmon & Davis. *Brady Skills Series: ALS*.

PARAMEDIC NATIONAL STANDARDS SELF-TEST
Miller. *Paramedic National Standards Self-Test*, 4th edition.

Companion Website (for students)   Additional review quizzes and links to EMS resources will contribute to further reinforcement of the chapter.

OneKey   On-line support is offered for this course on one of three platforms: CourseCompass, Blackboard, or Web CT. Includes the IRM, PowerPoints, TestGen, and Companion Website for instruction. Ask your local sales representative for more information.

Brady Skills Series: Advanced Life Skills (Video or CD)   Have your students watch the skills come to life on VHS or CD-ROM, or they can purchase the highly visual, full-color text with step-by-step procedures and rationales.

Handout 7-1

Student's Name _____

CHAPTER 7 OBJECTIVES CHECKLIST

PART 1: PRINCIPLES AND ROUTES OF MEDICATION ADMINISTRATION

Knowledge	Date Mastered
1. Review the specific anatomy and physiology pertinent to medication administration.	
2. Describe the indications, equipment needed, technique used, precautions, and general principles for the following • inhalation routes of medication administration. • parenteral routes of medication administration. • percutaneous routes of medication administration. • enteral routes of medication administration, including gastric tube administration and rectal administration.	
3. Describe the indications, contraindications, side effects, dosages, and routes of administration for medications commonly administered by paramedics.	
4. Discuss legal aspects affecting medication administration.	
5. Discuss the "six rights" of drug administration and correlate them with the principles of medication administration.	
6. Differentiate among the percutaneous routes of medication administration.	
7. Discuss medical asepsis and the differences between clean and sterile techniques.	
8. Describe uses of antiseptics and disinfectants.	
9. Describe the use of body substance isolation (BSI) procedures when administering a medication.	
10. Describe disposal of contaminated items and sharps.	
11. Synthesize a pharmacologic management plan including medication administration.	

HANDOUT 7-1 Continued

PART 2: INTRAVENOUS ACCESS, BLOOD SAMPLING, AND INTRAOSSEOUS INFUSION

Knowledge	Date Mastered
1. Review the specific anatomy and physiology pertinent to medication administration.	
2. Describe the indications, equipment needed, technique used, precautions, and general principles for the following: • peripheral venous or external jugular cannulation. • intraosseous needle placement and infusion. • obtaining a blood sample.	

PART 3: MEDICAL MATHEMATICS

Knowledge	Date Mastered
1. Review mathematical equivalents.	
2. Differentiate temperature readings between the centigrade and Fahrenheit scales.	
3. Discuss formulas as a basis for performing drug calculations.	
4. Describe how to perform mathematical conversions from the household system to the metric system.	

Handout 7-2

Student's Name _____

MEDICATION ADMINISTRATION

Charting Student Progress:
1. *Learning skill*
2. *Performs skill with direction*
3. *Performs skill independently*

PERIPHERAL INTRAVENOUS ACCESS

Procedure	1	2	3
1. Takes BSI precautions.			
2. Explains procedure to patient.			
3. Selects appropriate fluid, administration set, cannula.			
4. Examines fluid for clarity and expiration date.			
5. Assembles administration set and bag/bottle correctly.			
6. Selects venipuncture site.			
7. Places constricting band proximal to intended site of puncture.			
8. Cleanses venipuncture site.			
9. Inserts intravenous cannula into the vein.			
10. Slides Teflon catheter over needle into vein.			
11. Removes metal stylet and disposes of it in proper container.			
12. Removes constricting band.			
13. Attaches administration tubing to cannula.			
14. Applies antibiotic ointment to site; covers with adhesive bandage.			
15. Loops distal tubing and secures to patient with tape.			
16. Labels intravenous solution bag/bottle.			
17. Monitors patient and flow rate.			
18. Maintains aseptic technique throughout procedure.			

Comments:

HANDOUT 7-2 Continued

SUBCUTANEOUS INJECTION

Procedure	1	2	3
1. Takes BSI precautions.			
2. Elicits patient allergies; explains procedure.			
3. Selects correct medication.			
4. Checks label for correct name, concentration, expiration date.			
5. Inspects medication for discoloration, particles.			
6. Prepares correct amount of medication.			
7. Chooses and cleanses injection site appropriately.			
8. Rechecks correct drug and dose.			
9. Inserts needle at 45° angle, aspirates for blood return.			
10. If no blood return, injects medication at appropriate rate.			
11. Removes needle and disposes of it in proper container.			
12. Applies pressure to injection site.			
13. Monitors patient for effects of medication.			
14. Maintains aseptic technique throughout procedure.			

Comments:

INTRAMUSCULAR INJECTION

Procedure	1	2	3
1. Takes BSI precautions.			
2. Elicits patient allergies; explains procedure.			
3. Selects correct medication.			
4. Checks label for correct name, concentration, expiration date.			
5. Inspects medication for discoloration, particles.			
6. Prepares correct amount of medication.			
7. Chooses and cleanses injection site appropriately.			

HANDOUT 7-2 Continued

Procedure	1	2	3
8. Rechecks correct drug and dose.			
9. Inserts needle at 90° angle; aspirates for blood return.			
10. If no blood return, injects medication at appropriate rate.			
11. Disposes of needle and syringe in proper container.			
12. Applies gauze or adhesive bandage to site and massages.			
13. Monitors patient for desired or undesired effects.			
14. Maintains aseptic technique throughout procedure.			

Comments:

INTRAVENOUS MEDICATION ADMINISTRATION THROUGH EXISTING IV LINE

Procedure	1	2	3
1. Takes BSI precautions.			
2. Elicits patient allergies.			
3. Selects the correct medication and administration equipment.			
4. Checks label for correct name, concentration, expiration date.			
5. Inspects medication for discoloration, particles.			
6. Prepares correct dose. • Assembles prefilled syringe; expels air. • Draws up correct amount from ampule or vial.			
7. Cleanses injection site.			
8. Stops IV flow above injection site.			
9. Reaffirms correct medication, dose.			
10. Inserts needle; injects correct dose at appropriate rate.			
11. Opens and flushes IV line; readjusts IV flow rate.			
12. Disposes of needle and syringe in appropriate container.			

HANDOUT 7-2 Continued

Procedure	1	2	3
13. Observes patient for medication effects.			
14. Maintains aseptic technique throughout procedure.			

Comments:

IV PIGGYBACK

Procedure	1	2	3
1. Takes BSI precautions.			
2. Elicits possible allergies.			
3. Selects correct medication.			
4. Checks label for correct name, concentration, expiration date.			
5. Checks medication and IV bag for discoloration, particles.			
6. Injects correct amount of medication into IV bag; mixes it.			
7. Connects IV tubing to the bag and flushes line.			
8. Attaches needle to IV line.			
9. Cleanses medication port and inserts needle.			
10. Stops flow of primary IV.			
11. Sets infusion at desired rate and tapes line securely.			
12. Labels bag or bottle appropriately.			
13. Observes patient for effects of medication.			
14. Maintains aseptic technique throughout procedure.			

Comments:

HANDOUT 7-2 Continued

ENDOTRACHEAL DRUG ADMINISTRATION

Procedure	1	2	3
1. Takes BSI precautions.			
2. Selects correct medication.			
3. Checks label for correct name, concentration, expiration date.			
4. Inspects medication for discoloration, particles.			
5. Prepares correct amount of medication.			
6. Hyperventilates patient.			
7. Removes ventilation device.			
8. Administers the medication down the endotracheal tube.			
9. Replaces the ventilation device and hyperventilates patient.			
10. Monitors patient for desired and undesired effects.			

Comments:

HANDOUT 7-3

Student's Name _____

CHAPTER 7 QUIZ

PART 1: PRINCIPLES AND ROUTES OF MEDICATION ADMINISTRATION

Write the letter of the best answer in the space provided.

_____ 1. The six "rights" of drug administration include the:
   A. right person.
   B. right drug.
   C. right time.
   D. all of these

_____ 2. Drug administration by the paramedic should be done under a condition free of pathogens. This condition is called:
   A. sterile.
   B. medically clean.
   C. aseptic.
   D. antiseptic.

_____ 3. Medically clean refers to techniques involving:
   A. maintaining an aseptic environment.
   B. cleansing with disinfectants.
   C. careful handling of sterile equipment to prevent contamination.
   D. sterilizing equipment that comes in contact with a patient.

_____ 4. To minimize or eliminate the risk of accidental needle stick, precautions include:
   A. minimizing tasks in a moving ambulance.
   B. recapping needles immediately after use.
   C. placing all sharps in a red plastic bag with a biohazard label on it.
   D. avoiding the use of any needles in the prehospital setting.

_____ 5. Medications given by the transdermal route are:
   A. placed beneath the tongue.
   B. absorbed through the skin.
   C. injected into the subcutaneous layer.
   D. placed between the patient's cheek and gum.

_____ 6. Delivering medication through the mucous membranes of the ear is called the:
   A. buccal route.
   B. sublingual route.
   C. ocular route.
   D. aural route.

_____ 7. A metered dose inhaler is a(n):
   A. handheld device that produces a medicated spray for inhalation.
   B. inhalation aid that disperses liquid into aerosol spray or mist.
   C. regulator device that administers oxygen along with inhaled medication.
   D. specially designed regulator used for nitrous-oxide administration.

_____ 8. Which of the following is true regarding drug administration via a small-volume nebulizer?
   A. Set the oxygen source regulator for 10–15 liters per minute.
   B. If the patient's tidal volume is shallow, place twice the normal amount of medication into the nebulizer.
   C. It is important for the patient to exhale completely before inhaling medication.
   D. Attaching a nebulizer to an oxygen humidifier will enhance absorption of the medication.

250 ESSENTIALS OF PARAMEDIC CARE

HANDOUT 7-3 Continued

_____ 9. If you have not established an IV line, some medications can be given through an endotracheal tube. Which of the following is correct regarding drug administration through an ET tube?
   A. Dilute the medication in normal saline to create 10 mL of solution.
   B. Pulmonary absorption of drugs is much slower than the intravenous route.
   C. Lidocaine, atropine, and naloxone should not be given via ET tube.
   D. Use the same dose of medication for ET tube administration as you would for IV administration.

_____ 10. An example of an enteral route of drug administration is:
   A. rectal.
   B. intradermal.
   C. subcutaneous.
   D. intravenous.

_____ 11. Guidelines for oral administration of a medication include which of the following?
   A. Always administer oral medication on an empty stomach.
   B. Do not give any fluid by mouth for 20–30 minutes after oral administration of a medication.
   C. Never use household teaspoons to measure medications.
   D. Place the patient in the semi-Fowler's position when administering oral medications.

_____ 12. Rectal administration of medication:
   A. results in rapid drug absorption.
   B. is subject to hepatic alteration.
   C. has an unpredictable absorption rate.
   D. should not be used for Valium.

_____ 13. Some medications are packaged in a nonconstituted vial. This means:
   A. the medication is a highly concentrated solution, given in small doses.
   B. the vial has two containers; one holds the powdered medication and the other holds a liquid mixing solution.
   C. the medication is in powder form and placed in a nebulizer with normal saline.
   D. the medication is in a viscous liquid form and diluted with sterile water.

_____ 14. Steps in administering medication by subcutaneous injection include:
   A. gently rubbing the injection site to help initiate systemic absorption.
   B. inserting the needle at a 10°–15° angle, bevel up.
   C. pulling the patient's skin taut with your nondominant hand.
   D. using a 24- to 26-gauge needle, 1″–1 1/2″ long.

_____ 15. When administering medication by the intramuscular route, insert the needle at a:
   A. 10°–15° angle.
   B. 25° angle.
   C. 45° angle.
   D. 90° angle.

_____ 16. Intramuscular injection sites include which of the following muscles?
   A. gastrocnemius
   B. vastus lateralis
   C. psoas major
   D. biceps brachii

_____ 17. When administering medication by the subcutaneous injection route:
   A. correct placement of the needle is confirmed by a blood return when the plunger of the syringe is pulled back.
   B. do not rub or massage the site, as this promotes systemic absorption and nullifies the advantage of localized effect.
   C. you may use an air plug in the syringe, which pushes the medication further into the subcutaneous tissue.
   D. avoid pinching the skin at the injection site, as this will result in a slower absorption of the medication.

HANDOUT 7-3 Continued

_____ 18. When administering an intramuscular injection, you should:
  A. pinch the skin together gently at the site of the injection.
  B. choose a bruised area for the injection if possible.
  C. stretch the skin taut over the injection site.
  D. inject the medication rapidly.

_____ 19. Intradermal injection is particularly useful for:
  A. delivery of local anesthetics.
  B. insulin injection.
  C. epineprine injection.
  D. delivery of antiemetics.

_____ 20. The least expensive form of single-dose packaging of drugs for injection is the:
  A. vial.
  B. nonconstituted drug vial.
  C. prefilled syringe.
  D. glass ampule.

Handout 7-4

Student's Name _____

CHAPTER 7 QUIZ

PART 2: INTRAVENOUS ACCESS, BLOOD SAMPLING, AND INTRAOSSEOUS INFUSION

Write the letter of the best answer in the space provided.

_____ 1. Which of the following is true regarding intravenous access?
   A. Arterial access is preferable to venous access.
   B. Central venous access is most often performed in the prehospital setting.
   C. When establishing a peripheral IV, start at the distal end of an extremity.
   D. Peripheral IVs are used when medical conditions require repeated access for medication or fluid delivery.

_____ 2. Examples of colloid IV solutions include:
   A. lactated Ringer's solution.
   B. normal saline solution.
   C. salt-poor albumin.
   D. 5 percent dextrose in water.

_____ 3. One of the most common IV solutions used in the prehospital setting for fluid replacement is:
   A. Dextran.
   B. lactated Ringer's solution.
   C. plasmanate.
   D. hetastarch.

_____ 4. In standard microdrip administration tubing, 1 mL of fluid is:
   A. 10 gtts.
   B. 15 gtts.
   C. 45 gtts.
   D. 60 gtts.

_____ 5. A burette chamber on IV administration tubing is:
   A. a clear plastic chamber that allows visualization of the drip rate.
   B. the device that regulates the size of the drops.
   C. a calibrated chamber that enables precise measurement and delivery of fluids and medicated solutions.
   D. a device that contains a filter to prevent clots or other debris from entering the patient.

_____ 6. Hollow needle catheters do not have:
   A. a Teflon tube.
   B. a metal stylet.
   C. "wings" for guidance and securing.
   D. clear tubing.

_____ 7. Which of the following IV sites is NOT considered a peripheral site?
   A. antecubital fossa
   B. external jugular
   C. subclavian
   D. cephalic

_____ 8. Consider accessing the external jugular vein if a patient requires immediate fluid administration. When using this route, remember:
   A. to attach a 10-mL syringe with 3–5 mL of sterile saline to the cannula.
   B. you will need a larger constricting band than those used with arm or leg sites.
   C. to insert the catheter at a 45° angle, bevel up.
   D. to place the patient in the semi-Fowler's position during the procedure.

_____ 9. The most common cause of an IV not flowing properly is:
   A. the cannula abutting the vein wall or valve.
   B. leaving the constricting band in place.
   C. a completely filled drip chamber.
   D. edema at the puncture site.

©2007 Pearson Education, Inc.
Essentials of Paramedic Care, 2nd ed.

HANDOUT 7-4 Continued

_____ 10. If your patient develops an abrupt onset of fever, chills, backache, headache, nausea, and vomiting within 1/2 to 1 after an IV was started, the cause may be:
   A. local infection.
   B. thrombophlebitis.
   C. pyrogenic reaction.
   D. air embolism.

_____ 11. Catheter shear is caused by:
   A. pulling the Teflon catheter through or over the needle after you have advanced it into the vein.
   B. accidental arterial puncture.
   C. inflammation of the vein.
   D. a blood clot caused by the injury to the vessel wall.

_____ 12. Steps in changing an IV bag or bottle include:
   A. occluding the flow of solution from the depleted bag by moving the roller clamp on the IV administration tubing.
   B. cleansing the spike with a disinfectant before inserting it into the new bag.
   C. changing the administration set at the same time.
   D. flushing the IV site with a heparinized solution before attaching the new bag/bottle to the administration set.

_____ 13. When injecting an intravenous bolus of medication into an existing IV site:
   A. use a 14- to 16-gauge needle for rapid administration.
   B. flush the IV site with 20 cc of fluid before giving the medication.
   C. pinch the IV line above the medication port before giving the medication.
   D. open the flow regulator to allow a 1–2 minute fluid flush after giving the medication.

_____ 14. Some cardiac drugs and antibiotics are given as an intravenous infusion, or piggyback. When mixing an infusion, remember to:
   A. administer intravenous infusions as a primary IV line.
   B. gently agitate the bag or bottle to mix its contents.
   C. keep fluid flowing from the primary line as the medication infusion is administered.
   D. run the infusion in as rapidly as possible, then readjust the primary line to the desired drip rate.

_____ 15. Which of the following is true regarding drawing blood from your patient?
   A. Blood tubes may be used in any order, as long as all are filled.
   B. A green top on a blood tube indicates it has fluoride in it as an anticoagulant.
   C. Never place blood tubes into the vacutainer and leur lock until you are ready to draw blood.
   D. Veins on the back of the hand are your first choice when drawing a venous blood sample.

_____ 16. The bone most commonly used for intraosseous access is the:
   A. sternum.   C. femur.
   B. radius.   D. tibia.

_____ 17. Which of the following is true regarding intraosseous infusion?
   A. This procedure is performed only on pediatric patients.
   B. You may attempt intraosseous placement even if a peripheral IV line is in place.
   C. Periodic flushing of the needle is necessary to keep it from becoming occluded.
   D. Easy access of bone marrow and blood from the site into a syringe indicates incorrect placement of the needle.

HANDOUT 7-4 Continued

_____ **18.** Hemoconcentration occurs when:
   A. a constricting band is left in place too long while starting a peripheral IV.
   B. red blood cells are destroyed during vigorous shaking of blood tubes after they are filled.
   C. blood tubes are not agitated to mix blood with the anticoagulant in the tube.
   D. the wrong blood type is given to a patient.

_____ **19.** Which of the following is a contraindication for intraosseous placement?
   A. lordosis
   B. osteoporosis
   C. patient taking nitroglycerin
   D. kyphosis

_____ **20.** The color of the top of a blood tube containing the anticoagulant heparin is:
   A. gray
   B. purple
   C. blue
   D. green

HANDOUT 7-5

Student's Name _____

CHAPTER 7 QUIZ

PART 3: MEDICAL MATHEMATICS

Write the letter of the best answer in the space provided.

_____ 1. How many milligrams are in a gram?
  A. 10
  B. 100
  C. 1,000
  D. 10,000

_____ 2. How many milliliters are in a liter?
  A. 10
  B. 100
  C. 1,000
  D. 10,000

_____ 3. How many micrograms are in a gram?
  A. 100
  B. 1,000
  C. 10,000
  D. 1,000,000

_____ 4. A patient who weighs 70 kilograms weighs how many pounds?
  A. 32 pounds
  B. 105 pounds
  C. 140 pounds
  D. 154 pounds

_____ 5. Calculate the following: 1,600 micrograms = _____ gram.
  A. 0.16
  B. 0.016
  C. 0.0016
  D. 0.00016

_____ 6. Calculate the following: 5.6 milligrams = _____ micrograms.
  A. 56
  B. 560
  C. 5,600
  D. 56,000

_____ 7. One gallon, or four quarts, equals how many liters?
  A. 37.85
  B. 3.785
  C. 0.3785
  D. 0.03785

_____ 8. One teaspoon is equal to:
  A. 250 milliliters.
  B. 16 milliliters.
  C. 4–5 milliliters.
  D. 2–3 milliliters.

_____ 9. How many kilograms does a 182-lb. person weigh?
  A. 91 kilograms
  B. 82.7 kilograms
  C. 273 kilograms
  D. 151.1 kilograms

_____ 10. The amount of drug available in a solution is called the:
  A. volume on hand.
  B. desired dose.
  C. stock solution.
  D. dosage on hand.

_____ 11. The available amount of solution containing a medication is called the:
  A. volume on hand.
  B. desired dose.
  C. stock solution.
  D. dosage on hand.

_____ 12. How many mL of solution would you have to administer to give a patient 90 mg of oral acetaminophen using a concentration of 500 mg in 8 mL of solution?
  A. 14.4 mL
  B. 1.44 mL
  C. 0.144 mL
  D. 0.0144 mL

HANDOUT 7-5 Continued

_____ 13. Your orders are to give 250 mg of a drug via IV bolus. The multidose vial contains 2 grams of the drug in 10 mL of solution. How many mL will you administer?
   A. 125 mL
   B. 12.5 mL
   C. 1.25 mL
   D. 0.125 mL

_____ 14. You are going to administer 1.5 mg/kg of lidocaine, IV bolus, to a patient who has unstable ventricular tachycardia. The lidocaine concentration is 100 mg in a prefilled syringe of 10 mL. The patient weighs 158 pounds. How many mL of lidocaine will you administer?
   A. 10.8 mL
   B. 1.08 mL
   C. 0.108 mL
   D. 0.0108 mL

_____ 15. Your medical control physician orders an IV drip of lidocaine at 2 mg/minute. You mix 2 grams of lidocaine in 500 mL of D_5W. You are using a microdrip administration set delivering 60 gtts/mL. How many drops per minute will your infusion be?
   A. 15 gtts
   B. 30 gtts
   C. 45 gtts
   D. 60 gtts

HANDOUT 7-6

Student's Name _____

CHAPTER 7 SCENARIO

Review the following real-life situation. Then answer the question that follows.

At 2:00 A.M., Medic 12 receives a call for an elderly patient who is short of breath. The crew reaches the scene, a first-floor apartment in a small tenement building, in 4 minutes. They knock on the door of the apartment and hear a weak call to come in. Upon entering, they find a one-room apartment crammed with boxes, old newspapers, magazines, and heaps of old clothes. The patient, a 72-year-old man, is across the room in a recliner, where he apparently sleeps during the night. Upon taking the history, the crew learns that the patient has had several previous episodes of this problem and was last admitted to the hospital 4 months ago. The patient is in obvious respiratory distress with slight cyanosis in the lips.

The senior paramedic decides that interventions and transport are necessary but that the cramped conditions of the apartment are no place to work. He asks the patient to walk to the stretcher in the hall before beginning treatment.

Once the patient is lying on the stretcher, the crew continues the assessment and physical exam. The patient has significant jugular vein distention sitting upright, severe pitting edema, and profuse rales in the posterior bases of the lungs. The patient is supposed to take numerous medications but has not been doing so for the past week. The medications were digitalis, Tonocard, Lasix, and Ventolin. The ECG shows atrial fibrillation at a rate of 110 with frequent PVCs. Respirations are 20 and labored; the pulse is strong, but irregular, corresponding to the ECG; the BP is 160/100.

The crew places the patient on high-flow oxygen and establishes an IV of D_5W at a TKO rate. System protocols call for administration of 60 mg of Lasix. The medication is packaged as 100 mg/10 mL. The senior paramedic estimates that a bit more than half the syringe is appropriate and administers it via rapid IV push.

The patient experiences a dizzy spell shortly thereafter. The paramedic gives morphine via rapid IV push and the dizziness is more profound. The patient almost passes out. The crew lowers the patient's torso and raises his feet to reverse the profound vasodilation. The patient now experiences significant respiratory distress.

The patient is still experiencing frequent PVCs. Protocol permits administration of 1 mg/kg of lidocaine, and the paramedic administers the dose via IV push. The patient experiences some facial twitching a few minutes later, but by this time he is packaged and en route to the hospital. There the crew turns him over to the ED staff, and he is soon in the facility's critical care unit.

1. What faults can you find in Medic 12's handling of this case?

Handout 7-7

Student's Name _____

CHAPTER 7 REVIEW

PART 1: PRINCIPLES AND ROUTES OF MEDICATION ADMINISTRATION

Write the word or words that best complete each sentence in the space provided.

1. The six rights of drug administration are the right _____, the right _____, the right _____, the right _____, the right _____, and the right _____.

2. Measures to decrease your risk of exposure to blood and body fluids are called _____ _____ _____.

3. A condition in which a medical environment is free from pathogens is called _____.

4. _____ means limited to one area of the body.

5. _____ means throughout the body.

6. An environment that is free from all forms of life is _____.

7. _____ _____ techniques involve the careful handling of sterile equipment and supplies to prevent contamination.

8. A cleansing agent that is toxic to living tissue is called a(n) _____.

9. A cleansing agent that is not toxic to living tissue is called a(n) _____.

10. Percutaneous routes for medications include _____ administration and _____ administration.

11. Mucous membrane medication sites include the _____, _____, _____, _____, and _____.

12. The route of medication administration given beneath the tongue is called _____.

13. _____ refers to the route of medication administration between the cheek and gums.

14. Drugs administered through the mucous membranes of the eye are called _____ medications.

15. Medications are drawn into the lungs along with air while breathing during the process of _____.

16. _____ is the placement of medication in or under the skin with a needle and syringe.

17. A(n) _____ is an inhalation aid that disperses liquid into aerosol spray or mist.

18. A(n) _____ _____ _____ is a handheld device that produces a medicated spray for inhalation.

19. The delivery of any medication that is absorbed through the gastrointestinal tract is called _____ drug administration.

20. A concentrated mass of medication is called a(n) _____.

21. A change in a medication's chemical composition that occurs in the liver is called _____ _____.

22. A vial with two containers, one holding a powdered medication and the other holding a liquid mixing solution, is called a(n) _____ _____ _____.

23. When performing a subcutaneous injection, insert the needle at a _____ angle.

24. Intramuscular injection sites include the _____, _____ _____, _____ _____, and the _____ _____ muscles.

25. When performing an intramuscular injection, insert the needle at a _____ angle.

©2007 Pearson Education, Inc.
Essentials of Paramedic Care, 2nd ed.

HANDOUT 7-8

Student's Name _____

CHAPTER 7 REVIEW

PART 2: INTRAVENOUS ACCESS, BLOOD SAMPLING, AND INTRAOSSEOUS INFUSION

Write the word or words that best complete each sentence in the space provided.

1. The surgical puncture of a vein to deliver medication or withdraw blood is called _____ access.
2. Surgical puncture of a vein in the arm, leg, or neck is called _____ _____ _____.
3. Surgical puncture of the internal jugular, subclavian, or femoral vein is called _____ _____ _____.
4. Intravenous solutions containing large proteins that cannot pass through capillary membranes are called _____.
5. Intravenous solutions that contain electrolytes but lack the larger proteins are called _____.
6. _____ solutions are those that have a tonicity equal to blood plasma's.
7. _____ solutions have a higher solute concentration than do the cells.
8. _____ solutions have a lower solute concentration than do the cells.
9. _____ _____ _____ is an isotonic electrolyte solution containing sodium chloride, potassium chloride, calcium chloride, and sodium lactate in water.
10. A solution of 0.9 percent sodium chloride in water is also called _____ _____.
11. An IV administration tubing that delivers 60 gtts/mL is _____ tubing.
12. Administration tubing that delivers 10 gtts/mL is _____ tubing.
13. The sharp, pointed device inserted into the IV solution bag's administration set port is the _____.
14. The calibrated chamber on a specific type of IV administration tubing that enables precise measurement and delivery of fluids and medicated solutions is called the _____ _____.
15. IV administration tubing that contains a filter to prevent clots or other debris from entering the patient is _____ _____.
16. A hollow needle catheter does not have a _____ _____ but is itself inserted into the vein and secured there.
17. If you have exhausted other means of peripheral IV access or when a patient requires immediate fluid administration, consider accessing the _____ _____ _____.
18. The most common cause of an IV that does not flow properly is leaving the _____ _____ in place.
19. A foreign protein capable of producing fever is called a(n) _____.
20. An excess in intravascular fluid volume is called _____ _____.
21. Inflammation of a vein is called _____.
22. A(n) _____ _____ is a peripheral IV port that does not use a bag of fluid.
23. The term _____ means "outside the vein."
24. If the anticoagulant heparin is in a blood tube, the color of the top will be _____.
25. _____ infusions involve inserting a rigid needle into the cavity of a long bone.

HANDOUT 7-9

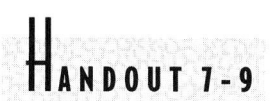

Student's Name _____

CHAPTER 7 REVIEW

PART 3: MEDICAL MATHEMATICS

Write the word or words that best complete each sentence in the space provided.

1. Fundamental metric units are _____, _____, and _____.
2. 3 grams equal _____ milligrams.
3. 5.39 liters is equal to _____ milliliters.
4. 7,000 micrograms is equal to _____ grams.
5. 1 gallon is equal to _____ quarts, or _____ liters.
6. 1 quart is equal to _____ liters.
7. 16 ounces is equal to approximately _____ pint, or _____ milliliters.
8. 1 teaspoon is equal to approximately _____ milliliters.
9. 1 kilogram is equal to _____ pounds.
10. Complete the equation, degrees Celsius = 5/9 (_____).
11. 98.2° Fahrenheit is equal to _____ Celsius.
12. 28.4° Celsius is equal to _____ Fahrenheit.
13. The standard concentration of routinely used medications is called the _____ _____.
14. Weight per volume is called _____.
15. The amount of a drug available in a solution is the _____ _____ _____.
16. The available amount of solution containing a medication is the _____ _____ _____.
17. To administer 120 mg of an oral medication supplied in a concentration of 1,000 mg in 16 mL, you would give _____ mL.
18. Your medical control orders administration of 125 mg of a drug via IV bolus. The multidose vial contains 5 grams of the drug in 15 mL of solution. You would administer _____ mL of solution.
19. Your 175-pound patient is to be given lidocaine via IV bolus at 1.5 mg/kg. The lidocaine is supplied in a 20-mL solution with 200 mg of the drug. You would administer _____ mL of lidocaine.
20. You are to start an IV infusion of lidocaine at 3 mg/min. The concentration is 2 grams of lidocaine in 250 mL of solution. You use a microdrip administration set delivering 60 gtts/mL. Your drip rate would be _____ gtts/min.

©2007 Pearson Education, Inc.
Essentials of Paramedic Care, 2nd ed.

HANDOUT 7-10

Student's Name _____

DRUG CALCULATIONS

Complete the following drug calculations.

1. A 154-pound patient needs Lasix. The physician orders 40 mg via IV push. Lasix is supplied as 100 mg/10 mL. How many mL will you give to deliver 40 mg as ordered?

   _____

2. You are to start an IV of normal saline with a 10 gtts/mL administration set and infuse 300 mL over 2 hours. At how many gtts/min. will you set your IV?

   _____

3. You are treating a patient for whom lidocaine is ordered at 1 mg/kg via IV push. The lidocaine is packaged as a 1 percent solution containing 100 mg/10 mL. The patient weighs 198 pounds. What is the patient's weight in kilograms? How many mL will you give? How many milligrams are contained in the amount of fluid given?

   _____

4. You are instructed to prepare and hang a lidocaine drip of 2 mg/min. The lidocaine is packaged as 1 g/250 mL. You will use a microdrip (60 gtts/mL) administration set. At how many drops per minute will you run the IV?

   _____

5. A dopamine drip is ordered at 5 mcg/kg/min. You are to set up your IV drip by injecting 400 mg of dopamine into a 500-mL IV bag of D_5W. Use a microdrip (60 gtts/mL) administration set. The patient weighs 176 pounds. What is the patient's weight in kilograms? At how many drops per minute will you run the IV?

   _____

6. Atropine is ordered for a symptomatic bradycardia. The desired dose is 0.5 mg. Atropine is packaged as 1 mg/10 mL. How many mL will you give to deliver 0.5 mg?

   _____

Chapter 7 Answer Key

Handout 7-3: Chapter 7 Quiz, Part 1

1. D	6. D	11. C	16. B
2. C	7. A	12. A	17. C
3. C	8. C	13. B	18. C
4. A	9. A	14. A	19. A
5. B	10. A	15. D	20. D

Handout 7-4: Chapter 7 Quiz, Part 2

1. C	6. A	11. A	16. D
2. C	7. C	12. A	17. C
3. B	8. A	13. C	18. A
4. D	9. B	14. B	19. B
5. C	10. C	15. C	20. D

Handout 7-5: Chapter 7 Quiz, Part 3

1. C	6. C	11. A
2. C	7. B	12. B
3. D	8. C	13. C
4. D	9. B	14. A
5. C	10. D	15. B

Handout 7-6: Chapter 7 Scenario

1. Students should find many errors here. Among them: history taking was out of order; requesting that the patient walk to the ambulance; having a patient with possible pulmonary edema lie down; estimating rather than calculating Lasix dose; no indication of checking any medications before administering them; administering Lasix via rapid, rather than slow, IV push; no indication of vital signs being checked after drug administration; no indication of consultation with medical control when problems were experienced; no altering of lidocaine dosage as would be appropriate for a patient over 70.

Handout 7-7: Chapter 7 Review, Part 1

1. person, drug, dose, time, route, documentation
2. body substance isolation
3. asepsis
4. Local
5. Systemic
6. sterile
7. Medically clean
8. disinfectant
9. antiseptic
10. transdermal, mucous membrane
11. tongue, cheek, eye, nose, ear
12. sublingual
13. Buccal
14. ocular
15. inhalation
16. Injection
17. nebulizer
18. metered dose inhaler
19. enteral
20. bolus
21. hepatic alteration
22. nonconstituted drug vial
23. 45°
24. deltoid, dorsal gluteal, vastus lateralis, rectus femoris
25. 90°

Handout 7-8: Chapter 7 Review, Part 2

1. intravenous
2. peripheral venous access
3. central venous access
4. colloids
5. crystalloids
6. Isotonic
7. Hypertonic
8. Hypotonic
9. Lactated Ringer's solution
10. normal saline
11. microdrip
12. macrodrip
13. spike
14. burette chamber
15. blood tubing
16. Teflon tube
17. external jugular vein
18. constricting band
19. pyrogen
20. circulatory overload
21. thrombophlebitis
22. heparin lock
23. extravascular
24. green
25. Intraosseous

Handout 7-9: Chapter 7 Review, Part 3

1. grams, meters, liters
2. 3,000
3. 5,390
4. 0.007
5. 4, 3.785
6. 0.946
7. 1, 473
8. 4–5
9. 2.2
10. degrees Fahrenheit − 32
11. 36.8
12. 83.1
13. stock solution
14. concentration
15. dosage on hand
16. volume on hand
17. 1.92
18. 0.375
19. 11.9
20. 22.5

Handout 7-10: Drug Calculations

1. 4 mL
2. 25 gtts/min
3. 90 kg, 9 mL, 90 mg of lidocaine
4. 30 gtts/min
5. 80 kg, 30 gtts/min
6. 5 Ml

Chapter 8

Airway Management and Ventilation

INTRODUCTION

Although all paramedic skills are important to master and maintain, none are more important than those associated with airway management and ventilation. Airway and breathing are the first and most critical steps in the initial assessment of every patient you care for. No matter what else you do, what other procedures you perform, or what medications you give, without adequate airway maintenance and ventilation, the patient will suffer brain injury or even death within as little as 6 to 10 minutes. This chapter will provide the information and skills you need to manage even the most difficult airway.

CHAPTER OBJECTIVES

After reading this chapter, you should be able to:

1. Describe the anatomy of the airway and the physiology of respiration. (see Chapter 3)
2. Explain the primary objective of airway maintenance. (p. 456)
3. Identify commonly neglected prehospital skills related to the airway. (p. 469)
4. Describe assessment of the airway and the respiratory system. (pp. 458–468)
5. Describe the modified forms of respiration and list the factors that affect respiratory rate and depth. (pp. 460–461)
6. Discuss the methods for measuring oxygen and carbon dioxide in the blood and their prehospital use. (pp. 462–468)
7. Define and explain the implications of partial airway obstruction with good and poor air exchange and complete airway obstruction. (pp. 456–457)
8. Describe the common causes of upper airway obstruction, including:
    - the tongue (p. 457)
    - foreign body aspiration (pp. 457, 458)
    - laryngeal spasm (pp. 457–458)

TOTAL TEACHING TIME: 22.46 HOURS
The total teaching time is only a guideline based on the didactic and practical lab averages in the National Standard Curriculum. Instructors should take into consideration such factors as the pace at which students learn, the size of the class, and breaks. The actual time devoted to teaching objectives is the responsibility of the instructor.

©2007 Pearson Education, Inc.
Essentials of Paramedic Care, 2nd ed.

- laryngeal edema (pp. 457–458)
- trauma (p. 457)

9. Describe complete airway obstruction maneuvers, including:
   - Heimlich maneuver (pp. 511–512)
   - removal with Magill forceps (pp. 511–512)

10. Describe causes of respiratory distress, including:
    - upper and lower airway obstruction (pp. 456–458)
    - inadequate ventilation (p. 458)
    - impairment of respiratory muscles (p. 458)
    - impairment of nervous system (p. 458)

11. Explain the risk of infection to EMS providers associated with airway management and ventilation. (pp. 456, 525–526)

12. Describe manual airway maneuvers, including:
    - head-tilt/chin-lift maneuver (p. 469)
    - jaw-thrust maneuver (pp. 469–470)
    - modified jaw-thrust maneuver (pp. 469–470)

13. Discuss the indications, contraindications, advantages, disadvantages, complications, special considerations, equipment, and techniques of the following:
    - upper airway and tracheobronchial suctioning (pp. 521–522)
    - nasogastric and orogastric tube insertion (pp. 522–523)
    - oropharyngeal and nasopharyngeal airway (pp. 471–474)
    - ventilating a patient by mouth-to-mouth, mouth-to-nose, mouth-to-mask, one/two/three-person bag-valve mask, flow-restricted oxygen-powered ventilation device, automatic transport ventilator (pp. 525–529)

14. Compare the ventilation techniques used for an adult patient to those used for pediatric patients, and describe special considerations in airway management and ventilation for the pediatric patient. (pp. 497–501, 527)

15. Identify types of oxygen cylinders and pressure regulators, and explain safety considerations of oxygen storage and delivery, including steps for delivering oxygen from a cylinder and regulator. (pp. 523–534)

16. Describe the indications, contraindications, advantages, disadvantages, complications, liter flow range, and concentration of delivered oxygen for the following supplemental oxygen delivery devices:
    - nasal cannula (pp. 524–525)
    - simple face mask (pp. 524–525)
    - partial rebreather mask (pp. 524–525)
    - nonrebreather mask (pp. 524–525)
    - Venturi mask (pp. 524–525)

17. Describe the use, advantages, and disadvantages of an oxygen humidifier. (p. 525)

18. Describe the indications, contraindications, advantages, disadvantages, complications, equipment, and technique for the following:
    - endotracheal intubation by direct laryngoscopy (pp. 483–486)
    - digital endotracheal intubation (pp. 489–491)
    - dual lumen airway (pp. 504–511)
    - nasotracheal intubation (pp. 501–503)
    - rapid-sequence intubation (pp. 494–497)

- endotracheal intubation using sedation (pp. 494–497)
- open cricothyrotomy (pp. 516–519)
- needle cricothyrotomy (translaryngeal catheter ventilation) (pp. 512–516)
- extubation (p. 504)

19. Describe the use of cricoid pressure during intubation. (pp. 470–471, 483, 484)
20. Discuss the precautions that should be taken when intubating the trauma patient. (pp. 492, 493)
21. Discuss agents used for sedation and rapid-sequence intubation. (pp. 494–497)
22. Discuss methods to confirm correct placement of the endotracheal tube. (pp. 486–489)

FRAMING THE LESSON

Begin the class by reviewing the important points from Chapter 7, "Medication Administration." Discuss any aspects of the chapter not understood by students. Then go on to Chapter 8. Ask students to recall from their CPR training the length of time a person may be in cardiac and/or respiratory arrest with no ventilation or oxygen flow to the brain before brain cells begin to die. Review the information that the brain is the most sensitive organ in the body to any reduction in oxygen delivery. Brain cells begin to die within 4 to 6 minutes if the brain is not perfused. Next, have students do two exercises. First, have them hold their breath as long as they can. Ask how they feel once they resume breathing. Then distribute a plastic coffee stirring stick to each student. Have them place the sticks in their mouth and breathe in and out only through their mouth. This will graphically depict how people in respiratory distress, such as asthma attacks, feel when they breathe. Stress that no matter what advanced skill or procedure is done for a patient, the patient will not survive if he does not have an adequate airway and ventilation.

TEACHING STRATEGIES

People learn in a variety of ways. Some do better with the spoken word, whereas others prefer the written. Some prefer to work alone, whereas others profit from working in groups. Recognizing these different ways of acquiring knowledge, the authors of this *Instructor's Resource Manual* have provided a variety of teaching strategies for the different types of learners. These strategies are intended to foster higher-level cognitive skills and encourage creative learning and problem solving. For greatest effectiveness, incorporate these strategies into your class lecture. Symbols in the Lecture Outline indicate the points at which various exercises might be most appropriate. Other strategies can be used to preview the lesson or to summarize it.

The following strategies are keyed to specific sections of the lesson.

1. ***Airway Familiarization.*** Ask your local butcher for a pig pluck, which is the trachea, esophagus, lungs, and heart of a pig. These can be kept without smelling for up to a week in the refrigerator. Let students intubate the trachea and ventilate the lungs. You will marvel at the wonderful demonstration of the alveoli, lung parenchyma, and even atelectasis. Because this specimen is fresh, it is even better than a human cadaver, which will lack the elasticity of the pig pluck. This activity is fun for your visual and kinesthetic learners but can be messy. Have lots of plastic bags, premoistened towelettes, and gloves on hand.

2. Pulse Oximeter Familiarization. Use the pulse oximeter on every student in class. Students love to learn what their own readings are, and you can even have contests for the lowest and highest pulse ox reading. This will be a great lead into a conversation about what conditions affect pulse oximeter readings. If your program does not have a pulse oximeter, arrange for an ambulance or rescue unit to stop by for an hour or so. Borrow the equipment without taking the vehicle out of service. Alternatively, borrow one from the ER.

3. Intubating the Class. Pass out six or seven endotracheal tubes to several students (or the whole class). Instruct them to breathe through the tubes for the duration of the class. The difficulties they will experience when breathing through a small-diameter tube should give students a new perspective and a greater empathy for what it is like to be an intubated patient.

4. Guest Speaker. Consider inviting the chief of anesthesiology from the local or regional hospital to the class. Such a speaker would have a wealth of stories about difficult intubations and how the problems that they posed were overcome.

5. Developing Suctioning Skills. Have a variety of actual substances for students to suction during this lab session. Practice with such materials can go a long way toward preparing them for managing a difficult airway with massive quantities of liquid or food. Pudding simulates mucus; apple juice simulates bile; tomato juice simulates blood; and soup looks like vomit. This activity helps add realism to your classroom lab activities. You might then test students' suctioning skills in a contest. Have a variety of suctioning devices available. Divide the class into groups. Assign students in the first group one of the suctioning devices. Then bring out bowls of cold oatmeal. Challenge students to see who can do the most efficient job of suctioning. Time their efforts. Repeat with other groups until all students have had a chance. Have a runoff among the group winners. You might use pea soup or a chunky barley soup, instead.

6. Ventilation Drills. Test students' grasp of some airway basics at this point. Have them practice ventilation drills using a recording Resusci-Annie. Ask for several students who think they "know how to bag." Do not use the intubation heads. These heads can be ventilated in almost any position. After 5 minutes, start recording the effectiveness of ventilations. This experiment can be very enlightening. Add to learning by showing how even one finger break in the seal can markedly decrease the ventilations' effectiveness. Also consider having a contest between teams. One team uses a bag-valve mask while the other uses a pocket mask. Again, let ventilations continue for 5 minutes before you start to record. The results often tell a great deal about the effectiveness of the bag-valve mask over the pocket mask.

The following strategies can be used at various points throughout the lesson or to help summarize and demonstrate what students have learned:

Airway Cam. The new "airway camera" technology provides amazing video of actual human airways during intubation. If this technology is not available to you for use by your students, purchase or borrow a video from one of the manufacturing companies or a university with a medical school. Although the technology is expensive, it is also relatively common. Demonstrations of "airway cam" have even been offered at EMS conferences around the country.

Cultural Considerations, Legal Notes, and Patho Pearls. The Student CD-ROM contains this series of informative features to enhance the student's understanding of the material covered in this chapter.

TEACHING OUTLINE

Chapter 8, "Airway Management and Ventilation," is the eighth lesson in Division 1, *Introduction to Advanced Prehospital Care*. Distribute Handout 8-1 so that students can familiarize themselves with the learning goals for this chapter. If students have any questions about the objectives, answer them at this time.

Then present the chapter. One possible lecture outline follows. In the outline, the parenthetical references in regular type are references to text pages; those in bold type are references to figures or tables.

I. Introduction. Airway management and ventilation skills are the first and most critical steps in the initial assessment of every patient paramedics will encounter. This chapter will provide the information and skills needed to manage even the most difficult airway. (p. 456)

II. Respiratory problems. Paramedics must calmly and quickly assess the severity of a patient's illness or injury while considering the potential causes of and treatment for his respiratory distress. (pp. 456–458)

A. Airway obstruction (pp. 456–458)
   1. The tongue (**Fig. 8-1, p. 547**)
   2. Foreign bodies
   3. Trauma
   4. Laryngeal spasm and edema
   5. Aspiration
B. Inadequate ventilation (p. 458)

III. Respiratory system assessment. Assessment of the respiratory system begins with the initial assessment and should continue through the focused history and physical exam and the ongoing assessment. (pp. 458–468)

A. Initial assessment (pp. 458–459) (**Fig. 8-2, p. 459**)
B. Focused history and physical examination (pp. 459–462)
   1. Focused history
   2. Physical exam
      a. Inspection
         i. Modified forms of respiration
            a) Coughing
            b) Sneezing
            c) Hiccoughing
            d) Sighing
            e) Grunting
         ii. Respiratory patterns
            a) Kussmaul's respirations
            b) Cheyne-Stokes respirations
            c) Biot's respirations
            d) Central neurogenic hyperventilation
            e) Agonal respirations
      b. Auscultation (**Fig. 8-3, p. 461**)
         i. Airflow compromise
            a) Snoring
            b) Gurgling
            c) Stridor
            d) Wheezing
            e) Quiet
         ii. Gaseous exchange compromise
            a) Crackles (rales)
            b) Rhonchi
      c. Palpation

HANDOUT 8-1
Chapter 8 Objectives Checklist

POWERPOINT PRESENTATION
Chapter 8 PowerPoint slides 3, 5–48

POWERPOINT PRESENTATION
Chapter 8 PowerPoint slides 49–53

TEACHING STRATEGY 1
Airway Familiarization

POWERPOINT PRESENTATION
Chapter 8 PowerPoint slides 54–73

TEACHING STRATEGY 2
Pulse Oximeter Familiarization

TEACHING TIP
Bring in to class models of pulse oximeters and end-tidal carbon dioxide detectors in use in your area. Demonstrate the operation of these devices. Let students take turns obtaining pulse oximetry readings on each other.

READING/REFERENCE
Krauss, B. "Capnography in EMS." *JEMS*, Jan. 2003.

Whitehead, S. "The Capnography Revolution Begins." *JEMS*, Jan. 2003.

Criss, E. "Portable End-Tidal Indicator." *JEMS*, May 2004.

POWERPOINT PRESENTATION
Chapter 8 PowerPoint slides 74–87

POINT TO EMPHASIZE
Your deliberate and precise use of simple, basic airway skills is the key to successful airway management and good patient outcome.

POWERPOINT PRESENTATION
Chapter 8 PowerPoint slides 88–178

TEACHING TIP
Have students practice manual airway maneuvers on each other. Mannequin practice is good, but nothing beats the feel of opening a human airway. Have students practice stabilizing the head and neck and using the jaw-thrust maneuver to simultaneously open the airway.

TEACHING STRATEGY 3
Intubating the Class

TEACHING STRATEGY 4
Guest Speaker

C. Noninvasive respiratory monitoring (pp. 462–468)
  1. Pulse oximetry (**Fig. 8-4, p. 463**)
     a. Hemoglobin oxygen saturation
     b. SpO_2 of 95 to 99 percent is normal
     c. SpO_2 of 91 to 94 percent indicates mild hypoxia
     d. SpO_2 of 86 to 91 percent indicates moderate hypoxia
     e. SpO_2 of 85 percent or lower indicates severe hypoxia
  2. Capnography (**Fig. 8-5, p. 464**) (**Table 8-1, p. 465**)
     a. Measurement of exhaled carbon dioxide concentration
     b. Terminology
        i. Capnometry
        ii. Capnography
        iii. Capnogram
        iv. End-tidal CO_2 ($ETCO_2$)
     c. Colormetric devices
     d. Electronic devices (**Fig. 8-6, p. 465; Figs. 8-7 and 8-8, p. 466**)
     e. Capnogram (**Figs 8-9 and 8-10, p. 467**)
     f. Clinical applications
  3. Esophageal detector device (EDD) (**Fig. 8-11, p. 468**)
  4. Peak expiratory flow testing

IV. Basic airway management. Once it is determined that intervention is needed, simple manual airway maneuvers and equipment should be used before proceeding with more advanced techniques. (pp. 469–474)

A. Manual airway maneuvers (pp. 469–471)
  1. Head-tilt/chin-lift
  2. Jaw-thrust maneuver
  3. Sellick's maneuver (**Figs. 8-12 and 8-13, p. 470**)
B. Basic mechanical airways (pp. 471–474)
  1. Nasopharyngeal airway (**Fig. 8-14, p. 472; Fig. 8-15, p. 472**)
  2. Oropharyngeal airway (**Figs. 8-16 and 8-17, p. 474**)

V. Advanced airway management. Inserting advanced mechanical airways requires special training; the preferred method of airway management is endotracheal intubation. (pp. 474–519)

A. Endotracheal intubation (pp. 475–501)
  1. Equipment
     a. Laryngoscope (**Figs. 8-18 and 8-19, p. 475; Figs. 8-20, 8-21, and 8-22, p. 476**)
     b. Endotracheal tubes (**Figs. 8-23 and 8-24, p. 477; Fig. 8-25, p. 477; Fig. 8-26, p. 478**)
     c. Stylet (**Fig. 8-27, p. 478; Fig. 8-28, p. 479**)
     d. Gum Elastic Bougie (**Fig. 8-29, p. 479**)
     e. 10-mL syringe
     f. Tube-holding devices
     g. Magill forceps (**Fig. 8-30, p. 480**)
     h. Lubricant
     i. Suction unit
     j. End-tidal CO_2 detector
     k. Additional airways
     l. Protective equipment
  2. Endotracheal intubation indications
     a. Respiratory or cardiac arrest
     b. Unconsciousness or obtusion with no gag reflex
     c. Risk of aspiration
     d. Obstruction

             e. Respiratory extremes due to disease
             f. Pneumothorax, hemothorax, or hemopneumothorax with breathing difficulty
         3. Advantages of endotracheal intubation
             a. Isolates trachea; permits complete control of airway
             b. Impedes gastric distention
             c. Eliminates need for mask seal
             d. Offers direct route for suctioning
             e. Permits administration of some medications
         4. Disadvantages of endotracheal intubation
             a. Requires considerable training and expertise
             b. Requires specialized equipment
             c. Requires direct visualization of vocal cords
             d. Bypasses upper airway warming, filtering, humidifying of air
         5. Complications of endotracheal intubation
             a. Equipment malfunction
             b. Teeth breakage and soft tissue lacerations
             c. Hypoxia
             d. Esophageal intubation
             e. Endobronchial intubation
             f. Tension pneumothorax
         6. Orotracheal intubation technique (**Fig. 8-31, p. 485**)
             a. Procedure (**Proc. 8-1, p. 484**)
             b. Verification of proper endotracheal tube placement
             c. Transillumination intubation (**Fig. 8-32, p. 487; Figs. 8-33 and 8-34, p. 488; Fig. 8-35, p. 489**)
             d. Digital intubation (**Fig. 8-36, p. 490; Figs. 8-37 and 8-38, p. 491; Fig. 8-39, p. 492**)
             e. Trauma patient intubation (**Proc. 8-2, p. 493**)
         7. Rapid-sequence intubation (**Tables 8-2 and 8-3, p. 496**)
             a. Equipment
             b. Procedure
         8. Pediatric intubation
             a. Equipment (**Table 8-4, p. 498**)
             b. Procedure (**Proc. 8-3, pp. 499–500**)
    B. Nasotracheal intubation (pp. 501–504)
         1. Indications
         2. Advantages
         3. Disadvantages
         4. Technique (**Fig. 8-40, p. 502**)
         5. Nasotracheal Tube Auscultation Device (**Fig. 8-41a, p. 503; Fig. 8-41b, p. 504**)
    C. Field extubation (p. 504)
    D. Esophageal Tracheal CombiTube (pp. 504–507)
         1. Advantages
         2. Disadvantages
         3. Insertion (**Fig. 8-42, p. 505; Fig. 8-43, p. 506**)
    E. Pharyngo-tracheal lumen airway (pp. 507–508) (**Fig. 8-44, p. 507**)
         1. Advantages
         2. Disadvantages
         3. Insertion
    F. Laryngeal mask airway (pp. 508–510) (**Fig. 8-45, p. 509**)
         1. Intubating LMA (**Fig. 8-46, p. 509**)
         2. Cobra Perilaryngeal Airway (**Fig. 8-47, p. 510**)
         3. Ambu Laryngeal Mask (**Fig. 8-48, p. 510**)
    G. Esophageal gastric tube airway and esophageal obturator airway (p. 511)

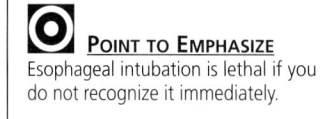

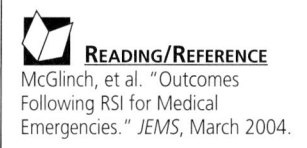

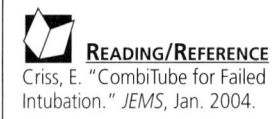

POINT TO EMPHASIZE
Esophageal intubation is lethal if you do not recognize it immediately.

READING/REFERENCE
Criss, E. "Validating ET Tube Placement." *JEMS*, March 2003.

READING/REFERENCE
McGlinch, et al. "Outcomes Following RSI for Medical Emergencies." *JEMS*, March 2004.

READING/REFERENCE
Criss, E. "CombiTube for Failed Intubation." *JEMS*, Jan. 2004.

POINT TO EMPHASIZE
The only indication for a surgical airway is the inability to establish an airway by any other method.

TEACHING STRATEGY 5
Developing Suctioning Skills

POWERPOINT PRESENTATION
Chapter 8 PowerPoint slide 179

POWERPOINT PRESENTATION
Chapter 8 PowerPoint slides 180–184

POWERPOINT PRESENTATION
Chapter 8 PowerPoint slides 185–187

POINT TO EMPHASIZE
Never withhold oxygen from any patient for whom it is indicated.

POWERPOINT PRESENTATION
Chapter 8 PowerPoint slides 188–191

TEACHING STRATEGY 6
Ventilation Drills

POWERPOINT PRESENTATION
Chapter 8 PowerPoint slides 192–196

POINT TO EMPHASIZE
If you do not correct any significant decrease in the patient's rate or depth of breathing, respiratory or cardiac arrest may occur.

POWERPOINT PRESENTATION
Chapter 8 PowerPoint slide 197

H. Foreign body removal under direct laryngoscopy (pp. 511–512) (**Fig. 8-49, p. 511**)
I. Surgical airways (pp. 512–519)
   1. Needle cricothyrotomy
      a. Complications
      b. Technique (**Figs. 8-50 and 8-58, p. 513; Figs. 8-52 and 8-53, p. 514; Figs. 8-54 and 8-55, p. 515**)
   2. Open cricothyrotomy
      a. Complications
      b. Technique (**Proc. 8-4, pp. 517–519**)

VI. Managing patients with stoma sites. A stoma is an opening in the anterior neck that connects the trachea with the ambient air; patients with stomas often have problems with excessive secretions. (pp. 520–521) (**Fig. 8-56, p. 520**)

VII. Suctioning. Paramedics must be prepared to suction all airways in order to remove blood or other secretions and patient vomitus. (pp. 521–522) (**Table 8-5, p. 521**)

A. Suctioning equipment (pp. 521–522)
B. Suctioning techniques (p. 522)
C. Tracheobronchial suctioning (p. 522)

VIII. Gastric distention and decompression. A common problem with ventilating a nonintubated patient is gastric distention, which occurs when the procedure's high pressures trap air in the stomach. (pp. 522–523)

A. Routes of decompression (pp. 522–523)
   1. Nasogastric
   2. Orogastric
B. Tube placement technique (p. 523)

IX. Oxygenation. Oxygen is an important drug, and its indications and precautions must be thoroughly understood. (pp. 523–525)

A. Oxygen supply and regulation (pp. 523–524)
B. Oxygen delivery devices (pp. 524–525)
   1. Nasal cannula
   2. Venturi mask
   3. Simple face mask
   4. Partial rebreather mask
   5. Nonrebreather mask
   6. Small-volume nebulizer
   7. Oxygen humidifier

X. Ventilation. Effective artificial ventilation requires a patent airway, an effective seal between the mask and the patient's face, and delivery of adequate ventilatory volumes. (pp. 525–529)

A. Mouth-to-mouth/mouth-to-nose ventilation (p. 525)
B. Mouth-to-mask ventilation (pp. 525–526)
C. Bag-valve devices (pp. 526–527) (**Fig. 8-57, p. 526**)
D. Demand valve device (pp. 527–528) (**Fig. 8-58, p. 528**)
E. Automatic transport ventilator (pp. 528–529) (**Fig. 8-59, p. 529**)

XI. Chapter Summary (p. 529). Airway assessment and maintenance is the most critical step in managing any patient. If you do not promptly establish a definitive airway and provide proper ventilation, the patient's outcome will be poor. Frequently reassessing the airway is mandatory to ensure that the patient has not decompensated, requiring additional airway procedures. Successful management of all airways requires the paramedic to follow the proper management sequence.

Basic airway and management skills can make the difference between a successful outcome and a poor patient prognosis. Once you have mastered these basic skills and made them a part of airway management in every patient, you should learn and utilize advanced skills such as intubation, RSI, and cricothyrotomy. You must maintain proficiency in all airway skills, especially the more advanced techniques, through ongoing continuing education, physician medical direction, and testing with each EMS service. If you cannot do this, it is in the patient's best interest to focus on less sophisticated airway skills. If you anticipate that every airway will be complicated, apply basic airway skills before using advanced procedures, and perform frequent reassessments, you will give the patient his best chance for meaningful survival.

SKILLS DEMONSTRATION AND PRACTICE

Divide the class into as many groups as appropriate. Have the groups circulate through the stations. Monitor the groups to be sure all groups have a chance to practice each of the skills. You may wish to have other instructors or qualified paramedics assist students in these activities.

Station	Equipment Needed	Activities
Adult Basic Airway Maneuvers	Adult ET head Adult CPR mannequin Airway management kit 1 instructor	Have students practice the following skills: manual airway maneuvers; insertion of oropharyngeal and nasopharyngeal airways; and oropharyngeal suctioning.
Pediatric Basic Airway Maneuvers	Infant ET head Child/infant CPR mannequins Airway management kit 1 instructor	Have students practice the following skills: manual airway maneuvers; insertion of oropharyngeal and nasopharyngeal airways; and oropharyngeal suctioning.
Ventilation and Oxygentaion Techniques	Adult/infant ET head Adult/child/infant CPR mannequins Airway management kit 1 instructor	Have students practice the following skills: ventilation using pocket mask, BVM, flow-restricted oxygen-powered ventilation device, autovent; oxygen administration via masks and cannulae.

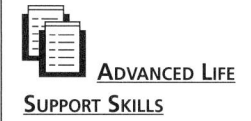

HANDOUTS 8-2 TO 8-16
Chapter 8 Skills Sheets

ADVANCED LIFE SUPPORT SKILLS
Larmon & Davis. *Advanced Life Support Skills.*

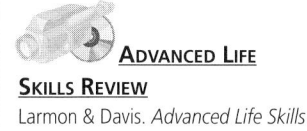

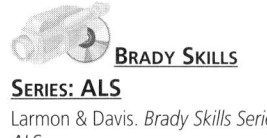

ADVANCED LIFE SKILLS REVIEW
Larmon & Davis. *Advanced Life Skills Review.*

BRADY SKILLS SERIES: ALS
Larmon & Davis. *Brady Skills Series: ALS.*

Foreign Body Removal	Adult/infant ET head Adult/child/infant CPR mannequins Airway management kit 1 instructor	Have students practice removing foreign bodies from the mannequins using AHA standards and Magill forceps.
Esophageal Airways	Adult ET head Airway management kit EOA, EGTA, PtL, ETC airways 1 instructor	Have students practice the following skills: EOA, EGTA, PtL, and ETC insertion.
Adult Endotracheal Intubation	Adult ET head Airway management kit 1 instructor	Have students practice orotracheal, digital, and trauma intubation on the adult mannequin.
Pediatric Intubation	Infant ET head Airway management kit 1 instructor	Have students practice orotracheal, digital, and trauma intubation on the infant mannequin.
Nasotracheal Intubation	Adult ET head Airway management kit 1 instructor	Have students practice nasotracheal intubation.
Rapid-Sequence Intubation	Adult ET head Airway management kit Medication kit 1 instructor	Have students practice rapid-sequence intubation with neuromuscular blockage.

WORKBOOK
Chapter 8 Activities

READING/REFERENCE
Textbook, pp. 532–544

HANDOUT 8-17
Chapter 8 Quiz

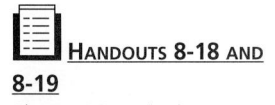

HANDOUTS 8-18 AND 8-19
Chapter 8 Scenarios

PARAMEDIC STUDENT CD
Student Activities

COMPANION WEBSITE
http://www.prenhall.com/bledsoe

TESTGEN
Chapter 8

ASSIGNMENTS

Assign students to complete Chapter 8, "Airway Management and Ventilation," of the workbook. Also assign them to read Chapter 9, "Therapeutic Communications," before the next class.

EVALUATION

Chapter Quiz and Scenario Distribute copies of the Chapter Quiz provided in Handout 8-17 to evaluate student understanding of this chapter. Make sure each student reads the scenarios to reinforce critical thinking on the scene. Remind students not to use their notes or textbooks while taking the quiz.

Student CD Quizzes for every chapter are contained on the dynamic and highly visual in-text student CD.

Companion Website Additional quizzes for every chapter are contained on this exciting website.

TestGen You may wish to create a custom-tailored test using *Prentice Hall TestGen for Essentials of Paramedic Care,* 2nd Edition to evaluate student understanding of this chapter.

On-line Test Preparation (for students and instructors)   Additional test preparation is available through Brady's new on-line product, *EMT Achieve: Paramedic Test Preparation* at *http://www.prenhall.com/emtachieve/*. Instructors can also monitor student mastery on-line.

Review Manual for the EMT-Paramedic   This comprehensive exam review contains hundreds of test questions and rationales, including scenarios, along with two 180-question practice tests on CD.

REINFORCEMENT

Handouts   If classroom discussion or performance on the quiz indicates that some students have not fully mastered the chapter content, you may wish to assign some or all of the Reinforcement Handouts for this chapter.

Student CD (for students)   A wide variety of material on this CD-ROM will reinforce and also expand student knowledge and skills.

PowerPoint Presentation (for instructors)   The PowerPoint material developed for this chapter offers useful reinforcement of chapter content.

Companion Website (for students)   Additional review quizzes and links to EMS resources will contribute to further reinforcement of the chapter.

OneKey   On-line support is offered for this course on one of three platforms: Course Compass, Blackboard, or Web CT. Includes the IRM, PowerPoints, TestGen, and Companion Website for instruction. Ask your local sales representative for more information.

Brady Skills Series: Advanced Life Skills (Video or CD)   Have your students watch the skills come to life on VHS or CD-ROM, or they can purchase the highly visual, full-color text with step-by-step procedures with rationales.

EMT ACHIEVE: PARAMEDIC TEST PREPARATION
Mistovich & Beasley. *EMT Achieve: Paramedic Test Preparation.*
www.prenhall.com/emtachieve/

REVIEW MANUAL FOR THE EMT-PARAMEDIC
Cherry & Mistovich. *Review Manual for the EMT-Paramedic,* 3rd edition.

HANDOUTS 8-20 TO 8-23
Reinforcement Activities

PARAMEDIC STUDENT CD
Student Activities

POWERPOINT PRESENTATION
Chapter 8

COMPANION WEBSITE
http://www.prenhall.com/bledsoe

ONEKEY
Chapter 8

ADVANCED LIFE SUPPORT SKILLS
Larmon & Davis. *Advanced Life Support Skills.*

ADVANCED LIFE SKILLS REVIEW
Larmon & Davis. *Advanced Life Skills Review.*

BRADY SKILLS SERIES: ALS
Larmon & Davis. *Brady Skills Series: ALS.*

PARAMEDIC NATIONAL STANDARDS SELF-TEST
Miller. *Paramedic National Standards Self-Test,* 4th edition.

OBJECTIVES

Handout 8-1

Student's Name _____

CHAPTER 8 OBJECTIVES CHECKLIST

Knowledge	Date Mastered
1. Describe the anatomy of the airway and the physiology of respiration.	
2. Explain the primary objective of airway maintenance.	
3. Identify commonly neglected prehospital skills related to the airway.	
4. Describe assessment of the airway and the respiratory system.	
5. Describe the modified forms of respiration and list the factors that affect respiratory rate and depth.	
6. Discuss the methods for measuring oxygen and carbon dioxide in the blood and their prehospital use.	
7. Define and explain the implications of partial airway obstruction with good and poor air exchange and complete airway obstruction.	
8. Describe the common causes of upper airway obstruction, including: • the tongue • foreign body aspiration • laryngeal spasm • laryngeal edema • trauma	
9. Describe complete airway obstruction maneuvers, including: • Heimlich maneuver • removal with Magill forceps	
10. Describe causes of respiratory distress, including: • upper and lower airway obstruction • inadequate ventilation • impairment of respiratory muscles • impairment of nervous system	
11. Explain the risk of infection to EMS providers associated with airway management and ventilation.	
12. Describe manual airway maneuvers, including: • head-tilt/chin-lift maneuver • jaw-thrust maneuver • modified jaw-thrust maneuver	

HANDOUT 8-1 Continued

Knowledge	Date Mastered
13. Discuss the indications, contraindications, advantages, disadvantages, complications, special considerations, equipment, and techniques of the following: • upper airway and tracheobronchial suctioning • nasogastric and orogastric tube insertion • oropharyngeal and nasopharyngeal airway • ventilating a patient by mouth-to-mouth, mouth-to-nose, mouth-to-mask, one/two/three-person bag-valve mask, flow-restricted oxygen-powered ventilation device, automatic transport ventilator	
14. Compare the ventilation techniques used for an adult patient to those used for pediatric patients, and describe special considerations in airway management and ventilation for the pediatric patient.	
15. Identify types of oxygen cylinders and pressure regulators, and explain safety considerations of oxygen storage and delivery, including steps for delivering oxygen from a cylinder and regulator.	
16. Describe the indications, contraindications, advantages, disadvantages, complications, liter flow range, and concentration of delivered oxygen for the following supplemental oxygen delivery devices: • nasal cannula • simple face mask • partial rebreather mask • nonrebreather mask • Venturi mask	
17. Describe the use, advantages, and disadvantages of an oxygen humidifier.	
18. Describe the indications, contraindications, advantages, disadvantages, complications, equipment, and technique for the following: • endotracheal intubation by direct laryngoscopy • digital endotracheal intubation • dual-lumen airway • nasotracheal intubation • rapid-sequence intubation • endotracheal intubation using sedation • open cricothyrotomy • needle cricothyrotomy (translaryngeal catheter ventilation) • extubation	
19. Describe the use of cricoid pressure during intubation.	
20. Discuss the precautions that should be taken when intubating the trauma patient.	
21. Discuss agents used for sedation and rapid-sequence intubation.	
22. Discuss methods to confirm correct placement of the endotracheal tube.	

Handout 8-2

Student's Name _____

MANUAL AIRWAY MANEUVERS

Charting Student Progress:
1. *Learning skill*
2. *Performs skill with direction*
3. *Performs skill independently*

HEAD-TILT/CHIN-LIFT

Procedure	1	2	3
1. Takes BSI precautions.			
2. Places patient supine and positions self at the side of the patient's head.			
3. Places one hand on the patient's forehead and, using firm downward pressure with the palm, tilts the head back.			
4. Puts two fingers of the other hand under the bony part of the chin and lifts the jaw anteriorly to open the airway.			

JAW-THRUST

Procedure	1	2	3
1. Takes BSI precautions.			
2. Places the patient supine and kneels at the top of his head.			
3. Applies fingers to each side of the jaw at the mandibular angles.			
4. Lifts the jaw forward (anteriorly) with a gentle tilting of the patient's head to open the airway.			

MODIFIED JAW-THRUST

Procedure	1	2	3
1. Takes BSI precautions.			
2. Places the patient supine and kneels at the top of his head.			
3. Applies fingers to each side of the jaw at the mandibular angles.			

HANDOUT 8-2 Continued

Procedure	1	2	3
4. Lifts the jaw using fingers behind the mandibular angles, without tilting the head.			
5. Jaw-thrust without head-tilt: lifts the jaw by grasping under the chin and behind the teeth, without tilting the head.			

Handout 8-3

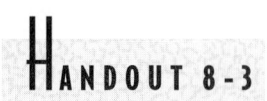

Student's Name _____

NASOPHARYNGEAL/OROPHARYNGEAL AIRWAYS

Charting Student Progress:
1. *Learning skill*
2. *Performs skill with direction*
3. *Performs skill independently*

NASOPHARYNGEAL AIRWAY

Procedure	1	2	3
1. Takes BSI precautions.			
2. Hyperextends patient's head and neck if no history of trauma.			
3. Hyperventilates with 100% oxygen.			
4. Measures tube from tip of nose to angle of jaw and the diameter of nostril.			
5. Lubricates exterior of the tube with water-soluble gel or lidocaine gel.			
6. Pushes gently up on tip of nose and passes tube into the right nostril, bevel toward septum.			
7. Verifies appropriate position of airway; clear breath sounds, chest rise, airflow at proximal end on expiration.			
8. Hyperventilates patient with 100% oxygen.			

OROPHARYNGEAL AIRWAY

Procedure	1	2	3
1. Takes BSI precautions.			
2. Hyperextends patient's head and neck if no history of trauma. Opens mouth and removes visible obstructions.			
3. Hyperventilates patient with 100% oxygen, if indicated.			
4. Measures airway from corner of mouth to earlobe.			
5. Grasps patient's jaw and lifts anteriorly.			
6. With other hand, holds airway at proximal end and inserts into patient's mouth, with curve reversed and tip pointing toward roof of mouth.			

HANDOUT 8-3 Continued

Procedure	1	2	3
7. As tip reaches level of soft palate, gently rotates airway 180° until it comes to rest over the tongue.			
8. Verifies appropriate position of airway; clear breath sounds, and chest rise.			
9. Hyperventilates patient with 100% oxygen.			

Handout 8-4

Student's Name _____

OROTRACHEAL INTUBATION

Charting Student Progress:
1. *Learning skill*
2. *Performs skill with direction*
3. *Performs skill independently*

Procedure	1	2	3
1. Takes BSI precautions.			
2. Places patient supine.			
3. Uses appropriate basic manual and adjunct airway maneuvers, hyperventilates with 100% oxygen.			
4. Assembles and checks equipment.			
5. Places head in sniffing position.			
6. Has partner apply Sellick's maneuver.			
7. Holds laryngoscope in the left hand; inserts it into the right side of mouth.			
8. Displaces tongue to the left and brings laryngoscope midline.			
9. Lifts laryngoscope forward to displace jaw without putting pressure on teeth.			
10. Suctions the hypopharynx as necessary.			
11. Places blade in proper position, visualizing tip of epiglottis.			
12. Lifts jaw at 45° angle to the ground, exposing glottis.			
13. Holds ETT in right hand and advances tube through right corner of patient's mouth.			
14. Directly visualizes vocal cords, passes ETT through the glottic opening until distal cuff disappears beyond vocal cords.			
15. Removes stylet, inflates distal cuff with 5–10 ml of air, attaches BVM with ETCO$_2$ detector to connector on ETT.			

HANDOUT 8-4 Continued

Procedure	1	2	3
16. Checks for proper tube placement; equal bilateral breath sounds, symmetrical rise and fall of chest.			
17. Hyperventilates patient with 100% oxygen.			
18. Secures ETT with tape or commercial device.			
19. Periodically rechecks tube placement.			

Handout 8-5

Student's Name _____

TRANSILLUMINATION INTUBATION

Charting Student Progress:
1. *Learning skill*
2. *Performs skill with direction*
3. *Performs skill independently*

Procedure	1	2	3
1. Takes BSI precautions.			
2. Hyperventilates patient with 100% oxygen.			
3. Assembles and checks equipment.			
4. Uses 7.5–8.5 mm ETT; cuts tube to 25–27 cm to accommodate stylet.			
5. Places stylet in tube, bending it proximal to the cuff.			
6. With patient supine and head in neutral position, kneels along either side of patient, facing patient's head, and turns on light.			
7. With index and middle fingers inserted deeply into patient's mouth and thumb under his chin, lifts his tongue and jaw forward.			
8. Inserts tube/stylet into patient's mouth; advances it through oropharynx into hypopharynx.			
9. Uses "hooking" action with tube/stylet to lift epiglottis out of the way.			
10. Holds stylet stationary when circle of light is visible at the level of the patient's Adam's apple.			
11. Advances tube off stylet into the larynx approximately 1–2 cm, while retracting internal wire from stylet using O-ring at proximal end.			
12. Holds tube in place with one hand and removes stylet.			
13. Inflates the cuff with 5–10 ml of air.			
14. Attaches BVM with $ETCO_2$ detector and delivers several breaths.			
15. Secures ETT with tape or commercial device.			
16. Periodically rechecks tube placement.			

HANDOUT 8-6

Student's Name _____

DIGITAL INTUBATION

Charting Student Progress:
1. *Learning skill*
2. *Performs skill with direction*
3. *Performs skill independently*

Procedure	1	2	3
1. Takes BSI precautions.			
2. Hyperventilates with 100% oxygen.			
3. Assembles and checks equipment.			
4. Instructs partner to stabilize head and neck as needed.			
5. Kneels at the left shoulder, facing patient.			
6. Places bite block between patient's molars to protect fingers.			
7. Inserts left middle and index fingers into patient's mouth; walks down midline tugging forward on the tongue.			
8. Palpates epiglottis with the middle finger.			
9. Presses epiglottis forward and inserts ETT anterior to fingers.			
10. Advances tube, pushing it with right hand, using index finger to maintain the tip of the tube against the middle finger, directing it to the epiglottis.			
11. Using middle and index fingers, directs the tube tip between the epiglottis and the fingers and advances the tube through the cords.			
12. Holds tube in place, attaches BVM with $ETCO_2$ detector, inflates cuff with 5–10 ml of air.			
13. Verifies tube placement; clear lung sounds bilaterally, symmetrical chest rise.			
14. Hyperventilates with 100% oxygen.			
15. Periodically rechecks tube placement.			

Handout 8-7

SKILLS

Student's Name _____

TRAUMA INTUBATION

Charting Student Progress:
1. *Learning skill*
2. *Performs skill with direction*
3. *Performs skill independently*

Procedure	1	2	3
1. Takes BSI precautions.			
2. One team member faces patient on one side, establishes cervical spine stabilization from the front.			
3. Intubating paramedic sits behind patient on the ground with legs straddling patient's shoulders, moves up until patient's head is secured, applies firm pressure to ensure immobilization.			
4. Hyperventilates patient with 100% oxygen.			
5. Assembles and checks equipment.			
6. Holds laryngoscope in left hand and inserts it into right side of the mouth, displacing tongue to the left, and brings laryngoscope to midline.			
7. Advances blade until it reaches the base of the tongue.			
8. Lifts laryngoscope forward to displace the jaw without putting pressure on front teeth.			
9. Looks for tip of epiglottis and places blade into proper position.			
10. Lifts jaw at 45° angle to the ground until glottis is exposed.			
11. Grasps tube with the right hand and advances it through right corner of patient's mouth.			
12. Advances the tube through the glottic opening until the distal cuff disappears past vocal cords.			
13. Removes stylet, inflates distal cuff with 5–10 ml of air, removes syringe.			
14. Verifies proper placement of tube; clear breath sounds, symmetrical chest rise.			
15. Hyperventilates patient with 100% oxygen.			
16. Periodically rechecks tube placement.			

Handout 8-8

Student's Name _____

RAPID-SEQUENCE INTUBATION WITH NEUROMUSCULAR BLOCKADE

Charting Student Progress:
1. *Learning skill*
2. *Performs skill with direction*
3. *Performs skill independently*

Procedure	1	2	3
1. Takes BSI precautions.			
2. Assembles required equipment.			
3. Ensures IV in place and running.			
4. Places patient on cardiac monitor and pulse oximeter.			
5. Hyperventilates patient with 100% oxygen.			
6. Considers premedicating as needed with Versed, atropine, lidocaine, and so on, per local protocols.			
7. Has assistant apply Sellick's maneuver until proper ETT placement is confirmed.			
8. Administers 1.5 mg/kg IV bolus of succinylcholine and continues oxygenation.			
9. Watches for apnea and jaw relaxation.			
10. Performs endotracheal intubation.			
11. Confirms proper placement of ETT, inflates distal cuff, ventilates with BVM with a CO_2 detector attached, watching for chest rise and fall with ventilations, bilateral breath sounds, no gastric sounds over the stomach.			
12. Releases Sellick's maneuver.			
13. Inserts bite block device, secures ETT in place, reconfirms ETT placement.			
14. Hyperventilates patient with 100% oxygen.			
15. Periodically rechecks tube placement.			

Handout 8-9

Student's Name _____

PEDIATRIC INTUBATION

Charting Student Progress:
1. *Learning skill*
2. *Performs skill with direction*
3. *Performs skill independently*

Procedure	1	2	3
1. Takes BSI precautions.			
2. Hyperventilates patient with 100% oxygen.			
3. Assembles and checks equipment.			
4. Places patient's head and neck in appropriate position.			
5. Has partner apply Sellick's maneuver.			
6. Holds laryngoscope in left hand and inserts into right side of mouth.			
7. Moves blade slightly toward midline, advancing it until the distal end reaches the base of the tongue.			
8. Looks for tip of epiglottis, and positions laryngoscope properly.			
9. Grasps ETT in right hand and, under direct visualization of the vocal cords, inserts it through the right corner of the patient's mouth into the glottic opening until distal 10 mm or distal cuff disappears 2–3 cm beyond the vocal cords.			
10. Holds tube in place with left hand and attaches infant- or child-size BVM to the connector with CO_2 detector.			
11. Delivers several breaths, checking for proper tube placement; symmetrical rise and fall of chest, equal bilateral breath sounds.			
12. Hyperventilates patient with 100% oxygen.			
13. Secures tube with tape or commercial device.			
14. Periodically rechecks tube placement.			

Handout 8-10

Student's Name _____

NASOTRACHEAL INTUBATION

Charting Student Progress:
1. *Learning skill*
2. *Performs skill with direction*
3. *Performs skill independently*

Procedure	1	2	3
1. Takes BSI precautions.			
2. Hyperventilates patient with 100% oxygen.			
3. Assembles and checks equipment.			
4. Inspects nose and selects the larger nostril as passageway.			
5. Applies topical anesthesia with Hurricane spray or topical lidocaine.			
6. Inserts the tube into the nostril with the bevel along the floor of the nostril or facing the nasal septum.			
7. As the tube drops into the posterior pharynx, listens closely at its proximal end for the patient's respiratory sounds.			
8. With the patient's next inhaled breath, advances the ETT quickly into the glottic opening and continues passing it until the cuff is just past the vocal cords.			
9. Watches for condensation in the clear tube, feels for exhaled air from the tube.			
10. Holding the ETT with one hand to prevent displacement, inflates the distal cuff with 5–10 ml of air and removes syringe.			
11. Verifies proper placement by observing chest rise, auscultating breath sounds, monitoring color change in end-tidal CO_2 detector.			
12. Secures tube with tape or commercial device.			
13. Hyperventilates patient with 100% oxygen.			
14. Periodically rechecks tube placement.			

Handout 8-11

Student's Name _____

ESOPHAGEAL TRACHEAL COMBITUBE AIRWAY

Charting Student Progress:
1. *Learning skill*
2. *Performs skill with direction*
3. *Performs skill independently*

Procedure	1	2	3
1. Takes BSI precautions.			
2. Hyperventilates patient with 100% oxygen.			
3. Assembles and checks equipment.			
4. Places the patient supine and kneels at the top of his head.			
5. Places patient's head in neutral position.			
6. Inserts ETC at midline through oropharynx, using a tongue-jaw-lift maneuver, advancing it past the hypopharynx to the depth indicated by the markings on the tube so that the black rings of the tube are between patient's teeth.			
7. Inflates pharyngeal cuff with 100 ml of air and distal cuff with 10–15 ml of air.			
8. Ventilates through the longer blue proximal port with BVM connected to 100% oxygen.			
9. Auscultates lungs and stomach.			
10. If gastric sounds are heard instead of breath sounds, changes ports and ventilates through the clear connector.			
11. Confirms bilateral lung sounds, visualizes chest rise, watches for color change in CO_2 detector.			
12. Secures tube and continues ventilating with 100% oxygen.			
13. Frequently reassesses airway and adequacy of ventilation.			

Handout 8-12

Student's Name _____

PTL AIRWAY

Charting Student Progress:
1. Learning skill
2. Performs skill with direction
3. Performs skill independently

Procedure	1	2	3
1. Takes BSI precautions.			
2. Hyperventilates patient with 100% oxygen.			
3. Assembles and checks equipment.			
4. Places patient's head in appropriate position.			
5. Inserts PtL gently, using the tongue-jaw-lift maneuver.			
6. Inflates distal cuffs of both PtL tubes simultaneously with sustained breath into inflation valve.			
7. Delivers breath into green tube and looks for chest rise.			
8. If chest rises, inflates pharyngeal balloon and continues ventilating through green tube, auscultating bilateral breath sounds.			
9. If chest does not rise and no breath sounds are audible with auscultation, removes stylet from clear tube and ventilates patient through that tube.			
10. Verifies proper placement by watching chest rise and auscultating lungs.			
11. Attaches BVM, secures tube, and hyperventilates patient with 100% oxygen.			
12. Frequently reassesses airway and adequacy of ventilation.			

Handout 8-13

Student's Name _____

FOREIGN BODY REMOVAL UNDER DIRECT LARYNGOSCOPY

Charting Student Progress:
1. Learning skill
2. Performs skill with direction
3. Performs skill independently

Procedure	1	2	3
1. Takes BSI precautions.			
2. Confirms airway obstruction and unsuccessful BLS procedures.			
3. Prepares equipment.			
4. Places head in sniffing position.			
5. Inserts laryngoscope and visualizes glottic opening.			
6. Identifies obstruction.			
7. Inserts Magill forceps in closed position.			
8. Opens forceps to grasp object and removes obstruction.			
9. Removes laryngoscope.			
10. Reassesses airway and breathing.			

HANDOUT 8-14

Student's Name _____

NEEDLE CRICOTHYROTOMY

Charting Student Progress:
1. Learning skill
2. Performs skill with direction
3. Performs skill independently

Procedure	1	2	3
1. Takes BSI precautions.			
2. Places patient supine and hyperextends head and neck.			
3. Positions at patient's side.			
4. Prepares equipment.			
5. Palpates inferior portion of thyroid cartilage and cricoid cartilage and identifies cricothyroid membrane.			
6. Cleanses site appropriately.			
7. Firmly grasps laryngeal cartilages and reconfirms site of cricothyroid membrane.			
8. Attaches large-bore IV needle with catheter to 10- or 20-ml syringe.			
9. Inserts needle into cricothyroid membrane at midline, directed 45° caudally.			
10. Advances needle no more than 1 cm and aspirates with syringe.			
11. Confirms placement and advances catheter, withdraws needle.			
12. Reconfirms placement and secures catheter in place.			
13. Checks adequacy of ventilations; chest rise, bilateral breath sounds.			
14. If spontaneous ventilations are absent or inadequate, begins transtracheal jet ventilation.			
15. Connects one end of oxygen tubing to catheter, other end to jet ventilator.			
16. Opens release valve and adjusts pressure to allow adequate lung expansion.			

HANDOUT 8-14 Continued

Procedure	1	2	3
17. Watches chest carefully, turning off release valve as soon as chest rises.			
18. Delivers at least 20 breaths per minute.			
19. Continues ventilatory support, assessing for adequacy of ventilations and watching for potential complications.			

HANDOUT 8-15

Student's Name _____

OPEN CRICOTHYROTOMY

Charting Student Progress:
1. *Learning skill*
2. *Performs skill with direction*
3. *Performs skill independently*

Procedure	1	2	3
1. Takes BSI precautions.			
2. Locates thyroid cartilage and the cricoid cartilage.			
3. Finds cricothyroid membrane.			
4. Cleanses site appropriately.			
5. Stabilizes the cartilages with one hand.			
6. Uses scalpel to make 1–2-cm vertical skin incision over membrane.			
7. Makes 1-cm incision in the horizontal plane through the membrane.			
8. Inserts curved hemostats into the membrane incision and spreads it open.			
9. Inserts either cuffed endotracheal tube (6.0 mm or 7.0 mm) or tracheostomy tube (6 or 8 Shiley), directing the tube into trachea.			
10. Inflates cuff and ventilates.			
11. Confirms placement with auscultation, end-tidal CO_2 detector, and chest rise.			
12. Secures tube in place.			

HANDOUT 8-16

Student's Name _____

SUCTIONING

Charting Student Progress:
1. *Learning skill*
2. *Performs skill with direction*
3. *Performs skill independently*

Procedure	1	2	3
1. Takes BSI precautions.			
2. Hyperventilates patient with 100% oxygen.			
3. Determines depth of catheter insertion by measuring from patient's earlobe to lips.			
4. With suction turned off, inserts catheter into patient's pharynx to the predetermined depth.			
5. Turns on suction unit and places thumb over suction control orifice.			
6. Suctions while withdrawing catheter, no more than 10 seconds.			
7. Hyperventilates patient with 100% oxygen.			

HANDOUT 8-17

Student's Name _____

CHAPTER 8 QUIZ

Write the letter of the best answer in the space provided.

_____ 1. The potentially most ominous finding of auscultation is:
   A. snoring.
   B. gurgling.
   C. wheezing.
   D. quiet.

_____ 2. Which manual maneuver should you use to open the airway of a patient with a suspected neck or head injury?
   A. jaw-thrust maneuver
   B. Sellick's maneuver
   C. modified jaw-thrust maneuver
   D. head-tilt/chin-lift maneuver

_____ 3. One advantage of the nasopharyngeal airway over the oropharyngeal is that the nasopharyngeal airway:
   A. may be used in the presence of a gag reflex.
   B. makes suctioning of the pharynx easier.
   C. isolates the trachea.
   D. eliminates the possibility of pressure necrosis.

_____ 4. The laryngoscope permits visualization of the vocal cords by lifting of the tongue and:
   A. soft palate.
   B. epiglottis.
   C. hyoid bone.
   D. none of these

_____ 5. The curved blade made for the laryngoscope is the:
   A. Miller.
   B. Wisconsin.
   C. Flagg.
   D. Macintosh.

_____ 6. The curved laryngoscope blade is designed to fit into the:
   A. pyriform fossa.
   B. vallecula.
   C. epiglottis.
   D. larynx.

_____ 7. The greatest advantage of a straight blade is:
   A. greater displacement of the tongue.
   B. indirect elevation of the epiglottis.
   C. lessened chance of stimulating the gag reflex.
   D. wider field of vision for intubation.

_____ 8. Stylets are a valuable asset when intubating a patient with a:
   A. short, fat neck.
   B. long, thin neck.
   C. posterior larynx.
   D. none of these

_____ 9. The dangers of movement of an endotracheal tube once it is positioned include:
   A. elevation of intracranial pressure.
   B. stimulation of the vallecula.
   C. cardiovascular depression.
   D. all of these

_____ 10. Potentially dangerous complications of improper endotracheal intubation include:
   A. esophageal intubation.
   B. pyriform sinus intubation.
   C. right mainstem intubation.
   D. all of these

_____ 11. Indications of proper endotracheal intubation include all of the following EXCEPT:
   A. the presence of bilateral breath sounds.
   B. the absence of abdominal sounds.
   C. phonation.
   D. the presence of condensation in the tube.

HANDOUT 8-17 Continued

_____ 12. Digital intubation can be useful in situations in which:
   A. a trauma patient has a suspected cervical spinal injury.
   B. entrapment prevents proper positioning.
   C. facial injuries distort the anatomy.
   D. all of these

_____ 13. All of the following statements about the pediatric airway are true EXCEPT:
   A. the tongue is larger in relation to the oropharynx than in adults.
   B. the glottic opening is lower and more posterior than in adults.
   C. the vocal cords slant upward.
   D. the narrowest part is the cricoid cartilage.

_____ 14. In patients with clenched teeth or who are awake or combative, the preferred method of intubation is:
   A. digital.
   B. lighted stylet.
   C. rapid-sequence with neuromuscular blockade.
   D. nasal.

_____ 15. Blind nasotracheal intubation is contraindicated if the patient:
   A. is apneic.
   B. has sustained a mandibular injury.
   C. is anorexic.
   D. is severely obese.

_____ 16. Both the PtL and the ETC airways:
   A. can be inserted into either the esophagus or trachea.
   B. can be used in patients under 16 years of age.
   C. can be used in patients with a gag reflex.
   D. all of these

_____ 17. The preferred point of entry when inserting a surgical airway is the:
   A. hyoid membrane.
   B. arytenoid folds.
   C. cricothyroid membrane.
   D. pyriform fossa.

_____ 18. An absolute contraindication to oxygen administration in hypoxic patients is:
   A. COPD.
   B. a premature infant.
   C. hyperventilation.
   D. none of these

_____ 19. To ventilate the patient with a stoma device, rescue personnel will generally use a:
   A. mouth-to-stoma technique.
   B. BVM device.
   C. demand valve device.
   D. automatic transport ventilator.

_____ 20. The minimum acceptable vacuum level in suctioning units for the prehospital setting is:
   A. 200 mmHg.
   B. 300 mmHg.
   C. 500 mmHg.
   D. 750 mmHg.

_____ 21. Both standard routes of gastric decompression put the patient at risk for all of the following EXCEPT:
   A. misplacement into the brain.
   B. vomiting.
   C. misplacement into the trachea.
   D. trauma or bleeding from poor technique.

_____ 22. The bag-valve device has an adjunct oxygen reservoir or corrugated tubing that can deliver _____ oxygen.
   A. 60 percent–70 percent
   B. 70 percent–75 percent
   C. 80 percent–90 percent
   D. 90 percent–95 percent

_____ 23. _____ is the measurement of expired CO_2.
   A. Capnography
   B. Capnograph
   C. Capnometry
   D. Capnogram

HANDOUT 8-17 Continued

_____ **24.** Decreased ETCO$_2$ levels can be found in
  A. shock.
  B. pulmonary embolism.
  C. cardiac arrest.
  D. all of these

_____ **25.** An esophageal detector device (EDD) uses the anatomic principle that the
  A. trachea is rigid and will collapse under negative pressure.
  B. trachea is rigid and will not collapse under negative pressure.
  C. esophagus is rigid and will collapse under negative pressure.
  D. esophagus is rigid and will not collapse under negative pressure.

HANDOUT 8-18

Student's Name _____

CHAPTER 8 SCENARIO 1

Review the following real-life situation. Then answer the questions that follow.

The call is for an unknown medical emergency, with a man down on the sidewalk in front of the county building. Medic 6 is literally around the corner from the call. The unit arrives to find a small crowd of people standing around the patient. The patient is well known to the crew as an alcoholic with a history of epileptic seizures.

In this case, the patient apparently fell and struck his head, as blood is still oozing from a laceration to his forehead. An EMT ensures stabilization of the head, while the paramedic tries to arouse the patient. Witnesses say that the patient had a seizure that lasted for "several minutes." None report that he turned cyanotic. After getting no response to his loud questions and commands, the paramedic attempts a painful stimulation. This effort produces only a groan from the patient. The paramedic attempts to insert an oral airway, but the patient gags and spits it out. The paramedic then tries a nasopharyngeal airway. The patient tolerates this, so the crew supplies oxygen and prepares to package the patient for transport.

When he is secured to the backboard, the patient suddenly seizes again. The crew rolls him onto his side while on the backboard, suctions his mouth, and reassesses his airway and breathing after he stops seizing. The seizure lasts less than 1 minute.

1. Why was the airway a concern in this patient?

2. What other causes of the seizure might be possible?

3. Why would the paramedic not immediately intubate this unconscious patient on scene?

HANDOUT 8-19

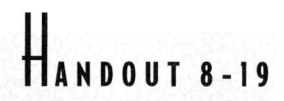

Student's Name _____

CHAPTER 8 SCENARIO 2

Review the following real-life situation. Then answer the questions that follow.

"Engine 5, Ambulance 3, respond to 7439 Burr Oak Rd. for a 21-year-old female experiencing an asthma attack. Time out 2230." Responding priority one, lights and siren, you arrive at the scene and are ushered into the kitchen. Even before you enter, you can hear wheezing through the doorway. Inside at the table, you find the patient, weighing approximately 100 kg, in obvious respiratory distress.

While the patient is conscious, she obviously is exhausted and is having trouble maintaining an upright posture. You assist her to the floor, where she leans against the wall. Asking others in the room to please put out their cigarettes, you proceed with your assessment.

The patient's respiratory rate is in the high 40s, with shallow, ineffective breaths. The BLS crew prepares to assist her with ventilations while you listen to the lungs. Wheezes in the upper lobes are present both with inspirations and expirations, but upon listening to her back you are alarmed to note that the bases are essentially silent. Despite assistance with the BVM, the patient is having trouble maintaining consciousness. You decide to intubate.

You explain to the patient that you intend to intubate her to make her breathing easier. As you do this, you proceed to prepare a number 7 endotracheal tube. Lubricating the nares with lidocaine gel, you slide the tube into the right nare. The tube meets slight resistance and then, after a slight turn downward, slides into the hypopharynx. The patient coughs for a second as the tube passes cleanly into the trachea. After confirming the placement, you secure the ETT and proceed with your examination.

The patient has a history of juvenile-onset asthma and two previous episodes requiring intubation and ventilation. She is on a theophylline compound as well as several inhalers. Just before your arrival, she had had an argument with her boyfriend about his smoking.

1. Why would early and aggressive intubation be indicated with this patient?

2. How can you confirm tube placement in this patient?

3. What are some of the dangers in intubating this patient?

©2007 Pearson Education, Inc.
Essentials of Paramedic Care, 2nd ed.

Handout 8-20

Student's Name _____

CHAPTER 8 REVIEW

Write the word or words that best complete the following sentences in the space provided.

1. The most common cause of airway obstruction is the _____.
2. _____ breathing is asymmetrical chest wall movement that lessens respiratory efficiency.
3. The measurement of exhaled carbon dioxide concentrations is called _____.
4. In the absence of cervical spine trauma, the _____ / _____ is the best technique for opening the airway of an unresponsive patient.
5. The _____ airway may be used for intubation in the presence of a gag reflex.
6. Once the tip of a(n) _____ airway reaches the level of the soft palate, gently rotate it 180 degrees.
7. Miller, Wisconsin, and Flagg are types of _____ laryngoscope blades.
8. Verification of proper endotracheal tube placement includes absence of _____ _____ over the epigastrium, the presence of _____ breath sounds (lungs), and the presence of _____ inside the tube.
9. Giving medications to sedate and temporarily paralyze a patient before performing orotracheal intubation is called _____ _____ _____.
10. Partial ingestion of caustic poisons is a contraindication to the use of the _____ _____ _____.
11. Often patients who have had a laryngectomy or tracheostomy breathe through a(n) _____, an opening in the anterior neck that connects the trachea with the ambient air.
12. Suctioning should be limited to _____ seconds.
13. In an awake patient with gastric distention, the _____ approach to decompression is generally preferred.
14. To calculate how many minutes the oxygen in a tank will last, multiply the psi in the tank by _____, then divide by _____ _____ _____.
15. The difference between a partial rebreather mask and a nonrebreather mask is that the nonrebreather mask has a(n) _____ _____ _____ attached.
16. The memory aid used to establish a rhythm for adequately ventilating a child is _____, _____, _____.
17. Most demand-valve devices have a(n) _____ _____ _____ that makes them useful in treating spontaneously breathing patients who need high oxygen concentrations.
18. The _____ _____ _____ is a dual lumen airway with a ventilation port for each lumen. The longer, blue port is the distal port; the shorter, clear port is the proximal port, which terminates in the hypopharynx.
19. The _____ _____ _____ has an inflatable distal end (similar to a face mask) which is placed in the hypopharynx and then inflated.
20. The compact ventilator typically comes with two or three controls: one for the _____ _____, the other for _____ _____.

Handout 8-21

Student's Name _____

ADVANCED AIRWAY MATCHING

Write the letter of the term in the space next to the appropriate description.

- **A.** Oropharyngeal airway
- **B.** Succinylcholine
- **C.** EOA
- **D.** PtL
- **E.** EGTA
- **F.** ETC
- **G.** Endotracheal tube
- **H.** Yankauer
- **I.** Macintosh
- **J.** Demand valve
- **K.** Wisconsin
- **L.** Nonrebreather
- **M.** Stylet
- **N.** Venturi
- **O.** Magill

_____ 1. Type of scissors-style clamps with circle-shaped tips.

_____ 2. Straight laryngoscope blade.

_____ 3. Airway designed for insertion into the esophagus.

_____ 4. Neuromuscular blocking agent.

_____ 5. Airway comprising a short, large-diameter, green tube and a longer, narrow-diameter clear tube.

_____ 6. Manually triggered, oxygen-powered breathing device.

_____ 7. Tonsil tip suction catheter.

_____ 8. Semicircular plastic and rubber device that conforms to the palate's curvature and lifts the base of the tongue.

_____ 9. Metal wire covered with plastic.

_____ 10. Esophageal airway that permits suctioning of the stomach.

_____ 11. Two-tube airway in which tubes are combined with lumens separated by a partition.

_____ 12. Oxygen administration device particularly useful with COPD patients.

_____ 13. Flexible, 35-37-cm tube with adapter at one end and inflatable cuff at the other.

_____ 14. Device consisting of tubing, reservoir bag, and inlet/outlet ports covered by thin rubber flaps.

_____ 15. Curved laryngoscope blade.

HANDOUT 8-22

Student's Name _____

AIRWAY MANAGEMENT INDICATIONS, CONTRAINDICATIONS, ADVANTAGES, AND DISADVANTAGES

Complete the following lists.

1. What are three advantages of the nasopharyngeal airway?

2. What are three indications of accidental esophageal intubation?

3. What are three contraindications for nasotracheal intubation?

4. What are three indications for rapid-sequence intubation?

5. What are three advantages of the PtL airway?

6. What are three potential complications of needle cricothyrotomy with transtracheal jet ventilation?

Handout 8-23

Student's Name _____

RAPID-SEQUENCE INTUBATION COMPLETION

Fill in the blanks to complete the steps in rapid sequence intubation with neuromuscular blockade.

1. Preoxygenate the patient with _____ _____ _____ using basic manual and adjunct maneuvers.

2. Be certain to have at least one secure and working _____ _____.

3. Place the patient on a cardiac monitor and a _____ _____.

4. If the patient is alert, administer a _____ agent such as _____ before administering any neuromuscular blocking agents.

5. Apply _____ _____ and maintain until you confirm proper ETT placement.

6. If the patient is a child, premedicate with _____ to prevent bradycardia.

7. _____ and _____ _____ are indications that the patient is sufficiently relaxed to proceed with endotracheal intubation.

8. If unable to pass the ETT after _____ seconds, stop and hyperventilate the patient for 2 minutes.

9. Confirm proper placement of the ETT by watching for chest _____ _____ _____ with ventilations, auscultate with each ventilation for _____ breath sounds over the chest, and no _____ _____ over the stomach.

10. The effects of succinylcholine should wear off in _____ _____.

Chapter 8 Answer Key

Handout 8-17: Chapter 8 Quiz

1.	D	8.	A	15.	A	22.	B
2.	C	9.	A	16.	A	23.	A
3.	A	10.	D	17.	C	24.	D
4.	B	11.	C	18.	D	25.	B
5.	D	12.	D	19.	B		
6.	B	13.	B	20.	B		
7.	A	14.	C	21.	A		

Handout 8-18: Chapter 8 Scenario 1

1. The unconscious patient has little, if any, control over the airway, and therefore aspiration becomes a very real threat.
2. Reasonably, the patient may have seized due to alcohol withdrawal, epilepsy, hypoglycemia, overdose of antifreeze or wood alcohol, closed head injuries such as a subdural hematoma, or from an infectious process.
3. The decision to intubate either the diabetic with hypoglycemia or the postictal epileptic patient must be made carefully. These patients often respond quickly to simple measures and without further complications that might result from the use of advanced airway control methods.

Handout 8-19: Chapter 8 Scenario 2

1. The patient was hypoxic and tiring rapidly. Respiratory and/or cardiac arrest are definite possibilities in this case. Note that deaths secondary to asthma are increasing in this country, while treatments have not made significant advances. This form of intubation is called for because the patient is still conscious. In addition, nasotracheal intubation is recommended with obese patients.
2. If the tube is correctly placed, it should fog up due to condensation from the patient's breath. The breath should also be felt coming from the proximal end of the tube. Placement should be confirmed by auscultation and by watching for chest rise and fall.
3. The most significant danger would be accidental esophageal intubation and ventilation. The resultant gastric distention would further lessen tidal volume and possibly cause the patient to regurgitate stomach contents into the airway. Blind nasotracheal intubation also risks lacerating the turbinates, causing bleeding into the hypopharynx and further compromising the respiratory tract.

Handout 8-20: Chapter 8 Review

1. tongue
2. Paradoxical
3. capnography
4. head-tilt, chin-lift
5. nasopharyngeal
6. oropharyngeal
7. straight
8. gastric sounds, bilateral, condensation
9. rapid sequence intubation
10. Esophageal Tracheal CombiTube
11. stoma
12. 10
13. nasogastric
14. 0.28, liters per minute
15. oxygen reservoir bag
16. squeeze, release, release
17. inspiratory release valve
18. Esophageal Tracheal CombiTube
19. Laryngeal Mask Airway
20. ventilatory rate, tidal volume

Handout 8-21: Advanced Airway Matching

1.	H	5.	J	9.	G	13.	D
2.	F	6.	M	10.	C	14.	N
3.	B	7.	L	11.	K	15.	E
4.	I	8.	A	12.	O		

Handout 8-22: Airway Management Indications, Contraindications, Advantages, and Disadvantages

1. Any three of the following:
   rapid insertion
   bypasses tongue
   can be used with gag reflex
   can be used in patients with oral cavity injury
   can be used when teeth are clenched
2. Any three of the following:
   absence of chest rise and breath sounds
   gurgling sounds over epigastrium
   absence of condensation in ETT
   persistent air leak
   cyanosis and worsening of patient's condition
   phonation
3. Any three of the following:
   nasal fractures
   basilar skull fractures
   significantly deviated nasal septum
   nasal obstruction
   cardiac or respiratory arrest
   unresponsive patient
4. Any three of the following:
   impending respiratory failure due to intrinsic pulmonary disease
   acute airway disorder that threatens airway patency
   altered mental status with significant risk of vomiting and aspiration
5. Any three of the following:
   functions in either trachea or esophagus
   no face mask to seal
   does not require visualization of the larynx
   can be used with trauma patients
   helps protect trachea from upper airway bleeding and secretions
6. Any three of the following:
   may lead to barotrauma
   excessive bleeding
   subcutaneous emphysema
   airway obstruction
   hypoventilation

Handout 8-23: Rapid Sequence Intubation Completion

1. 100 percent oxygen
2. IV line
3. pulse oximeter
4. sedative, midazolam (Versed)
5. Sellick's maneuver
6. atropine
7. apnea, jaw relaxation
8. 20–30
9. rise and fall, bilateral, gastric sounds
10. 3–5 minutes

Chapter 9

Therapeutic Communications

INTRODUCTION

Technically, communication is the exchange of common symbols through speaking, writing, or other methods such as signing and body language. But EMS providers have the difficult challenge of communicating with patients—strangers in crisis. Appropriate communication is an art form. Paramedics must pay attention to their words, tone of voice, facial expressions, and body language. Communications may be even more difficult when the patient is a child, an elderly person, from a different culture than the paramedic, or hostile. The paramedic's respect and empathy for patients, families, bystanders, and other EMS providers is vital to successful communications. This chapter will discuss various communication techniques.

CHAPTER OBJECTIVES

After reading this chapter, you should be able to:

1. Define communication. (p. 533)
2. Identify internal and external factors that affect an interview. (pp. 533–535, 539–540)
3. Identify strategies for developing rapport with the patient. (p. 534)
4. Discuss open-ended and closed questions. (pp. 537–538)
5. Discuss common errors made when interviewing patients. (pp. 539–540)
6. Identify the nonverbal skills used in patient interviewing. (pp. 535–536)
7. Identify interview methods used to assess mental status. (p. 538)
8. Discuss strategies for interviewing a patient who is not motivated to talk. (pp. 535, 538, 540)
9. Describe the use of, and differentiate between, facilitation, reflection, clarification, empathetic responses, confrontation, and interpretation. (p. 539)
10. Differentiate strategies used for interviewing hostile and cooperative patients. (pp. 538, 543)
11. Summarize developmental considerations that influence patient interviewing. (pp. 540–542)
12. Define the unique interviewing techniques for patients with special needs. (pp. 540–543)

TOTAL TEACHING TIME: 3.78 HOURS
The total teaching time is only a guideline based on the didactic and practical lab averages in the National Standard Curriculum. Instructors should take into consideration such factors as the pace at which students learn, the size of the class, and breaks. The actual time devoted to teaching objectives is the responsibility of the instructor.

13. Discuss cross-cultural interviewing considerations. (pp. 542–543)
14. Given several preprogrammed simulated patients, provide a patient interview using therapeutic communication. (pp. 533–543)

FRAMING THE LESSON

Begin the class by reviewing the important points from Chapter 8, "Airway Management and Ventilation." Discuss any aspects of the chapter not understood by students. Then go on to Chapter 9. Ask students to name the various cultures represented in your area. These might include nationalities, ethnic groups, religions, or other cultural groups. Ask if any of the students have visited a foreign country, especially one in which English was not the dominant language. Ask how they felt trying to communicate with people who did not speak their language. What worked, and what did not? Did they use any means of communication besides verbal? Next, ask students to write down phrases commonly used in communicating with and assessing patients. Then have them say the phrases in different tones and varying volumes. For example, demonstrate how many ways the question, "What's wrong with you?" can be asked. Stress how tone of voice, volume, and facial expression can change the meaning of similar phrases. Also emphasize that preconceptions and prejudices have no place in EMS. Every patient receives the same respect and quality patient care. Finally, ask if any students would like to relate an experience they have had when a salesperson was rude to them. If they received poor service from a store, even if prices were better, would they return there? Ask students to think about how patients might respond to EMS personnel who acted in a similar manner.

TEACHING STRATEGIES

People learn in a variety of ways. Some do better with the spoken word, whereas others prefer the written. Some prefer to work alone, whereas others profit from working in groups. Recognizing these different ways of acquiring knowledge, the authors of this *Instructor's Resource Manual* have provided a variety of teaching strategies for the different types of learners. These strategies are intended to foster higher-level cognitive skills and encourage creative learning and problem solving. For greatest effectiveness, incorporate these strategies into your class lecture. Symbols in the Lecture Outline indicate the points at which various exercises might be most appropriate. Other strategies can be used to preview the lesson or to summarize it.

The following strategies are keyed to specific sections of the lesson.

1. Recognizing Stereotyping. Brainstorm with students about the types of calls or dispatch information that are likely to be stereotyped. You can begin by asking something like, "Which calls make you sigh or groan?" or "What are your most frustrating calls?" By identifying the prejudices and stereotypes, you can begin to break down the negative behavior that often accompanies these types of calls. For instance, someone might complain about "nursing home calls." You can then have someone describe his very kind, intelligent grandparent who lives in an assisted living facility and show how not all elderly folks fit the stereotypical "nursing home call." Another example is a complaint about "snowboarders or surfers." Point out a prominent or respected member of your community who participates in one of these activities to begin breaking the stereotype.

2. Practicing Nonverbal Communication. Divide the class into pairs for this exercise. Have one make the other feel "cared for" without touching them or speaking to them. Give them some time to figure it out. Some will get down on the other person's level and just sit with the person; others will bring the person a pillow or offer the person food. Let them be creative. Afterward, allow students to discuss how they felt as both caregivers and care recipients. Unless they have previously developed these skills, many will feel frustrated by not being able to speak. Reinforce the power of nonverbal communication.

3. Understanding Interpersonal Zones. Divide the class into four groups. Then draw up a list of 5 to 10 questions you would like students to try to get answered by someone. Assign one group to each of the four interpersonal zones—the intimate zone, personal space, social distance, or public distance. Have them begin asking strangers (or nurses in the ER, students in an EMT class, or whoever else is handy) the predetermined questions from the distances represented by each zone. Have students keep track of how many questions they were able to get answered by each person they questioned and those people's responses to the student's behavior. You will likely find that the most information could be gained from the personal and social distances. This exercise again introduces the fun of classroom and EMS research while being kinesthetic as well. This is usually quite enjoyable for students.

4. Role-Playing. Develop scenarios designed to illustrate differences in ages and cultures and dealing with hostile patients. Stress that angry or hostile patients are not angry with paramedics as much as they are with their situation. Include patients, family, bystanders, and other EMS providers in the scenarios. Assign the parts students are to play. Make sure each student has the opportunity to play the part of a paramedic facing a difficult situation. Scenarios may include cultural differences, patients with nonemergency complaints, or patients who are prejudiced, have hearing difficulties, or do not speak English.

5. Guest Speakers. Invite representatives from various religions and cultures to talk to students about their beliefs, family structure, and so on. Make an effort to include people from minority cultures. Allow students to ask questions, and encourage those involving medical and prehospital care (such as herbalists, naturopaths, faith healers, and so on), customs, and problems encountered in dealing with people outside of their own culture.

6. Scene Safety Expert. Invite a representative from law enforcement to the class to discuss scene safety and personal protection in unsafe situations. Though we do not want paramedics to place themselves in harm's way, they sometimes inadvertently become involved in dangerous situations.

The following strategies can be used at various points throughout the lesson or to help summarize and demonstrate what students have learned.

Dealing with Distractions. To illustrate the importance of managing external distractions to obtain effective communication, be sure to program preplanned external distractions into your classroom scenarios and labs. Record traffic on your street or near the airport, a barking dog, or restaurant conversations. Play the radio, use sirens, and so on. When distractions are present, see if the students will act to remove them, or you can remind students to do so. Learning to deal with distractions will help prepare students for success in the field because they will be used to considering the effectiveness of their communication in practice. This concept is so important that it is even given point value on the National Registry Patient Assessment Skill Sheet.

HANDOUT 9-1
Chapter 9 Objectives Checklist

POINT TO EMPHASIZE
The prime component of communications is respect for the patient as an individual. Treat the patient as you would want your own family treated. The patient, family, bystanders, and other EMS providers will see this and appreciate it.

TEACHING TIP
Teach by example. Make sure you are completely free of prejudices and biases in your instruction of this course. You are in a position of authority, and students will emulate you.

POWERPOINT PRESENTATION
Chapter 9 PowerPoint slide 4

TEACHING STRATEGY 1
Recognizing Stereotyping

POINT TO EMPHASIZE
Make sure the first impression the patient receives from you is a positive one.

POWERPOINT PRESENTATION
Chapter 9 PowerPoint slides 5–13

TEACHING TIP
Establish a classroom culture that promotes the professional behaviors described in this section. Require a uniform and good hygiene. Discourage emotional outbursts and immature behaviors. Do not allow running or sitting on tables. The work and behavior ethics you instill in your students now will help to elevate the level of the paramedic profession. Employers will appreciate this type of employee. It only takes 28 days to create a habit. You usually will have your students for 6 months to 1 year. You have the power to create good habits or allow bad ones!

Improving Communications Skills. Several good videos exist in the human resources arena on interpersonal communication. Try to borrow some of these tapes. While individuals with poor communication skills rarely notice their own poor skills, they often can identify the troublesome behavior in a skit or on videotape. Play the videos and have students identify the behaviors that do not promote good communication. Discuss how to modify those behaviors.

Clinical Observation Locations. Have students schedule part of their clinical observation time at a nursing home or facility caring for people with special needs. At these locations, communicating appropriately is often more important than medical care.

Cultural Considerations, Legal Notes, and Patho Pearls. The Student CD-ROM contains this series of informative features to enhance the student's understanding of the material covered in this chapter.

TEACHING OUTLINE

Chapter 9, "Therapeutic Communications," is the ninth lesson in Division 1, *Introduction to Advanced Prehospital Care*. Distribute Handout 9-1 so that students can familiarize themselves with the learning goals for this chapter. If students have any questions about the objectives, answer them at this time.

Then present the chapter. One possible lecture outline follows. In the outline, the parenthetical references in regular type are references to text pages; those in bold type are references to figures or tables.

I. Introduction. Often, communicating with a patient is as important as the medical care the patient receives. (p. 533)

    A. Communication with (p. 533)
        1. Patient
        2. Patient's relatives
        3. Bystanders
        4. Other EMS providers

    B. Communication strategies (p. 533)
        1. Word choices
        2. Tone of voice
        3. Facial expressions
        4. Body language
        5. Minimize distractions
        6. Adjust personal communications style

    C. The paramedic must communicate with every patient in the same caring, professional, empathetic manner. (p. 533)

II. Basic elements of communication. Keep in mind that patience and flexibility are hallmarks of a good communicator. (pp. 533–535)

    A. Communication component (p. 533)
        1. Encoding
        2. Decoding
        3. Feedback

    B. Reasons for failing to communicate (p. 533)
        1. Prejudice
        2. Lack of privacy
        3. External distractions
        4. Internal distractions

    C. Trust and rapport (p. 533)

D. Professional behaviors (p. 534)
   1. Clean, neat uniform
   2. Good personal hygiene
   3. Physical fitness
   4. Overall professional demeanor
   5. Appropriate facial expression
   6. Confident stance
   7. Appropriate gait
   8. Consideration for the patient
E. Building trust and rapport in the patient interview (pp. 534–535)
   1. Use patient's name.
   2. Address patient properly.
   3. Modulate your voice.
   4. Use a professional but compassionate tone of voice.
   5. Explain what you are doing and why.
   6. Keep a kind, calm facial expression.
   7. Use appropriate style of communication.

III. Communication techniques. To get the information that you need from your patient, you must be consistently professional, nonjudgmental, and willing to talk about any concerns the patient might have. (pp. 535–543)

A. General guidelines (pp. 535–537)
   1. Nonverbal communication
      a. Distance (**Table 9-1, p. 535**)
      b. Relative level
      c. Stance (**Fig. 9-1, p. 536**)
   2. Eye contact
   3. Compassionate touch (**Fig. 9-2, p. 537**)
B. Interview techniques (pp. 537–540)
   1. Questioning techniques
      a. Continue to ask open-ended questions.
      b. Use direct questions.
      c. Do not ask leading questions.
      d. Ask only one question at a time, allowing complete answers.
      e. Listen to the patient's complete response before asking the next question.
      f. Use language the patient can understand.
      g. Do not allow interruptions.
   2. Observing the patient
   3. Effective listening and feedback techniques
      a. Silence
      b. Reflection
      c. Facilitation
      d. Empathy
      e. Clarification
      f. Confrontation
      g. Interpretation
      h. Explanation
      i. Summarization
   4. Common errors
      a. Providing false assurances
      b. Giving advice
      c. Authority
      d. Using avoidance language
      e. Distancing
      f. Professional jargon

TEACHING STRATEGY 2
Practicing Nonverbal Communication

POWERPOINT PRESENTATION
Chapter 9 PowerPoint slides 14–35

TEACHING TIP
Try this exercise with students: Have the class divide into pairs, one student playing the role of the paramedic, the other playing the patient. Have the paramedic conduct a patient assessment on the patient without using verbal communication, instead developing other ways to communicate.

TEACHING STRATEGY 3
Understanding Interpersonal Zones

TEACHING STRATEGY 4
Role-Playing

TEACHING STRATEGY 5
Guest Speakers

READING/REFERENCE
Keeland, B., and L. Jordan. CommuniMed: Multilingual Patient Assessment Manual. 3rd ed. St. Louis, MO: Mosby, 1994.

Periz-Sabido, J. Spanish-English Handbook for Medical Professionals. 4th ed. Los Angeles: Practice Management Information Corp., 1994.

READING/REFERENCE
Dernocoeur, K. B. *Streetsense Communication, Safety, and Control.* 3rd ed. Redmond, WA: Laing Research Services, 1996.

Federal Emergency Management Agency. "EMS Safety: Techniques and Applications." FA-144. Washington, DC: Author, FEMA 1994.

POWERPOINT PRESENTATION
Chapter 9 PowerPoint slide 36

TEACHING STRATEGY 6
Scene Safety Expert

WORKBOOK
Chapter 9 Activities

READING/REFERENCE
Textbook, pp. 546–563

HANDOUT 9-2
Chapter 9 Quiz

HANDOUT 9-3
Chapter 9 Scenario

PARAMEDIC STUDENT CD
Student Activities

COMPANION WEBSITE
http://www.prenhall.com/bledsoe

TESTGEN
Chapter 9

g. Talking too much
h. Interrupting
i. Using "why" questions
C. Patients with special needs (pp. 540–543)
   1. Children (**Fig. 9-3, p. 541**)
   2. Elderly patients
   3. Patients with sensory impairment
   4. Language and cultural considerations
      a. Guidelines for using interpreters
         i. If children are used, keep language to an appropriate level.
         ii. Recognize that the interpreter may be emotionally affected by the emergency.
         iii. Speak slowly.
         iv. Phrase questions carefully and clearly.
         v. Address both patient and interpreter.
         vi. Ask one question at a time; wait for response.
         vii. Understand that information received may not be reliable.
         viii. Have patience.
   5. Hostile or uncooperative patients
D. Transferring patient care (p. 543)

IV. Chapter summary (p. 542). The skills required to manage medical situations are obviously an important part of emergency care. Remember, much of the information you will gather from your patients is extremely personal. You will need an enormous degree of sensitivity to recognize and respond to the signs of suffering in order to create an ideal, individualized process of communication.

ASSIGNMENTS

Assign students to complete Chapter 9, "Therapeutic Communications," of the workbook. Also assign them to read Chapter 10, "History Taking," before the next class.

EVALUATION

Chapter Quiz and Scenario Distribute copies of the Chapter Quiz provided in Handout 9-2 to evaluate student understanding of this chapter. Make sure each student reads the scenario to reinforce critical thinking on the scene. Remind students not to use their notes or textbooks while taking the quiz.

Student CD Quizzes for every chapter are contained on the dynamic and highly visual in-text student CD.

Companion Website Additional quizzes for every chapter are contained on this exciting website.

TestGen You may wish to create a custom-tailored test using *Prentice Hall TestGen for Essentials of Paramedic Care*, 2nd Edition to evaluate student understanding of this chapter.

On-line Test Preparation (for students and instructors) Additional test preparation is available through Brady's new on-line product, *EMT Achieve: Paramedic Test Preparation* at *http://www.prenhall.com/emtachieve/*. Instructors can also monitor student mastery on-line.

Review Manual for the EMT-Paramedic   This comprehensive exam review contains hundreds of test questions and rationales, including scenarios, along with two 180-question practice tests on CD.

REINFORCEMENT

Handouts   If classroom discussion or performance on the quiz indicates that some students have not fully mastered the chapter content, you may wish to assign some or all of the Reinforcement Handouts for this chapter.

Student CD (for students)   A wide variety of material on this CD-ROM will reinforce and also expand student knowledge and skills.

PowerPoint Presentation (for instructors)   The PowerPoint material developed for this chapter offers useful reinforcement of chapter content.

Companion Website (for students)   Additional review quizzes and links to EMS resources will contribute to further reinforcement of the chapter.

OneKey   On-line support is offered for this course on one of three platforms: CourseCompass, Blackboard, or Web CT. Includes the IRM, PowerPoints, TestGen, and Companion Website for instruction. Ask your local sales representative for more information.

Brady Skills Series: Advanced Life Skills (Video or CD)   Have your students watch the skills come to life on VHS or CD-ROM, or they can purchase the highly visual, full-color text with step-by-step procedures and rationales.

EMT ACHIEVE: PARAMEDIC TEST PREPARATION
Mistovich & Beasley. *EMT Achieve: Paramedic Test Preparation.*
www.prenhall.com/emtachieve/

REVIEW MANUAL FOR THE EMT-PARAMEDIC
Cherry & Mistovich. *Review Manual for the EMT-Paramedic,* 3rd edition

HANDOUTS 9-4 AND 9-5
Reinforcement Activities

PARAMEDIC STUDENT CD
Student Activities

POWERPOINT PRESENTATION
Chapter 9

COMPANION WEBSITE
http://www.prenhall.com/bledsoe

ONEKEY
Chapter 9

ADVANCED LIFE SUPPORT SKILLS
Larmon & Davis. *Advanced Life Support Skills.*

ADVANCED LIFE SKILLS REVIEW
Larmon & Davis. *Advanced Life Skills Review.*

BRADY SKILLS SERIES: ALS
Larmon & Davis. *Brady Skills Series: ALS.*

PARAMEDIC NATIONAL STANDARDS SELF-TEST
Miller. *Paramedic National Standards Self-Test,* 4th edition.

HANDOUT 9-1

Student's Name _____

CHAPTER 9 OBJECTIVES CHECKLIST

Knowledge	Date Mastered
1. Define communication.	
2. Identify internal and external factors that affect an interview.	
3. Identify strategies for developing rapport with the patient.	
4. Discuss open-ended and closed questions.	
5. Discuss common errors made when interviewing patients.	
6. Identify the nonverbal skills used in patient interviewing.	
7. Identify interview methods used to assess mental status.	
8. Discuss strategies for interviewing a patient who is not motivated to talk.	
9. Describe the use of, and differentiate between, facilitation, reflection, clarification, empathetic responses, confrontation, and interpretation.	
10. Differentiate strategies used for interviewing hostile and cooperative patients.	
11. Summarize developmental considerations that influence patient interviewing.	
12. Define the unique interviewing techniques for patients with special needs.	
13. Discuss cross-cultural interviewing considerations.	
14. Given several preprogrammed simulated patients, provide a patient interview using therapeutic communication.	

HANDOUT 9-2

Student's Name _____

CHAPTER 9 QUIZ

Write the letter of the best answer in the space provided.

_____ 1. Identification with and understanding of another's situation, feelings, and motives is called:
   A. sympathy.
   B. empathy.
   C. internalization.
   D. advocacy.

_____ 2. The term *encode* means to:
   A. interpret a message.
   B. listen to or read a message.
   C. respond to a message.
   D. create a message.

_____ 3. Reasons for failing to communicate include:
   A. lack of privacy.
   B. feedback.
   C. nonverbal communication.
   D. decoding.

_____ 4. Ways to build trust and rapport with a patient, family, and bystanders include:
   A. using the patient's first name as soon as you learn it.
   B. strolling casually into the scene.
   C. modulating your voice appropriately.
   D. using a pleasant cologne or perfume.

_____ 5. Elements of nonverbal communication include all of the following EXCEPT:
   A. relative level.
   B. facial expression.
   C. stance.
   D. written questions.

_____ 6. In the United States, personal distance or "personal space" is considered to extend _____ from an individual.
   A. 12 feet or more
   B. 4–12 feet
   C. 1.5–4 feet
   D. 0–1.5 feet

_____ 7. Standing below the patient's eye level indicates:
   A. a willingness to let the patient have some control of the situation.
   B. equality.
   C. an air of authority.
   D. that you are completely confident and in control of the situation.

_____ 8. An open stance means that you are:
   A. vulnerable.
   B. off balance.
   C. confident.
   D. tense.

_____ 9. Which of the following statements about social distance is true?
   A. It is best for assessing breath and other body odors.
   B. It is best for performing patient assessment.
   C. It causes visual distortion.
   D. It is used for impersonal business transactions.

_____ 10. Questions framed to guide the direction of a patient's answer are called:
   A. leading questions.
   B. open-ended questions.
   C. closed questions.
   D. direct questions.

_____ 11. Appropriate questioning techniques include all of the following EXCEPT:
   A. asking only one question at a time.
   B. listening to the patient's complete response.
   C. using medical terminology as much as possible.
   D. using open-ended questions.

HANDOUT 9-2 Continued

_____ 12. Once the speaker has stopped talking, provide feedback to confirm that you understood the message. Feedback techniques include all of the following EXCEPT:
   A. evocation.
   B. clarification.
   C. interpretation.
   D. confrontation.

_____ 13. Effective communications with pediatric patients include all of the following EXCEPT:
   A. telling the child what you are doing and why.
   B. explaining your equipment.
   C. not telling the child if something will hurt.
   D. getting down to the child's eye level.

_____ 14. Characteristics of adolescents age 13–18 years include:
   A. being distrustful and uncooperative.
   B. seeing the world from their own perspective only.
   C. resenting being spoken to as if still a child.
   D. being scared and believing that what has happened is their own fault.

_____ 15. A guideline for dealing with pediatric patients is:
   A. keeping parents and children separated.
   B. choosing your words carefully.
   C. telling the child to stop crying if he is.
   D. using a firm, authoritative voice.

_____ 16. The term *ethnocentrism* means:
   A. viewing one's own lifestyle as the most desirable.
   B. viewing one's own lifestyle as being inferior.
   C. the interaction of one culture with another.
   D. the imposition of one's beliefs, values, and so forth on people of another culture.

_____ 17. An important principle to follow when using an interpreter is to:
   A. avoid using the children of immigrants as interpreters.
   B. address only the interpreter.
   C. ask only one question at a time.
   D. realize the interpreter will not show emotions.

_____ 18. When caring for elderly patients, it is important to remember:
   A. to be familiar with them, using their first names.
   B. to treat them similarly to the way you treat children.
   C. to use affectionate terms such as "honey," "missy," or "dude."
   D. that interviews may take longer.

_____ 19. If a patient is blatantly hostile, EMS personnel should:
   A. approach the patient cautiously but firmly.
   B. leave the patient alone.
   C. avoid making any show of force.
   D. be sure to maintain a clear path to an exit from the situation.

_____ 20. When transferring patient care to emergency department staff, the paramedic should:
   A. wait with the patient a maximum of 5 minutes before leaving the ED.
   B. leave the hand-off report at the receiving desk.
   C. introduce the patient by name to the receiving nurse or doctor and say good-bye to the patient before leaving.
   D. leave as soon as the receiving nurse or doctor looks at the patient.

Handout 9-3

Student's Name _____

CHAPTER 9 SCENARIO

Review the following real-life situation. Then answer the questions that follow.

On a cold November morning, Medic 3 responds to an elderly female having chest pain. It has been snowing and the roads are a little slick. The call comes in just before shift change. As Medic 3 arrives on scene, the fire department First Responders are already there. As the paramedic and his partner get out of the ambulance, he recognizes the house as one he has been to numerous times in the past. The patient often calls 911 for chest pain. The underlying cause usually turns out to be anxiety, as she has lived alone since her husband died 2 years ago. While the paramedic and his EMT-B partner walk up to the door, he complains rather loudly about having to come out in the cold, just before shift change, for a patient who probably has nothing wrong with her. The paramedic looks up and sees a concerned friend at the door, who has heard everything he has said.

The crew enters the living room of the small house to find fire department First Responders kneeling next to the seated patient, taking her vital signs. "So what is it this time, Hilda?" the paramedic asks the patient "The usual?" The patient and her friend who met the ambulance crew at the door look surprised. The First Responder taking the patient's blood pressure says, "She's complaining of crushing chest pain and short . . ." The paramedic interrupts the First Responder and says, "Yeah, I know. It's always the same." He sends his partner out to the ambulance for the stretcher and turns back to the First Responder. "Just jot down her vitals for me on some paper," he orders, "and we'll get her out of here." The First Responder complies. Because the stretcher is difficult to get down the narrow hall, the paramedic has the patient stand and walk to the stretcher at the front door.

The patient is transferred to the ambulance, and the paramedic gets into the patient compartment. He puts the patient on high flow, high concentration oxygen by nonrebreather mask and calls the hospital en route, giving them the vital signs obtained by the First Responder. Upon arrival at the hospital, the ambulance crew turns the patient over to the ER staff. The paramedic writes a quick prehospital care report, leaves a copy with the ER clerk, and quickly leaves.

1. What communication problems do you see in this situation?

2. What patient assessment and care problems do you see in this situation? What might be the consequences of such problems?

CHAPTER 9 REVIEW

Student's Name _____

Write the word or words that best complete the following sentences in the space provided.

1. _____ is the exchange of information using common symbols—written, spoken, or other forms such as signing or body language.

2. Identification with and understanding of another's situation, feelings, and motives is called _____.

3. To create a message is to _____.

4. To interpret a message is to _____.

5. A response to a message is _____.

6. Interaction with a patient for the purpose of obtaining in-depth information about the emergency and the patient's pertinent medical history is called a(n) _____ _____.

7. Gestures, mannerisms, and postures by which a person communicates with others are called _____ _____.

8. A posture or body position that is relaxed and suggests confidence, ease, warmth, and attentiveness is called a(n) _____ stance.

9. A posture or body position that is tense and suggests negativity, discomfort, fear, disgust, or anger is a(n) _____ stance.

10. The _____ zone ranges from 0 to 1.5 feet.

11. The _____ space ranges from 1.5 to 4 feet.

12. The area ranging from 4 to 12 feet around an individual is called _____ distance.

13. The area 12 feet or more away from a person is called _____ distance.

14. Questions framed to guide the direction of a patient's answers are called _____ questions.

15. Questions that permit unguided, spontaneous answers are _____-_____ questions.

16. Questions that ask for specific information and require only very short or yes-or-no answers are called _____ or _____ questions.

17. The feedback technique of echoing the speaker's message back to him in your own words is called _____.

18. A person who chooses to change the subject rather than discuss something difficult may be using _____ _____.

19. The imposition of one's beliefs, values, and patterns of behavior on people of another culture is called _____ _____.

20. Viewing one's own life as the most desirable, acceptable, or best and acting superior to another culture is called _____.

Handout 9-5

Student's Name _____

THERAPEUTIC COMMUNICATIONS LISTING

Complete the following lists.

1. Common reasons for failure of communication in EMS:
   A. _____
   B. _____
   C. _____
   D. _____

2. Techniques for building trust and rapport in the patient interview:
   A. _____
   B. _____
   C. _____
   D. _____
   E. _____
   F. _____
   G. _____

3. How to remember a name:
   A. _____
   B. _____
   C. _____

4. Interpersonal zones:
   A. Intimate zone: _____ feet
   B. Personal space: _____ feet
   C. Social distance: _____ feet
   D. Public distance: _____ feet

5. Feedback techniques:
   A. _____
   B. _____
   C. _____
   D. _____
   E. _____
   F. _____
   G. _____
   H. _____
   I. _____

Chapter 9 Answer Key

Handout 9-2: Chapter 9 Quiz

1. B	6. C	11. C	16. A
2. D	7. A	12. A	17. C
3. A	8. C	13. C	18. D
4. C	9. D	14. C	19.
5. D	10. A	15. B	20. C

Handout 9-3: Chapter 9 Scenario

1. The problems begin with the attitude of the paramedic who is complaining about having to take a call in the cold, right at shift change, to a location they have repeatedly been to. As he is stating his complaints, he notes a friend of the patient is standing at the door to meet them. He has already made a bad first impression on the friend who has heard his complaints. The paramedic is rude to the patient from the first contact, making an inappropriate statement about why she called the ambulance ("The usual?"). The paramedic has now made a bad first impression on the patient as well as on the friend. He then insults the First Responder by not listening to his report, saying, "Yeah, it's always the same."

2. The paramedic makes a major mistake in patient care by having a patient with chest pain walk to the stretcher by the front door. He does not perform a focused history or physical exam. Nor does he take an ECG, establish an IV, or even perform a good patient assessment. In his haste to get off work, the paramedic omits several steps in patient assessment and care. Just because the patient has frequently called 911 for chest pain that turns out to be anxiety, that does not mean she is not having a cardiac episode this time. A myocardial infarction could be taking place. Without the proper assessment and treatment, this patient could have increased damage to her heart muscle or even experience a cardiac arrest before her arrival at the hospital.

Handout 9-4: Chapter 9 Review

1. Communication
2. empathy
3. encode
4. decode
5. feedback
6. patient interview
7. nonverbal communication
8. open
9. closed
10. intimate
11. personal
12. social
13. public
14. leading
15. open-ended
16. closed, direct
17. reflection
18. avoidance language
19. cultural imposition
20. ethnocentrism

Handout 9-5: Therapeutic Communications Listing

1. **A.** Prejudice
   B. Lack of privacy
   C. External distractions
   D. Internal distractions
2. **A.** Use the patient's name.
   B. Address the patient appropriately.
   C. Modulate your voice.
   D. Use a professional but compassionate tone.
   E. Explain what you are doing and why.
   F. Keep a kind, calm expression.
   G. Use appropriate style of communication.
3. **A.** Say the name out loud three times.
   B. "See" the name in bold letters.
   C. "Feel" yourself writing the name.
4. **A.** 0–1.5
   B. 1.5–4
   C. 4–12
   D. 12 or more
5. **A.** Silence
   B. Reflection
   C. Facilitation
   D. Empathy
   E. Clarification
   F. Confrontation
   G. Interpretation
   H. Explanation
   I. Summarization

Essentials of Paramedic Care

Division 2

Patient Assessment

Chapter 10

History Taking

INTRODUCTION

Although patient history is an important component of any assessment, you may wish to stress to students that the history of a medical patient is more likely to yield information relevant to the emergency than in the trauma patient. They may learn more about a patient's condition by obtaining a history than by performing a physical exam. The areas of the body on which a physical exam is performed may be dictated by the history obtained from the patient. Frequently, the field diagnosis is based on the patient's medical history. Current chief complaints are often the manifestations of chronic or previous medical problems such as heart or respiratory diseases. This chapter focuses on how students can obtain a pertinent history of a patient. It begins by discussing appropriate interpersonal, communications, and questioning skills, then proceeds through an explanation of all the elements needed in a comprehensive patient history: preliminary data, chief complaint, present illness or injury, past history, current health status, and a review of the body systems. Special challenges to history taking are also discussed. Reiterate that obtaining a history is a skill as important as performing an assessment or providing treatment. Good history taking will result in good patient assessment and ultimately in good patient care and outcome.

TOTAL TEACHING TIME: 4.97 HOURS
The total teaching time is only a guideline based on the didactic and practical lab averages in the National Standard Curriculum. Instructors should take into consideration such factors as the pace at which students learn, the size of the class, and breaks. The actual time devoted to teaching objectives is the responsibility of the instructor.

CHAPTER OBJECTIVES

After reading this chapter, you should be able to:

1. Describe the techniques of history taking. (pp. 547–550)
2. Describe the structure, purpose, and how to obtain a comprehensive health history. (pp. 547–561)
3. List the components of a comprehensive history of an adult patient. (pp. 550–561)

FRAMING THE LESSON

Begin teaching of the lesson with a role-play scenario to engage students in the lesson. This 10-minute exercise is active (appeals to your kinesthetic learners) and interesting. It establishes the content of the lesson and may provide examples later in the lesson as students learn how to correct mistakes made here. For example, you play the role of a patient. Have one student or a team of students respond to you and attempt to gather a history. It is likely that the history they gather will not be perfect. Following their effort, ask the class as a whole to make a few notes about the content and quality of the history. You can refer back to these later. If students wrote that the history was very well developed, they may later wish to revise that statement when they learn how to do a proper history. If they thought it to be poor, they will find specific reasons for their feelings in the following lesson.

TEACHING STRATEGIES

People learn in a variety of ways. Some do better with the spoken word, whereas others prefer the written. Some prefer to work alone, whereas others profit from working in groups. Recognizing these different ways of acquiring knowledge, the authors of this *Instructor's Resource Manual* have provided a variety of teaching strategies for the different types of learners. These strategies are intended to foster higher-level cognitive skills and encourage creative learning and problem solving. For greatest effectiveness, incorporate these strategies into your class lecture. Symbols in the Lecture Outline indicate the points at which various exercises might be most appropriate. Other strategies can be used to preview the lesson or to summarize it.

The following strategies are keyed to specific sections of the lesson.

1. Working with the First Response Team. Discuss the importance of listening respectfully to the first response team's report and then gathering information from the patient himself. Disregarding the initial responders alienates them, making them feel they are not an important part of the health care team. Liken the first responder/paramedic interchange to the situation of a paramedic giving a report to the emergency department staff upon arrival.

2. Emphasizing a Professional Dress Code. Help students to look and feel professional by suggesting that a dress code be observed in class. People's behavior is influenced by how they look and feel. The dress code could be uniformlike clothing, such as will be required in the clinical and field settings, or the code could be less specific, such as "collared shirts required" or "no jeans." At the very least, you should be able to have visitors come to your classroom and feel that they have just met a group of professionals.

3. Illustrating Professional Appearance. Illustrate the idea that people make impressions based on appearance by showing your class a set of photographs of providers in different clothing. Ask students to rate the pictures on a scale of 1 (least professional) to 5 (most professional) on how the providers look. Show providers in scrubs, a department-issued T-shirt, a uniform with a badge, a polo-type shirt with a stethoscope around the neck, and so on. You could even ask students to describe the type of care (level, quality) the provider in each photograph provides. Discuss the findings as a group. It is likely that students will rate those in uniform more highly than those dressed more casually. This activity does more than illustrate the concept of professional appearance—it gives those who will eventually become managers and supervisors an important lesson when the issue of dress code or uniform is up for discussion at their service. In addition, this is a visual and verbal activity well-suited for your visual and oral learners.

4. Empathy Exercise. Pair students in the roles of patient and paramedic. Have the paramedic make the patient feel cared for without using words. To be successful, the students will have to employ the use of touch: Some will hold a hand; some will offer food; some will prop up the patient with pillows; some will cover the patient with a blanket. This activity illustrates the importance of touch and body language in patient care. It is both a creative-thinking exercise and a kinesthetic activity.

5. *Developing Skills in Asking Questions.* Arrange for three volunteers/students to play the roles of patients, and provide each with the same scenario/history. Divide the class into thirds. Have one third ask only open-ended questions, one third only closed-ended questions, and one third only multiple-choice questions. Have them time how long it takes to obtain standard history information such as SAMPLE, OPQRST, and AVPU. Then compare the information obtained by each group. The patient's history will probably seem different for each group, depending on the type of questions. The activity will emphasize that a good historian uses all types of questions, depending on the patient and situation. Additionally, this is an activity that helps to improve the language skills of your students.

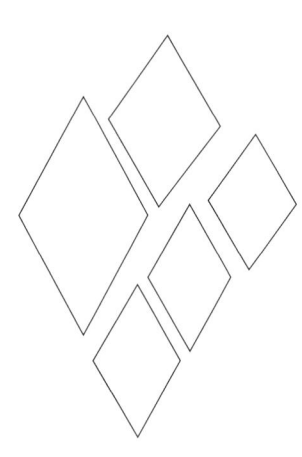

6. *Developing Communications Skills.* Help develop your students' communications skills with the "Diamond Description" activity. Pair students with their backs to one another. Those facing front will be the speakers, and those with their backs to the front will be those who draw. Put a picture of diamond shapes of various sizes on the overhead (such as the one that appears here). Have the speaker describe the shapes to the drawer. The drawer must follow the instructions and cannot ask for clarification. When everyone is done, let the drawers turn around and compare their drawings with the illustration on the overhead. Discuss the findings. This is both a right-brain (drawing and visualizing) and left-brain (speaking) activity.

7. *Interview Techniques.* Play audiotapes or videotapes of patient interviews, and ask students to identify the different types of interview techniques they hear or observe. Audiotapes can be created easily and inexpensively by your own staff simulating patient interviews. For videotapes, you could use commercial products such as Pulse tapes or video clips from documentary programs on the Learning Channel or a similar television station.

8. *Handling Sensitive Topics.* Unless you prepare your students with techniques for taking a history on sensitive topics such as physical deformities, violence and abuse, and sexual activity or dysfunction, it may take them years to become comfortable with these topics. The common approach for providers not skilled in this type of interview is to avoid sensitive topics altogether, possibly missing important information related to the patient's condition. Set up scenarios involving these difficult situations, and have students ask the pertinent questions as part of the history. If you do not feel skilled in asking the embarrassing and personal questions required for this type of interview, invite guests who have had such experience to help you. Consider employees from an AIDS clinic, a domestic violence shelter, or a veteran's hospital. Better yet, include a facility such as this in clinical rotations for your students. Make the interview a key part of the objectives for this clinical shift.

9. *Using a Flow Sheet.* Even your best student is not going to be able to make sense of and effectively use all the elements of inquiring into past medical history. Assign your students, working either individually or in groups, to develop their own flow sheets for this information. Have them use the flow sheet(s) during class simulations and perhaps even during clinical rotations until they can consistently employ the use of the elements of the past medical history.

10. Helping Patients with Special Challenges. Ask students to develop a tool to improve communications with a patient who has a special challenge. One example is a picture chart of common responses in place of words (used for hearing-impaired or non–English speakers). This exercise uses problem solving and allows the student to choose from a variety of media, for example, the written word, drawings, cutouts from magazines, music, computer programs. The classroom presentation of projects improves oral presentation skills and fosters self-esteem.

The following strategy can be used at various points throughout the lesson or to help summarize and demonstrate what students have learned.

Cultural Considerations, Legal Notes, and Patho Pearls. The Student CD-ROM contains this series of informative features to enhance the student's understanding of the material covered in this chapter.

TEACHING OUTLINE

Chapter 10, "History Taking," is the first lesson in Division 2, *Patient Assessment*. Distribute Handout 10-1 so that students can familiarize themselves with the learning goals for this chapter. If students have any questions about the objectives, answer them at this time.

Then present the chapter. One possible lecture outline follows. In the outline, the parenthetical references in regular type are references to text pages; those in bold type are references to figures, tables, or procedures.

I. Introduction. The ability to elicit a good history lays the foundation for quality patient care. (p. 547)

A. The history (p. 547)
  1. Chief complaint
  2. Past medical history
  3. Family and social history
  4. Lifestyle

B. The interview (p. 547)
  1. Establishes a bond between provider and patient
  2. May be altered by the patient's responses
  3. Differential field diagnosis

II. Establishing patient rapport. The care provider has only a few minutes to make a good impression on the patient. (pp. 547–550)

A. Setting the stage (pp. 547–548)
  1. When available, use the patient's chart
     a. Name
     b. Age
     c. Sex
     d. Race
     e. Marital status
     f. Address
     g. Occupation
     h. Past medical history
     i. Treatments rendered and effects
     j. Admitting diagnosis
  2. On emergency scenes, use the first responder's report
     a. Name
     b. Chief complaint

   c. Medication list
   d. Past medical history
   e. Initial vital signs
  3. Be sure not to be biased about the presenting problems based on the patient's chart, first responder report, past medical history, or dispatch information.
 B. The first impression (pp. 547–548)
  1. The first impression is based largely on appearance.
  2. Behaviors that reinforce these qualities
   a. Positioning oneself at eye level with the patient
   b. Giving the patient's requests high priority
   c. Using a calm, reassuring voice
   d. Nonverbal communication
 C. Asking questions (pp. 547–548)
  1. Open-ended questions
   a. Allow the most details
   b. Use patient's own words
   c. Are usually more accurate and complete
   d. May allow patients to wander off course
   e. Can be time-consuming
  2. Closed-ended questions
   a. Get short answers (one or two words)
   b. Are very direct questions
   c. Are appropriate for critical patients
   d. May mislead the patient
   e. Elicit limited information
  3. Multiple-choice questions
   a. Facilitate responses for patients having trouble describing their symptoms
 D. Language and communication (pp. 548–549)
  1. Good communication practices
   a. Avoid complicated medical terminology.
   b. Listen closely to the patient's responses.
   c. Watch for clues that the patient may not be telling the truth.
   d. Employ active listening.
  2. Facilitation
   a. Gestures or language that encourage the patient to talk
  3. Reflection
   a. Repeating the patient's words
  4. Clarification
   a. Asking for specific details to ensure the correct meaning
  5. Empathy
   a. Gestures or language that show an understanding or compassion for how the patient feels
  6. Confrontation
   a. Asking about inconsistencies in the patient's behavior or words
  7. Interpretation
   a. Questioning the patient about what the paramedic believes might be the problem based on the patient's actions or words
  8. Asking about feelings
   a. Questioning patients about how they are feeling about what they are experiencing
 E. Taking a history on sensitive topics (pp. 549–550)
  1. Some topics will be embarrassing or uncomfortable for both the provider and patient.
   a. Death and dying

TEACHING STRATEGY 2
Emphasizing a Professional Dress Code

TEACHING STRATEGY 3
Illustrating Professional Appearance

POINT TO EMPHASIZE
The paramedic has only a few minutes to make a positive first impression and gain the trust of the patient. Voice, body language, gestures, and eye contact should communicate caring, compassion, competence, and confidence.

TEACHING STRATEGY 4
Empathy Exercise

TEACHING STRATEGY 5
Developing Skills in Asking Questions

READING/REFERENCE
Coulehan, J. L., and M. R. Block. *The Medical Interview: Mastering Skills for Clinical Practice*. 4th ed. Philadelphia: F. A. Davis, 2001.

TEACHING STRATEGY 6
Developing Communications Skills

TEACHING STRATEGY 7
Interview Techniques

POINT TO EMPHASIZE
Listen to the patient. He will tell the caregiver what is wrong. Active listening is an important part of history taking. Active listening means responding to the patient's statements with words or gestures that demonstrate understanding.

TEACHING STRATEGY 8
Handling Sensitive Topics

    b. Sexual activity or dysfunction
    c. Physical deformities
    d. Violence and abuse
    e. Bodily functions

III. **The comprehensive patient history.** Common sense and clinical experience will determine how much of the following history to use. (pp. 550–558)
  A. Preliminary data (p. 550)
    1. Consider the source (patient, bystander, family member)
    2. Establish reliability of the information (medical record, first responder, other health care worker)
    3. Record information
      a. Date and time of exam
      b. Age
      c. Sex
      d. Race
      e. Birthplace
      f. Occupation
  B. The chief complaint (p. 551)
    1. The chief complaint is the reason EMS was called.
      a. Use open-ended questions.
      b. Document in patient's own words.
      c. Use your own observations of the presenting problem for the unconscious patient.
    2. The primary or presenting problem is the principal medical cause of the chief complaint.
  C. The present illness (pp. 551–552)
    1. Use the mnemonic OPQRST-ASPN to explore each complaint in greater detail.
      a. Onset
        i. How and when did the problem develop?
      b. Provocation/palliation
        i. What makes the symptoms better or worse?
      c. Quality
        i. Does the pain feel sharp, crushing, tearing, crampy?
      d. Region/radiation/referred
        i. Where is the symptom?
        ii. Does it go anywhere else?
        iii. Does the pain exist in a location away from its source?
      e. Severity
        i. How bad is the pain on a scale of 1 to 10?
      f. Time
        i. When did the symptom begin?
        ii. How long does it last?
      g. Associated symptoms
        i. What other symptoms commonly occurring with this chief complaint are present?
      h. Pertinent negatives
        i. Are other likely associated symptoms absent?
  D. The past history (p. 553)
    1. The past medical history may provide significant insight into the cause of the patient's chief complaint.
    2. Look in-depth at each of the following as they may relate to the patient
      a. General state of health
        i. How healthy does the patient describe himself or herself?

POWERPOINT PRESENTATION
Chapter 10, PowerPoint slides 14–24

TEACHING STRATEGY 9
Using a Flow Sheet

HANDOUT 10-2
Obtaining a Patient History

POINT OF INTEREST
Although there are several elements of the patient history, not every element may be appropriate or necessary for every patient. Common sense and clinical experience will determine which elements of the history to use.

  b. Childhood diseases
    i. What childhood diseases did the patient have (mumps, measles, rubella, chickenpox, rheumatic fever, polio)?
  c. Adult diseases
    i. Ask about preexisting medical conditions and their effect on the patient.
     a) Diabetes
     b) Hypertension
     c) Asthma
     d) COPD
     e) Seizures
     f) CAD
  d. Psychiatric illnesses
    i. Does the patient have a history of mental illnesses?
     a) Depression
     b) Mania
     c) Schizophrenia
  e. Accidents or injuries
    i. Has the patient had any major illness or injury that has required a hospital stay?
  f. Surgeries or hospitalizations
    i. Has the patient had any other hospitalizations or surgeries not already mentioned?
E. Current health status (pp. 554–556)
 1. The current health status assembles all of the factors of the patient's medical condition in an attempt to determine the presenting problem.
  a. Current medications
    i. What medications is the patient taking or supposed to be taking? (**Fig. 10-1, p. 554**)
     a) Prescription
     b) Over-the-counter
     c) Home remedies
     d) Vitamins
     e) Holistic preparations
  b. Allergies
    i. What allergies is the patient known to have?
     a) Medications
     b) Environment
     c) Food
  c. Tobacco
    i. Determine pack/year history by multiplying years smoked by packs per day.
  d. Alcohol, drug, or related substance abuse
    i. Quantify the use of alcohol and drugs by the patient without passing judgment.
    ii. Use the CAGE questionnaire to identify possible substance abuse:
     a) Have you ever felt the need to **Cut down** on your use?
     b) Have you ever felt **Annoyed** by criticism of your use?
     c) Have you ever had **Guilty** feelings about your use?
     d) Have you ever taken a drink/drugs first thing in the morning as an **Eye-opener**?
  e. Diet
    i. Determine normal input and output and any recent deviations.

- **f.** Screening tests
  - **i.** Ask about screening tests done for the patient, such as PPD, pap smear, mammograms, or occult blood tests.
- **g.** Immunizations
  - **i.** Ask about immunizations such as influenza, hepatitis, tetanus, and polio.
- **h.** Sleep patterns
  - **i.** Determine sleep patterns and variances.
- **i.** Exercise and leisure activities
  - **i.** Is the patient active or sedentary? Have there been any changes or limitations lately?
- **j.** Environmental hazards
  - **i.** Consider the possibility of hazardous materials in the patient's environment such as lead, air or water pollution, or toxic chemicals.
- **k.** Use of safety measures
  - **i.** Ask about helmets, pads, restraints, and even sunscreen.
- **l.** Family history
  - **i.** Determine any hereditary diseases experienced by parents, grandparents, siblings, aunts, and uncles, including:
    - **a)** Diabetes
    - **b)** Heart disease
    - **c)** Hypertension
    - **d)** Stroke
    - **e)** Kidney disease
    - **f)** Cancer
    - **g)** Seizures
    - **h)** Mental illness
    - **i)** Alcoholism
- **m.** Home situation and significant others
  - **i.** Determine the living conditions and support system of the patient.
- **n.** Daily life
  - **i.** Ask the patient to describe a typical day.
- **o.** Important experiences
  - **i.** Schooling
  - **ii.** Military experience
  - **iii.** Career
  - **iv.** Marital status
  - **v.** Hobbies
- **p.** Religious beliefs
  - **i.** Ask if the patient's religious beliefs place any limitations on the type of care he or she would want.
- **q.** The patient's outlook
  - **i.** Ask how the patient feels about the present and the future.

F. Review of systems (pp. 556–558)
  1. The review of systems should be tailored to the patient's complaint.
  2. General
     - **a.** Weight
     - **b.** Weakness
     - **c.** Fatigue
     - **d.** Fever
  3. Skin
     - **a.** Rashes
     - **b.** Lumps
     - **c.** Sores
     - **d.** Itching
     - **e.** Color changes

4. HEENT (Head, Eyes, Ears, Nose, and Throat)
    a. Headaches
    b. Visual disturbances
    c. Glasses or contact lenses
    d. Glaucoma or cataracts
    e. Hearing aids
    f. Tinnitus
    g. Vertigo
    h. Nasal discharge or stuffiness
    i. Nosebleeds
    j. Sinusitus
    k. Dentures
    l. Gum bleeding
    m. Sore throats
    n. Hoarseness
    o. Swollen glands
    p. Neck pain
    q. Aphagia
5. Respiratory
    a. Wheezing
    b. Coughing
    c. Hemoptysis
    d. Asthma
    e. Bronchitis
    f. Orthopnea
    g. Pneumonia
6. Cardiac
    a. Heart trouble
    b. Dysrhythmias
    c. Hypertension
    d. Chest pain
    e. Palpitations
    f. Dyspnea
    g. Edema
7. Gastrointestinal
    a. Aphagia
    b. Heartburn
    c. Anorexia
    d. Nausea
    e. Vomiting
    f. Hematemesis
    g. Indigestion
    h. Bowel movements
    i. Rectal bleeding
    j. Diarrhea
    k. Constipation
    l. Abdominal pain
    m. Flatulence
    n. Jaundice
    o. Gallbladder problems
8. Urinary
    a. Frequency
    b. Polyuria
    c. Nocturia
    d. Burning
    e. Pain
    f. Hematuria

     g. Urgency
     h. Incontinence
     i. Infection
     j. Stones
9. Male genitalia
     a. Hernia
     b. Discharge
     c. Sores
     d. Testicular pain
     e. STDs
10. Female genitalia
     a. Onset of menstruation
     b. Regularity and frequency of periods
     c. LMP
     d. Dysmenorrhea
     e. PMS
     f. Menopause
     g. Vaginal discharge
     h. Lumps
     i. Sores
     j. Itching
     k. STDs
     l. Gravida
     m. Para
     n. Abortions
     o. Living children
     p. Birth control
11. Peripheral vascular
     a. Calf pain
     b. Leg cramps
     c. Varicose veins
     d. Blood clots
12. Musculoskeletal
     a. Myalgia
     b. Joint pain
     c. Arthritis
     d. Gout
     e. Backaches
13. Neurologic
     a. Fainting
     b. Blackouts
     c. Seizures
     d. Aphasia
     e. Vertigo
     f. Weakness
     g. Headaches
     h. Paralysis
     i. Paresthesias
14. Hematologic
     a. Anemia
     b. Transfusions
     c. Bruising or bleeding
15. Endocrine
     a. Thyroid problems
     b. Heat or cold intolerance
     c. Excessive sweating
     d. Diabetes

           e. Polyuria
           f. Polyphagia
       16. Psychiatric
           a. Nervousness
           b. Tension
           c. Anxiety
           d. Stress
           e. Depression
           f. Attempted suicide

IV. Special challenges. Even the best paramedic will be occasionally challenged by certain patients. (pp. 558–562)

   A. Silence (p. 558)
       1. Is the patient in pain?
       2. Angry?
       3. Scared?
       4. Depressed?
       5. Offended?
   B. Overly talkative patients (p. 559)
       1. Is the patient nervous?
       2. Lonely?
       3. Excited?
   C. Patients with multiple symptoms (p. 559)
       1. Multiple disease states
       2. Psychosocial problem
       3. Confusion
   D. Anxious patients (p. 559)
       1. Tenseness
       2. Sweating
       3. Trembling
       4. Tachycardia
       5. Nausea
       6. Chest pain
       7. Hyperventilation
   E. Patients needing reassurance (p. 559)
   F. Anger and hostility (p. 559)
       1. Often the paramedic will be the target of someone's anger in a time of crisis.
       2. Protecting personal safety is the first priority.
   G. Intoxication (p. 560)
       1. Use police if necessary to ensure scene safety.
   H. Crying (p. 560)
       1. Be supportive and allow the patient to vent as necessary.
   I. Depression (p. 560)
       1. It is often misdiagnosed as insomnia or fatigue but can be life-threatening.
       2. Ask the patient specific questions about possible plans to hurt him- or herself.
   J. Sexually attractive patients (p. 560)
       1. Always be professional
       2. Keep a partner present to avoid accusations of improper behavior or touching.
   K. Confusing behavior or histories (pp. 560–561)
       1. Determine if dementia or delirium is the cause for inaccurate or inappropriate responses.

POWERPOINT PRESENTATION
Chapter 10, PowerPoint slides 25–27

TEACHING STRATEGY 10
Helping Patients with Special Challenges

POINT TO EMPHASIZE
Sometimes patients will present with special circumstances that challenge the skills of the paramedic. Remind students that time and experience will increase their ability to deal with patients who, for example, are silent, anxious, hostile, intoxicated, depressed, or speak a language they do not understand.

POINT OF INTEREST

AT&T has a service called "Language Line" that can provide an interpreter for any language. Determine the availability of this service in your area. A demonstration of how it works might be interesting for your students.

POWERPOINT PRESENTATION
Chapter 10, PowerPoint slide 28

WORKBOOK
Chapter 10 Activities

READING/REFERENCE
Textbook, pp. 564–650

HANDOUT 10-3
Chapter 10 Quiz

HANDOUT 10-4
Chapter 10 Scenario

PARAMEDIC STUDENT CD
Student Activities

COMPANION WEBSITE
http://www.prenhall.com/bledsoe

L. Limited intelligence (p. 561)
  1. Speak first to the patient; then fill in any gaps with history from family or friends.
M. Language barriers (p. 561)
  1. Use an interpreter if possible.
N. Hearing problems (p. 561)
  1. Handwriting responses
  2. Sign language
  3. Lip reading
O. Blindness (p. 561)
  1. Always identify yourself and other providers on scene.
  2. Allow the use of a cane or guide dog.
  3. Keep constant contact with the patient.
P. Talking with family or friends (pp. 561–562)
  1. Protect confidentiality at all costs when trying to supplement patient observations with information provided by family, friends, or bystanders. **(Fig. 10-2, p. 562)**

V. Chapter summary (p. 562). This chapter deals with taking a good history. Though it presents the patient history in its entirety, common sense will determine which parts are appropriate for a given situation. Most of a paramedic's work is patient contact. It is making a connection with people in crisis. Patients most often comment on the attitudes of their paramedics. How well did they relate to them? Did they make them feel at ease? Did they care for them? Patients rarely comment on a paramedic's technical skills. Top-notch paramedics are technically skillful and treat all their patients with dignity and compassion. This begins with the history.

Good patient interaction can lead to good patient outcomes, improved patient satisfaction, and better adherence to treatment. As a paramedic you may be your patient's first contact when he enters the health care world. Let his first impression of the health care industry be your caring, compassionate, professional demeanor. Conducting effective and efficient interviews and communicating with your patient are essential to good medical practice. Medical interviewing is a basic clinical skill that must be learned and practiced, much like airway management.

ASSIGNMENTS

Assign students to complete Chapter 10, "History Taking," of the workbook. Also assign them to read Chapter 11, "Physical Exam Techniques," before the next class.

EVALUATION

Chapter Quiz and Scenario Distribute copies of the Chapter Quiz provided in Handout 10-3 to evaluate student understanding of this chapter. Make sure each student reads the scenario to reinforce critical thinking on the scene. Remind students not to use their notes or textbooks while taking the quiz.

Student CD Quizzes for every chapter are contained on the dynamic and highly visual in-text student CD.

Companion Website Additional quizzes for every chapter are contained on this exciting website.

TestGen   You may wish to create a custom-tailored test using *Prentice Hall TestGen for Essentials of Paramedic Care*, 2nd Edition to evaluate student understanding of this chapter.

On-line Test Preparation (for students and instructors)   Additional test preparation is available through Brady's new on-line product, *EMT Achieve: Paramedic Test Preparation* at *http://www.prenhall.com/emtachieve/*. Instructors can also monitor student mastery on-line.

Review Manual for the EMT-Paramedic   This comprehensive exam review contains hundreds of test questions and rationales, including scenarios, along with two 180-question practice tests on CD.

REINFORCEMENT

Handouts   If classroom discussion or performance on the quiz indicates that some students have not fully mastered the chapter content, you may wish to assign some or all of the Reinforcement Handouts for this chapter.

Student CD (for students)   A wide variety of material on this CD-ROM will reinforce and also expand student knowledge and skills.

PowerPoint Presentation (for instructors)   The PowerPoint material developed for this chapter offers useful reinforcement of chapter content.

Companion Website (for students)   Additional review quizzes and links to EMS resources will contribute to further reinforcement of the chapter.

OneKey   On-line support is offered for this course on one of three platforms: CourseCompass, Blackboard, or Web CT. Includes the IRM, PowerPoints, TestGen, and Companion Website for instruction. Ask your local sales representative for more information.

Brady Skills Series: Advanced Life Skills (Video or CD)   Have your students watch the skills come to life on VHS or CD-ROM, or they can purchase the highly visual, full-color text with step-by-step procedures and rationales.

TestGen
Chapter 10

EMT Achieve: Paramedic Test Preparation
Mistovich & Beasley. *EMT Achieve: Paramedic Test Preparation*. www.prenhall.com/emtachieve/

Review Manual for the EMT-Paramedic
Cherry & Mistovich. *Review Manual for the EMT-Paramedic*, 3rd edition.

Handouts 10-5 through 10-7
Reinforcement Activities

Paramedic Student CD
Student Activities

PowerPoint Presentation
Chapter 10

Companion Website
http://www.prenhall.com/bledsoe

OneKey
Chapter 10

Advanced Life Support Skills
Larmon & Davis. *Advanced Life Support Skills*.

Advanced Life Skills Review
Larmon & Davis. *Advanced Life Skills Review*.

Brady Skills Series: ALS
Larmon & Davis. *Brady Skills Series: ALS*.

Paramedic National Standards Self-Test
Miller. *Paramedic National Standards Self-Test*, 4th edition.

Handout 10-1

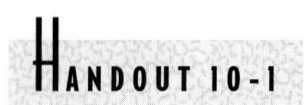

Student's Name _____

CHAPTER 10 OBJECTIVES CHECKLIST

Knowledge	Date Mastered
1. Describe the techniques of history taking.	
2. Describe the structure, purpose, and how to obtain a comprehensive health history.	
3. List the components of a comprehensive history of an adult patient.	

Handout 10-2

Student's Name _____

OBTAINING A PATIENT HISTORY

Charting Student Progress:
1. *Learning skill*
2. *Performs skill with direction*
3. *Performs skill independently*

Procedure	1	2	3
1. Establishes patient rapport and trust.			
2. Performs proper introductions.			
3. Asks appropriate open-ended and closed-ended questions.			
4. Demonstrates active listening skills.			
5. Obtains preliminary data.			
6. Obtains chief complaint.			
7. Obtains history of present illness or injury.			
8. Obtains information on pertinent past history.			
9. Obtains information on current health status.			
10. Performs a review of body systems.			
11. Handles special challenges appropriately.			

Comments:

HANDOUT 10-3

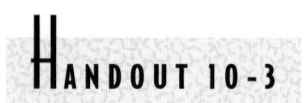

Student's Name _____

CHAPTER 10 QUIZ

Write the letter of the best answer in the space provided.

_____ 1. You are dispatched to an extended care facility for a 50-year-old male who is complaining of shortness of breath. When you arrive, staff tells you his name is Herman Baxter. As you approach him, you should call him by what name until told otherwise by the patient?
   A. Herman
   B. "Partner"
   C. Mr. Baxter
   D. any of these

_____ 2. Which of the following is an example of proper nonverbal communication used to gain the patient's trust?
   A. avoiding eye contact with the patient
   B. standing over the patient as you talk with him
   C. offering a comforting touch to the patient's arm or hand
   D. using slang terms or names, such as "Mack" or "Pops"

_____ 3. Within the first few minutes that you are on the scene, you will want to make a positive first impression. Which of the following is true regarding positive first impressions?
   A. Give the patient's requests and concerns high priority.
   B. Your physical appearance has little to do with the first impression.
   C. Direct eye contact with the patient will intimidate him.
   D. It is important to use a firm tone in your voice to keep control of the situation.

_____ 4. Which of the following is an example of a closed-ended question?
   A. "Tell me what your chest pain feels like."
   B. "Do you take any medication for your asthma?"
   C. "Where do you hurt?"
   D. "What were you doing just before you fell?"

_____ 5. The statement "You tell me that you are not short of breath, yet you cannot say more than two words without taking a breath" is an example of which type of active listening?
   A. facilitation
   B. clarification
   C. confrontation
   D. empathy

_____ 6. Which of the following illustrates the active listening skill of reflection?
   A. Patient: "I can't breathe." Paramedic: "You can't breathe?" Patient: "No, I can't take a full breath because my chest hurts." Paramedic: "Your chest hurts, too?"
   B. Paramedic: "Do you have any allergies?" Patient: "Yes, the last time I took codeine, I had a bad reaction." Paramedic: "Can you describe the reaction?" Patient: "I got really nauseated and had cold sweats."
   C. The paramedic maintains sincere eye contact and uses cues such as, "Mm-hmm," "Go on," and so on.
   D. Paramedic: "You say your chest doesn't hurt, but you keep rubbing it. Are you afraid you are having a heart attack but don't want to admit it?"

_____ 7. The patient's age, sex, race, birthplace, and occupation are included in which element of the comprehensive patient history?
   A. past history
   B. preliminary data
   C. current health status
   D. none of these

_____ 8. The mnemonic OPQRST-ASPN is a tool used during which element of the comprehensive patient history?
   A. chief complaint
   B. past history
   C. present illness/injury
   D. current health status

340 ESSENTIALS OF PARAMEDIC CARE

HANDOUT 10-3 Continued

_____ 9. Which of the following is true regarding the patient's chief complaint?
   A. The chief complaint is asked as a closed-ended question.
   B. The chief complaint is the reason EMS was called.
   C. An accurate chief complaint can always be determined from dispatch information.
   D. The chief complaint is the same as the primary problem.

_____ 10. In the OPQRST mnemonic, the "P" stands for:
   A. pertinent negatives.
   B. past medical history.
   C. prescription medications.
   D. provocative/palliative factors.

_____ 11. The term *referred pain* means pain that:
   A. is not really there, as in an amputated limb.
   B. is felt at a location away from its source.
   C. has been relieved or is not as severe as it previously was.
   D. is elicited through palpation.

_____ 12. Which of the following statements about obtaining a patient's past medical history is true?
   A. Your field diagnosis may be based primarily on the patient's past history.
   B. Asking about past medical history is a formality only and has little bearing on your care of the patient.
   C. Asking about childhood diseases is always relevant.
   D. Use the mnemonic OPQRST-ASPN when questioning about past history.

_____ 13. The patient's current health status should include questions regarding:
   A. surgeries and hospitalizations.
   B. the onset of the chief complaint.
   C. tobacco, alcohol, and drug use.
   D. childhood diseases.

_____ 14. The CAGE questionnaire should be employed when investigating:
   A. the patient's chief complaint.
   B. alcohol use.
   C. the history of the present illness/injury.
   D. tobacco (cigarette, cigar, smokeless) use.

_____ 15. The patient's home situation, daily life, and religious beliefs are among the elements that may be determined when investigating the patient's:
   A. current health status.   C. present illness.
   B. past medical history.   D. preliminary data.

_____ 16. Which of the following statements is true regarding the review of systems?
   A. Your history taking should begin with questions regarding the systems.
   B. The questions you ask will be determined by the patient's chief complaint, condition, and clinical status.
   C. It is important to ask all questions in the review of systems of each patient.
   D. The questions asked in the review of systems include sleep patterns and family history.

_____ 17. A sudden onset of shortness of breath at night is called:
   A. nocturia.
   B. hemoptysis.
   C. paroxysmal nocturnal dyspnea.
   D. chronic obstructive pulmonary disease.

HANDOUT 10-3 Continued

_____ 18. The term *gravida* refers to the number of:
   A. times a woman has been pregnant.
   B. viable births a woman has had.
   C. abortions a woman has had.
   D. living children the woman has.

_____ 19. A mood disorder characterized by hopelessness and malaise is known as:
   A. dementia.   C. depression.
   B. delirium.   D. dysmenorrhea.

_____ 20. Which of the following statements is true regarding history taking with patients who present with special circumstances?
   A. Crying should be accepted as a natural release, and not suppressed.
   B. Your first concern with a violent patient is your own safety.
   C. Always keep your relationship with the patient professional.
   D. All of these are true.

HANDOUT 10-4

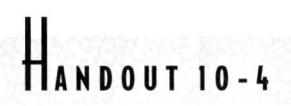

Student's Name _____

CHAPTER 10 SCENARIO

Review the following real-life situation. Then answer the questions that follow.

You receive an early-morning call to a residence for an elderly female who is complaining of chest tightness. While you are en route, the dispatcher advises you that you are responding to a 67-year-old female patient, conscious and breathing, who was awakened by chest pain this morning. When you arrive, fire department EMTs are on scene. The patient's daughter meets you at the door. She tells you her mother lives with her and woke up this morning with bad chest pain. The patient is very anxious. You find her lying in bed, clutching her chest, with labored breathing. It is obvious that she is alert and breathing, but you note sweating and pale skin.

The fire department EMTs have applied high-concentration oxygen and taken vital signs. Her respirations and pulse are rapid, and her blood pressure is lower than normal. You apply your cardiac monitor, which shows a rapid heart rate, but no other irregularities. As you start an IV of 5 percent dextrose solution, you obtain her history. She rates her chest pain as the worst she has ever had. She had a heart attack about 3 years ago and is on several medications. She has taken three nitroglycerin tablets in the past 10 minutes without relief. You contact medical control and receive permission to administer IV morphine for the pain. Within a few minutes, the patient's chest pain has lessened. You transfer the patient to your stretcher and move her to the ambulance. You continue your patient assessment while en route and arrive at the hospital without any further complications.

1. On your arrival at the scene, you note the patient is very anxious. What methods would you use to establish a rapport with her? How would you gain her confidence?

2. The patient is having difficulty describing exactly what she feels. She is using vague, generalized words. What type of active listening skill would work best in this situation?

3. Which elements of the comprehensive patient history would you use in this scenario?

4. Which elements of the review of systems would you ask about in this scenario?

HANDOUT 10-5

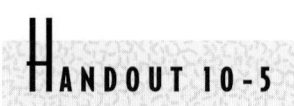

Student's Name _____

CHAPTER 10 REVIEW

Write the word or words that best complete the following sentences in the space provided.

1. The list of possible causes for your patient's symptoms is known as the _____ _____ _____.
2. The reason the ambulance was called to respond is known as the _____ _____.
3. The list of active listening skills includes _____, _____, _____, _____, _____, and _____.
4. Questions that elicit a one- or two-word answer are called _____-_____ questions.
5. Questions that allow your patient to answer in detail are called _____-_____ questions.
6. The underlying cause of a patient's symptoms is the _____ _____.
7. The use of a 1 to 10 scale is often helpful in determining the _____ of a patient's pain.
8. A practical template for exploring chief complaints is the mnemonic _____-_____.
9. The pain that is elicited through palpation is called _____.
10. The pain that is felt at a location away from its source is called _____ pain.
11. The absence of any likely associated symptom is known as a(n) _____ _____.
12. Your patient has a chief complaint of chest pain and also complains of shortness of breath, nausea, and vomiting. These latter complaints are known as _____ _____.
13. The acronym HEENT refers to the _____, _____, _____, _____, and _____.
14. The CAGE questionnaire is asked regarding the use of _____ or _____.
15. The list of questions categorized by body system is known as the _____ _____ _____.
16. Difficulty breathing while lying supine is called _____.
17. Coughing up blood is called _____.
18. Menstrual difficulties are called _____.
19. Polyuria is the name given to excessive _____.
20. A deterioration of mental status that is usually associated with structural neurological disease is called _____.

HANDOUT 10-6

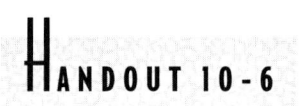

Student's Name _____

HISTORY MATCHING

Match the active listening skills with the appropriate examples.

A. Empathy
B. Facilitation
C. Interpretation
D. Reflection
E. Clarification
F. Confrontation
G. Asking about feelings

_____ 1. "I can't breathe."
"You can't breathe?"
"I can't take a full breath because my chest hurts."
"Your chest hurts, too?"

_____ 2. "Do you have any allergies?"
"Yes, the last time I ate peanuts, I had a bad reaction."
"Can you describe the reaction?"
"I got itchy all over with a rash."

_____ 3. "Mm-hmm." "Go on." "I'm listening."

_____ 4. "I understand." "That must have been very difficult."

_____ 5. "You say your chest doesn't hurt, but you keep rubbing it."

_____ 6. "You say your chest doesn't hurt, but you keep rubbing it. Are you afraid you are having a heart attack but don't want to admit it?"

_____ 7. "How do you feel about what's happening?"

HANDOUT 10-7

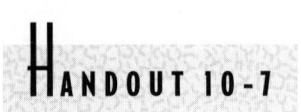

Student's Name _____

HISTORY LISTING

1. List five conditions that should lead you to consider the possibility of physical abuse when assessing a patient.
   _____
   _____
   _____
   _____
   _____

2. List the six elements of the comprehensive patient history.
   _____
   _____
   _____
   _____
   _____
   _____

3. List the four questions asked in the CAGE questionnaire.
   _____
   _____
   _____
   _____

Chapter 10 Answer Key

Handout 10-3 Chapter 10 Quiz

1. C	6. A	11. B	16. B
2. C	7. B	12. A	17. C
3. A	8. C	13. C	18. A
4. B	9. B	14. B	19. C
5. C	10. D	15. A	20. D

Handout 10-4: Chapter 10 Scenario

1. Present yourself as a caring, compassionate, competent, and confident health care professional. Use a calm, reassuring voice. Maintain eye contact with the patient. Introduce yourself, and ask the patient what she would like you to call her. Kneel or sit beside the patient, addressing her at eye level or lower. Make contact by offering a comforting touch.
2. In crisis, patients often cannot clearly describe what they feel. They use vague, general words. Do not hesitate to ask for clarification.
3. For documentation, always record preliminary data, such as date and time of the exam, the patient's age, sex, race, birthplace, and occupation. Then proceed to an open-ended question asking about your patient's chief complaint. Use the mnemonic OPQRST-ASPN and gather information on the present illness. The past history may provide significant insights into the patient's chief complaint and your field diagnosis. But, only parts of the past history may be pertinent. In this case, general state of health, adult diseases, and surgeries or hospitalizations would be appropriate questions to ask. Current health status questions should include current medications and allergies. Review of systems will most likely be limited to those suggested by the chief complaint. The respiratory and cardiac systems questions should be asked.
4. Review of systems will most likely be limited to those suggested by the chief complaint. The respiratory and cardiac systems questions should be asked.

Handout 10-5: Chapter 10 Review

1. differential field diagnosis
2. chief complaint
3. facilitation, reflection, clarification, empathy, confrontation, interpretation
4. closed-ended
5. open-ended
6. primary problem
7. severity
8. OPQRST-ASPN
9. tenderness
10. referred
11. pertinent negative
12. associated symptoms
13. head, eyes, ears, nose, throat
14. alcohol, drugs
15. review of systems
16. orthopnea
17. apoptosis
18. dysmenorrhea
19. urination
20. dementia

Handout 10-6: History Matching

1. D	3. B	5. F	7. G
2. E	4. A	6. C	

Handout 10-7: History Listing

1. Injuries that are inconsistent with the story given. Injuries that embarrass your patient. A delay between the time of the injury and seeking help. A past history of "accidents." Suspicious behavior of the supposed abuser.
2. Preliminary data, chief complaint, present illness/injury, past history, current health status, and review of systems.
3. Have you ever felt the need to *Cut* down on your drinking? Have you ever felt *Annoyed* by criticism of your drinking? Have you ever had *Guilty* feelings about drinking? Have you ever taken a drink first thing in the morning as an *Eye*-opener?

Chapter 11

Physical Exam Techniques

INTRODUCTION

Patient assessment is one of the most important, essential skills a paramedic will perform. Without an adequate, efficient physical assessment of a patient, important clues to the patient's condition may be missed. This can result in inadequate or improper patient care procedures. Although EMT-Basics are taught patient assessment, the assessments performed by the paramedic are more detailed and thorough because many of the ALS skills performed are potentially dangerous. The physical exam begins when the paramedic first sees the patient and may continue throughout the entire time the paramedic is with the patient. This chapter discusses the various physical exam techniques, gives an overview of a comprehensive examination, and explains each component of a physical exam in detail. This chapter also includes the special considerations for performing a physical exam on an infant or child.

CHAPTER OBJECTIVES

After reading this chapter, you should be able to:

1. Define and describe the techniques of inspection, palpation, percussion, and auscultation. (pp. 566–569)
2. Describe the evaluation of mental status. (pp. 629–632)
3. Evaluate the importance of a general survey. (pp. 576–584)
4. Describe the examination of the following body regions, differentiate between normal and abnormal findings, and define the significance of abnormal findings:
   - skin, hair, and nails (pp. 585–590)
   - head, scalp, and skull (pp. 590, 592)
   - eyes, ears, nose, mouth, and pharynx (pp. 590–603)
   - neck (pp. 603–604)
   - thorax (anterior and posterior) (pp. 605–609)
   - arterial pulse including rate, rhythm, and amplitude (pp. 609–612)
   - jugular venous pressure and pulsations (pp. 609–612)
   - heart and blood vessels (pp. 609–612)
   - abdomen (pp. 612–615)
   - male and female genitalia (p. 615)
   - anus and rectum (pp. 615–616)

TOTAL TEACHING TIME: 17.01 HOURS

The total teaching time is only a guideline based on the didactic and practical lab averages in the National Standard Curriculum. Instructors should take into consideration such factors as the pace at which students learn, the size of the class, and breaks. The actual time devoted to teaching objectives is the responsibility of the instructor.

©2007 Pearson Education, Inc.
Essentials of Paramedic Care, 2nd ed.

349

- peripheral vascular system (pp. 625, 627–629)
- musculoskeletal system (pp. 616–625)
- nervous system (pp. 629–642)
- cranial nerves (pp. 632–635)

5. Describe the assessment of visual acuity. (pp. 590–592)
6. Explain the rationale for the use of an ophthalmoscope and otoscope. (pp. 575, 593–596, 597–599)
7. Describe the survey of respiration. (pp. 570–572, 605–609)
8. Describe percussion of the chest. (pp. 567–568, 606, 607, 609)
9. Differentiate the percussion notes and their characteristics. (pp. 567–568)
10. Describe special examination techniques related to the assessment of the chest. (pp. 605–609)
11. Describe the auscultation of the chest, heart, and abdomen. (pp. 606–613)
12. Distinguish between normal and abnormal auscultation findings of the chest, heart, and abdomen and explain their significance. (pp. 606–613)
13. Describe special techniques of the cardiovascular examination. (pp. 609–612)
14. Describe the general guidelines of recording examination information. (p. 647)
15. Discuss the examination considerations for an infant or child. (pp. 642–647)

FRAMING THE LESSON

Begin the session with a review of anatomy and physiology of the human body and its systems to orient students to the scope of the physical examination. Using a mannequin or an outline of the human body on a flip chart or board, have the class identify the location and function of important body systems and individual organs. Then have the students describe the function of those organs and systems, as well as the signs and symptoms that might appear when each of these systems malfunctions or fails.

TEACHING STRATEGIES

People learn in a variety of ways. Some do better with the spoken word whereas others prefer the written. Some prefer to work alone, whereas others profit from working in groups. Recognizing these different ways of acquiring knowledge, the authors of this *Instructor's Resource Manual* have provided a variety of teaching strategies for the different types of learners. These strategies are intended to foster higher-level cognitive skills and encourage creative learning and problem solving. For greatest effectiveness, incorporate these strategies into your class lecture. Symbols in the Lecture Outline indicate the points at which various exercises might be most appropriate. Other strategies can be used to preview the lesson or to summarize it.

The following strategies are keyed to specific sections of the lesson.

1. Approaching the Patient. You can illustrate the idea that much is to be learned about your patient without actually speaking to him by flashing slides or photos of patients. Ask students what they "know" about the patient by just looking. They should be able to tell approximate age, gender, weight, physical conditioning or general health, grooming habits, level of distress, level of consciousness on the AVPU scale, position of comfort, mechanism of injury, and so on. This is particularly important when treating nonverbal, unconscious, or non–English-speaking patients. This is a visual activity.

2. ***Recognizing Exam Techniques.*** Create a list of physical findings and have students demonstrate how the information is obtained. For instance, a bruise is discovered by inspection. Chest wall instability is found on palpation. Rales are found by auscultation. This is a psychomotor activity that can be done during the course of lecturing on these techniques, rather than waiting for a skills lab.

3. ***Physical Examination Equipment.*** Bring examples of each type of examination equipment to class. Use class members as patients to demonstrate each piece of equipment's use, and then have one class member use that piece of equipment to examine another class member. Finally, have stations set up where students can work in pairs or teams to practice using each type of equipment.

4. ***Mastering Vital Signs.*** It is important to create challenging situations for students when teaching the measurement of vital signs. At this point in their careers, most paramedic students have taken literally hundreds of sets of vitals. They may become careless with these very important skills as they acquire seemingly more advanced lifesaving skills. Emphasize to students the importance of a complete, accurate set of vital signs. Use the following activities to aid in the practice of vital sign gathering:

- Place simulated patients in difficult positions, such as prone or fetal. Have some patients wear bulky or layered clothing. Have some be in a great deal of pain or distress. Then have students attempt to take vital signs.
- In pairs, have students locate as many pulses as possible on their partners. Mark the locations with washable marker. Offer a prize to the student who correctly locates the most pulse points. This is a psychomotor activity that can be done in less than 10 minutes in class, rather than waiting for lab time.
- Be sure to emphasize the importance of accurate blood pressure measurement. Do not allow students in class to palpate blood pressures. This is an inaccurate measurement and should be reserved for dire situations. Encourage good habits and skills by requiring students to actually take the victim's blood pressure in simulations before the scenario patient's blood pressure is given to the student. Don't forget to cover specifics of the equipment as well, such as how to size the cuff, how to calibrate it, and how to place it on the extremity. Preceptors, partners, employers, and patients will appreciate your diligence in creating good habits related to basic physical exam techniques.

5. ***Conducting Physical Exams of Infants and Children.*** Discuss how conducting a physical exam of a sick or injured child can challenge the paramedic. Have class members who are parents bring their children to class for students to practice history taking and physical exams. Attempt to have a wide age range of infants and children present so students may gain as much experience as possible with a variety of ages. Remember to have the parent present during the practice session to avoid frightening the infant or child.

6. ***Developing Reporting Skills.*** Develop or obtain textbooks of scenarios of various medical problems (for example, Braunworth and Howe's *Street Scenarios for the EMT and Paramedic* published by Brady), and have students role-play patients and paramedics. Based on information the students role-playing paramedics obtain from the history and physical exam of the patients, have them complete a patient care report. Obtain blank patient care reports from the local ambulance service or state EMS office for students to practice with.

7. Cultural Considerations: A Matter of Respect. Ask representatives from various cultures in your community to speak to the students about their beliefs and practices. There are a variety of practices that may affect your assessment and management of patients in your area. By understanding some basic principles of these cultures you will be able to obtain better patient information, avoid embarrassment and possibly insult, and better achieve the goal of providing the best patient care possible.

The following strategies can be used at various points throughout the lesson or to help summarize and demonstrate what the students have learned.

Role-Playing the Physical Exam. After discussing each component of the comprehensive physical examination in detail, have the students practice that particular component of the exam. When you have reached the end of the chapter, role-play a patient to combine all of the exam components. Have the students work as a group, first to obtain an appropriate history and then to perform a comprehensive physical examination based on your history.

Classroom Physical Exam Practice. Ask for help from members of ambulance crews, hospital staffs, EMS instructors, or other health care professionals in arranging to bring in volunteer patients ranging in age from young adults to the elderly. Give each patient a scenario, clinical findings, and instructions on how to act with his specific condition. You may also have a clinical instructor stationed with each patient. Have students rotate to each patient as if they were responding to EMS calls as paramedics. Have them obtain a history and perform an appropriate physical exam. This includes proper interaction with the patients.

Practice in the Field. A single day to practice the comprehensive patient assessment in a clinical setting would enhance students' skills in this area. Arrange time in a well-baby clinic, nursing home, or rehabilitation center where acuity is low and ample time can be spent on thorough assessments. Supervision by a nurse practitioner, physician assistant, or physician would be ideal because the average nurse or technician is less likely to conduct comprehensive physical examinations.

Guest Lecturer. Physicians specializing in internal medicine and physician assistants are very knowledgeable about patient assessment and can present and demonstrate a comprehensive patient assessment. Consider bringing one of these medical professionals to a class session during your instruction of patient assessment.

Cultural Considerations, Legal Notes, and Patho Pearls. The Student CD-ROM contains this series of informative features to enhance the student's understanding of the material covered in this chapter.

TEACHING OUTLINE

Chapter 11, "Physical Exam Techniques," is the second lesson in Division 2, *Patient Assessment*. Distribute Handout 11-1 so that students can familiarize themselves with the learning goals for this chapter. If students have any questions about the objectives, answer them at this time.

Then present the chapter. One possible lecture outline follows. In the outline, the parenthetical references in regular type are references to text pages; those in bold type are references to figures, tables, or procedures.

I. Introduction. The purpose of the physical exam is to investigate areas that you suspect are involved in your patient's primary problem. (p. 565)

II. Approach and overview (pp. 565-576)

  A. Examination techniques (pp. 566–573)

   1. Inspection (**Fig. 11-1, p. 566**)

HANDOUT 11-1
Chapter 11 Objectives Checklist

TEACHING STRATEGY 1
Approaching the Patient

POINT TO EMPHASIZE
Always take appropriate body substance isolation precautions, and assume every patient is infectious. If it's wet, and not yours, don't touch it without protection.

POWERPOINT PRESENTATION
Chapter 11 PowerPoint slide 4

POWERPOINT PRESENTATION
Chapter 11 PowerPoint slides 5–37

2. Palpation (**Fig. 11-2, p. 567**)
   3. Percussion (**Fig. 11-3, p. 568**) (**Table 11-1, p. 568**)
   4. Auscultation (**Fig. 11-4, p. 569**)
   5. Measurement of vital signs.
      a. Pulse (**Fig. 11-5, p. 570**)
         i. Rate
            a) Bradycardia
            b) Tachycardia
         ii. Rhythm
         iii. Quality
      b. Respiration (**Table 11-2, p. 572**)
         i. Rate
            a) Bradypnea
            b) Tachypnea
         ii. Effort
         iii. Quality
         iv. Tidal volume
      c. Blood pressure
         i. Systolic
         ii. Diastolic
         iii. Korotkoff's sounds
         iv. Pulse pressure
         v. Hypertension
         vi. Hypotension
      d. Body temperature
         i. Hyperthermia
         ii. Hypothermia
B. Equipment (pp. 573–575)
   1. Stethoscope (**Fig. 11-6, p. 573**)
      a. To auscultate most sounds
   2. Sphygmomanometer (**Fig. 11-7, p. 574**)
      a. To measure blood pressure
   3. Ophthalmoscope (**Fig. 11-8, p. 575**)
      a. To examine the interior of the eyes
   4. Otoscope (**Fig. 11-9, p. 575**)
      a. To inspect ear canal and tympanic membrane
   5. Scale (**Fig. 11-10, p. 575**)
      a. To weigh the patient
   6. Tongue blades (**Fig. 11-11, p. 576**)
      a. To inspect mouth and check gag reflexes
   7. Thermometer (**Fig. 11-11, p. 576**)
      a. To measure body temperature
   8. Penlight (**Fig. 11-11, p. 576**)
      a. To test pupillary response
   9. Visual acuity chart/card (**Fig. 11-11, p. 576**)
      a. To measure visual acuity
   10. Reflex hammer (**Fig. 11-11, p. 576**)
      a. To test deep tendon reflexes
D. General approach (pp. 575–576)
   1. How you approach your patient, both in the emergency setting and elsewhere, will set the stage for an efficient and effective patient assessment.

III. Overview of a comprehensive examination. You will determine which elements to use based on the patient's presenting problem and clinical status. (pp. 576–585)

TEACHING STRATEGY 2
Recognizing Exam Techniques

POINT TO EMPHASIZE
Repeat vital signs often and look for trends

POINT TO EMPHASIZE
Abnormal respirations require rapid intervention, which may save the patient's life.

TEACHING STRATEGY 3
Physical Examination Equipment

POINT TO EMPHASIZE
To make palpation therapeutic and respectful, keep your hands warm, keep your fingernails short, and be gentle.

READING/REFERENCE
Bates, B. L., L. S. Bickley, and R. A. Hoekelman. *A Guide to Physical Examination and History Taking.* 8th ed. Philadelphia: J. B. Lippincott, 2002.

Swartz, M. H. *Textbook of Physical Diagnosis, 4th Edition—History and Examination.* Philadelphia: Elsevier, 2002.

POWERPOINT PRESENTATION
Chapter 11, PowerPoint slides 38–58

TEACHING TIP
At the beginning of each session, have students assess vital signs on each other and record them.

TEACHING STRATEGY 4
Mastering Vital Signs

POINT OF INTEREST
Remember that the cardiac monitor shows only electrical, not mechanical, activity. Always compare what you see on the monitor with the patient's pulse.

TEACHING TIP
Include as much hands-on assessment practice with actual patients, real or simulated, as possible.

READING/REFERENCE
Bledsoe, B., and R. Martini. *Anatomy and Physiology for Emergency Care*. 1st ed. Upper Saddle River, NJ: Prentice Hall, 2002.

POWERPOINT PRESENTATION
Chapter 11, PowerPoint slides 59–151 (Part 1), 4–143 (Part 2)

TEACHING TIP
Don't allow your students to practice mistakes. Always have clinical instructors observe practice sessions so corrections can be made quickly.

A. The general survey (pp. 576–585)
  1. Appearance
      a. Level of consciousness
      b. Signs of distress
      c. Apparent state of health
      d. Vital statistics
      e. Sexual development
      f. Skin color and obvious lesions
      g. Posture, gait, and motor activity
      h. Dress, grooming, and personal hygiene
      i. Odors of breath and/or body
      j. Facial expression
  2. Vital signs (**Proc. 11-1, pp. 580–581**)
      a. Pulse
      b. Respiration
      c. Blood pressure
      d. Temperature
  3. Additional assessment techniques
      a. Pulse oximetry (**Fig. 11-12, p. 582**)
          i. Measure oxygen saturation of the blood
          ii. Reading 96 to 100 percent
              a) Normal
          iii. Below 95 percent
              a) Suspect shock, hypoxia, or respiratory compromise
              b) Provide appropriate airway management
              c) Provide supplemental oxygen
          iv. Below 90 percent
              a) Aggressive airway management
              b) Oxygen administration
              c) Positive pressure ventilation
      b. Capnography (**Fig. 11-13, p. 582; Fig. 11-14, p. 583; Fig. 11-15, p. 583**)
          i. Real-time measurement of exhaled CO_2 concentrations
          ii. Colormetric devices (**Fig. 11-13, p. 582**)
          iii. Electronic monitors (**Fig. 11-14, p. 583; Fig. 11-15, p. 583**)
          iv. Assists in confirmation of ETT placement
              a) CO_2 absence
                  1) Possible esophageal placement
                  2) "Purple" on colormetric device
              b) CO_2 presence
                  1) Proper ETT placement
                  2) "Yellow" on colormetric device
              c) $ETCO_2$ level falls precipitously during cardiac arrest.
                  1) These patients may not cause a color change on the $ETCO_2$ detector despite proper placement of the ETT.
      c. Cardiac monitoring (**Fig. 11-16, p. 584**)
          i. Observe the electrical activity of the heart.
          ii. Essential in assessing and managing a patient requiring ACLS
      d. Blood glucose determination (**Fig. 11-17, p. 585**)
          i. Usually performed on patients with altered mental status

IV. Anatomical regions. After you complete the general survey, you will examine the body regions and systems in more detail. (pp. 585–642)

A. Skin (pp. 585–589) (**Fig. 11-18, p. 586**)
  1. Color
  2. Moisture
  3. Temperature

  4. Texture
  5. Mobility and turgor
  6. Lesions (**Fig. 11-19, pp. 587–588; Fig. 11-20, p. 589**)
B. Hair
C. Nails (p. 590)
D. Head (p. 590) (**Proc. 11-2, p. 592**)
  1. Scalp (**Fig. 11-21, p. 590**)
  2. Skull
  3. Face
  4. Sinuses
E. Eyes (pp. 590–596) (**Proc. 11-3, pp. 592–593**)
  1. Visual acuity
  2. External eye
   a. Pupils
    i. Size
    ii. Shape
    iii. symmetry
  3. Internal eye (**Fig. 11-23a, p. 594**)
   a. Opthalmoscopic exam (**Proc. 11-3h, p. 593**)
    i. Opthalmoscope
    ii. Examination environment
    iii. Structures (**Fig. 11-23a, p. 594; Figs. 11-23b-c, p. 595**)
     a) Retina
     b) Retinal blood vessel (**Figs. 11-23d and 11-23e, p. 596**)
     c) Optic disc
     d) Fovea
F. Ears (pp. 596–599)
  1. Anatomy of the ear
   a. Outer ear
   b. Middle ear
   c. Inner ear
  2. Examining the ear (**Proc. 11-4, p. 597**)
   a. External ear
   b. Tuning fork
    i. Rinne test
    ii. Weber test
   c. Otoscope
    i. Structures
     a) Ear canal
     b) Cerumen
     c) Tympanic membrane (**Fig. 11-24a, p. 598; Figs. 11-24b, c & d, p. 599**)
G. Nose (pp. 600–601)
  1. External nose and nasal cavities
  2. Paranasal sinuses
  3. Examining the nose (**Proc. 11-5, p. 601**)
H. Mouth (pp. 600–603)
  1. Oral anatomy
  2. Salivary glands
  3. Oral examination (**Table 11-3, p. 600**) (**Proc. 11-6, p. 602**)
I. Neck (pp. 603–604)
  1. Neck anatomy
  2. Lymph nodes (**Table 11-4, p. 603**)
  3. Neck examination (**Proc. 11-7, p. 604**)
J. Chest and lungs (pp. 605–609)
  1. Thorax anatomy and physiology (**Fig. 11-25, p. 605**)
  2. Initial assessment of chest

TEACHING TIP
Remind students that in some people, unequal pupils are normal.

POINT TO EMPHASIZE
Pay special attention to anything in your patient's mouth that may become an airway obstruction.

SLIDES/VIDEOS
Dalton, T. *Advanced Medical Life Support, PowerPoint Slides*. 3rd ed. Upper Saddle River, NJ: Pearson Education, 2007.

3. Breath sounds (**Table 11-5, p. 606**)
   a. Normal
   b. Crackles (rales)
   c. Wheezes
   d. Rhonchi
   e. Pleural friction rubs
4. Posterior chest examination (**Proc. 11-8, p. 607**)
5. Anterior chest examination

K. Cardiovascular system (pp. 609–612)
   1. Cardiac anatomy and physiology (**Fig. 11-26, p. 610**)
   2. Cardiovascular assessment (**Proc. 11-9, p. 611**)
      a. Heart sounds
         i. S_1
            a) "Lub" in "lub-dub"
            b) Closing of tricuspid and mitral valves
         ii. S_2
            a) "Dub" in "lub-dub"
            b) Closing of pulmonic and aortic semilunar valves
         iii. S_3
            a) "Dee" in "lub-dub-dee"
            b) Kentucky
            c) Ventricular gallop
         iv. S_4
            a) "Dee" in "dee-lub-dub"
            b) Tennessee
            c) Arial gallop
         v. Additional sounds
            a) Clicks
               1) Stiff or stuck valve
            b) Snaps
               1) Abrupt recoil of stenotic mitral or tricuspid valve
            c) Friction rubs
               1) Rubbing of visceral and parietal surfaces
            d) Murmurs
               1) Turbulent blood flow
      b. Carotid bruits
      c. Jugular venous pressure
      d. Point of maximal impulse (PMI)

L. Abdomen (pp. 612–615)
   1. Abdominal quadrants
   2. Abdominal organs and systems
      a. Digestive organs
      b. Urinary organs
      c. Female reproductive organs
      d. Male reproductive organs
      e. Abdominal cardiovascular system
      f. Spleen
   3. Abdominal examination (**Proc. 11-10, p. 614**)
      a. Cullen's sign
         i. Discoloration over the umbilicus
      b. Grey Turner's sign
         i. Discoloration over the flanks
      c. Ascites
         i. Bulging caused by edema

M. Female genitalia (p. 615)
N. Male genitalia (p. 615)
O. Anus (pp. 615–616)

- **P.** Musculoskeletal system (pp. 616–625)
    1. Musculoskeletal anatomy and physiology
    2. Musculoskeletal assessment principles
    3. Extremities
        a. Wrists and hands (**Proc. 11-11, p. 618**)
        b. Elbows (**Proc. 11-12, p. 619**)
        c. Shoulders (**Proc. 11-13, p. 620**)
        d. Ankles and feet (**Proc. 11-14, p. 622**)
        e. Knees (**Proc. 11-15, p. 623**)
        f. Hips (**Proc. 11-16, p. 624**)
        g. Spine (**Table 11-6, p. 625**) (**Proc. 11-17, p. 626**)
- **Q.** Peripheral vascular system (pp. 625–629)
    1. Peripheral vascular anatomy and physiology
    2. Peripheral vascular assessment (**Table 11-7, p. 627; Table 11-18, p. 629**) (**Proc. 11-18, p. 628**) (**Fig. 11-27, p. 267**)
- **R.** Nervous system (pp. 629–642)
    1. Mental status and speech (**Table 11-9, p. 630**)
        a. Appearance and behavior
        b. Speech and language
        c. Mood
        d. Thought and perceptions
        e. Insight and judgment
        f. Memory and attention
    2. Cranial nerves (**Table 11-10, p. 632**) (**Proc. 11-19, p. 634**)
        a. CN-I: olfactory
            i. Smell
        b. CN-II: optic
            i. Sight
        c. CN-III: oculomotor; CN-IV: trochlear; and CN-VI: abducens
            i. Pupil constriction
            ii. Superior obliques
            iii. Lateral rectus
        d. CN-V: trigeminal
            i. Forehead
            ii. Cheek
            iii. Chin
            iv. Chewing muscles
        e. CN-VII: facial
            i. Tongue
            ii. Face
        f. CN-VIII: acoustic
            i. Hearing
            ii. Balance
        g. CN-IX: glossopharyngeal
            i. Posterior pharynx
            ii. Posterior palate taste
        h. CN-X: vagus
            i. Posterior tongue taste
            ii. Posterior palate
            iii. Pharynx
        i. CN-XI: accessory; CN-XII: hypoglossal
            i. Trapezius
            ii. Sternocleidomastoids
            iii. Tongue
    3. Motor system
        a. Motor system anatomy and physiology

b. Motor system assessment (**Table 11-11, p. 635; Table 11-12, p. 636; Table 11-13, p. 636**) (**Proc. 11-20, p. 637**)
4. Sensory system
   a. Sensory system anatomy and physiology
   b. Sensory system assessment (**Fig. 11-28, p. 638**)
5. Reflexes
   a. Reflex anatomy and physiology (**Fig. 11-29, p. 639**)
   b. Assessment principles (**Table 11-14, p. 639**)
   c. Assessing reflexes (**Proc. 11-21, pp. 640–641**)
      i. Biceps
      ii. Triceps
      iii. Brachioradialis
      iv. Quadriceps
      v. Achilles
      vi. Abdominal/plantar

V. Physical examination of infants and children. Conducting a physical exam on a sick or injured child can challenge the paramedic. (pp. 642–647)

A. Building patient and family rapport (pp. 642–643)
   1. Infants
   2. Toddlers
   3. Preschoolers
   4. School-age
   5. Adolescents

B. Anatomy and the physical exam (pp. 643–647) (**Fig. 11-30, p. 643**)
   1. General appearance (**Fig. 11-30, p. 643**)
   2. Head and neck (**Fig. 11-31, p. 644**)
   3. Chest and lungs (**Fig. 11-32, p. 645**) (**Table 11-15, p. 645**)
   4. Cardiovascular
   5. Abdomen (**Fig. 11-33, p. 646**)
   6. Musculoskeletal (**Fig. 11-34, p. 646**)
   7. Nervous system

VI. Recording examination findings. After performing the history and physical exam, record your findings on a patient's chart. (p. 647)

A. Purposes and principles (p. 647)
B. Completeness (p. 647)
   1. Pertinent negatives
C. SOAP format (p. 647)
   1. Subjective
   2. Objective
   3. Assessment
   4. Plan

VII. Chapter summary (p. 648). This chapter has presented both a regional and a systems approach to physical examination. The setting, chief complaint, and clinical status of your patient will dictate how much of the physical exam you actually use. For example, if you are hired to conduct preemployment physicals, you may decide to conduct a complete examination. If you are at the scene of a critically ill or injured patient, you will assess only those areas relevant to the situation. If your patient presents with a minor, isolated musculoskeletal injury, you may focus your exam on that area and system. As you become more experienced, making these decisions will become easier.

POWERPOINT PRESENTATION
Chapter 11, PowerPoint slides 144–164

TEACHING STRATEGY 5
Conducting Physical Exams of Infants and Children

POINT TO EMPHASIZE
Children are not little adults. Don't treat them as if they were.

POINT TO EMPHASIZE
The more invasive the procedure, the later in the exam of the child you should perform it.

POWERPOINT PRESENTATION
Chapter 11, PowerPoint slides 165–168

POINT TO EMPHASIZE
Tachycardia and bradycardia can both be the result of hypoxia in infants and children. Aggressive intervention is vital to the survival of the patient.

POWERPOINT PRESENTATION
Chapter 11, PowerPoint slide 169

TEACHING STRATEGY 6
Developing Reporting Skills

TEACHING STRATEGY 7
Cultural Considerations: A Matter of Respect

SKILLS DEMONSTRATION AND PRACTICE

Students can practice skills discussed in this chapter in the following settings.

Skills Lab: Divide the class into as many groups as appropriate. Have the groups circulate through the stations, and be sure each station is equipped with stethoscope, sphygmomanometer, opthalmoscope, otoscope, scale, tongue blades, penlight, visual acuity card or chart, reflex hammer, and thermometer. Monitor the groups to be sure all groups have a chance to practice each of the skills. You may wish to have other instructors or qualified paramedics assist students in these activities.

Station	Equipment and Personnel Needed	Activities
Examination Techniques	Assessment kits 1 victim 1 instructor	Have students practice the four examination techniques of inspection, palpation, percussion, and auscultation and the measurement of vital signs on a simulated patient.
Comprehensive Examination	Assessment kits 1 victim 1 instructor	Have students practice a comprehensive physical examination on a simulated patient.

Hospital: Begin patient assessments in the emergency department.

Field Internship: Begin patient assessments on simple emergency calls.

ASSIGNMENTS

Assign students to complete Chapter 11, "Physical Exam Techniques," of the workbook. Also assign them to read Chapter 12, "Patient Assessment in the Field," before the next class.

EVALUATION

Chapter Quiz and Scenario Distribute copies of the Chapter Quizzes provided in Handouts 11-3 through 11-5 to evaluate student understanding of this chapter. Make sure each student reads the scenario to reinforce critical thinking on the scene. Remind students not to use their notes or textbooks while taking the quiz.

Student CD Quizzes for every chapter are contained on the dynamic and highly visual in-text student CD.

Companion Website Additional quizzes for every chapter are contained on this exciting website.

TestGen You may wish to create a custom-tailored test using *Prentice Hall TestGen for Essentials of Paramedic Care*, 2nd Edition to evaluate student understanding of this chapter.

TEACHING TIP
Include practice written patient care reports when having your students practice patient assessment.

HANDOUT 11-2
Performing a General Survey

ADVANCED LIFE SUPPORT SKILLS
Larmon & Davis. *Advanced Life Support Skills.*

ADVANCED LIFE SKILLS REVIEW
Larmon & Davis. *Advanced Life Skills Review.*

BRADY SKILLS SERIES: ALS
Larmon & Davis. *Brady Skills Series: ALS.*

WORKBOOK
Chapter 11 Activities

READING/REFERENCE
Textbook, pp. 564–650

HANDOUTS 11-3 TO 11-5
Chapter 11 Quizzes

HANDOUT 11-6
Chapter 11 Scenario

PARAMEDIC STUDENT CD
Student Activities

COMPANION WEBSITE
http://www.prenhall.com/bledsoe

TESTGEN
Chapter 11

EMT ACHIEVE:
PARAMEDIC TEST PREPARATION
Mistovich & Beasley. *EMT Achieve: Paramedic Test Preparation.* www.prenhall.com/emtachieve/

REVIEW MANUAL FOR THE EMT-PARAMEDIC
Cherry & Mistovich. *Review Manual for the EMT-Paramedic,* 3rd edition.

HANDOUTS 11-7 TO 11-12
Reinforcement Activities

PARAMEDIC STUDENT CD
Student Activities

POWERPOINT PRESENTATION
Chapter 11

COMPANION WEBSITE
http://www.prenhall.com/bledsoe

ONEKEY
Chapter 11

ADVANCED LIFE SUPPORT SKILLS
Larmon & Davis. *Advanced Life Support Skills.*

ADVANCED LIFE SKILLS REVIEW
Larmon & Davis. *Advanced Life Skills Review.*

BRADY SKILLS SERIES: ALS
Larmon & Davis. *Brady Skills Series: ALS.*

PARAMEDIC NATIONAL STANDARDS SELF-TEST
Miller. *Paramedic National Standards Self-Test,* 4th edition.

On-line Test Preparation (for students and instructors). Additional test preparation is available through Brady's new on-line product, *EMT Achieve: Paramedic Test Preparation* at *http://www.prenhall.com/emtachieve/*. Instructors can also monitor student mastery on-line.

Review Manual for the EMT-Paramedic This comprehensive exam review contains hundreds of test questions and rationales, including scenarios, along with two 180-question practice tests on CD.

REINFORCEMENT

Handouts If classroom discussion or performance on the quizzes indicates that some students have not fully mastered the chapter content, you may wish to assign some or all of the Reinforcement Handouts for this chapter.

Student CD (for students). A wide variety of material on this CD-ROM will reinforce and also expand student knowledge and skills.

PowerPoint Presentation (for instructors). The PowerPoint material developed for this chapter offers useful reinforcement of chapter content.

Companion Website (for students). Additional review quizzes and links to EMS resources will contribute to further reinforcement of the chapter.

OneKey On-line support is offered for this course on one of three platforms: CourseCompass, Blackboard, or Web CT. Includes the IRM, PowerPoints, TestGen, and Companion Website for instruction. Ask your local sales representative for more information.

Brady Skills Series: Advanced Life Skills (Video or CD) Have your students watch the skills come to life on VHS or CD-ROM, or they can purchase the highly visual, full-color text with step-by-step procedures and rationales.

Handout 11-1

Student's Name _____

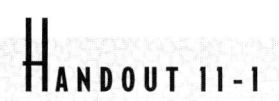

CHAPTER 11 OBJECTIVES CHECKLIST

Knowledge	Date Mastered
1. Define and describe the techniques of inspection, palpation, percussion, and auscultation.	
2. Describe the evaluation of mental status.	
3. Evaluate the importance of a general survey.	
4. Describe the examination of the following body regions, differentiate between normal and abnormal findings, and define the significance of abnormal findings: • skin, hair, and nails • head, scalp, and skull • eyes, ears, nose, mouth, and pharynx • neck • thorax (anterior and posterior) • arterial pulse including rate, rhythm, and amplitude • jugular venous pressure and pulsations • heart and blood vessels • abdomen • male and female genitalia • anus and rectum • peripheral vascular system • musculoskeletal system • nervous system • cranial nerves	
5. Describe the assessment of visual acuity.	
6. Explain the rationale for the use of an ophthalmoscope and otoscope.	
7. Describe the survey of respiration.	
8. Describe percussion of the chest.	
9. Differentiate the percussion notes and their characteristics.	
10. Describe special examination techniques related to the assessment of the chest.	
11. Describe the auscultation of the chest, heart, and abdomen.	

OBJECTIVES

HANDOUT 11-1 Continued

Knowledge	Date Mastered
12. Distinguish between normal and abnormal auscultation findings of the chest, heart, and abdomen and explain their significance.	
13. Describe special techniques of the cardiovascular examination.	
14. Describe the general guidelines of recording examination information.	
15. Discuss the examination considerations for an infant or child.	

OBJECTIVES

HANDOUT 11-2

Student's Name _____

PERFORMING A GENERAL SURVEY

Charting Student Progress:
1. *Learning skill*
2. *Performs skill with direction*
3. *Performs skill independently*

Procedure	1	2	3
1. Evaluate Appearance: • Level of consciousness • Signs of distress • Apparent state of health • Vital statistics • Sexual development • Skin color and obvious lesions • Posture, gait, and motor activity • Dress, grooming, and personal hygiene • Odors of breath or body • Facial expression			
2. Obtain Vital Signs: • Pulse • Respiration • Blood pressure • Temperature			
3. Use Additional Assessment Techniques:			
• Pulse oximetry • Cardiac monitoring • Blood glucose determination			

SKILLS

Comments:

Handout 11-3

Student's Name _____

CHAPTER 11 QUIZ, PART A

Write the letter of the best answer in the space provided.

_____ 1. The examination technique of informed observation is called:
   A. palpation.
   B. inspection.
   C. percussion.
   D. auscultation.

_____ 2. The production of sound waves by striking one object against another is called:
   A. palpation.
   B. inspection.
   C. percussion.
   D. auscultation.

_____ 3. The term *auscultation* refers to:
   A. using your sense of touch to gather information.
   B. listening with a stethoscope for sounds produced by the body.
   C. obtaining a blood pressure by feeling for the return of a pulse.
   D. using your sense of smell to detect any abnormal odors on the breath.

_____ 4. A pulse rate lower than 60 beats per minute is called:
   A. bradycardia.
   B. tachypnea.
   C. hypotension.
   D. hypoxia.

_____ 5. Which of the following is considered a normal adult vital sign?
   A. a pulse rate of 50 to 100 beats per minute
   B. a respiratory rate of 12 to 20 breaths per minute
   C. a body temperature of 98.4° to 99.0°F
   D. a systolic blood pressure of 110 to 140 mmHg in a postmenopausal woman

_____ 6. The amount of air one breath moves in and out of the lungs is called:
   A. minute volume.
   B. tidal volume.
   C. breath volume.
   D. inspired volume.

_____ 7. Your patient is experiencing rapid, deep respirations (gasps) with short pauses between sets. This is known as what type of respiration?
   A. Kussmaul's
   B. apneustic
   C. Cheyne-Stokes'
   D. Biot's

_____ 8. The difference between systolic and diastolic pressures is called:
   A. pulse pressure.
   B. orthostatic pressure.
   C. arterial resistance.
   D. pericardial range.

_____ 9. As the body temperature rises, it begins to threaten body processes. The neurons of the brain may denature at a temperature of:
   A. 100°F.
   B. 101°F.
   C. 102°F.
   D. 103°F.

_____ 10. Extreme cold affects body temperature. Shivering stops at a temperature of:
   A. 96°F.
   B. 94°F.
   C. 92°F.
   D. 90°F.

_____ 11. The device used to examine the interior of the eye is called a(n):
   A. otoscope.
   B. manometer.
   C. ophthalmoscope.
   D. Doppler.

HANDOUT 11-3 Continued

_____ **12.** A thorough evaluation of your patient's appearance can provide a great deal of valuable information about his health. This evaluation includes:
  A. odors of breath and body.
  B. temperature.
  C. pulse oximetry.
  D. cardiac monitoring.

_____ **13.** The noninvasive device that measures the oxygen saturation of your patient's blood is called a:
  A. sphygmomanometer.
  B. Doppler.
  C. glucometer.
  D. pulse oximeter.

_____ **14.** The most simple prehospital machines monitor the electrical activity of the heart in three "leads" or positions. These positions are called:
  A. limb leads.
  B. quick-look.
  C. rhythm leads.
  D. AV leads.

_____ **15.** Which of the following is true regarding cardiac monitors?
  A. The ECG reading shows the mechanical function of the heart.
  B. All monitor-defibrillators can deliver an unsynchronized countershock for unstable tachycardia.
  C. Some ECG machines have a "code summary" feature that prints out the electrical record of events and times.
  D. All of these statements are true.

HANDOUT 11-4

Student's Name _____

CHAPTER 11 QUIZ, PART B

Write the letter of the best answer in the space provided.

_____ 1. The skin is the largest organ in the human body, making up _____ of our total body weight.
   A. 10 percent
   B. 15 percent
   C. 20 percent
   D. 25 percent

_____ 2. The skin consists of three layers. They are, starting with the surface of the skin:
   A. dermis, epidermis, subcutaneous.
   B. epidermis, subcutaneous, dermis.
   C. epidermis, dermis, subcutaneous.
   D. none of these

_____ 3. The skin regulates body temperature through all of the following EXCEPT:
   A. radiation.
   B. ventilation.
   C. convection.
   D. conduction.

_____ 4. Poor skin turgor, or tenting, results from:
   A. malnutrition.
   B. obesity.
   C. liver dysfunction.
   D. dehydration.

_____ 5. Skin characteristics to assess include:
   A. color.
   B. moisture.
   C. texture.
   D. all of these

_____ 6. A skin lesion that is an elevated area, less than 1 cm in diameter, containing purulent fluid is called a:
   A. cyst.
   B. vesicle.
   C. pustule.
   D. bulla.

_____ 7. An inflammation of the proximal and lateral nail folds is called:
   A. a paronychia.
   B. an onycholysis.
   C. beau's lines.
   D. clubbing.

_____ 8. The scalp consists of five layers of tissue, including:
   A. mastoid tissue.
   B. periosteum.
   C. tight tissue.
   D. the sphenoid layer.

_____ 9. Which of the following bones is in the cranium?
   A. zygomatic
   B. maxillary
   C. ethmoid
   D. styloid

_____ 10. In the depression just in front of the ear is the:
   A. zygomatic arch.
   B. temporal bone.
   C. temporomandibular joint.
   D. external auditory canal.

_____ 11. The ocular muscles control eye movement and are innervated by three cranial nerves. These nerves are:
   A. CN-I, CN-III, CN-IV.
   B. CN-III, CN-IV, CN-VI.
   C. CN-I, CN-II, CN-V.
   D. CN-II, CN-III, CN-IV.

_____ 12. The internal eye includes the:
   A. sclera.
   B. conjunctiva.
   C. lacrimal gland.
   D. ocular muscles.

HANDOUT 11-4 Continued

_____ 13. The optic nerve senses light and is one of the 12 cranial nerves. It is:
   A. CN-I.
   B. CN-II.
   C. CN-III.
   D. CN-IV.

_____ 14. Pupils react sluggishly when intracranial pressure increases because of:
   A. decreased perfusion to the ocular muscles.
   B. decreased oxygen supply to the eyeball.
   C. increased pressure inside the eyeball.
   D. pressure on the oculomotor nerve.

_____ 15. Which of the following is true regarding the mastoid bone?
   A. An inner ear infection often presents with tenderness in the mastoid area.
   B. The mastoid bone contains fluid-filled cells that carry sound waves to the eardrum.
   C. The mastoid process is part of the occipital bone.
   D. The mastoid bone is palpable just in front of the earlobe.

_____ 16. Cyanosis of the lips may be caused by:
   A. anemia.
   B. allergic reaction.
   C. respiratory or cardiac insufficiency.
   D. dehydration.

_____ 17. The structure of the neck commonly called the "Adam's apple" is the:
   A. cricoid cartilage.
   B. thyroid cartilage.
   C. hyoid bone.
   D. tonsillar cartilage.

_____ 18. The major arteries in the neck that carry blood to the brain are the:
   A. carotid arteries.
   B. subclavian arteries.
   C. jugular arteries.
   D. supraclavicular arteries.

_____ 19. Neck wounds should be covered immediately with an occlusive dressing because occlusive dressings:
   A. control bleeding better than gauze dressings.
   B. prevent the blood vessels from collapsing.
   C. prevent air from entering the jugular vein.
   D. are not as bulky as large gauze dressings.

_____ 20. Which of the following is true regarding the chest?
   A. The right chest contains three lung lobes and the left contains only two.
   B. When the chest walls contract, a vacuum draws air into the lungs.
   C. The visceral layer of the pleura lines the inner chest wall.
   D. During inhalation, the diaphragm relaxes and moves downward.

_____ 21. Paradoxical movement of the chest caused by multiple rib fractures is called a:
   A. pneumothorax.
   B. sucking chest wound.
   C. flail chest.
   D. funnel chest.

_____ 22. Light crackling, popping, nonmusical sounds heard during inspiration are called:
   A. wheezes.
   B. rhonchi.
   C. stridor.
   D. rales.

_____ 23. Bronchovesicular lung sounds are heard:
   A. over the manubrium.
   B. over the trachea.
   C. between the scapulae and the 2nd and 3rd ICS lateral to the sternum.
   D. at the lung periphery.

_____ 24. Predominantly inspiratory wheezes associated with laryngeal obstruction are called:
   A. rhonchi.
   B. crackles.
   C. rales.
   D. stridor.

HANDOUT 11-4 Continued

_____ 25. To help determine whether underlying tissues of the anterior chest are air-filled, fluid-filled, or solid, use the examination technique known as:
   A. auscultation.
   B. percussion.
   C. palpation.
   D. inspection.

_____ 26. Systole is:
   A. the phase of the cardiac cycle when the ventricles contract.
   B. the term for constriction of the arteries in response to shock.
   C. the measurement of the strength of a cardiac contraction.
   D. one of the "heart sounds."

_____ 27. Blood traveling through the heart follows which of the following routes?
   A. left atrium, left ventricle, lungs, right atrium, right ventricle, aorta
   B. aorta, right atrium, right ventricle, pulmonary vein, pulmonary artery, left atrium, left ventricle
   C. vena cava, right atrium, right ventricle, lungs, left atrium, left ventricle
   D. right atrium, right ventricle, pulmonary artery, pulmonary vein, left atrium, left ventricle, aorta

_____ 28. Assessment of the cardiovascular system includes auscultating for bruits. This means:
   A. listening for an abnormal heart sound that indicates congestive heart failure.
   B. listening to the carotid arteries for turbulent blood flow around a partial obstruction.
   C. listening to the heart sounds for leaking valves.
   D. listening to the lungs for air flow around mucus plugs.

_____ 29. The organs in the right upper abdominal quadrant include the:
   A. liver.
   B. spleen.
   C. descending colon.
   D. appendix.

_____ 30. If your patient is complaining of abdominal pain, you should:
   A. examine the painful areas first.
   B. place a pillow under the patient's knees.
   C. place the patient in the left lateral recumbent position for the exam.
   D. conduct your exam as quickly as possible.

_____ 31. Cullen's sign is a discoloration around the umbilicus suggestive of:
   A. hypoxia.
   B. hypoperfusion.
   C. congestive heart failure.
   D. intraabdominal hemorrhage.

_____ 32. While assessing your patient's abdomen, you note the presence of ascites. These are bulges at the flanks and across the abdomen and indicate:
   A. internal hemorrhage.
   B. congestive heart failure.
   C. liver dysfunction.
   D. COPD.

_____ 33. The muscles of the rotator cuff include the:
   A. supraspinatus.
   B. deltoid.
   C. coracobrachialis.
   D. teres major.

_____ 34. When you assess your patient's range of motion by raising both arms forward and then straight overhead, you should expect to see forward flexion of:
   A. 45 degrees.
   B. 90 degrees.
   C. 130 degrees.
   D. 180 degrees.

_____ 35. The first cervical vertebra supports the head and is named after a mythical character who supported the world. It is called the:
   A. hercules.
   B. zeus.
   C. atlas.
   D. auricle.

HANDOUT 11-4 Continued

_____ 36. The vertebral sections of the spine, in order from top to bottom, are:
   A. cervical, thoracic, lumbar, sacral, and coccygeal.
   B. cervical, lumbar, thoracic, sacral, and coccygeal.
   C. cervical, lumbar, thoracic, coccygeal, and sacral.
   D. cervical, thoracic, lumbar, coccygeal, and sacral.

_____ 37. The most massive vertebrae, due to the amount of weight they bear, are the:
   A. thoracic.   C. cervical.
   B. lumbar.   D. sacral.

_____ 38. An exaggerated lumbar concavity is known as:
   A. lordosis.   C. scoliosis.
   B. kyphosis.   D. perosis.

_____ 39. The aorta branches into two main arteries leading to the legs, which are called the:
   A. femoral arteries.   C. common iliac arteries.
   B. popliteal arteries. D. peroneal arteries.

_____ 40. A pitting depression results from pressure against the skin when pitting edema is present. Using a scale, pitting edema of 1/2 to 1 inch is classified as:
   A. 1+.   C. 3+.
   B. 2+.   D. 4+.

HANDOUT 11-5

Student's Name _____

CHAPTER 11 QUIZ, PART C

Write the letter of the best answer in the space provided.

_____ 1. The areas of a neurologic exam include all of the following EXCEPT:
   A. mental status.
   B. cranial nerves.
   C. spinal curvatures.
   D. motor system.

_____ 2. The portion of the brain that is the center for conscious thought is the:
   A. frontal lobe.
   B. occipital lobe.
   C. cerebral cortex.
   D. cerebellum.

_____ 3. Singing, dancing, and expansive movements are possible signs of _____ behavior.
   A. anxious
   B. agitated
   C. depressed
   D. manic

_____ 4. Defective language caused by neurologic damage to the brain is termed:
   A. dysarthria.
   B. dysphonia.
   C. aphasia.
   D. dyslexia.

_____ 5. Assessing your patient's mental status and speech includes evaluating your patient's insight and judgment. This is accomplished by:
   A. asking if the patient knows the time of day, day of week, and year.
   B. noting if the patient's speech is inflected, clear, and strong.
   C. asking him what he would do if he cut himself shaving.
   D. noting if the patient organizes his thoughts as he speaks.

_____ 6. You would test your patient's second cranial nerve (CN-II) by:
   A. performing a pupil reaction test.
   B. compressing one nostril and presenting him with a variety of common odors.
   C. having the patient assume a variety of facial expressions.
   D. using visual acuity and visual field tests.

_____ 7. The eighth cranial nerve (CN-VIII) relates to:
   A. hearing.
   B. tasting.
   C. smelling.
   D. seeing.

_____ 8. The major extensor muscles of the elbow are the:
   A. biceps.
   B. triceps.
   C. pronator quadratus.
   D. brachialis.

_____ 9. While assessing your patient's muscle tone, you note spasticity. This is:
   A. increased rigidity throughout movement.
   B. sudden changes in tone with passive movement.
   C. loss of muscle tone causing the limb to be loose.
   D. increased tone when passive movement is applied.

_____ 10. Which nerve affects the quadriceps' strength?
   A. L3
   B. L5
   C. S1
   D. S2

_____ 11. The _____ test asks the patient to stand with his feet together and his eyes open, and then to close his eyes for 20 to 30 seconds.
   A. pronator drift
   B. tandem walking
   C. Romberg
   D. Altman

HANDOUT 11-5 Continued

_____ 12. You can test your patient's abdominal reflexes by:
  A. palpating all four quadrants.
  B. having the patient tense his abdominal muscles.
  C. stroking each side with an irregular object.
  D. lightly pricking the abdomen with a sterile pin.

_____ 13. Which of the following techniques is appropriate for the assessment of an infant or child?
  A. Position yourself above the child's eye level.
  B. Use a strong, authoritative voice.
  C. Separate the child from his parents to reduce distractions.
  D. Allow the child to handle diagnostic equipment before you use it.

_____ 14. Which of the following is NOT an age-group classification?
  A. infant   C. preschooler
  B. toddler   D. grade schooler

_____ 15. One sign of dehydration in an infant is:
  A. sunken fontanelles.
  B. increased urine output.
  C. a soft bulging spot on the head.
  D. stiff neck and fever.

_____ 16. Relative to adults, infants and children have a:
  A. slower respiratory rate.
  B. longer neck.
  C. proportionally smaller tongue.
  D. proportionally larger spleen and liver.

_____ 17. When associated with fever, neck stiffness in a pediatric patient suggests:
  A. meningitis.   C. otitis media.
  B. lymphadenopathy.   D. encephalitis.

_____ 18. A good indication of a child's peripheral perfusion status is:
  A. blood pressure.   C. capillary refill.
  B. pulse rate.   D. respiratory rate.

_____ 19. Which of the following is true regarding patient care reports?
  A. Including any "negative" findings of your assessment is not necessary.
  B. The patient care report is a legal document.
  C. General adjectives such as _good_, _normal_, and _poor_ are suitable for prehospital care.
  D. Paramedics should document their interpretation of what the patient tells them.

_____ 20. Which is NOT an element of the SOAP format for patient charts?
  A. Subjective   C. Assessment
  B. Objective   D. Progression

EVALUATION

HANDOUT 11-6

Student's Name _____

CHAPTER 11 SCENARIO

Review the following real-life situation. Then answer the questions that follow.

You and your EMT-Basic partner, Bill Niles, are at breakfast when your pagers go off, and you are dispatched to 345 Edna Place, one of the newer residential subdivisions in town. The dispatcher states that you are responding to a 27-year-old male who has fallen into a hole at a new house construction site. He is conscious and breathing, and complaining of right hip pain. When you arrive at the scene, coworkers have already gotten the patient out of the hole. He is lying supine on the ground with several people standing around him. He is in obvious pain. As you approach the patient, Mr. Hammond, you introduce yourself and your partner and obtain consent to treat the patient. You assign your partner to obtain a set of vital signs while you conduct your interview of the patient. You learn that Mr. Hammond slipped on some wet ground and fell into a hole approximately 4 feet deep. He says he landed on his right hip, which is very painful now, especially if he tries to move it. You note no respiratory distress as the patient talks to you, and no serious external hemorrhage is evident.

1. Based on his condition and chief complaint, describe your physical examination of the patient.

2. Based on the mechanism of injury, what other areas of the body would you examine?

HANDOUT 11-7

Student's Name _____

CHAPTER 11 REVIEW, PART A

Write the word or words that best complete the following sentences in the space provided.

1. _____ is the process of informed observation.
2. _____ is using your sense of touch to gather information.
3. _____ is the production of sound waves by striking one object against another.
4. _____ is listening with a stethoscope for sounds produced by the body.
5. The loud, high-pitched, drumlike sound heard when the stomach is percussed is called _____.
6. The loud, low-pitched, booming sound heard when a hyperinflated lung is percussed is called _____.
7. The loud, low-pitched, hollow sound heard when the normal lung is percussed is called _____.
8. The pattern and equality of intervals between pulses is called pulse _____.
9. The strength of a pulse, which can be weak, thready, strong, or bounding, is called pulse _____.
10. A pulse rate lower than 60 beats per minute is called _____.
11. A pulse rate higher than 100 beats per minute is called _____.
12. The term used for rapid breathing is _____.
13. The term used for slow breathing is _____.
14. How hard the patient works to breathe is called _____ _____.
15. The depth and pattern of breathing is called _____ _____ _____.
16. The amount of air one breath moves in and out of the lungs is called _____ _____.
17. The force of blood against arteries when ventricles contract is called _____ _____ _____.
18. The force of blood against arteries when ventricles relax is called _____ _____ _____.
19. _____ _____ are sounds of blood hitting arterial walls.
20. The normal breathing rate and pattern is called _____.
21. Breathing at a normal rate, but with deep respirations is called _____.
22. Gradual increases and decreases in respirations with periods of apnea are called _____-_____ _____.
23. Tachypnea and hyperpnea are called _____ _____.
24. The passage of blood through an organ or tissue is called _____.
25. The difference between a patient's systolic and diastolic blood pressure is called _____ _____.
26. Blood pressure that is higher than normal is called _____.
27. Blood pressure that is lower than normal is called _____.
28. An increase in the body's core temperature is called _____.

REINFORCEMENT

HANDOUT 11-7 Continued

29. A decrease in the body's core temperature is called _____.
30. The blood-pressure measuring device comprising a bulb, a cuff, and a manometer is a(n) _____.
31. A handheld device used to examine the interior of the eye is a(n) _____.
32. A handheld device used to examine the interior of the ears and nose is a(n) _____.
33. A(n) _____ _____ is a device that measures an infant's length and provides information concerning drug dosages, airway management adjuncts, and intravenous calculations.
34. _____-_____ _____ _____ are essential in gathering data to confirm a myocardial infarction.
35. The device used to check a patient's blood glucose levels is a(n) _____.

HANDOUT 11-8

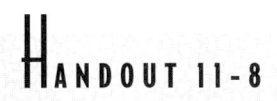

Student's Name _____

CHAPTER 11 REVIEW, PART B

Write the word or words that best complete the following sentences in the space provided.

1. The general survey begins with noting your patient's _____ and goes on to include _____ _____ and _____ _____.

2. Your patient's vital statistics are his _____ and _____.

3. Vital signs include _____, _____, _____ _____ and _____.

4. Normal oxygen saturation at sea level should be between _____ and _____.

5. Any disruption in normal tissue is a(n) _____.

6. Failure to develop normal hair growth during puberty may indicate a(n) _____ or _____ problem.

7. Depressions that appear in all nails are usually caused by _____ _____.

8. The acronym SCALP stands for _____, _____, _____, _____, _____ and _____.

9. Discharge from the ear canal is called _____.

10. Epistaxis means _____.

11. The smell of acetone on a patient's breath often indicates _____ _____.

12. Hard or fixed lymph nodes suggest a(n) _____.

13. The _____ attaches the lungs to the inner chest wall.

14. Soft, swishy, low-pitched sounds at the lung periphery are _____ sounds.

15. The squeaking or grating sounds of the pleural linings rubbing together are _____ _____ _____.

16. The apical impulse at the 5th intercostal space, near the midclavicular line, is the _____ _____ _____ _____.

17. In _____ _____ the amplitude of the pulse diminishes with inspiration and increases with exhalation.

18. The abdomen contains major organs of the _____, _____, _____, _____, and _____ systems.

19. Loud, prolonged, gurgling abdominal sounds are known as _____.

20. _____-_____-_____ joints such as the hip and shoulder allow rotation and a wide range of motion.

21. The crunching sound of unlubricated parts of a joint or broken bones rubbing against each other is called _____.

22. Hand pain and numbness, especially at night, suggests _____ _____ _____.

23. The _____ _____ runs through the bicipital groove between the greater and lesser tubercles.

24. Acute inflammation of the metatarsophalangeal joints suggests _____.

25. The _____ test is useful in evaluating the anterior and posterior cruciate ligaments in the knee.

HANDOUT 11-8 Continued

26. The degree of hip abduction is normally _____.
27. The spinal cord runs through the _____, the opening in the center of each vertebra.
28. _____ is a lateral curvature of the spine.
29. A score of 3+ indicates a(n) _____ peripheral pulse.
30. Unilateral coldness in a patient's feet and legs suggests a(n) _____ _____.

Handout 11-9

Student's Name _____

CHAPTER 11 REVIEW, PART C

Write the word or words that best complete the following sentences in the space provided.

1. The five areas of a neurologic exam include _____ _____ _____ _____, _____ _____, _____ _____, _____ _____, and _____.
2. The motor strip that controls voluntary skeletal muscle movement is located in the _____ _____ of the brain.
3. In amnesia cases, you may see _____, a condition in which the patient makes up facts and events in response to questions.
4. If you shine a light obliquely into a patient's pupil and the pupil in the eye opposite constricts, it is called _____ _____.
5. _____ is a loss of muscle tone, causing a limb to be loose.
6. A ratchet-like jerkiness in a patient's resistance to passive stretching in the extremities is known as _____-_____ rigidity.
7. Abnormalities in a patient's sense of position suggest _____ _____.
8. An abnormality in a patient's sense of light touch suggests _____ _____.
9. If the big toe dorsiflexes while the other toes fan out during a plantar reflex assessment, the patient has a positive _____ _____.
10. The absence of abdominal reflexes can suggest either a(n) _____ or _____ nervous system disorder.
11. Infants recognize their parents' faces and voices at about _____ months.
12. Toddlers should be able to walk by their _____ month.
13. Bulging sutures in an infant's skull indicate _____ _____ _____.
14. Normal heart rate for a toddler ranges from _____ to _____.
15. Normal systolic pressure for a school-age child ranges from _____ to _____.
16. The child's _____ _____ is a better guide to pain than his words.
17. The most important characteristic of a physical assessment is _____.
18. In the SOAP format for patient charts, _____ _____ includes what your patient tells you.
19. In the SOAP format for patient charts, _____ _____ includes the data collected from the head-to-toe anatomical exam.
20. In the SOAP format, the plan outlines your management strategy in three categories: _____, _____, and _____.

REINFORCEMENT

HANDOUT 11-10

Student's Name _____

IDENTIFYING PULSE LOCATIONS

Write the correct name of each of the pulses indicated on the diagram in the space provided.

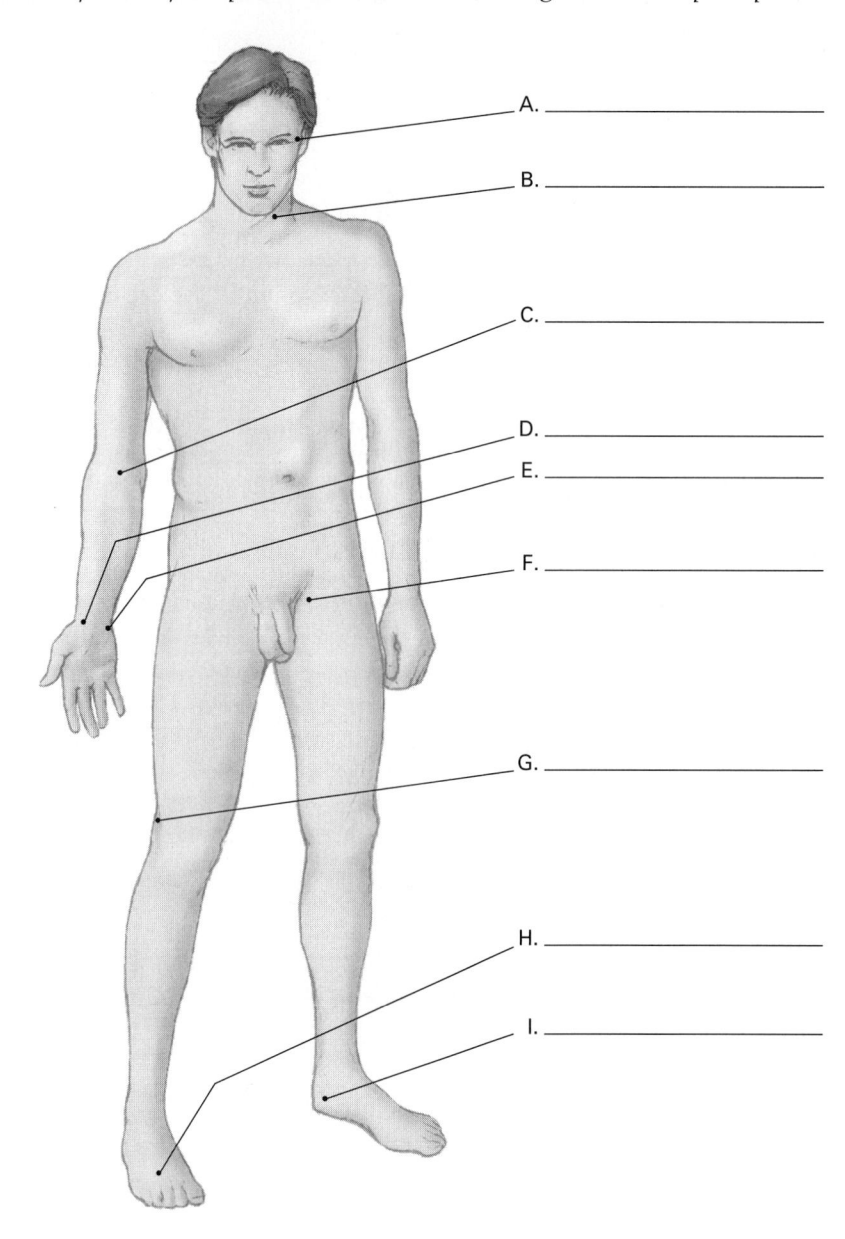

A. _____

B. _____

C. _____

D. _____
E. _____

F. _____

G. _____

H. _____
I. _____

1. In an adult patient, the most common pulse to palpate is the _____.
2. In an unconscious patient, first palpate for a(n) _____ pulse.
3. In infants and small children, palpate for a(n) _____ pulse.

378 ESSENTIALS OF PARAMEDIC CARE

©2007 Pearson Education, Inc.
Essentials of Paramedic Care, 2nd ed.

HANDOUT 11-11

Student's Name _____

CRANIAL NERVE ASSESSMENT IDENTIFICATION

Fill in the number of the cranial nerve you would be testing with each of the following assessments. There may be more than one correct answer for each assessment.

_____ 1. Assess your patient's face at rest and during conversation. Note any asymmetry, eyelid drooping, or abnormal movements such as tics. Have the patient assume a variety of facial expressions.

_____ 2. Evaluate your patient's speech articulation. Ask him to stick out his tongue, and watch for midline projection. Have your patient move his tongue from side to side.

_____ 3. Ask the patient to follow your finger with only his eyes as you move it through the six cardinal positions of gaze.

_____ 4. Have your patient close his eyes and compress one nostril while you present him with a variety of common, nonirritating odors.

_____ 5. Ask your patient to occlude one ear with a finger. Then whisper something softly into the other ear. Ask him to repeat what you said.

_____ 6. Ask your patient to clench his teeth while you palpate the temporal and masseter muscles. Note the strength of the muscle contraction.

_____ 7. Listen to your patient's voice. Hoarseness suggests a vocal cord problem; a nasal quality suggests a palate problem. Ask your patient to swallow; note any difficulties. Ask him to open his mouth and say, "aaahhhh."

_____ 8. Inspect the upper portions of your patient's trapezius muscles and sternocleidomastoid muscles for symmetry at rest.

_____ 9. Perform pupil reaction tests on your patient. Inspect the size and shape of your patient's pupils, and compare one side to the other.

_____ 10. Perform visual acuity and visual field tests.

HANDOUT 11-12

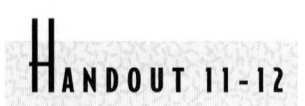

Student's Name _____

ASSESSMENT IDENTIFICATION

Complete the following lists.

1. What are the four basic physical exam techniques?
   _____
   _____
   _____
   _____

2. What are the five percussion sounds and their descriptions?
   _____
   _____
   _____
   _____

3. What are the normal adult vital signs?

   Pulse rate: _____   Systolic blood pressure ranges:

   Respiratory rate: _____   Male: _____

   Body temperature: _____   Female (premenopause): _____

   Female (postmenopause): _____

4. What are the nine breathing patterns and the causes of the abnormal patterns?
   _____
   _____
   _____
   _____
   _____
   _____
   _____
   _____
   _____

5. What are the four muscle tone findings and their descriptions?
   _____
   _____
   _____
   _____

Chapter 11 Answer Key

Handout 11-3: Chapter 11 Quiz, Part A

1. B
2. C
3. B
4. A
5. B
6. B
7. D
8. A
9. D
10. D
11. C
12. A
13. D
14. A
15. C

Handout 11-4: Chapter 11 Quiz, Part B

1. B
2. C
3. B
4. D
5. D
6. C
7. A
8. B
9. C
10. C
11. B
12. A
13. B
14. D
15. A
16. C
17. B
18. A
19. C
20. A
21. C
22. D
23. C
24. D
25. B
26. A
27. D
28. B
29. A
30. B
31. D
32. B
33. A
34. D
35. C
36. A
37. B
38. A
39. C
40. C

Handout 11-5: Chapter 11 Quiz, Part C

1. C
2. C
3. D
4. C
5. C
6. D
7. A
8. B
9. D
10. A
11. C
12. C
13. D
14. C
15. A
16. D
17. A
18. C
19. B
20. D

Handout 11-6: Chapter 11 Scenario

1. First, of course, you will assess the patient's level of consciousness, airway, breathing, and circulation. This patient is obviously alert and breathing normally. Because the patient appears stable and has an isolated traumatic injury, you may conduct a focused physical exam of the area that is causing the pain. You begin your exam of the hip by visualizing the area. Inspect the hip for deformity, discoloration, symmetry with the uninjured hip, and swelling. Carefully palpate for tenderness all around the joint, including the three bursa and the greater trochanter of the femur. If the palpation causes increased pain, you do not need to palpate the area again. You may consider testing the hip's range of motion if this movement does not cause increased pain; however, if movement causes additional pain, this should be avoided. You should also check pulses, such as the popliteal and dorsalis pedis pulses, to assess distal circulation.

2. Because the mechanism of injury was a fall, with the patient falling on the right hip, you would also examine the leg and foot for deformity, discoloration, symmetry with the uninjured side, and swelling. Palpate the leg, ankle, and foot for tenderness. Assess distal pulses. Look for any shortening or rotation of the leg. Assess the range of motion of the knee and ankle. You would also consider the possibility of spine injury resulting from energy transmitted from the hip to the back.

Handout 11-7: Chapter 11 Review, Part A

1. Inspection
2. Palpation
3. Percussion
4. Auscultation
5. tympany
6. hyperresonance
7. resonance
8. rhythm
9. quality
10. bradycardia
11. tachycardia
12. tachypnea
13. bradypnea
14. respiratory effort
15. quality of respirations
16. tidal volume
17. systolic blood pressure
18. diastolic blood pressure
19. Korotkoff sounds
20. eupnea
21. hyperpnea
22. Cheyne-Stokes respirations
23. Kussmaul's respirations
24. perfusion
25. pulse pressure
26. hypertension
27. hypotension
28. hyperthermia
29. hypothermia
30. sphygmomanometer
31. ophthalmoscope
32. otoscope
33. Broselow tape
34. 12-lead heart monitors (or ECGs)
35. glucometer

Handout 11-8: Chapter 11 Review, Part B

1. appearance, vital signs, additional assessments
2. height, weight
3. pulse, respiration, blood pressure, temperature
4. 96 percent, 100 percent
5. lesion
6. pituitary, hormonal
7. systemic disease
8. skin, connective tissue, apneurosis, loose tissue, periosteum
9. otorrhea
10. nosebleed
11. diabetic ketoacidosis
12. malignancy
13. pleura
14. vesicular
15. pleural friction rubs
16. point of maximal impulse (PMI)
17. pulsus paradoxus
18. digestive, urinary, reproductive, cardiovascular, lymphatic
19. boborygmi
20. Ball-and-socket
21. crepitus
22. carpal tunnel syndrome
23. biceps tendon
24. gout
25. drawer
26. 90°

27. foramen
28. Scoliosis
29. bounding
30. arterial occlusion

Handout 11-9: Chapter 11 Review, Part C

1. mental status and speech, cranial nerves, motor system, sensory system, reflexes
2. frontal lobe
3. confabulation
4. consensual reaction
5. Flaccidity
6. cog-wheel
7. cerebellar disease
8. peripheral neuropathy
9. Babinski response
10. central, peripheral
11. two
12. 18th
13. increased intracranial pressure
14. 80, 110
15. 97, 112
16. facial expression
17. thoroughness
18. subjective information
19. objective information
20. diagnostic, therapeutic, educational

Handout 11-10: Identifying Pulse Locations

A. Temporal
B. Carotid
C. Brachial
D. Radial
E. Ulnar
F. Femoral
G. Popliteal
H. Dorsal pedis
I. Posterior tibial
1. radial
2. carotid
3. brachial

Handout 11-11: Cranial Nerve Assessment Identification

1. CN-VII
2. CN-XII
3. CN-III, CN-IV, CN-VI
4. CN-I
5. CN-VIII
6. CN-V
7. CN-IX, CN-X
8. CN-XI
9. CN-III
10. CN-II

Handout 11-12: Assessment Identification

1. Inspection, palpation, percussion, and auscultation
2. *Tympany:* drumlike
   Hyperresonance: booming
   Resonance: hollow
   Dull: thud
   Flat: extremely dull
3. *Pulse rate:* 60–100
   Respiratory rate: 12–20
   Body temperature: 98.6°F (37°C)
   Systolic blood pressure ranges:
   Male: 120–150
   Female (premenopause): 110–140
   Female (postmenopause): 120–150
4. *Eupnea* (normal)
   Tachypnea (increased respirations): fever, anxiety, exercise, shock
   Bradypnea (decreased respirations): sleep, drugs, metabolic disorder, head injury, stroke
   Apnea (no breathing): deceased patient, head injury, stroke
   Hyperpnea (normal rate, but deep): emotional stress, diabetic ketoacidosis
   Cheyne-Stokes (gradual increases and decreases in rate with periods of apnea): increased intracranial pressure, brainstem injury
   Biots (rapid, deep gasps, with pauses): spinal meningitis, many CNS causes, head injury
   Kussmauls (rapid and deep): renal failure, metabolic acidosis, diabetic ketoacidosis
   Apneustic (prolonged inspirations, shortened expirations): lesion in brainstem
5. *Spasticity:* increased tone when passive movement applied
   Rigidity: increased rigidity throughout movement
   Flaccidity: loss of muscle tone causing limb to be loose
   Paratonia: sudden changes in tone with passive movement

Chapter 12 Patient Assessment in the Field

INTRODUCTION

In the previous chapters, students studied the techniques of performing a comprehensive history and physical exam. Paramedics will rarely, if ever, perform such complete exams in the prehospital setting; however, based on the patient's chief complaint and condition, the paramedic will decide which components of the comprehensive exam pertain to each particular acute situation. In this chapter, students will study how to perform an assessment in the field. That performance will depend, in large part, on the classification of patients as either trauma or medical patients. The chapter further classifies trauma patients as either having a significant mechanism of injury or having minor, isolated injuries and medical patients as either responsive or unresponsive. Based on the patient's category, the paramedic will decide which type of assessment is most appropriate, what interventions are needed, and when the interventions should be performed.

TOTAL TEACHING TIME: 13.17 HOURS
The total teaching time is only a guideline based on the didactic and practical lab averages in the National Standard Curriculum. Instructors should take into consideration such factors as the pace at which students learn, the size of the class, and breaks. The actual time devoted to teaching objectives is the responsibility of the instructor.

CHAPTER OBJECTIVES

After reading this chapter, you should be able to:

1. Recognize hazards/potential hazards associated with the medical and trauma scene. (pp. 654–660)
2. Identify unsafe scenes and describe methods for making them safe. (pp. 654–660)
3. Discuss common mechanisms of injury/nature of illness. (pp. 662–663)
4. Predict patterns of injury based on mechanism of injury. (pp. 662–663, 673–675)
5. Discuss the reason for identifying the total number of patients at the scene. (p. 661)
6. Organize the management of a scene following size-up. (pp. 654–660)
7. Explain the reasons for identifying the need for additional help or assistance during the scene size-up. (pp. 654, 656–660)
8. Summarize the reasons for forming a general impression of the patient. (pp. 664–665)
9. Discuss methods of assessing mental status/levels of consciousness in the adult, infant, and child patient. (pp. 665–666)

10. Discuss methods of assessing and securing the airway in the adult, child, and infant patient. (pp. 666–667)
11. State reasons for cervical spine management for the trauma patient. (pp. 664–665)
12. Analyze a scene to determine if spinal precautions are required. (pp. 664–665, 673–675)
13. Describe methods for assessing respiration in the adult, child, and infant patient. (pp. 667–668)
14. Describe the methods used to locate and assess a pulse in an adult, child, and infant patient. (pp. 668–669, 670–671)
15. Discuss the need for assessing the patient for external bleeding. (p. 669)
16. Describe normal and abnormal findings when assessing skin color, temperature, and condition. (p. 669)
17. Explain the reason and process for prioritizing a patient for care and transport. (pp. 669, 672–673)
18. Use the findings of the initial assessment to determine the patient's perfusion status. (pp. 668–672)
19. Describe orthostatic vital signs and evaluate their usefulness in assessing a patient in shock. (pp. 688–689)
20. Describe the medical patient physical examination. (pp. 685–689)
21. Differentiate between the assessment for an unresponsive, altered mental status, and alert medical patients. (pp. 683–691)
22. Discuss the reasons for reconsidering the mechanism of injury. (pp. 673–675)
23. Recite examples and explain why patients should receive a rapid trauma assessment. (p. 675)
24. Describe the trauma patient physical examination. (pp. 675–682)
25. Describe the elements of the rapid trauma assessment and discuss their evaluation. (pp. 675–682)
26. Identify cases when the rapid assessment is suspended to provide patient care. (p. 675)
27. Discuss the reason for performing a focused history and physical exam. (pp. 673, 682, 683–684)
28. Describe when and why a detailed physical examination is necessary. (p. 692)
29. Discuss the components of the detailed physical examination. (pp. 692–698)
30. Explain what additional care is provided while performing the detailed physical exam. (pp. 692–698)
31. Distinguish between the detailed physical exam that is performed on a trauma patient and that of the medical patient. (pp. 692–698)
32. Differentiate between patients requiring a detailed physical exam and those who do not. (p. 692)
33. Discuss the rationale for repeating the initial assessment as part of the ongoing assessment. (pp. 698–699, 700)
34. Describe the components of the ongoing assessment. (pp. 698–701)
35. Describe trending of assessment components. (pp. 698–701)
36. Discuss medical identification devices/systems. (p. 680)
37. Given several preprogrammed and moulaged medical and trauma patients, provide the appropriate scene survey, initial assessment, focused assessment, detailed assessment, and ongoing assessments. (pp. 653–701)

FRAMING THE LESSON

Begin the lesson with a brief review of the previous chapter. Then present students with four scenario stations: (1) a trauma patient with a significant mechanism of injury; (2) a trauma patient with a minor, isolated injury; (3) a responsive medical patient; and (4) an unresponsive medical patient. You can draw these scenarios from the case studies that open chapters in other volumes of this series or from your personal experience. Divide the students into four groups, and have every group rotate through each of the four stations. A clinical instructor or one of the students will read the scenario. Then have each group "voice" perform an appropriate assessment on the patient, making notes as to which components of the comprehensive physical exam they used and the order in which they performed them. Compare the results of the different groups, and tell students that in this lesson they will learn the most effective and efficient ways of gathering information from a variety of patients. After you have presented the lesson, have students rotate through the same four scenario stations and note any differences in their assessment.

TEACHING STRATEGIES

People learn in a variety of ways. Some do better with the spoken word, whereas others prefer the written. Some prefer to work alone, whereas others profit from working in groups. Recognizing these different ways of acquiring knowledge, the authors of this *Instructor's Resource Manual* have provided a variety of teaching strategies for the different types of learners. These strategies are intended to foster higher-level cognitive skills and encourage creative learning and problem solving. For greatest effectiveness, incorporate these strategies into your class lecture. Symbols in the Lecture Outline indicate the points at which various exercises might be most appropriate. Other strategies can be used to preview the lesson or to summarize it.

The following strategies are keyed to specific sections of the lesson.

1. Practicing Personal Safety. To illustrate the importance of proper hand washing, have students handle objects that have been covered in glitter. The glitter simulates germs. Then dismiss students to go wash their hands. When they return, have them examine each other for traces of glitter left after the hand washing. The glitter will likely be all over the tables, pencils, books, floor, light switches, and so on. The concept of cross-contamination is also illustrated well with this activity. Likewise, a product named Glo Germ may be used to illustrate hand washing technique. A small amount of Glo Germ is rubbed onto the student's hands. After a thorough washing, the student holds his hands under a black light, which reveals the Glo Germ remaining on the student's hands, especially around the fingernails. A similar activity places shaving cream on gloved hands. You can have students practice taking off their gloves without contaminating their hands. To do this, cover the gloves with shaving cream, which simulates blood. Shaving cream also illuminates under black light, to highlight trace amounts of "blood." These are kinesthetic activities.

2. Identifying Scene Hazards. Although it is difficult to simulate all potential hazards in the classroom, you do not want the internship to be the first time your students have given any thought to scene size-up. One suggestion is to cut clips of popular TV shows, such as *Third Watch*, *ER*, *Cops*, and so on, and show those clips to your class. *Brady's Paramedic Student CD* is also another good source for this activity. Have students determine all potential scene hazards they observe in the clips, from chemical spills to fires to violence. This is a visual activity.

3. Managing Scene Hazards. Have students, working together as a class, make a comprehensive list of possible scene hazards. Help them identify the resource(s) needed to safely manage the scene in each situation. For example, the hazards list should include: downed wires, gun, oil spill, unstable vehicle, water main break, snake, cliff, and so on. The list of possible resources could include: electric or public utility company, law enforcement, hazmat team, fire department, animal control, and search and rescue, for example. Help students to identify what hazards and resources are located in their response areas. This is a discussion activity that improves verbal communication and problem-solving skills.

4. Personal Protective Equipment. Bring examples of personal protective equipment to class, and explain their proper use, either by demonstrating them yourself or by demonstrating them with volunteers from the class.

5. Scene Size-up Practice. With the help of other instructors, develop a scenario to give students practice in scene size-up. Set up the scene in a room other than the students' usual classroom. If space is available, you may set up more than one room, with different scenarios in each room. You may simulate an incident requiring special attention to body substance isolation and others with various scene safety concerns. Make the scene as realistic as possible, including moulaging patients with injuries. Students may enter the scenes alone or with a partner. Stress to students not to discuss the scenarios with each other until all have rotated through them.

6. Evaluating Scene Size-ups. Have students recollect and share times when they or others have mismanaged the scene size-up. They will likely be able to recall times when they underestimated the intoxicated patient, or failed to manage a large crowd, or did not notice a weapon with which they were later threatened. This activity requires reflection and visualization, which are right-brain activities.

7. Using a Flow Sheet. Assign students individually or in groups to develop a flow sheet for patient assessment information. Have them include components of the initial assessment and physical exam. Reinforce the importance of pertinent negatives. Have students use the flow sheets during class simulations and clinical rotations until they can consistently perform the elements of patient assessment.

8. Identifying Mechanisms of Injury. Show slides or photos of many different scenes and ask students to identify the mechanism of injury or nature of illness in each scene. More sophisticated students may be able to make multiple observations about the patient from a single, static photo. Be able to point out elements that students missed during their scene size-up. You could use photographs from magazines, books, or even videos to set up this exercise. This activity gets students thinking about personal and scene safety, as well as the MOI analysis, early in their education.

9. Determining Patient Priority. Give students practice in determining priority by having them categorize a list of patients. Give only the chief complaint, pertinent history, and findings of the primary survey. Additionally, help students to determine if the patient should be stabilized on scene or rapidly transported with ALS procedures done en route. (Insert this after priority determination.) You might use descriptions of patients from chapter-opening case studies in this book or other volumes in this series, from collections of case studies like Brady's *Street Scenarios for the EMT and Paramedic,* or your own records (with identities of people involved in the cases concealed).

The following strategy can be used at various points throughout the lesson or to help summarize and demonstrate what students have learned.

Cultural Considerations, Legal Notes, and Patho Pearls. The Student CD-ROM contains this series of informative features to enhance the student's understanding of the material covered in this chapter.

TEACHING OUTLINE

Chapter 12, "Patient Assessment in the Field," is the third lesson in Division 2, *Patient Assessment*. Distribute Handout 12-1 so that students can familiarize themselves with the learning goals for this chapter. If students have any questions about the objectives, answer them at this time.

Then present the chapter. One possible lecture outline follows. In the outline, the parenthetical references in regular type are references to text pages; those in bold type are references to figures, tables, or procedures.

I. Introduction. Patient assessment is the problem-oriented evaluation of the patient and establishment of priorities based on existing and potential threats to human life. (p. 653)

  A. Importance of thorough, accurate patient assessment (p. 653)
  B. Components of patient assessment (p. 653)
    1. Initial assessment
    2. Focused history and physical exam
    3. Detailed physical exam
    4. Ongoing assessment

II. Scene size-up. Scene size-up is both the essential first step at any emergency and an ongoing process. (pp. 654–663) **(Fig. 12-1, p. 654)**

  A. Components of scene size-up (p. 654)
    1. Body substance isolation
    2. Scene safety
    3. Location of all patients
    4. Mechanism of injury
    5. Nature of illness
  B. Body substance isolation (pp. 655–656)
    1. Personal protective equipment (PPE) **(Fig. 12-2, p. 655; Figs. 12-4 and 12-5, p. 656)**
    2. Hand washing **(Fig. 12-3, p. 655)**
  C. Scene safety (pp. 656–660)
    1. Priorities for scene safety **(Fig. 12-6, p. 657)**
    2. Potential hazards **(Fig. 12-7, p. 657)**
    3. Crime scenes **(Fig. 12-8, p. 658)**
    4. Crash scenes **(Fig. 12-9, p. 658)**
    5. Minimum rescue operations equipment **(Fig. 12-10, p. 659; Fig. 12-11, p. 659; Fig. 12-12, p. 660)**
      a. Four-point suspension helmets
      b. Eye goggles and industrial safety glasses
      c. High-quality hearing protection
      d. Leather work gloves
      e. High-top steel-toed boots
      f. Insulated coveralls
      g. Turnout gear
    6. Minimum patient safety equipment for rescue operations
      a. Construction-type hard hats
      b. Eye goggles
      c. Hearing and respiratory protection

HANDOUT 12-1
Chapter 12 Objectives Checklist

TEACHING TIP
Patient assessment is the one important skill that the paramedic uses on every call and with every patient. It is vital that students practice the various types of assessments as often as possible. Consider setting aside some time in every class session for skills practice.

POWERPOINT PRESENTATION
Chapter 12, PowerPoint slides 4–5

HANDOUT 12-2
Performing a Scene Size-up and Initial Assessment

POWERPOINT PRESENTATION
Chapter 12, PowerPoint slides 6–32

TEACHING STRATEGY 1
Practicing Personal Safety

POINT TO EMPHASIZE
Because there are no reliable ways to determine which patients are infectious, take commonsense body substance isolation precautions on all patient contacts. If it is wet and not yours, don't touch it without protection.

TEACHING STRATEGY 2
Identifying Scene Hazards

TEACHING STRATEGY 3
Managing Scene Hazards

TEACHING STRATEGY 4
Personal Protective Equipment

TEACHING STRATEGY 5
Scene Size-up Practice

TEACHING STRATEGY 6
Evaluating Scene Size-ups

TEACHING STRATEGY 7
Using a Flow Sheet

TEACHING TIP
Impress upon your students to adopt a hands-on philosophy with regard to their future patients. They should be assessing everything with every patient during training. Even an ankle fracture gets a chest auscultation. Only by repeatedly assessing normal patient findings will they become able to recognize abnormal findings.

POWERPOINT PRESENTATION
Chapter 12, PowerPoint slides 33–75

SLIDES/VIDEOS
Brady. *Patient Assessment* (Video).

   d. Protective blankets
   e. Protective shielding (**Fig. 12-13, p. 660; Fig. 12-14, p. 660**)
D. Location of all patients (pp. 661–662)
   1. Searching for all patients
   2. Calling for assistance early
   3. Mass casualty incidents and triage (**Fig. 12-15, p. 661; Fig. 12-16, p. 661; Fig. 12-17, p. 662**)
E. Mechanism of injury (pp. 662–663) (**Fig. 12-18, p. 662**)
   1. Combined strength, direction, and nature of forces that injured patient
   2. Index of suspicion
   3. May be only clue to possibility of serious injury
F. Nature of illness (p. 663)
   1. Determine from patient, family, bystanders, clues at scene
   2. Often not readily apparent
   3. May be different from chief complaint

III. Initial assessment. Its goal is to identify and correct immediately life-threatening conditions of the patient's airway, breathing, or circulation. (pp. 663–673)

A. Identify and correct immediately life-threatening conditions (ABCs) (p. 663)
B. Components of initial assessment (p. 663)
   1. Forming a general impression
   2. Stabilizing the cervical spine, as needed
   3. Assessing a baseline mental status
   4. Assessing the airway
   5. Assessing breathing
   6. Assessing circulation
   7. Determining priority
C. Form general impression (pp. 664–665)
   1. Initial, intuitive evaluation of patient
   2. Age, gender, race
   3. Trauma/medical problem
D. Stabilize cervical spine as needed (pp. 664–665) (**Fig. 12-19a, p. 664; Fig. 12-19b, p. 665**)
   1. Significant mechanism of injury
   2. Unresponsive patient
E. Mental status (pp. 665–666)
   1. Importance
   2. AVPU
      a. Alert
      b. Verbal
      c. Painful stimuli
      d. Unresponsive
F. Airway assessment (pp. 666–667)
   1. Manual maneuvers
      a. Head-tilt/chin lift
      b. Jaw thrust
   2. Chest rise
   3. Air movement
   4. Quality of breathing
      a. Suctioning (**Fig. 12-20, p. 667**)
      b. Abnormal sounds
      c. Ventilation

        5. Airway adjuncts
            a. Oropharyngeal airway
            b. Nasopharyngeal airway
            c. Endotracheal intubation
            d. Multi-lumen airways
            e. Needle and surgical cricothyrotomy
    G. Breathing assessment (pp. 667–668)
        1. Normal respiratory rates (Table 12-1, p. 668)
        2. Signs of inadequate breathing
            a. Altered mental status
            b. Shortness of breath while speaking
            c. Retractions
            d. Asymmetric chest wall movement
            e. Accessory muscle use
            f. Cyanosis
            g. Audible sounds
            h. Abnormal rate or depth
            i. Nasal flaring
        3. Chest injuries
            a. Sucking chest wound
            b. Flail chest
            c. Pneumothorax
    H. Circulation assessment (pp. 668–671) (Proc. 12-1, pp. 670–671)
        1. Normal pulse rates (Table 12-2, p. 669)
        2. Pulse quality
        3. External bleeding
        4. Skin temperature, color, condition
        5. Capillary refill
    I. Priority determination (pp. 669–673)
        1. High-priority patients (Fig. 12-21, p. 672)
            a. Poor general impression
            b. Altered mental status
            c. Airway compromise
            d. Abnormal breathing
            e. Poor circulation
            f. Obvious serious or multiple injuries

IV. Focused history and physical exam. The second stage of patient assessment is a problem-oriented process based on your initial assessment and your patient's chief complaint. (pp. 673–691)

    A. Types of patients (p. 673)
        1. Trauma patient with significant mechanism of injury
        2. Trauma patient with isolated injury
        3. Responsive medical patient
        4. Unresponsive medical patient
    B. Major trauma patients (pp. 673–682)
        1. Mechanism of injury (Fig. 12-22, p. 674; Fig. 12-23, p. 675)
            a. Ejection from vehicle
            b. Death in same passenger compartment
            c. Fall from higher than 20 feet
            d. Rollover of vehicle
            e. High-speed vehicle collision
            f. Vehicle-pedestrian collision
            g. Motorcycle crash
            h. Penetration of head, chest, or abdomen

POINT OF INTEREST
The American Heart Association has excellent handouts and charts showing breathing rates for adults, infants, and children.

POWERPOINT PRESENTATION
Chapter 12, PowerPoint slides 76–136

TEACHING STRATEGY 8
Identifying Mechanisms of Injury

HANDOUT 12-3
Performing a Rapid Trauma Assessment

READING/REFERENCE
Parsons, P. E., and J. P. Weiner-Kronish. *Critical Care Secrets*. 3rd ed. Elsevier, 2003.

POINT TO EMPHASIZE
Never allow the patient's clothing to get in the way of your assessment, yet always try to protect your patient's privacy and dignity.

POINT TO EMPHASIZE
For medical emergencies, the history becomes the most vital component of the focused history and physical exam and should come immediately after the initial assessment. Probably 95 percent of your diagnoses will come from the history.

POINT TO EMPHASIZE
Listen to your patient. He is trying to tell you what is wrong. There are no poor historians, only poor history takers.

POINT TO EMPHASIZE
If your patient says, "I think I'm going to die," take him very seriously.

READING/REFERENCE
Carpenito-Moyet, L. J. *Nursing Diagnosis: Application to Clinical Practice*. 10th ed. Philadelphia: Lippincott, 2003.

    2. Additional predictors of serious internal injury for infants and children
       a. Fall from higher than 10 feet
       b. Bicycle collision
       c. Medium-speed vehicle collision
    3. Initial assessment
    4. Rapid trauma assessment
       a. Fast, systematic head-to-toe assessment for signs of serious injury
       b. Patients with
          i. Significant mechanism of injury
          ii. Altered mental status
          iii. Multiple body system trauma
       c. DCAP-BTLS
          i. Deformities
          ii. Contusions
          iii. Abrasions
          iv. Penetrations
          v. Burns
          vi. Tenderness
          vii. Lacerations
          viii. Swelling
       d. Head
       e. Neck (Proc. 12-2, p. 677)
       f. Chest (Proc. 12-3, p. 679)
       g. Abdomen
       h. Pelvis
       i. Extremities (Fig. 12-24, p. 680) (Proc. 12-4, p. 681)
       j. Posterior body (Fig. 12-25, p. 682)
    5. Vital signs
    6. History (SAMPLE)
       a. Signs and symptoms
       b. Allergies
       c. Medications
       d. Pertinent past medical history
       e. Last oral intake
       f. Events preceding the incident
  C. The isolated-injury trauma patient (pp. 682–683)
    1. Focus assessment on the specific injury.
    2. DCAP-BTLS
    3. Vital signs
    4. SAMPLE history
  D. Responsive medical patient (pp. 683–690) (Fig. 12-26, p. 684)
    1. History
       a. Chief complaint
       b. History of present illness (OPQRST-ASPN)
          i. Onset
          ii. Provocation/palliation
          iii. Quality
          iv. Region/radiation
          v. Severity
          vi. Time
          vii. Associated symptoms
          viii. Pertinent negatives
       c. Past medical history
       d. Current health status
    2. Focused physical exam (Fig. 12-27, p. 686)

   a. Chest pain/respiratory distress
    i. HEENT
    ii. Neck
    iii. Chest
    iv. Cardiovascular
    v. Abdomen
    vi. Extremities
   b. Altered mental status (1-minute cranial nerve exam) (**Table 12-3, p. 688**)
    i. HEENT
    ii. Chest
    iii. Abdomen
    iv. Pelvis
    v. Extremities
    vi. Posterior body
    vii. Neuro
   c. Acute abdomen
    i. HEENT
    ii. Chest
    iii. Abdomen
    iv. Posterior body
  3. Baseline vital signs
   a. Blood pressure
   b. Pulse
   c. Respiration
   d. Temperature
   e. Basic pupil assessment
   f. Importance
    i. Capsule assessment of clinical status, indicate severity of illness, urgency to intervene, changes in condition
     a) Deteriorating
     b) Responding to therapy
   g. Orthostatic vital signs
  4. Additional assessment techniques
   a. Pulse oximetry
   b. Capnography
   c. Cardiac monitoring
   d. Blood glucose determination
  5. Emergency medical care (**Fig. 12-28, p. 690**)
   a. Care authorized by standing orders
   b. Online medical direction's further orders
   c. Appropriate advanced assessment techniques
 E. Unresponsive medical patient (pp. 690–691)
  1. Initial assessment
  2. Rapid medical assessment
  3. Brief history
  4. Expedite transport, performing ongoing assessment every 5 minutes en route

V. Detailed physical exam. More detailed and slower than the focused history and physical exam, the detailed physical exam is a luxury, designed for use en route to the hospital, if time allows, for patients with significant trauma or serious medical illness. (pp. 692–698)

A. Components of the comprehensive exam (pp. 692–698) (**Proc. 12-5, pp. 694–695**)

POWERPOINT PRESENTATION
Chapter 12, PowerPoint slides 137–145

1. Head
   a. Tenderness
   b. Deformities
   c. Areas of unusual warmth
   d. Stability of facial bones
   e. Discoloration
      i. Periorbital ecchymosis
      ii. Battle's sign
   f. Temporomandibular joint
2. Eyes
   a. External structures
   b. Pupils
   c. Movement
3. Ears
   a. Deformities
   b. Lumps
   c. Lesions
   d. Tenderness
   e. Erythema
   f. Drainage
   g. Hearing acuity
4. Nose and sinuses
   a. Depressions
   b. Deformities
   c. Tenderness
   d. Nasal flaring
   e. Drainage
   f. Nasal obstruction
5. Mouth and pharynx
   a. Lips
   b. Oral mucosa
   c. Tongue
   d. Uvula
   e. Odors
   f. Fluids
6. Neck (pp. 000–000)
   a. Symmetry
   b. Deformity
   c. Deviation
   d. Tugging
   e. Masses
   f. Surgical scars
   g. Gland enlargement
   h. Lymph nodes
   i. Penetrating injuries
   j. Jugular veins
   k. Trachea
   l. Carotid arteries
7. Chest and lungs (**Proc. 12-6, p. 697**)
   a. Breathing
   b. Inspect
   c. Palpate
   d. Percuss
   e. Auscultate
8. Cardiovascular system
   a. Skin
   b. Carotid arteries

            c. PMI
            d. Heart sounds
        9. Abdomen
            a. Scars
            b. Dilated veins
            c. Stretch marks
            d. Rashes
            e. Lesions
            f. Pigmentation changes
                i. Cullen's sign
                ii. Grey-Turner's sign
            g. Size, shape, and symmetry
            h. Palpate last
            i. Tenderness
            j. Muscular rigidity
            k. Superficial organs and masses
        10. Pelvis (pain, instability, crepitus, immobilization)
        11. Genitalia (hemorrhage, priapism, rape or sexual abuse)
        12. Anus and rectum (rectal bleeding)
        13. Peripheral vascular system
            a. Size
            b. Symmetry
            c. Peripheral pulses
            d. Temperature
            e. Moisture
            f. Color
            g. Capillary refill
        14. Musculoskeletal system
            a. Inspect
            b. Palpate
            c. Test range of motion
            d. Crepitation
            e. Distal neurovascular checks
        15. Nervous system exam
            a. Mental status and speech
            b. Cranial nerves
            c. Motor system
            d. Reflexes
            e. Sensory system
    B. Vital signs (p. 698)
        1. Trending
    C. Recording exam findings (p. 698)

VI. Ongoing assessment. Because patient condition can change suddenly, you must repeatedly reassess mental status, ABCs, and any deterioration in areas already compromised. (pp. 698–701) (**Proc. 12-7, p. 700**)

    A. Mental status (p. 698)
        1. AVPU
        2. Deterioration
    B. Airway patency (p. 699)
        1. Deterioration
        2. Treatment
    C. Breathing rate and quality (p. 699)
        1. Signs of deteriorating conditions
    D. Pulse rate and quality (p. 699)
        1. Signs of deteriorating conditions

POWERPOINT PRESENTATION
Chapter 12, PowerPoint slides 146–150

TEACHING STRATEGY 9
Determining Patient Priority

E. Skin condition (p. 699)
   1. Signs of deteriorating conditions
F. Transport priorities (p. 699)
   1. Revise according to changes in patient's condition
G. Vital signs (p. 701)
   1. Signs of deteriorating conditions
H. Focused assessment (p. 701)
   1. Repeat as chief complaint dictates
I. Effects of interventions (p. 701)
J. Management plans (p. 701)
   1. Ability to reassess patient
   2. Reevaluate field diagnosis
   3. Alter management plan to optimizes patient care

VII. Chapter summary (pp. 701–702). Patient assessment is the key to providing effective prehospital emergency medical care. Its components include the initial assessment, the focused history and physical exam, vital signs, ongoing assessment, and the detailed physical exam. The initial assessment is designed to identify life-threatening airway, breathing, and circulation problems. The focused history and physical exam is designed to identify the signs and symptoms surrounding your patient's chief complaint. It is a problem-oriented approach that is easily modified to match your patient's clinical situation. The ongoing assessment is designed to reevaluate your patient for changes in status en route to the hospital. The detailed physical exam is a comprehensive head-to-toe evaluation designed to identify any conditions not already found. Although more suited to a clinical setting, it is intended to be done en route to the hospital if time allows.

The four general types of patients require distinctly different assessment approaches. The trauma patient with a significant mechanism of injury should receive an initial assessment, a rapid trauma assessment, and rapid transport. The patient with isolated, minor trauma, such as a cut finger or sprained ankle, should receive a physical exam focused on his particular problem or area. The responsive medical patient requires an initial assessment, a history and physical exam that focuses on his chief complaint, and vital signs. The unresponsive medical patient requires an initial assessment, followed by a rapid head-to-toe medical assessment and rapid transport. You will perform detailed history and physical exam techniques en route to the hospital if time and your patient's condition allow.

SKILLS DEMONSTRATION AND PRACTICE

The following activities reinforce different assessment skills that students will practice in the field.

Vital Signs Practice: At the beginning of the class session, distribute stethoscopes and blood pressure cuffs to students. Have each student check vital signs on another student and record them on Handout 12-10. Encourage students to pair with a different student each class. (Make sure the students record their own vital signs on their handout.)

Physical Assessment and Transport Decision Practice: Use students or paper cutouts as patients. Print scene size-up and initial assessment findings on a 3 × 5 card, and place it on the patient. Develop cards for several patients and number them. Have each student rotate through all patients, carrying a clipboard with Handout 12-11, "Initial Assessment Identification." Have students circle the appropriate type of physical assessment they would use and note whether this patient is a high priority for rapid transport.

Cranial Nerve Exam: Distribute copies of Handout 12-12. Then have students choose partners and perform on each other the One-Minute Cranial Nerve Exam on text page 688 and summarized in the handout. Students should then choose new partners and again perform the exam on each other. Have students continue to trade partners until they have completed the exam on five other students. (This may be done on a continual basis along with practicing vital signs at the beginning of each class.)

HANDOUT 12-12
One-Minute Cranial Nerve Exam

WORKBOOK
Chapter 12 Activities

ASSIGNMENTS

Assign students to complete Chapter 12, "Patient Assessment in the Field," of the workbook. Also assign them to read Chapter 13, "Clinical Decision Making," before the next class.

READING/REFERENCE
Textbook, pp. 704–715

HANDOUTS 12-4 AND 12-5
Chapter 12 Quizzes

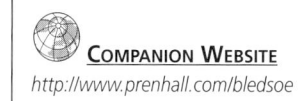

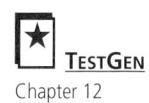

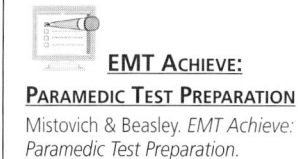

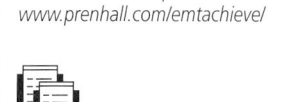

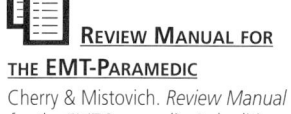

EVALUATION

HANDOUT 12-6
Chapter 12 Scenario

Chapter Quiz and Scenario   Distribute copies of the Chapter Quizzes provided in Handouts 12-4, 12-5 to evaluate student understanding of this chapter. Make sure each student reads the scenario to reinforce critical thinking on the scene. Remind students not to use their notes or textbooks while taking the quiz.

Student CD   Quizzes for every chapter are contained on the dynamic and highly visual in-text student CD.

PARAMEDIC STUDENT CD
Student Activities

Companion Website   Additional quizzes for every chapter are contained on this exciting website.

COMPANION WEBSITE
http://www.prenhall.com/bledsoe

TestGen   You may wish to create a custom-tailored test using *Prentice Hall TestGen for Essentials of Paramedic Care,* 2nd Edition to evaluate student understanding of this chapter.

TESTGEN
Chapter 12

On-line Test Preparation (for students and instructors)   Additional test preparation is available through Brady's new on-line product, *EMT Achieve: Paramedic Test Preparation* at *http://www.prenhall.com/emtachieve/.* Instructors can also monitor student mastery on-line.

EMT ACHIEVE: PARAMEDIC TEST PREPARATION
Mistovich & Beasley. *EMT Achieve: Paramedic Test Preparation.*
www.prenhall.com/emtachieve/

Review Manual for the EMT-Paramedic   This comprehensive exam review contains hundreds of test questions and rationales, including scenarios, along with two 180-question practice tests on CD.

REVIEW MANUAL FOR THE EMT-PARAMEDIC
Cherry & Mistovich. *Review Manual for the EMT-Paramedic,* 3rd edition.

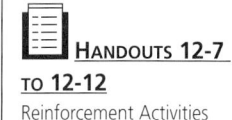

REINFORCEMENT

Handouts   If classroom discussion or performance on the quizzes indicates that some students have not fully mastered the chapter content, you may wish to assign some or all of the Reinforcement Handouts for this chapter.

HANDOUTS 12-7 TO 12-12
Reinforcement Activities

Student CD (for students)   A wide variety of material on this CD-ROM will reinforce and also expand student knowledge and skills.

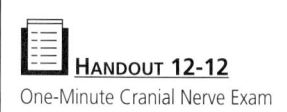

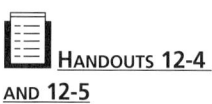

PARAMEDIC STUDENT CD
Student Activities

PowerPoint Presentation (for instructors)   The PowerPoint material developed for this chapter offers useful reinforcement of chapter content.

Companion Website (for students)   Additional review quizzes and links to EMS resources will contribute to further reinforcement of the chapter.

OneKey   On-line support is offered for this course on one of three platforms: CourseCompass, Blackboard, or Web CT. Includes the IRM, PowerPoints, TestGen, and Companion Website for instruction. Ask your local sales representative for more information.

Brady Skills Series: Advanced Life Skills (Video or CD)   Have your students watch the skills come to life on VHS or CD-ROM, or they can purchase the highly visual, full-color text with step-by-step procedures and rationales.

POWERPOINT PRESENTATION
Chapter 12

COMPANION WEBSITE
http://www.prenhall.com/bledsoe

ONEKEY
Chapter 12

ADVANCED LIFE SUPPORT SKILLS
Larmon & Davis. *Advanced Life Support Skills.*

ADVANCED LIFE SKILLS REVIEW
Larmon & Davis. *Advanced Life Skills Review.*

BRADY SKILLS SERIES: ALS
Larmon & Davis. *Brady Skills Series: ALS.*

PARAMEDIC NATIONAL STANDARDS SELF-TEST
Miller. *Paramedic National Standards Self-Test*, 4th edition.

HANDOUT 12-1

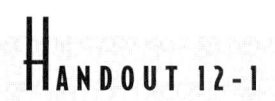

Student's Name _____

CHAPTER 12 OBJECTIVES CHECKLIST

Knowledge	Date Mastered
1. Recognize hazards/potential hazards associated with the medical and trauma scene.	
2. Identify unsafe scenes and describe methods for making them safe.	
3. Discuss common mechanisms of injury/nature of illness.	
4. Predict patterns of injury based on mechanism of injury.	
5. Discuss the reason for identifying the total number of patients at the scene.	
6. Organize the management of a scene following size-up.	
7. Explain the reasons for identifying the need for additional help or assistance during the scene size-up.	
8. Summarize the reasons for forming a general impression of the patient.	
9. Discuss methods of assessing mental status/levels of consciousness in the adult, infant, and child patient.	
10. Discuss methods of assessing and securing the airway in the adult, child, and infant patient.	
11. State reasons for cervical spine management for the trauma patient.	
12. Analyze a scene to determine if spinal precautions are required.	
13. Describe methods for assessing respiration in the adult, child, and infant patient.	
14. Describe the methods used to locate and assess a pulse in an adult, child, and infant patient.	
15. Discuss the need for assessing the patient for external bleeding.	
16. Describe normal and abnormal findings when assessing skin color, temperature, and condition.	
17. Explain the reason and process for prioritizing a patient for care and transport.	
18. Use the findings of the initial assessment to determine the patient's perfusion status.	
19. Describe orthostatic vital signs and evaluate their usefulness in assessing a patient in shock.	

OBJECTIVES

©2007 Pearson Education, Inc.
Essentials of Paramedic Care, 2nd ed.

CHAPTER 12 *Patient Assessment in the Field* 397

HANDOUT 12-1 Continued

Knowledge	Date Mastered
20. Describe the medical patient physical examination.	
21. Differentiate between the assessment for an unresponsive, altered mental status, and alert medical patients.	
22. Discuss the reasons for reconsidering the mechanism of injury.	
23. Recite examples and explain why patients should receive a rapid trauma assessment.	
24. Describe the trauma patient physical examination.	
25. Describe the elements of the rapid trauma assessment and discuss their evaluation.	
26. Identify cases when the rapid assessment is suspended to provide patient care.	
27. Discuss the reason for performing a focused history and physical exam.	
28. Describe when and why a detailed physical examination is necessary.	
29. Discuss the components of the detailed physical examination.	
30. Explain what additional care is provided while performing the detailed physical exam.	
31. Distinguish between the detailed physical exam that is performed on a trauma patient and that of the medical patient.	
32. Differentiate between patients requiring a detailed physical exam and those who do not.	
33. Discuss the rationale for repeating the initial assessment as part of the ongoing assessment.	
34. Describe the components of the ongoing assessment.	
35. Describe trending of assessment components.	
36. Discuss medical identification devices/systems.	
37. Given several preprogrammed and moulaged medical and trauma patients, provide the appropriate scene survey, initial assessment, focused assessment, detailed assessment, and ongoing assessments.	

Handout 12-2

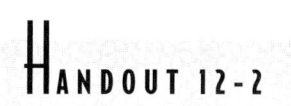

Student's Name _____

PERFORMING A SCENE SIZE-UP AND INITIAL ASSESSMENT

Charting Student Progress:
1. *Learning skill*
2. *Performs skill with direction*
3. *Performs skill independently*

Procedure	1	2	3
Scene size-up			
1. Takes body substance isolation precautions.			
2. Ensures scene safety.			
3. Locates all patients.			
4. Determines mechanism of injury/nature of illness.			
Initial assessment			
1. Forms general impression.			
2. Stabilizes cervical spine as needed.			
3. Assesses baseline level of response.			
Airway			
1. Opens airway with appropriate maneuver.			
2. Looks, listens, and feels for air movement.			
3. Immediately corrects obstructed airway.			
4. Inserts oral or nasal airway adjunct as needed.			
Breathing			
1. Assesses breathing rate and quality.			
2. Inspects chest and back.			
3. Palpates chest and back.			
4. Auscultates bilaterally for equality/adequacy of ventilation.			
5. Immediately corrects injuries that may compromise airway/breathing.			
6. Administers oxygen; assists ventilations.			

SKILLS

©2007 Pearson Education, Inc.
Essentials of Paramedic Care, 2nd ed.

HANDOUT 12-2 Continued

Procedure	1	2	3
Circulation			
1. Checks radial pulses for rate and quality.			
2. Checks skin color, temperature, and condition.			
3. Checks capillary refill time in children.			
4. Controls gross hemorrhage.			
5. Elevates legs; keeps patient warm, as needed.			
6. Applies and inflates PASG as needed.			
7. Assigns priority for rapid transport.			

Comments:

Handout 12-3

Student's Name _____

PERFORMING A RAPID TRAUMA ASSESSMENT

Charting Student Progress:
1. *Learning skill*
2. *Performs skill with direction*
3. *Performs skill independently*

Procedure	1	2	3
Head: DCAP-BTLS and crepitation			
1. Palpates the head.			
2. Periodically examines gloves for blood.			
Neck: DCAP-BTLS and crepitation			
1. Inspects and palpates the anterior neck.			
2. Checks for tracheal deviation.			
3. Checks for subcutaneous emphysema.			
4. Checks for jugular vein distention.			
Chest: DCAP-BTLS and crepitation			
1. Inspects and palpates the chest.			
2. Checks for subcutaneous emphysema.			
3. Auscultates both lungs.			
Abdomen: DCAP-BTLS and crepitation			
1. Inspects and palpates abdomen.			
Pelvis: DCAP-BTLS and crepitation			
1. Evaluates the pelvic ring.			
Extremities: DCAP-BTLS and crepitation			
1. Inspects and palpates all four extremities.			
2. Evaluates distal neurovascular functions (pulse, sensation, movement).			
Posterior: DCAP-BTLS and crepitation			
1. Inspects and palpates posterior trunk, buttocks.			

SKILLS

Comments:

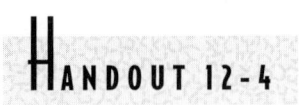

CHAPTER 12 QUIZ, PART A

Write the letter of the best answer in the space provided.

_____ 1. The problem-oriented evaluation of a patient with establishment of priorities based on existing and potential threats to human life is called:
   A. rapid trauma assessment.
   B. patient assessment.
   C. focused physical assessment.
   D. detailed physical exam.

_____ 2. The purpose of the initial assessment is to identify and correct:
   A. scene safety concerns.
   B. serious injuries such as fractures and dislocations.
   C. immediately life-threatening conditions.
   D. minor injuries.

_____ 3. Which of the following problems would you be likely to note during your scene size-up of a situation?
   A. You palpate several possible rib fractures in the patient's chest.
   B. The patient's pulse pressure is narrowing.
   C. The patient is complaining of chest pain.
   D. The patient is bradycardic.

_____ 4. Body substance isolation is a component of:
   A. scene size-up.
   B. initial assessment.
   C. focused history and physical exam.
   D. detailed physical exam.

_____ 5. In a medical emergency, you can sometimes determine the nature of your patient's illness from clues at the scene. These would include:
   A. the smell of a lower gastrointestinal bleed.
   B. the sound of a hissing oxygen tank.
   C. the sight of drug paraphernalia.
   D. all of these

_____ 6. The most effective method of preventing disease transmission between you and your patients is:
   A. always wearing appropriate eye protection.
   B. wearing a surgical mask when treating any patient.
   C. washing your hands before and after patient contact.
   D. wearing an HEPA filter mask whenever caring for a patient with breathing difficulty.

_____ 7. Which of the following is true regarding scene safety?
   A. Your personal safety is the top priority at any emergency scene.
   B. If your scene is unsafe, enter cautiously.
   C. All medical scenes may be considered safe.
   D. It is expected of you, as a paramedic, to risk your life to care for a patient if necessary.

_____ 8. The nature of the patient's illness:
   A. is always the same as his chief complaint.
   B. is always readily apparent.
   C. can only be obtained from the patient himself.
   D. may be evident from clues you find at the scene.

_____ 9. Determining the patient's priority for transport is a component of the:
   A. scene size-up.
   B. initial assessment.
   C. ongoing assessment.
   D. detailed assessment.

HANDOUT 12-4 Continued

_____ 10. Components of the initial assessment include:
   A. assessment of the patient's airway, breathing, and circulation.
   B. baseline vital signs.
   C. assessing the body for DCAP-BTLS.
   D. location of medic alert tags or other forms of medical information.

_____ 11. While performing the initial assessment of a patient, you note an open wound to the chest. This injury should be treated:
   A. during the focused physical examination.
   B. during the rapid trauma assessment.
   C. during the initial assessment.
   D. during the detailed physical exam.

_____ 12. If the mechanism of injury is significant or if your patient is unresponsive:
   A. immediately apply high-concentration oxygen by nonrebreather mask.
   B. have your partner manually stabilize the patient's head and neck.
   C. immediately transport the patient after completing the initial assessment.
   D. apply a cervical collar after completing the initial assessment.

_____ 13. Serious external hemorrhage should be controlled:
   A. during the initial assessment.   C. during the detailed physical exam.
   B. before beginning the initial assessment. D. during the scene size-up.

_____ 14. If you suspect a possible cervical spine injury, you should open the patient's airway with:
   A. a nasopharyngeal airway.   C. the head-tilt/chin-tilt method.
   B. an oropharyngeal airway.   D. the jaw-thrust maneuver.

_____ 15. To record your patient's mental status, use the acronym AVPU. Which of the following is true?
   A. A stands for awake.   C. P stands for painful stimuli.
   B. V stands for visual.   D. U stands for unilateral.

_____ 16. Signs of inadequate breathing in the adult patient include:
   A. symmetrical chest wall movement.   C. a pulse rate over 100.
   B. a respiratory rate over 24.   D. swelling or edema in the patient's lips.

_____ 17. If your patient has a radial pulse, you can assume that the systolic blood pressure is at least:
   A. 100.   C. 90.
   B. 95.   D. 60.

_____ 18. Mottled, cyanotic, pale, or ashen skin may indicate:
   A. hypertension.   C. shock.
   B. stroke.   D. sepsis.

_____ 19. Which of the following statements regarding assessment of an infant's or small child's circulation is true?
   A. Assess the carotid pulse of an infant first; then check the brachial pulse.
   B. Capillary refill time is a reliable indicator of perfusion in the infant patient.
   C. If an infant or small child is hypotensive, wrap his entire body in one leg of the PASG.
   D. A pulse rate over 100 in an infant or small child indicates circulatory compromise.

_____ 20. A patient is considered a top priority for rapid transport if:
   A. the patient has chest pain and a B/P of 120 systolic.
   B. the patient is pregnant and delivery is imminent.
   C. you have an extended en route time to the hospital.
   D. you have a poor general impression of the patient.

EVALUATION

©2007 Pearson Education, Inc.
Essentials of Paramedic Care, 2nd ed.   **CHAPTER 12** *Patient Assessment in the Field*   403

HANDOUT 12-5

Student's Name _____

CHAPTER 12 QUIZ, PART B

Write the letter of the best answer in the space provided.

_____ 1. How the focused history and physical exam are performed is based on the initial assessment and:
   A. the patient's chief complaint.
   B. local protocols.
   C. consultation with medical direction.
   D. the patient's vital signs.

_____ 2. One subclassification of trauma patients includes those:
   A. with an isolated injury.
   B. who are responsive.
   C. who have either internal or external bleeding.
   D. who are a high priority for rapid transport.

_____ 3. Predictors of serious internal injury of a patient include:
   A. traumatic amputation of a limb.
   B. airbag inflation during a vehicle collision.
   C. death in any of the vehicles involved in a collision.
   D. motorcycle crash.

_____ 4. The predictors of serious internal injury for infants and children that differ from those for adults include:
   A. a fall from higher than 10 feet.
   B. a slow-speed collision.
   C. the injury of another in the same passenger compartment.
   D. an unrestrained passenger.

_____ 5. The mnemonic DCAP-BTLS is helpful in conducting a rapid trauma assessment. The letters represent:
   A. the patient's level of consciousness.
   B. a score based on the assessment findings that predicts survival.
   C. common signs of injury for which you are looking.
   D. conditions that cause the patient to be a high priority for rapid transport.

_____ 6. The C in the mnemonic DCAP-BTLS stands for:
   A. cuts.
   B. concussion.
   C. consciousness.
   D. contusions.

_____ 7. The P in the mnemonic DCAP-BTLS stands for:
   A. penetration.
   B. pertinent history.
   C. percussion.
   D. pulse oximetry.

_____ 8. Subcutaneous emphysema is:
   A. fluid in the lungs causing severe respiratory distress.
   B. fluid or blood under the skin from damaged blood vessels.
   C. air just under the skin, causing a crackling sensation.
   D. a type of pulmonary embolism caused by an air bubble.

_____ 9. Treatment for a tension pneumothorax includes:
   A. stabilizing the injured side of the chest with a bulky dressing.
   B. needle cricothyrotomy.
   C. minimal supplemental oxygen administration to prevent an increase in pressure in the chest.
   D. needle decompression.

HANDOUT 12-5 Continued

_____ 10. A patient with a _____ fracture or dislocation risks lacerating the iliac arteries and veins, through which he can lose a significant amount of blood.
   A. vertebral
   B. pelvic
   C. cranial
   D. rib

_____ 11. When assessing the trauma patient with an isolated injury, you most likely will not need to perform a(n):
   A. scene size-up.
   B. initial assessment.
   C. SAMPLE history.
   D. detailed physical exam.

_____ 12. The history for a responsive medical patient should include the:
   A. chief complaint, history of the present illness, and current health status.
   B. chief complaint, history of the present illness, past history, and current health status.
   C. chief complaint, history of the present illness, current health status, and 1-minute cranial nerve exam.
   D. chief complaint and DCAP-BTLS.

_____ 13. Once you have obtained a chief complaint from a responsive medical patient, you should next:
   A. perform the initial assessment.
   B. perform a detailed physical exam.
   C. obtain a history of present illness.
   D. perform a focused physical exam.

_____ 14. In the acronym OPQRST-ASPN, ASPN stands for:
   A. amplified sounds, positional nystagmus.
   B. allergies, skin, pupils, neurologic status.
   C. associated symptoms, pertinent negatives.
   D. abdomen, sigmoid (colon), plantar reflex, nervous system.

_____ 15. To quickly test the seventh cranial nerve (CN-VII), you should have your patient:
   A. stand on one foot.
   B. close his eyes and touch his nose.
   C. stick out his tongue.
   D. show his teeth with his finger.

_____ 16. After completing the initial assessment of an unresponsive medical patient, you should next:
   A. obtain a brief history from family or bystanders.
   B. perform a detailed physical exam.
   C. immediately transport the patient.
   D. perform a rapid medical assessment.

_____ 17. After conducting the focused physical exam for a responsive medical patient, you should next:
   A. provide necessary emergency medical care authorized by standing orders.
   B. contact on-line medical direction to request further orders.
   C. immediately transport the patient to the correct facility.
   D. conduct a detailed physical exam.

_____ 18. The detailed physical exam is designed for use:
   A. on all trauma patients.
   B. on patients en route to the hospital.
   C. on all responsive medical patients.
   D. on patients prior to transport.

_____ 19. The ongoing assessment:
   A. detects trends.
   B. determines changes.
   C. assesses intervention effects.
   D. all of these

_____ 20. The ongoing assessment should be conducted every _____ minutes for stable patients and every _____ minutes for unstable patients.
   A. 15, 10
   B. 15, 5
   C. 10, 5
   D. 10, 3

EVALUATION

HANDOUT 12-6

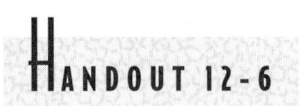

Student's Name _____

CHAPTER 12 SCENARIO

Review the following real-life situation. Then answer the questions that follow.

A 5-year-old boy playing on his front lawn is startled when a stray dog runs up to him. When he puts out his hand to pet the dog, the dog lunges for the boy's throat. Shocked by the attack, the child falls unconscious. The dog releases his grip and runs off as neighbors who have witnessed the attack call 911 and rush to the child's aid.

The local volunteer BLS quick response team arrives and quickly assesses the boy. His airway is compromised by blood from multiple puncture wounds. He is ashen and pale. He is barely moving air. His radial pulses are weak and rapid. As the crew assesses him, they treat him with suction, insertion of an oral airway, oxygen via a nonrebreather mask, and spinal immobilization. When the paramedic ambulance arrives, the QRT crew chief gives his report to the paramedic, who decides to rapidly transport the child to the regional trauma center.

En route, the paramedic performs a more detailed examination of the boy. She notes the airway difficulty and elects to intubate the child immediately because swelling and discoloration around the throat suggest his airway could collapse despite vigorous suctioning. The child has subcutaneous emphysema around his clavicles. The paramedic is somewhat relieved when auscultation reveals clear breath sounds bilaterally. Nevertheless, she requests pulse oximetry. Meanwhile, the child's color is visibly improving.

The paramedic is also concerned for the child's cervical spine and assesses the distal neurological functions, but not before obtaining a set of vital signs. Content that the child was hypoxic and not hypovolemic, she begins to evaluate the child's mental status. The child is conscious but is "in shock" from the attack. The best that can be determined is that he is verbal; he will follow commands such as grasping fingers or moving toes.

Upon arrival at the trauma center, the paramedic gives a detailed report of her assessment findings to the surgeons. Rapidly stabilized in the emergency department, the boy is rushed to the operating suite for exploration and repair of his injuries. He has a puncture to the larynx and requires multiple sutures but is otherwise stable.

1. Based on the initial dispatch information, what problems might you anticipate regarding scene size-up and initial assessment findings?

2. Why did this patient warrant rapid transport to a trauma center?

3. What critical interventions did the BLS quick response team members and the paramedic provide to correct immediate life threats?

4. What were the treatment priorities for this patient?

HANDOUT 12-7

Student's Name _____

CHAPTER 12 REVIEW, PART A

Write the word or words that best complete the following sentences in the space provided.

1. The components of patient assessment include the initial assessment, focused history and physical exam, _____ _____ _____, and _____ _____.
2. The essential first step at any emergency involves taking time to judge the situation, which is called the _____ _____-_____.
3. The most effective method of preventing disease transmission between you and your patients is _____ _____ _____.
4. The combined strength, direction, and nature of forces that injured your patient are called the _____ _____ _____.
5. Your anticipation of possible injuries based upon your analysis of the event is the _____ _____ _____.
6. The first step of the initial assessment is _____ _____ _____ _____.
7. The purpose of the initial assessment is to identify and correct _____ _____ _____-_____.
8. Determining the patient's priority for transport is a step in the _____ _____.
9. The acronym used to record your patient's mental status is _____.
10. Your unresponsive patient has his arms flexed and legs extended. This is known as _____ posturing.
11. If your unresponsive patient has both arms and legs extended, this is known as _____ posturing.
12. If you suspect a cervical spine injury, you should open your patient's airway using the _____ _____ maneuver.
13. When using the head-tilt/chin-lift maneuver on an infant, it is important not to _____ the head and neck.
14. Unconscious patients without a gag reflex will tolerate an airway adjunct known as a(n) _____ airway.
15. Signs of inadequate breathing include the use of _____ muscles to breathe.
16. When assessing an adult patient's circulation, you should feel for a(n) _____ pulse first.
17. Assess an infant's circulation at the _____ artery.
18. _____ _____ _____ provides important information about the circulatory status of infants and young children.
19. If a patient shows signs of circulatory compromise, consider _____ his legs to encourage venous return.
20. Top-priority patients include those with poor _____ _____, complicated _____, and chest pain with a systolic B/P of less than _____.

REINFORCEMENT

©2007 Pearson Education, Inc.
Essentials of Paramedic Care, 2nd ed.

CHAPTER 12 *Patient Assessment in the Field* 407

Handout 12-8

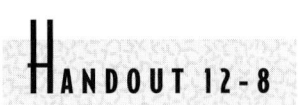

Student's Name _____

CHAPTER 12 REVIEW, PART B

Write the word or words that best complete the following sentences in the space provided.

1. Trauma patients are classified as one of two types: patients with a(n) _____ _____ _____ _____ and patients with a(n) _____ _____ _____ _____.

2. Medical patients are classified as either _____ or _____ .

3. Predictors of serious internal injury include _____ from a vehicle, _____ in the same passenger compartment, and _____ of the vehicle.

4. After the initial assessment of a major trauma patient, the paramedic should perform a(n) _____ _____ assessment.

5. The T in DCAP-BTLS stands for _____ .

6. In the semi-Fowler's position, jugular venous distention beyond _____ degrees is significant.

7. The fracture of two or more adjacent ribs in two or more places causes an unstable flail (floating) segment that may be evidenced by _____ chest wall movement.

8. Occlusive dressings to seal open chest wounds should be applied at the _____ of exhalation and taped on _____ sides.

9. The _____ _____ _____ may be used as a splint to immobilize an unstable pelvic fracture.

10. Weakness or disability in the extremities on only one side of the body suggests brain injury due to _____ or _____ _____ .

11. For major trauma cases when time is critical, you should use the _____ history format.

12. When caring for an isolated-injury trauma patient, paramedics should avoid _____ _____ and develop a(n) _____ threshold for suspecting other injuries.

13. In the _____ _____ patient, the history takes precedence over the physical exam.

14. _____ _____ and the seriousness of your patient's condition will determine which exam techniques you use for your responsive medical patient.

15. When inspecting your patient's chest, you should look for the typical bulge that indicates a(n) _____ _____ or _____ .

16. To test your patient's 12th cranial nerve (CN-12) using the 1-minute cranial nerve exam, you should ask him to _____ _____ _____ _____ .

17. To identify the presence and location of a possible myocardial infarction, you should perform _____-_____ _____ monitoring.

18. Always base your emergency care on your patient's _____ and _____ as obtained through a thorough focused history and physical exam.

19. The steps in assessing unresponsive medical patients include (1) _____ _____ , (2) _____ _____ _____ , and (3) _____ _____ .

20. The detailed physical exam is a more focused exam using components of the _____ _____ _____ .

21. The three goals of an ongoing assessment are to _____ _____ , _____ _____ , and _____ _____ _____ .

Handout 12-9

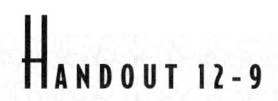

Student's Name _____

ACRONYM COMPLETION

Complete the mnemonics and acronyms for different phases of the assessment process.

1. Mental status
   - A _____
   - V _____
   - P _____
   - U _____

2. Initial assessment
   - A _____
   - B _____
   - C _____

3. Rapid trauma assessment
   - D _____
   - C _____
   - A _____
   - P _____
   - B _____
   - T _____
   - L _____
   - S _____

4. History
   - S _____
   - A _____
   - M _____
   - P _____
   - L _____
   - E _____

5. History of present illness
   - O _____
   - P _____
   - Q _____
   - R _____
   - S _____
   - T _____
   - AS _____
   - PN _____

REINFORCEMENT

©2007 Pearson Education, Inc.
Essentials of Paramedic Care, 2nd ed.

CHAPTER 12 *Patient Assessment in the Field* 409

Handout 12-10

Student's Name _____

VITAL SIGNS PRACTICE

REINFORCEMENT

Date	Pulse/Location	Respirations	B/P Auscultation	B/P Palpation

HANDOUT 12-10 Continued

Date	Pulse/Location	Respirations	B/P Auscultation	B/P Palpation

REINFORCEMENT

HANDOUT 12-11

Student's Name _____

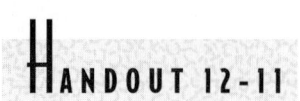

INITIAL ASSESSMENT IDENTIFICATION

For each simulated patient, you will be given a scenario and initial assessment findings. Based on the information given, indicate the appropriate type of physical exam you would perform and whether the patient is a high priority for transport or not.

Pt. #	Type of Physical Exam	Detailed Exam	High Priority, Rapid Transport
1	Rapid Trauma Assessment Focused Physical Exam	Yes No	Yes No
2	Rapid Trauma Assessment Focused Physical Exam	Yes No	Yes No
3	Rapid Trauma Assessment Focused Physical Exam	Yes No	Yes No
4	Rapid Trauma Assessment Focused Physical Exam	Yes No	Yes No
5	Rapid Trauma Assessment Focused Physical Exam	Yes No	Yes No
6	Rapid Trauma Assessment Focused Physical Exam	Yes No	Yes No
7	Rapid Trauma Assessment Focused Physical Exam	Yes No	Yes No
8	Rapid Trauma Assessment Focused Physical Exam	Yes No	Yes No
9	Rapid Trauma Assessment Focused Physical Exam	Yes No	Yes No
10	Rapid Trauma Assessment Focused Physical Exam	Yes No	Yes No
11	Rapid Trauma Assessment Focused Physical Exam	Yes No	Yes No
12	Rapid Trauma Assessment Focused Physical Exam	Yes No	Yes No
13	Rapid Trauma Assessment Focused Physical Exam	Yes No	Yes No
14	Rapid Trauma Assessment Focused Physical Exam	Yes No	Yes No
15	Rapid Trauma Assessment Focused Physical Exam	Yes No	Yes No
16	Rapid Trauma Assessment Focused Physical Exam	Yes No	Yes No
17	Rapid Trauma Assessment Focused Physical Exam	Yes No	Yes No
18	Rapid Trauma Assessment Focused Physical Exam	Yes No	Yes No
19	Rapid Trauma Assessment Focused Physical Exam	Yes No	Yes No
20	Rapid Trauma Assessment Focused Physical Exam	Yes No	Yes No

REINFORCEMENT

HANDOUT 12-12

Student's Name _____

ONE-MINUTE CRANIAL NERVE EXAM

Cranial Nerves	Test
I	Normally not tested in the field
II, III	Direct response to light
III, IV, VI	"H" test for extraocular movements
V	Clench teeth; palpate masseter and temporal muscles. Test sensory to forehead, cheek, and tongue.
VII	Show teeth.
IX, X	Say "aaahhh"; watch uvula movement. Test gag reflex.
XII	Stick out tongue.
VIII	Test balance (Romberg test) and hearing.
XI	Shrug shoulders, turn head.

Chapter 12 Answer Key

Handout 12-4: Chapter 12 Quiz, Part A

1. B	6. C	11. C	16. B
2. C	7. A	12. B	17. D
3. C	8. D	13. A	18. C
4. A	9. B	14. D	19. B
5. D	10. A	15. C	20. D

Handout 12-5: Chapter 12 Quiz, Part B

1. D	6. D	11. D	16. D
2. A	7. A	12. B	17. A
3. D	8. C	13. C	18. B
4. A	9. D	14. C	19. D
5. C	10. B	15. D	20. B

Handout 12-6: Chapter 12 Scenario

1. Safety is an immediate concern in this scenario. Where is the dog? Are the police or animal control officer en route? Could the dog have rabies? Body substance isolation precautions must be taken. Is the child becoming hypovolemic or hypoperfused? Because the injuries are on and around the neck, is there any airway compromise? Cervical spine injuries may also be present. There may be problems with all the ABCs. This child may be a high priority for rapid transport to the hospital.
2. The patient is a high priority for rapid transport for a number of reasons. First would be a poor general impression. His level of consciousness is altered, and he is having obvious airway and respiratory difficulty. He is also showing some signs of possible hypoperfusion during the initial assessment. The serious multiple wounds to the neck also would be a reason for rapid transport.
3. The BLS crew immediately recognized the airway problem, suctioned the patient, inserted an oropharyngeal airway, and applied high-concentration oxygen by nonrebreather mask. The crew also immobilized the patient due to possible cervical spine injuries. The paramedic continued treatment of the patient's airway by performing an endotracheal intubation.
4. As with all patients, treatment began with correcting life-threatening problems found during the initial assessment. The BLS crew maintained the airway and applied oxygen. They completed the initial assessment by assessing breathing and circulation. Considering the patient's condition and the location of his wounds, his airway was of primary concern.

Handout 12-7: Chapter 12 Review, Part A

1. detailed physical exam, ongoing assessment
2. scene size-up
3. washing your hands
4. mechanism of injury
5. index of suspicion
6. forming a general impression
7. immediately life-threatening conditions
8. initial assessment
9. AVPU
10. decorticate
11. decerebrate
12. jaw thrust
13. overextend
14. oropharyngeal
15. accessory
16. radial
17. brachial
18. Capillary refill time
19. elevating
20. general impression, childbirth, 100

Handout 12-8: Chapter 12 Review, Part B

1. significant mechanism of injury, isolated mechanism of injury (any order)
2. responsive, unresponsive (any order)
3. ejection, death, rollover
4. rapid trauma
5. tenderness
6. 45
7. paradoxical
8. end, three
9. pneumatic antishock garment
10. stroke, head injury
11. SAMPLE
12. tunnel vision, low
13. responsive medical
14. Clinical judgment
15. implanted pacemaker, defibrillator
16. stick out his tongue
17. 12-lead ECG
18. signs, symptoms
19. (1) initial assessment, (2) rapid medical assessment, (3) brief history
20. comprehensive physical exam
21. detect trends, determine changes, assess intervention effects

Handout 12-9: Acronym Completion

1. **A** Alert
   V Verbal
   P Painful
   U Unresponsive
2. **A** Airway
   B Breathing
   C Circulation
3. **D** Deformities
   C Contusions
   A Abrasions
   P Penetration
   B Burns
   T Tenderness
   L Lacerations
   S Swelling
4. **S** Symptoms
   A Allergies
   M Medications
   P Past medical history
   L Last oral intake
   E Events preceding the incident
5. **O** Onset
   P Provocation/Palliation
   Q Quality
   R Region/Radiation
   S Severity
   T Time
   AS Associated Symptoms
   PN Pertinent Negatives

Chapter 13

Clinical Decision Making

INTRODUCTION

Emphasize to students that as paramedics they will confront situations that require them to make critical decisions on which a patient's life may depend. More than merely acting as technicians, they must be able to gather information, analyze it, form a field diagnosis, and devise a management plan. They must often perform these functions before contacting a medical direction physician. They may be faced with several options regarding a field diagnosis. Their ability to make correct clinical decisions will determine their strength as prehospital practitioners of emergency medicine. They will base their decisions not only on training and knowledge but also on experience. Listening to hospital and field preceptors is a vital part of this process.

TOTAL TEACHING TIME:
5.21 HOURS
The total teaching time is only a guideline based on the didactic and practical lab averages in the National Standard Curriculum. Instructors should take into consideration such factors as the pace at which students learn, the size of the class, and breaks. The actual time devoted to teaching objectives is the responsibility of the instructor.

CHAPTER OBJECTIVES

After reading this chapter, you should be able to:

1. Compare the factors influencing medical care in the out-of-hospital environment to other medical settings. (p. 706)
2. Differentiate between critical life-threatening, potentially life-threatening, and non-life-threatening patient presentations. (p. 706)
3. Evaluate the benefits and shortfalls of protocols, standing orders, and patient care algorithms. (pp. 706–707)
4. Define the components, stages, and sequences of the critical thinking process for paramedics. (pp. 708–714)
5. Apply the fundamental elements of critical thinking for paramedics. (pp. 711–714)
6. Describe the effects of the fight-or-flight response and its positive and negative effects on a paramedic's decision making. (p. 710)
7. Summarize the "six Rs" of putting it all together: *R*ead the patient, *R*ead the scene, *R*eact, *R*eevaluate, *R*evise the management plan, *R*eview performance. (pp. 713–714)
8. Given several preprogrammed and moulaged trauma and medical patients, demonstrate clinical decision making. (pp. 705–714)

©2007 Pearson Education, Inc.
Essentials of Paramedic Care, 2nd ed.

FRAMING THE LESSON

Begin the class by having each student write down several reasons and symptoms for which people call an ambulance. Guide them in listing both specific and vague problems. Stress that not all calls to 911 are true emergencies and even fewer are true life-threatening emergencies. After you have compiled several different reasons for EMS calls, have the students discuss the possible causes of the symptoms presented in the list. Next, have the students categorize them into true life-threats, potential life-threats, and non-life-threatening calls. You may also include a brief review of anatomy and physiology. If a specific area of the body is painful, what organs lie in the area or could be causing the pain? If a particular portion of the body is injured as a result of trauma, what systems or organs may be affected?

TEACHING STRATEGIES

People learn in a variety of ways. Some do better with the spoken word, whereas others prefer the written. Some prefer to work alone, whereas others profit from working in groups. Recognizing these different ways of acquiring knowledge, the authors of this *Instructor's Resource Manual* have provided a variety of teaching strategies for the different types of learners. These strategies are intended to foster higher-level cognitive skills and encourage creative learning and problem solving. For greatest effectiveness, incorporate these strategies into your class lecture. Symbols in the Lecture Outline indicate the points at which various exercises might be most appropriate. Other strategies can be used to preview the lesson or to summarize it.

The following strategies are keyed to specific sections of the lesson.

1. Thinking about Problems. This first problem-solving activity is sure to be appreciated by employers and improve conditions within your own classroom. Have students create a "gripe" list or list of complaints. Divide the class into work groups and assign one of the complaints to each group. Have the groups create at least three possible, realistic solutions to the problem. Have them address finances, time, obstacles to implementation, benefits, and so on. From this point forward, you could establish a policy in your classroom or institution that states, "Every problem must be accompanied by two possible solutions." This is a cooperative learning exercise that emphasizes teamwork, verbal communication, and problem solving.

2. Patient Acuity Practice. Have each student write a scenario of a patient injury or illness. Make sure they include scene and physical exam findings, including vital signs. First, have each student read the dispatch information that would be given to the responders. Have students classify the situation as a critical life-threat, potential life-threat, or non-life-threat. Next, add the scene size-up information, and have students determine whether they would change the classification. Finally, give the physical exam findings and have students reevaluate their classification.

3. Algorithm Development. Have students create algorithms for common activities such as tying tennis shoes, making chicken noodle soup, or making a bed. Have them sketch and label their algorithms. Then discuss the ultimate outcome of following the procedures in the algorithm and alternative ways to reach the goal. The class can identify hazards or benefits to methods not included in the algorithm. This will help students to realize that algorithms and protocols are only guidelines that suffice in most but not all situations and sometimes need revision based on individual circumstances.

*4. **Thinking about Differential Diagnoses.*** Though students will not be able to formulate differential diagnoses for sophisticated medical problems, you can draw an analogy between diagnosis formulation and the process of cooking. Give students a list of ingredients, such as hamburger, pasta, and tomato sauce. Have them determine all the possible entrées they could create with these items. This is similar to encountering a patient who complains of headache, weakness, and nausea. He or she could be suffering a brain injury, migraine headache, flu, and so forth. The idea is to associate symptomatologies with diagnoses (or ingredients with recipes).

*5. **"Six Rs" Scenarios.*** Set up scenarios for your students to practice the "six Rs" of decision making, either through role-play or case study slides. Unlike the procedures in other scenario practices, stop students throughout the progression of the scenario to complete each step of the decision-making process. For instance, give them a COPD patient who is short of breath. Likely, they will apply high-flow oxygen. Have the patient's distress level increase, requiring a decrease in the flow of oxygen. Or, if they initially placed a nasal cannula, have the patient's distress level increase to require high-flow oxygen. Most students will know *what* to do but will not have thought about *why* until you stop them and make them think about it.

The following strategies can be used at various points throughout the lesson or to help summarize and demonstrate what students have learned.

Practice in the Field. Have students do clinical rotations in which they see the patient initially in the prehospital setting and then follow that same patient through the emergency department, lab tests, X-rays, and other diagnostic procedures and on through hospital admission, if applicable. Have students report on their field diagnosis, the patient's evaluation at the hospital, and subsequent admitting diagnosis. Encourage students to participate as much as allowable in patient assessment and history taking.

Cultural Considerations, Legal Notes, and Patho Pearls. The Student CD-ROM contains this series of informative features to enhance the student's understanding of the material covered in this chapter.

TEACHING OUTLINE

Chapter 13, "Clinical Decision Making," is the fourth lesson in Division 2, *Patient Assessment*. Distribute Handout 13-1 so that students can familiarize themselves with the learning goals for this chapter. If students have any questions about the objectives, answer them at this time.

Then present the chapter. One possible lecture outline follows. In the outline, the parenthetical references in regular type are references to text pages; those in bold type are references to figures, tables, or procedures.

I. Introduction. As a paramedic you will confront a situation that requires you to make a critical decision. (p. 705)

A. Paramedics as prehospital practitioners of emergency medicine (p. 705)
   1. Need for critical decision making
   2. Situations will appear totally unfamiliar
   3. The adage, "Patients do not read the textbooks"
B. Clinical judgment (p. 705)
   1. The use of knowledge and experience to diagnose patients and plan their treatment

HANDOUT 13-1
Chapter 13 Objectives Checklist

TEACHING STRATEGY 1
Thinking about Problems

POINT TO EMPHASIZE
Twenty-first-century paramedics are prehospital practitioners of emergency medicine—not field technicians.

POWERPOINT PRESENTATION
Chapter 13, PowerPoint slides 4–7

POINT OF INTEREST
Patients who fall between minor medical and life-threatening on the acuity spectrum pose the greatest challenge to your critical-thinking abilities.

TEACHING STRATEGY 2
Patient Acuity Practice

POWERPOINT PRESENTATION
Chapter 13, PowerPoint slides 8–21

TEACHING STRATEGY 3
Algorithm Development

TEACHING TIP
Walk your class through the algorithm for cardiac arrest shown in Figure 13-1 on text page 707. Bring copies or transparencies of one or two other algorithms to class; walk the class through each algorithm, and discuss instances in which a patient might not match the algorithm.

POWERPOINT PRESENTATION
Chapter 13, PowerPoint slides 22–26

POINT TO EMPHASIZE
Do not allow the linear thinking that protocols promote to restrain you from consulting with your medical direction physician.

TEACHING STRATEGY 4
Thinking about Differential Diagnoses

POINT TO EMPHASIZE
Except for safety concerns, never allow anything to distract you from your most important job—assessing and caring for your patient.

POINT TO EMPHASIZE
Whenever possible, anticipate problems and act before they occur.

POINT TO EMPHASIZE
Maintaining your composure is key to developing a management plan for the best patient outcome.

POWERPOINT PRESENTATION
Chapter 13, PowerPoint slides 27–28

II. Paramedic practice. As a paramedic, you must gather, evaluate, and synthesize information. (pp. 705–708)

   A. Field diagnosis (p. 705)
      1. Prehospital evaluation of the patient's condition and its causes
   B. Developing and implementing management plan (pp. 705–706)
   C. Patient acuity (p. 706)
      1. Obvious critical life threats
      2. Potential life threats
      3. Non-life-threatening presentations
   D. Protocols and algorithms (pp. 706–708) (**Fig. 13-1, p. 707**)
      1. Protocols
         a. General and specific procedures for managing certain patient conditions
      2. Standing orders
         a. Certain procedures that can be performed prior to contacting medical direction
      3. Algorithms
         a. Patient care schematic flow charts

III. Critical-thinking skills. The ability to think under pressure and make decisions cannot be taught; it must be developed. (pp. 708–710)

   A. Fundamental knowledge and abilities (pp. 708–709)
      1. Knowing anatomy, physiology, and pathophysiology
      2. Focusing on large amounts of data
      3. Organizing information
      4. Identifying and dealing with medical ambiguity
      5. Differentiating between relevant and irrelevant data
      6. Analyzing and comparing similar situations
      7. Explaining decisions and constructing logical arguments
      8. Differential field diagnosis
         a. The list of possible causes of your patient's symptoms
   B. Useful thinking styles (pp. 709–710)
      1. Reflective versus impulsive
         a. Reflective
            i. Acting thoughtfully, deliberately, and analytically
         b. Impulsive
            i. Acting instinctively, without stopping to think
      2. Divergent versus convergent
         a. Divergent
            i. Taking into account all aspects of a complex situation
         b. Convergent
            i. Focusing on only the most important aspect of a critical situation
      3. Anticipatory versus reactive
         a. Anticipatory
            i. Looking ahead proactively to potential ramifications of actions
         b. Reactive
            i. Responding to events after they occur

IV. Thinking under pressure. When you must make a critical decision, physical influences may help or hinder your ability to think clearly. (pp. 710–711)

   A. Autonomic nervous system (pp. 710–711)
      1. "Fight-or-flight" hormones

B. Pseudo-instinctive (p. 711)
1. Learned actions that are practiced until they can be done without thinking
C. Mental checklist (p. 711)
1. Scan the situation
2. Stop and think
3. Decide and act
4. Maintain control
5. Reevaluate

V. The critical decision process. Your ability to analyze data effectively and devise a practical management plan optimizes patient care. (pp. 711–714)

A. Form a concept. (p. 712)
1. Scene size-up and initial assessment
2. Focused history and physical exam
B. Interpret the data. (p. 712)
1. Consider the most serious condition that fits your patient's situation.
2. When clear diagnosis is elusive, base treatment on presenting signs and symptoms.
C. Apply the principles. (pp. 712–713)
1. Devise management plan that covers all contingencies.
D. Evaluate the results. (p. 713)
1. Ongoing assessment
E. Reflect on the incident. (p. 713)
1. Consult emergency physician.
2. Consult crew.
F. Putting it all together. The six Rs. (pp. 713–714)
1. Read the scene.
   a. Observe general environmental conditions.
   b. Observe immediate surroundings.
   c. Observe mechanism of injury.
2. Read the patient.
   a. Observe level of consciousness.
   b. Observe skin color.
   c. Observe patient's position, location.
   d. Observe any obvious deformity or asymmetry.
   e. Determine chief complaint.
   f. Touch patient to evaluate skin temperature and condition.
   g. Touch patient to evaluate pulse rate and quality.
   h. Auscultate for problems with upper and lower airways.
   i. Identify life-threats with ABCs.
   j. Take full set of vital signs.
3. React
   a. Address life-threats as found.
   b. Determine most common and serious existing conditions.
   c. Treat patient accordingly.
4. Reevaluate
   a. Conduct focused and detailed physical assessment.
   b. Note response to initial management interventions.
   c. Discover other, less obvious problems.
5. Revise
   a. Change or stop interventions that are not working.
   b. Try new interventions as appropriate.
6. Review
   a. Be honest and critical in your run critique.
   b. Look for ways to improve patient management.

POINT TO EMPHASIZE
Make every patient contact a learning experience.

POWERPOINT PRESENTATION
Chapter 13, PowerPoint slides 29–30

TEACHING TIP
Stress that clinical decision making is not a perfectible skill but an art that paramedics must continue to develop throughout their careers, based on their accumulated knowledge and experience.

TEACHING STRATEGY 5
Six Rs Scenarios

HANDOUT 13-2
Clinical Decision Making

READING/REFERENCE
Damjanov, I. *Pathology for the Health-Related Professions.* 2nd ed. Philadelphia: W. B. Saunders, 2000.

POWERPOINT PRESENTATION
Chapter 13, PowerPoint slide 30

WORKBOOK
Chapter 13 Activities

READING/REFERENCE
Textbook, pp. 716–734

HANDOUT 13-3
Chapter 13 Quiz

HANDOUT 13-4
Chapter 13 Scenario

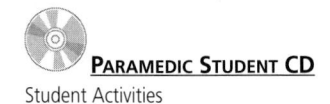

PARAMEDIC STUDENT CD
Student Activities

COMPANION WEBSITE
http://www.prenhall.com/bledsoe

TESTGEN
Chapter 13

EMT ACHIEVE: PARAMEDIC TEST PREPARATION
Mistovich & Beasley. EMT Achieve: Paramedic Test Preparation. www.prenhall.com/emtachieve/

VI. Chapter summary (p. 714). Clinical decision making is an essential paramedic skill that you will develop with time and experience. The prehospital environment is unlike any other medical care setting and you will have to make decisions in less-than-optimal and sometimes dangerous conditions. Most times you will have the benefit of consulting with your medical direction physician in difficult and unusual situations; other times you may not. Your ability to gather information, analyze it, and make a critical decision may someday be the difference between your patient's life and death. This is inevitable. How well you prepare for that challenge will determine your ultimate success. The process begins in your paramedic training program. You must develop a good working knowledge of anatomy, physiology, pathophysiology, and the principles of emergency medicine. In time, through repeated patient contacts, you will develop the clinical judgment you need to make effective patient care decisions.

The critical decision-making process involves a series of steps that experienced clinicians do almost unconsciously. First you gather information (history and physical exam) to form an initial impression and then interpret it against your knowledge and experience to develop a working field diagnosis. You next apply the principles of emergency medicine to devise and implement a management plan and evaluate the effects of your treatments. Then you reevaluate and revise your plan as necessary. Finally you compare your findings with the emergency physician's diagnosis and discuss alternate ways to manage similar patients. With every patient contact, your experience grows and your clinical judgment improves. This is the essence of paramedic practice.

ASSIGNMENTS

Assign students to complete Chapter 13, "Clinical Decision Making," of the workbook. Also assign them to read Chapter 14, "Communications," before the next class.

EVALUATION

Chapter Quiz and Scenario Distribute copies of the Chapter Quiz provided in Handout 13-3 to evaluate student understanding of this chapter. Make sure each student reads the scenario to reinforce critical thinking on the scene. Remind students not to use their notes or textbooks while taking the quiz.

Student CD Quizzes for every chapter are contained on the dynamic and highly visual in-text student CD.

Companion Website Additional quizzes for every chapter are contained on this exciting website.

TestGen You may wish to create a custom-tailored test using *Prentice Hall TestGen for Essentials of Paramedic Care,* 2nd Edition to evaluate student understanding of this chapter.

On-line Test Preparation (for students and instructors) Additional test preparation is available through Brady's new on-line product, *EMT Achieve: Paramedic Test Preparation* at http://www.prenhall.com/emtachieve/. Instructors can also monitor student mastery on-line.

Review Manual for the EMT-Paramedic   This comprehensive exam review contains hundreds of test questions and rationales, including scenarios, along with two 180-question practice tests on CD.

REINFORCEMENT

Handouts   If classroom discussion or performance on the quiz indicates that some students have not fully mastered the chapter content, you may wish to assign some or all of the Reinforcement Handouts for this chapter.

Student CD (for students)   A wide variety of material on this CD-ROM will reinforce and also expand student knowledge and skills.

PowerPoint Presentation (for instructors)   The PowerPoint material developed for this chapter offers useful reinforcement of chapter content.

Companion Website (for students)   Additional review quizzes and links to EMS resources will contribute to further reinforcement of the chapter.

OneKey   On-line support is offered for this course on one of three platforms: CourseCompass, Blackboard, or Web CT. Includes the IRM, PowerPoints, TestGen, and Companion Website for instruction. Ask your local sales representative for more information.

Brady Skills Series: Advanced Life Skills (Video or CD)   Have your students watch the skills come to life on VHS or CD-ROM, or they can purchase the highly visual, full-color text with step-by-step procedures and rationales.

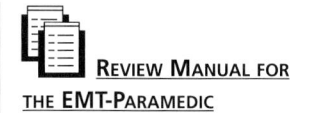

REVIEW MANUAL FOR THE EMT-PARAMEDIC
Cherry & Mistovich. *Review Manual for the EMT-Paramedic,* 3rd edition.

HANDOUTS 13-5 AND 13-6
Reinforcement Activities

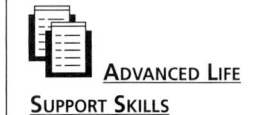

PARAMEDIC STUDENT CD
Student Activities

POWERPOINT PRESENTATION
Chapter 13

COMPANION WEBSITE
http://www.prenhall.com/bledsoe

ONEKEY
Chapter 13

ADVANCED LIFE SUPPORT SKILLS
Larmon & Davis. *Advanced Life Support Skills.*

ADVANCED LIFE SKILLS REVIEW
Larmon & Davis. *Advanced Life Skills Review.*

BRADY SKILLS SERIES: ALS
Larmon & Davis. *Brady Skills Series: ALS.*

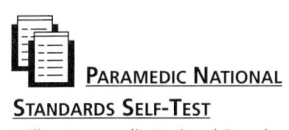

PARAMEDIC NATIONAL STANDARDS SELF-TEST
Miller. *Paramedic National Standards Self-Test,* 4th edition.

Handout 13-1   Student's Name _____

CHAPTER 13 OBJECTIVES CHECKLIST

Knowledge	Date Mastered
1. Compare the factors influencing medical care in the out-of-hospital environment to other medical settings.	
2. Differentiate between critical life-threatening, potentially life-threatening, and non-life-threatening patient presentations.	
3. Evaluate the benefits and shortfalls of protocols, standing orders, and patient care algorithms.	
4. Define the components, stages, and sequences of the critical thinking process for paramedics.	
5. Apply the fundamental elements of critical thinking for paramedics.	
6. Describe the effects of the fight-or-flight response and its positive and negative effects on a paramedic's decision making.	
7. Summarize the "six *R*s" of putting it all together: *R*ead the patient, *R*ead the scene, *R*eact, *R*eevaluate, *R*evise the management plan, and *R*eview performance.	
8. Given several preprogrammed and moulaged trauma and medical patients, demonstrate clinical decision making.	

HANDOUT 13-2

Student's Name _____

CLINICAL DECISION MAKING

Charting Student Progress:
1. *Learning skill*
2. *Performs skill with direction*
3. *Performs skill independently*

Procedure	1	2	3
Read the scene			
1. Observes general environmental conditions.			
2. Observes immediate surroundings.			
3. Observes mechanism of injury.			
Read the patient			
1. Observes level of consciousness.			
2. Observes skin color.			
3. Observes patient's position, location.			
4. Observes any obvious deformity or asymmetry.			
5. Determines chief complaint.			
6. Touches patient to evaluate skin temperature and condition.			
7. Touches patient to evaluate pulse rate and quality.			
8. Auscultates for problems with upper and lower airways.			
9. Identifies life-threats with ABCs.			
10. Takes full set of vital signs.			
React			
1. Addresses life-threats as found.			
2. Determines most common and serious existing conditions.			
3. Treats patient accordingly.			

HANDOUT 13-2 Continued

Procedure	1	2	3
Reevaluate			
1. Conducts focused and detailed physical assessment.			
2. Notes response to initial management interventions.			
3. Discovers other, less obvious problems.			
Revise			
1. Changes or stops interventions that are not working.			
2. Tries new interventions as appropriate.			
Review			
1. Run critique is honest and critical.			
2. Looks for ways to improve patient management.			

Comments:

HANDOUT 13-3

Student's Name _____

CHAPTER 13 QUIZ

Write the letter of the best answer in the space provided.

_____ 1. The use of knowledge and experience to diagnose patients and plan their treatment is called:
   A. field diagnostics.
   B. clinical judgment.
   C. patient acuity.
   D. critical thinking.

_____ 2. Critically life-threatening, potentially life-threatening, and non-life-threatening are classes of:
   A. patient acuity.
   B. clinical judgment.
   C. field diagnosis.
   D. critical thinking.

_____ 3. Which patient conditions pose the greatest challenge to a paramedic's critical-thinking abilities?
   A. major medical
   B. major trauma
   C. those between potentially life-threatening and life-threatening
   D. those between minor medical and life-threatening

_____ 4. A standard that includes general and specific principles for managing certain patient conditions is called a(n):
   A. algorithm.
   B. standing order.
   C. protocol.
   D. advanced directive.

_____ 5. A standing order is a:
   A. standard that includes general and specific principles for managing certain types of patients.
   B. treatment you can perform before contacting medical control.
   C. schematic flow chart that outlines appropriate care for specific signs and symptoms.
   D. direct order or permission obtained from medical control by phone or radio before performing a treatment.

_____ 6. Which of the following statements about standing orders, protocols, and algorithms is true?
   A. They cover patients with multiple disease etiologies.
   B. They cover multiple treatment situations.
   C. They eliminate the need for paramedics to make clinical judgments.
   D. They cover "classic patients."

_____ 7. A differential field diagnosis is the:
   A. list of possible causes of your patient's symptoms.
   B. one final diagnosis you decide on to guide you in your treatment.
   C. diagnosis jointly arrived at by the paramedic and the medical control physician.
   D. diagnosis of the patient after all labs, X-rays, and other diagnostic procedures have been evaluated.

_____ 8. The term that describes acting thoughtfully, deliberately, and analytically is:
   A. reflective.
   B. divergent.
   C. impulsive.
   D. convergent.

_____ 9. The divergent approach to situation analysis means:
   A. acting instinctively without stopping to think.
   B. focusing on only the most important aspect of a critical situation.
   C. taking into account all aspects of a complex situation.
   D. anticipating the possible ramifications of your actions in a proactive way.

HANDOUT 13-3 Continued

_____ 10. Which approach is most appropriate if your patient presents apneic and pulseless?
   A. divergent
   B. anticipatory
   C. impulsive
   D. reflective

_____ 11. Facilitating behaviors include:
   A. anticipating problems and acting before they occur.
   B. taking into account all aspects of a complex situation.
   C. learning actions that are practiced until they can be done without thinking.
   D. staying calm.

_____ 12. The part of the nervous system that controls involuntary actions is the:
   A. sympathetic nervous system.
   B. autonomic nervous system.
   C. parasympathetic nervous system.
   D. pseudo-instinctive nervous system.

_____ 13. Your mental checklist as a paramedic should include:
   A. acting quickly and instinctively.
   B. scanning the situation.
   C. interpreting the data.
   D. forming a concept.

_____ 14. Steps in critical decision making include:
   A. applying the principles.
   B. maintaining control.
   C. planning for the worst.
   D. knowing anatomy, physiology, and pathophysiology.

_____ 15. The six Rs include all of the following EXCEPT:
   A. Read the scene.
   B. Reevaluate.
   C. Reflect.
   D. Review performance.

HANDOUT 13-4

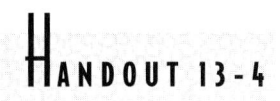

Student's Name _____

CHAPTER 13 SCENARIO

Review the following real-life situation. Then answer the questions that follow.

A 68-year-old female has called 911 to request an ambulance. The only chief complaint the dispatcher can obtain from the woman is that she "just doesn't feel right." She cannot give any specific problem. You and your EMT-Basic partner, Beth Lynch, are dispatched to the scene. When you arrive, the local fire department quick response team is on scene. They have done an initial assessment and taken vitals. They report that everything seems normal. You note that the patient is conscious and breathing normally, and skin color is good. Her vital signs are a pulse of 86, respirations of 18, and blood pressure of 146/78. You kneel next to her chair and take her hand. It feels slightly cool. The woman is obviously anxious. You begin a SAMPLE history and learn that your patient has "an upset stomach" and a slight headache that began earlier in the morning. She is allergic to an antibiotic but does not know which one. She takes a "water" pill and something for her heart but cannot recall its name. She had a heart attack about 4 years ago. She hasn't eaten since last night, when she ate some home-canned peaches. The sensation came on about an hour ago while she was doing the laundry in the basement. You perform a physical exam without finding anything pertinent. You assist her to the stretcher and move her to the ambulance. Once in the ambulance, you apply supplemental oxygen and begin an IV of D_5W, TKO. You gently transport her to the hospital and release her to the emergency department staff.

1. What style of situational analysis would you use, reflective or impulsive? Explain why.

2. Taking your physical assessment and history findings into account, what would be your differential field diagnosis for this patient?

3. What is your patient's acuity?

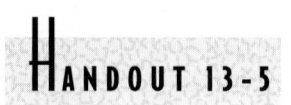

CHAPTER 13 REVIEW

Write the word or words that best complete the following sentences in the space provided.

1. The severity or acuteness of your patient's condition is called the patient's _____.
2. The use of knowledge and experience to diagnose patients and plan their treatment is called _____ _____.
3. Prehospital evaluation of the patient's condition and its causes is the _____ _____.
4. The schematic flow chart that outlines appropriate care for specific signs and symptoms is called a(n) _____.
5. Treatments you can perform before contacting the medical control physician for permission are called _____ _____.
6. Differentiating between relevant and irrelevant data is one of the _____-_____ requirements.
7. The list of possible causes of your patient's symptoms is called a(n) _____ _____ _____.
8. Two of the facilitating behaviors a paramedic needs include planning for the _____ and working _____.
9. Acting instinctively without stopping to think is being _____.
10. The _____ approach focuses on only the most important aspects of a critical situation.
11. Learned actions that are practiced until they can be done without thinking are called _____-_____.
12. Forming a concept, interpreting the data, and reflecting are steps in _____ _____ _____.
13. The thought process used to analyze and evaluate is called _____ _____.
14. Your mental checklist as a paramedic should include maintaining _____.
15. After a call, you should discuss your field diagnosis with the _____ _____ _____ and conduct a(n) _____ _____ with your crew.

Handout 13-6

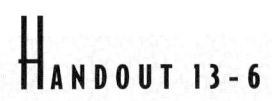

Student's Name _____

LISTING KEY IDEAS

Fill in the blanks to complete the clinical decision-making list.

1. Classes of patient acuity
   A. _____
   B. _____
   C. _____

2. Decision-making requirements
   A. _____
   B. _____
   C. _____
   D. _____
   E. _____
   F. _____
   G. _____

3. Facilitating behaviors
   A. _____
   B. _____
   C. _____
   D. _____

4. Mental checklist
   A. _____
   B. _____
   C. _____
   D. _____
   E. _____

5. Steps in critical decision making
   A. _____
   B. _____
   C. _____
   D. _____
   E. _____

6. The six Rs
   A. _____
   B. _____
   C. _____
   D. _____
   E. _____
   F. _____

REINFORCEMENT

Chapter 13 Answer Key

Handout 13-3: Chapter 13 Quiz

1. C	5. B	9. C	13. C
2. A	6. D	10. B	14. A
3. D	7. A	11. D	15. B
4. B	8. A	12. B	

Handout 13-4: Chapter 13 Scenario

1. Your situational analysis should be reflective. The patient does not appear to have an immediate life-threatening problem. Her only chief complaint at this time is an "upset stomach." Her vitals appear normal, and her skin color is good. She is in no real distress and is hemodynamically stable, so you can take the time to determine her primary problem. There is no need for immediate action.
2. A number of causes are possible for this patient not feeling well. Because you must consider the worst, you should think about a possible cardiac problem. Especially in elderly patients, a heart attack may not present with the typical chest pain. It may manifest itself with breathing difficulty, nausea, vague shoulder pain, or even with the patient's "just not feeling well." Other considerations may be food poisoning, possible toxic fumes in the basement, or the flu. Because of the possibility of a cardiac problem, you should treat the patient with high-concentration oxygen, a prophylactic IV, and cardiac monitor.
3. At this time, the patient appears to have a non-life-threatening condition. Naturally, this may change if the heart monitor reveals an abnormal heart rhythm.

Handout 13-5: Chapter 13 Review

1. acuity
2. clinical judgment
3. field diagnosis
4. algorithm
5. standing orders
6. decision-making
7. differential field diagnosis
8. worst, systematically
9. impulsive
10. convergent
11. pseudo-instinctive
12. critical decision making
13. critical thinking
14. control
15. emergency department physician, run critique

Handout 13-6: Listing Key Ideas

1. **A.** Critically life-threatening
   B. Potentially life-threatening
   C. Non-life-threatening

2. **A.** Knowing anatomy, physiology, and pathophysiology
   B. Focusing on large amounts of data
   C. Organizing information
   D. Identifying and dealing with medical ambiguity
   E. Differentiating between relevant and irrelevant data
   F. Analyzing and comparing similar situations
   G. Explaining decisions and constructing logical arguments

3. **A.** Stay calm.
   B. Plan for the worst.
   C. Work systematically.
   D. Remain adaptable.

4. **A.** Scan the situation.
   B. Stop and think.
   C. Decide and act.
   D. Maintain control.
   E. Reevaluate.

5. **A.** Form a concept.
   B. Interpret the data.
   C. Apply the principles.
   D. Evaluate.
   E. Reflect.

6. **A.** Read the scene.
   B. Read the patient.
   C. React.
   D. Reevaluate.
   E. Revise the management plan.
   F. Review your performance.

Chapter 14 Communications

INTRODUCTION

The communications network is the heart of any EMS system. Coordinating the components of the system to provide an organized response to urgent medical situations requires a comprehensive, flexible communications plan. The paramedic must interact effectively with everyone involved in the call, including the emergency medical dispatcher (EMD), the patient and family, bystanders, personnel from other agencies such as police and fire departments, responders from other EMS agencies, physicians, and allied health staff at the hospital. This chapter provides an overview of the equipment and procedures needed to establish a vital communications link in the EMS system.

CHAPTER OBJECTIVES

After reading this chapter, you should be able to:

1. Identify the role and importance of verbal, written, and electronic communications in the provision of EMS. (pp. 718–719, 726–730)
2. Describe the phases of communications necessary to complete a typical EMS response. (pp. 720–726)
3. List factors that impede and enhance effective verbal and written communications. (pp. 718–719)
4. Explain the value of data collection during an EMS response. (pp. 718–719, 730)
5. Recognize the legal status of verbal, written and electronic communications related to an EMS response. (pp. 718–719, 730)
6. Identify current technology used to collect and exchange patient and/or scene information electronically. (pp. 726–730)
7. Identify the various components of the EMS communications system and describe their function and use. (pp. 717–718, 720–726)
8. Identify and differentiate among the following communications systems:
   - Simplex (p. 727)
   - Duplex (p. 727)
   - Multiplex (p. 727)
   - Trunked (p. 728)
   - Digital communications (p. 728)
   - Cellular telephone (pp. 728–729)

TOTAL TEACHING TIME:
4.95 HOURS
The total teaching time is only a guideline based on the didactic and practical lab averages in the National Standard Curriculum. Instructors should take into consideration such factors as the pace at which students learn, the size of the class, and breaks. The actual time devoted to teaching objectives is the responsibility of the instructor.

- Facsimile (p. 729)
- Computer (p. 729)

9. Describe the functions and responsibilities of the Federal Communications Commission. (pp. 732–733)
10. Describe the role of emergency medical dispatch and the importance of prearrival instructions in a typical EMS response. (pp. 724–725)
11. List appropriate caller information gathered by the Emergency Medical Dispatcher. (p. 724)
12. Describe the structure and importance of verbal patient information communication to the hospital and medical direction. (pp. 730–732)
13. Diagram a basic communications system. (pp. 718–719)
14. Given several narrative patient scenarios, organize a verbal radio report for electronic transmission to medical direction. (pp. 717–733)

FRAMING THE LESSON

At the beginning of class, distribute copies of prehospital care reports obtained from your local EMS agencies. Be sure that identifying information, such as the patient's name and address, has been deleted or blacked out. Give one report to each student. Role-play the part of the physician at the receiving hospital, and have each student give you a verbal patient report as he would on the radio when transporting. If possible, obtain a set of inexpensive walkie-talkies to use for the report. Ask other students to critique the reports, noting strengths and weaknesses in them. Once the lesson has been completed, repeat this exercise and note improvement in reporting format and radio technique.

TEACHING STRATEGIES

People learn in a variety of ways. Some do better with the spoken word, whereas others prefer the written. Some prefer to work alone, whereas others profit from working in groups. Recognizing these different ways of acquiring knowledge, the authors of this *Instructor's Resource Manual* have provided a variety of teaching strategies for the different types of learners. These strategies are intended to foster higher-level cognitive skills and encourage creative learning and problem solving. For greatest effectiveness, incorporate these strategies into your class lecture. Symbols in the Lecture Outline indicate the points at which various exercises might be most appropriate. Other strategies can be used to preview the lesson or to summarize it.

The following strategies are keyed to specific sections of the lesson.

1. Recognizing Specialized Terminology. Show clips of video from programs that use specialized technical language, such as those dealing with politics, science, auto mechanics, or music. Ask students to share a time when they felt uncomfortable or embarrassed because they could not understand what was being said about or around them. Now ask them to consider how their patients feel when they are speaking to other members of the health care team in medical jargon. This is an affective domain activity.

2. Raising Public Awareness of EMS. Have students create a public education piece about the proper use and benefits of 911. They may work individually or in groups. They may create poster presentations, billboards, radio or

TV public service announcements, newspaper ads, and so on. Have them demonstrate their projects in class. This is both a creative problem-solving exercise and an opportunity to practice speaking in front of groups.

3. Recognizing Communications Technology. Avoid the temptation to assume that everyone in class is familiar with communications technology. Many people know how to use a cellular telephone but have no concept of how it actually works. Bring examples of every piece of hardware you can acquire from biotelemetry to portable radio to cell phone and so on, and show how they are used. Many students may not understand how these devices work and may be reluctant to ask because the devices are now common. This is a kinesthetic activity.

4. Hospital Radio Monitoring. Have students monitor patient reports at a base station hospital. Give the students templates of what radio reports should include. Have them record the information from the reports on the template forms.

5. Audiotape Reports. Obtain several tape-recorded copies of actual dispatches and patient reports to hospitals from your local EMS agencies. Have students listen to these tapes as a group. Using the standard format, have students write the information from the report and discuss whether the report was complete and efficient. Have them determine which information was relevant and which was irrelevant. This activity will reinforce what a good report sounds like.

6. Organizing Radio Reports. No matter how many times you describe the standard format for radio communication, students will be unable to give radio reports clearly and concisely until you create a "flow sheet" or "cheat sheet" for them. Do so and distribute it, encouraging students to use the sheet when giving radio reports on all scenario patients from this point forward in class. With enough practice in class, radio communication will be much easier in the field, where the stress involved with a real patient will be experienced. Additionally, organizing the radio report helps students to organize their assessments. This is an oral presentation activity.

The following strategies can be used at various points throughout the lesson or to help summarize and demonstrate what students have learned.

Guest Lecturers. Invite guest lecturers to the class, including a radio technician to explain the radio equipment and a dispatcher to discuss his role in the EMS system. Arrange for groups of students to spend observation time at a busy dispatch center in your area.

Dispatch Center Observation. Have students schedule observation time at an emergency dispatch center. Have them pay special attention to the use of prearrival instructions given by the emergency medical dispatcher to callers and the interaction of EMS, fire, and police departments.

Field Internship. Have students begin giving patient reports during field runs with their preceptors. Also, students can begin writing reports on actual runs with their preceptors.

Cultural Considerations, Legal Notes, and Patho Pearls. The Student CD-ROM contains this series of informative features to enhance the student's understanding of the material covered in this chapter.

HANDOUT 14-1
Chapter 14 Objectives Checklist

POWERPOINT PRESENTATION
Chapter 14, PowerPoint slides 4–7

POINT TO EMPHASIZE
Communication is the key link in the chain that results in the best possible patient outcome.

POWERPOINT PRESENTATION
Chapter 14, PowerPoint slides 8–11

POINT TO EMPHASIZE
Your communications network must consist of reliable equipment designed to afford clear communication among all agencies within the system.

POWERPOINT PRESENTATION
Chapter 14, PowerPoint slides 12–13

TEACHING STRATEGY 1
Recognizing Specialized Terminology

TEACHING OUTLINE

Chapter 14, "Communications," is the fifth lesson in Division 2, *Patient Assessment*. Distribute Handout 14-1 so that students can familiarize themselves with the learning goals for this chapter. If students have any questions about the objectives, answer them at this time.

Then present the chapter. One possible lecture outline follows. In the outline, the parenthetical references in regular type are references to text pages; those in bold type are references to figures, tables, or procedures.

I. Introduction to communication. All aspects of prehospital care require effective, efficient communication. (pp. 717–718)

  A. Emergency medical dispatcher (EMD) (p. 717)
    1. Manages entire system of EMS response and readiness
  B. Patient, family, bystanders (p. 717)
    1. May become obstructive
    2. Try to keep them well informed.
  C. Personnel from other responding agencies (p. 717)
    1. May not share paramedic's priorities
    2. Coordinating and implementing effective treatment requires effective communication.
  D. Health care staff from physicians' offices, nursing homes, and other health care facilities (p. 717)
  E. Medical direction physician (pp. 717–718)
    1. Resource to paramedic during call
    2. Can prepare for patient's arrival

II. Verbal communication. Semantic and technical factors can enhance or impede effective communication. (p. 718)

  A. Semantic (p. 718)
    1. Related to the meaning of words
  B. Technical (p. 718)
    1. Related to communications hardware
    2. Reliable equipment (**Fig. 14-1, p. 719**)
    3. Radio band
      a. Range of radio frequencies
    4. Radio frequency
      a. Number of times per minute a radio wave oscillates
      b. Ultrahigh frequency
        i. Radio frequency band from 300 to 3,000 megahertz

III. Written communication. Written records are an important aspect of EMS communications. (pp. 718–719) (**Fig. 14-2, p. 719**)

  A. Prehospital care report (pp. 718–719)
    1. Written record of EMS response
    2. Used by
      a. Hospital staff
      b. Agency administrators
      c. System quality assurance/improvement committees
      d. Insurance and billing departments
      e. Researchers
      f. Educators
      g. Lawyers
    3. Legal record of the incident

B. Terminology. Developing its own terminology makes communications within an industry more clear, concise, and unambiguous. (pp. 719–720) (Table 14-1, p. 720)

IV. The EMS response. Your ability to communicate effectively during a stressful EMS response will determine the success or failure of your efforts. (pp. 720–726)

A. Response sequence (pp. 720–726)
   1. Detection and citizen access (**Fig. 14-3, p. 721**)
      a. Basic 911 versus Enhanced 911
      b. Public Safety Answering Point (PSAP)
      c. Automatic Number Identification (ANI)
      d. Automatic Location Identification (ALI)
      e. Emergency Medical Dispatcher (EMD)
      f. Wireless 911
         i. Call routing
         ii. Terrestrial-based triangulation
         iii. Global positioning (GPS)
   2. Automatic Collision Notification (ACN)
   3. Call taking and emergency response (**Fig. 14-4, p. 724; Fig. 14-5, p. 725**)
      a. Priority dispatching
   4. Prearrival instructions
   5. Call coordination and incident recording
   6. Discussion with medical direction physician (**Fig. 14-6, p. 726**)
   7. Transfer communications (**Fig. 14-7, p. 726**)
   8. Back in service, ready for next call

V. Communications technology. EMS systems can use all of today's various communications technologies. (pp. 726–730)

A. Radio communications (pp. 726–728)
   1. Simplex (**Fig. 14-8, p. 727**)
      a. Transmits and receives on same frequency
   2. Duplex (**Fig. 14-9, p. 727**)
      a. Two frequencies for each channel
   3. Multiplex (**Fig. 14-10, p. 728**)
      a. Duplex system that can also transmit voice and data simultaneously
   4. Trunking
      a. Computer routes transmissions to next available frequency in group
   5. Digital communications
      a. Clearer transmissions
      b. Less overcrowding of radio frequencies
      c. More secure than radio
   6. Mobile data terminals (MDT)
B. Alternative technologies (pp. 728–729)
   1. Cellular phones (**Fig. 14-11, p. 728**)
      a. Need for recorded communication lines
   2. Facsimile
   3. Computer
C. New technology (pp. 729–730)
   1. Electronic documentation
   2. Legal concerns
      a. Patient confidentiality

POWERPOINT PRESENTATION
Chapter 14, PowerPoint slides 14–21

TEACHING STRATEGY 2
Raising Public Awareness of EMS

TEACHING TIP
Bring in a tape of an entire ALS call that illustrates each stage of response communications, from citizen access through taking the call, dispatch, prearrival instructions, on-scene and hospital communications, and the back-in-service call.

POWERPOINT PRESENTATION
Chapter 14, PowerPoint slides 22–27

POINT OF INTEREST
Transmitting clear, concise, controlled reports will encourage your medical direction physicians to trust your assessments and on-scene treatment plans.

TEACHING TIP
Bring in examples of radio equipment (portable, pagers, and so on), or show pictures of local hardware.

TEACHING TIP
Have students complete an inventory of frequencies used by the public safety agencies in your EMS system using Handout 14-8.

TEACHING STRATEGY 3
Recognizing Communications Technology

PowerPoint Presentation
Chapter 14, PowerPoint slides 28–33

Point to Emphasize
One of your most important skills will be gathering essential patient information, organizing it, and relaying it to the medical direction physician.

Teaching Strategy 4
Hospital Radio Monitoring

Teaching Strategy 5
Audiotape Reports

Teaching Strategy 6
Organizing Radio Reports

Teaching Tip
Turn on a scanner, tune in the local EMS frequency, and listen to various types of communications—good and bad. Let your students critique and evaluate what they hear.

Teaching Tip
Distribute copies of Handout 14-2 so that students can chart their progress in communicating required information about patients.

PowerPoint Presentation
Chapter 14, PowerPoint slides 34–35

---

   b. Slander
   c. Libel

VI. Reporting procedures. Paramedics must effectively relay all relevant medical information to the receiving hospital staff. (pp. 730–732)
   A. Standard format (pp. 730–731)
      1. Identification of unit and provider
      2. Description of scene
      3. Patient's age, sex, approximate weight
      4. Patient's chief complaint and severity
      5. Brief, pertinent history of the present illness or injury (OPQRST)
      6. Pertinent past medical history, medications, and allergies (SAMPLE)
      7. Pertinent physical exam findings
      8. Treatment given so far/request for orders (protocols)
      9. Estimated time of arrival at the hospital
      10. Other pertinent information
   B. General radio reporting procedures (p. 731) (**Fig. 14-12, p. 731**)
      1. Listen to the channel before transmitting.
      2. Press the transmit button for 1 second before speaking.
      3. Speak at close range, approximately 2 to 3 inches, directly into or across the face of the microphone.
      4. Speak slowly and clearly. Pronounce each word distinctly, avoiding words that are difficult to understand.
      5. Speak in a normal pitch, keeping your voice free of emotion.
      6. Be brief. Know what you are going to say before you press the transmit button.
      7. Avoid codes unless they are part of your EMS system.
      8. Do not waste air time with unnecessary information.
      9. Protect your patient's privacy. When appropriate
         a. Use telephone rather than radio.
         b. Turn off external speaker.
         c. Do not use your patient's name; doing so violates FCC regulations.
      10. Use proper unit or hospital numbers and correct names or titles.
      11. Do not use slang or profanity.
      12. Use standard formats for transmission.
      13. Be concise in order to hold the attention of the person receiving your radio report.
      14. Use the echo procedure when receiving directions from the dispatcher or orders from the physician.
         a. Immediately repeating each statement will confirm accurate reception and understanding.
      15. Always write down addresses, important dispatch communications, and physician orders.
      16. When completing a transmission, obtain confirmation that your message was received and understood.
   C. Model verbal reports

VII. Regulation. The Federal Communications Commission (FCC) requires all EMS communications systems to follow appropriate governmental regulations and laws. (pp. 732–733)
   A. The FCC controls and regulates all nongovernmental communications in the United States. (pp. 732–733)
   B. Primary functions (p. 733)
      1. Licensing and allocating radio frequencies
      2. Establishing technical standards for radio equipment

3. Licensing and regulating personnel who repair and operate radio equipment
   4. Monitoring frequencies to ensure appropriate use
   5. Spot-checking base stations and dispatch centers for licenses and records

VIII. Chapter Summary (p. 733). As one of the fundamental aspects of prehospital care, accurate communications help ensure an EMS system's efficiency. Communications begin when the citizen accesses the EMS system and end when you complete your patient report. Your spoken messages must be understandable, and your written messages must be legible. All of your communications must be concise and complete and conform to national and local protocols. The more sophisticated and advanced your EMS system grows, the more sophisticated and advanced its communications—and, accordingly, your communications skills—must become.

POWERPOINT PRESENTATION
Chapter 14, PowerPoint slide 36

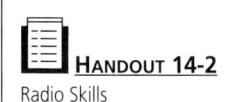

SKILLS DEMONSTRATION AND PRACTICE

Set up the two stations described in the accompanying table. Then divide the class into two groups. Have the groups circulate through the two stations. Monitor the groups to be sure all students have a chance to practice each of the skills. You may wish to have other instructors or qualified paramedics assist students in these activities.

You may base the descriptions of patients on the chapter-opening case studies in this or other volumes in this series, on collections of case studies like Brady's *Street Scenarios for the EMT and Paramedic;* "Street Scenarios" from Brady's *Paramedic Student CD*, or actual cases drawn from your own records (with the identities of the people involved in the case concealed).

HANDOUT 14-2
Radio Skills

ADVANCED LIFE SUPPORT SKILLS
Larmon & Davis. *Advanced Life Support Skills.*

ADVANCED LIFE SKILLS REVIEW
Larmon & Davis. *Advanced Life Skills Review.*

Station	Equipment Needed	Activities
General radio reports	Two-way radios, simplex mode Handout 14-2: Radio Skills	Have students transmit simple radio reports to an instructor in another room.
Written reports	Local prehospital emergency care forms	Have students practice filling out copies of local prehospital care reports (PCR).

BRADY SKILLS SERIES: ALS
Larmon & Davis. *Brady Skills Series: ALS.*

ASSIGNMENTS

Assign students to complete Chapter 14, "Communications," of the workbook. Also assign them to read Chapter 15, "Documentation," before the next class.

WORKBOOK
Chapter 14 Activities

READING/REFERENCE
Textbook, pp. 735–757

EVALUATION

HANDOUT 14-3
Chapter 14 Quiz

Chapter Quiz and Scenario Distribute copies of the Chapter Quiz provided in Handout 14-3 to evaluate student understanding of this chapter. Make sure each student reads the scenario to reinforce critical thinking on the scene. Remind students not to use their notes or textbooks while taking the quiz.

HANDOUT 14-4
Chapter 14 Scenario

Student CD Quizzes for every chapter are contained on the dynamic and highly visual in-text student CD.

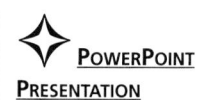

PARAMEDIC STUDENT CD
Student Activities

Companion Website Additional quizzes for every chapter are contained on this exciting website.

TestGen You may wish to create a custom-tailored test using *Prentice Hall TestGen for Essentials of Paramedic Care,* 2nd Edition, to evaluate student understanding of this chapter.

On-line Test Preparation (for students and instructors) Additional test preparation is available through Brady's new on-line product, *EMT Achieve: Paramedic Test Preparation* at *http://www.prenhall.com/emtachieve/.* Instructors can also monitor student mastery on-line.

Review Manual for the EMT-Paramedic This comprehensive exam review contains hundreds of test questions and rationales, including scenarios, along with two 180-question practice tests on CD.

REINFORCEMENT

Handouts If classroom discussion or performance on the quiz indicates that some students have not fully mastered the chapter content, you may wish to assign some or all of the Reinforcement Handouts for this chapter.

Student CD (for students) A wide variety of material on this CD-ROM will reinforce and also expand student knowledge and skills.

PowerPoint Presentation (for instructors) The PowerPoint material developed for this chapter offers useful reinforcement of chapter content.

Companion Website (for students) Additional review quizzes and links to EMS resources will contribute to further reinforcement of the chapter.

OneKey On-line support is offered for this course on one of three platforms: CourseCompass, Blackboard, or Web CT. Includes the IRM, PowerPoints, TestGen, and Companion Website for instruction. Ask your local sales representative for more information.

Brady Skills Series: Advanced Life Skills (Video or CD) Have your students watch the skills come to life on VHS or CD-ROM, or they can purchase the highly visual, full-color text with step-by-step procedures and rationales.

COMPANION WEBSITE
http://www.prenhall.com/bledsoe

TESTGEN
Chapter 14

EMT ACHIEVE: PARAMEDIC TEST PREPARATION
Mistovich & Beasley. *EMT Achieve: Paramedic Test Preparation.*
www.prenhall.com/emtachieve/

REVIEW MANUAL FOR THE EMT-PARAMEDIC
Cherry & Mistovich. *Review Manual for the EMT-Paramedic,* 3rd edition.

HANDOUTS 14-5 TO 14-8
Reinforcement Activities

PARAMEDIC STUDENT CD
Student Activities

POWERPOINT PRESENTATION
Chapter 14

COMPANION WEBSITE
http://www.prenhall.com/bledsoe

ONEKEY
Chapter 14

ADVANCED LIFE SUPPORT SKILLS
Larmon & Davis. *Advanced Life Support Skills.*

ADVANCED LIFE SKILLS REVIEW
Larmon & Davis. *Advanced Life Skills Review.*

BRADY SKILLS SERIES: ALS
Larmon & Davis. *Brady Skills Series: ALS.*

PARAMEDIC NATIONAL STANDARDS SELF-TEST
Miller. *Paramedic National Standards Self-Test,* 4th edition.

HANDOUT 14-1

Student's Name _____

CHAPTER 14 OBJECTIVES CHECKLIST

Knowledge	Date Mastered
1. Identify the role and importance of verbal, written, and electronic communications in the provision of EMS.	
2. Describe the phases of communications necessary to complete a typical EMS response.	
3. List factors that impede and enhance effective verbal and written communications.	
4. Explain the value of data collection during an EMS response.	
5. Recognize the legal status of verbal, written, and electronic communications related to an EMS response.	
6. Identify current technology used to collect and exchange patient and/or scene information electronically.	
7. Identify the various components of the EMS communications system and describe their function and use.	
8. Identify and differentiate among the following communications systems: • Simplex • Duplex • Multiplex • Trunked • Digital communications • Cellular telephone • Facsimile • Computer	
9. Describe the functions and responsibilities of the Federal Communications Commission.	
10. Describe the role of emergency medical dispatch and the importance of prearrival instructions in a typical EMS response.	
11. List appropriate caller information gathered by the Emergency Medical Dispatcher.	

OBJECTIVES

HANDOUT 14-1 Continued

Knowledge	Date Mastered
12. Describe the structure and importance of verbal patient information communication to the hospital and medical direction.	
13. Diagram a basic communications system.	
14. Given several narrative patient scenarios, organize a verbal radio report for electronic transmission to medical direction.	

Handout 14-2

Student's Name _____

RADIO SKILLS

Charting Student Progress:
1. *Learning skill*
2. *Performs skill with direction*
3. *Performs skill independently*

Skill/Behavior	1	2	3
1. Verifies open channel before speaking.			
2. Presses transmit button 1 second before speaking.			
3. Holds microphone 2 to 3 inches from mouth.			
4. Speaks slowly and clearly.			
5. Speaks in a normal pitch, avoiding emotion.			
6. Is brief, knows what to say before transmitting.			
7. Does not waste air time.			
8. Protects privacy of patient.			
9. Echoes dispatch information or physician's orders.			
10. Writes down dispatch information and physician's orders.			
11. Confirms that message is received.			
12. Demonstrates ability to troubleshoot basic equipment malfunction.			

Comments:

CHAPTER 14 QUIZ

Write the letter of the best answer in the space provided.

_____ 1. The process of exchanging information between individuals is called:
   A. transmitting.
   B. communication.
   C. verbal skills.
   D. sending and receiving.

_____ 2. In the basic communications model, the:
   A. sender gives feedback to the receiver.
   B. receiver requests contact with the sender.
   C. sender encodes message.
   D. receiver decodes feedback to sender.

_____ 3. The term _____ can be defined as "related to the meaning of words."
   A. technical
   B. semantic
   C. encoded
   D. mutual

_____ 4. The number of times per minute a radio wave oscillates is its:
   A. encoding.
   B. frequency.
   C. band.
   D. carrier.

_____ 5. A radio band is:
   A. the number of times per minute a radio wave oscillates.
   B. a frequency at which a transmission is sent.
   C. a transmission signal sent by a radio.
   D. a range of radio frequencies.

_____ 6. _____ radio waves penetrate concrete and steel well and are less susceptible to interference.
   A. VHF
   B. UHF
   C. Low-band
   D. CB

_____ 7. The common radio term *stage* means:
   A. do not respond, but be aware you might be dispatched.
   B. wait before entering the scene.
   C. listen carefully to this.
   D. establish a landing zone.

_____ 8. The first link in the chain of events of an EMS response is:
   A. call taking and emergency response.
   B. prearrival instructions.
   C. detection and citizen access.
   D. call coordination and incident recording.

_____ 9. A dispatcher's telling callers how to perform appropriate emergency measures is called:
   A. priority drill.
   B. prearrival instructions.
   C. call coaching.
   D. medical direction.

_____ 10. A(n) _____ communications system allows simultaneous two-way communications by using two frequencies for each channel but does not allow simultaneous transmission of voice messages and data.
   A. simplex
   B. duplex
   C. multiplex
   D. trunking

HANDOUT 14-3 Continued

_____ 11. Oral defamation of another person is:
   A. slander.
   B. libel.
   C. negligence.
   D. malpractice.

_____ 12. Predetermined, written guidelines for patient care are:
   A. standing orders.
   B. procedures.
   C. protocols.
   D. policies.

_____ 13. The standard format for reporting patient and scene information to the hospital includes:
   A. patient's marital status.
   B. patient's name.
   C. patient's age, sex, and weight.
   D. patient's Social Security number.

_____ 14. General radio procedures include:
   A. using codes whenever possible to shorten transmissions.
   B. giving patient's name so hospital can look up admission records.
   C. not waiting for confirmation that your message was received, to shorten transmission time.
   D. being concise in order to hold the attention of the person receiving your radio report.

_____ 15. The elements of a medical patient radio report to the hospital include:
   A. mechanism of injury.
   B. patient's name, age, and sex.
   C. subjective data.
   D. date of patient's last visit to the hospital.

Handout 14-4

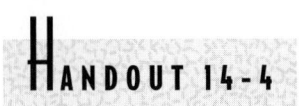

Student's Name _____

CHAPTER 14 SCENARIO

Review the following real-life situation. Then answer the questions that follow.

A woman walking down a city side street notices a man lying on the sidewalk. He appears to be having a seizure. The woman runs to a nearby pay phone and dials 911. The dispatcher asks the woman to describe the problem and to give her location. The woman describes the man's condition to the best of her ability, but she is a visitor to the area and does not know the street's name or her exact location. The dispatcher, through an enhanced 911 system, locates the site of the pay phone and dispatches an ALS ambulance and police to the scene.

The EMS unit arrives and begins patient care. The paramedics recognize the patient as an individual with diabetes-related problems whom they have assisted in the past. After managing the patient's airway and taking cervical spinal precautions, the paramedics initiate an IV, complete a rapid test for blood glucose, and administer 50 percent dextrose solution. They contact the hospital, report their findings and treatment to the emergency room physician, and continue on to the hospital. There, the paramedics turn the patient over to the emergency room staff, complete the prehospital care report, clean and restock the ambulance, and inform EMS dispatch that they are back in service.

1. List the EMS response communications chain of events illustrated in this scenario.

2. Why was the local 911 system of great importance in this scenario?

3. What tasks did the dispatcher perform?

4. What information about the patient and the situation should the paramedics have conveyed to the emergency room physician?

5. Why is a written prehospital care report important in a case like this?

HANDOUT 14-5

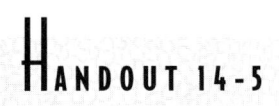

Student's Name _____

CHAPTER 14 REVIEW

Write the word or words that best complete the following sentences in the space provided.

1. _____ barriers to effective communication are those related to the meanings of words.
2. The _____ radio frequency band ranges from 300 to 3,000 megahertz.
3. The written report of an EMS response is a(n) _____ _____ _____.
4. The radio term meaning "end of transmission" is _____.
5. In radio terminology, *LZ* means _____ _____.
6. The public's first contact with the EMS system is the _____ _____ _____.
7. The dispatcher's directions to a caller for appropriate emergency measures are known as _____ instructions.
8. A medical dispatcher's interrogating a distressed caller and following established guidelines to determine the appropriate level of response is called _____ dispatching.
9. A(n) _____ communications system transmits and receives on the same frequency.
10. A(n) _____ communications system can transmit voice and data simultaneously.
11. A(n) _____ communications system pools all frequencies and routes transmissions to the next available frequency.
12. A vehicle-mounted computer keyboard with display is called a(n) _____ _____ _____.
13. Oral defamation of another person is _____.
14. Written defamation of another person is _____.
15. Predetermined written guidelines for patient care are called _____.
16. A SAMPLE history is used to determine the patient's _____ past medical history.
17. OPQRST is used to obtain the pertinent history of the _____ illness or injury.
18. Using your patient's _____ on the radio violates FCC regulations.
19. A patient's complaint of sudden onset of substernal chest pain is an example of _____ data.
20. The patient's vital signs are an example of _____ data.

ORGANIZING THE PATIENT MEDICAL REPORT

Below are elements of the patient report given by a paramedic to the hospital physician. Place the elements in correct order by writing a 1 next to the information that should be given first, a 2 next to the information that should be given second, and so on.

_____ Past medical history

_____ Vital signs; level of consciousness, general appearance/degree of distress; ECG findings; glucose testing results; trauma index/Glasgow Coma Scale score; other pertinent physical findings

_____ Scene description/mechanism of injury

_____ Associated symptoms

_____ Brief history of present illness

_____ Chief complaint

_____ Patient's age, sex, weight

_____ Agency, unit designation, paramedic's name and level of certification

HANDOUT 14-7

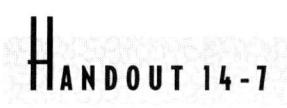

Student's Name _____

COMPOSING THE PATIENT MEDICAL REPORT

Listed below are elements of a patient report for a call by Medic Unit 4, with a crew of one paramedic and one EMT-Basic. The information is not necessarily in the proper order for a radio report, nor is all of the information relevant to the present circumstances. Use the information to assemble a clear, concise, and orderly radio report to the hospital on this patient. The unit is about 5 minutes' traveling time from the hospital.

- Patient is an 83-year-old female patient.
- Patient states she became dizzy and fell on the floor in her hallway.
- Lungs are clear bilaterally.
- Patient complains of pain to her left hip and leg.
- Patient lives by herself and has four cats.
- Distal pulses are present in the left leg.
- Patient denies shortness of breath.
- Daughter lives three blocks away and is not on the scene.
- Patient appears confused and not totally aware of her surroundings.
- Skin of the left leg is warm and pink.
- Patient's physician is Dr. Allen Miller.
- Patient has been immobilized to backboard.
- Daughter says patient has cardiac history and takes digoxin and Lasix daily.
- IV has been established.
- ECG shows atrial fibrillation.
- There is lateral rotation and shortening of the patient's left leg.
- Supplemental oxygen is being provided.
- Vital signs are: B/P—110/70; pulse—136, weak; respirations—28, shallow.

REINFORCEMENT

Handout 14-8

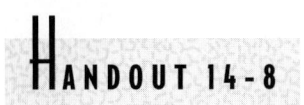

Student's Name _____

SPECIAL PROJECT: RADIO INVENTORY

Complete this radio inventory for the EMS vehicles and agencies in your area. Indicate each channel, its designated frequency, and what it is used for.

BASE STATION RADIOS

Location	Channel	Frequency	Use

MOBILE RADIOS

Location	Channel	Frequency	Use

HANDOUT 14-8 Continued

PORTABLE RADIOS

Channel	Frequency	Use

Chapter 14 Answer Key

Handout 14-3: Chapter 14 Quiz

1. B
2. C
3. B
4. B
5. D
6. B
7. B
8. C
9. B
10. B
11. A
12. C
13. C
14. D
15. C

Handout 14-4: Chapter 14 Scenario

1. Detection and citizen access, call taking and emergency response, prearrival instructions, call coordination and incident recording, discussion with medical direction physician, transfer communications, back in service, ready for next call.
2. The enhanced 911 system permitted the dispatcher to recognize the location of the call and dispatch the EMS unit to the proper site.
3. The dispatcher obtained basic information about the call, directed the appropriate vehicles to it, and noted the unit's return to service.
4. The paramedics should have conveyed the following: their unit and paramedic identifications; scene description; patient's age, sex, and weight; patient's chief complaint, associated symptoms, history of present illness, pertinent past medical history, physical exam findings, ECG results, and Glasgow Coma Scale score, if appropriate; treatment rendered; ETA at the hospital; name of the patient's physician, if known.
5. The written record helps ensure a continuum of care for the patient and can help provide legal protection for the paramedics should any legal issues arise.

Handout 14-5: Chapter 14 Review

1. Semantic
2. UHF
3. patient care report
4. clear
5. landing zone
6. emergency medical dispatcher
7. prearrival
8. priority
9. simplex
10. multiplex
11. trunking
12. mobile data terminal
13. slander
14. libel
15. protocols
16. pertinent
17. present
18. name
19. subjective
20. objective

Handout 14-6: Organizing the Patient Medical Report

Numbers reading from top to bottom should be 7, 8, 2, 6, 5, 4, 3, 1.

Handout 14-7: Composing the Patient Medical Report

One suggested example follows; variations are acceptable.

Medical control, this is Unit 4, paramedic _____. We are en route to your location with an 83-year-old female who states that she became weak and dizzy and fell at home. Her chief complaint is pain to her left leg and hip. She appears rather confused and is not oriented to time or place. Current vitals are B/P 110/70, pulse 136 and weak, respirations 28 and shallow. Her left leg is laterally rotated and shortened. Distal pulses to the leg are present, and the skin is warm and pink. She has a cardiac history and takes digoxin and Lasix daily. Patient denies chest pain or shortness of breath. Her ECG reads atrial fibrillation, and her lungs are clear bilaterally. We have immobilized the patient on a backboard, applied oxygen, have an IV in place, and will continue to monitor. Our ETA is 5 minutes. Patient's physician is Dr. Allen Miller.

Chapter 15

Documentation

INTRODUCTION

Documentation is an essential element of prehospital care. Written information on the prehospital care report (PCR) should accurately and completely describe the scene, the patient, all care provided, and the effects of the care or treatments delivered. Other members of the health care team use prehospital care reports for further patient care, administrators use them for billing and record keeping, and lawyers use them for litigation. The quality of the PCR is often considered an indicator of the quality of care provided. This chapter examines the uses of the PCR and the elements of proper documentation.

CHAPTER OBJECTIVES

After reading this chapter, you should be able to:

1. Identify the general principles regarding the importance of EMS documentation and ways in which documents are used. (pp. 736–738)
2. Identify and properly use medical terminology, medical abbreviations, and acronyms. (pp. 738, 740–743)
3. Explain the role of documentation in agency reimbursement. (p. 737)
4. Identify and eliminate extraneous or nonprofessional information. (pp. 747–748)
5. Describe the differences between subjective and objective elements of documentation. (pp. 748–749)
6. Evaluate a finished document for errors and omissions and proper use and spelling of abbreviations and acronyms. (pp. 745, 747–748)
7. Evaluate the confidential nature of an EMS report. (p. 756)
8. Describe the potential consequences of illegible, incomplete, or inaccurate documentation. (pp. 745, 747–748)
9. Describe the special documentation considerations concerning patient refusal of care and/or transport. (pp. 753–754)
10. Demonstrate how to properly record direct patient or bystander comments. (p. 744)
11. Describe the special considerations concerning mass casualty incident documentation. (p. 755)
12. Demonstrate proper document revision and correction. (p. 747)

TOTAL TEACHING TIME:
4.54 HOURS
The total teaching time is only a guideline based on the didactic and practical lab averages in the National Standard Curriculum. Instructors should take into consideration such factors as the pace at which students learn, the size of the class, and breaks. The actual time devoted to teaching objectives is the responsibility of the instructor.

13. Given a prehospital care report form and a narrative patient care scenario, record all pertinent administrative information using a consistent format, identify and record the pertinent, reportable clinical data for each patient, correct errors and omissions, using proper procedures, and note and record "pertinent negative" clinical findings. (pp. 736–756)

FRAMING THE LESSON

Begin with a scenario to engage the students in today's lesson. For example, ask for a volunteer to be "on the stand" during litigation about a patient involved in an altercation. Provide the student with a prewritten patient care report, and give him a minute to become familiar with its content. Then question the student about the incident, the patient, the scene, comments made by the patient, care provided, transportation destination, and so forth. The student will quickly become uncomfortable when he cannot find the information in the PCR provided. This will powerfully demonstrate to the entire class the principle that "if it is not written down, it did not happen." During this exercise, have the other students jot down elements that they discover are important in a PCR's content. Afterward, ask students to share their responses. They will likely be able to create a comprehensive list of elements to include in their own documentation.

TEACHING STRATEGIES

People learn in a variety of ways. Some do better with the spoken word, whereas others prefer the written. Some prefer to work alone, whereas others profit from working in groups. Recognizing these different ways of acquiring knowledge, the authors of this *Instructor's Resource Manual* have provided a variety of teaching strategies for the different types of learners. These strategies are intended to foster higher-level cognitive skills and encourage creative learning and problem solving. For greatest effectiveness, incorporate these strategies into your class lecture. Symbols in the Lecture Outline indicate the points at which various exercises might be most appropriate. Other strategies can be used to preview the lesson or to summarize it.

The following strategies are keyed to specific sections of the lesson:

1. ***Legal Critiques.*** Search PCRs from prehospital care agencies for judgmental statements, subjective opinions, and cases of libel. Omitting or blocking out any patient identifying information, make overhead transparencies of these PCRs. Ask students to identify the inappropriate comments in the PCRs. This activity operates in the affective domain, helping students to see how the patient would feel if he read the comments.

2. ***Medical "Pictionary."*** Play "Pictionary" with medical terms. Have one student draw the meaning of the word and other students on his team try to guess the meaning. Consider offering small prizes for the winning team such as candy or key chains. Drawing is a right-brain activity, but vocabulary and speech are left-brain functions. Additionally, this activity is fun, which helps students to relax and learn more. It has team-building benefits as well.

3. ***Abbreviation Quizzes.*** Present medical terminology and abbreviations in blocks to facilitate learning. In abbreviations alone there are nearly 300 terms to memorize. Consider quizzing students on the information every day to reinforce their studying.

4. Abbreviation Exercises. Use a variety of exercises to help make mastering the information in Table 15-1 enjoyable. For example, have students make flash cards of common abbreviations from the table. Or write a number of complete medical terms on a large poster board, and place 3 × 5 cards with abbreviations over the complete terms; have students take turns giving the word or words associated with the abbreviations. Divide the students into groups, and assign point values for each correct answer. Or have students revise for brevity. Give them copies of a long patient report that uses no medical abbreviations. Ask them to rewrite the report with as many abbreviations and acronyms as possible. Have a contest and give a small prize, such as a pocket mask, pouch, or penlight, for the most concise report. This activity builds written communication skills and provides the added bonus of friendly competition.

5. Scenarios for Approaches to Documentation. Present two scenarios, either verbally or by acting them out in class. Have students document both, using first the head-to-toe approach and then the body systems approach to documentation. Share with them the "correct" way, and let them identify which method they did better or more completely. Most students will immediately take to one method or the other. Encourage them to stay with this approach until they are accurately and completely documenting each call. Encouraging proper documentation in class facilitates good communication habits that students will carry with them after the course. These habits can help them avoid disciplinary and legal problems in the future.

6. Mass Casualty Incident Simulation. A mass casualty incident (MCI) documentation exercise is a must in class! Students will not likely encounter this type of situation during internship, and if they do, they will probably be performing patient care, not documentation. Create "paper patients" if limited by resources to stage an MCI. Have pairs of students or teams triage and complete the tags for each of the patients. Have another crew follow them and try to make treatment and transport decisions based on the documentation on the first group's triage tags. This is a kinesthetic exercise that is fast moving and fun. It can also be a springboard to additional discussion.

The following strategies can be used at various points throughout the lesson or to help summarize and demonstrate what students have learned.

Field Internship. Consider assigning documentation during clinical and field internships as well as the classroom. Have students document three patients per shift, or whatever is reasonable for your area. Be sure to grade or critique the documentation either in class or privately so that their documentation improves throughout the hospital and field experiences. Poor documentation is a frequent complaint among employers who hire new graduates. This exercise gives your students an edge in the marketplace.

Cultural Considerations, Legal Notes, and Patho Pearls. The student CD-ROM contains this series of informative features to enhance the student's understanding of the material covered in this chapter.

HANDOUT 15-1
Chapter 15 Objectives Checklist

TEACHING TIP
Bring examples to class of various documentation forms such as reports with check boxes, bubble sheets, and computer-scannable reports from different systems.

TEACHING OUTLINE

Chapter 15, "Documentation," is the sixth lesson in Division 2, *Patient Assessment*. Distribute Handout 15-1 so that students can familiarize themselves with the learning goals for this chapter. If students have any questions about the objectives, answer them at this time.

POINT TO EMPHASIZE
Your PCR reflects your professionalism.

POWERPOINT PRESENTATION
Chapter 15, PowerPoint slides 4–7

POWERPOINT PRESENTATION
Chapter 15, PowerPoint slides 8–10

POINT TO EMPHASIZE
Your PCR is an important document that helps ensure your patient's continuity of care.

TEACHING TIP
Ask students to give functional examples of each of the four uses for PCRs (medical, administrative, research, legal). For example, one system collects information on the use of bike helmets in certain zip codes. They share that information with the county health department, which can then conduct free bike helmet give-aways at day care centers and schools in those zip codes.

POINT TO EMPHASIZE
A complete, accurate, and objective account of the emergency call may be your best and only defense in court.

TEACHING STRATEGY 1
Legal Critiques

TEACHING STRATEGY 2
Medical "Pictionary"

POWERPOINT PRESENTATION
Chapter 15, PowerPoint slides 11–16

POINT TO EMPHASIZE
If you do not know how to spell a word, look it up or use another word.

TEACHING STRATEGY 3
Abbreviation Quizzes

TEACHING STRATEGY 4
Abbreviation Exercises

Then present the chapter. One possible lecture outline follows. In the outline, the parenthetical references in regular type are references to text pages; those in bold type are references to figures, tables, or procedures.

I. Introduction. A comprehensive, well-written patient care report (PCR) reflects the provider's professionalism. (p. 736)

    A. The PCR records events. (p. 736)
    B. The PCR records care provided. (p. 736)
    C. The PCR records time of interventions, arrivals, and departures. (p. 736)
    D. The PCR records effects of interventions. (p. 736)

II. Uses for documentation. The PCR is a valuable resource for medical professionals, EMS administrators, researchers, and lawyers. (pp. 736–738)

    A. Medical (p. 736) (**Fig. 15-1, p. 736**)
        1. Establishes a baseline for assessment findings
        2. Provides information in your absence
        3. Will likely be the only account of the scene and bystander information
        4. Can be used by other hospital services, such as ICU, physical therapy, social services, and so on, to improve patient care
    B. Administrative (p. 737)
        1. Quality improvement
        2. System or resource management
        3. Community needs
        4. Risk management
        5. Patient billing
        6. Insurance claims processing
        7. Allocation of funds
    C. Research (p. 737) (**Fig. 15-2, p. 737**)
        1. Analyze response times.
        2. Adjust staffing patterns.
        3. Determine efficacy of interventions.
        4. Evaluate and revise protocols.
    D. Legal (pp. 737–738)
        1. Permanent part of the patient's medical record
        2. Legal uses for the PCR
            a. May be sole evidence in your own defense
            b. May determine the accused's innocence or guilt
        3. Desirable traits of PCR for legal purposes
            a. Complete and accurate
            b. Consistent and unambiguous
            c. Objective

III. General considerations. Specific requirements for data collection on the PCR vary by system, but all documentation should be complete and accurate. (pp. 738–745) (**Fig. 15-3, p. 739**)

    A. Medical terminology (p. 738)
        1. Use accepted universal language in medicine.
        2. Accuracy is important to the meanings.
        3. Use correct spelling.
        4. Use plain English if you do not know the correct term or its spelling.
    B. Abbreviations and acronyms (pp. 738–743) (**Table 15-1, pp. 740–743**)
        1. Allow more information to be conveyed in less space
        2. Can have multiple accepted meanings

      3. Need for familiarity with local accepted abbreviations
      4. Agencies or hospital reference guides to accepted abbreviations
  C. Times (pp. 743–744)
      1. Record the following times related to your response
          a. Dispatch time
          b. Time en route
          c. Arrival at scene
          d. Arrival at patient's side
          e. Departure from scene
          f. Arrival at hospital
          g. Back in service
      2. Record the following times related to your patient care
          a. Vital sign checks
          b. Medication administration
          c. Procedures
          d. Changes in patient condition
      3. Whenever possible, record all times from same clock.
      4. Explain any inconsistencies in times in your narrative.
  D. Communications (p. 744)
      1. Record advice or orders from medical control on the PCR.
      2. Document changes in patient condition that result from the ordered interventions.
      3. If possible, have the physician sign the PCR to verify treatments.
  E. Pertinent negatives (p. 744)
      1. Document all assessment findings, including both positive and negative
  F. Oral statements (p. 744)
      1. Document bystanders' statements.
      2. Include disposition of valuables.
      3. Include disposition of weapons.
      4. Quote directly.
      5. Identify sources of statements.
  G. Additional resources (pp. 744–745)
      1. Identify all agencies assisting on scene such as law enforcement, air-medical service, and fire-suppression agencies.
      2. Identify what was done and by whom.
      3. Identify physicians on scene by name and credentials.
      4. Identify names, credentials, and care provided by other qualified medical personnel on scene.

IV. Elements of good documentation. A well-written PCR is accurate, legible, timely, unaltered, and professional. (pp. 745–748)

  A. Completeness and accuracy (p. 745) (**Fig. 15-4, p. 746**)
      1. Include all pertinent information.
      2. Exclude superfluous information.
      3. Complete every section of the PCR.
      4. Use the narrative section for further explanation or details.
      5. Assure consistency between check boxes and narrative.
      6. Be sure spelling is correct.
      7. Be sure all abbreviations and acronyms are correct and understandable.
  B. Legibility (p. 745)
      1. Handwriting must be neat and legible by all, not just you.
      2. Press hard enough for all carbon copies.
      3. Black ballpoint pen is best.

POINT TO EMPHASIZE
Document any medical advice or orders you receive and the results of implementing that advice and those orders.

POINT TO EMPHASIZE
Document all findings of your assessment, even those that are normal.

POWERPOINT PRESENTATION
Chapter 15, PowerPoint slides 17–21

TEACHING TIP
Employers frequently complain about poor documentation by new graduates. One study demonstrated that students were not as weak in documentation technique as in basic grammar, spelling, and handwriting. *Insist* that spelling counts! The examples set in your classroom quickly become the work habits of your graduates.

POINT TO EMPHASIZE
Your handwriting must be neat enough that other people can read and understand the report.

POINT TO EMPHASIZE
Never try to hide an error.

POINT TO EMPHASIZE
Write cautiously and avoid any remarks that might be construed as derogatory.

POWERPOINT PRESENTATION
Chapter 15, PowerPoint slides 22–26

READING/REFERENCE
McClincy, W. D. *Instructional Methods in Emergency Services with CD-ROM*. Upper Saddle River, NJ: Brady, 2002.

TEACHING STRATEGY 5
Scenarios for Approaches to Documentation

C. Timeliness (p. 747)
   1. Do not neglect ongoing assessments during transport to finish documentation.
   2. Complete the PCR at the hospital immediately after the run.
   3. Check with partner or patient if you have questions.
   4. Leave a copy of the PCR at the hospital to be included in the patient's medical record.
D. Absence of alterations (p. 747)
   1. Draw a single line through errors. (**Fig. 15-5, p. 747**)
   2. Initial and possibly date the error.
   3. Use an addendum as necessary.
      a. Use an addendum when you cannot correct an error right away.
      b. Use an addendum when you need additional information or explanation.
      c. Write the addendum as soon as you realize you made the mistake or need additional information.
      d. Record the purpose of the addendum.
      e. Sign and date the addendum.
E. Professionalism (pp. 747–748)
   1. Write cautiously.
   2. Avoid derogatory remarks.
   3. Avoid slang and jargon.
   4. Use only objective, factual statements.
   5. Be cautious of slander and libel.

V. Narrative writing. The narrative section of the report allows freedom to describe and explain your patient's situation in detail. (pp. 748–753)

A. Narrative sections (pp. 748–750)
   1. Subjective narrative
      a. Chief complaint
      b. History of present illness
      c. Past medical history
      d. Current health status
      e. Review of systems
   2. Objective narrative
      a. Head-to-toe
         i. General impression
         ii. Vital signs
         iii. HEENT
         iv. Neck
         v. Chest
         vi. Abdomen
         vii. Pelvis
         viii. Extremities
         ix. Posterior
         x. Lab or diagnostic tests
      b. Body systems
         i. General
         ii. Vital signs
         iii. HEENT
         iv. Respiratory
         v. Peripheral vascular
         vi. Lab or diagnostic tests
   3. Assessment and management
      a. Document field diagnosis or impression
      b. On scene
         i. Extrication

    ii. Airway
    iii. Breathing
    iv. Circulation
    v. Management
   c. During transport
    i. Ongoing assessment
    ii. Management
    iii. Arrival at facility
 B. General formats (pp. 750–751)
  1. SOAP
   a. Subjective
   b. Objective
   c. Assessment
   d. Plan
  2. CHART
   a. Chief complaint
   b. History
   c. Assessment
   d. Rx
   e. Transport
  3. Other formats (pp. 752–753)
   a. Patient management
    i. Chronological order of events
    ii. Time and interventions
   b. Call incident
    i. Emphasizes
     a) Mechanism of injury
     b) Surrounding circumstances
     c) How the incident occurred
    ii. Subjective information
    iii. Objective information

VI. Special considerations. Patient refusals, calls where transport is not necessary, multiple patients, and mass casualties are among the circumstances that create special problems for EMS documentation. (pp. 753–755)

 A. Patient refusals (pp. 753–754)
  1. Patients with minor illnesses or injuries may refuse care because it is simply not needed.
  2. Patients may refuse care against medical advice (AMA).
   a. High incidence of bad outcomes in AMA refusals
   b. Refusal of care documentation checklist (**Table 15-2, p. 753**)
  3. Complete a thorough assessment.
  4. Determine mental competence of patient.
  5. Advise patient.
   a. Field diagnosis
   b. Recommendation for care and transport
   c. Discuss alternative treatments
  6. Explain possible consequences of not seeking treatment.
  7. Offer other suggestions for accessing care.
  8. Offer to return if patient changes his mind.
  9. Document patient's understanding of statements and suggestions and apparent competence to refuse care based on that understanding.
  10. Refusal of care form (**Fig. 15-6, p. 754**)
 B. Services not needed (p. 755)
  1. Document if canceled en route, and by whom.
  2. Document if no patients were found.

POINT TO EMPHASIZE
No single narrative format is ideal for all situations.

POINT TO EMPHASIZE
Most patient refusals require thorough documentation because the opportunity for and consequences of abandonment charges are tremendous.

POWERPOINT PRESENTATION
Chapter 15, PowerPoint slides 27–32

TEACHING TIP
Bring examples to class of PCRs documenting patient refusals of care against medical advice; discuss their strengths and weaknesses and their conformity to the refusal-of-care documentation checklist shown in Table 15-2.

POINT TO EMPHASIZE
The risks of denying transport are even greater than those of patient refusals.

POINT TO EMPHASIZE
Whatever your local policies regarding multiple patients and mass casualties, document as completely and accurately as possible without detracting from patient care.

TEACHING STRATEGY 6
Mass Casualty Incident Simulation

TEACHING TIP
Bring examples to class of various triage tags from different systems. Point out which items they all have in common, as well as their differences.

POWERPOINT PRESENTATION
Chapter 15, PowerPoint slides 33–34

POINT TO EMPHASIZE
Poor, incomplete, or inaccurate documentation encourages frivolous lawsuits; good documentation discourages them.

POWERPOINT PRESENTATION
Chapter 15, PowerPoint slide 35

TEACHING TIP
Many schools help students assemble a portfolio of their accomplishments and competencies. Examples of excellent documentation are a perfect item to include in such a job placement tool.

---

   3. Document if canceled by a first responder agency.
   4. Document if you did not make contact with any patients.
   5. If you did make patient contact, assess and document each patient thoroughly.
C. Mass casualty incidents (p. 755)
   1. Obtaining complete information on every patient may be impossible.
   2. Providing care may supersede the need to document thoroughly.
   3. Add to the PCR using an addendum.
   4. If your documentation is incomplete, include a description of the circumstances.
   5. Triage tags
      a. Use
      b. Tag documentation
         i. Patient name
         ii. Major injuries
         iii. Vital signs
         iv. Treatment
         v. Priority

VII. **Consequences of inappropriate documentation.** Inappropriate documentation can have both medical and legal consequences. (pp. 755–756)

A. Medical consequences (p. 755)
   1. Inaccurate or incomplete reports can harm the patient for hours or days to come.
   2. Nurses, physicians, and therapists rely on the PCR to create treatment plans and begin their assessments.
   3. Some omissions, such as allergies, could be life-threatening.
B. Legal consequences (pp. 755–756)
   1. Liability is possible if poor documentation results in improper care.
   2. Inappropriate documentation can result in encouragement of litigation.
   3. Inaccurate, incomplete, or illegible documentation reflects poorly on the provider writing the report.
   4. If you did not write it, you did not do it.

VIII. **Closing.** Although documentation is often a begrudged task, it is one of the most important parts of an EMS call. (p. 756)

A. Ensure that your documentation is (p. 756)
   1. Complete
   2. Accurate
   3. Legible
   4. Appropriate
B. Patient confidentiality (p. 756)
C. Computer charting (p. 756)

IX. **Chapter summary** (p. 756). Regardless of the system you use for documentation, all EMS records should possess the same basic attributes. Appropriate terminology, proper spelling, accepted abbreviations and acronyms, and accurate times are essential. A description of the patient assessment and interventions, including pertinent negatives and communications with on-line physicians, is equally important. Finally, all of the personnel and resources involved in a call must be documented. The record must be accurate and precise, free of jargon, and neatly written. Corrections should be made properly, including the use of an addendum when appropriate.

Prehospital care providers may use many systems of documentation, including the CHART and SOAP formats. Whatever system you use, it is best if you use the same one consistently. This results in more reliable, complete documentation and reduces the chances of omitting important information. Any of the existing documentation systems can incorporate a head-to-toe assessment of the patient. Special situations such as multiple patients and refusals of transportation require extra attention. They are often the most difficult calls to document, yet they are also the calls for which good documentation can be most valuable. A complete narrative—in addition to any check boxes or filled-in "bubble" sheets—is the best way to ensure that all the necessary information is documented.

Although EMS providers frequently dislike documentation, it is one of the most important parts of the EMS call. Ensuring that the documentation is complete, accurate, legible, and appropriate is one of an EMS provider's professional responsibilities. Your PCR is the only permanent record of the ambulance call and the only permanent reflection of your professionalism.

SKILLS

Give students a chance to apply what they have learned to a real-life situation by using a contest to prepare the best prehospital care report. To conduct the contest, obtain enough copies of the PCRs used in your area and give each student two copies of the PCR. Students will use one for the contest and keep the other for reference. Then either read or distribute copies of a case history to students. For the case history, you might use one of the chapter-opening case studies from this volume or from other volumes in this series, from a collection of case studies such as Brady's *Street Scenarios for the EMT and Paramedic,* "Street Scenarios" from *Brady's Paramedic Student CD,* or actual cases drawn from your own records (with the identities of the people involved in the case concealed). When you have chosen the case and presented the facts about it, give students 10 minutes to complete their PCRs. Remind them to fill out the entire form—the check boxes as well as the narrative. When students have finished, call on each one to read the narrative portion of the form aloud. Have the rest of the class take notes to answer these questions: What were the strengths of the narrative? How could the narrative have been improved? After each report is read, have students use their notes to provide constructive feedback. When all class members have presented their narratives, instruct students to write on separate slips of paper who they think wrote the best narrative. Tally the votes and provide the winner with a small prize, such as a pen with the insignia of a local EMS unit.

ASSIGNMENTS

Assign students to complete Chapter 15, "Documentation," of the workbook. Also assign them to read Chapter 16, "Trauma and Trauma Systems," before the next class.

EVALUATION

Chapter Quiz and Scenario Distribute copies of the Chapter Quiz provided in Handout 15-3 to evaluate student understanding of this chapter. Make sure each student reads the scenario to reinforce critical thinking on the scene. Remind students not to use their notes or textbooks while taking the quiz.

HANDOUT 15-2
Documentation Skills

ADVANCED LIFE SUPPORT SKILLS
Larmon & Davis. *Advanced Life Support Skills.*

ADVANCED LIFE SKILLS REVIEW
Larmon & Davis. *Advanced Life Skills Review.*

BRADY SKILLS SERIES: ALS
Larmon & Davis. *Brady Skills Series: ALS.*

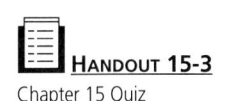

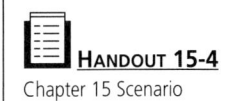

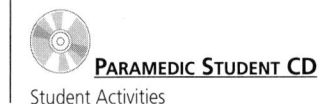

WORKBOOK
Chapter 15 Activities

READING/REFERENCE
Textbook, pp. 759–769

HANDOUT 15-3
Chapter 15 Quiz

HANDOUT 15-4
Chapter 15 Scenario

PARAMEDIC STUDENT CD
Student Activities

COMPANION WEBSITE
http://www.prenhall.com/bledsoe

TESTGEN
Chapter 15

EMT ACHIEVE: PARAMEDIC TEST PREPARATION
Mistovich & Beasley. *EMT Achieve: Paramedic Test Preparation.* www.prenhall.com/emtachieve/

REVIEW MANUAL FOR THE EMT-PARAMEDIC
Cherry & Mistovich. *Review Manual for the EMT-Paramedic,* 3rd edition.

HANDOUTS 15-5 AND 15-6
Reinforcement Activities

PARAMEDIC STUDENT CD
Student Activities

POWERPOINT PRESENTATION
Chapter 15

COMPANION WEBSITE
http://www.prenhall.com/bledsoe

ONEKEY
Chapter 15

ADVANCED LIFE SUPPORT SKILLS
Larmon & Davis. *Advanced Life Support Skills.*

ADVANCED LIFE SKILLS REVIEW
Larmon & Davis. *Advanced Life Skills Review.*

BRADY SKILLS SERIES: ALS
Larmon & Davis. *Brady Skills Series: ALS.*

PARAMEDIC NATIONAL STANDARDS SELF-TEST
Miller. *Paramedic National Standards Self-Test,* 4th edition.

Student CD Quizzes for every chapter are contained on the dynamic and highly visual in-text student CD.

Companion Website Additional quizzes for every chapter are contained on this exciting website.

TestGen You may wish to create a custom-tailored test using *Prentice Hall TestGen for Essentials of Paramedic Care,* 2nd Edition to evaluate student understanding of this chapter.

On-line Test Preparation (for students and instructors) Additional test preparation is available through Brady's new on-line product, *EMT Achieve: Paramedic Test Preparation* at *http://www.prenhall.com/emtachieve/.* Instructors can also monitor student mastery on-line.

Review Manual for the EMT-Paramedic This comprehensive exam review contains hundreds of test questions and rationales, including scenarios, along with two 180-question practice tests on CD.

REINFORCEMENT

Handouts If classroom discussion or performance on the quiz indicates that some students have not fully mastered the chapter content, you may wish to assign some or all of the Reinforcement Handouts for this chapter.

Student CD (for students) A wide variety of material on this CD-ROM will reinforce and also expand student knowledge and skills.

PowerPoint Presentation (for instructors) The PowerPoint material developed for this chapter offers useful reinforcement of chapter content.

Companion Website (for students) Additional review quizzes and links to EMS resources will contribute to further reinforcement of the chapter.

OneKey On-line support is offered for this course on one of three platforms: CourseCompass, Blackboard, or Web CT. Includes the IRM, PowerPoints, TestGen, and Companion Website for instruction. Ask your local sales representative for more information.

Brady Skills Series: Advanced Life Skills (Video or CD) Have your students watch the skills come to life on VHS or CD-ROM, or they can purchase the highly visual, full-color text with step-by-step procedures and rationales.

HANDOUT 15-1

Student's Name _____

CHAPTER 15 OBJECTIVES CHECKLIST

Knowledge	Date Mastered
1. Identify the general principles regarding the importance of EMS documentation and ways in which documents are used.	
2. Identify and properly use medical terminology, medical abbreviations, and acronyms.	
3. Explain the role of documentation in agency reimbursement.	
4. Identify and eliminate extraneous or nonprofessional information.	
5. Describe the differences between subjective and objective elements of documentation.	
6. Evaluate a finished document for errors and omissions and proper use and spelling of abbreviations and acronyms.	
7. Evaluate the confidential nature of an EMS report.	
8. Describe the potential consequences of illegible, incomplete, or inaccurate documentation.	
9. Describe the special documentation considerations concerning patient refusal of care and/or transport.	
10. Demonstrate how to properly record direct patient or bystander comments.	
11. Describe the special considerations concerning mass casualty incident documentation.	
12. Demonstrate proper document revision and correction.	
13. Given a prehospital care report form and a narrative patient care scenario, record all pertinent administrative information using a consistent format, identify and record the pertinent, reportable clinical data for each patient, correct errors and omissions, using proper procedures, and note and record "pertinent negative" clinical findings.	

OBJECTIVES

Handout 15-2

Student's Name _____

DOCUMENTATION SKILLS

Charting Student Progress:
1. *Learning skill*
2. *Performs skill with direction*
3. *Performs skill independently*

SKILLS

Skill/Behavior	1	2	3
1. Records all pertinent administrative information using a consistent format.			
2. Identifies and records all pertinent, reportable clinical data for each patient, including pertinent negatives.			
3. Uses appropriate medical terminology, abbreviations, and acronyms.			
4. Records accurate, consistent times.			
5. Includes relevant oral statements of witnesses, bystanders, and patient.			
6. Completely identifies all additional resources and personnel.			
7. Uses correct spelling and grammar.			
8. Writes legibly.			
9. Uses appropriate narrative format and includes all appropriate information.			
10. Thoroughly documents patient refusals, denials of transport, and call cancellations.			
11. Properly corrects errors and omissions.			
12. Writes cautiously, and avoids jargon, inferences, or any remarks that might be construed as derogatory or libelous.			
13. Completes report as soon as possible after the call.			

Comments:

HANDOUT 15-3

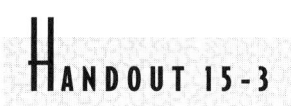

Student's Name _____

CHAPTER 15 QUIZ

Write the letter of the best answer in the space provided.

_____ 1. Uses for prehospital care reports include:
  A. medical.
  B. administrative.
  C. research.
  D. all of these

_____ 2. The time elapsed between a unit's being alerted and its arrival on the scene is the:
  A. en route time.
  B. response time.
  C. on-scene time.
  D. time of call.

_____ 3. Analyzing data from a prehospital care report to determine the efficacy of certain medical devices or interventions such as drugs is a(n) _____ use.
  A. administrative
  B. medical
  C. legal
  D. research

_____ 4. A scannable run sheet on which you fill in boxes to record assessment and care information is known as a:
  A. bubble sheet.
  B. narrative report.
  C. fill-in-the-dot report.
  D. check-box report.

_____ 5. Which of the following is a characteristic of a well-written PCR?
  A. deletion of any negative findings
  B. times approximated by the paramedics
  C. complete identification of all additional resources and personnel
  D. use of as much medical terminology as possible, even if the spelling is not accurate

_____ 6. A patient who has a history of CABG in 1978 has had a:
  A. coronary artery bypass graft.
  B. chronic abdominal growth.
  C. calcium arterial blockage.
  D. cardiac artery balloon geoplasty.

_____ 7. The abbreviation for paroxysmal nocturnal dyspnea is:
  A. PXD.
  B. PND.
  C. PNOCD.
  D. PXNOCD.

_____ 8. If a medication is labeled to be taken pc, it should be taken:
  A. on an empty stomach.
  B. with a full glass of water.
  C. after eating.
  D. before bed.

_____ 9. The letter *a* in the abbreviation a.c. means:
  A. before.
  B. after.
  C. when needed.
  D. in the morning.

_____ 10. The route of administration of a medication abbreviated po means:
  A. injected in the muscle.
  B. orally.
  C. rectally.
  D. under the tongue.

_____ 11. Physical assessment findings that are normal are known as:
  A. nonrelevant.
  B. positive findings.
  C. pertinent negatives.
  D. relevant nominals.

_____ 12. Additional or supplemental information to the original PCR is called a(n):
  A. epilog.
  B. postscript.
  C. supplement.
  D. addendum.

HANDOUT 15-3 Continued

_____ 13. To make a correction on a PCR you have written:
   A. completely black out the error before making the correction.
   B. destroy the PCR and rewrite it, making the correction.
   C. cross out the error with red ink, and write the correction above it.
   D. draw a single line through the error and initial it.

_____ 14. An example of subjective information written in the narrative portion of your PCR is:
   A. blood glucose of 102 mg/dL.
   B. chief complaint of chest pain.
   C. cardiac monitor showing 1st-degree block.
   D. trachea deviated to the left.

_____ 15. The initials of the SOAP format of organizing a narrative report include:
   A. symptoms.
   B. overall impression.
   C. assessment.
   D. past medical history.

_____ 16. The initials of the CHART format of organizing a narrative report include:
   A. chief complaint.
   B. abnormalities.
   C. relevant history.
   D. time.

_____ 17. The refusal of care documentation checklist includes:
   A. contacting the patient's family and advising of his refusal.
   B. having a police officer present to witness the refusal.
   C. assessing the competency of the patient.
   D. elimination of the need for a completed PCR.

_____ 18. Which statement about denying transport is true?
   A. People with even the most minor injuries should be evaluated if they refuse transport.
   B. The risks of patient refusals are greater than those of denying transport.
   C. If a call is cancelled en route, completing a PCR is optional but not necessary.
   D. The difference between "no patients found" and "only minor injuries, patients refusing transport" is relatively insignificant in documentation.

_____ 19. Which of the following is true regarding mass casualty incidents?
   A. A complete PCR must be done on each patient.
   B. If you cannot remember details to include on your PCR, make an educated guess.
   C. Proper documentation takes precedence over patient care.
   D. Completing documentation for one patient before going on to care for others might be impractical.

_____ 20. Which statement about inappropriate documentation is true?
   A. High-pressure, fast-paced situations eliminate the need for neatness.
   B. An inaccurate report can affect patient care days after the ambulance call ends.
   C. Paramedics are legally excused for any harmful consequences of poor documentation.
   D. Misspelled words do not reflect on the care provider's professionalism.

HANDOUT 15-4

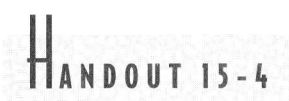

Student's Name _____

CHAPTER 15 SCENARIO

Review the following real-life situation. Then answer the questions that follow.

You were dispatched to a senior citizens' high-rise complex for a "diabetic emergency." On arrival, you find your patient, 74-year-old Mr. Herbert, seated in the lobby. One of the other residents reports that he is an insulin-dependent diabetic. Mr. Herbert complains that he has a headache and feels nauseated. His skin is pale, cool, and diaphoretic. Vital signs are as follows: B/P 100/80, pulse 64 and irregular, respirations 22 and shallow. Pulse oximetry shows an oxygen saturation of 96 percent on room air. You place him on high-flow, high-concentration oxygen via a nonrebreather mask. Your partner obtains a blood sample and determines the blood glucose to be 50 mg/dL. You start an IV and administer 50 milligrams of 50 percent dextrose. You contact medical direction and prepare to transport. Mr. Herbert reports that he is feeling much better now but has been having problems with his blood sugar for the past several days. You complete a focused physical exam and find no other acute problems. The ECG monitoring shows atrial fibrillation with a slow ventricular response.

By the time you arrive at the hospital, they have obtained Mr. Herbert's medical records. After giving your report and restocking your unit, you stop at the desk to look at his medical records. You read the following:

74 y/o WM with long history of CAD. CABG × 5 in 1986. Angina controlled with NTG PRN. DD insulin-dependent DM in 1980. Diabetic retinopathy and neuropathy. Meds: dig 0.25 mg q day, Semi-Lente insulin 25 units subcutaneous daily.

Rewrite this paragraph, spelling out the acronyms and abbreviations.

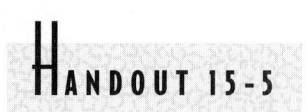

CHAPTER 15 REVIEW

Write the word or words that best complete the following sentences in the space provided.

1. Providing hospital staff such as nurses and physicians with information regarding the patient is a(n) _____ use for PCRs.

2. Gathering information for quality improvement and system management is a(n) _____ use for PCRs.

3. One characteristic of a well-written PCR is the inclusion of _____ negatives.

4. If you do not know how to spell a word, _____ _____ _____ or use _____ _____.

5. Whenever possible, record all times from the _____ _____.

6. An element of good documentation is the absence of _____.

7. Because many people must be able to read your PCR, one element of good documentation is _____.

8. Ideally, PCRs should be completed _____ _____ the call.

9. If you find an error after you've already written several more sentences, submit a(n) _____ to the PCR.

10. If you make a mistake writing your report, simply cross out the error with a(n) _____ _____.

11. "The patient is a 58-year-old male, conscious and breathing, complaining of shortness of breath" is an example of the _____ part of your narrative.

12. Vital signs, physical exam findings, and tests are examples of the _____ part of your narrative.

13. The two common patterns of organizing a narrative report are known by the mnemonics _____ and _____.

14. If your patient refuses care, you should explain to the patient about the possible _____ of refusing care.

15. _____ _____ affixed to patients at a mass casualty incident contain vital patient information.

Handout 15-6

Student's Name _____

STANDARD CHARTING ABBREVIATIONS

Write the standard abbreviation for each word or phrase listed in the space provided.

_____ 1. Chief complaint
_____ 2. Private medical doctor
_____ 3. Abdomen
_____ 4. Ear, nose, and throat
_____ 5. No apparent distress
_____ 6. Chronic obstructive pulmonary disease
_____ 7. Coronary artery disease
_____ 8. Insulin-dependent diabetes mellitus
_____ 9. Upper respiratory infection
_____ 10. Aspirin
_____ 11. Nitroglycerin
_____ 12. Nonsteroidal antiinflammatory agent
_____ 13. Sodium bicarbonate
_____ 14. Antecubital
_____ 15. Arterial blood gas
_____ 16. Complete blood count
_____ 17. Computerized tomography
_____ 18. Electrocardiogram
_____ 19. Palpation
_____ 20. After (post-)
_____ 21. As needed
_____ 22. Nothing by mouth
_____ 23. Drop(s)
_____ 24. Millimeters of mercury
_____ 25. Premature ventricular contraction

REINFORCEMENT

Chapter 15 Answer Key

Handout 15-3: Chapter 15 Quiz

1. D
2. B
3. D
4. A
5. C
6. A
7. B
8. C
9. A
10. B
11. C
12. D
13. D
14. B
15. C
16. A
17. C
18. A
19. D
20. B

Handout 15-4: Chapter 15 Scenario

74-year-old white male with long history of coronary artery disease. Five coronary artery bypass grafts in 1986. Angina controlled with nitroglycerin as needed. Differential diagnosis insulin-dependent diabetes mellitus in 1980. Diabetic retinopathy and neuropathy. Medications: digoxin 0.25 mg every day, semilente insulin 25 units subcutaneously daily.

Handout 15-5: Chapter 15 Review

1. medical
2. administrative
3. pertinent
4. look it up, another word
5. same clock
6. alterations
7. legibility
8. immediately after
9. addendum
10. single line
11. subjective
12. objective
13. SOAP, CHART
14. consequences
15. Triage tags

Handout 15-6: Standard Charting Abbreviations

1. CC
2. PMD
3. Abd
4. ENT
5. NAD
6. COPD
7. CAD
8. IDDM
9. URI
10. ASA
11. NTG
12. NSAID
13. $NaHCO_3$
14. AC
15. ABG
16. CBC
17. CT
18. ECG, EKG
19. Palp
20. $\bar{p}$
21. prn
22. NPO
23. gtt(s)
24. mmHg
25. PVC

Essentials of Paramedic Care

Division 3

Trauma Emergencies

Chapter 16

Trauma and Trauma Systems

INTRODUCTION

Trauma is a physical injury caused by an external force. It is the number one killer of persons under the age of 44, and therefore steals the greatest number of productive years from its victims. Trauma accounts for about 150,000 deaths per year, including motor vehicle crashes and gunshot wounds. As a paramedic, you must understand the structure and objectives of the trauma care system; promote injury prevention; and provide the seriously injured trauma patient with proper assessment, aggressive care, and rapid transport to the most appropriate facility.

TOTAL TEACHING TIME: 5.50 HOURS
The total teaching time is only a guideline based on the didactic and practical lab averages in the National Standard Curriculum. Instructors should take into consideration such factors as the pace at which students learn, the size of the class, and breaks. The actual time devoted to teaching objectives is the responsibility of the instructor.

CHAPTER OBJECTIVES

After reading this chapter, you should be able to:

1. Describe the prevalence and significance of trauma. (pp. 761–762)
2. List the components of a comprehensive trauma system. (pp. 762–764)
3. Identify the characteristics of community, area, and regional trauma centers. (pp. 762–763)
4. Identify the trauma triage criteria and apply them to narrative descriptions of trauma patients. (pp. 764–766)
5. Describe how trauma emergencies differ from medical emergencies in the scene size-up, assessment, prehospital emergency care, and transport. (pp. 764–766)
6. Explain the "Golden Hour" concept, and describe how it applies to prehospital emergency medical service. (pp. 765–766)
7. Explain the value of air medical service in trauma patient care and transport. (pp. 765–766)

FRAMING THE LESSON

Begin class with an open discussion about situations students have been in or have seen that caused serious trauma. Discuss the types of situations that lead to major trauma: motor vehicle collisions, assaults, stabbings, and gunshots. Discuss the level of care available in your community for serious trauma patients. Through discussion, determine the answers to the following questions: What level of trauma center is available in the area? What level of EMS care is available? Is there a helicopter available for scene responses? How is care for the trauma patient different from care for a medical patient? Why is definitive care for the trauma patient so time dependent? Why are severe trauma cases often very emotional?

TEACHING STRATEGIES

People learn in a variety of ways. Some do better with the spoken word, whereas others prefer the written. Some prefer to work alone, whereas others profit from working in groups. Recognizing these different ways of acquiring knowledge, the authors of this *Instructor's Resource Manual* have provided a variety of teaching strategies for the different types of learners. These strategies are intended to foster higher-level cognitive skills and encourage creative learning and problem solving. For greatest effectiveness, incorporate these strategies into your class lecture. Symbols in the Lecture Outline indicate the points at which various exercises might be most appropriate. Other strategies can be used to preview the lesson or to summarize it.

The following strategies are keyed to specific sections of the lesson.

1. Brainstorming and Classifying Trauma Calls. Have students brainstorm the types of trauma calls to which they have responded (or for an inexperienced class, calls they have seen on TV). Make a big list on the board or poster paper. Now, have students take turns indicating "P" for penetrating trauma or "B" for blunt mechanisms. This activity encourages group participation during the brainstorming portion of the exercise. Additionally, it requires students to get out of their chairs to participate and maintains individual accountability when trying to decide blunt versus penetrating mechanism of injury.

2. Scenario Writing. Allow students to have some fun with this exercise. It is an opportunity to facilitate discussion and encourage students to use critical thinking skills in a nonthreatening classroom environment.

Divide the class into groups of three or four students. Next, ask each group to write one major trauma scenario. However (and this is the fun part), ask the groups to build into their scenarios situations that will involve as many mechanisms of injury, along with the appropriate physical findings, as they can for one patient. Have each group work together at creating its scenario without referring to the text.

Next, have each group select one person to read its scenario before the class. Ask the class to identify as many of the mechanisms of injury and physical finding indicators as possible. Write them on the board. The group that has created the scenario with the most major trauma indicators wins.

3. Trauma Center Tour. The resources of a Level I trauma center are awesome. Arrange for a tour of the trauma center, even if you have to travel some distance to get there, and especially if students will not do clinical time at that hospital. Seeing the trauma team respond to a patient will leave a lasting impression on the students and will reinforce the need to transport patients to the most appropriate receiving facility. Bypassing one hospital for another is an uncomfortable decision for most prehospital providers. Seeing the advanced technology and resources of a Level I trauma center will help students recognize the benefit provided to the major trauma patient and will likely increase the number of times the provider appropriately transports patients to the trauma center.

4. Local Trauma Center Locations. Get a map of your area and pinpoint the locations of all trauma centers in your area. Then, indicate their designations,

I–IV. Make a key or legend explaining the differences in resources available for each designation. During scenarios and classroom skills labs, refer to the map when asking students to make appropriate transport decisions for their patients. This requires students to be familiar with their local hospital resources and requires clinical decision making during scenarios.

5. *Simulations and Scenarios.* Be sure to specifically design simulations and scenarios in your class to depict patients who meet trauma guidelines and criteria. Students need practice making clinical decisions based on physical findings they determine themselves. Do not allow students to end their scenarios without making determinations of transport destinations and scene times based on trauma triage criteria. If you find students having a hard time remembering the criteria, make posters with the information to hang in your skills lab rooms.

6. *Vehicle Junkyard Tour.* Take a tour of your local junk or salvage yard to examine wrecked vehicles. Have students reconstruct in their heads the collisions that caused the damage to the vehicles seen there. This kinesthetic activity develops an index of suspicion in an interactive and creative way.

The following strategies can be used at various points throughout the lesson or to help summarize and demonstrate what students have learned.

Guest Speakers: Case Histories from the Field. Invite local paramedics to talk about interesting trauma cases they have encountered. Ask the paramedics to describe what happened in these cases and, further, to give their emotional reactions to some of the cases. Also, invite a local trauma surgeon to talk to the class about cases he has had. Ask the surgeon to bring pertinent X-rays, scans, and so on.

In the News. Have students collect newspaper articles on incidents involving major trauma for a week prior to class. Try to obtain newspapers from other cities as well. Then have students read the articles aloud to the class. Hold a class discussion on the possible mechanisms of injury, physical findings, and appropriate treatments that might have been called for in the incidents.

Brady Trauma Slides. Use the Brady Trauma Slides to show various mechanisms of injury (MOI). Ask students to predict what injuries they would expect to see based on the MOI. This activity helps students to develop an index of suspicion. Additionally, it encourages teamwork by creating and adding onto lists as a class.

Cultural Considerations, Legal Notes, and Patho Pearls. The Student CD-ROM contains this series of informative features to enhance the student's understanding of the material covered in this chapter.

TEACHING OUTLINE

Chapter 16, "Trauma and Trauma Systems," is the first lesson in Division 3, *Trauma Emergencies*. Distribute Handout 16-1 so that students can familiarize themselves with the learning goals for this chapter. If students have any questions about the objectives, answer them at this time.

Then present the chapter. One possible lecture outline follows. In the outline, the parenthetical references in regular type are references to text pages; those in bold type are references to figures, tables, or procedures.

I. Introduction. Trauma is the fourth leading cause of death in the United States. The paramedic's role in trauma care includes proper assessment, care,

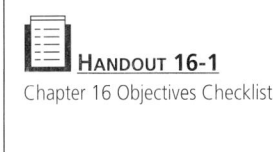

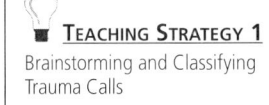

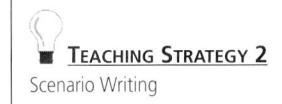

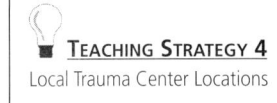

HANDOUT 16-1
Chapter 16 Objectives Checklist

TEACHING STRATEGY 1
Brainstorming and Classifying Trauma Calls

TEACHING STRATEGY 2
Scenario Writing

TEACHING STRATEGY 3
Trauma Center Tour

TEACHING STRATEGY 4
Local Trauma Center Locations

Sidebar

TEACHING STRATEGY 5
Simulations and Scenarios

POWERPOINT PRESENTATION
Chapter 16 PowerPoint slides 4–5

TEACHING STRATEGY 6
Vehicle Junkyard Tour

POWERPOINT PRESENTATION
Chapter 16 PowerPoint slide 6

POWERPOINT PRESENTATION
Chapter 16 PowerPoint slides 7–12

READING/REFERENCE
Baird, J. "Taking the Tricks Out of Trauma." *JEMS*, March 2003.

Criss, E. "Rural Hospitals and Trauma Survival." *JEMS*, Sept. 2002.

Ottaway, M. "Twenty Trauma Traps to Avoid." *JEMS*, Feb. 2000.

POWERPOINT PRESENTATION
Chapter 16 PowerPoint slides 13–22

WORKBOOK
Chapter 16 Activities

READING/REFERENCE
Textbook, pp. 770–801

POWERPOINT PRESENTATION
Chapter 16 PowerPoint slide 23

HANDOUT 16-2
Chapter 16 Quiz

HANDOUT 16-3
Chapter 16 Scenario

PARAMEDIC STUDENT CD
Student Activities

COMPANION WEBSITE
http://www.prenhall.com/bledsoe

---

and transport. This chapter will increase understanding of the structure and objectives of the trauma care system as it defines trauma, explains the components of the trauma care system, identifies the capabilities of different levels of trauma centers, and more fully defines the paramedic's role as a care provider in the trauma system. (p. 761)

II. Trauma (pp. 761–762)

  A. Penetrating trauma (p. 761)
  B. Blunt trauma (p. 761)
  C. Serious life-threatening conditions (pp. 761–762)
  D. Non-life-threatening conditions (p. 762) (**Fig. 16-1, p. 761**)

III. The trauma care system (p. 762)

  A. Trauma Care System Planning and Development Act of 1990 (p. 762)
  B. Trauma is a surgical disease. (p. 762)
  C. Serious trauma. (p. 762)

IV. Trauma center designation (pp. 762–764) (**Table 16-1, p. 763**)

  A. Level I regional trauma center (p. 762) (**Fig. 16-2, p. 763**)
  B. Level II area trauma center (pp. 762–763)
  C. Level III community trauma center (p. 763)
  D. Level IV trauma facility (pp. 763–764)
  E. Specialty centers (p. 764)
   1. Neurocenters
   2. Burn centers
   3. Pediatric trauma centers
   4. Microsurgery/hand and limb reimplantation centers
   5. Hyperbaric oxygenation

V. Your role as an EMT-Paramedic (pp. 764–767) (**Fig. 16-3, p. 764**)

  A. Mechanism of injury analysis (p. 765)
  B. Index of suspicion (p. 765)
  C. The Golden Hour (pp. 765–766)
  D. The decision to transport (p. 766) (**Fig. 16-4, p. 766**) (**Table 16-2, p. 767**)
   1. Mechanism of injury
   2. Physical findings
  E. Injury prevention (pp. 766–767)
  F. Data and the trauma registry (p. 767)
  G. Quality improvement (p. 767)

VI. Summary (p. 768). Trauma remains one of the greatest tragedies of our modern society. It accounts for large numbers of deaths and disabling injuries and often affects individuals who are in their most productive years of life. A well-designed and well-implemented trauma system offers a way of lessening the impact of these traumas.

As a paramedic, you are a part of the trauma system. You are charged with evaluating trauma patients by comparing their mechanisms of injury and the physical signs of their injuries to preestablished trauma triage criteria in order to determine which patients should enter the trauma system and which could be best cared for at a general hospital. In the presence of severe, life-threatening trauma, you must assure rapid assessment, on-scene care, and appropriate transport to provide your patients with the best chances for survival.

ASSIGNMENTS

Assign students to complete Chapter 16, "Trauma and Trauma Systems," of the workbook. Also assign them to read Chapter 17, "Blunt Trauma," before the next class.

EVALUATION

Chapter Quiz and Scenario Distribute copies of the Chapter Quiz provided in Handout 16-2 to evaluate student understanding of this chapter. Make sure each student reads the scenario to reinforce critical thinking on the scene. Remind students not to use their notes or textbooks while taking the quiz.

Student CD Quizzes for every chapter are contained on the dynamic and highly visual in-text student CD.

Companion Website Additional quizzes for every chapter are contained on this exciting website.

TestGen You may wish to create a custom-tailored test using *Prentice Hall TestGen for Essentials of Paramedic Care*, 2nd Edition to evaluate student understanding of this chapter.

On-line Test Preparation (for students and instructors) Additional test preparation is available through Brady's new on-line product, *EMT Achieve: Paramedic Test Preparation* at *http://www.prenhall.com/emtachieve/*. Instructors can also monitor student mastery on-line.

Review Manual for the EMT-Paramedic This comprehensive exam review contains hundreds of test questions and rationales, including scenarios, along with two 180-question practice tests on CD.

REINFORCEMENT

Handouts If classroom discussion or performance on the quiz indicates that some students have not fully mastered the chapter content, you may wish to assign some or all of the Reinforcement Handouts for this chapter.

Student CD (for students) A wide variety of material on this CD-ROM will reinforce and also expand student knowledge and skills.

PowerPoint Presentation (for instructors) The PowerPoint material developed for this chapter offers useful reinforcement of chapter content.

Companion Website (for students) Additional review quizzes and links to EMS resources will contribute to further reinforcement of the chapter.

OneKey On-line support is offered for this course on one of three platforms: CourseCompass, Blackboard, or Web CT. Includes the IRM, PowerPoints, TestGen, and Companion Website for instruction. Ask your local sales representative for more information.

Brady Skills Series: Advanced Life Skills (Video or CD) Have your students watch the skills come to life on VHS or CD-ROM, or they can purchase the highly visual, full-color text with step-by-step procedures with rationales.

TESTGEN
Chapter 16

EMT ACHIEVE: PARAMEDIC TEST PREPARATION
Mistovich & Beasley. *EMT Achieve: Paramedic Test Preparation.* www.prenhall.com/emtachieve/

REVIEW MANUAL FOR THE EMT-PARAMEDIC
Cherry & Mistovich. *Review Manual for the EMT-Paramedic,* 3rd edition.

HANDOUT 16-4
Reinforcement Activities

PARAMEDIC STUDENT CD
Student Activities

POWERPOINT PRESENTATION
Chapter 16

COMPANION WEBSITE
http://www.prenhall.com/bledsoe

ONEKEY
Chapter 16

ADVANCED LIFE SUPPORT SKILLS
Larmon & Davis. *Advanced Life Support Skills.*

ADVANCED LIFE SKILLS REVIEW
Larmon & Davis. *Advanced Life Skills Review.*

BRADY SKILLS SERIES: ALS
Larmon & Davis. *Brady Skills Series: ALS.*

PARAMEDIC NATIONAL STANDARDS SELF-TEST
Miller. *Paramedic National Standards Self-Test,* 4th edition.

Handout 16-1

Student's Name _____

CHAPTER 16 OBJECTIVES CHECKLIST

Knowledge	Date Mastered
1. Describe the prevalence and significance of trauma.	
2. List the components of a comprehensive trauma system.	
3. Identify the characteristics of community, area, and regional trauma centers.	
4. Identify the trauma triage criteria and apply them to narrative descriptions of trauma patients.	
5. Describe how trauma emergencies differ from medical emergencies in the scene size-up, assessment, prehospital emergency care, and transport.	
6. Explain the "Golden Hour" concept, and describe how it applies to prehospital emergency medical service.	
7. Explain the value of air medical service in trauma patient care and transport.	

OBJECTIVES

HANDOUT 16-2

Student's Name _____

CHAPTER 16 QUIZ

Write the letter of the best answer in the space provided.

_____ 1. A physical injury or wound caused by an external force or violence is known as a:
   A. mechanism.
   B. trauma.
   C. directed injury.
   D. forceful entry.

_____ 2. An injury caused by the collision of an object with the body in which the object does not enter the body is called a(n):
   A. internal injury.
   B. surgical trauma.
   C. closed injury.
   D. blunt trauma.

_____ 3. Penetrating trauma refers to an injury in which a(n):
   A. projectile is forced through the tissue and embedded in an organ.
   B. object enters and exits the body, resulting in two wounds.
   C. object breaks the skin and enters the body.
   D. object is impaled in the body.

_____ 4. The proper care for serious trauma is:
   A. aggressive resuscitation on scene.
   B. transport to the closest medical facility.
   C. fluid replacement on scene.
   D. immediate surgical intervention.

_____ 5. A medical facility that commits resources to address the most common trauma emergencies with surgical capability available 24 hours a day, 7 days a week, is classified as a:
   A. Level I trauma center.
   B. Level II trauma center.
   C. Level III trauma center.
   D. Level IV trauma center.

_____ 6. Neurocenters, burn centers, and pediatric trauma centers are examples of:
   A. Level II trauma centers.
   B. clinics.
   C. specialty centers.
   D. community medical centers.

_____ 7. Guidelines to aid prehospital personnel in determining which trauma patients require urgent transportation to a trauma center are called:
   A. trauma triage criteria.
   B. trauma transport protocols.
   C. prehospital standing orders.
   D. trauma system triage.

_____ 8. The force or process that causes trauma is known as the:
   A. nature of injury.
   B. force of trauma.
   C. compression factor.
   D. mechanism of injury.

_____ 9. The anticipation of injury to a body region, organ, or structure based on analysis of the mechanism of injury is called:
   A. suspicion of trauma.
   B. index of suspicion.
   C. mechanism index.
   D. consideration of injury.

_____ 10. The Golden Hour is the 60-minute period:
   A. after arrival at the hospital.
   B. after arrival of EMS on the trauma scene.
   C. after a severe injury.
   D. after surgery, in recovery.

HANDOUT 16-2 Continued

_____ 11. Initial patient assessment, stabilization, packaging, and initiation of transport should ideally take less than:
   A. 5 minutes.
   B. 10 minutes.
   C. 15 minutes.
   D. 20 minutes.

_____ 12. A mechanism of injury indicating the need for immediate transport is a(n):
   A. fall 6 to 8 feet for an adult.
   B. "T-bone" motor vehicle collision.
   C. ejection from a vehicle.
   D. auto crash with a speed at impact of 20 mph.

_____ 13. Physical findings that would indicate the need for immediate transport include:
   A. long bone fracture.
   B. pulse greater than 120 or less than 50.
   C. burns to more than 10 percent of body surface area.
   D. systolic blood pressure less than 100.

_____ 14. The data retrieval system for trauma patient information, used to evaluate and improve the trauma system, is called the trauma:
   A. triage criteria.
   B. database.
   C. associated statistics.
   D. registry.

_____ 15. The leading killer of persons under 44 years of age in the United States is:
   A. cardiovascular disease.
   B. trauma.
   C. stroke.
   D. cancer.

HANDOUT 16-3

Student's Name _____

CHAPTER 16 SCENARIO

Review the following real-life situation. Then answer the questions that follow.

Lowell Medic One is dispatched to a construction site where they are met by the site safety manager. He tells them an employee has fallen off some scaffolding. When the paramedics reach the base of the scaffolding, they see a middle-aged man holding the right side of his head. The man turns and walks away from the paramedics. The safety manager shouts out his name, "George!" but the man continues to walk away. The paramedics hurry to him and, when they reach his side, ask him what has happened. He says, "I just bumped my head and I want to be left alone." Both paramedics notice a hematoma on his forehead and believe they smell alcohol on the patient's breath. The patient continues to refuse treatment from the paramedics but finally agrees to be transported. He is taken to the nearest hospital where he is admitted for overnight observation.

1. What other information about the mechanism of injury should the paramedics have tried to obtain from the site manager or patient?

2. What type of traumatic injury does the patient have, blunt or penetrating?

3. Do you feel the patient should be transported? Why?

4. When should stabilization occur? In the field or en route to the hospital? Why?

5. What are at least three injuries or medical conditions that may have led to the fall or been incurred as a result of it?

HANDOUT 16-4

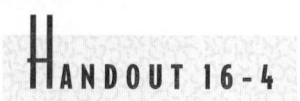

Student's Name _____

CHAPTER 16 REVIEW

Write the word or words that best complete the following sentences in the space provided.

1. A physical injury or wound caused by external force or violence is called _____.

2. _____ is the leading killer of persons under age 44 in the United States.

3. An injury caused by an object breaking the skin and entering the body is called _____ _____.

4. An injury caused by the collision of an object with the body in which the object does not enter the body is called _____ _____.

5. Serious trauma is a(n) _____ disease.

6. A Level _____, or _____ trauma center commits resources to address all types of specialty trauma 24 hours a day, 7 days a week.

7. A Level _____, or _____ trauma center commits resources to the most common trauma emergencies with surgical capability available 24 hours a day, 7 days a week.

8. A Level _____, or _____ trauma center commits to special emergency department training and has some surgical capability.

9. Certain medical facilities such as neurocenters and burn centers may be classified as _____ centers.

10. _____ _____ _____ are the guidelines to aid prehospital personnel in determining which trauma patients require urgent transportation to a trauma center.

11. The force or process that causes trauma is called the _____ _____ _____ .

12. The _____ _____ _____ is the anticipation of injury to a body region, organ, or structure based on analysis of the mechanism of injury.

13. The 60-minute period after a severe injury is called the _____ Hour.

14. A mechanism of injury indicating the need for immediate transport is a fall greater than _____ feet for an adult, and greater than _____ feet for an infant or child.

15. A physical finding indicating the need for immediate transport is a pulse rate greater than _____ or less than _____.

Chapter 16 Answer Key

Handout 16-2: Chapter 16 Quiz

1. B
2. D
3. C
4. D
5. B
6. C
7. A
8. D
9. B
10. C
11. B
12. C
13. B
14. D
15. B

Handout 16-3: Chapter 16 Scenario

1. The height of the fall. Was it greater than 20 feet?
2. Blunt.
3. Yes, since there appears to be at least the possibility of a fall greater than 20 feet; if in doubt, transport.
4. Because the patient refuses in-field treatment, the best thing to do is to provide rapid and safe transport to the hospital and hope that personnel there can convince him to accept treatment.
5. Possible injuries/conditions include intracranial bleeding, diabetes, alcohol intoxication, neck injury; possible internal injuries if fall was greater than 20 feet.

Handout 16-4: Chapter 16 Review

1. trauma
2. Trauma
3. penetrating trauma
4. blunt trauma
5. surgical
6. I, regional
7. II, area
8. III, community
9. specialty
10. Trauma triage criteria
11. mechanism of injury
12. index of suspicion
13. Golden
14. 20, 10
15. 120, 50

Chapter 17

Blunt Trauma

INTRODUCTION

The most common cause of trauma death and disability is blunt trauma, or the energy exchange between an object and the human body, without intrusion of the object through the skin. Blunt trauma can be deceptive because serious internal injury may be hidden, and the signs and symptoms of the injury may be subtle or slow to present. This chapter will look at the kinetics of blunt trauma (the injury process and its results), vehicular collisions, blast injuries, and other types of blunt trauma to better understand the mechanisms of injury and the resulting effects on the body systems.

CHAPTER OBJECTIVES

After reading this chapter, you should be able to:

1. Identify, and explain by example, the laws of inertia and conservation of energy. (pp. 771–772)
2. Define kinetic energy and force as they relate to trauma. (pp. 772–773)
3. Compare and contrast the types of vehicle impacts and their expected injuries. (pp. 774–777, 779–790)
4. Discuss the benefits of auto restraint and motorcycle helmet use. (pp. 777–779, 788)
5. Describe the mechanisms of injury associated with falls, crush injuries, and sports injuries. (pp. 796–799)
6. Identify the common blast injuries and any special considerations regarding their assessment and proper care. (pp. 790–796)
7. Identify and explain any special assessment and care considerations for patients with blunt trauma. (pp. 779–799)
8. Given several preprogrammed and moulaged blunt trauma patients, provide the appropriate scene size-up, initial assessment, rapid trauma or focused physical exam and history, detailed exam, and ongoing assessment and provide appropriate patient care and transportation. (pp. 771–799)

TOTAL TEACHING TIME

There is no specific time requirement for this topic in the National Standard Curriculum. Instructors should take into consideration such factors as the pace at which students learn, the size of the class, and breaks. The actual time devoted to teaching objectives is the responsibility of the instructor.

FRAMING THE LESSON

Begin by reviewing the important points of Chapter 16, "Trauma and Trauma Systems." Use this time to answer any questions about the previous chapter and to discuss any items not completely understood by students. Then begin the discussion of Chapter 17.

On a flip chart or chalkboard, draw an outline of the human body. Or ask for a student volunteer to stand in front of the class in the anatomical position. Point to each major body division, such as chest, abdomen, pelvis, head, and so on, and ask the class to name the major organs or systems contained within that division. Quickly review the positions and functions of major organs and describe them as solid or hollow. Discuss the result of trauma to the organ and what signs and symptoms might be seen. Stress the importance of knowing the location of the organs to better anticipate injuries to them, based on the mechanism of injury. Remind students that internal injuries may not show immediate signs or symptoms and stress the importance of watching for trends in patients' vital signs and general condition.

TEACHING STRATEGIES

People learn in a variety of ways. Some do better with the spoken word, whereas others prefer the written. Some prefer to work alone, whereas others profit from working in groups. Recognizing these different ways of acquiring knowledge, the authors of this *Instructor's Resource Manual* have provided a variety of teaching strategies for the different types of learners. These strategies are intended to foster higher-level cognitive skills and encourage creative learning and problem solving. For greatest effectiveness, incorporate these strategies into your class lecture. Symbols in the Lecture Outline indicate the points at which various exercises might be most appropriate. Other strategies can be used to preview the lesson or to summarize it.

The following strategies are keyed to specific sections of the lesson.

1. Car Crash Physics. To illustrate the physics involved in blunt trauma, use short clips from popular movies involving car crashes or other traumatic incidents. After each clip, discuss the kinetic energy, acceleration, and deceleration involved in each. Using popular culture in the classroom helps add relevance and reality to the education of adult learners. Additionally, this activity is highly visual.

2. Saturday Morning Cartoons. Saturday morning cartoons ought to give students great examples of trauma. Wile E. Coyote was famous for falling great distances, using explosives, and experiencing sudden decelerations. Either tape the cartoons for class, or make a homework assignment out of them. Ask students to describe the trauma, classify as blunt or penetrating, and list at least three injuries that would be possible from that particular mechanism. Using popular culture in the classroom helps add relevance and reality to the education of adult learners. Additionally, this activity is highly visual and will surely stimulate classroom discussion.

3. Solid and Hollow Organ Demonstration. Demonstrate the difference in damage to solid and hollow organs using a melon and a water balloon. First, use a hammer to smash a water-filled balloon. This will simulate a hollow organ such as the bladder. The balloon will, of course, rupture or burst, spilling its contents onto the floor, the instructor, and first row of students. Then, use the hammer to smash a cantaloupe or similar melon. The melon will fracture into pieces, simulating the damage done to solid organs from blunt trauma. The sights and sounds associated with this demonstration will make a lasting impression on students, further reinforcing their index of suspicion for injuries following trauma.

4. Sliced Liver Demonstration. Use a wire cheese cutter and brick of cheese to demonstrate the way the liver is sliced by the ligamentum teres. Dental floss works well also. Slice a piece of the liver (cheese) for each student. Alternately, have students work the example themselves, using dental floss to cut the cheese. This way, students handle their own cheese slice and may eat it afterward.

5. Egg Crash-Dummy Demonstration. Draw a face on an egg and place it in the driver's position of a child's toy car, or make a simple toy car using a flat piece of wood as a frame with four wheels attached, one at each corner (see diagram on this page). On top of the piece of wood, attach a smaller piece to represent the dash and a fifth wheel attached to the dashboard to represent the steering wheel. Make a seat for the car by cutting out one side of a paper cup.

Place the car at the top of a ramp, allowing it to crash into a wall at the bottom of the ramp. The car will hit the wall, the egg will hit the steering wheel, and the organs (yolk) of the egg will hit the eggshell. You can even crack open the egg to show that the yolk has been broken.

This visual activity clearly demonstrates the vehicle-body-organ collision concept presented in this chapter. The injuries will be obvious. Stress, however, that blunt trauma injuries in humans are not nearly as obvious.

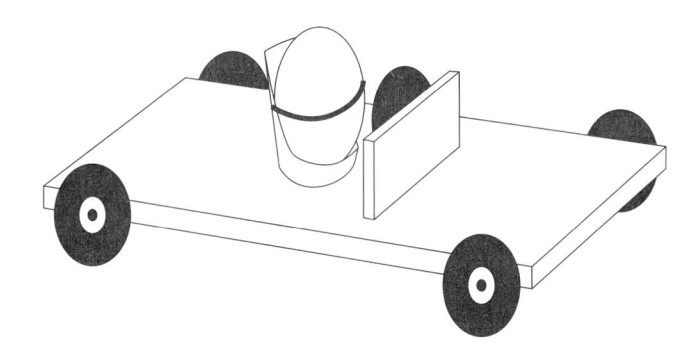

Make a seat belt for the egg and reconstruct your collision. The organs and eggshell will be spared this time, thus illustrating the powerful protection afforded by a seat belt. Your seat belt can be made out of a rubber band or strip of fabric.

The following strategies can be used at various points throughout the lesson or to help summarize and demonstrate what students have learned.

Mechanism of Injury Scenarios. Divide the class into small groups. Give each group a page with an outline of the human body on it. Prior to handing out the pages, make a small circle on each body outline—on a different portion of the body for each—indicating an area of injury or impact. Assign each group to develop a scenario for a mechanism of injury that would result in an injury to the area marked. Then, have the group develop a patient report of signs and symptoms of injury they would expect to find based on injury to that specific site. After the scenarios have been completed, have a member of each group present the patient and information to the class.

Guest Lecturer: Trauma Surgeon. Invite a local trauma surgeon to class and ask him to bring photos of blunt trauma injuries, either from his personal experience or other sources. With each photo shown, have the surgeon describe the type of internal

HANDOUT 17-1
Chapter 17 Objectives Checklist

TEACHING TIP
Have some fun demonstrating Newton's law with some common household items. Bring in toy vehicles and let your students see for themselves how increasing the speed of these vehicles leads to increased damage in staged "crashes."

TEACHING STRATEGY 1
Car Crash Physics

POWERPOINT PRESENTATION
Chapter 17 PowerPoint slide 4

TEACHING STRATEGY 2
Saturday Morning Cartoons

POWERPOINT PRESENTATION
Chapter 17 PowerPoint slides 5–7

TEACHING STRATEGY 3
Solid and Hollow Organ Demonstration

TEACHING STRATEGY 4
Sliced Liver Demonstration

POWERPOINT PRESENTATION
Chapter 17 PowerPoint slides 8–32

READING/REFERENCE
Goss, J. "Complexities of Blunt Chest Trauma." *JEMS*, Nov. 2004.

Phrampus, P. et al. "Danger Zone (Blunt & Penetrating Neck Trauma)." *JEMS*, Nov. 2002.

POINT TO EMPHASIZE
Know the indicators for decision to transport rapidly. Always err on the side of precaution. Look for subtle signs of serious injury and deterioration and expect the worst.

POINT TO EMPHASIZE
Everything and everyone in a moving ambulance should be secured in some way. In a deceleration collision, anything not secured to the vehicle becomes a rapidly moving projectile.

injuries he found and what was necessary to repair them. Graphic photos of actual injuries will help students recognize potential internal injuries in the field.

Cultural Considerations, Legal Notes, and Patho Pearls. The Student CD-ROM contains this series of informative features to enhance the student's understanding of the material covered in this chapter.

TEACHING OUTLINE

Chapter 17, "Blunt Trauma," is the second lesson in Division 3, *Trauma Emergencies*. Distribute Handout 17-1 so that students can familiarize themselves with the learning goals for this chapter. If students have any questions about the objectives, answer them at this time.

Then present the chapter. One possible lecture outline follows. In the outline, the parenthetical references in regular type are references to text pages; those in bold type are references to figures, tables, or procedures.

I. Introduction to kinetics. Blunt trauma is the most common cause of trauma death and disability. Blunt trauma can be deceptive because the true nature of the injury is often hidden and evidence of the serious injury is very subtle or even absent. (p. 771)

II. Kinetics of blunt trauma (pp. 771–773) (**Fig. 17-1, p. 771**)
  A. Inertia (pp. 771–772)
  B. Conservation of energy (p. 772)
  C. Kinetic energy (pp. 772–773) (**Fig. 17-2, p. 772**)
    1. Mass
    2. Velocity
  D. Force (p. 773) (**Fig. 17-3, p. 773**)
    1. Acceleration
    2. Deceleration

III. Blunt trauma (pp. 774–799)
  A. Automobile collisions (pp. 774–787)
    1. Events of impact (**Fig. 17-4, pp. 775–776**)
       a. Vehicle collision
       b. Body collision
       c. Organ collision
       d. Secondary collisions
       e. Additional collisions
    2. Restraints
       a. Seat belts
       b. Airbags (**Fig. 17-5, p. 778**)
       c. Child safety seats
    3. Types of impact (**Fig. 17-6, p. 779**)
       a. Frontal (**Fig. 17-7, p. 780; Fig. 17-9, p. 781; Fig. 17-10, p. 781**)
          i. Up-and-over pathway (**Fig. 17-8, p. 780**)
          ii. Down-and-under pathway
          iii. Ejection
       b. Lateral (**Fig. 17-11, p. 782; Fig. 17-12, p. 783**)
       c. Rotational (**Fig. 17-13, p. 783**)
       d. Rear-end (**Fig. 17-14, p. 784; Fig. 17-15, p. 784**)
       e. Rollover (**Fig 17-16, p. 785**)

486 ESSENTIALS OF PARAMEDIC CARE

  4. Vehicle collision analysis (**Fig. 17-17, p. 785**)
    a. Intoxication
    b. Vehicular mortality (**Table 17-1, p. 786**)
    c. Collision evaluation
 B. Motorcycle collisions (pp. 787–788) (**Fig. 17-18, p. 787**)
  1. Frontal
  2. Angular
  3. Sliding
  4. Ejection
 C. Pedestrian collisions (p. 788) (**Fig. 17-19, p. 789; Fig. 17-20, p. 789**)
 D. Recreational vehicle collisions (pp. 788–790)
  1. Snowmobiles
  2. Watercraft (**Fig 17-21, p. 790**)
  3. All-terrain vehicles (ATVs) (**Fig. 17-22 p. 790**)
 E. Blast injuries (pp. 790–796)
  1. Explosion
    a. Fuel and oxidizing agent instantly combine
    b. Chemical bonds are broken down and reestablished
    c. Resultant heat and pressure differential produce several mechanisms of injury
     i. Pressure wave
     ii. Blast wind
     iii. Projectiles
     iv. Heat (**Fig. 17-23, p. 791**)
     v. Displacement
  2. Pressure wave
    a. Overpressure
    b. Compression
    c. Decompression
    d. Victim's orientation
  3. Blast wind
  4. Projectiles
    a. Ordnance
    b. Flechettes
  5. Personnel displacement
  6. Confined space explosions and structural collapses
  7. Burns
  8. Blast injury phases (**Fig. 17-24, p. 794**)
    a. Primary
    b. Secondary
    c. Tertiary
  9. Blast injury assessment
  10. Blast injury care
    a. Lungs
    b. Abdomen
    c. Ears
    d. Penetrating wounds
    e. Burns
 F. Other types of blunt trauma (pp. 796-799)
  1. Falls (**Fig. 17-25, p. 797**)
  2. Sports injuries (**Fig. 17-26, p. 798**)
  3. Crush injuries

IV. Chapter summary (p. 799). Blunt trauma accounts for most injury deaths and disabilities. While vehicle collisions are the most frequent cause of blunt trauma, blast injuries, sports injuries, crush injuries, and falls also ac-

---

TEACHING STRATEGY 5
Egg Crash-Dummy Demonstration

POINT TO EMPHASIZE
Patients experiencing a loss of consciousness resulting from blunt trauma should be seen by a physician, no matter how good their condition seems.

POINT TO EMPHASIZE
In adult vehicle versus pedestrian collisions there are actually three collisions. The bumper hits the patient, the patient hits the hood or windshield, and the patient hits the ground. Account for all three in forming your index of suspicion.

POWERPOINT PRESENTATION
Chapter 17 PowerPoint slide 33

count for significant mortality and morbidity. Blunt trauma is difficult to assess accurately so you, as the care provider, must look carefully at the mechanism of injury and subtle physical signs to help anticipate serious internal injury. Careful analysis of the mechanism of injury, followed by development of indices of suspicion for injury can help guide you to recognize those patients needing rapid entry into the trauma system and those best served by on-scene care and transport to the nearest appropriate care facility.

ASSIGNMENTS

Assign students to complete Chapter 17, "Blunt Trauma," of the workbook. Also assign them to read Chapter 18, "Penetrating Trauma," before the next class.

EVALUATION

Chapter Quiz and Scenario Distribute copies of the Chapter Quiz provided in Handout 17-2 to evaluate student understanding of this chapter. Make sure each student reads the scenario to reinforce critical thinking on the scene. Remind students not to use their notes or textbooks while taking the quiz.

Student CD Quizzes for every chapter are contained on the dynamic and highly visual in-text student CD.

Companion Website Additional quizzes for every chapter are contained on this exciting website.

TestGen You may wish to create a custom-tailored test using *Prentice Hall TestGen for Essentials of Paramedic Care*, 2nd Edition to evaluate student understanding of this chapter.

On-line Test Preparation (for students and instructors) Additional test preparation is available through Brady's new on-line product, *EMT Achieve: Paramedic Test Preparation* at *http://www.prenhall.com/emtachieve/*. Instructors can also monitor student mastery on-line.

Review Manual for the EMT-Paramedic This comprehensive exam review contains hundreds of test questions and rationales, including scenarios, along with two 180-question practice tests on CD.

REINFORCEMENT

Handouts If classroom discussion or performance on the quiz indicates that some students have not fully mastered the chapter content, you may wish to assign some or all of the Reinforcement Handouts for this chapter.

Student CD (for students) A wide variety of material on this CD-ROM will reinforce and also expand student knowledge and skills.

PowerPoint Presentation (for instructors) The PowerPoint material developed for this chapter offers useful reinforcement of chapter content.

Companion Website (for students) Additional review quizzes and links to EMS resources will contribute to further reinforcement of the chapter.

WORKBOOK
Chapter 17 Activities

READING/REFERENCE
Textbook, pp. 802–820

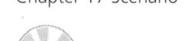

HANDOUT 17-2
Chapter 17 Quiz

HANDOUT 17-3
Chapter 17 Scenario

PARAMEDIC STUDENT CD
Student Activities

COMPANION WEBSITE
http://www.prenhall.com/bledsoe

TESTGEN
Chapter 17

EMT ACHIEVE: PARAMEDIC TEST PREPARATION
Mistovich & Beasley. *EMT Achieve: Paramedic Test Preparation.* www.prenhall.com/emtachieve/

REVIEW MANUAL FOR THE EMT-PARAMEDIC
Cherry & Mistovich. *Review Manual for the EMT-Paramedic,* 3rd edition.

HANDOUTS 17-4 AND 17-5
Reinforcement Activities

PARAMEDIC STUDENT CD
Student Activities

POWERPOINT PRESENTATION
Chapter 17

COMPANION WEBSITE
http://www.prenhall.com/bledsoe

OneKey On-line support is offered for this course on one of three platforms: CourseCompass, Blackboard, or Web CT. Includes the IRM, PowerPoints, TestGen, and Companion Website for instruction. Ask your local sales representative for more information.

Brady Skills Series: Advanced Life Skills (Video or CD) Have your students watch the skills come to life on VHS or CD-ROM, or they can purchase the highly visual, full-color text with step-by-step procedures and rationales.

ONEKEY
Chapter 17

ADVANCED LIFE SUPPORT SKILLS
Larmon & Davis. *Advanced Life Support Skills.*

ADVANCED LIFE SKILLS REVIEW
Larmon & Davis. *Advanced Life Skills Review.*

BRADY SKILLS SERIES: ALS
Larmon & Davis. *Brady Skills Series: ALS.*

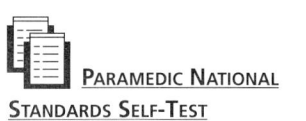

PARAMEDIC NATIONAL STANDARDS SELF-TEST
Miller. *Paramedic National Standards Self-Test,* 4th edition.

Handout 17-1

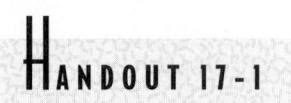

Student's Name _____

CHAPTER 17 OBJECTIVES CHECKLIST

Knowledge	Date Mastered
1. Identify, and explain by example, the laws of inertia and conservation of energy.	
2. Define kinetic energy and force as they relate to trauma.	
3. Compare and contrast the types of vehicle impacts and their expected injuries.	
4. Discuss the benefits of auto restraint and motorcycle helmet use.	
5. Describe the mechanisms of injury associated with falls, crush injuries, and sports injuries.	
6. Identify the common blast injuries and any special considerations regarding their assessment and proper care.	
7. Identify and explain any special assessment and care considerations for patients with blunt trauma.	
8. Given several preprogrammed and moulaged blunt trauma patients, provide the appropriate scene size-up, initial assessment, rapid trauma or focused physical exam and history, detailed exam, and ongoing assessment and provide appropriate patient care and transportation.	

HANDOUT 17-2

Student's Name _____

CHAPTER 17 QUIZ

Write the letter of the best answer in the space provided.

_____ 1. The branch of physics dealing with forces affecting objects in motion and the energy exchanges that occur as objects collide is called:
  A. conservation of energy.
  B. inertia.
  C. kinetics.
  D. kinematics.

_____ 2. The capacity to do work in the strict physical sense is:
  A. inertia.
  B. motion.
  C. velocity.
  D. energy.

_____ 3. Kinetic energy is:
  A. a measure of the matter that an object contains.
  B. the energy an object has while it is in motion.
  C. the rate of motion in a particular direction.
  D. the rate at which speed or velocity changes.

_____ 4. The formula "mass multiplied by velocity squared, divided by 2" equals:
  A. acceleration.
  B. force.
  C. deceleration.
  D. kinetic energy.

_____ 5. When specific kinetic energy is applied to human anatomy, it is called:
  A. trauma.
  B. velocity.
  C. mass.
  D. force.

_____ 6. When an object or force impacts the body and kinetic energy is transferred through body tissues the result is called:
  A. penetrating trauma.
  B. blunt trauma.
  C. exsanguination.
  D. internal trauma.

_____ 7. One of the five events of every vehicle collision is the:
  A. object collision.
  B. primary collision.
  C. organ collision.
  D. tertiary collision.

_____ 8. When a vehicle occupant strikes the vehicle's interior, it is called a(n):
  A. vehicle collision.
  B. body collision.
  C. secondary collision.
  D. additional collision.

_____ 9. Which of the following is TRUE regarding the use of seat belts?
  A. Due to the security of the ambulance patient compartment, it is not necessary for EMS personnel to wear seat belts while caring for the patient.
  B. Lap belts alone will effectively restrain the torso, neck, and head.
  C. In some cases, a shoulder strap may induce chest contusions and rib fractures.
  D. The combination of seat belt and shoulder strap protects the occupant against intrusions into the passenger compartment.

_____ 10. Which of the following is TRUE regarding airbags?
  A. Child carriers should be secured in the back seat because airbag inflation may push the carrier into the seat with tremendous force, causing serious injury or death to the child.
  B. Airbags have, overall, had little effect in reducing injury and death in vehicular crashes.
  C. If an airbag has deployed, there is no need to check the steering wheel for deformity.
  D. The airbag must be triggered by the driver to deploy.

EVALUATION

HANDOUT 17-2 Continued

_____ 11. The frontal impact is the most common type of impact in motor vehicle crashes. One of the pathways of patient travel during a frontal impact is:
  A. around-and-through.
  B. down-and-under.
  C. through-and-out.
  D. up-and-out.

_____ 12. An injury process frequently associated with steering column impact is the "paper bag" syndrome in which the:
  A. driver yells just before impact, and the impact with the steering wheel presses all of the residual air from the lungs.
  B. driver "gulps" air into the stomach, and the stomach ruptures when the abdomen impacts the steering wheel.
  C. driver takes a deep breath in anticipation of the collision, and lung tissue ruptures when the chest impacts the steering wheel.
  D. car seat breaks loose and comes forward, crushing the patient between the seat and the steering wheel much like an inflated paper bag caught between clapping hands.

_____ 13. Your patient was involved in a frontal impact collision when his car hit a tree. He was ejected from the vehicle. An important point to remember when assessing this patient is that:
  A. the ejection was the result of the down-and-under pathway.
  B. ejected victims experience two impacts.
  C. older cars may have a "crumple zone" that allows energy to pass easily to the vehicle interior from the point of impact.
  D. due to advanced vehicle design, ejection is responsible for very few vehicular fatalities.

_____ 14. Rotational impact injuries are often less than vehicle damage might suggest, because the:
  A. occupant's stopping distance is much greater, and deceleration is more gradual.
  B. collision force pushes the auto forward, actually causing an acceleration in speed.
  C. amount of structural steel between the impact site and the vehicle interior is increased.
  D. rotational force of the vehicle tends to keep the occupants stationary in the vehicle instead of being thrown to the front, back, or side.

_____ 15. An important point to remember when analyzing vehicle crashes is that:
  A. alcohol intoxication is not present in most serious crashes.
  B. head trauma accounts for a small number of deaths in vehicle crashes.
  C. you should examine both the interior and exterior of a vehicle to identify forces expressed to the patient.
  D. you should stay focused on analyzing the mechanisms of injury, not on the cause of the crash.

_____ 16. Which of the following is TRUE regarding motorcycle crashes?
  A. Helmets have greatly reduced the incidence of spinal trauma.
  B. "Laying the bike down" results in the bike absorbing much of the energy.
  C. Actual ejection during a motorcycle crash is uncommon.
  D. Leather clothing and boots protect the rider against fractures and dislocations.

_____ 17. When responding to a vehicle versus pedestrian collision, remember that:
  A. adults tend to turn away from the oncoming vehicle, while children turn toward it.
  B. because of their lower centers of gravity, children are often thrown onto the hood and into the windshield.
  C. adults are frequently thrown in front of vehicles, and then run over by them.
  D. children will usually be hit by the vehicle first in the leg.

_____ 18. The most lethal explosions are those:
  A. causing structural collapses.
  B. in confined spaces.
  C. involving volatile chemicals.
  D. creating a blast wind.

HANDOUT 17-2 Continued

_____ **19.** The most common and serious trauma associated with explosions is:
   A. head injuries.
   B. abdominal injuries.
   C. lung injuries.
   D. airway blockages.

_____ **20.** A severe fall for an adult is from a height of:
   A. 6 feet or more.
   B. 10 feet or more.
   C. 20 feet or more.
   D. twice the patient's own height.

Handout 17-3

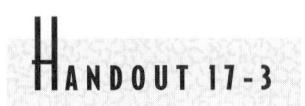

Student's Name _____

CHAPTER 17 SCENARIO

Review the following real-life situation. Then answer the questions that follow.

Medic 3 responds to a motor-vehicle collision at a busy intersection. The paramedics are met by a police officer, who tells them, "It looks like a real nasty T-bone crash." The paramedics notice two vehicles. One is a small sports car, which appears to have struck the driver's side of an older station wagon. The front end of the sports car is heavily damaged. The station wagon's door is caved in.

The paramedics see that the driver of the sports car is slumped over the steering wheel. The driver of the station wagon is sitting motionless. One paramedic assesses the driver of the sports car and finds an unconscious patient with respirations of 30 and a pulse of 130. The other paramedic checks on the driver of the station wagon and finds the patient is conscious and complaining of slight chest pain. His respirations are 12 and his pulse is 98. A BLS unit arrives. Both patients are extricated from their vehicles. The patient from the sports car is immobilized and intubated, and two large-bore IVs are established. The patient is then transported to the trauma center where, following emergency department evaluation, he is sent to the operating room. Later he is admitted to the intensive care unit.

Against the paramedics' advice, the patient from the station wagon refuses transportation. However, a couple of hours later he arrives at the emergency department by private vehicle. At this time, his BP is 80/60, his pulse is 160, and his respiratory rate is 32. He is rushed into the operating room for surgical repair to his aortic arch. After a period of hospitalization, he recovers.

1. What types of auto impacts are present in this scenario?

2. Besides the obvious vehicle deformity to both cars, what other indicator would it have been helpful to know?

3. Based on the mechanism of injury and physical findings of the patient taken from the sports car, when should the IVs have been started?

4. List at least five types of traumatic injuries you might expect to find in the patient taken from the sports car.

5. List at least five types of traumatic injuries you might expect to find in the patient taken from the station wagon.

HANDOUT 17-4

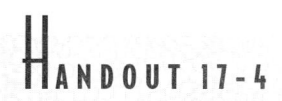

Student's Name _____

CHAPTER 17 REVIEW

Write the word or words that best complete the following sentences in the space provided.

1. _____ trauma is the most common cause of trauma death and disability.
2. _____ is the branch of physics that deals with motion, taking into consideration mass and force.
3. The tendency of an object to remain at rest or remain in motion unless acted upon by an external force is called _____.
4. _____ is the process of changing place.
5. The capacity to do work in the strict physical sense is called _____.
6. The energy an object has while it is in motion is called _____ energy.
7. _____ is the rate of motion in a particular direction in relation to time.
8. _____ is the rate at which speed increases, and _____ is the rate at which speed decreases.
9. Trauma can be categorized as either _____ or _____.
10. _____ is the draining of blood to the point at which life cannot be sustained.
11. The five types of vehicle impacts are _____, _____, _____, _____-_____, and _____.
12. The five events of vehicle collision are _____ collision, _____ collision, _____ collision, _____ collisions, and _____ impacts.
13. Parents should secure child carriers in the _____ seat when a passenger _____ system is in place.
14. Mechanisms associated with frontal impacts include _____-and-_____ pathway, _____-and-_____ pathway, and _____.
15. The _____-_____-_____ pathway accounts for over half of the deaths in vehicular crashes.
16. The _____ _____ syndrome results from compression of the chest against the steering column.
17. _____ _____ is the application of the forces of trauma along the axis of the spine.
18. The region of a vehicle designed to absorb the energy of impact is called the _____ _____.
19. Due to the deflection of impact, the occupant's stopping distance being greater, and the deceleration being more gradual, injuries are generally less serious in _____ impact collisions.
20. _____ and _____ _____ trauma account for 85 percent of deaths in vehicular crashes.
21. Helmets reduce the incidence and severity of _____ injuries in motorcycle crashes.
22. In pedestrian versus automobile crashes, adults tend to turn _____ from the oncoming vehicle, while children turn _____ it.
23. A(n) _____ is an agent that combines oxygen with a fuel.
24. Breaking glass and parts of collapsing walls propelled outward with the release of the blast energy are called _____.
25. A rapid increase then decrease in atmospheric pressure created by an explosion is called _____.
26. Mechanisms associated with blasts include _____ wave, _____ wind, _____, _____ displacement, _____ spaces and _____ collapses, and _____.

REINFORCEMENT

HANDOUT 17-4 Continued

27. The three blast injury phases are _____, _____, and _____.
28. _____ injuries are the most common and serious trauma associated with explosions.
29. A(n) _____ is a collection of air or gas in the pleural cavity between the chest wall and lung.
30. A serious fall for an adult is one that is from _____ feet or higher, or _____ times the patient's own height.

Handout 17-5

Student's Name _____

BLUNT TRAUMA LISTS

1. List the five events of vehicle collision and give a brief definition of each.

2. List the five types of vehicle impact and give a brief definition of each.

3. List the three mechanisms associated with frontal impacts.

4. List the six mechanisms associated with blasts.

5. List the three blast injury phases.

REINFORCEMENT

Chapter 17 Answer Key

Handout 17-2: Chapter 17 Quiz

1. C
2. D
3. B
4. D
5. A
6. B
7. C
8. B
9. C
10. A
11. B
12. C
13. B
14. A
15. C
16. B
17. A
18. A
19. C
20. C

Handout 17-3: Chapter 17 Scenario

1. Frontal and lateral.
2. Knowing the approximate speed of the sports car when it struck the station wagon would be useful because impacts at speeds greater than 20 mph are significant mechanisms of injury.
3. Because the vehicle deformity indicated the likelihood of severe internal trauma, initiation of the IVs should have been attempted en route.
4. Possible injuries include: myocardial contusion, flail chest, aortic tear, pneumothorax, cervical spine injury.
5. Expected injuries might include: cervical spine injury; internal head injuries; clavicle, pelvis, and femur fractures; diaphragmatic rupture; and aortic tear.

Handout 17-4: Chapter 17 Review

1. Blunt
2. Kinetics
3. inertia
4. Motion
5. energy
6. kinetic
7. Velocity
8. Acceleration, deceleration
9. blunt, penetrating
10. Exsanguination
11. frontal, lateral, rotational, rear-end, rollover
12. vehicle, body, organ, secondary, additional
13. back, airbag
14. down, under; up, over; ejection
15. up-and-over
16. paper bag
17. Axial loading
18. crumple zone
19. rotational
20. Head, body cavity
21. head
22. away, toward
23. oxidizer
24. projectiles
25. overpressure
26. pressure, blast, projectiles, personnel, confined, structural, burns
27. primary, secondary, tertiary
28. Lung
29. pneumothorax
30. 20, three

Handout 17-5: Blunt Trauma Lists

1. Vehicle collision—auto strikes an object; Body collision—vehicle occupant strikes the vehicle's interior; Organ collision—tissues behind contacting surface collide as the body halts; Secondary collisions—vehicle occupant impacted by objects within auto; Additional impacts—vehicle receives a second impact
2. frontal, lateral, rotational, rear-end, rollover
3. down-and-under pathway; up-and-over pathway; ejection
4. pressure wave, blast wind, projectiles, personnel displacement, confined spaces and structural collapses, burns
5. primary, secondary, tertiary

Chapter 18

Penetrating Trauma

INTRODUCTION

About 28,000 deaths occur each year as a result of gunshot wounds. Deaths from penetrating trauma, as a whole, are increasing. Penetrating wounds may be caused by knives, arrows, nails, and pieces of glass or wire. The basic laws of physics in blunt trauma discussed in Chapter 17 also apply to penetrating trauma. This chapter will help you anticipate potential injuries and adequately assess and care for victims of penetrating trauma.

CHAPTER OBJECTIVES

After reading this chapter, you should be able to:

1. Explain the energy exchange process between a penetrating object or projectile and the object it strikes. (pp. 803–806)
2. Determine the effects that profile, yaw, tumble, expansion, and fragmentation have on projectile energy transfer. (pp. 804–806)
3. Describe elements of the ballistic injury process including direct injury, cavitation, temporary cavity, permanent cavity, and zone of injury. (pp. 804–806, 809–811)
4. Identify the relative effects a penetrating object or projectile has when striking various body regions and tissues. (pp. 811–816)
5. Anticipate the injury types and the extent of damage associated with high-velocity/high-energy projectiles, such as rifle bullets; with medium-energy/medium-velocity projectiles such as handgun and shotgun bullets, slugs, or pellets; and with low-energy/low-velocity penetrating objects, such as knives and arrows. (pp. 806–809)
6. Identify important elements of the scene size-up associated with shootings or stabbings. (pp. 816–817)
7. Identify and explain any special assessment and care considerations for patients with penetrating trauma. (pp. 817–818)
8. Given several preprogrammed and moulaged penetrating trauma patients, provide the appropriate scene size-up, initial assessment, rapid trauma or focused physical exam and history, detailed exam, and ongoing assessment and provide appropriate patient care and transportation. (pp. 803–818)

TOTAL TEACHING TIME

There is no specific time requirement for this topic in the National Standard Curriculum. Instructors should take into consideration such factors as the pace at which students learn, the size of the class, and breaks. The actual time devoted to teaching objectives is the responsibility of the instructor.

FRAMING THE LESSON

Begin by reviewing the important points of Chapter 17, "Blunt Trauma." Use this time to answer any questions about the previous chapter and to discuss any items not completely understood by students. Then begin the discussion of Chapter 18.

For approximately 1 week before the lesson, cut out as many newspaper articles as you can find that involve penetrating trauma to a victim. This would include shootings, stabbings, collisions, and so on. Paste each article on a page of a flip chart. It should not be difficult to cover one full page with articles. Also, obtain statistics from your local trauma center and law enforcement agencies of the numbers of gunshots and stabbings that occured over a specific period. Present this information to students. There are often more penetrating trauma cases than students may realize. Invite a member of local law enforcement or an area trauma surgeon to present information on the various calibers and types of bullets and how they react when fired, when they enter the body, and so on.

TEACHING STRATEGIES

People learn in a variety of ways. Some do better with the spoken word, whereas others prefer the written. Some prefer to work alone, whereas others profit from working in groups. Recognizing these different ways of acquiring knowledge, the authors of this *Instructor's Resource Manual* have provided a variety of teaching strategies for the different types of learners. These strategies are intended to foster higher-level cognitive skills and encourage creative learning and problem solving. For greatest effectiveness, incorporate these strategies into your class lecture. Symbols in the Lecture Outline indicate the points at which various exercises might be most appropriate. Other strategies can be used to preview the lesson or to summarize it.

The following strategies are keyed to specific sections of the lesson.

1. ***Demonstration of Trajectory and Drag with Darts.*** To demonstrate trajectory and drag, mount a dartboard in class. Allow students to throw darts of varying types and from various distances. The two concepts will become clear quickly. This kinesthetic activity will be fun for students. Be sure to exercise caution when using darts in the classroom to avoid injury.

2. ***Demonstration of Trajectory and Drag with Paintball Guns.*** While you may not want students to fire real firearms, you could use paintball guns to demonstrate the principles of a bullet's travel. These guns use compressed air or CO_2 to discharge the paint bullet. They are not lethal and could effectively demonstrate trajectory, drag, and the kick of the gun. Most cities and suburbs have both indoor and outdoor paintball ranges.

3. ***Guest Speaker: Ballistics Expert.*** Invite an expert to teach ballistics for your class. Few instructors will have the experience or resources to teach this section themselves. An expert from law enforcement will be able to bring sample firearms and ammunition as well as photos and video footage of the concepts to be explained.

4. ***Practical Demonstration.*** Arrange for students to take a field trip to a local gun range. Have an instructor discuss firearm safety with the students and demonstrate various calibers of weapons. This should instill a new understanding of and respect for a weapon. This is also an excellent opportunity to stress scene safety.

5. Law Enforcement Training Videos. Often, law enforcement agencies or the coroner's office have training videos or films dealing with ballistics and gunshot wounds. Many of these videos have segments appropriate for EMS courses dealing with the damage caused by various calibers and styles of bullets. A classic training film demonstrates damage done by bullets by having various sizes and types shot through large blocks of gelatin, simulating human tissue. If possible, have a police officer or representative of the coroner's office bring one of these videos or films to class and answer questions students may have.

The following strategies can be used at various points throughout the lesson or to help summarize and demonstrate what students have learned.

Epidemiology of Trauma. Be sure you have the most recent information about the epidemiology of trauma and, specifically, penetrating trauma in the United States and your specific state. You can request this information from both the Department of Transportation and the Centers for Disease Control. Discuss with students the reasons for increases or decreases in incident levels of trauma. Discuss prevention programs or the lack thereof in your neighborhoods. Using local data increases the relevance of the material to your adult learners.

Autopsy Videos. Law enforcement or the coroner's office may have videos or films of autopsies of people killed by penetrating trauma, such as gunshots or stabbings. Or a trauma surgeon may have photos taken of penetrating trauma and the resulting damage found during surgery. Ask them to bring photos or videos with them and address the class regarding their experiences.

Guest Speaker: Gun Safety Instructor. Promote gun safety in your classroom by inviting a gun safety instructor. This way, students will be prepared to handle and secure a weapon should they find one on scene. You could find an instructor from a local gun club, fish and game office, firing range, military base, or law enforcement agency.

Brady Trauma Slides: Penetrating Trauma. Use the Brady Trauma Slides to illustrate penetrating trauma to each body area listed under "Specific Tissue/Organ Injuries." It will improve students' response to these injuries if they have previewed them, as the sight of some of these injuries can be grotesque. Using the slides can help students get past the visual shock and key into the assessment of life threats.

Cultural Considerations, Legal Notes, and Patho Pearls. The Student CD-ROM contains this series of informative features to enhance the student's understanding of the material covered in this chapter.

TEACHING OUTLINE

Chapter 18, "Penetrating Trauma," is the third lesson in Division 3, *Trauma Emergencies*. Distribute Handout 18-1 so that students can familiarize themselves with the learning goals for this chapter. If students have any questions about the objectives, answer them at this time.

Then present the chapter. One possible lecture outline follows. In the outline, the parenthetical references in regular type are references to text pages; those in bold type are references to figures, tables, or procedures.

I. Introduction. The numbers and severities of cases of penetrating trauma have greatly increased, especially injuries from gunshots. Other mechanisms include knives, arrows, nails, and pieces of glass and wire. The types of

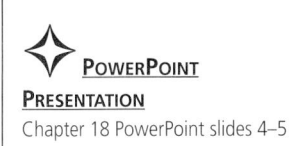

HANDOUT 18-1
Chapter 18 Objectives Checklist

POWERPOINT PRESENTATION
Chapter 18 PowerPoint slides 4–5

TEACHING STRATEGY 1
Demonstration of Trajectory and Drag with Darts

POWERPOINT PRESENTATION
Chapter 18 PowerPoint slides 6–39

TEACHING STRATEGY 2
Demonstration of Trajectory and Drag with Paintball Guns

READING/REFERENCE
Porter, R. "Ballistics: The Hole Story." *JEMS*, Sept. 1999.

TEACHING STRATEGY 3
Guest Speaker: Ballistics Expert

TEACHING STRATEGY 4
Practical Demonstration

TEACHING STRATEGY 5
Law Enforcement Training Videos

POINT OF INTEREST
Twenty-five percent of abdominal knife wounds involve the diaphragm and chest.

POWERPOINT PRESENTATION
Chapter 18 PowerPoint slides 40–44

POINT TO EMPHASIZE
Primary injuries are the most often overlooked, while secondary and tertiary injuries are the most often treated.

TEACHING TIP
Demonstrate, and have students practice, decompression of a tension pneumothorax by placing pork or beef ribs over an inner tube.

weapons and projectiles involved and the characteristics of the tissue they impact affect the severity of the injury. It is important to understand the principles of energy exchange and projectile travel to adequately assess and care for patients of penetrating trauma. (p. 803)

II. Physics of penetrating trauma (pp. 803–811)
   A. Kinetic energy (pp. 803–804) (Fig 18-1, p. 803)
      1. Mass
      2. Velocity
      3. Conservation of energy
   B. Ballistics (pp. 804–806)
      1. Trajectory
      2. Drag
      3. Cavitation
      4. Profile (**Fig. 18-2, p. 805**)
         a. Caliber
      5. Stability (**Fig. 18-3, p. 805**)
         a. Yaw
      6. Expansion and fragmentation (**Fig. 18-4, p. 806**)
      7. Secondary impacts
      8. Shape
   C. Specific weapon characteristics (pp. 806–809) (**Fig. 18-5, p. 807**)
      1. Handgun (**Fig. 18-6, p. 807**)
      2. Rifle (**Fig. 18-7, p. 808**)
      3. Assault rifle
      4. Shotgun (**Fig. 18-8, p. 808**)
      5. Knives and arrows
   D. Damage pathway (pp. 809–811)
      1. The projectile injury process (**Fig. 18-9, p. 809**)
      2. Direct injury
      3. Pressure shock wave (**Fig. 18-10, p. 810**)
      4. Temporary cavity
      5. Permanent cavity
      6. Zone of injury
   E. Low-velocity wounds (p. 811) (**Fig. 18-11, p. 811**)

III. Specific tissue/organ injuries (pp. 811–816)
   A. Connective tissue (pp. 811–812)
   B. Organs (p. 812)
      1. Solid organs
      2. Hollow organs (**Fig. 18-12, p. 812**)
   C. Lungs (pp. 812–813)
   D. Bone (p. 813)
   E. General body regions (pp. 813–816) (**Fig. 18-13, p. 813**)
      1. Extremities
      2. Abdomen
      3. Thorax
      4. Neck
      5. Head
      6. Entrance wound (**Fig. 18-14, p. 815**)
      7. Exit wound (**Fig. 18-15, p. 815**)

IV. Special concerns with penetrating trauma (pp. 816–818)

   A. Scene size-up (pp. 816–817) (**Fig. 18-16, p. 816**)
   B. Penetrating wound assessment (p. 817)
   C. Penetrating wound care (pp. 817–818)
      1. Facial wounds (**Fig. 18-17, p. 817**)
      2. Chest wounds (**Fig. 18-18, p. 818**)
      3. Impaled objects

V. Chapter summary (pp. 818–819). Penetrating injuries, especially those associated with gunshot wounds, are responsible for a high incidence of prehospital trauma and death. Your understanding of the mechanisms of injury that produce these wounds and an understanding of the types of injuries caused by these mechanisms (index of suspicion) can help you rapidly identify serious life threats and assure these patients receive rapid transport to a trauma center. Special prehospital care techniques such as sealing an open pneumothorax and managing a difficult airway can also help you stabilize the patient in the field and help assure that he safely reaches definitive care.

POWERPOINT PRESENTATION
Chapter 18 PowerPoint slides 45–48

POINT TO EMPHASIZE
Stress the Golden Hour principle.

POWERPOINT PRESENTATION
Chapter 18 PowerPoint slide 49

ASSIGNMENTS

Assign students to complete Chapter 18, "Penetrating Trauma," of the workbook. Also assign them to read Chapter 19, "Hemorrhage and Shock," before the next class.

WORKBOOK
Chapter 18 Activities

READING/REFERENCE
Textbook, pp. 821–851

EVALUATION

Chapter Quiz and Scenario   Distribute copies of the Chapter Quiz provided in Handout 18-2 to evaluate student understanding of this chapter. Make sure each student reads the scenario to reinforce critical thinking on the scene. Remind students not to use their notes or textbooks while taking the quiz.

Student CD   Quizzes for every chapter are contained on the dynamic and highly visual in-text student CD.

Companion Website   Additional quizzes for every chapter are contained on this exciting website.

TestGen   You may wish to create a custom-tailored test using *Prentice Hall TestGen for Essentials of Paramedic Care*, 2nd Edition to evaluate student understanding of this chapter.

On-line Test Preparation (for students and instructors)   Additional test preparation is available through Brady's new on-line product, *EMT Achieve: Paramedic Test Preparation* at *http://www.prenhall.com/emtachieve/*. Instructors can also monitor student mastery on-line.

Review Manual for the EMT-Paramedic   This comprehensive exam review contains hundreds of test questions and rationales, including scenarios, along with two 180-question practice tests on CD.

HANDOUT 18-2
Chapter 18 Quiz

HANDOUT 18-3
Chapter 18 Scenario

PARAMEDIC STUDENT CD
Student Activities

COMPANION WEBSITE
http://www.prenhall.com/bledsoe

TESTGEN
Chapter 18

EMT ACHIEVE: PARAMEDIC TEST PREPARATION
Mistovich & Beasley. *EMT Achieve: Paramedic Test Preparation.*
www.prenhall.com/emtachieve/

REVIEW MANUAL FOR THE EMT-PARAMEDIC
Cherry & Mistovich. *Review Manual for the EMT-Paramedic*, 3rd edition.

HANDOUTS 18-4 AND 18-5
Reinforcement Activities

PARAMEDIC STUDENT CD
Student Activities

POWERPOINT PRESENTATION
Chapter 18

COMPANION WEBSITE
http://www.prenhall.com/bledsoe

ONEKEY
Chapter 18

ADVANCED LIFE SUPPORT SKILLS
Larmon & Davis. *Advanced Life Support Skills.*

ADVANCED LIFE SKILLS REVIEW
Larmon & Davis. *Advanced Life Skills Review.*

BRADY SKILLS SERIES: ALS
Larmon & Davis. *Brady Skills Series: ALS.*

PARAMEDIC NATIONAL STANDARDS SELF-TEST
Miller. *Paramedic National Standards Self-Test*, 4th edition.

REINFORCEMENT

Handouts If classroom discussion or performance on the quiz indicates that some students have not fully mastered the chapter content, you may wish to assign some or all of the Reinforcement Handouts for this chapter.

Student CD (for students) A wide variety of material on this CD-ROM will reinforce and also expand student knowledge and skills.

PowerPoint Presentation (for instructors) The PowerPoint material developed for this chapter offers useful reinforcement of chapter content.

Companion Website (for students) Additional review quizzes and links to EMS resources will contribute to further reinforcement of the chapter.

OneKey On-line support is offered for this course on one of three platforms: CourseCompass, Blackboard, or Web CT. Includes the IRM, PowerPoints, TestGen, and Companion Website for instruction. Ask your local sales representative for more information.

Brady Skills Series: Advanced Life Skills (Video or CD) Have your students watch the skills come to life on VHS or CD-ROM, or they can purchase the highly visual, full-color text with step-by-step procedures and rationales.

HANDOUT 18-1

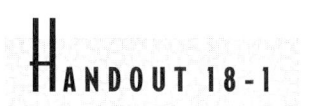

Student's Name _____

CHAPTER 18 OBJECTIVES CHECKLIST

Knowledge	Date Mastered
1. Explain the energy exchange process between a penetrating object or projectile and the object it strikes.	
2. Determine the effects that profile, yaw, tumble, expansion, and fragmentation have on projectile energy transfer.	
3. Describe elements of the ballistic injury process including direct injury, cavitation, temporary cavity, permanent cavity, and zone of injury.	
4. Identify the relative effects a penetrating object or projectile has when striking various body regions and tissues.	
5. Anticipate the injury types and the extent of damage associated with high-velocity/high-energy projectiles, such as rifle bullets; with medium-energy/medium-velocity projectiles such as handgun and shotgun bullets, slugs, or pellets; and with low-energy/low-velocity penetrating objects, such as knives and arrows.	
6. Identify important elements of the scene size-up associated with shootings or stabbings.	
7. Identify and explain any special assessment and care considerations for patients with penetrating trauma.	
8. Given several preprogrammed and moulaged penetrating trauma patients, provide the appropriate scene size-up, initial assessment, rapid trauma or focused physical exam and history, detailed exam, and ongoing assessment and provide appropriate patient care and transportation.	

CHAPTER 18 QUIZ

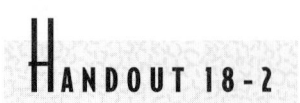

Student's Name _____

Write the letter of the best answer in the space provided.

_____ 1. When recalling the physics of penetrating trauma, remember that:
   A. wounds from rifle bullets are two to four times more lethal than wounds from handgun bullets.
   B. if you double the speed of an object, its kinetic energy also doubles.
   C. handguns and shotguns are considered low-energy/low-velocity weapons.
   D. the trajectory of a bullet is a straight line until it reaches its target.

_____ 2. The formation of a partial vacuum and subsequent cavity within a semifluid medium is called:
   A. trajectory.
   B. drag.
   C. cavitation.
   D. expansion.

_____ 3. A bullet's profile is the:
   A. diameter of a bullet expressed in hundredths of an inch.
   B. size and shape of a projectile as it contacts a target.
   C. swing or wobble around the axis of a projectile's travel.
   D. path a projectile follows.

_____ 4. Which of the following is TRUE regarding bullets?
   A. Handgun bullets generally deform significantly upon impact with soft tissue.
   B. Most military ammunition seldom deforms solely with soft-tissue collision.
   C. Some bullets are designed to mushroom on impact, decreasing their profile and energy exchange rate.
   D. Some firearm projectiles fragment, which decreases their profile and damage potential.

_____ 5. Knives and arrows are objects that:
   A. cause low-energy/low-velocity wounds.
   B. are considered medium-velocity projectiles.
   C. produce pressure shock waves and cavitation just as bullets do.
   D. generally cause little internal damage.

_____ 6. One of the three factors associated with the results inflicted by the damage pathway of a projectile wound is:
   A. indirect injury.
   B. secondary impact.
   C. creation of a temporary cavity.
   D. fragmentation.

_____ 7. The damage done as a projectile strikes tissue, contuses and tears that tissue, and pushes the tissue out of its way is called:
   A. the pressure shock wave.
   B. direct injury.
   C. cavitation.
   D. zone of injury.

_____ 8. Tissue cells in front of bullets are pushed forward and to the side. They, in turn, push adjacent cells forward and outward. This is known as:
   A. the pressure shock wave.
   B. direct injury.
   C. cavitation.
   D. zone of injury.

_____ 9. Damage caused by low-velocity objects:
   A. can create a pressure shock wave.
   B. is usually limited to the object's path of travel.
   C. may include creation of an exit wound with a "blown-out" appearance.
   D. is usually very obvious by the size of the entrance wound.

HANDOUT 18-2 Continued

_____ 10. The extent of damage that a penetrating projectile causes varies with the particular type of tissue it encounters. One important point to remember about tissues in relation to penetrating wounds is that:
   A. solid organs have the resiliency of muscle and other connective tissues.
   B. muscles, the skin, and other connective tissues are thin, delicate tissues.
   C. when muscle tissue is penetrated, the wound track closes and serious injury is limited.
   D. penetrating injury to lung tissue is generally less extensive than can be expected with any other body tissue.

_____ 11. Hollow organs are muscular containers holding fluid. When considering a penetrating injury to a hollow organ, remember that:
   A. if the container is filled with fluid at the time of impact, the energy can tear the organ apart explosively.
   B. if the container is filled with fluid at the time of impact, the energy is dispersed in the fluid, and little damage is done to the organ.
   C. a penetrating wound to the heart may result in pericardial tamponade, which results in a sudden release of blood into the thorax.
   D. if a hollow organ holds air, the air compresses with the passage of the pressure, resulting in explosive tissue damage and hemorrhage.

_____ 12. When caring for a patient with a penetrating injury to the abdomen, keep in mind that:
   A. the area is well protected by skeletal structures.
   B. the passage of a projectile through the abdominal cavity produces little cavitational wave.
   C. the bowel is very tolerant of compression and stretching.
   D. if the small or large bowel is perforated by a penetrating injury, serious peritoneal irritation may result, with signs and symptoms developing almost immediately.

_____ 13. The appearance of the entrance wound caused by a bullet:
   A. is usually the size of the bullet's profile.
   B. will often have a "blown-out" look.
   C. may indicate signs of subcutaneous emphysema if the shot was fired at very close range.
   D. may accurately reflect the potential for damage caused by the bullet's passage.

_____ 14. When arriving at the scene of a shooting or stabbing, your first priority is:
   A. the patient's airway.
   B. your safety.
   C. removing any weapons from the patient's reach.
   D. the preservation of evidence.

_____ 15. Your patient has been shot in the chest with a handgun. Care would include all of the following EXCEPT:
   A. high-flow, high-concentration oxygen by nonrebreather mask.
   B. sealing the wound with an occlusive dressing secured on all four sides.
   C. consideration of needle decompression for tension pneumothorax.
   D. preparation for endotracheal intubation if breathing becomes inadequate.

EVALUATION

HANDOUT 18-3

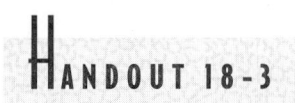

Student's Name _____

CHAPTER 18 SCENARIO

Review the following real-life situation. Then answer the questions that follow.

The emergency medical dispatch center sends Medic 7 to the Wilson High School parking lot. As the unit arrives, a police officer directs the paramedics to a far corner of the lot where, she tells them, a student has just been stabbed. As paramedics approach, they see a young male lying prone on the asphalt near a pickup truck. He yells, "I know who did this, and I'm going to get him!" There is blood seeping through the patient's shirt. The paramedics notice the blood is coming from the patient's left posterior chest. The paramedics cut away the patient's shirt and see a small round wound near the spine at approximately T-4.

1. At this point in the scenario, what is a question the paramedics should ask to determine the mechanism of injury?

Next, the paramedics place the patient on a long backboard. They decide to provide care en route to the hospital. While en route, the patient tells the paramedics he was stabbed with an ice pick.

2. Was this a high-velocity or low-velocity wound?

3. If the ice pick were still in the patient's back, should the paramedics remove it? Why or why not?

4. If the patient's injury had been caused by a bullet, what sort of signs might the paramedics have seen near the site of the wound?

5. Was the paramedics' decision to transport the patient rather than provide field treatment the correct choice?

6. What types of injuries might the patient have sustained?

EVALUATION

HANDOUT 18-4

Student's Name _____

CHAPTER 18 REVIEW

Write the word or words that best complete the following sentences in the space provided.

1. Wounds from _____ bullets are from two to four times more lethal than wounds from _____ bullets.
2. _____ is the study of projectile motion and its interactions with the gun, the air, and the object it contacts.
3. The path a projectile follows is its _____.
4. _____ is the forces acting on a projectile in motion to slow its progress.
5. Factors affecting energy exchange between a projectile and body tissue are _____, _____, _____, expansion and _____, _____ impacts, and _____.
6. The formation of a partial vacuum and subsequent cavity within a semifluid medium is called _____.
7. The size and shape of a projectile as it contacts a target is called its _____.
8. The _____ of a bullet is its diameter expressed in hundredths of an inch.
9. _____ is the swing or wobble around the axis of a projectile's travel.
10. The location of a bullet's center of mass affects its _____.
11. Some bullets are designed to mushroom on impact, thus increasing their _____, _____ exchange rate, and _____ potential.
12. The handgun is a(n) _____ velocity weapon, while the rifle is a(n) _____ velocity weapon.
13. The damage pathway that a high-velocity projectile inflicts results from three specific factors: _____ injury, the _____ _____ wave, and _____.
14. The connective strength and elasticity of an object or material is called its _____.
15. _____ organs have the density but not the resiliency of muscle.
16. The filling of the pericardial sac with fluid is called pericardial _____.
17. The _____ is the largest body cavity and contains most of the internal organs.
18. Monitor the _____ closely of any patient with a penetrating wound to the neck.
19. A(n) _____ wound may more accurately reflect the potential damage caused by a bullet's pathway through the body than a(n) _____ wound.
20. If a call involves a knifing injury, attempt to determine the _____ and approximate _____ of the attacker and the _____ of the blade.
21. _____ is the surgical incision to provide an emergency airway.
22. _____ is the introduction of a needle to provide an emergency airway.
23. The anticipated outcome of a disease or injury is the _____.
24. Seal open chest wounds with a(n) _____ dressing.
25. Unless the impaled object is in the cheek and interfering with the patient's airway, you should _____ impaled objects in place.

REINFORCEMENT

©2007 Pearson Education, Inc.
Essentials of Paramedic Care, 2nd ed.

Handout 18-5

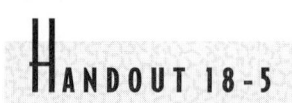

Student's Name _____

PENETRATING TRAUMA TRUE OR FALSE

Indicate whether the following statements are true or false by writing T or F in the space provided.

_____ 1. Wounds from handguns are just as lethal as those from rifles.

_____ 2. Bullets follow a curved path once fired from a gun.

_____ 3. To prevent tumbling, bullets are sent spinning through the air by the gun barrel's rifling.

_____ 4. When bullets mushroom, their profile, energy exchange rate, and damage potential increase.

_____ 5. Handguns and rifles are considered medium-velocity weapons.

_____ 6. The damage caused by high-energy bullets rarely extends beyond the actual track of the projectile.

_____ 7. Low-velocity projectiles do not produce either a pressure shock wave or cavitation.

_____ 8. The pressure shock wave is the damage done as the projectile strikes tissue, contuses and tears that tissue, and pushes the tissue out of its way.

_____ 9. Damage caused by low-velocity wounds is limited to the object's path of travel.

_____ 10. Muscles, the skin, and other connective tissues are dense, elastic, and very well held together.

_____ 11. Solid organs have the same density and resiliency as muscle.

_____ 12. If a high-velocity bullet impacts the heart immediately after a cardiac contraction, rupture and exsanguination may occur.

_____ 13. Penetrating injury to lung tissue is generally less extensive than can be expected with any other body tissue.

_____ 14. The passage of a projectile through the abdominal cavity does not produce a significant cavitational wave.

_____ 15. Impaled objects in the chest should be removed and an occlusive dressing applied.

_____ 16. Entrance wounds will often have a "blown-out" appearance.

_____ 17. If you arrive at the scene of a shooting or stabbing before law enforcement, make every effort to secure the scene.

_____ 18. The presence of frothy blood from a gunshot wound to the chest may indicate a developing tension pneumothorax.

_____ 19. Seal open chest wounds with a moist, sterile dressing.

_____ 20. An impaled object may obstruct blood vessels, thereby restricting blood loss.

Chapter 18 Answer Key

Handout 18-2: Chapter 18 Quiz

1. A
2. C
3. B
4. C
5. A
6. C
7. B
8. A
9. B
10. D
11. A
12. C
13. C
14. B
15. B

Handout 18-3: Chapter 18 Scenario

1. "What caused the wound?"
2. Low-velocity.
3. Except in the case of an object lodged in a cheek, impaled objects should not be removed since removal may cause further injury.
4. Residue from the blast, powder burns (tattooing), abrasions from muzzle exhaust.
5. Yes. Penetrating wounds either anterior or posterior have a high mortality rate. Remember the Golden Hour.
6. Possibilities include spinal cord injury, pulmonary contusion, pneumothorax, pericardial tamponade, hemothorax.

Handout 18-4: Chapter 18 Review

1. rifle, handgun
2. Ballistics
3. trajectory
4. Drag
5. velocity, profile, stability, fragmentation, secondary, shape
6. cavitation
7. profile
8. caliber
9. Yaw
10. stability
11. profile, energy, damage
12. medium-, high-
13. direct, pressure shock, cavitation
14. resiliency
15. Solid
16. tamponade
17. abdomen
18. airway
19. exit, entrance
20. gender, weight, length
21. Cricothyrotomy
22. Cricothyrostomy
23. prognosis
24. occlusive
25. stabilize

Handout 18-5: Penetrating Trauma True or False

1. F
2. T
3. T
4. T
5. F
6. T
7. T
8. F
9. T
10. T
11. F
12. F
13. T
14. F
15. F
16. F
17. F
18. T
19. F
20. T

Chapter 19

Hemorrhage and Shock

INTRODUCTION

Acute and continuous loss of blood decreases the ability of the body to provide oxygen and nutrients to, and to remove waste products from, the body's cells. Without adequate perfusion, or circulating oxygenated blood, the cells, organs, and eventually the body itself, die. The transition between the normally functioning body and death is shock. It is vital that the paramedic recognizes hemorrhage and shock, and provides care to the patient in a timely manner. This chapter provides students with an understanding of the cardiovascular system as it relates to hemorrhage and shock, and describes how to recognize and care for the life-threatening symptoms.

TOTAL TEACHING TIME: 18.63 HOURS

The total teaching time is only a guideline based on the didactic and practical lab averages in the National Standard Curriculum. Instructors should take into consideration such factors as the pace at which students learn, the size of the class, and breaks. The actual time devoted to teaching objectives is the responsibility of the instructor.

CHAPTER OBJECTIVES

After reading this chapter, you should be able to:

1. Describe the epidemiology, including the morbidity/mortality and prevention strategies, for shock and hemorrhage. (pp. 829–831, 837–841)
2. Discuss the anatomy, physiology, and pathophysiology of the cardiovascular system. (see Chapters 3 and 4)
3. Define shock based on aerobic and anaerobic metabolism. (see Chapter 4)
4. Describe the body's physiological response to changes in blood volume, blood pressure, and perfusion. (pp. 837–841)
5. Describe the effects of decreased perfusion at the capillary level. (pp. 838–839)
6. Discuss the cellular ischemic, capillary stagnation, and capillary washout phases related to hemorrhagic shock. (pp. 838–839)
7. Discuss the various types and degrees of shock and hemorrhage. (pp. 829–831, 837–841)
8. Predict shock and hemorrhage based on mechanism of injury. (pp. 832, 841–842)
9. Identify the need for intervention and transport of the patient with hemorrhage or shock. (pp. 831–834, 841–843)
10. Discuss the assessment findings and management of internal and external hemorrhage and shock. (pp. 831–834, 841–843)
11. Differentiate between the administration rate and volume of IV fluid in patients with controlled versus uncontrolled hemorrhage. (pp. 844–846)

©2007 Pearson Education, Inc.
Essentials of Paramedic Care, 2nd ed.

12. Relate pulse pressure and orthostatic vital sign changes to perfusion status. (pp. 834, 843)
13. Define and differentiate between compensated and decompensated hemorrhagic shock. (pp. 839–840)
14. Discuss the pathophysiological changes, assessment findings, and management associated with compensated and decompensated shock. (pp. 839–840)
15. Identify the need for intervention and transport of patients with compensated and decompensated shock. (pp. 841–849)
16. Differentiate among normotensive, hypotensive, or profoundly hypotensive patients. (pp. 841–849)
17. Describe differences in administration of intravenous fluid in normotensive, hypotensive, or profoundly hypotensive patients. (pp. 844–846)
18. Discuss the physiologic changes associated with application and inflation of the pneumatic antishock garment (PASG). (pp. 846–847)
19. Discuss the indications and contraindications for the application and inflation of the PASG. (pp. 846–847)
20. Given several preprogrammed and moulaged hemorrhage and shock patients, provide the appropriate scene size-up, initial assessment, rapid trauma or focused physical exam and history, detailed exam, and ongoing assessment and provide appropriate patient care and transportation. (pp. 822–849)

FRAMING THE LESSON

Begin by reviewing the important points of Chapter 18, "Penetrating Trauma." Use this time to answer any questions about the previous chapter and to discuss any items not completely understood by students. Then begin the discussion of Chapter 19.

Review the "Golden Hour" concept from previous chapters. Review the signs and symptoms of shock that EMS personnel look for, especially the early signs of increased breathing and pulse and cool, clammy skin. Discuss how these signs are actually the body's response to a decrease in perfusion or compensation for it. Ask students to pick a sign or symptom of shock and then tell the class why it is occurring. You can graphically demonstrate how increased cardiac output from an increased heart rate and stronger contractions compensate for a decrease in fluid (blood) by filling a balloon with water. Place a tiny pinhole in the balloon so the water streams out. Note that as the amount of water decreases, the stream is shortened and not as strong. But by squeezing the balloon (increasing the cardiac output), you can keep the water stream at the same strength (compensated shock). But when the amount of water in the balloon is significantly decreased, increasing the pressure no longer works. This demonstrates decompensated shock.

Stress that without adequate blood pressure, oxygen-carrying red blood cells do not enter the tiny capillaries. Cells are not only deprived of oxygen and nutrients, but also cannot give off carbon dioxide and waste products, thereby becoming toxic. Remind students that this is the reason tourniquets are no longer advised, as they cut off all blood and oxygen flow to cells.

TEACHING STRATEGIES

People learn in a variety of ways. Some do better with the spoken word, whereas others prefer the written. Some prefer to work alone, whereas others profit from working in groups. Recognizing these different ways of acquiring knowledge, the authors of this *Instructor's Resource Manual* have provided a variety of teaching strategies for the different types of learners. These strategies are intended to foster higher-level cognitive skills and encourage creative learning and problem solving. For greatest effectiveness, incorporate these strategies into your class lecture. Symbols in the Lecture Outline indicate the points at which various exercises might be most appropriate. Other strategies can be used to preview the lesson or to summarize it.

The following strategies are keyed to specific sections of the lesson.

1. Angiogram Video. To view the entire circulatory system, arrange for a video of an angiogram. Using today's technology, students will be allowed to view the "inside" of the body. Vessel sizes, spasms, decreased circulation, and other findings will be obvious on the tape. Contact your hospital's radiology or nuclear medicine department for this request. Requesting a tape, rather than taking a field trip to the hospital for this lesson, will ensure you have a means to demonstrate the flow of blood in a human to subsequent classes.

2. Estimating Blood Loss. Practice estimating blood loss by placing pools of simulated blood in and on different surfaces. Be sure to measure it out beforehand so that you know exactly how much blood exists in your experiments. Put the same amount on the carpet and tile and they will likely look different. Blood mixed with water tends to look grossly more than it is. Place the same amount in the sink and the toilet bowl. Estimating blood loss accurately helps the paramedic anticipate shock in the patient who is hemorrhaging. Additionally, it aids the hospital in their assessment since the paramedic functions as the hospital staff's "eyes and ears" on scene.

3. Arterial Blood Pumping Simulation. You can simulate the pumping action of arterial blood by using an IV bag full of simulated blood, blood pump tubing, and a pressure infuser. Run the tubing through the "patient's" pant leg or sleeve, placing the ball of the infuser under their buttocks so that a slight rocking motion will produce the desired spurt of blood. When the paramedic has successfully attended to the bleeding, the patient can simply release pressure on the bag, which will stop the flow. The sight of blood is distracting for many students. Being able to practice hemorrhage management with the sight, feel, and mess of blood will put your students at a distinct advantage on their first major bleeding call.

4. Six-Pack Blood Loss Simulation. A six-pack can help you illustrate the effect of major bleeding on your patient. This lesson will stick with your students, but is messy, so be prepared! Start with a full six-pack of soda. As you discuss the effects on the patient after each liter of blood loss, spray or dump out a can of soda, reducing your six-pack by one can as you go. Students will soon realize that unless they intervene with IV fluid and eventually blood at the hospital, the fluid is forever lost.

The following strategies can be used at various points throughout the lesson or to help summarize and demonstrate what students have learned.

Calculating IV Flow Rates. Paramedics will need to decide IV flow rates for patients depending on their condition. While a wide-open rate is appropriate for a patient showing the signs of shock or the patient whose condition is deteriorating, patients with stable vital signs will not require such large amounts of fluid. Calculating drip rates for IVs is an important skill for paramedics. Give students an extra opportunity to practice this skill.

Start by noting that there are three pieces of information needed to correctly calculate an IV drip rate. They are (1) the desired amount of fluid to be given,

(2) the conversion factor of the IV drip to be used, and (3) the time over which the fluid is to be administered. To determine the flow rate, multiply the desired dose of fluid to be given by the conversion value of the administration set and divide the result by the time over which the dose is to be administered. The equation is as follows:

$$\frac{\text{Volume of Fluid to Be Given} \times \text{IV Drip Set Conversion Factor}}{\text{Time}}$$

Amounts of fluid should be expressed in the same unit of measure. IV infusion rates are calculated in drops (gtt) per volume of fluid to be given per minute. The length of time over which the desired dose is to be administered should be converted to minutes.

Illustrate by showing how to calculate the drip rate for an IV to administer 300 mL over 2 hours, using a macrodrip set (10 gtt/mL).

$$\frac{300 \text{ mL} \times 10 \text{ gtt/mL}}{2 \text{ hr}}$$

Convert the hours to minutes.

$$\frac{300 \text{ mL} \times 10 \text{ gtt/mL}}{120 \text{ min}}$$

Cancel out the label mL, and multiply the 300 by the 10, then divide by 120.

$$\frac{300 \times 10}{120} = \frac{3000}{120} = 25 \text{ gtt/min}$$

Have each student make up a calculation problem. Collect these problems and return them to other students in the class for practice.

Guest Speakers: Local Paramedics and Physicians. Invite local paramedics and physicians to present some cases from their own experience demonstrating the signs and symptoms of shock and the dramatic effects that untreated shock can produce on the body. Especially stress the cases in which the Golden Hour was apparent.

Cultural Considerations, Legal Notes, and Patho Pearls. The Student CD-ROM contains this series of informative features to enhance the student's understanding of the material covered in this chapter.

TEACHING OUTLINE

Chapter 19, "Hemorrhage and Shock," is the fourth lesson in Division 3, *Trauma Emergencies*. Distribute Handout 19-1 so that students can familiarize themselves with the learning goals for this chapter. If students have any questions about the objectives, answer them at this time.

Then present the chapter. One possible lecture outline follows. In the outline, the parenthetical references in regular type are references to text pages; those in bold type are references to figures, tables, or procedures.

I. Introduction. This lesson is on hemorrhage and shock. Hemorrhage is the loss of the body's most important medium, blood. Shock, or decreased perfusion to the body's cells, is the transition between normal function and death. Signs and symptoms we see in patients "going into shock" are actually the body's compensatory mechanisms to maintain perfusion to the body's cells and organs. This chapter will provide an understanding of the cardiovascular

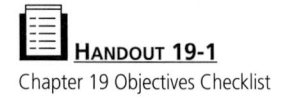

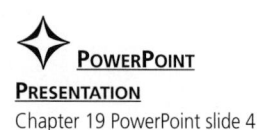

HANDOUT 19-1
Chapter 19 Objectives Checklist

POWERPOINT PRESENTATION
Chapter 19 PowerPoint slide 4

system, hemorrhage, shock, and the treatment and care of patients with this life-threatening condition. (p. 822)

II. Hemorrhage (pp. 822–837)

A. Hemorrhage classification (pp. 822–823)
   1. Capillary
   2. Venous
   3. Arterial
B. Clotting (pp. 823–824) (**Fig. 19-1, p. 823; Fig. 19-2, p. 824**)
   1. Vascular phase
   2. Platelet phase
   3. Coagulation
C. Factors affecting the clotting process (p. 825)
   1. Movement of the wound site
   2. Aggressive fluid therapy
   3. Body temperature
   4. Medications such as aspirin, ibuprofen, and other NSAIDs; heparin; and Coumadin
D. Hemorrhage control (pp. 825–829)
   1. External hemorrhage
      a. Direct pressure (**Figs. 19-3a through 19-3d, p. 826**)
      b. Elevation
      c. Pressure points
      d. Tourniquet as a last resort (**Fig. 19-4, p. 827**)
   2. Internal hemorrhage
      a. Fascia
      b. Hematoma
      c. Epistaxis (**Figs. 19-5a and 19-5b, p. 828**)
      d. Hemoptysis
      e. Esophageal varices
      f. Melena
      g. Anemia
E. Stages of hemorrhage (pp. 829–831) (**Table 19-1, p. 829**)
   1. Stage 1
      a. Blood loss to 15 percent
      b. Nervousness
      c. Marginally cool skin
      d. Slight pallor
   2. Stage 2
      a. Blood loss 15–25 percent
      b. Thirst
      c. Anxiety, restlessness
      d. Cool, clammy skin
   3. Stage 3
      a. Blood loss 25–35 percent
      b. Hunger
      c. Dyspnea
      d. Severe thirst
      e. Anxiety, restlessness
      f. Survival unlikely without rapid intervention
   4. Stage 4
      a. Blood loss greater than 35 percent
      b. Pulse barely palpable
      c. Respirations ineffective
      d. Lethargy
      e. Confused

POWERPOINT PRESENTATION
Chapter 19 PowerPoint slides 5–117

TEACHING STRATEGY 1
Angiogram Video

TEACHING STRATEGY 2
Estimating Blood Loss

TEACHING STRATEGY 3
Arterial Blood Pumping Simulation

TEACHING STRATEGY 4
Six-Pack Blood Loss Simulation

    f. Moving toward unresponsiveness
    g. Survival unlikely
  5. Special cases
    a. Pregnant women
    b. Athletes
    c. Obese patients
    d. Infants and children
      i. Suspect hemorrhage early and treat aggressively.
    e. Elderly
F. Hemorrhage assessment (pp. 831–834) (**Fig. 19-6, p. 832**)
 1. Scene size-up
 2. Initial assessment
 3. Focused history and physical exam
   a. Rapid trauma assessment
   b. Focused physical exam
   c. Additional assessment considerations
     i. Hematochezia
     ii. Orthostatic hypotension
     iii. Tilt test
 4. Injuries that can cause significant blood loss
   a. Fractured pelvis (2,000 mL)
   b. Fractured femur (1,500 mL)
   c. Fractured tibia (750 mL)
   d. Fractured humerus (750 mL)
   e. Large contusion (500 mL)
 5. Early signs and symptoms of internal hemorrhage
   a. Pain, tenderness, swelling, or discoloration of injury site
   b. Bleeding from mouth, rectum, vagina, or other orifice
   c. Vomiting of bright red blood or blood the color of coffee grounds
   d. Tender, rigid, or distended abdomen
 6. Late signs and symptoms of internal hemorrhage
   a. Anxiety, restlessness, or combativeness
   b. Altered mental status
   c. Weakness, faintness, dizziness
   d. Thirst
   e. Shallow, rapid breathing
   f. Rapid, weak pulse
   g. Pale, cool, clammy skin
   h. Capillary refill greater than 2 seconds
     i. Most reliable in infants and children under 6 years of age
   i. Dropping blood pressure
   j. Dilated pupils, sluggishness in responding to light
   k. Nausea and vomiting
 7. Ongoing assessment
G. Hemorrhage management (pp. 834–837)
 1. During initial assessment, care for serious hemorrhage only after airway and breathing problems are corrected.
 2. Direct pressure (**Fig. 19-7, p. 835**)
 3. PASG and fluid therapy; do not delay transport
 4. Pressure dressing
 5. Elevation
 6. Arterial pulse pressure point (**Fig. 19-8, p. 836**)
 7. Splinting and pneumatic splints
 8. Tourniquet as a last resort only (BP cuff)
 9. Specific wound considerations
   a. Head wounds
     i. Do not attempt to stop blood or fluid flow from nose or ears.

POINT TO EMPHASIZE

Inflating the abdominal section of the PASG may cause up to 50 percent reduction in diaphragm movement; watch closely for signs of respiratory distress.

POINT TO EMPHASIZE

There are more complications from IVs started in the field than from those started in the hospital. Pay attention to aseptic technique.

      b. Neck wounds
          i. Occlusive dressing
      c. Large, gaping wounds
      d. Crush injuries
  10. Transport considerations (p. 837)

III. Shock (pp. 837–849)

A. A state of inadequate tissue perfusion (pp. 837–838)
B. The body's response to blood loss (pp. 838–839)
  1. Cellular ischemia
  2. Capillary microcirculation
    a. Hydrostatic pressure
    b. Rouleaux
  3. Capillary washout
C. Stages of shock (pp. 839–841) (**Table 19-2, p. 840**)
  1. Compensated shock (**Fig. 19-9, p. 840**)
    a. Increased pulse rate
    b. Decreased pulse strength
    c. Cool, clammy skin
    d. Progressing anxiety, restlessness, combativeness
    e. Thirst, weakness, eventual air hunger
  2. Decompensated shock
    a. Pulse becomes unpalpable
    b. Blood pressure drops precipitously
    c. Patient becomes unconscious
    d. Respirations slow or cease
  3. Irreversible shock
    a. Irreversible cell damage
    b. Cell death
    c. Tissue dysfunction
    d. Organ dysfunction
    e. Patient dies
D. Shock assessment (pp. 841–843) (**Fig. 19-10, p. 842**)
  1. Scene size-up
  2. Initial assessment
  3. Focused history and physical exam
    a. Rapid trauma assessment
  4. Detailed physical exam
  5. Ongoing assessment
E. Shock management (pp. 843–849) (**Fig. 19-11, p. 844**)
  1. Airway and breathing management
    a. Overdrive respirations
    b. Positive end-expiratory pressure (PEEP)
    c. Continuous positive airway pressure (CPAP)
    d. Capnography
  2. Hemorrhage control
  3. Fluid resuscitation (**Fig. 19-13, p. 845**)
    a. Fluid
      i. Polyhemoglobins
      ii. 20 mL/kg infusion in children
    b. Catheter size (**Fig. 19-12, p. 845**)
  4. Temperature control
  5. Pneumatic antishock garment (**Proc. 19-1, p. 848**)
  6. Pharmacological intervention (**Fig. 19-14, p. 849**)

POWERPOINT PRESENTATION
Chapter 19 PowerPoint slides 118–124

POINT OF INTEREST
Shock has been described as "a momentary pause in the act of death."

TEACHING TIP
When discussing perfusion, compare the circulatory system to a closed plumbing system: a pump, pipes, and fluid. If there are any problems with the system, such as a problem with the pump, or a leak in the pipes, the pressure in the system drops.

READING/REFERENCE
Phrampus, P. "Concepts in Shock." *JEMS*, March 2004.

SLIDES/VIDEOS
"Shock Syndrome," *24-7 EMS*, Summer 2004.

READING/REFERENCE
Criss, E. "Comparison of Isotonic and Hypertonic Saline." *JEMS*, Nov. 2003.

Criss, E. "Fluid Resuscitation I—Blunt Trauma Victim." *JEMS* Jan. 2003.

PowerPoint Presentation
Chapter 19 PowerPoint slide 125

Advanced Life Support Skills
Larmon & Davis. *Advanced Life Support Skills.*

Advanced Life Skills Review
Larmon & Davis. *Advanced Life Skills Review.*

Brady Skills Series: ALS
Larmon & Davis. *Brady Skills Series: ALS.*

IV. Chapter summary (p. 849). Significant hemorrhage and its serious consequence, shock, are genuine threats to the trauma patient's life. The signs of these threats are often subtle or hidden, especially if bleeding is internal. Only through careful analysis of the mechanism of injury during the scene size-up and careful evaluation of the patient during the assessment process can you recognize and then treat these life-threatening problems. Treatment often involves rapidly bringing the patient to the services of a trauma center and, while doing so, providing aggressive care—supplemental oxygen, positive pressure ventilations, fluid resuscitation, and use of a PASG as necessary—aimed at maintaining vital signs, not necessarily improving them. With this approach, you afford your patient the best chance for survival.

SKILLS DEMONSTRATION AND PRACTICE

Students can practice skills discussed in this chapter in the following settings:

Skills Lab: Divide the class into as many groups as appropriate. Have the groups circulate through the stations. Monitor the groups to be sure all groups have a chance to practice each of the skills. You may wish to have other instructors or qualified paramedics assist students in these activities.

Station	Equipment Needed	Activities
Hemorrhage Control	Dressings and bandages 1 instructor	Have students practice hemorrhage control by direct pressure and pulse pressure points.
Pneumatic Antishock Garment	Full-body mannequin PASG 1 instructor	Have students practice applying the PASG.
Peripheral IV Insertion	IV administration kits IV trainer 1 instructor	Have students practice starting peripheral IVs on the IV arm.

Scenario Lab: Divide the class into teams. Have the teams circulate through the stations. Monitor the groups to be sure all groups have a chance to manage each of the cases and so that every student has the opportunity to be team leader. You may wish to have other instructors or qualified paramedics assist students in these activities.

Station	Equipment Needed	Activities
Hypovolemic Shock	Long spine board C-spinal immobilization device Airway management kit Trauma bag IV administration kit 1 victim 1 instructor	Have students practice assessing and managing patients in hypovolemic shock.
Distributive Shock	Long spine board C-spinal immobilization device Airway management kit Trauma bag	Have students practice assessing and managing patients in distributive shock.

	IV administration kit 1 victim 1 instructor	
Neurogenic Shock	Long spine board C-spinal immobilization device Airway management kit Trauma bag IV administration kit 1 victim 1 instructor	Have students practice assessing and managing patients in neurogenic shock.

Hospital:

- Practice IV therapy rotation.
- Practice IVs in the ED.
- Draw venous blood samples in the ED.

ASSIGNMENTS

Assign students to complete Chapter 19, "Hemorrhage and Shock," of the workbook. Also assign them to read Chapter 20, "Soft-Tissue Trauma," before the next class.

EVALUATION

Chapter Quiz and Scenario   Distribute copies of the Chapter Quiz provided in Handout 19-2 to evaluate student understanding of this chapter. Make sure each student reads the scenario to reinforce critical thinking on the scene. Remind students not to use their notes or textbooks while taking the quiz.

Student CD   Quizzes for every chapter are contained on the dynamic and highly visual in-text student CD.

Companion Website   Additional quizzes for every chapter are contained on this exciting website.

TestGen   You may wish to create a custom-tailored test using *Prentice Hall TestGen for Essentials of Paramedic Care*, 2nd Edition to evaluate student understanding of this chapter.

On-line Test Preparation (for students and instructors)   Additional test preparation is available through Brady's new on-line product, *EMT Achieve: Paramedic Test Preparation* at *http://www.prenhall.com/emtachieve/*. Instructors can also monitor student mastery on-line.

Review Manual for the EMT-Paramedic   This comprehensive exam review contains hundreds of test questions and rationales, including scenarios, along with two 180-question practice tests on CD.

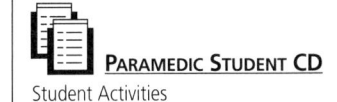

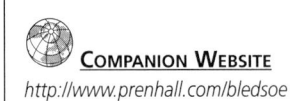

WORKBOOK
Chapter 19 Activities

READING/REFERENCE
Textbook, pp. 852–890

HANDOUT 19-2
Chapter 19 Quiz

HANDOUT 19-3
Chapter 19 Scenario

PARAMEDIC STUDENT CD
Student Activities

COMPANION WEBSITE
http://www.prenhall.com/bledsoe

TESTGEN
Chapter 19

EMT ACHIEVE:
PARAMEDIC TEST PREPARATION
Mistovich & Beasley. *EMT Achieve: Paramedic Test Preparation.*
www.prenhall.com/emtachieve/

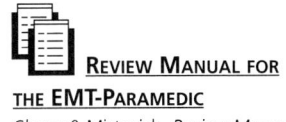

REVIEW MANUAL FOR the EMT-PARAMEDIC
Cherry & Mistovich. *Review Manual for the EMT-Paramedic,* 3rd edition.

Sidebar

HANDOUTS 19-4 AND 19-5
Reinforcement Activities

PARAMEDIC STUDENT CD
Student Activities

POWERPOINT PRESENTATION
Chapter 19

COMPANION WEBSITE
http://www.prenhall.com/bledsoe

ONEKEY
Chapter 19

ADVANCED LIFE SUPPORT SKILLS
Larmon & Davis. *Advanced Life Support Skills.*

ADVANCED LIFE SKILLS REVIEW
Larmon & Davis. *Advanced Life Skills Review.*

BRADY SKILLS SERIES: ALS
Larmon & Davis. *Brady Skills Series: ALS.*

PARAMEDIC NATIONAL STANDARDS SELF-TEST
Miller. *Paramedic National Standards Self-Test,* 4th edition.

REINFORCEMENT

Handouts If classroom discussion or performance on the quiz indicates that some students have not fully mastered the chapter content, you may wish to assign some or all of the Reinforcement Handouts for this chapter.

Student CD (for students)   A wide variety of material on this CD-ROM will reinforce and also expand student knowledge and skills.

PowerPoint Presentation (for instructors)   The PowerPoint material developed for this chapter offers useful reinforcement of chapter content.

Companion Website (for students)   Additional review quizzes and links to EMS resources will contribute to further reinforcement of the chapter.

OneKey   On-line support is offered for this course on one of three platforms: CourseCompass, Blackboard, or Web CT. Includes the IRM, PowerPoints, TestGen, and Companion Website for instruction. Ask your local sales representative for more information.

Brady Skills Series: Advanced Life Skills (Video or CD)   Have your students watch the skills come to life on VHS or CD-ROM, or they can purchase the highly visual, full-color text with step-by-step procedures and rationales.

HANDOUT 19-1

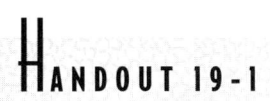

Student's Name _____

CHAPTER 19 OBJECTIVES CHECKLIST

Knowledge	Date Mastered
1. Describe the epidemiology, including the morbidity/mortality and prevention strategies, for shock and hemorrhage.	
2. Discuss the anatomy, physiology, and pathophysiology of the cardiovascular system.	
3. Define shock based on aerobic and anaerobic metabolism.	
4. Describe the body's physiological response to changes in blood volume, blood pressure, and perfusion.	
5. Describe the effects of decreased perfusion at the capillary level.	
6. Discuss the cellular ischemic, capillary stagnation, and capillary washout phases related to hemorrhagic shock.	
7. Discuss the various types and degrees of shock and hemorrhage.	
8. Predict shock and hemorrhage based on mechanism of injury.	
9. Identify the need for intervention and transport of the patient with hemorrhage or shock.	
10. Discuss the assessment findings and management of internal and external hemorrhage and shock.	
11. Differentiate between the administration rate and volume of IV fluid in patients with controlled versus uncontrolled hemorrhage.	
12. Relate pulse pressure and orthostatic vital sign changes to perfusion status.	
13. Define and differentiate between compensated and decompensated hemorrhagic shock.	
14. Discuss the pathophysiological changes, assessment findings, and management associated with compensated and decompensated shock.	
15. Identify the need for intervention and transport of patients with compensated and decompensated shock.	
16. Differentiate among normotensive, hypotensive, or profoundly hypotensive patients.	
17. Describe differences in administration of intravenous fluid in normotensive, hypotensive, or profoundly hypotensive patients.	

HANDOUT 19-1 Continued

Knowledge	Date Mastered
18. Discuss the physiologic changes associated with application and inflation of the pneumatic antishock garment (PASG).	
19. Discuss the indications and contraindications for the application and inflation of the PASG.	
20. Given several preprogrammed and moulaged hemorrhage and shock patients, provide the appropriate scene size-up, initial assessment, rapid trauma or focused physical exam and history, detailed exam, and ongoing assessment and provide appropriate patient care and transportation.	

OBJECTIVES

HANDOUT 19-2

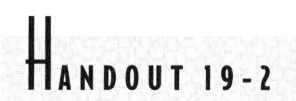

Student's Name _____

CHAPTER 19 QUIZ

Write the letter of the best answer in the space provided.

_____ 1. Venous bleeding is usually:
   A. bright red and spurting in nature.
   B. dark red and flowing.
   C. oozing and quick-clotting.
   D. dark red, forming droplets on the skin.

_____ 2. The step in the clotting process in which the smooth blood vessel muscle contracts, reducing the vessel lumen, is called the:
   A. platelet phase.
   B. vascular phase.
   C. coagulation phase.
   D. aggregate phase.

_____ 3. The network that forms around a wound to stop the bleeding, ward off infection, and lay a foundation for healing and repair of the wound is made up of:
   A. platelets.
   B. hemoglobin.
   C. fibrin.
   D. plasma.

_____ 4. One of the factors that can hinder the clotting process is:
   A. immobilization.
   B. dehydration.
   C. fever.
   D. medications such as aspirin.

_____ 5. The method most commonly used to control external bleeding is:
   A. a tourniquet.
   B. pulse pressure points.
   C. direct pressure.
   D. elevation.

_____ 6. If a decision is made to use a tourniquet to stop external hemorrhage, an important point to remember is that:
   A. the accumulation of lactic acid, potassium, and anaerobic metabolites can occur with tourniquet use.
   B. the tourniquet should be released every 10 minutes to maintain circulation.
   C. you should use a thin or narrow constricting device to avoid tissue damage.
   D. you should apply the tourniquet properly so that arterial blood flow remains intact.

_____ 7. One of the best early indicators of internal hemorrhage is:
   A. a decrease in blood pressure.
   B. the mechanism of injury.
   C. the patient's capillary refill time.
   D. unconsciousness.

_____ 8. Treatment of epistaxis includes:
   A. tilting the patient's head back.
   B. placement of gauze into the nasal cavity.
   C. pinching the fleshy part of the patient's nostrils together.
   D. any of these

_____ 9. Your patient has lost approximately 20 percent of his total blood volume. He is anxious, restless, and has cool, clammy skin. Which stage of hemorrhage is he in?
   A. Stage 1
   B. Stage 2
   C. Stage 3
   D. Stage 4

_____ 10. During Stage 2 hemorrhage, the patient's pulse pressure will:
   A. remain constant.
   B. be noticeably narrower.
   C. be noticeably wider.
   D. widen briefly, but return to normal.

EVALUATION

©2007 Pearson Education, Inc.
Essentials of Paramedic Care, 2nd ed.

HANDOUT 19-2 Continued

_____ 11. The blood volume of an infant or young child is proportionally:
   A. about 20 percent greater than that of an adult.
   B. about 20 percent less than that of an adult.
   C. about the same as that of an adult.
   D. varies from 10–20 percent less than that of an adult.

_____ 12. One step in the initial assessment of a hemorrhage/shock patient is:
   A. application of individual splints for suspected injuries.
   B. initiation of IV fluid resuscitation.
   C. checking skin color and condition.
   D. obtaining baseline vitals.

_____ 13. If a patient's blood pressure decreases when he is moved from a supine to a sitting position, he is said to have:
   A. postural vitals.
   B. orthostatic hypotension.
   C. supine hypotension.
   D. a negative "tilt test."

_____ 14. If you notice blood or fluid flowing from the nose or ear canal of a head-injured patient, you should:
   A. cover the area with an occlusive dressing.
   B. cover the area with a porous dressing and bandage loosely.
   C. pack the nose or ear canal with a sterile dressing to stop the flow.
   D. use a bulb syringe or other suction device to clean out the nose or ear canal.

_____ 15. Acidosis, due to lack of perfusion, causes relaxation of post-capillary sphincters, releasing lactic acid, carbon dioxide, and columns of coagulated red blood cells into the venous circulation. This is known as:
   A. a rouleaux.
   B. hydrostatic pressure.
   C. capillary washout.
   D. angiotensin flow.

_____ 16. As decompensated shock sets in, one of the signs and symptoms you will see is:
   A. an increase in pulse rate.
   B. a drop in blood pressure.
   C. anxiety and restlessness.
   D. cool, clammy skin.

_____ 17. Cell death and tissue dysfunction occur during which stage of shock?
   A. compensated
   B. decompensated
   C. irreversible
   D. any of these

_____ 18. Entry into decompensated shock is indicated by:
   A. unconsciousness.
   B. thready pulse.
   C. bradypnea.
   D. a precipitous drop in blood pressure.

_____ 19. Hypovolemic shock may be caused by:
   A. severe hemorrhage.
   B. granulating wounds.
   C. protracted vomiting.
   D. any of these

_____ 20. The object of prehospital fluid resuscitation is:
   A. the stabilization of vital signs until the patient reaches the hospital.
   B. the return of normal vital signs.
   C. the increase of glucose in the bloodstream.
   D. electrolyte balance.

_____ 21. Which of the following statements is TRUE regarding the use of the PASG?
   A. Inflation of the PASG returns about 1 liter of blood to the central circulation.
   B. The PASG has been found not to increase peripheral vascular resistance.
   C. Inflation of the PASG reduces venous capacitance by as much as 1 liter.
   D. Inflation of the PASG pressurizes the abdominal cavity and may reduce chest excursion.

HANDOUT 19-2 Continued

_____ 22. Pharmacological intervention in patients in hypovolemic shock:
   A. has not been shown to be effective in the prehospital setting.
   B. should include dopamine along with a fluid challenge.
   C. should occur as soon as IV lines are placed.
   D. should be given through an IV line of normal saline, not lactated Ringer's solution.

_____ 23. When using a blood pressure cuff as a tourniquet, you should place the cuff:
   A. distal to the hemorrhage and inflate to 20–30 mmHg above the systolic BP.
   B. proximal to the hemorrhage and inflate to 20–30 mmHg above the systolic BP.
   C. distal to the hemorrhage and inflate to 30–40 mmHg above the systolic BP.
   D. proximal to the hemorrhage and inflate to 30–40 mmHg above the systolic BP.

_____ 24. An expiratory CO_2 level _____ suggests hypoventilation and the need for faster or deeper ventilations.
   A. below 30 mmHg
   B. below 40 mmHg
   C. above 30 mmHg
   D. above 40 mmHg

_____ 25. Maintain the blood pressure at a steady level once it has dropped below 80 mmHg; however, do not let the pressure drop below _____ nor below _____ for head-injury patient with a GCS of 8 or less.
   A. 50 mmHg; 100 mmHg
   B. 50 mmHg; 90 mmHg
   C. 50 mmHg; 80 mmHg
   D. 80 mmHg; 100mmHg

HANDOUT 19-3

Student's Name _____

CHAPTER 19 SCENARIO

Review the following real-life situation. Then answer the questions that follow.

Late one Thursday night, Medic 6 is returning to quarters after transporting a patient with "chest pains" to the hospital. It has been raining heavily for a little while and the roads are very slick. Wendi, the driver, has slowed and is proceeding cautiously along a twisty stretch of Kuna Road when Mark, her partner, yells, "Slow down!" Up ahead, a stretch of guard rail is missing at a point where the land falls away sharply toward a creek. Wendi turns on the warning flashers and pulls to a stop. Mark gets out and reports that a car has gone off the road.

The vehicle did not get very far. It hit a large oak just a short way beyond the guard rail and is badly damaged. Wendi notifies dispatch, while Mark gathers the gear. After surveying the scene, the crew decides it is safe to approach the car. Once there, they find only one person, a male about 25 years old who appears to have been ejected when the car door flew open on impact. He is unconscious, with difficulty breathing.

Wendi maintains cervical spinal immobilization, while Mark completes the initial assessment. He discovers an airway partially obstructed with blood and teeth. The airway is suctioned and secured. The rest of the initial assessment reveals the following: respirations, 44 and labored; no radial pulse but a carotid pulse rate of 132; capillary refill time of 4 seconds; responsive only to pain; there is a large laceration on the patient's forehead; skin turgor is good, skin is pale, cool, diaphoretic. The patient's weight is estimated to be 175 pounds.

1. What immediate problems should the crew suspect with this patient?

2. What should their next actions be?

Handout 19-4

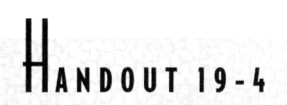

Student's Name _____

CHAPTER 19 REVIEW

Write the word or words that best complete the following sentences in the space provided.

1. Abnormal internal or external discharge of blood is called _____.
2. _____ means inadequate tissue perfusion.
3. The three phases of the clotting process are the _____ phase, the _____ phase, and _____.
4. _____ acid is a byproduct of anaerobic metabolism.
5. Bleeding from the nose is called _____.
6. The difference between the systolic and diastolic blood pressures is the _____ _____.
7. A drop in systolic blood pressure of 20 mmHg or an increase in pulse rate of 20 beats per minute when a patient is moved from a supine to a sitting position is called a positive _____ _____.
8. A decrease in blood pressure that occurs when a person moves from a supine or sitting position to an upright position is called _____ hypotension.
9. _____ _____ controls all but the most persistent hemorrhage.
10. The second stage of metabolism, requiring the presence of oxygen, is called _____ metabolism.
11. The blood flow in the arterioles, capillaries, and venules is called the _____.
12. _____ shock is the stage of shock in which we see increased pulse rate, cool clammy skin, and anxiety and restlessness.
13. Cells die, tissues dysfunction, organs dysfunction, and the patient dies in the _____ stage of shock.
14. _____ _____ solution is the most practical choice for prehospital fluid resuscitation.
15. _____ _____ _____, _____ _____, and _____ _____ are contraindications to PASG application and inflation.

HANDOUT 19-5

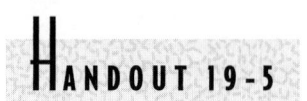

Student's Name _____

SHOCK MATCHING

Write the letter of the term in the space provided next to the appropriate description.

A. decompensated shock
B. platelet phase
C. pulse pressure
D. lactic acid
E. coagulation
F. compensated shock
G. clotting
H. direct pressure
I. anemia
J. fibrin
K. hematochezia
L. epistaxis
M. homeostasis
N. shock
O. vascular phase
P. irreversible shock
Q. orthostatic hypotension
R. rouleaux
S. overdrive respiration
T. hemorrhage

_____ 1. final stage of shock in which organs and cells are so damaged that recovery is impossible.

_____ 2. method of hemorrhage control that relies on the application of pressure to the actual site of the bleeding.

_____ 3. an abnormal internal or external discharge of blood.

_____ 4. passage of stools containing red blood.

_____ 5. continuing hemodynamic insult to the body in which the compensatory mechanisms break down. The signs and symptoms become very pronounced, and the patient moves rapidly toward death.

_____ 6. compound produced from pyruvic acid during anaerobic glycolyis.

_____ 7. a state of inadequate tissue perfusion.

_____ 8. second step in the clotting process in which platelets adhere to blood vessel walls and to each other.

_____ 9. group of red blood cells that are stuck together.

_____ 10. bleeding from the nose resulting from injury, disease, or environmental factors; a nosebleed.

_____ 11. hemodynamic insult to the body in which the body responds effectively. Signs and symptoms are limited, and the human system functions normally.

_____ 12. a decrease in blood pressure that occurs when a person moves from a supine or sitting to an upright position.

_____ 13. the natural tendency of the body to maintain a steady and normal internal environment.

_____ 14. difference between the systolic and diastolic blood pressures.

HANDOUT 19-5 Continued

_____ 15. step in the clotting process in which smooth blood vessel muscle contracts, reducing the vessel lumen and the flow of blood through it.

_____ 16. a reduction in the hemoglobin content in the blood to a point below that required to meet the oxygen requirements of the body.

_____ 17. positive pressure ventilation supplied to a breathing patient.

_____ 18. the third step in the clotting process, which involves the formation of a protein called fibrin that forms a network around a wound to stop bleeding, ward off infection, and lay a foundation for healing and repair of the wound.

_____ 19. the body's three-step response to stop the loss of blood.

_____ 20. protein fibers that trap red blood cells as part of the clotting process.

Chapter 19 Answer Key

Handout 19-2: Chapter 19 Quiz

1. B	8. C	15. C	22. A
2. B	9. B	16. B	23. B
3. C	10. B	17. C	24. D
4. D	11. A	18. D	25. B
5. C	12. C	19. D	
6. A	13. B	20. A	
7. B	14. B	21. D	

Handout 19-3: Chapter 19 Scenario

1. Immediate problems to be dealt with include airway compromise, shock, and cardiorespiratory collapse.
2. The crew should act to maintain ABCs; provide positive-pressure ventilation with 100 percent oxygen; provide full spinal immobilization; and provide rapid transport to a trauma center. En route, they can initiate large-bore IVs with NS or LR run wide open.

Handout 19-4: Chapter 19 Review

1. hemorrhage
2. Shock
3. vascular, platelet, coagulation
4. Lactic
5. epistaxis
6. pulse pressure
7. tilt test
8. orthostatic
9. Direct pressure
10. aerobic
11. microcirculation
12. Compensated
13. irreversible
14. Lactated Ringer's
15. Penetrating chest trauma, pulmonary edema, cardiogenic shock

Handout 19-5: Shock Matching

1. P	6. D	11. F	16. I
2. H	7. N	12. Q	17. S
3. T	8. B	13. M	18. E
4. K	9. R	14. C	19. G
5. A	10. L	15. O	20. J

Chapter 20

Soft-Tissue Trauma

INTRODUCTION

Soft-tissue injuries are among the most common problems encountered by paramedics.

Trauma to the skin and underlying tissues seldom poses a direct life threat, but such injuries may endanger blood vessels, nerves, connective tissue, and other internal structures. This chapter deals with the assessment and management of soft-tissue injuries.

CHAPTER OBJECTIVES

After reading this chapter, you should be able to:

1. Describe the incidence, morbidity, and mortality of soft-tissue injuries. (p. 854)
2. Describe the anatomy and physiology of the integumentary system, including epidermis, dermis, and subcutaneous tissue. (see Chapter 3)
3. Identify the skin tension lines of the body. (pp. 857–858)
4. Predict soft-tissue injuries based on mechanism of injury. (pp. 872–874)
5. Discuss blunt and penetrating trauma. (pp. 854–860)
6. Discuss the pathophysiology of soft-tissue injuries. (pp. 854–860)
7. Differentiate among the following types of soft-tissue injuries:
    - Closed (pp. 855–856)
        - Contusion
        - Hematoma
        - Crush injuries
    - Open (pp. 857–860)
        - Abrasions
        - Lacerations
        - Incisions
        - Avulsions
        - Impaled objects
        - Amputations
        - Punctures

TOTAL TEACHING TIME:
5.26 HOURS
The total teaching time is only a guideline based on the didactic and practical lab averages in the National Standard Curriculum. Instructors should take into consideration such factors as the pace at which students learn, the size of the class, and breaks. The actual time devoted to teaching objectives is the responsibility of the instructor.

8. Discuss the assessment and management of open and closed soft-tissue injuries. (pp. 871–888)
9. Discuss the incidence, morbidity, and mortality of crush injuries. (pp. 856, 884–886)
10. Define the following conditions:
    - Crush injury (pp. 856, 867–868, 884–886)
    - Crush syndrome (pp. 856, 868, 884–886)
    - Compartment syndrome (pp. 866–867, 886)
11. Discuss the mechanisms of injury, assessment findings, and management of crush injuries. (pp. 856, 867–868, 884–886)
12. Discuss the effects of reperfusion and rhabdomyolysis on the body. (pp. 868, 885–886)
13. Discuss the pathophysiology, assessment, and care of hemorrhage associated with soft-tissue injuries, including: (pp. 861, 875–878)
    - Capillary bleeding
    - Venous bleeding
    - Arterial bleeding
14. Describe and identify the indications for and application of the following dressings and bandages: (pp. 869–871)
    - Sterile/nonsterile dressing
    - Occlusive/nonocclusive dressing
    - Adherent/nonadherent dressing
    - Absorbent/nonabsorbent dressing
    - Wet/dry dressing
    - Self-adherent roller bandage
    - Gauze bandage
    - Adhesive bandage
    - Elastic bandage
15. Predict the possible complications of an improperly applied dressing or bandage. (pp. 869–871, 881–882)
16. Discuss the process of wound healing, including:
    - Hemostasis (pp. 862–863)
    - Inflammation (p. 863)
    - Epithelialization (p. 863)
    - Neovascularization (p. 863)
    - Collagen synthesis (p. 864)
17. Discuss the assessment and management of wound healing. (pp. 861–868)
18. Discuss the pathophysiology, assessment, and management of wound infection. (pp. 864–866)
19. Formulate treatment priorities for patients with soft-tissue injuries in conjunction with:
    - Airway/face/neck trauma (pp. 886–887)
    - Thoracic trauma (open/closed) (pp. 887–888)
    - Abdominal trauma (p. 888)
20. Given several preprogrammed and moulaged soft-tissue trauma patients, provide the appropriate scene size-up, initial assessment, rapid trauma or focused physical exam and history, detailed exam, and ongoing assessment and provide appropriate patient care and transportation. (pp. 854–888)

FRAMING THE LESSON

Begin by reviewing the important points of Chapter 19, "Hemorrhage and Shock." Use this time to answer any questions about the previous chapter and to discuss any items not completely understood by students. Then begin the discussion of Chapter 20.

Begin with a review of the anatomy and physiology of the integumentary system. Using models or charts, display the three layers of skin and have students describe each of the three layers and what structures, if any, are contained within them. Briefly discuss what signs and symptoms might be found for various trauma and medical problems when examining the skin. This would include skin color, temperature, and condition. Also, review gross anatomy, highlighting what major organs lie beneath the skin in various portions of the body. Discuss the frequency of soft-tissue injuries by asking students when they received their last soft-tissue injury. Lacerations? Bruises? Ask a paramedic from a local or nearby EMS system to come to class and discuss protocols for soft-tissue injuries, including those for amputations. Have students locate the nearest facility capable of performing the reattachment of amputated parts.

TEACHING STRATEGIES

People learn in a variety of ways. Some do better with the spoken word, whereas others prefer the written. Some prefer to work alone, whereas others profit from working in groups. Recognizing these different ways of acquiring knowledge, the authors of this *Instructor's Resource Manual* have provided a variety of teaching strategies for the different types of learners. These strategies are intended to foster higher-level cognitive skills and encourage creative learning and problem solving. For greatest effectiveness, incorporate these strategies into your class lecture. Symbols in the Lecture Outline indicate the points at which various exercises might be most appropriate. Other strategies can be used to preview the lesson or to summarize it.

The following strategies are keyed to specific sections of the lesson.

1. Playground Safety Program. Rural/Metro Corporation (8401 E. Indian School Road, Scottsdale, AZ 85252; 1-800-421-5718) has designed a playground safety program for paramedics to teach to students, staff, and parents at local elementary schools. The program educates parents on the proper types of equipment and ground surfaces that they should request when playgrounds are being built or remodeled. Involve students in a community education program in your school's neighborhood. In cooperation with your research lecture, you could then track the number of playground injuries reported at the school where your students are involved in safety education. This type of community service project not only reinforces the trauma lesson, but helps to develop your students into productive, respected members of the community.

2. Guest Speaker: Dermatologist. Consider inviting a dermatologist to class to discuss the various layers of skin and care of the skin.

3. Suture Experience. While not within the paramedic scope of practice, students may be interested in learning the basics of suturing. Invite a surgeon to class to demonstrate the skill. Issue gloves and suturing material to students, along with a banana. "Lacerate" the skin of the banana and have students suture the "wound."

4. Brady Trauma Slides: Gaping Wounds. Your Brady Trauma Slides will illustrate gaping wounds. From those graphic illustrations you can discuss skin tension lines. This is a very visual introduction to an otherwise routine discussion.

5. *Brady Trauma Slides: Wound Type ID.* Using your Brady Trauma Slides, show injuries and request students to classify the injury as open or closed. Additionally, students can label the photos as one of the following: amputation, avulsion, crush injury, puncture, abrasion, laceration, incision, and impaled object. It will not matter if your students have seen these photos repeatedly by now. Each time you show the slides you are requesting them to look at or process a different element of the injury.

6. *Show and Tell.* Ask students for volunteers to show the class any sites of scars or previous injuries, describe how they received the injuries, and what treatment was done. Bandaging? Sutures?

7. *Brainstorming Mechanisms of Injury.* Divide students into teams. Each team is charged with making the longest possible list of causes or mechanisms of injury for each injury you name. Use the following injuries: hematoma, amputation, avulsion, crush injury, puncture, abrasion, laceration, and contusion. The team with the longest list for each wins. This activity uses the student's visual mind to create possibilities that may be encountered in the future. It is a right-brain activity. Additionally, it fosters teamwork and healthy competition.

8. *Microsurgical Limb Attachment Video.* The Discovery Channel offers a video on microsurgery and limb reattachment. It is available from its stores and mail order catalog. Use the video to discuss prehospital management of an amputation, as well as to help students understand how their proper management of an extremity could improve the patient's outcome significantly. This video is less than $30 and will appeal to your visual learners.

The following strategies can be used at various points throughout the lesson or to help summarize and demonstrate what students have learned.

Wound Care Grab Bag. Create a wound care grab bag. Put the numerous wound care items in a pillowcase. Have students draw an item out and describe it and its use. If the student is correct, he wins a small prize. If not, the item goes back into the pillowcase. Continue until all items are properly identified.

Guest Speaker: Nurse from Wound Clinic. A nurse from a wound clinic will be able to discuss the process of wound healing with ease and expertise. Invite the nurse to your class for a 45-minute discussion of wound management and wound care. Additionally, you might obtain observation clinical time in the guest's wound care clinic.

Guest Speaker: Orthopedic Surgeon on Amputation. Consider inviting an orthopedic surgeon to class to discuss care of the major trauma patient, including field care of the patient with an amputation. Discuss the field care of the amputated part and, if possible, the reattachment process.

Guest Speaker: Plastic Surgeon. Consider having a plastic surgeon speak to the class on the care of soft-tissue injuries and wounds from his perspective. Slides or photos of major injuries before and after treatment will impress students.

Cultural Considerations, Legal Notes, and Patho Pearls. The student CD-ROM contains this series of informative features to enhance the student's understanding of the material covered in this chapter.

TEACHING OUTLINE

Chapter 20, "Soft-Tissue Trauma," is the fifth lesson in Division 3, *Trauma Emergencies*. Distribute Handout 20-1 so that students can familiarize themselves with the learning goals for this chapter. If students have any questions about the objectives, answer them at this time.

Then present the chapter. One possible lecture outline follows. In the outline, the parenthetical references in regular type are references to text pages; those in bold type are references to figures, tables, or procedures.

I. Introduction. The skin is one of the largest organs of the body, composing 16 percent of total body weight. It protects the body from invading pathogens and contains the body's substances and fluid. It also helps the body regulate temperature. Injuries to the body, such as penetrating and blunt trauma, must pass through the skin first before impacting internal structures. The skin is of great significance at all stages of the patient assessment process, as we examine it for color, temperature, and condition. (p. 854)

A. Epidemiology (p. 854)
B. Most wounds require simple care. (p. 854)
C. Significant injuries include damaged arteries, nerves, and tendons. (p. 854)
D. Uncontrolled hemorrhage (p. 854)
E. Closed wounds, "bumps and bruises" (p. 854)
F. Risk factors include age, alcohol or drug abuse, and occupation. (p. 854)
G. Risk reduction (p. 854)

II. Pathophysiology of soft-tissue injury (pp. 854–869) (**Fig. 20-1, p. 855**)

A. Closed wounds (pp. 855–857)
  1. Contusions (**Fig. 20-2, p. 856**)
  2. Hematomas
  3. Crush injuries (**Fig. 20-3, p. 856**)
B. Open wounds (pp. 857–861)
  1. Abrasions (**Fig. 20-4, p. 857**)
  2. Lacerations (**Fig. 20-5, p. 857; Fig. 20-6, p. 858**)
  3. Incisions
  4. Punctures (**Fig. 20-7, p. 859**)
  5. Impaled objects (**Fig. 20-8, p. 859**)
  6. Avulsions (**Fig. 20-9, p. 860; Fig. 20-10, p. 860**)
  7. Amputations (**Fig. 20-11, p. 861**)
C. Hemorrhage (p. 861) (**Fig. 20-12, p. 861**)
D. Wound healing (pp. 861–864) (**Fig. 20-13, p. 862**)
  1. Hemostasis
  2. Inflammation
  3. Epithelialization
  4. Neovascularization
  5. Collagen synthesis
E. Infection (pp. 864–866)
  1. Infection risk factors
  2. Infection management
    a. Gangrene
    b. Tetanus

HANDOUT 20-1
Chapter 20 Objectives Checklist

TEACHING TIP
Take this opportunity to have a student review the basic circulatory system. Have him/her trace a drop of blood from the aorta to the tip of one finger and back to the vena cava.

POWERPOINT PRESENTATION
Chapter 20 PowerPoint slides 4–11

TEACHING STRATEGY 1
Playground Safety Program

TEACHING STRATEGY 2
Guest Speaker: Dermatologist

TEACHING STRATEGY 3
Suture Experience

POWERPOINT PRESENTATION
Chapter 20 PowerPoint slides 12–23

TEACHING STRATEGY 4
Brady Trauma Slides: Gaping Wounds

POINT TO EMPHASIZE
On average, an adult has about 2.4 square yards of skin, weighing about 9 pounds.

TEACHING STRATEGY 5
Brady Trauma Slides: Wound Type ID

TEACHING STRATEGY 6
Show and Tell

TEACHING STRATEGY 7
Brainstorming Mechanisms of Injury

TEACHING TIP
Bring in some various meat products from the butcher and demonstrate soft-tissue injury patterns, such as contusions, abrasions, lacerations, incisions, punctures, avulsions, and amputations.

TEACHING TIP

Have examples of a number of types of dressing and bandaging supplies available. Moulage various types of soft-tissue injuries on some students and have other students practice applying dressings and bandages. Use scenarios that will require students to apply specific dressings, such as occlusive dressings. Use appropriate parts of "Skills Demonstration and Practice" from Chapter 19.

POWERPOINT PRESENTATION
Chapter 20 PowerPoint slides 24–25

POWERPOINT PRESENTATION
Chapter 20 PowerPoint slide 26

POWERPOINT PRESENTATION
Chapter 20 PowerPoint slides 27–47

F. Other wound complications (pp. 866–867)
  1. Impaired hemostasis
  2. Re-bleeding
  3. Delayed healing
  4. Compartment syndrome (Fig. 20-14, p. 867)
  5. Abnormal scar formation
  6. Pressure injuries
G. Crush injury (pp. 867–868)
  1. Associated injury
  2. Crush syndrome (p. 868)
     a. Necrosis
     b. Rhabdomyolysis
H. Injection injury (pp. 868–869) (Fig. 20-15, p. 869)

III. **Dressing and bandage materials** (pp. 869–871) (Fig. 20-16, p. 869)

A. Types of dressings and bandages (pp. 869–871)
  1. Sterile/nonsterile dressings
  2. Occlusive/nonocclusive dressings
  3. Adherent/nonadherent dressings
  4. Absorbent/nonabsorbent dressings
  5. Wet/dry dressings
  6. Self-adherent roller bandages (Fig. 20-17, p. 870)
  7. Gauze bandages
  8. Adhesive bandages
  9. Elastic (Ace) bandages
  10. Triangular bandages

IV. **Assessment of soft-tissue injuries** (pp. 871–875)

A. Scene size-up (pp. 871–872) (Fig. 20-18, p. 872)
B. Initial assessment (p. 872)
C. Focused history and physical exam (pp. 872–874) (Fig. 20-19, p. 873)
  1. Significant mechanism of injury
     a. Rapid trauma assessment
  2. No significant mechanism of injury
     a. Focused trauma assessment
D. Detailed physical exam (p. 874)
E. Assessment techniques (pp. 874–875)
  1. Inquiry
  2. Inspection
  3. Palpation
F. Ongoing assessment (p. 875)

V. **Management of soft-tissue injury** (pp. 875–888)

A. Objectives of wound dressing and bandaging (pp. 875–879)
  1. Hemorrhage control (Proc. 20-1, p. 876)
     a. Direct pressure
     b. Elevation
     c. Additional dressings as needed
     d. Digital pressure with a gloved hand
     e. Bandage dressing in place
     f. Digital pressure to proximal artery
     g. Tourniquet as last resort (Fig. 20-20, p. 878)
  2. Sterility
  3. Immobilization
  4. Pain and edema control

538 ESSENTIALS OF PARAMEDIC CARE

B. Anatomical considerations for bandaging (pp. 879–881) (**Fig. 20-21, p. 880**)
   1. Scalp
   2. Face
   3. Ear or mastoid
   4. Neck
   5. Shoulder
   6. Trunk (**Fig. 20-22, p. 881**)
   7. Groin and hip
   8. Elbow and knee
   9. Hand and finger
   10. Ankle and foot
C. Complications of bandaging (pp. 881–882)
D. Care of specific wounds (pp. 882–886)
   1. Amputations (**Fig. 20-23, p. 882; Fig. 20-24, p. 883**)
   2. Impaled objects (**Fig. 20-25, p. 883; Fig. 20-26, p. 884**)
   3. Crush syndrome (**Fig. 20-27, p. 885**)
   4. Compartment syndrome
E. Special anatomical sites (pp. 886–888)
   1. Face and neck (**Fig. 20-28, p. 887**)
   2. Thorax
   3. Abdomen
F. Wounds requiring transport (p. 888)
G. Soft-tissue treatment and refer/release (p. 888)

VI. Summary (p. 889). Soft-tissue injury may compromise the skin—the envelope that protects and contains the human body. Any trauma must penetrate the skin before it can harm the interior organs and threaten life. Any damage to the skin may interfere with its ability to contain water and blood and to prevent damaging agents from entering. For these reasons, the assessment and care of soft-tissue injuries are important parts of prehospital care.

Assess wounds carefully because they may provide the only overt signs of serious internal injury. Realize that discoloration and swelling take time to develop and may not be as apparent in the field as when you present the patient at the emergency department. Look carefully for the early signs of wounds, and use the mechanism of injury to locate potential trauma sites. When caring for soft-tissue injuries, keep in mind the basic goals: controlling hemorrhage, keeping the wound as clean as possible, and immobilizing the injury site.

ASSIGNMENTS

Assign students to complete Chapter 20, "Soft-Tissue Trauma," of the workbook. Also assign them to read Chapter 21, "Burns," before the next class.

EVALUATION

Chapter Quiz and Scenario Distribute copies of the Chapter Quiz provided in Handout 20-2 to evaluate student understanding of this chapter. Make sure each student reads the scenario to reinforce critical thinking on the scene. Remind students not to use their notes or textbooks while taking the quiz.

Student CD Quizzes for every chapter are contained on the dynamic and highly visual in-text student CD.

TEACHING STRATEGY 8
Microsurgical Limb Attachment Video

READING/REFERENCE
Raynovich, W. "Crush Syndrome." *JEMS*, Jan. 2000.

POWERPOINT PRESENTATION
Chapter 20 PowerPoint slide 48

WORKBOOK
Chapter 20 Activities

READING/REFERENCE
Textbook, pp. 891–923

HANDOUT 20-2
Chapter 20 Quiz

HANDOUT 20-3
Chapter 20 Scenario

PARAMEDIC STUDENT CD
Student Activities

COMPANION WEBSITE
http://www.prenhall.com/bledsoe

TestGen
Chapter 20

EMT Achieve: Paramedic Test Preparation
Mistovich & Beasley. *EMT Achieve: Paramedic Test Preparation.* www.prenhall.com/emtachieve/

Review Manual for the EMT-Paramedic
Cherry & Mistovich. *Review Manual for the EMT-Paramedic,* 3rd edition.

Handouts 20-4 and 20-5
Reinforcement Activities

Paramedic Student CD
Student Activities

PowerPoint Presentation
Chapter 20

Companion Website
http://www.prenhall.com/bledsoe

OneKey
Chapter 20

Advanced Life Support Skills
Larmon & Davis. Advanced Life Support Skills.

Advanced Life Skills Review
Larmon & Davis. Advanced Life Skills Review.

Brady Skills Series: ALS
Larmon & Davis. Brady Skills Series: ALS.

Paramedic National Standards Self-Test
Miller. *Paramedic National Standards Self-Test,* 4th edition.

Companion Website   Additional quizzes for every chapter are contained on this exciting website.

TestGen   You may wish to create a custom-tailored test using *Prentice Hall TestGen for Essentials of Paramedic Care,* 2nd Edition to evaluate student understanding of this chapter.

On-line Test Preparation (for students and instructors)   Additional test preparation is available through Brady's new on-line product, *EMT Achieve: Paramedic Test Preparation* at *http://www.prenhall.com/emtachieve/*. Instructors can also monitor student mastery on-line.

Review Manual for the EMT-Paramedic   This comprehensive exam review contains hundreds of test questions and rationales, including scenarios, along with two 180-question practice tests on CD.

REINFORCEMENT

Handouts   If classroom discussion or performance on the quiz indicates that some students have not fully mastered the chapter content, you may wish to assign some or all of the Reinforcement Handouts for this chapter.

Student CD (for students)   A wide variety of material on this CD-ROM will reinforce and also expand student knowledge and skills.

PowerPoint Presentation (for instructors)   The PowerPoint material developed for this chapter offers useful reinforcement of chapter content.

Companion Website (for students)   Additional review quizzes and links to EMS resources will contribute to further reinforcement of the chapter.

OneKey   On-line support is offered for this course on one of three platforms: CourseCompass, Blackboard, or Web CT. Includes the IRM, PowerPoints, TestGen, and Companion Website for instruction. Ask your local sales representative for more information.

Brady Skills Series: Advanced Life Skills (Video or CD)   Have your students watch the skills come to life on VHS or CD-ROM, or they can purchase the highly visual, full-color text with step-by-step procedures with rationales.

HANDOUT 20-1

Student's Name _____

CHAPTER 20 OBJECTIVES CHECKLIST

Knowledge	Date Mastered
1. Describe the incidence, morbidity, and mortality of soft-tissue injuries.	
2. Describe the anatomy and physiology of the integumentary system, including epidermis, dermis, and subcutaneous tissue.	
3. Identify the skin tension lines of the body.	
4. Predict soft-tissue injuries based on mechanism of injury.	
5. Discuss blunt and penetrating trauma.	
6. Discuss the pathophysiology of soft-tissue injuries.	

7. Differentiate among the following types of soft-tissue injuries:
• Closed
  • Contusion
  • Hematoma
  • Crush injuries
• Open
  • Abrasions
  • Lacerations
  • Incisions
  • Avulsions
  • Impaled objects
  • Amputations
  • Punctures	

8. Discuss the assessment and management of open and closed soft-tissue injuries.	
9. Discuss the incidence, morbidity, and mortality of crush injuries.	
10. Define the following conditions: • Crush injury • Crush syndrome • Compartment syndrome	
11. Discuss the mechanisms of injury, assessment findings, and management of crush injuries.	
12. Discuss the effects of reperfusion and rhabdomyolysis on the body.	

OBJECTIVES

HANDOUT 20-1 Continued

Knowledge	Date Mastered
13. Discuss the pathophysiology, assessment, and care of hemorrhage associated with soft-tissue injuries, including: • Capillary bleeding • Venous bleeding • Arterial bleeding	
14. Describe and identify the indications for and application of the following dressings and bandages: • Sterile/nonsterile dressing • Occlusive/nonocclusive dressing • Adherent/nonadherent dressing • Absorbent/nonabsorbent dressing • Wet/dry dressing • Self-adherent roller bandage • Gauze bandage • Adhesive bandage • Elastic bandage	
15. Predict the possible complications of an improperly applied dressing or bandage.	
16. Discuss the process of wound healing, including: • Hemostasis • Inflammation • Epithelialization • Neovascularization • Collagen synthesis	
17. Discuss the assessment and management of wound healing.	
18. Discuss the pathophysiology, assessment, and management of wound infection.	
19. Formulate treatment priorities for patients with soft-tissue injuries in conjunction with: • Airway/face/neck trauma • Thoracic trauma (open/closed) • Abdominal trauma	
20. Given several preprogrammed and moulaged soft-tissue trauma patients, provide the appropriate scene size-up, initial assessment, rapid trauma or focused physical exam and history, detailed exam, and ongoing assessment and provide appropriate patient care and transportation.	

OBJECTIVES

Handout 20-2

Student's Name _____

CHAPTER 20 QUIZ

Write the letter of the best answer in the space provided.

_____ 1. The skin, as one of the largest organs of the body, comprises what percentage of total body weight?
   A. 5 percent
   B. 9 percent
   C. 16 percent
   D. 21 percent

_____ 2. The skin is known collectively as the:
   A. integumentary system.
   B. inanition system.
   C. indagation system.
   D. inductotherm system.

_____ 3. Which of the following is TRUE regarding soft-tissue injuries?
   A. Soft-tissue injuries are one of the least common types of trauma.
   B. Most open wounds require only simple care and limited suturing.
   C. The majority of soft-tissue injuries involve damage to arteries, nerves, or tendons.
   D. Of the open wounds presenting to the emergency department, nearly half will eventually become infected.

_____ 4. The outermost layer of skin is the:
   A. epidermis.
   B. dermis.
   C. subcutaneous tissue.
   D. sebum.

_____ 5. The glands within the dermis that secrete a lubricant are called the:
   A. lymph glands.
   B. subcutaneous glands.
   C. sebaceous glands.
   D. soporiferous glands.

_____ 6. The tunica intima, tunica media, and tunica adventitia are found in all blood vessels except for the:
   A. arteries.
   B. veins.
   C. capillaries.
   D. aorta.

_____ 7. Thick, fibrous, inflexible membranes surrounding muscle that help bind muscle groups together are called:
   A. tendons.
   B. fascia.
   C. tension lines.
   D. ligaments.

_____ 8. One type of closed wound is the:
   A. crush injury.
   B. laceration.
   C. avulsion.
   D. abrasion.

_____ 9. Blunt, nonpenetrating injuries that crush and damage small blood vessels are called:
   A. hematomas.
   B. erythema.
   C. contusions.
   D. crush injuries.

_____ 10. A hematoma or collection of blood beneath the skin:
   A. is most commonly caused by injury to an artery.
   B. is difficult to identify in cases of head trauma because of the underlying skull.
   C. in the thigh, can contain nearly 2 liters of blood before swelling becomes noticeable.
   D. in the thigh, leg, or arm is very pronounced but rarely contains significant hemorrhage

_____ 11. The mechanism of trauma injury in which tissue is locally compressed by high-pressure forces is called:
   A. crush syndrome.
   B. traumatic asphyxiation.
   C. crush injury.
   D. compartment syndrome.

©2007 Pearson Education, Inc.
Essentials of Paramedic Care, 2nd ed.

CHAPTER 20 *Soft-Tissue Trauma* 543

HANDOUT 20-2 Continued

_____ 12. One type of open wound is the:
   A. abrasion.
   B. crush injury.
   C. contusion.
   D. hematoma.

_____ 13. An injury in which the mechanism of injury tears the skin off the underlying muscle, tissue, blood vessels, and bone is called a(n):
   A. amputation.
   B. degloving injury.
   C. compartment injury.
   D. complete avulsion.

_____ 14. The stage of wound healing in which you will see arterial constriction and longitudinal muscle contraction is:
   A. hemostasis.
   B. inflammation.
   C. epithelialization.
   D. neovascularization.

_____ 15. Minor bleeding associated with capillary wounds often continues because:
   A. blood in capillaries is under a great deal of pressure.
   B. capillaries dilate in response to the injury to cleanse the area.
   C. muscles around the injury become flaccid.
   D. capillaries cannot contract and thus continue to bleed.

_____ 16. During the inflammation process, a specific type of cell arrives at the injury site that can engulf bacteria, debris, and foreign material. These cells are called:
   A. granulocytes.
   B. chemotactic factors.
   C. phagocytes.
   D. lymphocytes.

_____ 17. The result of the inflammation stage of healing is:
   A. cushioning of the injury site to reduce pain.
   B. clearing away of dead tissue and removal of bacteria.
   C. increased red blood cell production at the injury site.
   D. pain on movement of the injury site to expedite healing.

_____ 18. Which of the following is TRUE regarding infection?
   A. Infection is a rare complication of open wounds.
   B. Noticeable signs of infection usually develop within hours of the injury.
   C. Signs of infection include lymphangitis and warmth.
   D. The general health of the host has little to do with the risk of infection.

_____ 19. Several circumstances or conditions can interfere with normal wound healing. One of these is the fact that:
   A. fibrinolytics interfere with or break down protein fibers that form clots.
   B. penicillins may decrease clotting times and increase red cell production.
   C. compartment syndrome is a likely complication with closed abdominal wounds.
   D. an excess of serous fluid may result in overproduction of scar tissue.

_____ 20. Crush syndrome can be a very serious complication of soft-tissue injuries. Crush syndrome occurs when:
   A. bones are "crushed," resulting in multiple fractures.
   B. body parts are trapped for 4 hours or longer.
   C. a sudden impact damages internal organs.
   D. the body is trapped under pressure, resulting in decreased respiratory function.

_____ 21. A bandage is used to hold a dressing in place. One fact to keep in mind about dressings is that:
   A. even nonsterile dressings are free of microscopic contamination and microorganisms.
   B. nonadherent dressings promote clot formation, thus reducing hemorrhage.
   C. dry dressings are often applied to small burns and abdominal eviscerations.
   D. elastic bandages are not commonly used in prehospital care.

HANDOUT 20-2 Continued

_____ 22. A rapid trauma assessment should be performed on:
   A. all patients with traumatic injuries.
   B. any patient with a significant mechanism of injury.
   C. only patients who are actually showing signs and symptoms of severe trauma.
   D. any patient with external hemorrhage.

_____ 23. Use of the "inquiry" assessment technique:
   A. may employ the AVPU mnemonic to elicit information about the patient's signs and symptoms.
   B. is performed after the "palpation" portion of the assessment.
   C. allows the paramedic to question the patient about signs and symptoms before touching an area.
   D. is used to identify discolorations, deformities, or open wounds.

_____ 24. An important point to remember regarding the management of soft-tissue injuries is that:
   A. all wounds should be dressed and bandaged prior to transport and are a high priority for treatment.
   B. the three objectives of dressing and bandaging a wound are control of hemorrhage, keeping the wound clean, and applying an antibiotic solution to prevent infection.
   C. when using a tourniquet to control hemorrhage, apply just enough pressure to halt venous return while permitting arterial blood flow to continue.
   D. elevation of the injury can reduce edema and increase blood flow through the wound and injured extremity.

_____ 25. In order of preference, the methods of controlling external hemorrhage are:
   A. direct pressure with a dressing; elevation of the injury site; exposure of the wound and placement of digital pressure on the site; application of digital pressure to a proximal artery.
   B. digital pressure with a gloved hand on the site; direct pressure with a dressing; elevation of the injury site; application of a pressure bandage over the dressing.
   C. digital pressure to a proximal artery; direct pressure with a dressing; elevation of the injury site; application of a cold pack.
   D. digital pressure with a gloved hand on the site; elevation of the injury site; direct pressure with a dressing; application of digital pressure to a proximal artery.

_____ 26. Whenever you consider using a tourniquet, one precaution to keep in mind is that:
   A. if pressure is applied insufficiently, arterial blood may continue to flow.
   B. when the tourniquet is applied properly, the entire limb distal to the device is without circulation.
   C. when circulation is restored, the blood flows and pools in the extremity, adding to hypovolemia.
   D. all of these

_____ 27. Pain and edema control are best handled by:
   A. application of heat to the injury site.
   B. application of cold packs and moderate-pressure bandages.
   C. application of an elastic or Ace bandage.
   D. keeping the injury site below heart level.

_____ 28. Complications of bandaging include the fact that:
   A. bandages that are too loose may lead to decreased blood flow and ischemia.
   B. bandages and dressings left on too long can become soaked with blood and body fluid and serve as incubators for infection.
   C. large, bulky dressings are not as effective in controlling hemorrhage as one or two layers of gauze dressings.
   D. all of these

©2007 Pearson Education, Inc.
Essentials of Paramedic Care, 2nd ed.

CHAPTER 20 Soft-Tissue Trauma 545

HANDOUT 20-2 Continued

_____ 29. Current recommendations for managing amputated body parts include:
  A. immersing the amputated part in ice water.
  B. wrapping the part in sterile gauze and placing it in a plastic bag.
  C. placing the part in a plastic bag and immersing the bag in cold water.
  D. placing the part in a plastic bag and covering the bag with ice.

_____ 30. Impaled objects should not be removed unless the object is impaled in:
  A. an extremity and movement is impaired.
  B. the neck and the patient must be immobilized.
  C. the central chest of a patient who needs CPR.
  D. the head and increased intracranial pressure is a concern.

Handout 20-3

Student's Name _____

CHAPTER 20 SCENARIO

Review the following real-life situation. Then answer the questions that follow.

Only one-half mile and her daily jog would be complete. To cool off, the woman slows down her pace. Suddenly and without warning, a large dog leaps over a nearby hedge and bites her right calf and then her right mid-thigh. The dog's owner comes rushing to the woman's aid and pulls the dog away. The owner then calls 911. Rescue 8 responds within 10 minutes and begins assessment of the patient.

As the paramedics assess the jogger's anterior right mid-thigh, they see a torn flap of skin approximately 4 inches long. There is a moderate amount of oozing red blood. They also notice flowing dark red blood.

1. What type of injury has the woman sustained? What are the origins of the hemorrhage?

2. What method of bleeding control should the paramedics use first? Briefly, describe how this first choice of bleeding control would be accomplished.

3. What happens if the paramedic does not apply pressure to the exact site of blood loss?

4. If the first choice for bleeding control was unsuccessful, what method of bleeding control would be the second choice? Briefly, describe how this second choice of bleeding control would be accomplished.

5. What are the benefits of the second choice of bleeding control?

6. If the first two attempts at hemorrhage control were not successful, what would be the next action?

HANDOUT 20-3 Continued

With successful reduction of bleeding from the right mid-thigh, the paramedics assess the right calf and find a deep, narrow wound surrounded by black-and-blue skin.

7. What is the medical term for this type of wound? What is the medical term for the skin discoloration, and what is the underlying pathophysiology of this wound?

8. What is the potential long-term medical complication that might result from the wound to the patient's right calf?

9. What are the three objectives of bandaging soft-tissue injuries?

EVALUATION

As the paramedics prepare the patient for transport, her vital signs are BP 132/78, pulse 110, and respirations 14. She complains only of slight pain to her leg.

10. Is this patient a candidate for a trauma center? Why or why not?

HANDOUT 20-4

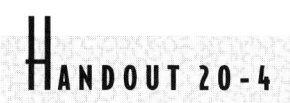

Student's Name _____

CHAPTER 20 REVIEW

Write the word or words that best complete the following sentences in the space provided.

1. The three layers of the skin, beginning with the outermost, are the _____, the _____, and the _____ layers.

2. Collectively, the skin is known as the _____ system.

3. The fatty secretion that helps keep the skin pliable and waterproof is called _____.

4. A(n) _____ is a white blood cell that specializes in humoral immunity and antibody formation.

5. The natural patterns in the surface of the skin are called _____ lines.

6. General reddening of the skin due to dilation of the superficial capillaries is called _____.

7. Blue-black discoloration of the skin due to leakage of blood into the tissues is called _____.

8. A(n) _____ is a closed wound in which the skin is unbroken, although damage has occurred to the tissue immediately beneath.

9. _____ is a collection of blood beneath the skin or trapped within a body compartment.

10. A(n) _____ _____ is a mechanism of injury in which tissue is locally compressed by high-pressure forces.

11. _____ _____ is the systemic disorder of severe metabolic disturbances resulting from the crushing of a limb or other body part.

12. The natural tendency of the body to maintain its normal functions is called _____.

13. _____ is tough, strong protein that comprises most of the body's connective tissue.

14. _____ is the most common complication of open wounds.

15. _____ are the visible red streaks extending from a wound and are an indication of infection.

16. The new growth of capillaries in response to healing is called _____.

17. Some medications, like aspirin, warfarin, and heparin, can interfere with the _____ process.

18. Muscle ischemia caused by rising pressures within an anatomic fascial space is called _____ syndrome.

19. Perform a(n) _____ _____ assessment on patients with a significant mechanism of injury.

20. Perform a(n) _____ _____ assessment on patients who have no significant mechanism of injury.

21. Three assessment techniques used during the assessment of a trauma patient are _____, _____, and _____.

22. The three objectives of dressing and bandaging wounds are _____ _____, _____, and _____.

23. A(n) _____ is used to control hemorrhage as a last resort.

24. Current recommendations for managing amputated body parts include dry _____ and _____ transport.

25. Do not remove _____ objects because of the risk of serious, uncontrollable bleeding.

REINFORCEMENT

Handout 20-5

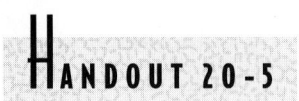

Student's Name _____

SOFT-TISSUE INJURIES MATCHING

Write the letter of the term in the space provided next to the appropriate description.

A. Incision
B. Laceration
C. Degloving injury
D. Subcutaneous tissue
E. Epidermis
F. Hematoma
G. Dermis
H. Direct pressure
I. Infection
J. Inflammation
K. Ecchymosis
L. Compartment syndrome

_____ **1.** Outermost layer of the skin.

_____ **2.** Layer of adipose and connective tissue.

_____ **3.** Layer of tissue producing the epidermis and consisting of blood vessels, nerves, and glands.

_____ **4.** A collection of blood trapped within a body compartment.

_____ **5.** Open wound, normally with jagged borders.

_____ **6.** Smooth, surgical-type open wound.

_____ **7.** Blue-black discoloration of the skin due to leakage of blood into the tissues.

_____ **8.** The most common and, next to hemorrhage, the most serious complication of open wounds.

_____ **9.** Wound in which the skin is torn off the underlying muscle, blood vessels, and bone.

_____ **10.** The primary, and most effective method, of controlling hemorrhage.

_____ **11.** Process of local cellular and biochemical changes as a consequence of injury or infection.

_____ **12.** Muscle ischemia that is caused by rising pressures within an anatomic fascia space.

Chapter 20 Answer Key

Handout 20-2: Chapter 20 Quiz

1. C	9. C	17. B	25. A
2. A	10. A	18. C	26. D
3. B	11. C	19. A	27. B
4. A	12. A	20. B	28. B
5. C	13. B	21. D	29. C
6. C	14. A	22. B	30. C
7. B	15. D	23. C	
8. A	16. A	24. D	

Handout 20-3: Chapter 20 Scenario

1. The mid-thigh wound is an avulsion. The bleeding is venous and capillary.
2. First choice for bleeding control would be to apply direct pressure with surgical trauma dressings or several 4 × 4 pads.
3. Hemorrhage may continue because pressure is distributed throughout the wound site, rather than directly to the wound source.
4. The second choice would be to elevate the leg while continuing to maintain direct pressure.
5. Elevation reduces bleeding. Elevation also reduces extremity arterial pressure and increases venous return while minimizing potential edema.
6. The next choice would be the use of a pressure point, accomplished by locating the pulse point proximal to the wound and applying firm pressure to it. In this case, the femoral artery would be the pressure point. Continue alternating among all three techniques to control hemorrhage.
7. The calf wound is a puncture and the discoloration is ecchymosis, which is caused by leakage of blood into the tissues.
8. Infection.
9. The three objectives are hemorrhage control, immobilization, and sterility.
10. This patient is probably not a candidate for a trauma center. However, it is important that you know and learn your local protocols regarding destination of the trauma patient.

Handout 20-4: Chapter 20 Review

1. epidermis, dermis, subcutaneous
2. integumentary
3. sebum
4. lymphocyte
5. tension
6. erythema
7. ecchymosis
8. contusion
9. Hematoma
10. crush injury
11. Crush syndrome
12. homeostasis
13. Collagen
14. Infection
15. Lymphangitis
16. neovascularization
17. clotting
18. compartment
19. rapid trauma
20. focused trauma
21. inquiry, inspection, palpation
22. hemorrhage control, sterility, immobilization
23. tourniquet
24. cooling, rapid
25. impaled

Handout 20-5: Soft-Tissue Injuries Matching

1. E	4. F	7. K	10. H
2. D	5. B	8. I	11. J
3. G	6. A	9. C	12. L

Chapter 21

Burns

INTRODUCTION

Although the number of burn injuries in the United States is declining, 1.25 to 2 million Americans are treated for burns each year. Of these burns, 3 to 5 percent are considered life-threatening. The decline in burn injuries can be attributed to safer buildings, smoke detectors, and educational campaigns. This chapter discusses the pathologic effects of burns on the tissues and the body in general and the effective assessment and treatment of burns.

CHAPTER OBJECTIVES

After reading this chapter, you should be able to:

1. Describe the anatomy and physiology of the skin and remaining human anatomy as they pertain to thermal burn injuries. (see Chapter 3)
2. Describe the epidemiology, including incidence, mortality, morbidity, and risk factors, for thermal burn injuries as well as strategies to prevent such injuries. (p. 892)
3. Describe the local and systemic complications of a thermal burn injury. (pp. 893–894, 904–906)
4. Identify and describe the depth classifications of burn injuries, including superficial burns, partial-thickness burns, and full-thickness burns. (pp. 902–903)
5. Describe and apply the "rule of nines" and the "rule of palms" methods for determining body surface area percentage of a burn injury. (pp. 903–904)
6. Identify and describe the severity of a burn including a minor burn, a moderate burn, and a critical burn. (pp. 909–912)
7. Describe the effects age and preexisting conditions have on burn severity and a patient's prognosis. (pp. 905–906, 910–911)
8. Discuss complications of burn injuries caused by trauma, blast injuries, airway compromise, respiratory compromise, and child abuse. (pp. 901–902, 906–909, 914–915)
9. Describe thermal burn management including considerations for airway and ventilation, circulation, pharmacological and nonpharmacological measures, transport decisions, and psychological support/communication strategies. (pp. 906–915)

TOTAL TEACHING TIME:
9.31 HOURS
The total teaching time is only a guideline based on the didactic and practical lab averages in the National Standard Curriculum. Instructors should take into consideration such factors as the pace at which students learn, the size of the class, and breaks. The actual time devoted to teaching objectives is the responsibility of the instructor.

10. Describe special considerations for a pediatric patient with a burn injury and describe the criteria for determining pediatric burn severity. (pp. 903–904, 905–906, 910–911)
11. Describe the specific epidemiologies, mechanisms of injury, pathophysiologies, and severity assessments for inhalation, chemical, and electrical burn injuries and for radiation exposure. (pp. 914–921)
12. Discuss special considerations that impact the assessment, management, and prognosis of patients with inhalation, chemical, and electrical burn injuries and with exposure to radiation. (pp. 914–921)
13. Differentiate between supraglottic and subglottic inhalation burn injuries. (pp. 901–902)
14. Describe the special considerations for a chemical burn injury to the eye. (p. 919)
15. Given several preprogrammed, simulated thermal, inhalation, electrical, and chemical burn injury and radiation exposure patients, provide the appropriate scene size-up, initial assessment, rapid trauma or focused physical exam and history, detailed exam, and ongoing assessment and provide appropriate patient care and transportation. (pp. 892–921)

FRAMING THE LESSON

Begin by reviewing the important points of Chapter 20, "Soft-Tissue Trauma." Use this time to answer any questions about the previous chapter and to discuss any items not completely understood by students. Then begin the discussion of Chapter 21.

Begin by reviewing the layers of the skin. Knowing what the layers are and what is contained in them will help students understand the classification of burns and the resulting complications. If you have access to a burn center, you may consider inviting a burn specialist to class to discuss burn injury and care and to show photos or slides of various classifications of burn injuries. You may also want to consider covering the protocols of the local paramedic service regarding burn care. Have students list as many specific types of burn injuries as they can think of. This could include specific burns from stoves, fires, chemicals, inhalation, and so on. Discuss also the various "old wives' tales" treatments for burns that students have heard over the years: applying butter, ice, lotions, and so on.

TEACHING STRATEGIES

People learn in a variety of ways. Some do better with the spoken word, whereas others prefer the written. Some prefer to work alone, whereas others profit from working in groups. Recognizing these different ways of acquiring knowledge, the authors of this *Instructor's Resource Manual* have provided a variety of teaching strategies for the different types of learners. These strategies are intended to foster higher-level cognitive skills and encourage creative learning and problem solving. For greatest effectiveness, incorporate these strategies into your class lecture. Symbols in the Lecture Outline indicate the points at which various exercises might be most appropriate. Other strategies can be used to preview the lesson or to summarize it.

The following strategies are keyed to specific sections of the lesson.

1. ***Rule of Nines with Paper Dolls.*** Use paper dolls to teach the rule of nines. Each section of the body should represent 9 percent of the body surface

  b. Ionization
    i. Alpha radiation
    ii. Beta radiation
    iii. Gamma radiation
    iv. Neutron radiation
  c. Effects of radiation on the body (**Fig. 21-6, p. 899**)
    i. Radiation absorbed dose (rad)
    ii. Roentgen equivalent in man (rem)
  d. Principles of safety
    i. Time
    ii. Distance
    iii. Shielding
 5. Inhalation injury (**Fig. 21-7, p. 901**)
  a. Toxic inhalation
  b. Carbon monoxide
  c. Airway thermal burn

B. Depth of burn (pp. 902–903) (**Fig. 21-8, p. 903**)
 1. Superficial burn
 2. Partial-thickness burn
 3. Full-thickness burn

C. Body surface area (pp. 903–904)
 1. Rule of nines (**Fig. 21-9, p. 904**)
 2. Rule of palms (**Fig. 21-10, p. 904**)

D. Systemic complications (pp. 904–906)
 1. Hypothermia
 2. Hypovolemia
 3. Eschar (**Fig. 21-11, p. 905**)
 4. Infection
 5. Organ failure
 6. Special factors
 7. Physical abuse (**Fig. 21-12, p. 906**)

III. Assessment of thermal burns (pp. 906–912)

A. Scene size-up (pp. 906–908) (**Fig. 21-13, p. 907**)
B. Initial assessment (pp. 908–909) (**Fig. 21-14, p. 908**)
C. Focused and rapid trauma assessment (pp. 909–912) (**Fig. 21-15, p. 909; Figs. 21-16 and 21-17, p. 910**)
 1. Characteristics of various depths of burns (**Table 21-1, p. 911**)
  a. Superficial
  b. Partial-thickness
  c. Full-thickness
 2. Burn severity (**Table 21-2, p. 911**)
  a. Local
  b. Moderate
  c. Critical
 3. Injuries that benefit from burn center care (**Table 21-3, p. 912**)
  a. Partial-thickness greater than 15 percent BSA
  b. Full-thickness greater than 5 percent
  c. Significant burns to face, feet, hands, perineal area
  d. High-voltage electrical burns
  e. Inhalation injuries
  f. Chemical burns causing progressive tissue destruction
  g. Associated significant injuries
D. Ongoing assessment (p. 912)

TEACHING STRATEGY 1
Rule of Nines with Paper Dolls

TEACHING STRATEGY 2
Rule of Palms with Paint

POINT OF INTEREST
When you arrive at a fire scene, try to find out what is burning. In the Cleveland Clinic fire of 1929, 123 deaths were linked to poisoning from oxides of nitrogen released by the burning of nitrocellulose X-ray films.

POINT TO EMPHASIZE
Sometimes a physical exam won't help in diagnosing respiratory burns. Sooty sputum is present in only 50 percent of cases, hoarseness in less than 25 percent, and singed nasal hairs in only 13 percent. Mechanism of injury may be a better determinant.

POWERPOINT PRESENTATION
Chapter 21 PowerPoint slides 45–49

TEACHING STRATEGY 3
Kitchen Medicine

READING/REFERENCE
Danks, R. "Burn Management." *JEMS*, May 2003.

TEACHING STRATEGY 4
Application of Parkland Formula

POINT TO EMPHASIZE
At the scene, the burn injury is the least priority. Remember the ABCs.

POWERPOINT PRESENTATION
Chapter 21 PowerPoint slides 50–54

POWERPOINT PRESENTATION
Chapter 21 PowerPoint slides 55–64

IV. Management of thermal burns (pp. 912–915)
  A. Local and minor burns (pp. 912–913)
  B. Moderate to severe burns (pp. 913–914) (Fig. 21-18, p. 913)
     1. Intravenous fluids
     2. Medications
  C. Inhalation injury (pp. 914–915) (Fig. 21-19, p. 915)

V. Assessment and management of electrical, chemical, and radiation burns (pp. 915–921)
  A. Electrical injuries (pp. 915–917)
     1. Lightning strikes (Fig. 21-20, p. 916)
  B. Chemical burns (pp. 917–919) (Fig. 21-21, p. 918)
     1. Phenol
     2. Dry lime
     3. Sodium
     4. Riot control agents
  C. Radiation burns: dose-effect relationships to ionizing radiation (pp. 919–921) (Table 21-4, p. 920)
     1. Park the rescue vehicle upwind to minimize contamination.
     2. Look for signs of radiation exposure. Radioactive packages are marked by clearly identifiable color-coded labels (Fig. 21-22, p. 921)
     3. If you are trained and equipped with appropriate gear, consider using portable instruments to measure the level of radioactivity. If dose estimates are significant, rotate rescue personnel.
     4. Apply normal principles of emergency care, for example, ABCs, shock management, and trauma care.
     5. Once they are decontaminated as necessary, externally radiated patients pose little danger to rescue personnel. Initiate normal care procedures for injuries other than radiation.
     6. Internally contaminated patients (who have ingested or inhaled radioactive particles) pose little danger to rescue personnel. Normal care procedures should be undertaken. Collect body wastes. If assisted ventilation is required, use a bag-valve-mask unit or demand valve. If radioactive particles are inhaled, swab the nasal passages and save the swabs.
     7. Externally contaminated patients (liquids, dirt, smoke) require decontamination. Following decontamination, initiate normal emergency care procedures. Decontamination of paramedic personnel and equipment is required after the call is completed.
     8. Patients with open, contaminated wounds require normal emergency care procedures. Avoid cross-contamination of wounds.
  D. Ongoing assessment (p. 921)

POWERPOINT PRESENTATION
Chapter 21 PowerPoint slide 65

VI. Chapter summary (pp. 921–922). Burn injuries may compromise the skin—the protective envelope that protects and contains the human body. Burn damage to the skin may interfere with its ability to contain water within the body and to prevent damaging agents from entering. For these reasons, assessment and care of these soft-tissue injuries are important.

Assess the burn to determine its depth and the extent of the body surface area it involves. Be sensitive to any respiratory, joint, hand, foot, or circumferential regions affected by the burn. Give special consideration to pediatric and geriatric burn patients and to burn patients who are also ill or otherwise injured. Consider all these factors in determining the overall severity of a burn. If the patient's condition warrants, institute aggressive care. Anticipate airway compromise and fluid loss. Secure the airway very early in prehospital care. Initiate IV access, and begin fluid administration. Electrical, chemical, or radiation burns require special care and assessment. An electrical burn requires careful assessment to determine the area and depth of burn involvement and should be followed by wound site dressing and cardiac monitoring. Chemical burns need rapid and effective decontamination. Radiation burns call for extreme care in removing the patient from the radiation source and in providing decontamination and supportive care.

ASSIGNMENTS

Assign students to complete Chapter 21, "Burns," of the workbook. Also assign them to read Chapter 22, "Musculoskeletal Trauma," before the next class.

EVALUATION

Chapter Quiz and Scenario   Distribute copies of the Chapter Quiz provided in Handout 21-2 to evaluate student understanding of this chapter. Make sure each student reads the scenario to reinforce critical thinking on the scene. Remind students not to use their notes or textbooks while taking the quiz.

Student CD   Quizzes for every chapter are contained on the dynamic and highly visual in-text student CD.

Companion Website   Additional quizzes for every chapter are contained on this exciting website.

TestGen   You may wish to create a custom-tailored test using *Prentice Hall TestGen for Essentials of Paramedic Care,* 2nd Edition to evaluate student understanding of this chapter.

On-line Test Preparation (for students and instructors)   Additional test preparation is available through Brady's new on-line product, *EMT Achieve: Paramedic Test Preparation* at *http://www.prenhall.com/emtachieve/*. Instructors can also monitor student mastery on-line.

Review Manual for the EMT-Paramedic   This comprehensive exam review contains hundreds of test questions and rationales, including scenarios, along with two 180-question practice tests on CD.

REINFORCEMENT

Handouts   If classroom discussion or performance on the quiz indicates that some students have not fully mastered the chapter content, you may wish to assign some or all of the Reinforcement Handouts for this chapter.

Student CD (for students)   A wide variety of material on this CD-ROM will reinforce and also expand student knowledge and skills.

PowerPoint Presentation (for instructors)   The PowerPoint material developed for this chapter offers useful reinforcement of chapter content.

Companion Website (for students)   Additional review quizzes and links to EMS resources will contribute to further reinforcement of the chapter.

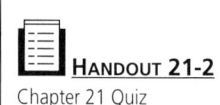

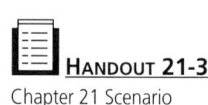

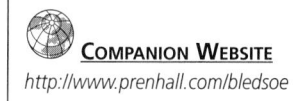

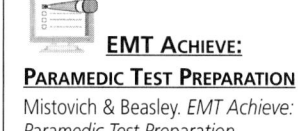

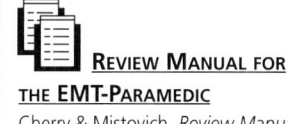

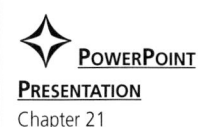

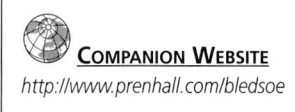

WORKBOOK
Chapter 21 Activities

READING/REFERENCE
Textbook, pp. 924–957

HANDOUT 21-2
Chapter 21 Quiz

HANDOUT 21-3
Chapter 21 Scenario

PARAMEDIC STUDENT CD
Student Activities

COMPANION WEBSITE
http://www.prenhall.com/bledsoe

TESTGEN
Chapter 21

EMT ACHIEVE: PARAMEDIC TEST PREPARATION
Mistovich & Beasley. *EMT Achieve: Paramedic Test Preparation.* www.prenhall.com/emtachieve/

REVIEW MANUAL FOR THE EMT-PARAMEDIC
Cherry & Mistovich. *Review Manual for the EMT-Paramedic,* 3rd edition.

HANDOUTS 21-4 AND 21-5
Reinforcement Activities

PARAMEDIC STUDENT CD
Student Activities

POWERPOINT PRESENTATION
Chapter 21

COMPANION WEBSITE
http://www.prenhall.com/bledsoe

OneKey On-line support is offered for this course on one of three platforms: CourseCompass, Blackboard, or Web CT. Includes the IRM, PowerPoints, TestGen, and Companion Website for instruction. Ask your local sales representative for more information.

Brady Skills Series: Advanced Life Skills (Video or CD) Have your students watch the skills come to life on VHS or CD-ROM, or they can purchase the highly visual, full-color text with step-by-step procedures and rationales.

OneKey
Chapter 21

Advanced Life Support Skills
Larmon & Davis. *Advanced Life Support Skills.*

Advanced Life Skills Review
Larmon & Davis. *Advanced Life Skills Review.*

Brady Skills Series: ALS
Larmon & Davis. *Brady Skills Series: ALS.*

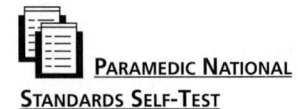

Paramedic National Standards Self-Test
Miller. *Paramedic National Standards Self-Test*, 4th edition.

HANDOUT 21-1

Student's Name _____

CHAPTER 21 OBJECTIVES CHECKLIST

Knowledge	Date Mastered
1. Describe the anatomy and physiology of the skin and remaining human anatomy as they pertain to thermal burn injuries.	
2. Describe the epidemiology, including incidence, mortality, morbidity, and risk factors, for thermal burn injuries as well as strategies to prevent such injuries.	
3. Describe the local and systemic complications of a thermal burn injury.	
4. Identify and describe the depth classifications of burn injuries, including superficial burns, partial-thickness burns, and full-thickness burns.	
5. Describe and apply the "rule of nines" and the "rule of palms" methods for determining body surface area percentage of a burn injury.	
6. Identify and describe the severity of a burn including a minor burn, a moderate burn, and a critical burn.	
7. Describe the effects age and preexisting conditions have on burn severity and a patient's prognosis.	
8. Discuss complications of burn injuries caused by trauma, blast injuries, airway compromise, respiratory compromise, and child abuse.	
9. Describe thermal burn management including considerations for airway and ventilation, circulation, pharmacological and nonpharmacological measures, transport decisions, and psychological support/communication strategies.	
10. Describe special considerations for a pediatric patient with a burn injury and describe the criteria for determining pediatric burn severity.	
11. Describe the specific epidemiologies, mechanisms of injury, pathophysiologies, and severity assessments for inhalation, chemical, and electrical burn injuries and for radiation exposure.	
12. Discuss special considerations that impact the assessment, management, and prognosis of patients with inhalation, chemical, and electrical burn injuries and with exposure to radiation.	
13. Differentiate between supraglottic and subglottic inhalation burn injuries.	

©2007 Pearson Education, Inc.
Essentials of Paramedic Care, 2nd ed.

HANDOUT 21-1 Continued

Knowledge	Date Mastered
14. Describe the special considerations for a chemical burn injury to the eye.	
15. Given several preprogrammed, simulated thermal, inhalation, electrical, and chemical burn injury and radiation exposure patients, provide the appropriate scene size-up, initial assessment, rapid trauma or focused physical exam and history, detailed exam, and ongoing assessment and provide appropriate patient care and transportation.	

OBJECTIVES

HANDOUT 21-2

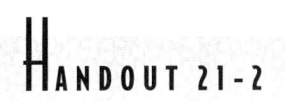

Student's Name _____

CHAPTER 21 QUIZ

Write the letter of the best answer in the space provided.

_____ 1. Burns resulting from exposure to heat are called:
   A. thermal burns.
   B. electrical burns.
   C. chemical burns.
   D. radiation burns.

_____ 2. The effects of heat, according to Jackson's theory of thermal wounds, cause structural proteins to break down. The term for this altering of the usual substance of something is:
   A. mutating.
   B. exacerbating.
   C. deteriorating.
   D. denaturing.

_____ 3. The area nearest the heat source that suffers the most damage is called the zone of:
   A. hyperemia.
   B. stasis.
   C. coagulation.
   D. denaturing.

_____ 4. The stage of the burn process characterized by catecholamine and pain-mediated reaction is called the:
   A. emergent phase.
   B. fluid shift phase.
   C. hypermetabolic phase.
   D. resolution phase.

_____ 5. Which of the following is TRUE regarding the fluid shift phase of the burn process?
   A. This phase includes a pain response as well as the outpouring of catecholamines.
   B. Chemicals are released to initiate an inflammatory response.
   C. Body metabolism increases to begin healing the burn.
   D. The capillaries begin leaking fluid and red blood cells.

_____ 6. The "pressure" of the electric flow is known as:
   A. amperage.
   B. current.
   C. ohmage.
   D. voltage.

_____ 7. In electrical burn injuries, the highest heat occurs at the points of greatest resistance. The area of the body that has the lowest resistance, allowing even small currents to pass, is:
   A. wet skin.
   B. mucous membranes.
   C. dry, callused skin.
   D. the palm of the hand.

_____ 8. Electrical burns are considered very serious because:
   A. the burn heats the victim from the inside out.
   B. serious vascular and nervous injury may occur.
   C. resulting tissue death causes the release of toxic materials.
   D. all of these

_____ 9. When caring for a patient with a chemical burn, it is important to know if the chemical is an acid or an alkali because:
   A. the skin is highly resistant to acids, so minimal surface damage is done.
   B. alkalis continue to destroy cell membranes through liquefaction necrosis.
   C. acids are difficult to neutralize and may continue to burn hours after the exposure.
   D. alkalis form a thick, insoluble mass where they contact tissue, limiting burn damage.

_____ 10. One type of radiation is only a significant hazard if the patient inhales or ingests contaminated material. This type of radiation is:
   A. alpha.
   B. beta.
   C. gamma.
   D. neutron.

HANDOUT 21-2 Continued

_____ 11. If a burn injury occurred in an enclosed space, always consider the possibility of:
   A. electrical burns.
   B. inhalation injury.
   C. circumferential burns.
   D. explosion.

_____ 12. Because very moist mucosa lines the airway:
   A. significant thermal burns of the lower airway are common.
   B. hot, dry air often causes lower airway burns.
   C. supraglottic structures may absorb heat and prevent lower airway burns.
   D. hot air produces "steam" from the moisture, causing burning of the entire airway.

_____ 13. Burns are classified by their depth. The classification in which you would expect to see blisters, intense pain, white to red skin, and moist and mottled skin is a:
   A. superficial burn.
   B. partial-thickness burn.
   C. full-thickness burn.
   D. any of these

_____ 14. When caring for a patient with a full-thickness burn, remember that:
   A. full-thickness burns are very painful.
   B. blisters are the hallmark of a full-thickness burn.
   C. full-thickness burns are characterized by eschar and areas that are white and dry.
   D. the skin will be bright red and warm to the touch.

_____ 15. When using the "rule of nines" to determine the total body surface area burned, the difference between infants and adults includes the recognition that the:
   A. anterior trunk of the adult is proportionally larger than that of an infant.
   B. legs of an adult are proportionally smaller than that of an infant.
   C. head of an infant is nearly twice as large proportionally as the head of an adult.
   D. neck of an adult is included in the percentage assigned to the head, while the neck of an infant is an additional 1 percent.

_____ 16. When estimating the size of a small burn, the best method to use is the:
   A. rule of nines.
   B. rule of palms.
   C. rule of 1 percent.
   D. rule of thumb.

_____ 17. The most persistent killer of burn victims is:
   A. shock.
   B. organ failure.
   C. infection.
   D. related traumatic injuries.

_____ 18. The scene size-up when responding to burn patients should include:
   A. early intubation.
   B. extinguishing smoldering shoes, belts, or watchbands.
   C. the standard ABCs.
   D. a rapid trauma assessment.

_____ 19. When considering intubation of the burn patient, an important point to remember is:
   A. to use succinylcholine for rapid sequence intubation, as this drug will not effect the body's calcium level.
   B. to administer high-flow, high-concentration oxygen to reduce the half-life of any carbon monoxide inhaled.
   C. to initially use the smallest endotracheal tube possible, as the airway may be swollen.
   D. to recognize that all patients with inhalation burns will show obvious symptoms such as sooty sputum, singed nasal hairs, hoarseness, and so on.

_____ 20. Your burn injury patient's skin is white and parchment-like, and he complains of little pain. This burn would be classified as what type of burn?
   A. superficial
   B. partial-thickness
   C. full-thickness
   D. none of these

HANDOUT 21-2 Continued

_____ 21. Your patient is a 3-year-old child, with partial-thickness burns over 20 percent of his body. This burn would be considered a:
   A. minor burn.
   B. moderate burn.
   C. serious burn.
   D. critical burn.

_____ 22. Patients who would benefit from care at a burn center include those who have:
   A. full-thickness burns greater than 2 percent BSA.
   B. significant burns to the face, feet, hands, or perineal area.
   C. partial-thickness burns greater than 10 percent BSA.
   D. patients with acute medical problems.

_____ 23. Use dry, sterile dressings to cover:
   A. partial-thickness burns of more than 15 percent BSA.
   B. all full-thickness burns.
   C. superficial burns of more than 25 percent BSA.
   D. any classification of burn covering more than 10 percent BSA.

_____ 24. Fluid resuscitation is an important part of treating serious burns. The formula for the amount of IV fluid needed to be infused includes:
   A. running in a liter of fluid during the first hour.
   B. 4 mL × patient weight (kg) × BSA burned.
   C. half of the fluid needed given within the first 4 hours after the burn.
   D. 1 liter × patient weight (kg) × BSA burned.

_____ 25. Management of patients with electrical burns includes ECG monitoring because:
   A. the patient may still be electrified even if disconnected from the power.
   B. electrolyte imbalance from the serious burn may cause cardiac dysrhythmias.
   C. electrical current may induce any number of cardiac dysrhythmias.
   D. decreased oxygenation due to airway problems may cause cardiac dysrhythmias.

EVALUATION

©2007 Pearson Education, Inc.
Essentials of Paramedic Care, 2nd ed.

Handout 21-3

Student's Name _____

CHAPTER 21 SCENARIO

Review the following real-life situation. Then answer the questions that follow.

Sitting on their bunk beds late at night, Jack knew Tommy shouldn't be playing with their father's cigarette lighter. Tommy was on the upper bunk, while Jack was on the lower bunk. Before Tommy knew what happened, a flame caught the corner of his pillow, which exploded into a ball of fire. Tommy kicked the pillow, and it fell onto Jack's bed, igniting the blankets. Jack screamed as flames erupted around him. Luckily, the boy's father came just in time to extinguish the flames with water from a nearby bathroom. The father called 911. Tommy was unhurt, but Jack needed immediate emergency medical care.

Jackson City Medic 5 is dispatched along with the fire department and arrives at the boy's home approximately 5 minutes after the incident. As paramedics Robert and Christy begin their assessment of Jack, they see blistering around his face and mottled, red skin on his chest and both arms. Bits and pieces of Jack's pajamas and blanket are embedded in his skin and still smoldering.

EVALUATION

1. What is the paramedics' immediate concern? Why?

2. What degree of burn has the child sustained?

3. What is the approximate total percentage of body surface area burned?

4. How would you manage the burns around the child's face?

5. How would you manage the burns to the child's chest and arms?

6. Would you use local cooling methods for burns to the child's chest and arms? Why or why not?

7. Is this patient a candidate for burn center care? Why or why not?

HANDOUT 21-4

Student's Name _____

CHAPTER 21 REVIEW

Write the word or words that best complete the following sentences in the space provided.

1. The four types of burns are _____, _____, _____, and _____.
2. As molecular speed increases from a burn injury, the cell components begin to break down, or _____.
3. The area of a burn most damaged and nearest the heat source is called the zone of _____.
4. The area of a burn adjacent to the most-damaged region, where you will see inflammation and a decrease in blood flow, is called the zone of _____.
5. The first stage of the burn process, characterized by a catecholamine and pain-mediated reaction, is the _____ phase.
6. The stage of the burn process in which there is increased body metabolism in an attempt by the body to heal the burn is called the _____ phase.
7. _____ usually continue to destroy cell membranes through liquefaction necrosis, allowing them to penetrate underlying tissue and causing deeper burns.
8. X-rays are _____ radiation.
9. _____ radiation is uncommon outside of nuclear reactors and bombs.
10. Suspect _____ _____ poisoning in any patient who was in an enclosed space during combustion.
11. _____ _____ has greater heat content than hot, dry air.
12. Burns involving only the epidermis are called _____ burns.
13. Burns involving the epidermis and the dermis are called _____-_____ burns.
14. Burns that damage all the layers of the skin are called _____-_____ burns.
15. Use the rule of _____ when estimating the size of a large burn.
16. Use the rule of _____ when estimating the size of a small burn.
17. Dead and denatured skin resulting from a full-thickness burn is called _____.
18. When considering rapid sequence intubation, use succinylcholine cautiously as it may worsen the _____ sometimes associated with severe burns.
19. Full-thickness burns greater than 10 percent BSA are considered _____ burns.
20. A full-thickness burn covering less than 2 percent BSA is considered a(n) _____ burn.
21. Separate burned _____ and _____ with dry, sterile gauze.
22. _____ _____ may induce dysrhythmias such as bradycardias, tachycardias, v-fib, and asystole.
23. Irrigate chemical splashes to the eye with large volumes of _____.
24. _____ (Do/Do not) attempt to neutralize chemicals splashed on the skin.
25. _____ _____, and _____ are important factors in determining dose of radiation exposure.

REINFORCEMENT

©2007 Pearson Education, Inc.
Essentials of Paramedic Care, 2nd ed.

CHAPTER 21 Burns 567

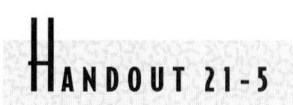

BURNS TRUE OR FALSE

Indicate whether the following statements are true or false by writing T or F in the space provided.

_____ 1. Burn injuries carry an increased danger of infection.

_____ 2. A burn is a progressive process.

_____ 3. Thermal and chemical burns are the only types of burns known to cause soft-tissue injury.

_____ 4. Electrical injury usually does very little damage to muscle tissue.

_____ 5. Respiratory arrest from an electrical burn is due to the immobilization of the muscles from prolonged exposure to an electrical current.

_____ 6. The human body offers little resistance to the flow of electricity.

_____ 7. A superficial, or first-degree burn, involves only the upper layers of the epidermis and dermis.

_____ 8. The presence of blisters is one way to differentiate between a superficial and partial-thickness burn.

_____ 9. Full-thickness burns involve injury to blood vessels, nerves, muscle tissue, bone, and sometimes internal organs.

_____ 10. A sunburn, resulting in red, painful skin, is an example of a partial-thickness burn.

_____ 11. A partial-thickness burn to the entire right leg of an infant represents approximately 9 percent of the child's total BSA.

_____ 12. A partial-thickness burn to an adult's upper and lower back represents approximately 18 percent total BSA.

_____ 13. During a burn, loss of plasma protein will reduce the body's ability to draw fluids from uninjured tissues.

_____ 14. Hypovolemia is an early sign of a partial-thickness burn.

_____ 15. A dry lime burn should first be flushed with water and then dried off.

Chapter 21 Answer Key

Handout 21-2: Chapter 21 Quiz

1.	A	8.	D	15.	C	22.	B
2.	D	9.	B	16.	B	23.	A
3.	C	10.	A	17.	C	24.	B
4.	A	11.	B	18.	B	25.	C
5.	B	12.	C	19.	B		
6.	D	13.	B	20.	C		
7.	B	14.	C	21.	D		

Handout 21-3: Chapter 21 Scenario

1. Smoldering pieces of clothing and bedding are immediate concerns. Any smoldering clothing or linens should be extinguished to stop the burning process. Airway management is also of concern because of the signs of burn injury to the child's face.
2. Second-degree burn.
3. Approximately 45 percent.
4. Airway burns are possible, but hot air or flame inspiration rarely has enough heat energy to cause significant laryngeal edema. Nonetheless, observe the child closely for signs of breathing difficulty, apply nonrebreather mask, and administer high-flow, high-concentration oxygen. Apply dry, sterile dressings to the child's face.
5. Once again, make certain all smoldering clothing and bed linen is extinguished. Apply dry, sterile dressings. Establish two large-bore IV routes and administer either normal saline or lactated Ringer's solution at a rate determined by local protocols.
6. Local cooling is not recommended since the body surface area burned is greater than 10 percent. Cooling of burns that involve 10 percent BSA or greater may result in hypothermia.
7. Yes. Second-degree burns greater than 15 percent of BSA necessitate burn center care.

Handout 21-4: Chapter 21 Review

1. thermal, electrical, chemical, radiation
2. denature
3. coagulation
4. stasis
5. emergent
6. hypermetabolic
7. Alkalis
8. gamma
9. Neutron
10. carbon monoxide
11. Superheated steam
12. superficial
13. partial-thickness
14. full-thickness
15. nines
16. palms
17. eschar
18. hyperkalemia
19. critical
20. moderate
21. toes, fingers
22. Electrical burns
23. water
24. Do not
25. Duration, distance, shielding

Handout 21-5: Burns True or False

1.	T	5.	T	9.	T	13.	T
2.	T	6.	F	10.	F	14.	F
3.	F	7.	T	11.	F	15.	F
4.	F	8.	T	12.	T		

Chapter 22

Musculoskeletal Trauma

INTRODUCTION

Musculoskeletal injuries usually result from direct or transmitted kinetic forces requiring only basic care. Assessment and management of musculoskeletal injuries for the unstable patient differ from those for the stable patient. Knowledge of the anatomy and physiology of the musculoskeletal system helps guide the paramedic in the effective management of these injuries. This chapter discusses the assessment and management of patients with musculoskeletal injuries.

CHAPTER OBJECTIVES

After reading this chapter, you should be able to:

1. Describe the incidence, morbidity, and mortality of musculoskeletal injuries. (p. 925)
2. Discuss the anatomy and physiology of the muscular and skeletal systems. (See Chapter 3)
3. Predict injuries based on the mechanism of injury, including: (pp. 926–931, 933)
   - Direct
   - Indirect
   - Pathologic
4. Discuss the types of musculoskeletal injuries, including:
   - Fractures (open and closed) (pp. 928–931)
   - Dislocations/fractures (pp. 927–928)
   - Sprains (p. 928)
   - Strains (p. 927)
5. Describe the six "Ps" of musculoskeletal injury assessment. (p. 935)
6. List the primary signs and symptoms of extremity trauma. (pp. 933–937)
7. List other signs and symptoms that can indicate less obvious extremity injury. (pp. 935–937)
8. Discuss the need for assessment of pulses, motor function, and sensation before and after splinting. (p. 940)

TOTAL TEACHING TIME:
7.84 HOURS
The total teaching time is only a guideline based on the didactic and practical lab averages in the National Standard Curriculum. Instructors should take into consideration such factors as the pace at which students learn, the size of the class, and breaks. The actual time devoted to teaching objectives is the responsibility of the instructor.

9. Identify the circumstances requiring rapid intervention and transport when dealing with musculoskeletal injuries. (pp. 933–934)
10. Discuss the general guidelines for splinting. (pp. 938–942)
11. Explain the benefits of the application of cold and heat for musculoskeletal injuries. (pp. 944–945)
12. Describe age-associated changes in the bones. (p. 931)
13. Discuss the pathophysiology, assessment findings, and management of open and closed fractures. (pp. 928–931, 933–948)
14. Discuss the relationship between the volume of hemorrhage and open or closed fractures. (pp. 934, 945–946)
15. Discuss the indications and contraindications for use of the pneumatic antishock garment (PASG) in the management of fractures. (pp. 945–946)
16. Describe the special considerations involved in femur fracture management. (pp. 945–947)
17. Discuss the pathophysiology, assessment findings, and management of dislocations. (pp. 928, 948–949, 949–950, 951)
18. Discuss the out-of-hospital management of dislocations/fractures, including splinting and realignment. (pp. 942–952)
19. Explain the importance of manipulating a knee dislocation/fracture with an absent distal pulse. (pp. 949–950)
20. Describe the procedure for reduction of a shoulder, finger, or ankle dislocation/fracture. (pp. 950, 951, 952)
21. Discuss the pathophysiology, assessment findings, and management of sprains, strains, and tendon injuries. (pp. 927, 928, 952)
22. Differentiate among musculoskeletal injuries based on the assessment findings and history. (pp. 933-938)
23. Given several preprogrammed and moulaged musculoskeletal trauma patients, provide the appropriate scene size-up, initial assessment, rapid trauma or focused physical exam and history, detailed exam, and ongoing assessment and provide appropriate patient care and transportation. (pp. 925–955)

FRAMING THE LESSON

Begin by reviewing the important points of Chapter 21, "Burns." Use this time to answer any questions about the previous chapter and to discuss any items not completely understood by students. Then begin the discussion of Chapter 22.

Ask students how many of them have ever had a musculoskeletal injury. Most people have had some type of fracture, sprain, dislocation, or strain, especially during childhood. Compare the various injuries described by students, noting that some are minor and some are more serious. Discuss how the seriousness of the injury often depends on the area of the body in which it occurs. For example, finger fractures or ankle strains are far less serious than, say, femoral fractures. Musculoskeletal injuries may be more serious if they occur in an area of the body that has large blood vessels and nerves running through it. Stress that injuries that take place in areas of the body containing large blood vessels, such as the femur and pelvic area, may result in severe internal bleeding and hypovolemia. Mention that the body does an excellent job of caring for itself. For example, in most cases, musculoskeletal injuries should not be moved until EMS arrival. If a patient has a leg fracture, and it hurts to move it, he/she will not move it. The body has effectively "splinted" itself. If possible, have on hand several X-rays to illustrate various musculoskeletal injuries.

TEACHING STRATEGIES

People learn in a variety of ways. Some do better with the spoken word, whereas others prefer the written. Some prefer to work alone, whereas others profit from working in groups. Recognizing these different ways of acquiring knowledge, the authors of this *Instructor's Resource Manual* have provided a variety of teaching strategies for the different types of learners. These strategies are intended to foster higher-level cognitive skills and encourage creative learning and problem solving. For greatest effectiveness, incorporate these strategies into your class lecture. Symbols in the Lecture Outline indicate the points at which various exercises might be most appropriate. Other strategies can be used to preview the lesson or to summarize it.

The following strategies are keyed to specific sections of the lesson.

*1. **Brainstorming Occupational Injuries.*** To facilitate a discussion about prevention, have the class brainstorm common and possible occupational injuries associated with EMS. Next, assign two or three injuries to small work groups. Together, they can create prevention strategies and share them with the class. Excellent ideas could also be shared with local employers. This activity feels "real" to your adult learners who will need to be informed well enough to protect their own health as EMS professionals. Additionally, it improves oral communication skills.

*2. **X-rays.*** Few visuals will be as effective as X-rays for demonstrating dislocations and fractures. Borrow films from your local hospital, sports medicine clinic, physician's office, or rehabilitation center. When possible, ask for duplicate copies so that you can build your own radiograph library.

*3. **Chicken Bone Fracture Demonstration.*** Save chicken bones for demonstrating types of fractures. If you have enough bones, give several to each lab group with some basic tools such as a hammer and gloves. Instruct each group to attempt to create the fractures listed in the text: comminuted, impacted, greenstick, oblique, spiral, and transverse. By creating the injuries, students will gain a better understanding of the forces involved in each type of injury, as well as the kinetic energy required to create such an injury. This activity will appeal to your kinesthetic learners. It develops a deeper appreciation of the forces of trauma because the students will be creating the injury right before their own eyes.

The following strategies can be used at various points throughout the lesson or to help summarize and demonstrate what students have learned.

Clinical Time with Orthopedic Patients. Caring for patients with orthopedic injuries will help students understand the pain and disability associated with seemingly minor injuries. When caring for serious patients, providers tend to minimize their care of extremities to attend to the life threats. However, it is often the extremity injury that is most painful to the patient. Arrange for clinical time in orthopedic surgery, the orthopedic ward of the hospital, a sports medicine clinic, physical therapy office, or other venue specifically designed for the care of orthopedic patients. This clinical time will help students improve their handling techniques of orthopedic patients, as well as help them appreciate the long-term disability often associated with what we classify as "minor injuries."

Guest Speaker: Orthopedic Surgeon. Orthopedic surgeons are an excellent source of information and visual aids for this chapter. Invite an orthopedic surgeon to

HANDOUT 22-1
Chapter 22 Objectives Checklist

POINT TO EMPHASIZE
How strong are your bones? For its weight, bone is as strong as steel and four times stronger than the same amount of reinforced concrete.

TEACHING STRATEGY 1
Brainstorming Occupational Injuries

POINT TO EMPHASIZE
You have about 650 muscles, with over 50 muscles in the face alone. You use 17 muscles to smile but over 40 to frown.

TEACHING TIP
Have a lean, muscular student or model display and demonstrate the anatomy and physiology of the musculoskeletal system. This is much more interesting than showing slides or transparencies. If possible, use body paint to highlight certain muscles or areas.

TEACHING TIP
If you have a model skeleton, demonstrate contusions, strains, muscle cramps, muscle spasms, and penetrating muscle injury. Show how the range of motion is extended beyond normal.

POWERPOINT PRESENTATION
Chapter 22 PowerPoint slides 4–14

POINT OF INTEREST
The smallest bone in the body is the stirrup, which is located inside the ear. It is only 0.12 inch long and weighs about 0.0001 ounce. The largest bone is the femur.

TEACHING TIP
To show the wide range of motion of the upper extremities, demonstrate what a baseball pitcher does to throw a curveball. Break down each twist and turn of the shoulder, elbow, and wrist required to throw the pitch.

POWERPOINT PRESENTATION
Chapter 22 PowerPoint slides 15–19

---

class to discuss assessment and management of musculoskeletal injuries. Specifically ask the surgeon to discuss the following:

- The appropriateness of the use of the PASG for pelvic and lower extremity fractures.
- Which pain medications are appropriate for musculoskeletal injuries and why.
- The appropriateness of realigning a femoral fracture while pulling contaminated bone ends back into the injury site.
- The appropriateness of shoulder reductions for patients with long transport times and absent distal pulses.

Guest Speaker: ED Paramedic. Invite a local paramedic or emergency department physician to class to discuss challenging musculoskeletal injury cases they have dealt with. If a paramedic visits the class, ask him/her to discuss splinting challenges experienced.

Cultural Considerations, Legal Notes, and Patho Pearls. The Student CD-ROM contains this series of informative features to enhance the student's understanding of the material covered in this chapter.

TEACHING OUTLINE

Chapter 22, "Musculoskeletal Trauma," is the seventh lesson in Division 3, *Trauma Emergencies*. Distribute Handout 22-1 so that students can familiarize themselves with the learning goals for this chapter. If students have any questions about the objectives, answer them at this time.

Then present the chapter. One possible lecture outline follows. In the outline, the parenthetical references in regular type are references to text pages; those in bold type are references to figures, tables, or procedures.

I. Introduction. In trauma, musculoskeletal injury occurrences are second in frequency only to soft-tissue injuries. They are usually the result of significant direct or transmitted blunt kinetic forces. Mechanisms of injury include sports injuries, motor vehicle crashes, falls, and acts of violence. Injuries may cause damage to bones, cartilage, ligaments, muscles, or tendons. Upper extremity injuries are painful, but not usually life-threatening. Lower extremity injuries, however, are generally associated with a greater magnitude of force and greater secondary blood loss, and more often constitute threats to life or limb. Musculoskeletal injuries may also damage internal organs. (p. 925)

II. Prevention strategies (p. 926)

  A. Modern vehicle and highway designs (p. 926)
  B. Safe driving practices (p. 926)
  C. Workplace safety standards (p. 926)
  D. Protective athletic gear (p. 926)
  E. Household safety practices (p. 926)

III. Pathophysiology of the musculoskeletal system (pp. 926–933)

  A. Muscular injury (pp. 926–927)
     1. Contusion
     2. Compartment syndrome
     3. Penetrating injury

4. Fatigue
   5. Muscle cramp
   6. Muscle spasm
   7. Strain
 B. Joint injury (pp. 927–928)
   1. Sprain
   2. Subluxation
   3. Dislocation (Fig. 22-1, p. 928)
 C. Bone injury (pp. 928–931)
   1. Fractures (Fig. 22-3, p. 930)
      a. Open (Fig. 22-2, p. 929)
      b. Closed (Fig. 22-2, p. 929)
      c. Hairline
      d. Impacted
      e. Transverse
      f. Oblique
      g. Comminuted
      h. Spiral
      i. Fatigue
   2. Pediatric considerations
      a. Greenstick
      b. Epiphyseal
   3. Geriatric considerations
      a. Osteoporosis
   4. Pathological fractures
 D. General considerations with musculoskeletal injuries (pp. 931–932)
 E. Bone repair cycle (p. 932)
 F. Inflammatory and degenerative conditions (pp. 932–933)
   1. Bursitis
   2. Tendonitis
   3. Arthritis
      a. Osteoporosis
      b. Rheumatoid arthritis
      c. Gout

IV. **Musculoskeletal injury assessment** (pp. 933–938)
 A. Scene size-up (p. 933)
 B. Initial assessment (pp. 933–934) (Fig. 22-4, p. 934)
   1. Classification of patients with musculoskeletal injuries
      a. Life- and limb-threatening injuries
      b. Life-threatening injuries, minor musculoskeletal injuries
      c. Non-life-threatening injuries, serious limb-threatening injuries
      d. Non-life-threatening injuries, isolated minor musculoskeletal injuries
 C. Rapid trauma assessment (pp. 934–935)
 D. Focused history and physical exam (pp. 935–937) (Fig. 22-5, p. 935)
   1. Pain (Fig. 22-6, p. 936)
   2. Pallor
   3. Paralysis
   4. Paresthesia
   5. Pressure
   6. Pulses
 E. Detailed physical exam (p. 937)
 F. Ongoing assessment (p. 937)
 G. Sports injury considerations (pp. 937–938)

POINT OF INTEREST
The range of motion of a joint depends on the number and size of the ligaments surrounding the joint. The shoulder, having few ligaments, allows for a very wide range, while the pelvis, having many large ligaments, is restricted. People with very loose joints are sometimes referred to as being "double-jointed" because their range of motion is greater than that of the average person.

POINT OF INTEREST
Mechanical receptors are found in muscles, tendons, and ligaments. They are nerve cells that send messages to the brain when your joints are bent and your muscles are stretched. This means you always know the position of your arms and legs without having to look at them.

TEACHING STRATEGY 2
X-rays

TEACHING TIP
Bring in a fresh tree limb and a dry one. Then demonstrate the greenstick fracture and its splintering effect.

POINT TO EMPHASIZE
Size for size, the strongest muscle in your body is the masseter. One masseter is located on each side of the mouth. Working together, the masseters give the biting force of about 150 lbs.

POWERPOINT PRESENTATION
Chapter 22 PowerPoint slides 20–22

POINT OF INTEREST
Sprains and strains can be classified according to the severity of injury: first-degree—microscopic tears of tendon or ligament fibers; second-degree—partial tear of the ligament or tendon; third-degree—complete tear of the ligament or tendon.

POINT OF INTEREST
Some 90 percent of hip dislocations are posterior, usually with the patient having followed the down-and-under pathway during a frontal MVC.

TEACHING STRATEGY 3
Chicken Bone Fracture Demonstration

> **POWERPOINT**
> **PRESENTATION**
> Chapter 22 PowerPoint slides 23–44
>
> **SLIDES/VIDEOS**
> "Musculoskeletal Emergencies," *24-7 EMS*, First Quarter 2005.
>
> **POINT OF INTEREST**
> The most common ankle fracture is of the distal fibula.
>
> **? WHAT WOULD YOU DO**
> Your patient's knee has locked in a flexed position. He cannot straighten the leg and complains of a great deal of pain when he tries. What is the problem?
>
> **? WHAT WOULD YOU DO**
> Your elderly stroke patient cannot speak and cannot complain. She is lying on the floor. What should you check for? (Ask yourself: How did she get to the floor? Check her wrists for a Colles' fracture from trying to break her fall. It is very embarrassing to arrive at the hospital and have missed it.)
>
> **? WHAT WOULD YOU DO**
> Your patient has a badly dislocated elbow with no signs of circulation at the wrist. Do you attempt to align the limb or not? What are the dangers? What factors should be considered in the decision?
>
> **POINT TO EMPHASIZE**
> Whether you are immobilizing the finger or the entire body, the principles are identical: Align the bone ends with a rigid splint; immobilize the adjacent joints; perform distal neurovascular checks on all extremities before and after all splinting.
>
> **POWERPOINT**
> **PRESENTATION**
> Chapter 22 PowerPoint slide 45

V. Musculoskeletal injury management (pp. 938–955)

    A. General principles of musculoskeletal injury management (pp. 938–940)
        1. Protecting open wounds
        2. Positioning the limb (**Fig. 22-7, p. 939**)
        3. Immobilizing the injury
        4. Checking neurovascular function

    B. Splinting devices (pp. 940–942) (**Fig. 22-8, p. 941**)
        1. Rigid splints
        2. Formable splints (**Fig 22-9, p. 941**)
        3. Soft splints
        4. Traction splints (**Fig. 22-10, p. 943**)
        5. Other splinting aids

    C. Fracture care (pp. 942–944)
    D. Joint care (p. 944)
    E. Muscular and connective tissue care (pp. 944–945)
    F. Care for specific fractures (pp. 945–948)
        1. Pelvis (**Fig. 22-11, p. 945**)
        2. Femur (**Fig. 22-12, p. 946**)
        3. Tibia/fibula (**Fig. 22-13, p. 947**)
        4. Clavicle
        5. Humerus
        6. Radius/ulna (**Fig. 22-14, p. 948**)

    G. Care for specific joint injuries (pp. 948–952)
        1. Hip
        2. Knee (**Fig. 22-15, p. 949**)
        3. Ankle (**Fig. 22-16, p. 950**)
        4. Foot
        5. Shoulder
        6. Elbow (**Fig. 22-17, p. 951**)
        7. Wrist/hand
        8. Finger

    H. Connective and soft-tissue injuries (p. 952)
    I. Medications (pp. 953–954)
        1. Often used to relieve pain and to premedicate
        2. Sedatives/analgesics
            a. Nitrous oxide
            b. Diazepam
            c. Morphine
            d. Fentanyl
            e. Nalbuphine

    J. Other musculoskeletal injury considerations (pp. 954–955)
        1. Pediatric musculoskeletal injury
        2. Athletic musculoskeletal injuries
            a. Rest
            b. Ice
            c. Compress
            d. Elevate
        3. Patient refusals and referral
        4. Psychological support for the musculoskeletal injury patient

VI. Chapter summary (p. 955). Injuries to the bones, ligaments, tendons, and muscles of the extremities rarely threaten your patient's life. Major exceptions to this statement are pelvic and serious or bilateral femur fractures, in which associated hemorrhage can contribute significantly to hypovolemia and shock. In addition, serious musculoskeletal trauma suggests the possibility of other, life-threatening trauma and, in fact, occurs in about 80 percent of cases of major multisystem trauma. The presence of serious musculoskeletal trauma should increase your index of suspicion for other serious internal injuries.

Care for isolated musculoskeletal trauma is usually delayed until the ABCs and other patient life threats are stabilized. The goals of the care are to protect any open wounds, position affected limbs properly, immobilize the area of injury, and carefully monitor distal extremities to assure neurovascular function.

Pelvic and bilateral femur fractures are immobilized through application of the PASG. This device both provides splinting for the pelvis and upper portion of the lower extremity and helps control internal blood loss in the region. Manage other fractures by aligning the extremity with gentle traction and immobilizing it by splinting. In cases where you discover a loss of distal neurovascular function, move the extremity slightly to restore distal neurovascular function and then splint.

Joint injuries carry a greater risk of damage to distal circulation, sensation, and motor function. Splint these injuries as you find them unless there is distal neurovascular compromise. If that is the case, employ gentle manipulation to restore circulation, motor function, or sensation. If gentle manipulation is unsuccessful and transport is to be delayed, attempt reduction of dislocations for the hip, knee, ankle, shoulder, or finger as permitted by local protocol.

Care for injuries to connective and muscular tissues by immobilizing the area of injury in the position of function. Evaluate distal extremities for pulse, capillary refill, color, temperature, sensation, and motor function before, during, and after any immobilization or movement of a limb and provide frequent monitoring thereafter.

SKILLS DEMONSTRATION AND PRACTICE

Students can practice skills discussed in this chapter in the following settings.

Skills Lab: The following stations will be part of a larger trauma skills lab. Divide the class into as many groups as appropriate. Have the groups circulate through the stations. Monitor the groups to be sure all groups have a chance to practice each of the skills. You may wish to have other instructors or qualified paramedics assist students in these activities.

Station	Equipment Needed	Activities
Fixation Splinting	Assorted fixation splinting devices Handout 22-2 1 instructor	Have students practice fixation splinting on all extremities.
Traction Splinting	Traction splints Handout 22-3 1 instructor	Have students practice traction splinting.

Scenario Lab: The following stations will be part of a larger trauma scenario lab. Divide the class into teams. Have the teams circulate through the stations. Monitor the groups to be sure all groups have a chance to manage each of the cases and so that every student has the opportunity to be team leader. You may wish to have other instructors or qualified paramedics assist students in these activities.

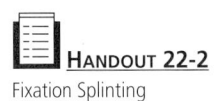

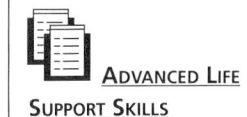

HANDOUT 22-2
Fixation Splinting

HANDOUT 22-3
Traction Splinting

ADVANCED LIFE SUPPORT SKILLS
Larmon & Davis. *Advanced Life Support Skills.*

ADVANCED LIFE SKILLS REVIEW
Larmon & Davis. *Advanced Life Skills Review.*

BRADY SKILLS SERIES: ALS
Larmon & Davis. *Brady Skills Series: ALS.*

Station	Equipment Needed	Activities
Isolated Femoral Fracture versus Bilateral Femoral Fracture with Shock	Traction splints PASG 1 patient 1 instructor	Have students practice assessing and managing patients with isolated femoral fractures versus bilateral femoral fractures with shock.
Multiple trauma	Long spine board Cervical immobilization devices Airway management kit Assorted splints PASG 1 patient 1 Instructor	Have students practice assessing and managing patients with various musculoskeletal injuries.

Hospital:
- Observe orthopedic surgery.
- Assist in assessment and management of orthopedic injuries in the ED.

Field Internship: Assist in assessment and management of orthopedic injuries in the field.

ASSIGNMENTS

Assign students to complete Chapter 22, "Musculoskeletal Trauma," of the workbook. Also assign them to read Chapter 23, "Head, Facial, and Neck Trauma," before the next class.

EVALUATION

Chapter Quiz and Scenario Distribute copies of the Chapter Quiz provided in Handout 22-4 to evaluate student understanding of this chapter. Make sure each student reads the scenario to reinforce critical thinking on the scene. Remind students not to use their notes or textbooks while taking the quiz.

Student CD Quizzes for every chapter are contained on the dynamic and highly visual in-text student CD.

Companion Website Additional quizzes for every chapter are contained on this exciting website.

TestGen You may wish to create a custom-tailored test using *Prentice Hall TestGen for Essentials of Paramedic Care*, 2nd Edition to evaluate student understanding of this chapter.

On-line Test Preparation (for students and instructors) Additional test preparation is available through Brady's new on-line product, *EMT Achieve: Paramedic Test Preparation* at *http://www.prenhall.com/emtachieve/*. Instructors can also monitor student mastery on-line.

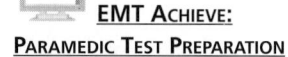

Review Manual for the EMT-Paramedic This comprehensive exam review contains hundreds of test questions and rationales, including scenarios, along with two 180-question practice tests on CD.

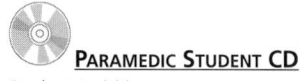

REINFORCEMENT

Handouts If classroom discussion or performance on the quiz indicates that some students have not fully mastered the chapter content, you may wish to assign some or all of the Reinforcement Handouts for this chapter.

Student CD (for students) A wide variety of material on this CD-ROM will reinforce and also expand student knowledge and skills.

PowerPoint Presentation (for instructors) The PowerPoint material developed for this chapter offers useful reinforcement of chapter content.

Companion Website (for students) Additional review quizzes and links to EMS resources will contribute to further reinforcement of the chapter.

OneKey On-line support is offered for this course on one of three platforms: CourseCompass, Blackboard, or Web CT. Includes the IRM, PowerPoints, TestGen, and Companion Website for instruction. Ask your local sales representative for more information.

Brady Skills Series: Advanced Life Skills (Video or CD) Have your students watch the skills come to life on VHS or CD-ROM, or they can purchase the highly visual, full-color text with step-by-step procedures and rationales.

HANDOUTS 22-6 TO 22-8
Reinforcement Activities

PARAMEDIC STUDENT CD
Student Activities

POWERPOINT PRESENTATION
Chapter 22

COMPANION WEBSITE
http://www.prenhall.com/bledsoe

ONEKEY
Chapter 22

ADVANCED LIFE SUPPORT SKILLS
Larmon & Davis. *Advanced Life Support Skills.*

ADVANCED LIFE SKILLS REVIEW
Larmon & Davis. *Advanced Life Skills Review.*

BRADY SKILLS SERIES: ALS
Larmon & Davis. *Brady Skills Series: ALS.*

PARAMEDIC NATIONAL STANDARDS SELF-TEST
Miller. *Paramedic National Standards Self-Test,* 4th edition.

Handout 22-1

Student's Name _____

CHAPTER 22 OBJECTIVES CHECKLIST

Knowledge	Date Mastered
1. Describe the incidence, morbidity, and mortality of musculoskeletal injuries.	
2. Discuss the anatomy and physiology of the muscular and skeletal systems.	
3. Predict injuries based on the mechanism of injury, including: • Direct • Indirect • Pathologic	
4. Discuss the types of musculoskeletal injuries, including: • Fractures (open and closed) • Dislocations/fractures • Sprains • Strains	
5. Describe the six "Ps" of musculoskeletal injury assessment.	
6. List the primary signs and symptoms of extremity trauma.	
7. List other signs and symptoms that can indicate less obvious extremity injury.	
8. Discuss the need for assessment of pulses, motor function, and sensation before and after splinting.	
9. Identify the circumstances requiring rapid intervention and transport when dealing with musculoskeletal injuries.	
10. Discuss the general guidelines for splinting.	
11. Explain the benefits of the application of cold and heat for musculoskeletal injuries.	
12. Describe age-associated changes in the bones.	
13. Discuss the pathophysiology, assessment findings, and management of open and closed fractures.	
14. Discuss the relationship between the volume of hemorrhage and open or closed fractures.	
15. Discuss the indications and contraindications for use of the pneumatic antishock garment (PASG) in the management of fractures.	

HANDOUT 22-1 Continued

Knowledge	Date Mastered
16. Describe the special considerations involved in femur fracture management.	
17. Discuss the pathophysiology, assessment findings, and management of dislocations.	
18. Discuss the out-of-hospital management of dislocations/fractures, including splinting and realignment.	
19. Explain the importance of manipulating a knee dislocation/fracture with an absent distal pulse.	
20. Describe the procedure for reduction of a shoulder, finger, or ankle dislocation/fracture.	
21. Discuss the pathophysiology, assessment findings, and management of sprains, strains, and tendon injuries.	
22. Differentiate among musculoskeletal injuries based on the assessment findings and history.	
23. Given several preprogrammed and moulaged musculoskeletal trauma patients, provide the appropriate scene size-up, initial assessment, rapid trauma or focused physical exam and history, detailed exam, and ongoing assessment and provide appropriate patient care and transportation.	

OBJECTIVES

HANDOUT 22-2

Student's Name _____

FIXATION SPLINTING

Charting Student Progress:
1. *Learning skill*
2. *Performs skill with direction*
3. *Performs skill independently*

Skill/Behavior	1	2	3
1. Takes BSI precautions.			
2. Directs application of manual stabilization.			
3. Assesses pulse, temperature, color, sensation, and capillary refill of distal extremity.			
4. Prepares splint.			
5. Applies splint.			
6. Immobilizes joint above and below the fracture site.			
7. Secures entire injured extremity.			
8. Reassesses pulse, temperature, color, sensation, and capillary refill.			

Comments:

Handout 22-3

Student's Name _____

TRACTION SPLINTING

Charting Student Progress:
1. *Learning skill*
2. *Performs skill with direction*
3. *Performs skill independently*

Skill/Behavior	1	2	3
1. Takes BSI precautions.			
2. Directs manual stabilization of injured leg.			
3. Assesses pulse, temperature, color, sensation, and capillary refill of distal extremity.			
4. Applies ankle hitch device.			
5. Directs application of manual traction.			
6. Prepares and adjusts splint to proper length.			
7. Positions splint at injured leg.			
8. Applies proximal securing device.			
9. Applies mechanical traction.			
10. Positions and secures supporting straps.			
11. Reassesses pulse, temperature, color, sensation, and capillary refill of distal extremity.			
12. Immobilizes hip joint on long board.			
13. Secures splint on long board.			

Comments:

HANDOUT 22-4

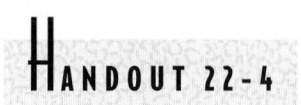

Student's Name _____

CHAPTER 22 QUIZ

Write the letter of the best answer in the space provided.

_____ 1. Fatigue, cramps, spasms, and strains are types of injuries to:
   A. tendons.
   B. muscles.
   C. ligaments.
   D. bones.

_____ 2. Severe trauma that crushes muscles between a blunt force and the skeletal structure beneath, resulting in damage to both the muscle cells and the blood vessels that supply them, is called:
   A. a muscle strain.
   B. compartment syndrome.
   C. contusion.
   D. concussion.

_____ 3. "Angina" of the muscle tissue is also known as muscle:
   A. sprain.
   B. strain.
   C. cramp.
   D. fatigue.

_____ 4. Grade I, Grade II, and Grade III are used to classify types of:
   A. fractures.
   B. strains.
   C. sprains.
   D. dislocations.

_____ 5. The complete displacement of a bone end from its position in a joint capsule is called a:
   A. fracture.
   B. strain.
   C. sprain.
   D. dislocation.

_____ 6. A fracture in which a bone is broken into several pieces is known as a(n):
   A. transverse fracture.
   B. comminuted fracture.
   C. oblique fracture.
   D. fatigue fracture.

_____ 7. A break in a bone involving a twisting motion may result in a(n):
   A. spiral fracture.
   B. oblique fracture.
   C. comminuted fracture.
   D. stress fracture.

_____ 8. Greenstick fractures are usually found in:
   A. elderly patients.
   B. patients with chronic medical conditions.
   C. pediatric patients.
   D. patients with bleeding disorders, such as hemophilia.

_____ 9. Internal bleeding from a femoral fracture may reach as much as _____ of blood loss.
   A. 250 mL
   B. 500 mL
   C. 1,000 mL
   D. 1,500 mL

_____ 10. The six "Ps" in evaluating a limb injury include:
   A. position.
   B. pallor.
   C. passivity.
   D. prognosis.

_____ 11. Evaluate the distal extremity for:
   A. pulse.
   B. color.
   C. sensation.
   D. all of these

_____ 12. A complication of musculoskeletal injury is compartment syndrome, caused by:
   A. air trapped in the muscle tissue of the chest wall resulting from a crushing injury.
   B. bleeding into, or edema within, a muscle mass surrounded by fasciae that do not stretch.
   C. a comminuted fracture causing multiple internal bleeding sites from sharp bone fragments.
   D. absence of blood supply, resulting in a buildup of carbon dioxide and waste products in the cells.

HANDOUT 22-4 Continued

_____ 13. General principles of musculoskeletal injury management include:
   A. not attempting to realign any dislocation.
   B. attempting to manipulate dislocations that are within 3 inches of a joint.
   C. considering manipulation of dislocations if distal circulation is compromised.
   D. not attempting to realign fractures of the midshaft femur, tibia/fibula, humerus, or radius/ulna.

_____ 14. The basics of musculoskeletal injury care include:
   A. pain medication.
   B. alignment of all fractures and dislocations.
   C. monitoring of neurovascular function.
   D. applying an elastic bandage to joint injuries.

_____ 15. Guidelines for immobilizing an injury include:
   A. immobilizing the bone above and the bone below the injury.
   B. immobilizing the joint above and the joint below the injury.
   C. application of traction to the injury prior to immobilization.
   D. all of these

_____ 16. It is necessary to check pulses, motor function, and sensation in the distal extremity:
   A. prior to splinting.   C. during splinting.
   B. after splinting.   D. all of these

_____ 17. Traction splints are applied to injuries to the:
   A. humerus.   C. tibia/fibula.
   B. femur.   D. cervical spine.

_____ 18. An injury closer than 3 inches from a joint should be considered, and treated as, a:
   A. strain.   C. joint injury.
   B. sprain.   D. fracture.

_____ 19. The PASG may be used as a soft splint for:
   A. femoral fractures.   C. hip dislocations.
   B. pelvic fractures.   D. tibial/fibular fractures.

_____ 20. A fractured humerus is best immobilized using a:
   A. cardboard splint.   C. sling and swathe.
   B. traction splint.   D. vacuum splint.

_____ 21. Angulated knee dislocations can be immobilized with:
   A. the PASG.   C. two padded board splints.
   B. a traction splint.   D. a full-leg air splint.

_____ 22. The best choice for immobilizing a possible ankle dislocation injury is a(n):
   A. traction splint.   C. elastic bandage.
   B. padded board splint.   D. pillow.

_____ 23. Contraindications to the use of nitrous oxide as an analgesic include:
   A. pregnancy.   C. age less than 8 years.
   B. pneumothorax.   D. cardiac history.

_____ 24. All of the following are advantages of Fentanyl EXCEPT:
   A. more rapid onset of action than morphine.
   B. considerably less potent than morphine.
   C. does not cause hypotension to the same degree as morphine.
   D. considerably more potent than morphine.

_____ 25. The RICE procedure for strains, sprains, and soft-tissue injuries includes:
   A. reposition.   C. cold.
   B. ice.   D. examination.

Handout 22-5

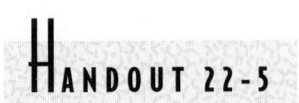

Student's Name _____

CHAPTER 22 SCENARIO

Review the following real-life situation. Then answer the questions that follow.

Nathan rounds first base on the way to second. He knows he'll need to run faster if he is to beat the throw from the center fielder to second. He runs a little harder and decides to slide into second. As he begins his slide, the cleat in his right shoe digs into the earth and his right ankle suddenly twists. He feels intense pain, but he's safe at second base.

    Paramedics George and Elizabeth are on standby at the Placerville Little League baseball game. They both saw Nathan twist his ankle and now see him sitting down, unable to move. The umpire calls time-out and motions for the paramedics to come onto the field to assess Nathan. You and your partner grab the stretcher and several different splints and head toward Nathan.

1. What types of musculoskeletal injuries could Nathan have sustained?

2. What are three types of splints you might bring to manage Nathan's injury?

You arrive to find Nathan clutching his right ankle. You complete your initial assessment.

3. What steps would you take to perform a musculoskeletal assessment of a lower extremity?

You note that Nathan's foot has good distal pulses and sensation, but there is swelling, some deformity, and warmth to the medial ankle.

4. What steps would you take to manage Nathan's injury?

Handout 22-6

Student's Name _____

CHAPTER 22 REVIEW

Write the word or words that best complete the following sentences in the space provided.

1. About _____ percent of patients who suffer multisystem trauma experience significant musculoskeletal injuries.

2. The types of muscular injuries are contusion, _____ syndrome, _____ injury, muscle _____, muscle _____, muscle _____, and muscle _____.

3. Muscle _____ occurs as the muscles reach their limit of performance.

4. A minor and incomplete capsule tear is called a Grade _____ sprain; significant but incomplete tear is a Grade _____; complete tear is a Grade _____.

5. The complete displacement of a bone end from its position in a joint capsule is called a(n) _____.

6. A broken bone in which the bone ends or the forces that caused the fracture do not penetrate the skin is called a(n) _____ fracture. A broken bone in which the bone ends or the forces that caused it penetrate the surrounding skin is called a(n) _____ fracture.

7. A fracture in which the bone is broken into several pieces is a(n) _____ fracture.

8. Softening of bone tissue due to loss of essential minerals, especially calcium, is known as _____.

9. A partial fracture of a child's bone is known as a(n) _____ fracture.

10. A pelvic fracture may account for hemorrhage of more than _____ liters.

11. A femoral fracture may account for as much as _____ mL of blood loss.

12. The six "Ps" in evaluating limb injury are _____, _____, _____, _____, _____, and _____.

13. Evaluate the distal extremity for _____, _____, _____, _____, and _____ refill.

14. _____ syndrome results from bleeding into, or edema within, a muscle mass surrounded by fasciae that do not stretch.

15. The basics of musculoskeletal injury care include protecting _____ wounds, proper _____, _____, and monitoring of _____ function.

16. Do not attempt alignment of dislocations and serious injuries within _____ inches of a joint.

17. The traction splint is used for care of the isolated traumatic _____ fracture.

18. When splinting a fracture, immobilize the joint _____ and _____ the injury site.

19. Begin fracture care by assuring distal _____, _____, and _____ function.

20. The PASG is an effective splint for traumatic _____ fractures and helps control internal _____.

21. The most effective splinting technique for a humeral fracture is to apply a(n) _____ and a(n) _____ to immobilize the bent limb.

22. A(n) _____ splint can be used with injuries to the ankles and feet.

23. _____ _____ is an analgesic used in a gaseous state.

24. _____ is an opiate narcotic, chemically unrelated to morphine, that provides immediate and effective pain control.

25. Recent studies have questioned the effectiveness of _____ as a prehospital analgesic, and it has fallen into relative disuse.

©2007 Pearson Education, Inc.
Essentials of Paramedic Care, 2nd ed.

Handout 22-7

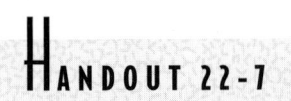

Student's Name _____

MUSCULOSKELETAL TRUE OR FALSE

Indicate whether the following statements are true or false by writing T or F in the space provided.

_____ 1. A dislocation is a displacement of bones from a joint.

_____ 2. The chance of blood vessel damage is much greater with long bone fractures than with injuries to the joint.

_____ 3. Pelvic fractures, though painful, seldom result in loss of circulation to the lower extremities.

_____ 4. A hip fracture will sometimes present with a lateral rotation of the foot and knee.

_____ 5. Fractures of the humerus, pelvis, and femur seldom contribute to hypovolemia.

_____ 6. Dislocations of the knee are only rarely accompanied by fractures at the same injury site.

_____ 7. Treat any fracture within 3 inches of the knee as you would a dislocation.

_____ 8. The fibula is more likely to fracture than the tibia in cases of lower-leg fracture.

_____ 9. With an unstable trauma patient, all fractures should be splinted prior to transport.

_____ 10. If distal pulses are absent due to a fractured elbow, gently manipulate the limb until a pulse returns.

_____ 11. Compartment syndrome occurs most often in hip dislocations.

_____ 12. You should immobilize a hand injury in the position of comfort.

_____ 13. A greenstick fracture disrupts only one side of a long bone.

_____ 14. Knee dislocations normally present with the knee at an angle and firmly fixed in place.

_____ 15. An anterior shoulder displacement presents with a prominent shoulder and with the arm close to the chest.

HANDOUT 22-8

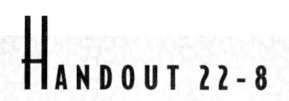

Student's Name _____

MANAGING MUSCULOSKELETAL INJURIES

1. Circle all of the following that are signs and symptoms of knee dislocation/fracture.
   A. Angulated knee, firmly fixed in place
   B. Deformity
   C. Discoloration
   D. Usually painless
   E. Pain
   F. Warmth or coolness
   G. Pain-free while attempting to move injury site

2. Circle all of the following that apply to the appropriate management of a pelvic fracture.
   A. Use of the PASG
   B. Naloxone for pain relief
   C. Nitronox for pain relief
   D. Morphine sulfate for pain relief
   E. Establishment of two large-bore IVs run TKO for hemodynamically stable patients
   F. Administration of oxygen
   G. Use of the traction splint
   H. Use of the vacuum splint
   I. Psychological support

3. Describe how you would manage a hemodynamically stable patient with an open femoral fracture and exposed bone ends.

4. Your patient has a dislocated elbow with absent distal pulses. Describe how you would immobilize the patient.

5. Describe how you would manage the patient with a knee dislocation in which you are not able to regain a distal pulse.

Chapter 22 Answer Key

Handout 22-4: Chapter 22 Quiz

1. B	8. C	15. B	22. D
2. C	9. D	16. D	23. B
3. C	10. B	17. B	24. B
4. C	11. D	18. C	25. B
5. D	12. B	19. B	
6. B	13. C	20. C	
7. A	14. C	21. C	

Handout 22-5: Chapter 22 Scenario

1. Possible injuries include ankle sprain, dislocation, tibial and fibular fracture, knee dislocation/fracture, and foot/ankle fracture.
2. Types of splints include full-leg air splint, pillow splint, and vacuum splint.
3. Put on disposable gloves. Gently expose the injury site. Avoid manipulation of the injury site. Look for deformity, discoloration, or other signs of injury. Question the patient about pain and the ability to move. Palpate for instability, deformity, crepitation. Feel for unusual warmth or coolness over the entire lateral and medial surfaces, then the anterior and posterior surfaces. Assess for presence or absence of distal pedal pulses bilaterally. Check skin for blanching. Evaluate sensation distal to injury site.
4. Administer oxygen, if needed. Apply either a vacuum, air, or pillow splint. Check for distal pulses, motor function, and sensation before and after the splinting. Apply cold packs to the injury site. Elevate the extremity and transport.

Handout 22-6: Chapter 22 Review

1. 80
2. compartment, penetrating, fatigue, cramp, spasm, strain
3. fatigue
4. I, II, III
5. dislocation
6. closed, open
7. comminuted
8. osteoporosis
9. greenstick
10. 2
11. 1,500
12. pain, pallor, paralysis, paresthesia, pressure, pulses
13. pulse, temperature, color, sensation, capillary
14. Compartment
15. open, positioning, immobilization, neurovascular
16. 3
17. femur
18. above, below
19. pulses, sensation, motor
20. pelvic, hemorrhage
21. sling, swathe
22. pillow
23. Nitrous oxide
24. Fentanyl
25. nalbuphine

Handout 22-7: Musculoskeletal True or False

1. T	5. F	9. F	13. T
2. F	6. F	10. T	14. T
3. F	7. T	11. F	15. T
4. T	8. F	12. F	

Handout 22-8: Managing Musculoskeletal Injuries

1. A, B, C, E, F
2. A, C, D, E, F, I
3. Administer oxygen; apply distal traction; irrigate exposed bone ends with normal saline; cover injury with a moist dressing; apply traction splint; place patient on a long spine board and start two large-bore IVs en route. Give pain medications according to local protocols (Nitrox, MS, and so on).
4. Gently move the limb while palpating for the return of a distal pulse. Then apply a vacuum, air, or padded board splint.
5. If you cannot regain a distal pulse after gentle movement of the extremity, then splint and transport without delay.

Chapter 23

Head, Facial, and Neck Trauma

INTRODUCTION

Head, facial, and neck injuries are common with major trauma. Head injury is the most frequent cause of trauma death. The signs and symptoms of head injuries are often difficult to recognize in the prehospital setting. As a result, subtle and unforeseen problems associated with injuries to the head, face, and neck too often cause the patient to quietly deteriorate while caregivers direct attention toward more obvious injuries. To lessen the chances of death and disability, the paramedic must learn to recognize the signs and symptoms of these injuries early in the patient assessment, to maintain a clear airway, adequate respirations, and the patient's blood pressure and to provide rapid transport to an appropriate facility. This chapter will consider injuries to the head, the facial region, and the neck.

TOTAL TEACHING TIME: 7.51 HOURS
The total teaching time is only a guideline based on the didactic and practical lab averages in the National Standard Curriculum. Instructors should take into consideration such factors as the pace at which students learn, the size of the class, and breaks. The actual time devoted to teaching objectives is the responsibility of the instructor.

CHAPTER OBJECTIVES

After reading this chapter, you should be able to:

1. Describe the incidence, morbidity, and mortality of head, facial, and neck injuries. (pp. 959–960)
2. Explain head and facial anatomy and physiology. (see Chapter 3)
3. Differentiate between the following types of facial injuries, highlighting the defining characteristics of each:
   - Eye (pp. 975–977)
   - Ear (pp. 974–975)
   - Nose (pp. 973–974)
   - Throat (pp. 977–978)
   - Mouth (p. 973)
4. Predict head, facial, and other related injuries based on mechanism of injury. (pp. 960–961)
5. Differentiate between facial injuries based on the assessment and history. (pp. 972–977)
6. Explain the pathophysiology, assessment, and management for patients with eye, ear, nose, throat, and mouth injuries. (pp. 972–997)
7. Explain anatomy and relate physiology of the CNS to head injuries. (pp. 966–972)

©2007 Pearson Education, Inc.
Essentials of Paramedic Care, 2nd ed.

8. Distinguish between facial, head, and brain injuries. (pp. 961–977)
9. Explain the pathophysiology of head/brain injuries. (pp. 960–972)
10. Explain the concept of increasing intracranial pressure (ICP). (pp. 969–970)
11. Explain the effect of increased and decreased carbon dioxide on ICP. (pp. 969–970)
12. Define and explain the process involved with each of the levels of increasing ICP. (pp. 969–970)
13. Relate assessment findings associated with head/brain injuries to the pathophysiologic process. (pp. 961–972)
14. Classify head injuries (mild, moderate, severe) according to assessment findings. (pp. 966–970)
15. Identify the need for rapid intervention and transport of the patient with a head/brain injury. (pp. 978, 984)
16. Describe and explain the general management of the head/brain injury patient, including pharmacological and nonpharmacological treatment. (pp. 985–996)
17. Analyze the relationship between carbon dioxide concentration in the blood and management of the airway in the head/brain-injured patient. (pp. 969–970)
18. Explain the pathophysiology, assessment, and management of a patient with:
    - Scalp injury (pp. 961–962, 980–981, 985–996)
    - Skull fracture (pp. 962–965, 980–981, 985–996)
    - Cerebral contusion (pp. 966–967, 985–996)
    - Intracranial hemorrhage (including epidural, subdural, subarachnoid, and intracerebral hemorrhage) (pp. 967–968, 985–996)
    - Axonal injury (including concussion and moderate and severe diffuse axonal injury) (pp. 968, 985–996)
    - Facial injury (pp. 972–977, 985–996)
    - Neck injury (pp. 977–978, 982, 985–996)
19. Develop a management plan for the removal of a helmet for a head-injured patient. (p. 979)
20. Differentiate between the types of head/brain injuries based on the assessment and history. (pp. 960–985)
21. Given several preprogrammed and moulaged head, face, and neck trauma patients, provide the appropriate scene size-up, initial assessment, rapid trauma or focused physical exam and history, detailed exam, and ongoing assessment and provide appropriate patient care and transportation. (pp. 959–997)

FRAMING THE LESSON

Begin by reviewing the important points of Chapter 22, "Musculoskeletal Trauma." Use this time to answer any questions about the previous chapter and to discuss any items not completely understood by students. Then begin the discussion of Chapter 23.

Discuss with students not only the deaths caused by injuries to the head and neck, but also the disability associated with these injuries. Discuss the importance of the recognition of injuries to these areas, stressing that treatment for such injuries may be based solely on mechanism of injury and a high index of suspicion. Review the anatomy of the head, face, and neck, paying special attention to the many major components found in this area, such as the brain and spinal cord, airway, and major blood vessels. An anatomical model or chart is helpful in visualizing this area of the body. Photos and X-rays of actual patients graphically illustrate injuries. This is also a good time to review basic immobilization equipment and skills.

TEACHING STRATEGIES

People learn in a variety of ways. Some do better with the spoken word, whereas others prefer the written. Some prefer to work alone, whereas others profit from working in groups. Recognizing these different ways of acquiring knowledge, the authors of this *Instructor's Resource Manual* have provided a variety of teaching strategies for the different types of learners. These strategies are intended to foster higher-level cognitive skills and encourage creative learning and problem solving. For greatest effectiveness, incorporate these strategies into your class lecture. Symbols in the Lecture Outline indicate the points at which various exercises might be most appropriate. Other strategies can be used to preview the lesson or to summarize it.

The following strategies are keyed to specific sections of the lesson.

1. Apples to Demonstrate Scalp Injury. An apple can be used to illustrate the types of scalp injuries described in the book. The juice of the apple will usually fill bruised or depressed areas of injury to the fruit. The skin can be fractured or pulled back like an avulsion. And certainly bruises to the flesh itself resemble scalp contusions. Pass around an apple or two labeled with each type of injury inflicted upon the apple for students to see and feel.

2. Immobilization Practice. Have students break into teams of four and practice spinal immobilization. Students should immobilize patients found standing, sitting, prone, and in supine positions. To make the drill more realistic, try adding all or a few of the following to the practice session:

- Ask other students to act as concerned bystanders.
- Set the room up so that it is dark, and ask students to use penlights and flashlights during patient assessment and treatment.
- Play a tape recording of siren sounds, radio transmissions, honking horns, and so on to simulate an actual call.
- Ask one student to pretend to be a physician who offers on-scene assistance.
- Practice removal of patients from as many different types of vehicles as possible.
- Have groups of students intentionally immobilize spinal cord injury patients the wrong way. Then ask the class as a whole to identify the improper immobilization procedures.

The following strategies can be used at various points throughout the lesson or to help summarize and demonstrate what students have learned.

Brain Injury Public Education. Direct students toward brain injury associations in gathering information on brain injury. (The same can be done for spinal cord injury.) Have them create a public education tool for some section of the population such as kids, elderly, high school students, and so on. Using the literature from national organizations, have them create a meaningful flyer, handout, video, or other educational medium and deliver the information to the intended audience. Schools usually welcome safety information, and community service is the backbone of the public service professions such as EMS and firefighting. Additionally, the demonstration will improve public speaking skills and later help with patient education.

Clinical Time in a Brain Injury Rehab Center. The profound, often permanent disability associated with brain injury will surprise some students. For many students who still feel immortal in this job, the reality of brain injury will be sobering. Clinical time in a brain injury rehabilitation center is extremely valuable. In one or two shifts the student will be exposed to issues of long-term care beyond the brain injury itself. These issues include such things as toileting and feeding, difficulties with speech and communication, problems with ambulation, bed sores, stress and boredom, the cost of care, and the social impact on families affected by brain injury. This type of affective yet clinical activity builds understanding and compassion that is likely to transfer directly to your students' patient care.

Guest Speaker: Neurologist or Radiologist. Invite a neurologist or radiologist to talk to your class about spinal cord and head injuries. Ask the neurologist or radiologist to present the information in a case-review format.

Guest Speaker: Rehabilitation Specialist. Invite a rehabilitation specialist to talk to your class about the importance of effective spinal immobilization and care of the head injury patient. If possible, ask the rehabilitation specialist to invite a patient to the class to discuss what it's like to live with a spinal cord or head injury.

Cultural Considerations, Legal Notes, and Patho Pearls. The student CD-ROM contains this series of informative features to enhance the student's understanding of the material covered in this chapter.

TEACHING OUTLINE

Chapter 23, "Head, Facial, and Neck Trauma," is the eighth lesson in Division 3, *Trauma Emergencies*. Distribute Handout 23-1 so that students can familiarize themselves with the learning goals for this chapter. If students have any questions about the objectives, answer them at this time.

Then present the chapter. One possible lecture outline follows. In the outline, the parenthetical references in regular type are references to text pages; those in bold type are references to figures, tables, or procedures.

I. Introduction. Approximately 4 million people experience significant head impact each year, with 1 in 10 requiring hospitalization. Head, facial, and neck injuries are common with major trauma. Head injuries are the most frequent cause of trauma death. Significant injuries include gunshot wounds and motor vehicle crashes. The severity of head, facial, and neck injuries is often difficult to recognize in the prehospital setting. To lessen the chances of death and disability, paramedics must learn to recognize the signs and symptoms of these injuries. Providing rapid transport to an appropriate facility and maintaining a clear airway, adequate respirations, and blood pressure are vital. (pp. 959–960)

II. Pathophysiology of head, facial, and neck injury (pp. 960–978)

    A. Mechanisms of injury (pp. 960–961)
        1. Blunt injury (**Fig. 23-1, p. 960**)
        2. Penetrating injury
    B. Head injury (pp. 961–972)
        1. Scalp injury (**Fig. 23-2, p. 962; Fig 23-3, p. 963**)
        2. Cranial injury (**Fig. 23-4, p. 964; Fig. 23-5, p. 965; Fig. 23-6, p. 965**)
        3. Brain injury

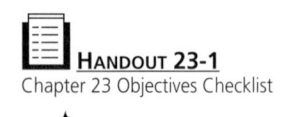

HANDOUT 23-1
Chapter 23 Objectives Checklist

TEACHING TIP
The skull is thick except in the temporal region. Bring in a skull and emphasize that the index of suspicion for blows to the side of the head should be high.

POWERPOINT PRESENTATION
Chapter 23 PowerPoint slides 4–60

POINT TO EMPHASIZE
How many times have you arrived on the scene to meet someone who looks like he has just come from the make-up room for the next Halloween movie to find only a small scalp laceration? Why do scalp lacerations seem to bleed so profusely?

POWERPOINT PRESENTATION
Chapter 23 PowerPoint slides 61–101

TEACHING STRATEGY 1
Apples to Demonstrate Scalp Injury

POINT OF INTEREST
The classic elements in traffic fatality with head injury include a single car, high speed, a head-on collision on a dark rural road, and a young, intoxicated driver. The greatest number of spinal cord injuries occurs among males age 16 to 20.

- a. Direct injury
    - i. Coup injury (**Fig. 23-7, p. 966**)
    - ii. Contrecoup injury
    - iii. Focal injuries
- b. Cerebral contusion
- c. Intracranial hemorrhage
    - i. Epidural hematoma (**Fig. 23-8, p. 967**)
    - ii. Subdural hematoma (**Fig. 23-9, p. 967**)
    - iii. Intracerebral hemorrhage
    - iv. Diffuse injury
- d. Concussion
- e. Moderate diffuse axonal injury
- f. Severe diffuse axonal injury
- g. Indirect injury
- h. Intracranial perfusion (**Fig. 23-10, p. 969**)
- i. Pressure and structural displacement
4. Signs and symptoms of brain injury (**Fig. 23-11, p. 971**)
    - a. Retrograde amnesia
    - b. Anterograde amnesia
    - c. Cheyne-Stokes respirations
    - d. Cushing's triad
5. Recognition of herniation
6. Pediatric head trauma
7. Glasgow Coma Scale
8. Eye signs

C. Facial injury (pp. 972–977)
1. Facial soft-tissue injury
2. Facial dislocations and fractures (**Fig. 23-12, p. 974**)
3. Nasal injury
4. Ear injury (**Fig. 23-13, p. 975**)
5. Eye injury (**Figs. 23-14 and 23-15, p. 976**)

D. Neck injury (pp. 977–978)
1. Blood vessel trauma (**Fig. 23-16, p. 977**)
2. Airway trauma
3. Cervical spine trauma
4. Other neck trauma

III. Assessment of head, facial, and neck injuries (pp. 978–985)

A. Scene size-up (p. 978)
B. Initial assessment (pp. 979–980) (**Fig. 23-17, p. 979**)
1. Airway
2. Breathing
3. Circulation
C. Rapid trauma assessment (pp. 980–984)
1. Head (**Fig. 23-18, p. 981**)
2. Face (**Fig. 23-19, p. 981**)
3. Neck
4. Glasgow Coma Scale score (**Tables 23-1 and 23-2, p. 983**)
5. Vital signs
D. Focused history and physical exam (p. 984)
E. Detailed assessment (p. 985)
F. Ongoing assessment (p. 985)

IV. Head, facial, and neck injury management (pp. 985–997)

A. Airway (pp. 985–990)
1. Suctioning

POINT TO EMPHASIZE
If the patient with a subdural hematoma is comatose, mortality is 60 to 90 percent.

POINT OF INTEREST
Often the patient with CSF in the mouth complains of a "salty" taste.

POINT TO EMPHASIZE
Cervical spine injuries are present in approximately 1 to 2 percent of all blunt trauma patients and in 5 to 10 percent of patients with head trauma.

POINT TO EMPHASIZE
The classic case of epidural hematoma is a blow to the side of the head with a brief loss of consciousness, followed by a lucid interval, followed by a decreasing level of consciousness.

POINT TO EMPHASIZE
Your patient can feel his legs but cannot move them. What may be wrong?

POINT OF INTEREST
Recreational road bicycling is increasing in popularity, particularly among adults 40 to 60 years old. During a collision, recreational bicyclists can and do suffer head and brain injuries, even when wearing ANSI- or SNELL-approved cycling helmets. Look on the outside of the victim's helmet for a medical symbol. If there is such a symbol, the victim's identification and medical and insurance information may be found in a folded packet stuck between the helmet's vent holes or inside the helmet.

POWERPOINT PRESENTATION
Chapter 23 PowerPoint slides 102–106

READING/REFERENCE
Cross, E. "Glasgow Coma Scale Score and Head Injury." *JEMS*, Sep. 2004.

POINT TO EMPHASIZE
The decision to immobilize the victim can be made by the mechanism of injury alone. Absence of clinical findings (pain) does not rule out significant spinal injuries, even in the ambulatory patient.

POWERPOINT PRESENTATION
Chapter 23 PowerPoint slides 107–126

> **POINT TO EMPHASIZE**
> C-1 got its name from Atlas, a character from Greek mythology, who was punished by the gods and forced to hold up the pillars separating Heaven from Earth.

> **TEACHING STRATEGY 2**
> Immobilization Practice

  2. Patient positioning
  3. Oropharyngeal and nasopharyngeal airways
  4. Endotracheal intubation (**Fig. 23-20, p. 987**)
   a. Orotracheal intubation
   b. Digital intubation
   c. Nasotracheal intubation
   d. Retrograde intubation
   e. Directed intubation
   f. Rapid-sequence intubation
   g. Confirmation of tube placement
  5. Cricothyrotomy (**Fig. 23-21, p. 990**)
 B. Breathing (p. 990)
  1. Oxygen
  2. Ventilations
 C. Circulation (p. 991)
  1. Hemorrhage control
  2. Blood pressure maintenance
 D. Hypoxia (p. 991)
 E. Hypovolemia (p. 992)
 F. Medications (pp. 992–995)
  1. Oxygen
  2. Diuretics
   a. Furosemide
  3. Paralytics
   a. Succinylcholine
   b. Atracurium and vecuronium
  4. Sedatives
   a. Diazepam
   b. Etomidate (Amidate)
   c. Midazolam
   d. Morphine
   e. Fentanyl
  5. Atropine
  6. Dextrose
  7. Thiamine
  8. Topical anesthetic spray
 G. Transport considerations (p. 995)
 H. Emotional support (pp. 995–996)
 I. Special injury care (pp. 996–997)
  1. Scalp avulsion
  2. Pinna injury
  3. Eye injury (**Fig. 23-22, p. 997**)
  4. Dislodged teeth
  5. Impaled objects

> **POWERPOINT PRESENTATION**
> Chapter 23 PowerPoint slide 127

V. Chapter summary (p. 998). The head, face, and neck contain very special and important structures—key elements of the central nervous system, the airway, the alimentary canal, and major organs of sensation. Serious trauma to the region endangers these structures and demands special assessment and care. During the scene size-up, identify possible mechanisms of injury and the injuries they suggest. Confirm the injuries during the initial and rapid trauma assessments. Identify your patient's level of consciousness and orientation early, and watch the eyes carefully for signs of cerebral hypoxia and increasing intracranial pressure. Assure that the spine is immobilized and the airway is clear and protected from aspiration and physical obstruction. Administer high-flow, high-concentration oxygen and ventilate, as necessary, being careful not to under- or overventilate the patient. Secure rapid transport for the patient with possible intracranial hemorrhage or serious lesion. Once the central nervous system, the airway, and breathing are protected, address skeletal structure fractures, minor bleeding, and open wounds. During all your care for the patient with injury to the head, face, or neck, provide emotional support.

ASSIGNMENTS

Assign students to complete Chapter 23, "Head, Facial, and Neck Trauma," of the workbook. Also assign them to read Chapter 24, "Spinal Trauma," before the next class.

EVALUATION

Chapter Quiz and Scenario Distribute copies of the Chapter Quiz provided in Handout 23-2 to evaluate student understanding of this chapter. Make sure each student reads the scenario to reinforce critical thinking on the scene. Remind students not to use their notes or textbooks while taking the quiz.

Student CD Quizzes for every chapter are contained on the dynamic and highly visual in-text student CD.

Companion Website Additional quizzes for every chapter are contained on this exciting website.

TestGen You may wish to create a custom-tailored test using *Prentice Hall TestGen for Essentials of Paramedic Care*, 2nd Edition to evaluate student understanding of this chapter.

On-line Test Preparation (for students and instructors) Additional test preparation is available through Brady's new on-line product, *EMT Achieve: Paramedic Test Preparation* at *http://www.prenhall.com/emtachieve/*. Instructors can also monitor student mastery on-line.

Review Manual for the EMT-Paramedic This comprehensive exam review contains hundreds of test questions and rationales, including scenarios, along with two 180-question practice tests on CD.

REINFORCEMENT

Handouts If classroom discussion or performance on the quiz indicates that some students have not fully mastered the chapter content, you may wish to assign some or all of the Reinforcement Handouts for this chapter.

Student CD (for students) A wide variety of material on this CD-ROM will reinforce and also expand student knowledge and skills.

PowerPoint Presentation (for instructors) The PowerPoint material developed for this chapter offers useful reinforcement of chapter content.

Companion Website (for students) Additional review quizzes and links to EMS resources will contribute to further reinforcement of the chapter.

WORKBOOK
Chapter 23 Activities

READING/REFERENCE
Textbook, pp. 1000–1029

HANDOUT 23-2
Chapter 23 Quiz

HANDOUT 23-3
Chapter 23 Scenario

PARAMEDIC STUDENT CD
Student Activities

COMPANION WEBSITE
http://www.prenhall.com/bledsoe

TESTGEN
Chapter 23

EMT ACHIEVE: PARAMEDIC TEST PREPARATION
Mistovich & Beasley. *EMT Achieve: Paramedic Test Preparation.*
www.prenhall.com/emtachieve/

REVIEW MANUAL FOR THE EMT-PARAMEDIC
Cherry & Mistovich. *Review Manual for the EMT-Paramedic,* 3rd edition.

HANDOUTS 23-4 AND 23-5
Reinforcement Activities

PARAMEDIC STUDENT CD
Student Activities

POWERPOINT PRESENTATION
Chapter 23

COMPANION WEBSITE
http://www.prenhall.com/bledsoe

OneKey
Chapter 23

ADVANCED LIFE SUPPORT SKILLS
Larmon & Davis. *Advanced Life Support Skills.*

ADVANCED LIFE SKILLS REVIEW
Larmon & Davis. *Advanced Life Skills Review.*

BRADY SKILLS SERIES: ALS
Larmon & Davis. *Brady Skills Series: ALS.*

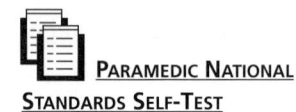

PARAMEDIC NATIONAL STANDARDS SELF-TEST
Miller. *Paramedic National Standards Self-Test,* 4th edition.

OneKey On-line support is offered for this course on one of three platforms: CourseCompass, Blackboard, or Web CT. Includes the IRM, PowerPoints, TestGen, and Companion Website for instruction. Ask your local sales representative for more information.

Brady Skills Series: Advanced Life Skills (Video or CD) Have your students watch the skills come to life on VHS or CD-ROM, or they can purchase the highly visual, full-color text with step-by-step procedures and rationales.

HANDOUT 23-1

Student's Name _____

CHAPTER 23 OBJECTIVES CHECKLIST

Knowledge	Date Mastered
1. Describe the incidence, morbidity, and mortality of head, facial, and neck injuries.	
2. Explain head and facial anatomy and physiology.	
3. Differentiate between the following types of facial injuries, highlighting the defining characteristics of each: • Eye • Ear • Nose • Throat • Mouth	
4. Predict head, facial, and other related injuries based on mechanism of injury.	
5. Differentiate between facial injuries based on the assessment and history.	
6. Explain the pathophysiology, assessment, and management for patients with eye, ear, nose, throat, and mouth injuries.	
7. Explain the anatomy and relate the physiology of the CNS to head injuries.	
8. Distinguish between facial, head, and brain injuries.	
9. Explain the pathophysiology of head/brain injuries.	
10. Explain the concept of increasing intracranial pressure (ICP).	
11. Explain the effect of increased and decreased carbon dioxide on ICP.	
12. Define and explain the process involved with each of the levels of increasing ICP.	
13. Relate assessment findings associated with head/brain injuries to the pathophysiologic process.	
14. Classify head injuries (mild, moderate, severe) according to assessment findings.	
15. Identify the need for rapid intervention and transport of the patient with a head/brain injury.	

HANDOUT 23-1 Continued

Knowledge	Date Mastered
16. Describe and explain the general management of the head/brain injury patient, including pharmacological and nonpharmacological treatment.	
17. Analyze the relationship between carbon dioxide concentration in the blood and management of the airway in the head/brain-injured patient.	
18. Explain the pathophysiology, assessment, and management of a patient with: • Scalp injury • Skull fracture • Cerebral contusion • Intracranial hemorrhage (including epidural, subdural, subarachnoid, and intracerebral hemorrhage) • Axonal injury (including concussion and moderate and severe diffuse axonal injury) • Facial injury. • Neck injury	
19. Develop a management plan for the removal of a helmet for a head-injured patient.	
20. Differentiate between the types of head/brain injuries based on the assessment and history.	
21. Given several preprogrammed and moulaged head, face, and neck trauma patients, provide the appropriate scene size-up, initial assessment, rapid trauma or focused physical exam and history, detailed exam, and ongoing assessment and provide appropriate patient care and transportation.	

HANDOUT 23-2

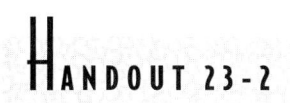

Student's Name _____

CHAPTER 23 QUIZ

Write the letter of the best answer in the space provided.

_____ 1. Which one of the following is the most frequent cause of death following a motor vehicle crash?
  A. abdominal injury
  B. neck injury
  C. chest injury
  D. head injury

_____ 2. The most common penetrating injuries to the head, face, and neck are:
  A. glass from windshields.
  B. gunshot wounds.
  C. stabbings (attacks).
  D. "clothesline" impacts.

_____ 3. When caring for a patient with a scalp injury, important points to remember include:
  A. scalp wounds rarely result in heavy bleeding.
  B. blood vessels in the scalp tend to constrict very effectively.
  C. scalp wounds do not heal well.
  D. the scalp's blood vessels may bleed into a depressed skull fracture.

_____ 4. The "halo sign" is most reliable when checking fluid from the:
  A. ear.
  B. eye.
  C. nose.
  D. mouth.

_____ 5. A contrecoup injury to the brain occurs:
  A. during a frontal impact to the skull.
  B. on the opposite side of impact.
  C. when the skull receives multiple fractures.
  D. to the brainstem when ICP increases.

_____ 6. Blunt trauma to local brain tissue that produces capillary bleeding into the substance of the brain is called a(n):
  A. epidural hemorrhage.
  B. cerebral contusion.
  C. subdural hematoma.
  D. intracerebral hemorrhage.

_____ 7. Elderly and alcoholic patients are more at risk for subdural hematoma because:
  A. these patients have a decreased amount of CSF in their central nervous system.
  B. the size of their brains is reduced.
  C. these patients tend to fall more.
  D. the skull becomes thinner in these patients.

_____ 8. A mild to moderate form of diffuse axonal injury, and the most common outcome of blunt head trauma, is:
  A. intracerebral hemorrhage.
  B. concussion.
  C. contusion.
  D. subdural hemorrhage.

_____ 9. Cushing's response is seen in patients with head injury. In Cushing's response, you will see:
  A. a decrease in blood pressure.
  B. deep, regular respirations.
  C. a slowing pulse rate.
  D. all of these

_____ 10. The head injury patient you are caring for is showing an irregular respiratory pattern, alternating periods of apnea and tachypnea. This is known as:
  A. Biot's respirations.
  B. Cheyne-Stokes respirations.
  C. paradoxical respirations.
  D. Kussmaul's respirations.

EVALUATION

HANDOUT 23-2 Continued

_____ 11. When increased ICP begins to affect the middle brainstem, you may see:
  A. a narrowing pulse pressure.
  B. tachycardia.
  C. deep, rapid respirations.
  D. dilated pupils.

_____ 12. Trauma to the head of a very young pediatric patient is much different than that to the older patient. Differences to keep in mind include:
  A. the skull of a pediatric patient will distort more easily with the force of an impact.
  B. the "soft spots" of the skull permit some intracranial expansion.
  C. internal hemorrhage in the cranium may significantly contribute to hypovolemia.
  D. all of these

_____ 13. Pay close attention to the eyes when evaluating a patient with possible head trauma. Which of the following is true?
  A. If perfusion is diminished, the eyes lose their luster quickly.
  B. Extreme hypoxia causes pupils to be constricted and fixed.
  C. An expanding cranial lesion causes the pupil on the opposite side of the head to become sluggish.
  D. As increasing pressure interferes with the cranial nerves, the pupil constricts and is unable to open.

_____ 14. When assessing a patient with a possible head injury, remember:
  A. that the mechanism of injury can often give a better indication of the seriousness of the injury than the patient's signs and symptoms.
  B. to maintain manual stabilization of the head until a cervical collar is applied.
  C. always to remove the patient's helmet prior to immobilization.
  D. that bilateral periorbital ecchymosis is a rapidly developing sign of basilar skull fracture.

_____ 15. Increasing intracranial pressure results in a(n):
  A. rapid, weak pulse rate.
  B. increasing systolic blood pressure.
  C. slow, regular respirations.
  D. narrowing pulse pressure.

_____ 16. The management of a patient with suspected head/brain injury includes:
  A. placing the patient in the Trendelenburg position.
  B. use of an oropharyngeal airway to reduce transient increases in intracranial pressure.
  C. elevating the head of the spine board about 30 degrees.
  D. administration of supplemental oxygen via nasal cannula, 1.5–2 liters/min.

_____ 17. Medications may be useful in the management of a patient with a head/brain injury. You may consider using:
  A. vecuronium as a diuretic.
  B. pancuronium bromide as a paralytic.
  C. furosemide as a sedative/amnesiac.
  D. diazepam as a diuretic.

_____ 18. The drug used during rapid-sequence intubation to reduce oral and airway secretions and limit the fasciculations associated with administration of succinylcholine is:
  A. diazepam.
  B. mannitol.
  C. atropine sulfate.
  D. thiamine hydrochloride.

_____ 19. Transport recommendations for the patient with a serious head injury include:
  A. limiting external stimulation, such as the use of lights and siren.
  B. avoiding air medical service transport, as altitude may increase ICP.
  C. answering the patient's questions only once, as it does no good to repeat them.
  D. loosening restraints and immobilization devices during transport for comfort.

HANDOUT 23-2 Continued

_____ 20. Your patient has an impaled object in his head. Management includes:
   A. immediate removal of any impaled object in the head.
   B. low concentration oxygen to keep CO_2 levels slightly elevated.
   C. leaving the object in place while stabilizing it with bulky dressings.
   D. placing the patient in the Trendelenburg position.

_____ 21. All of the following may be seen in a patient with cerebral herniation EXCEPT:
   A. singular or bilaterally dilated and fixed pupils.
   B. posturing (decerebrate or decorticate) or no movement with noxious stimuli.
   C. increasing pulse rate and decreasing blood pressure.
   D. decreasing level of consciousness.

_____ 22. Ventilation rates for a head-injury patient without signs of herniation should be to maintain an end-tidal CO_2 reading of:
   A. between 35 and 40 mmHg.
   B. between 25 and 30 mmHg.
   C. at least 40 mmHg.
   D. at least 60 mmHg.

_____ 23. Oxygen saturation in any patient with a serious head injury should be maintained at:
   A. at least 85 percent.
   B. at least 90 percent.
   C. at least 95 percent.
   D. at least 98 percent.

_____ 24. You should evaluate a head-injury patient's blood glucose to assure it is above:
   A. 60 mg/dL.
   B. 70 mg/dL.
   C. 80 mg/dL.
   D. 90 mg/dL.

_____ 25. Systolic blood pressure in a young child (2–5 years old) who has a head injury should be maintained to at least:
   A. 65 mmHg.
   B. 75 mmHg.
   C. 80 mmHg.
   D. 90 mmHg.

EVALUATION

Handout 23-3

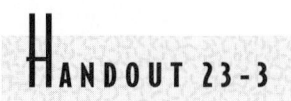

Student's Name _____

CHAPTER 23 SCENARIO

Review the following real-life situation. Then answer the questions that follow.

You are called to the scene of a bicycle crash. During your rapid scene size-up, you see a young male patient lying on his side next to a bicycle. He is conscious. You see he is not wearing a helmet. Bystanders tell you the cyclist struck the curb and immediately fell to the pavement.

1. The patient wants to get up. Will you let him? Why or why not?

2. As you begin your assessment, a bystander tells you that the cyclist had been unconscious. At this time, what is your general impression? What else should you ask the bystanders about the situation?

3. Bystanders tell you that just before the bicycle struck the curb, the cyclist was acting "strange." He was riding in front of traffic and weaving across the center line. Now what is your impression?

4. As you conduct your assessment, you note a hematoma to the patient's forehead but see no other signs of injury. His vital signs are stable. His Glasgow Coma Scale score is 14. Should you transport? Why or why not?

5. You decide to transport. How would you immobilize the patient?

6. En route, the patient tells you he forgot to take his medication. What might be the patient's underlying medical condition and what medication might your patient have forgotten to take?

7. Now that you know the patient has an underlying medical condition, do you still feel you made the correct decision to transport the patient for evaluation of a possible head injury? Why or why not?

HANDOUT 23-4

Student's Name _____

CHAPTER 23 REVIEW

Write the word or words that best complete the following sentences in the space provided.

1. Severe _____ injury is the most frequent cause of trauma death.
2. The pressure exerted on the brain by the blood and cerebrospinal fluid is known as _____ pressure.
3. The _____ _____ is the critical conduit for nervous signals between the brain and the body.
4. The _____ bone is one of the thinnest and most frequently fractured cranial bones.
5. The "_____ sign" is most reliable when associated with fluid leaking from the ear.
6. A(n) _____ injury is an injury to the brain occurring on the same side as the site of impact. A(n) _____ injury is one occurring on the opposite side of the impact.
7. An accumulation of blood between the dura mater and the cranium is called a(n) _____ _____ and causes ICP to build rapidly.
8. A(n) _____ is a transient period of unconsciousness, usually followed by a complete return of function.
9. The inability to remember events that occurred before the trauma that caused the condition is called _____ amnesia. The inability to remember events that occurred after the trauma that caused the condition is called _____ amnesia.
10. _____ reflex is a response due to cerebral ischemia that causes an increase in systemic blood pressure, which maintains cerebral perfusion during increased intracranial pressure.
11. _____ drugs or _____ hypoxia will reduce pupillary responsiveness.
12. Fractures involving the maxilla are classified using the _____ _____ criteria.
13. _____ or _____ draining from a patient's ear suggests basilar skull fracture.
14. If spinal injury is suspected, immediately _____ the head and neck.
15. _____ Volume = Tidal Volume × Respiratory Rate.
16. A slow, strong pulse may be an early sign of building _____ _____.
17. Raccoon eyes and Battle's sign are very _____ indications of basilar skull fracture.
18. Dull, lackluster eyes are a sign of _____ hypoxia.
19. Position the patient with potential brain injury by _____ the head of the spine board.
20. Any patient who has sustained a significant head injury or who displays any indication of lowered level of consciousness, orientation, or arousal is a candidate for _____ - _____, _____ - _____ oxygen.
21. _____ is the primary first-line drug used in the care of the patient with suspected head injury.
22. Diuretics used in the management of the head/brain injury patient are _____ and _____. Paralytics include _____ chloride. _____ sulfate is used as a sedative/amnestic.
23. _____ _____ is an anticholinergic agent sometimes used during rapid-sequence intubation.
24. When transporting head-injury patients, limit _____ stimulation such as the use of lights and siren.
25. Rinse dislodged teeth in _____ _____ and wrap them in _____ -soaked gauze for transport to the emergency department.

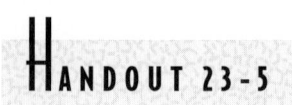

HEAD, FACIAL, AND NECK TRAUMA TRUE OR FALSE

Indicate whether the following statements are true or false by writing T or F in the space provided.

_____ 1. Severe head trauma is the most frequent cause of trauma death.

_____ 2. Any expanding lesion within the cranium results in a decrease in intracranial pressure.

_____ 3. Penetrating objects into the skull should be immediately removed and a pressure dressing placed on the wound.

_____ 4. Because of the rich circulation to the area, scalp wounds tend to heal well.

_____ 5. Sutures are small cracks in the cranium and represent about 80 percent of all skull fractures.

_____ 6. The temporal bone is one of the thickest cranial bones.

_____ 7. The "halo sign" is most reliable when associated with fluid leaking from the ear.

_____ 8. A coup injury is a brain injury occurring on the same side as the site of impact.

_____ 9. An epidural hematoma is a collection of blood directly beneath the dura mater.

_____ 10. A transient period of unconsciousness followed by a complete return to function is known as a concussion.

_____ 11. Hypertension, in the brain-injured patient with increasing ICP, may contribute to poor perfusion pressure.

_____ 12. The response to cerebral ischemia that causes an increase in systemic blood pressure, a decrease in pulse rate, and erratic respirations is known as Cushing's response.

_____ 13. Stimulant drugs or extreme cerebral hypoxia will cause the pupils to dilate and fix.

_____ 14. Blood or fluid draining from a patient's ear suggests basilar skull fracture.

_____ 15. Head-injury patients may need oxygen to overcome the effects of hypoxia and CO_2 retention, and hyperventilation of the patient is vital.

_____ 16. Raccoon eyes and Battle's sign are early indications of basilar skull fracture.

_____ 17. A Glasgow Coma Scale score of 12 or less indicates a severe head injury.

_____ 18. One hazard of nasal airway use is the possible insertion of the tube directly into the cranium through a fracture of the posterior nasal border.

_____ 19. Narcan is used to reverse the effects of diazepam, which is used during rapid-sequence intubation.

_____ 20. Patients who have received a needle cricothyrotomy require less time to exhale.

_____ 21. The drug mannitol is especially effective in drawing fluid from the brain.

_____ 22. Atropine sulfate is sometimes used during rapid-sequence intubation to reduce oral and airway secretions and limit the fasciculations associated with the administration of succinylcholine.

_____ 23. Xylocaine or benzocaine will anesthetize the oral and pharyngeal mucosa, making endotracheal intubation easier.

_____ 24. With a tearing or avulsion to the pinna, bandage the damaged tissue in the position found.

_____ 25. Rinse dislodged teeth in milk and wrap in sterile gauze.

Chapter 23 Answer Key

Handout 23-2: Chapter 23 Quiz

1.	D	8.	B	15.	B	22.	B
2.	B	9.	C	16.	C	23.	C
3.	D	10.	B	17.	B	24.	A
4.	A	11.	C	18.	C	25.	B
5.	B	12.	A	19.	A		
6.	B	13.	A	20.	C		
7.	B	14.	A	21.	C		

Handout 23-3: Chapter 23 Scenario

1. You should not allow the patient to get up until you have completed your assessment. You should maintain a high index of suspicion for head, neck, and spinal cord injury.
2. The patient may have sustained a concussion. At this point in the scenario, you would want to know how long the patient was unconscious. You may also want to learn more about the mechanism of injury. Was he wearing a helmet at the time of the crash? Approximately how fast was he riding the bicycle at the time of the crash? Also, what was he doing just prior to the crash?
3. The patient may have some other underlying condition that caused his "strange" behavior prior to the incident—for example, epilepsy, diabetes, or acute alcohol intoxication.
4. In most systems this patient would be transported. Patients with possible concussion deserve further definitive care and assessment. Additionally, the patient's behavior prior to the crash warrants further evaluation.
5. Based on the mechanism of injury, complete spinal immobilization is appropriate.
6. The patient may have suffered a seizure, or the patient may suffer from diabetes. It is possible that he forgot to take his seizure medication (e.g., Dilantin), or insulin for the diabetes.
7. The decision to transport continues to be the correct decision. The mechanism of injury and the fact that the patient was not wearing a helmet warrant further physician assessment.

Handout 23-4: Chapter 23 Review

1. head
2. intracranial
3. spinal cord
4. temporal
5. halo
6. coup, contrecoup
7. epidural hematoma
8. concussion
9. retrograde, anterograde
10. Cushing's
11. Depressant, cerebral
12. Le Fort
13. Blood, fluid
14. immobilize
15. Minute
16. intracranial pressure
17. late
18. cerebral
19. elevating
20. high-flow, high-concentration
21. Oxygen
22. mannitol, furosemide, succinylcholine, Morphine
23. Atropine sulfate
24. external
25. normal saline, saline

Handout 23-5: Head, Facial, and Neck Trauma True or False

1.	T	8.	T	15.	F	22.	T
2.	F	9.	F	16.	F	23.	T
3.	F	10.	T	17.	F	24.	F
4.	T	11.	T	18.	T	25.	F
5.	F	12.	T	19.	F		
6.	F	13.	T	20.	F		
7.	T	14.	T	21.	T		

Chapter 24

Spinal Trauma

INTRODUCTION

Each year more than 15,000 permanent spinal cord injuries occur. Injuries most commonly occur in males age 16 to 30. Motor vehicle crashes account for almost half of all spinal injuries, followed by falls, penetrating trauma, and sports-related injuries. Permanent spinal injuries affect the body's major communications pathway and control over either the lower extremities or both upper and lower extremities. Spinal cord injuries also affect the body's control over internal organs and the internal environment. As with most trauma, the best care is prevention. Reports indicate that as many as 25 percent of all spinal cord injuries result from improper handling of the spinal column after an injury.

This chapter discusses the anatomy and physiology of the structures related to spinal injuries, the pathophysiology of traumatic spinal injury, assessment findings, and the management of spinal injury patients.

TOTAL TEACHING TIME:
6.64 HOURS
The total teaching time is only a guideline based on the didactic and practical lab averages in the National Standard Curriculum. Instructors should take into consideration such factors as the pace at which students learn, the size of the class, and breaks. The actual time devoted to teaching objectives is the responsibility of the instructor.

CHAPTER OBJECTIVES

After reading this chapter, you should be able to:

1. Describe the incidence, morbidity, and mortality of spinal injuries in the trauma patient. (p. 1001)
2. Describe the anatomy and physiology of spinal structures and structures related to the spine, including the cervical spine, thoracic spine, lumbar spine, sacrum, coccyx, spinal cord, nerve tracts, and dermatomes. (see Chapter 3)
3. Predict spinal injuries based on mechanism of injury. (pp. 1001–1004)
4. Describe the pathophysiology of spinal injuries. (pp. 1004–1007)
5. Identify the need for rapid intervention and transport of the patient with spinal injuries. (pp. 1007–1012)
6. Describe the pathophysiology of traumatic spinal injury related to:
   - Spinal shock (p. 1006)
   - Neurogenic shock (p. 1006)
   - Quadriplegia/paraplegia (p. 1005)
   - Incomplete and complete cord injury (pp. 1005–1006)
   - Cord syndromes:
     - Central cord syndrome (p. 1006)
     - Anterior cord syndrome (p. 1005)
     - Brown-Séquard syndrome (p. 1006)
7. Describe the assessment findings associated with and management for traumatic spinal injuries. (pp. 1007–1027)

©2007 Pearson Education, Inc.
Essentials of Paramedic Care, 2nd ed.

8. Describe the various types of helmets and their purposes. (p. 1019)
9. Relate the priorities of care to factors determining the need for helmet removal in various field situations, including sports-related incidents. (pp. 1019–1020)
10. Given several preprogrammed and moulaged spinal trauma patients, provide the appropriate scene size-up, initial assessment, rapid trauma or focused physical exam and history, detailed exam, and ongoing assessment and provide appropriate patient care and transportation. (pp. 1001–1027)

FRAMING THE LESSON

Begin by reviewing the important points of Chapter 23, "Head, Facial, and Neck Trauma." Use this time to answer any questions about the previous chapter and to discuss any items not completely understood by students. Then begin the discussion of Chapter 24.

If there is a spinal trauma center or rehabilitation clinic in the area, arrange for a representative from the center to come to class and present case reviews of various spinal trauma patients. X-rays of injured spines will dramatically illustrate the cases. If possible, either have spinal injury patients attend the class, or have students meet patients in a spinal trauma care center to discuss their injuries and how such injuries have affected their lives. Bring to class any special utensils or equipment used by people with permanent spinal injuries and demonstrate their uses. Have students use the various pieces of equipment, including utensils and mobilization devices such as wheelchairs. This is also a good opportunity to review basic immobilization skills and to practice with immobilization equipment.

TEACHING STRATEGIES

People learn in a variety of ways. Some do better with the spoken word, whereas others prefer the written. Some prefer to work alone, whereas others profit from working in groups. Recognizing these different ways of acquiring knowledge, the authors of this *Instructor's Resource Manual* have provided a variety of teaching strategies for the different types of learners. These strategies are intended to foster higher-level cognitive skills and encourage creative learning and problem solving. For greatest effectiveness, incorporate these strategies into your class lecture. Symbols in the Lecture Outline indicate the points at which various exercises might be most appropriate. Other strategies can be used to preview the lesson or to summarize it.

The following strategies are keyed to specific sections of the lesson.

1. Spinal Injury Prevention Materials. Spinal injury prevention has become more common in the past 5 years. Have students gather warnings or precautions about spinal injury that they see around town or in the media. They could photograph billboards or posted signs or bring in newspaper articles or magazine ads. Discuss how such public education contributes to a decreasing incidence of spinal injury in a given population. An activity such as this encourages students to be aware of and active within their communities. It also helps to demonstrate the real benefits of prevention programs.

2. Mechanism of Injury Posters. With the diagrams in Figure 24-1 of the textbook as inspiration, have groups of students expand this diagram. Each group can create a poster depicting mechanisms of injury causing the types of injury they have been assigned. Have them draw their diagrams or clip pictures from magazines. Post their posters around the classroom during the trauma unit. This type of activity involves the right brain (for drawing) and ensures that the student's thinking will not be limited to the one visual image supplied by the book. For instance, for the flexion-rotation injury, students will now have the fall depicted in the book as well as a visual image of a football player being tackled as he turns to run, a person rotating while lifting a heavy box, and a lateral impact car crash.

3. Oreos to Demonstrate Ruptured Discs. Use Double-Stuffed Oreos to demonstrate a ruptured or bulging disc. Apply pressure to the chocolate cookie parts, similar to the vertebrae, and squeeze. The "stuffing," much like the disc, will begin to bulge out, revealing its vulnerability to injury. Next, apply pressure to one side or the other, noticing how the morphology of the bulging "disc" changes. Allow students to eat their Oreos when finished.

4. Mechanical Stabilization. Knowing that 25 percent of spinal injuries are caused or exacerbated by improper handling by medical professionals, the concept of manual stabilization supplied immediately and continued until full mechanical immobilization is achieved is paramount to quality care and minimal litigation on behalf of your students. NEVER allow spinal immobilization to be carried out by an imaginary or "ghost" partner during simulations and skills lab sessions. Students will perform as they have practiced. If you allow or encourage release of manual stabilization after initial contact with the patient, your students will allow this in the field. ALWAYS provide enough help (other students, bystanders, or instructors) so that manual immobilization can be established and maintained throughout the call until full mechanical immobilization is complete.

5. Immobilization Practice. Bring several types of immobilization devices to class, such as long spine boards, full body vacuum mattress, short spine boards, KEDs, cervical collars, and cravats. Break up students into groups for practice with applying each of the types of devices. You may wish to pay special attention to the short spine board. This is an underused device, but paramedics should be skilled in its application. Many EMT-Basics are proficient with long spine boards and KEDs but have little experience with short spine boards.

6. Helmet Removal Decisions. Helmet removal has long been, and continues to be, controversial and very confusing to students. Practicing the procedure is not enough. You must provide practice on the decision making required during potential helmet-removal calls as well. Use video clips of sports injuries (ask your local athletic trainer) or video clips from movies involving sports, motorcycles, and use of other recreational vehicles to help students create a decision-making model for helmet removal. Clinical decision making in the classroom is imperative to translation of these skills in the field. Use whatever medium is available to make your skills practice patient-based. In the absence of real patients, video can work well.

The following strategies can be used at various points throughout the lesson or to help summarize and demonstrate what students have learned.

Guest Speaker: Chiropractor. A chiropractor would serve as a great guest speaker for this unit. While there are few other opportunities to involve this member of the health care community in your classroom, the chiropractor does know a great deal about spinal anatomy and physiology. Additionally, he will be seeing many patients who suffer from chronic back pain or are rehabilitating from spinal injury.

Field Trip. Arrange for a field trip to an area spinal rehabilitation center or clinic. Have students interview patients regarding their injuries, what caused them, what symptoms developed, and how the injury has affected their lifestyle.

Guest Speakers. Invite a neurologist or radiologist to talk to the class about spinal cord injuries. Ask them to present information in a case-review format.

Cultural Considerations, Legal Notes, and Patho Pearls. The Student CD-ROM contains this series of informative features to enhance the student's understanding of the material covered in this chapter.

TEACHING OUTLINE

Chapter 24, "Spinal Trauma," is the ninth lesson in Division 3, *Trauma Emergencies*. Distribute Handout 24-1 so that students can familiarize themselves with the learning goals for this chapter. If students have any questions about the objectives, answer them at this time.

Then present the chapter. One possible lecture outline follows. In the outline, the parenthetical references in regular type are references to text pages; those in bold type are references to figures, tables, or procedures.

I. Introduction. A spinal cord injury can both threaten life and induce serious, lifelong disability. Each year more than 11,000 permanent spinal cord injuries occur, most commonly in men age 16 to 30. Auto and other vehicle crashes account for almost half these spinal cord injuries (48 percent) with falls (21 percent), intentional injuries (15 percent), and sports-related injuries (14 percent) also contributing significantly to the total. Further, of all patients who suffer neurologic deficit from trauma, some 40 percent have experienced cord injury. The remaining patients with neurologic deficits have suffered injuries that disrupt the spinal or peripheral nerve roots along their course. The spinal cord consists of highly specialized central nervous system tissue and does not repair itself when seriously injured. Prevention is the best form of care. Recent advances in motor vehicle and highway design have helped reduce the incidence of spine injury, as do educational programs to reduce drinking and driving and safe practices to reduce the potential for spinal cord injury. It is vital to assure that patients with mechanisms of injury or any signs or symptoms that suggest potential spinal cord or column injuries receive immediate and continuing manual spinal stabilization, followed rapidly by mechanical immobilization during prehospital assessment, care, and transport. (p. 1001)

II. Pathophysiology of spinal injury (pp. 1001–1007)
  A. Mechanisms of spinal injury (pp. 1001–1004) (**Fig. 24-1, p. 1002**)
    1. Extremes of motion
       a. Flexion
       b. Compression
       c. Hyperextension
       d. Flexion-rotation
       e. Distraction
       f. Penetration
    2. Axial stress
    3. Other mechanisms of injury
  B. Results of trauma to the spinal column (pp. 1004–1007)
    1. Column injury
    2. Cord injury
       a. Concussion
       b. Contusion
       c. Compression
       d. Laceration

HANDOUT 24-1
Chapter 24 Objectives Checklist

TEACHING STRATEGY 1
Spinal Injury Prevention Materials

POINT TO EMPHASIZE
Because of their position, curvature, and lack of protection, the most susceptible, and most often fractured, vertebrae are C-5, C-6, T-12, and L-1.

POWERPOINT PRESENTATION
Chapter 24, PowerPoint slides 4–31

POINT OF INTEREST
The spinal cord is about 17 inches long and weighs less than an ounce. It is a column of nervous tissue that acts like a relay station, connecting the brain with all the other parts of the body.

POINT TO EMPHASIZE
Your patient can feel his legs but cannot move them. What may be wrong?

POWERPOINT PRESENTATION
Chapter 24 PowerPoint slides 32–45

SLIDES/VIDEOS
"Spinal Injuries," *24-7 EMS*, Winter 2004.

POINT TO EMPHASIZE
The nervous system is a communications network for the body. It helps all body parts work together effectively.

TEACHING STRATEGY 2
Mechanism of Injury Posters

TEACHING STRATEGY 3
Oreos to Demonstrate Ruptured Discs

e. Hemorrhage
   f. Transection
   g. Anterior cord syndrome
   h. Central cord syndrome
   i. Brown-Séquard syndrome
  3. Spinal shock
  4. Neurogenic shock
  5. Autonomic hyperreflexia syndrome
  6. Other causes of neurologic dysfunction

III. **Assessment of the spinal injury patient** (pp. 1007–1014)

  A. Scene size-up (pp. 1007–1008) (**Fig. 24-2, p. 1007**)
  B. Initial assessment (pp. 1008–1010)
  C. Rapid trauma assessment (pp. 1010–1013) (**Figs 24-4 through 24-6, p. 1011**)
    1. Signs and symptoms of possible spinal injury (**Fig. 24-3, p. 1010**)
       a. Pain
       b. Tenderness
       c. Deformity
       d. Soft-tissue injury
       e. Paralysis
       f. Painful movement
       g. Loss of bowel or bladder control
       h. Priapism
       i. Impaired breathing
    2. Discontinuing spinal precautions (**Fig. 24-7, p. 1013**)
    3. Vital signs (pp. 1013–1014)
  D. Ongoing assessment (pp. 1013–1014) (**Fig. 24-8, p. 1014**)

IV. **Management of the spinal injury patient** (pp. 1014–1027)

  A. Spinal alignment (p. 1015)
  B. Manual cervical immobilization (pp. 1016–1018) (**Figs. 24-19 and 24-10, p. 1016; Fig. 24-11, p. 1017**)
  C. Cervical collar application (p. 1018) (**Fig. 24-12, p. 1018**)
  D. Standing takedown (pp. 1018–1019) (**Fig. 24-13, p. 1019**)
  E. Helmet removal (pp. 1019–1020) (**Fig. 24-14, p. 1020**)
  F. Moving the spinal injury patient (pp. 1020–1026)
    1. Log roll (**Fig. 24-15, p. 1021**)
    2. Straddle slide
    3. Rope-sling slide
    4. Orthopedic stretcher
    5. Vest-type immobilization device (and short spine board) (**Fig. 24-16, p. 1023; Fig. 24-17, p. 1023**)
    6. Rapid extrication (**Fig. 24-18, p. 1024**)
    7. Final patient positioning
    8. Long spine board (**Fig. 24-19, p. 1024**)
    9. Full-body vacuum mattress (**Fig 24-20, p. 1026**)
    10. Diving injury immobilization
  G. Medications (pp. 1026–1027)
    1. Medications and spinal cord injury
    2. Medications and neurogenic shock (**Fig. 24-21, p. 1027**)
    3. Medications and the combative patient

V. **Chapter summary** (p. 1028). Spinal injury is a frequent consequence of serious trauma and is likely to induce serious disability or death. Injury to the spinal column may occur with only minimal signs and patient symptoms. Thus, prehospital care for any patient with a significant mechanism of injury or any trauma patient with a reduced level of consciousness must include

---

TEACHING STRATEGY 4
Mechanical Stabilization

POINT TO EMPHASIZE
The decision to immobilize the victim can be made by the mechanism of injury alone. Absence of clinical findings (pain) does not rule out significant spinal injuries, even in the ambulatory patient.

POWERPOINT PRESENTATION
Chapter 24 PowerPoint slides 46–53

TEACHING STRATEGY 5
Immobilization Practice

POWERPOINT PRESENTATION
Chapter 24 PowerPoint slides 54–65

READING/REFERENCE
Platt, T. et al., "Prehospital Comparison of Head Immobilization Devices." *JEMS*, March 2004.

TEACHING STRATEGY 6
Helmet Removal Decisions

POWERPOINT PRESENTATION
Chapter 24 PowerPoint slide 66

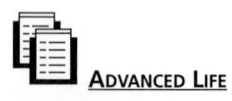

spinal precautions. Throughout patient care, provide emotional support and calming reassurance to help alleviate your patient's anxiety.

SKILLS DEMONSTRATION AND PRACTICE

Students can practice skills discussed in this chapter in the following settings.

Skills Lab: The following stations will be part of a larger trauma skills lab. Divide the class into as many groups as appropriate. Have the groups circulate through the stations. Monitor the groups to be sure that all groups have a chance to practice each of the skills. You may wish to have other instructors or qualified paramedics assist students in these activities.

Station	Equipment Needed	Activities
Spinal Immobilization	Car or car seat Short spine board or vest-type device Long spine board Cervical immobilization devices 1 patient 1 instructor	Have students practice extricating the patient from the car using the short spine board or vest-type device.
Rapid Extrication	Car or car seat Long spine board Cervical immobilization devices 1 patient 1 instructor	Have students practice rapid extrication technique.
Standing Takedown	Long spine board Cervical immobilization devices 1 patient 1 instructor	Have students practice standing takedown technique

Scenario Lab: The following stations will be part of a larger trauma scenario lab. Divide the class into teams. Have the teams circulate through the stations. Monitor the groups to be sure that all groups have a chance to manage each of the cases and that every student has the opportunity to be team leader. You may wish to have the other instructors or qualified paramedics assist students in these activities.

Station	Equipment Needed	Activities
Rapid extrication versus Short Board Extrication	Car or car seat Short spine board Long spine board Cervical immobilization devices 1 patient 1 instructor	Have students determine whether to perform rapid or slow extrication based on primary assessment of patient.
Neurogenic Shock	Long spine board Cervical immobilization devices	Have students practice assessing and managing a

ADVANCED LIFE SUPPORT SKILLS
Larmon & Davis. *Advanced Life Support Skills.*

ADVANCED LIFE SKILLS REVIEW
Larmon & Davis. *Advanced Life Skills Review.*

BRADY SKILLS SERIES: ALS
Larmon & Davis. *Brady Skills Series: ALS.*

	Airway management kit PASG 1 patient 1 instructor	patient in neurogenic shock following spinal cord injury.
Multitrauma	Long spine board Cervical immobilization devices Airway management kit PASG 1 patient 1 instructor	Have students practice assessing and managing a patient with spinal injury and hypovolemic shock.

Field Internship: Assist in assessment and management of head and spinal injuries in the field.

ASSIGNMENTS

Assign students to complete Chapter 24, "Spinal Trauma," of the workbook. Also assign them to read Chapter 25, "Thoracic Trauma," before the next class.

EVALUATION

Chapter Quiz and Scenario   Distribute copies of the Chapter Quiz provided in Handout 24-2 to evaluate student understanding of this chapter. Make sure each student reads the scenario to reinforce critical thinking on the scene. Remind students not to use their notes or textbooks while taking the quiz.

Student CD   Quizzes for every chapter are contained on the dynamic and highly visual in-text student CD.

Companion Website   Additional quizzes for every chapter are contained on this exciting website.

TestGen   You may wish to create a custom-tailored test using *Prentice Hall TestGen for Essentials of Paramedic Care,* 2nd Edition to evaluate student understanding of this chapter.

On-line Test Preparation (for students and instructors)   Additional test preparation is available through Brady's new on-line product, *EMT Achieve: Paramedic Test Preparation* at *http://www.prenhall.com/emtachieve/*. Instructors can also monitor student mastery on-line.

Review Manual for the EMT-Paramedic   This comprehensive exam review contains hundreds of test questions and rationales, including scenarios, along with two 180-question practice tests on CD.

REINFORCEMENT

Handouts   If classroom discussion or performance on the quiz indicates that some students have not fully mastered the chapter content, you may wish to assign some or all of the Reinforcement Handouts for this chapter.

Student CD (for students)   A wide variety of material on this CD-ROM will reinforce and also expand student knowledge and skills.

WORKBOOK
Chapter 24 Activities

READING/REFERENCE
Textbook, pp. 1030–1060

HANDOUT 24-2
Chapter 24 Quiz

HANDOUT 24-3
Chapter 24 Scenario

PARAMEDIC STUDENT CD
Student Activities

COMPANION WEBSITE
http://www.prenhall.com/bledsoe/

TESTGEN
Chapter 24

EMT ACHIEVE:
PARAMEDIC TEST PREPARATION
Mistovich & Beasley. *EMT Achieve: Paramedic Test Preparation.*
www.prenhall.com/emtachieve/

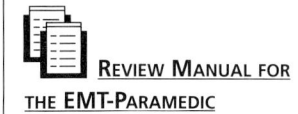

REVIEW MANUAL FOR THE EMT-PARAMEDIC
Cherry & Mistovich. *Review Manual for the EMT-Paramedic,* 3rd edition.

HANDOUT 24-4
Reinforcement Activity

PARAMEDIC STUDENT CD
Student Activities

POWERPOINT PRESENTATION
Chapter 24

COMPANION WEBSITE
http://www.prenhall.com/bledsoe

ONEKEY
Chapter 24

ADVANCED LIFE SUPPORT SKILLS
Larmon & Davis. *Advanced Life Support Skills.*

ADVANCED LIFE SKILLS REVIEW
Larmon & Davis. *Advanced Life Skills Review.*

BRADY SKILLS SERIES: ALS
Larmon & Davis. *Brady Skills Series: ALS.*

PARAMEDIC NATIONAL STANDARDS SELF-TEST
Miller. *Paramedic National Standards Self-Test*, 4th edition.

PowerPoint Presentation (for instructors)   The PowerPoint material developed for this chapter offers useful reinforcement of chapter content.

Companion Website (for students)   Additional review quizzes and links to EMS resources will contribute to further reinforcement of the chapter.

OneKey   On-line support is offered for this course on one of three platforms: CourseCompass, Blackboard, or Web CT. Includes the IRM, PowerPoints, Test-Gen, and Companion Website for instruction. Ask your local sales representative for more information.

Brady Skills Series: Advanced Life Skills (Video or CD)   Have your students watch the skills come to life on VHS or CD-ROM, or they can purchase the highly visual, full-color text with step-by-step procedures and rationales.

HANDOUT 24-1

Student's Name _____

CHAPTER 24 OBJECTIVES CHECKLIST

Knowledge	Date Mastered
1. Describe the incidence, morbidity, and mortality of spinal injuries in the trauma patient.	
2. Describe the anatomy and physiology of spinal structures and structures related to the spine, including the cervical spine, thoracic spine, lumbar spine, sacrum, coccyx, spinal cord, nerve tracts, and dermatomes.	
3. Predict spinal injuries based on mechanism of injury.	
4. Describe the pathophysiology of spinal injuries.	
5. Identify the need for rapid intervention and transport of the patient with spinal injuries.	

6. Describe the pathophysiology of traumatic spinal injury related to:
• Spinal shock
• Neurogenic shock
• Quadriplegia/paraplegia
• Incomplete and complete cord injury
• Cord syndromes:
  • Central cord syndrome
  • Anterior cord syndrome
  • Brown-Séquard syndrome	

7. Describe the assessment findings associated with and management for traumatic spinal injuries.	
8. Describe the various types of helmets and their purposes.	
9. Relate the priorities of care to factors determining the need for helmet removal in various field situations, including sports-related incidents.	
10. Given several preprogrammed and moulaged spinal trauma patients, provide the appropriate scene size-up, initial assessment, rapid trauma or focused physical exam and history, detailed exam, and ongoing assessment and provide appropriate patient care and transportation.	

OBJECTIVES

HANDOUT 24-2

Student's Name _____

CHAPTER 24 QUIZ

Write the letter of the best answer in the space provided.

_____ 1. A distraction injury occurs as a result of:
  A. bending the head forward.
  B. bending the head backwards.
  C. hanging.
  D. a penetrating object.

_____ 2. Bruising of the spinal cord is called a:
  A. concussion.
  B. contusion.
  C. compression.
  D. transection.

_____ 3. The condition caused by partial cutting of one side of the spinal cord resulting in sensory and motor loss to that side of the body is called:
  A. central cord syndrome.
  B. Brown-Séquard syndrome.
  C. anterior cord syndrome.
  D. posterior cord syndrome.

_____ 4. A temporary insult to the spinal cord that induces effects in the body below the level of injury is called:
  A. syndrome.
  B. spinal shock.
  C. neurogenic shock.
  D. autonomic hyperreflexia syndrome.

_____ 5. Provide any patient sustaining a serious injury with immediate:
  A. manual spinal traction.
  B. endotracheal intubation.
  C. manual spinal immobilization.
  D. application of a cervical immobilization device.

_____ 6. Neurogenic injury and possible shock secondary to spinal cord damage may be indicated by:
  A. tachycardia in the presence of low blood pressure.
  B. bradycardia in the presence of hypovolemia.
  C. warm, dry skin in the upper portions of the body with cool, clammy skin in the lower extremities.
  D. the rise and fall of the chest and abdomen together during respirations.

_____ 7. Well after the initial spinal injury, as the body begins to adapt to the problems associated with loss of neurologic control below the injury, a condition develops known as:
  A. anterior cord syndrome.
  B. Brown-Séquard syndrome.
  C. autonomic hyperreflexia syndrome.
  D. central cord syndrome.

_____ 8. Autonomic hyperreflexia syndrome presents with:
  A. sudden hypotension.
  B. tachycardia.
  C. warm, dry skin above the point of injury.
  D. pounding headache.

_____ 9. When evaluating the vital signs of a patient, spinal cord injury may be reflected by:
  A. abnormally high blood pressure.
  B. tachycardia.
  C. diaphragmatic breathing.
  D. all of these

618 ESSENTIALS OF PARAMEDIC CARE

HANDOUT 24-2 Continued

_____ 10. Do not align the spine of the potential spine injury patient if:
   A. movement causes a noticeable increase in pain.
   B. you meet with noticeable resistance during the procedure.
   C. you identify an increase in neurologic signs as you move the head.
   D. any of these

_____ 11. Once manual stabilization of the head and neck is established, it should not be released until:
   A. a cervical immobilization device is applied.
   B. the patient is placed on a long spine board.
   C. the head, neck, and spine are mechanically immobilized.
   D. the initial assessment has been completed.

_____ 12. If you find a patient walking around after a vehicle crash, remember:
   A. it is too late to immobilize the patient.
   B. apply a cervical immobilization device and place the patient supine on the stretcher.
   C. apply a cervical immobilization device and transport the patient in the seated position.
   D. bring the patient to a fully supine position, immobilize, and transport.

_____ 13. If your patient with a potential spinal injury is wearing a helmet, remove it if:
   A. the patient is alert and the neurological assessment is normal.
   B. the helmet does not immobilize the patient's head within.
   C. the patient is to be immobilized on a long spine board.
   D. you suspect a cervical spine injury.

_____ 14. When using the log-roll method to move a patient, be sure to:
   A. place both of the patient's arms at the patient's sides.
   B. place a bulky blanket between the patient's legs.
   C. place four care givers: one at the patient's shoulders, one at the hips, one at the knees, and one at the feet.
   D. never use any padding on the long spine board, to ensure proper support.

_____ 15. When using a long spine board, remember:
   A. the head should be elevated about 1 to 2 inches above the board's surface.
   B. no padding should be used on the board, maintaining neutral alignment of the spine.
   C. elevate the foot end of the board about 18 inches if you suspect a head injury.
   D. the long spine board has been shown to be more effective than a full-body vacuum splint.

EVALUATION

Handout 24-3

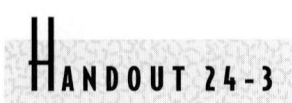

Student's Name _____

CHAPTER 24 SCENARIO

Review the following real-life situation. Then answer the questions that follow.

A Basic Life Support unit requests the assistance of Medic Rescue 8 at a college wrestling match. Paramedics Joyce and Alan are met by the wrestling coach, who tells them that one of his athletes was "thrown head first into the mat." As the paramedics enter the gymnasium, they see a student lying supine on the mat. An EMT tells Joyce that the patient is conscious and complaining of cervical spine pain.

1. What is the first step Joyce and Alan should perform during their rapid scene size-up?

2. Alan notices that the patient is experiencing breathing difficulty. How should he manage the patient's airway? Why?

3. Alan has difficulty managing the patient's airway. Should he continue with his assessment? Why or why not?

4. Joyce has suctioned and intubated the patient. What should she do next?

5. List at least five systemic signs of spinal cord injury.

6. Alan notices that the patient's skin is cool to the touch. Why? What should he do?

HANDOUT 24-4

Student's Name _____

CHAPTER 24 REVIEW

Write the word or words that best complete the following sentences in the space provided.

1. Because of the structure of the spine, the forces necessary to induce injury from _____ _____ are generally less that those needed to cause _____ / _____ injury.
2. A temporary and transient disruption of cord function is called a(n) _____.
3. A bruising of the cord is called a(n) _____.
4. A cutting across a long axis is called a(n) _____.
5. _____ - _____ syndrome is a condition caused by partial cutting of one side of the spinal cord, resulting in sensory and motor loss to that side of the body.
6. The condition usually related to hyperflexion of the cervical spine that results in motor weakness is called _____ _____ syndrome.
7. Put special emphasis on your analysis of the _____ _____ _____ with a potential spinal injury patient.
8. Provide any patient sustaining a serious injury with immediate _____ _____ _____.
9. Be very watchful of patients with _____ heart rates, especially when it is likely that they may be experiencing hypovolemia and shock.
10. Stroking the lateral aspect of the bottom of the foot and watching for movement of the toes is called testing for _____ sign.
11. _____ and _____ are the most commonly used steroids in the prehospital setting for spinally injured patients.
12. Consider using _____ or _____ to calm a patient.
13. A specialized piece of EMS equipment that may be used with some patients is the _____ - _____ _____ _____.
14. _____ _____ _____ is a condition caused by bony fragments or pressure compressing the arteries of the anterior spinal cord and resulting in loss of motor function and sensation to pain, light touch, and temperature below the injury site.
15. _____ _____ _____ is a condition usually related to hyperflexion of the cervical spine that results in motor weakness, usually in the upper extremities, and possible bladder dysfunction.

REINFORCEMENT

Chapter 24 Answer Key

Handout 24-2: Chapter 24 Quiz

1. C	6. B	11. C
2. B	7. C	12. B
3. B	8. D	13. B
4. B	9. C	14. B
5. C	10. D	15. A

Handout 24-3: Chapter 24 Scenario

1. The paramedics should first determine the mechanism of injury. Were there forces involved that might have caused head or spinal cord injury? Was the patient at any time unconscious? Was the patient's neck hyperextended or flexed? Are there any obvious outward signs of head injury such as hematomas, black-and-blue discoloration, bleeding?
2. Use the modified jaw thrust. The modified jaw thrust should be used on all patients suspected of having a spinal cord injury.
3. No. Managing the patient's airway is Alan's highest priority. Joyce may continue the assessment while Alan manages the airway.
4. Joyce should maintain in-line manual stabilization. She should apply a rigid cervical collar, use a cervical immobilization device, and secure the patient and it to a long spine board.
5. Systemic signs include bilateral paresthesia, anesthesia, weakness, paralysis, and priapism.
6. Patients with spinal injury may suffer from hypothermia. The nervous system sometimes loses its ability to maintain core temperature and control heat loss. Alan should keep the patient warm.

Handout 24-4: Chapter 24 Review

1. lateral bending, flexion/extension
2. concussion
3. contusion
4. transection
5. Brown-Séquard
6. central cord
7. mechanism of injury
8. manual spinal immobilization
9. bradycardic
10. Babinski's
11. Methylprednisolone, dexamethasone
12. meperidine, diazepam
13. vest-type immobilization device
14. Anterior cord syndrome
15. Central cord syndrome

Chapter 25

Thoracic Trauma

INTRODUCTION

Thoracic trauma can lead to a life-threatening event. The thoracic cavity contains many vital structures, including the heart, great vessels, esophagus, tracheobronchial tree, and the lungs. Twenty-five percent, or about 16,000, of U.S. motor vehicle deaths are due to thoracic trauma. The development of the modern automobile and the increase in penetrating trauma due to violent crime have added to the incidence of thoracic trauma. The incidence of mortality, however, has decreased due to advances in treatment and prevention measures. This chapter will discuss thoracic trauma in relation to penetrating and blunt injury, mechanism of injury, understanding the pathology of injuries, and the patient's physical signs of injury.

TOTAL TEACHING TIME:
7.54 HOURS
The total teaching time is only a guideline based on the didactic and practical lab averages in the National Standard Curriculum. Instructors should take into consideration such factors as: the pace at which students learn, the size of the class, and breaks. The actual time devoted to teaching objectives is the responsibility of the instructor.

CHAPTER OBJECTIVES

After reading this chapter, you should be able to:

1. Describe the incidence, morbidity, and mortality of thoracic injuries in the trauma patient. (pp. 1031–1032)
2. Discuss the anatomy and physiology of the thoracic organs and structures. (see Chapter 3)
3. Predict thoracic injuries based on mechanism of injury. (pp. 1032–1034)
4. Discuss the pathophysiology of, assessment findings with, and the management and need for rapid intervention and transport of the patient with chest wall injuries, including:
   - Rib fracture (pp. 1035–1036, 1054–1055)
   - Flail segment (pp. 1037–1038, 1055)
   - Sternal fracture (pp. 1036–1037)
5. Discuss the pathophysiology of, assessment findings with, and management and need for rapid intervention and transport of the patient with injury to the lung, including:
   - Simple pneumothorax (pp. 1038–1039)
   - Open pneumothorax (pp. 1039–1040, 1055–1056)
   - Tension pneumothorax (pp. 1040–1041, 1056–1057)
   - Hemothorax (pp. 1041–1042, 1057)
   - Hemopneumothorax (pp. 1041–1042)
   - Pulmonary contusion (pp. 1042–1043)

©2007 Pearson Education, Inc.
Essentials of Paramedic Care, 2nd ed.

6. Discuss the pathophysiology of, findings of assessment with, and management and need for rapid intervention and transport of the patient with myocardial injuries, including:
   - Myocardial contusion (pp. 1043–1044, 1057–1058)
   - Pericardial tamponade (pp. 1044–1045, 1058)
   - Myocardial rupture (p. 1046)

7. Discuss the pathophysiology of, findings of assessment with, and management and need for rapid intervention and transport of the patient with vascular injuries, including injuries to:
   - Aorta (pp. 1046–1047, 1058)
   - Vena cava (p. 1047)
   - Pulmonary arteries/veins (p. 1047)

8. Discuss the pathophysiology of, findings of assessment with, and management and need for rapid intervention and transport of patients with diaphragmatic, esophageal, and tracheobronchial injuries. (pp. 1047–1048, 1058)

9. Discuss the pathophysiology of, findings of assessment with, and management and need for rapid intervention and transport of the patient with traumatic asphyxia. (pp. 1048, 1058)

10. Differentiate between thoracic injuries based on the assessment and history. (pp. 1048–1053)

11. Given several preprogrammed and moulaged thoracic trauma patients, provide the appropriate scene size-up, initial assessment, rapid trauma or focused physical exam and history, detailed exam, and ongoing assessment and provide appropriate patient care and transportation. (pp. 1031–1058)

FRAMING THE LESSON

Begin by reviewing the important points of Chapter 24, "Spinal Trauma." Use this time to answer any questions about the previous chapter and to discuss any items not completely understood by students. Then begin the discussion of Chapter 25.

Begin by reviewing the anatomy of the thorax, especially the major organs contained therein. Stress the importance of these organs, such as the heart and lungs, and the great potential for serious, even life-threatening injuries to these organs. If possible, obtain a cow's or pig's heart and lungs to graphically present these organs. Also, obtain photos and X-rays of thoracic injuries if possible and review signs and symptoms of shock from the previous chapter. Invite a thoracic surgeon to class to make the presentation. When reviewing the anatomy of the thorax, be sure to discuss how the body protects the vital organs there with bone and muscle.

Based on the knowledge the students have so far, ask them to identify the various organs in the thorax and to develop a simple scenario relating how that specific organ may be injured and what signs and symptoms might be seen as a result of that injury.

TEACHING STRATEGIES

People learn in a variety of ways. Some do better with the spoken word, whereas others prefer the written. Some prefer to work alone, whereas others profit from working in groups. Recognizing these different ways of acquiring knowledge, the authors of this *Instructor's Resource Manual* have provided a variety of teaching strategies for the different types of learners. These strategies are intended to foster higher-level cognitive skills and encourage creative learning and problem solving. For greatest effectiveness, incorporate these strategies into your class lecture. Symbols in the Lecture Outline indicate the points at which various exercises might be most appropriate. Other strategies can be used to preview the lesson or to summarize it.

The following strategies are keyed to specific sections of the lesson.

1. Los Angeles F. D. Airbag Inflation Video. To illustrate both the protective function of airbags and the potential danger when an airbag is not handled properly, borrow a videotape created by the Los Angeles City Fire Department (www.lafd.org). Available from their training division, the tape was made while filming an extrication. Remarkably, the airbag deploys on a still vehicle while a firefighter is leaning in front of the steering wheel caring for the patient. This video emphasizes the benefits of safety devices such as airbags, but underscores the need for extreme caution and provider safety at all times.

2. Animal Bone and Food Organ Simulations. The sharp, jagged edges of fractured bones are rarely felt by students. To illustrate their significant cutting ability, use fractured chicken or beef bones to simulate the potential damage to other organs that may be caused by fractured ribs. Cooked pasta simulates blood vessels, raw beef simulates muscle, and chicken or beef fat easily simulates the omentum or subcutaneous tissue. This laboratory display will help students respect the potential for trauma to other organs caused by fractures.

3. Paper Bag Demonstration. Demonstrate the "paper bag effect" in class. Give each student a brown lunch sack. Have them blow into it, close off the top, and pop it using both hands. This will be a loud auditory and visual reminder of the effect of trauma on fully expanded lungs against a closed glottis.

4. Movie Clips. The movie *Three Kings* has an excellent digitally enhanced illustration of penetrating chest trauma. The clip is able to show cavitation, penetration, and even the development of a tension pneumothorax from a simple pneumothorax. Consider editing the movie down to this clip. The few minutes of tape will be memorable and lend visual imagery to your description of these injuries.

5. Gourds and Pumpkins to Demonstrate Percussion. Percussion is difficult to teach. Try practicing on a gourd to simulate hyperresonance and a pumpkin or other squash to simulate dull sounds similar to a hemothorax. Your auditory learners will appreciate hearing the difference in these "lung sounds."

6. Needle Decompression Practice. Here's a variant method of teaching needle decompression. You'll need:
- Hog ribs
- Car or bicycle inner tube(s)
- Tire pump
- IV tape or tire patch kit
- 10–14-gauge over-the-needle catheter

Place hog ribs over inflated automobile tire tube. Then ask students to demonstrate the mid-clavicular and mid-axillary approach to needle decompression. Have students describe each of the necessary steps to both techniques. Holes in the tube can be quickly patched with either tape or self-stick inner tube patches so that the tube may be reused.

HANDOUT 25-1
Chapter 25 Objectives Checklist

TEACHING STRATEGY 1
Los Angeles F.D. Airbag Inflation Video

POINT OF INTEREST
There is a 50 percent mortality within the first hour for patients with bronchial rupture.

POINT OF INTEREST
Most tension pneumothoraces are caused by overuse of positive-pressure ventilation with positive end-expiratory pressure valves (PEEPs) and by failure to seal open wounds.

POWERPOINT PRESENTATION
Chapter 25 PowerPoint slides 4–22

TEACHING STRATEGY 2
Animal Bone and Food Organ Simulations

POWERPOINT PRESENTATION
Chapter 25 PowerPoint slides 23–24

POINT TO EMPHASIZE
Four things can happen with a flail chest: decreased vital lung capacity, increased labored breathing, decreased tidal volume from pain, lung contusions. All four are bad.

POINT TO EMPHASIZE
Paradoxical chest wall movement is a poor prehospital discriminator. Normally the intercostal muscles will splint the flail segment, leaving only a slight movement, if any.

TEACHING STRATEGY 3
Paper Bag Demonstration

TEACHING STRATEGY 4
Movie Clips

The following strategies can be used at various points throughout the lesson or to help summarize and demonstrate what students have learned.

Guest Speakers. Invite emergency department physicians, surgeons, and radiologists to talk to your class about chest and abdominal trauma patients they have treated.

Cultural Considerations, Legal Notes, and Patho Pearls. The Student CD-ROM contains this series of informative features to enhance the student's understanding of the material covered in this chapter.

TEACHING OUTLINE

Chapter 25, "Thoracic Trauma," is the tenth lesson in Division 3, *Trauma Emergencies*. Distribute Handout 25-1 so that students can familiarize themselves with the learning goals for this chapter. If students have any questions about the objectives, answer them at this time.

Then present the chapter. One possible lecture outline follows. In the outline, the parenthetical references in regular type are references to text pages; those in bold type are references to figures, tables, or procedures.

I. Introduction. The thoracic cavity contains the heart, great vessels, esophagus, tracheobronchial tree, and the lungs. Twenty-five percent of all motor vehicle deaths are due to thoracic trauma. The incidence of blunt thoracic trauma has increased with the development of the modern automobile. An increase in penetrating trauma due to violent crime has been seen. Prevention efforts such as gun control legislation, firearm safety courses, seat-belt laws, and better design of automobiles have diminished the occurrence of injuries and the related morbidity and mortality. (pp. 1031–1032) (**Fig. 25-1, p. 1032**)

II. Pathophysiology of thoracic trauma (pp. 1032–1048)
  A. Blunt trauma (pp. 1032–1033) (**Fig. 25-2, p. 1033**)
  B. Penetrating trauma (pp. 1033–1034) (**Fig. 25-3, p. 1034**) (**Table 25-1, p. 1034**)
  C. Chest wall injuries (pp. 1035–1038)
    1. Chest wall contusion
    2. Rib fracture (**Fig. 25-4, p. 1036**)
    3. Sternal fracture and dislocation
    4. Flail chest (**Fig. 25-5, p. 1037; Fig. 25-6, p. 1038**)
  D. Pulmonary injuries (pp. 1038–1043)
    1. Simple pneumothorax (**Fig. 25-7, p. 1039**)
      a. Signs and symptoms of pneumothorax
        i. Trauma to chest
        ii. Chest pain on inspiration
        iii. Hyperinflation of chest
        iv. Diminished breath sounds on affected side
    2. Open pneumothorax (**Fig. 25-8, p. 1040**)
      a. Signs and symptoms of open pneumothorax
        i. Penetrating trauma
        ii. Sucking chest wound
        iii. Frothy blood at wound site
        iv. Severe dyspnea
        v. Hypovolemia
    3. Tension pneumothorax (**Fig. 25-9, p. 1041**)
      a. Signs and symptoms of tension pneumothorax
        i. Chest trauma

626 ESSENTIALS OF PARAMEDIC CARE

        ii. Dyspnea
       iii. Ventilation/perfusion mismatch
       iv. Hypoxemia
        v. Hyperinflation of affected side of chest
       vi. Hyperresonance of affected side of chest
     vii. Diminished, then absent, breath sounds
    viii. Cyanosis
       ix. Diaphoresis
        x. Altered mental status
       xi. Jugular venous distention
      xii. Hypotension
     xiii. Hypovolemia
   4. Hemothorax (**Fig. 25-10, p. 1042**)
      a. Signs and symptoms of hemothorax
         i. Blunt or penetrating chest trauma
        ii. Signs and symptoms of shock
       iii. Dyspnea
       iv. Dull percussive sounds over site of injury
   5. Pulmonary contusion
      a. Signs and symptoms of pulmonary contusion
         i. Blunt or penetrating chest trauma
        ii. Increasing dyspnea
       iii. Hypoxia
       iv. Increasing crackles
        v. Diminishing breath sounds
      vi. Hemoptysis
     vii. Signs and symptoms of shock
E. Cardiovascular injuries (pp. 1043–1047)
  1. Myocardial contusion (**Fig. 25-11, p. 1044**)
     a. Signs and symptoms of myocardial contusion
        i. Injury to chest
       ii. Bruising of chest wall
      iii. Weakness; rapid heart rate—may be irregular
      iv. Possible sweating
       v. Severe nagging pain not relieved with rest but may be relieved with oxygen
  2. Pericardial tamponade (**Fig. 25-12, p. 1045**)
     a. Signs and symptoms of pericardial tamponade
        i. Cardiac contusion
       ii. Blunt trauma to anterior chest
      iii. Penetrating chest wound
      iv. Recent cardiac surgery
       v. Tamponade may follow CPR
      vi. Dyspnea and possible cyanosis
     vii. Jugular venous distention
    viii. Weak, thready pulse
      ix. Decreasing blood pressure
       x. Shock
      xi. Narrowing pulse pressure
  3. Myocardial aneurysm or rupture
  4. Traumatic aneurysm or rupture of the aorta
F. Other vascular injuries (p. 1047) (**Table 25-2, p. 1046**)
G. Other thoracic injuries (pp. 1047–1048)
  1. Traumatic rupture or perforation of the diaphragm
  2. Traumatic esophageal rupture
  3. Tracheobronchial injury (disruption)
  4. Traumatic asphyxia

POINT TO EMPHASIZE

The classic "Beck's triad" includes muffled heart sounds, decreasing pulse pressure, and jugular venous distention. Once again, if the neck veins are flat, what is the problem?

TEACHING STRATEGY 5

Gourds and Pumpkins to Demonstrate Percussion

POINT TO EMPHASIZE

Look for the classic "hood sign" with traumatic asphyxia. This is caused by the bursting of capillary beds from extreme pressure. It appears from the nipple line up.

POWERPOINT PRESENTATION
Chapter 25 PowerPoint slides 26–32

POINT TO EMPHASIZE
As baseball philosopher Yogi Berra would say, "You can observe a lot by watching." Never let the patient's clothing get in the way of your assessment. Be naturally inquisitive and snoopy—look for injuries and subtle signs of internal damage.

POWERPOINT PRESENTATION
Chapter 25 PowerPoint slides 33–134

POINT TO EMPHASIZE
Severe force is required to fracture ribs 1, 2, and 3 because they are so well protected by surrounding structures. If they are fractured, expect severe underlying injuries and a high mortality rate (up to 30 percent). There is no such thing as a simple rib fracture. Any person with a fractured rib should be suspected of having associated lung tissue damage.

POWERPOINT PRESENTATION
Chapter 25 PowerPoint slide 135

READING/REFERENCE
Cross, E. "Needle Thoracostomy and Trauma," *JEMS*, March 2002.

TEACHING STRATEGY 6
Needle Decompression Practice

ADVANCED LIFE SUPPORT SKILLS
Larmon & Davis. *Advanced Life Support Skills.*

ADVANCED LIFE SKILLS REVIEW
Larmon & Davis. *Advanced Life Skills Review.*

BRADY SKILLS SERIES: ALS
Larmon & Davis. *Brady Skills Series: ALS.*

III. Assessment of the thoracic trauma patient (pp. 1048–1053)
   A. Scene size-up (p. 1049)
   B. Initial assessment (p. 1049)
   C. Rapid trauma assessment (pp. 1049–1053)
      1. Observe
      2. Question
      3. Palpate (**Fig. 25-13, p. 1050; Fig 25-14, p. 1050**)
      4. Auscultate (**Fig. 25-15, p. 1051**)
      5. Percuss (**Fig. 25-16, p. 1051**)
      6. Blunt trauma assessment
      7. Penetrating trauma assessment (**Figs. 25-17 and 25-18, p. 1053**)
   D. Ongoing assessment (p. 1053)

IV. Management of the chest injury patient (pp. 1053–1058) (**Fig. 25-19, p. 1054**)
   A. Rib fractures (pp. 1054–1055)
   B. Sternoclavicular dislocation (p. 1055)
   C. Flail chest (p. 1055) (**Fig. 25-20, p. 1055**)
   D. Open pneumothorax (pp. 1055–1056) (**Fig. 25-21, p. 1056**)
   E. Tension pneumothorax (pp. 1056–1057) (**Fig. 25-22, p. 1057**)
   F. Hemothorax (p. 1057)
   G. Myocardial contusion (pp. 1057–1058)
   H. Pericardial tamponade (p. 1058)
   I. Aortic aneurysm (p. 1058)
   J. Tracheobronchial injury (p. 1058)
   K. Traumatic asphyxia (p. 1058)

V. Chapter summary (p. 1059). Thoracic trauma by either blunt or penetrating mechanisms has a great potential for posing a threat to a patient's life. In fact, 25 percent of all traumatic deaths are secondary to injuries in this region. In assessing these patients, the mechanism of injury, when considered along with the clinical findings, may help in differentiating among the many possible injuries. The assessment, in turn, helps guide your interventions and determines the need for rapid extrication and transport. Aggressive airway management, oxygenation, ventilation, and fluid resuscitation, when indicated, can make the difference between the patient's survival or death. Specific interventions, such as pleural decompression or stabilization of a flail segment, can also affect mortality and morbidity from chest trauma. Understanding the pathological processes affecting the chest during trauma and employing proper assessment and care measures will assure the best possible outcome for your patients.

SKILLS DEMONSTRATION AND PRACTICE

Students can practice skills discussed in this chapter in the following settings.

Skills Lab: The following station will be part of a larger trauma skills lab. Divide the class into as many groups as appropriate. Have the groups circulate through the stations. Monitor the groups to be sure all groups have a chance to practice each of the skills. You may wish to have other instructors or qualified paramedics assist students in these activities.

Station	Equipment Needed	Activities
Needle Decompression	Decompression manikin or other model for practicing skill Handout 25-2 1 instructor	Have students practice needle decompression on the model.

HANDOUT 25-2
Chest Decompression

Scenario Lab: The following stations will be part of a larger trauma scenario lab. Divide the class into teams. Have the teams circulate through the stations. Monitor the groups to be sure that all groups have a chance to manage each of the cases and that every student has the opportunity to be team leader. You may wish to have other instructors or qualified paramedics assist students in these activities.

Station	Equipment Needed	Activities
Tension Pneumothorax versus Hemothorax	Long spine board Cervical immobilization devices Airway management kit 1 patient 1 instructor	Have students practice assessing and managing patients with hemothorax and tension pneumothorax.
Multitrauma	Long spine board Cervical immobilization Devices Airway management kit PASG 1 patient 1 instructor	Have students practice assessing and managing patients with various thoracic and abdominal injuries.

Hospital: Assist in assessment and management of chest and abdominal trauma in the ED.

Field Internship: Assist in assessment and management of chest and abdominal trauma in the field.

ASSIGNMENTS

Assign students to complete Chapter 25, "Thoracic Trauma," of the workbook. Also assign them to read Chapter 26, "Abdominal Trauma," before the next class.

EVALUATION

Chapter Quiz and Scenario Distribute copies of the Chapter Quiz provided in Handout 25-3 to evaluate student understanding of this chapter. Make sure each student reads the scenario to reinforce critical thinking on the scene. Remind students not to use their notes or textbooks while taking the quiz.

Student CD Quizzes for every chapter are contained on the dynamic and highly visual in-text student CD.

Companion Website Additional quizzes for every chapter are contained on this exciting website.

TestGen You may wish to create a custom-tailored test using *Prentice Hall TestGen for Essentials of Paramedic Care,* 2nd Edition to evaluate student understanding of this chapter.

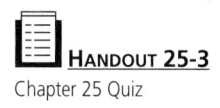

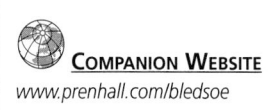

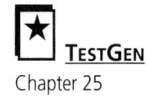

WORKBOOK
Chapter 25 Activities

READING/REFERENCE
Textbook, pp. 1061–1078

HANDOUT 25-3
Chapter 25 Quiz

HANDOUT 25-4
Chapter 25 Scenario

PARAMEDIC STUDENT CD
Student Activities

COMPANION WEBSITE
www.prenhall.com/bledsoe

TESTGEN
Chapter 25

EMT ACHIEVE: PARAMEDIC TEST PREPARATION
Mistovich & Beasley. *EMT Achieve: Paramedic Test Preparation.*
www.prenhall.com/emtachieve/

REVIEW MANUAL FOR THE EMT-PARAMEDIC
Cherry & Mistovich. *Review Manual for the EMT-Paramedic,* 3rd edition.

HANDOUTS 25-5 AND 25-7
Reinforcement Activities

PARAMEDIC STUDENT CD
Student Activities

POWERPOINT PRESENTATION
Chapter 25

COMPANION WEBSITE
http:/www/prenhall.com/bledsoe

ONEKEY
Chapter 25

ADVANCED LIFE SUPPORT SKILLS
Larmon & Davis. *Advanced Life Support Skills.*

ADVANCED LIFE SKILLS REVIEW
Larmon & Davis. *Advanced Life Skills Review.*

BRADY SKILLS SERIES: ALS
Larmon & Davis. *Brady Skills Series: ALS.*

PARAMEDIC NATIONAL STANDARDS SELF-TEST
Miller. *Paramedic National Standards Self-Test,* 4th edition.

On-line Test Preparation (for students and instructors)   Additional test preparation is available through Brady's new on-line product, *EMT Achieve: Paramedic Test Preparation* at *http://www.prenhall.com/emtachieve*. Instructors can also monitor student mastery on-line.

Review Manual for the EMT-Paramedic   This comprehensive exam review contains hundreds of test questions and rationales, including scenarios, along with two 180-question practice tests on CD.

REINFORCEMENT

Handouts   If classroom discussion or performance on the quiz indicates that some students have not fully mastered the chapter content, you may wish to assign some or all of the Reinforcement Handouts for this chapter.

Student CD (for students)   A wide variety of material on this CD-ROM will reinforce and also expand student knowledge and skills.

PowerPoint Presentation (for instructors)   The PowerPoint material developed for this chapter offers useful reinforcement of chapter content.

Companion Website (for students)   Additional review quizzes and links to EMS resources will contribute to further reinforcement of the chapter.

OneKey   On-line support is offered for this course on one of three platforms: CourseCompass, Blackboard, or Web CT. Includes the IRM, PowerPoints, TestGen, and Companion Website for instruction. Ask your local sales representative for more information.

Brady Skills Series: Advanced Life Skills (Video or CD)   Have your students watch the skills come to life on VHS or CD-ROM, or they can purchase the highly visual, full-color text with step-by-step procedures and rationales.

Handout 25-1

Student's Name _____

CHAPTER 25 OBJECTIVES CHECKLIST

Knowledge	Date Mastered
1. Describe the incidence, morbidity, and mortality of thoracic injuries in the trauma patient.	
2. Discuss the anatomy and physiology of the thoracic organs and structures.	
3. Predict thoracic injuries based on mechanism of injury.	
4. Discuss the pathophysiology of, assessment findings with, and the management and need for rapid intervention and transport of the patient with chest wall injuries, including: • Rib fracture • Flail segment • Sternal fracture	
5. Discuss the pathophysiology of, assessment findings with, and management and need for rapid intervention and transport of the patient with injury to the lung, including: • Simple pneumothorax • Open pneumothorax • Tension pneumothorax • Hemothorax • Hemopneumothorax • Pulmonary contusion	
6. Discuss the pathophysiology of, findings of assessment with, and management and need for rapid intervention and transport of the patient with myocardial injuries, including: • Myocardial contusion • Pericardial tamponade • Myocardial rupture	
7. Discuss the pathophysiology of, findings of assessment with, and management and need for rapid intervention and transport of the patient with vascular injuries, including injuries to: • Aorta • Vena cava • Pulmonary arteries/veins	
8. Discuss the pathophysiology of, findings of assessment with, and management and need for rapid intervention and transport of patients with diaphragmatic, esophageal, and tracheobronchial injuries.	

OBJECTIVES

HANDOUT 25-1 Continued

Knowledge	Date Mastered
9. Discuss the pathophysiology of, findings of assessment with, and management and need for rapid intervention and transport of the patient with traumatic asphyxia.	
10. Differentiate between thoracic injuries based on the assessment and history.	
11. Given several preprogrammed and moulaged thoracic trauma patients, provide the appropriate scene size-up, initial assessment, rapid trauma or focused physical exam and history, detailed exam, and ongoing assessment and provide appropriate patient care and transportation.	

OBJECTIVES

Handout 25-2

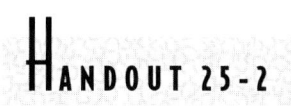

Student's Name _____

CHEST DECOMPRESSION

Charting Student Progress:
1. *Learning skill*
2. *Performs skill with direction*
3. *Performs skill independently*

Skill/Behavior	1	2	3
1. Takes BSI precautions.			
2. Recognizes indications for procedure.			
3. Prepares equipment.			
4. Palpates site at 2nd intercostal space, mid-clavicular line.			
5. Cleanses site appropriately.			
6. Inserts needle at superior border of third rib until air is released.			
7. Checks for improvement in clinical status.			
8. Applies flutter valve, tapes in place.			
9. Reassesses ventilations.			

Comments:

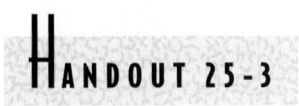

CHAPTER 25 QUIZ

Write the letter of the best answer in the space provided.

_____ 1. The term *comorbidity* refers to:
   A. at least two victims dying of the same injury or illness at the same time.
   B. an associated disease process; that is, the cause of death being two injuries or illnesses.
   C. a victim dying as the result of a multiple-patient incident.
   D. a patient dying after receiving an organ transplant from another person.

_____ 2. Thoracic trauma is classified by mechanism into two major categories, which are:
   A. crush and impact.
   B. flat and sharp.
   C. blunt and penetrating.
   D. sudden and prolonged.

_____ 3. Deceleration injuries occur when the body is in motion and:
   A. suddenly accelerates at a high rate of speed.
   B. impacts a fixed object.
   C. gradually slows to a stop.
   D. partially impacts an object, causing it to drastically change direction.

_____ 4. The age of the blunt trauma victim may affect the trauma received and its seriousness. Which of the following is TRUE?
   A. The elderly thorax is often soft, resulting in fewer rib fractures.
   B. Pediatric patients have fewer rib fractures but a greater incidence of serious internal injury.
   C. Preexisting disease has been shown to have little effect on the elderly response to trauma.
   D. The cartilaginous nature of the elderly thorax results in greater incidence of rib fracture.

_____ 5. Which of the following is TRUE regarding chest wall contusion?
   A. Chest wall contusion is the most common injury encountered in penetrating chest trauma.
   B. The most noticeable sign/symptom of chest wall contusion is rib fracture.
   C. The pain from a chest wall contusion does not change with inspiration.
   D. In the pediatric patient, you may find chest wall contusion and internal injury without rib fracture.

_____ 6. The most commonly fractured ribs are the:
   A. 1st through 4th.
   B. 4th through 9th.
   C. 5th through 8th.
   D. 9th through 12th.

_____ 7. Paradoxical chest wall motion is seen in the patient with:
   A. COPD.
   B. pneumothorax.
   C. flail chest.
   D. dislocation at the sternoclavicular joint.

_____ 8. The primary difference between a simple pneumothorax and a tension pneumothorax is that the:
   A. tension pneumothorax is caused by an open chest wound.
   B. simple pneumothorax must be treated by insertion of a large catheter into the chest.
   C. simple pneumothorax does not result in dyspnea, whereas the tension pneumothorax does.
   D. tension pneumothorax generates and maintains a pressure greater than atmospheric pressure within the thorax.

_____ 9. Signs and symptoms of a tension pneumothorax include:
   A. hyperresonance of the uninjured side of the chest.
   B. flat jugular veins.
   C. hypertension.
   D. ventilation/perfusion mismatch.

HANDOUT 25-3 Continued

_____ 10. Your patient has sustained a blunt trauma to the chest. He is dyspneic and is showing signs and symptoms of shock. You note dull percussive sounds over the site of the injury. You suspect:
   A. hemothorax.
   B. simple pneumothorax.
   C. tension pneumothorax.
   D. traumatic asphyxia.

_____ 11. Signs and symptoms including bruising to the chest wall; a weak, rapid, irregular heart rate; sweating; and a severe nagging pain not relieved by rest are indicative of:
   A. hemothorax.
   B. tension pneumothorax.
   C. pulmonary contusion.
   D. cardiac contusion.

_____ 12. Coughing up blood is called:
   A. hemothorax.
   B. hemoptysis.
   C. hematuria.
   D. hematemesis.

_____ 13. Blood or other fluid in the pericardial sac is called:
   A. hemothorax.
   B. cardiac contusion.
   C. pleural effusion.
   D. pericardial tamponade.

_____ 14. Your patient exhibits a drop of greater than 10 mmHg in the systolic blood pressure during inspiration. This condition is known as:
   A. pulsus paradoxus.
   B. narrowing pulse pressure.
   C. orthostatic hypotension.
   D. the tilt test.

_____ 15. Aortic aneurysm and rupture are extremely life-threatening injuries. When caring for a patient with either of these, you would expect:
   A. that the aorta is most commonly injured by penetrating trauma.
   B. aortic injury carries an overall mortality of 85 to 95 percent.
   C. unlike myocardial rupture, very few, possibly as little as 5 percent, of the victims will survive the initial insult and aneurysm.
   D. that the aorta is relatively fixed at only one point, the aortic annulus.

_____ 16. When caring for the patient with thoracic injuries, you should remember that:
   A. diaphragmatic rupture presents with signs and symptoms similar to tension pneumothorax.
   B. traumatic esophageal rupture is a common complication of blunt thoracic trauma.
   C. intermittent positive-pressure ventilation will greatly improve the condition of the patient with disruption of the trachea.
   D. traumatic asphyxia occurs when severe compressive force is applied to the trachea, crushing the structure.

_____ 17. Your primary concern when responding to a call of a gunshot wound to the chest is:
   A. the patient's mental status.
   B. airway control.
   C. hemorrhage control.
   D. personal safety.

_____ 18. During the rapid trauma assessment of the patient with a thoracic injury, you should:
   A. splint all suspected fractures.
   B. auscultate all lung lobes, both anteriorly and posteriorly.
   C. administer positive-pressure ventilations with 100 percent oxygen.
   D. initiate two large-bore IV lines and run wide open.

_____ 19. Management of the chest injury patient includes:
   A. the use of sandbags to support a flail segment.
   B. the administration of nitrous oxide for pain control of rib fractures.
   C. the application of an occlusive dressing to an open pneumothorax, completely sealing it on all four sides to prevent tension pneumothorax.
   D. placement of a second or third catheter to more rapidly decompress a tension pneumothorax if the patient remains symptomatic.

HANDOUT 25-3 Continued

_____ 20. Management of the patient with traumatic asphyxia includes:
   A. consideration of administering sodium bicarbonate if the patient remains entrapped for a prolonged time.
   B. establishing two large-bore IV lines for rapid infusion of crystalloid in anticipation of hypovolemia.
   C. preparation for immediate transport after release from entrapment.
   D. all of these

Handout 25-4

Student's Name _____

CHAPTER 25 SCENARIO

Review the following real-life situation. Then answer the questions that follow.

Ambulance 73 is dispatched to a woman who has been kicked in the chest by a horse. The injury occurred while the woman was filing and beveling the horse's left rear hoof. Her young son ran into the house to call 911. Paramedics David and Michael turn onto a dirt road leading to a farmhouse. The young boy is running toward the ambulance. "She's over here! Please hurry!" David grabs the trauma kit while Michael grabs the soft pack of portable oxygen supplies. The paramedics find the woman lying in the pasture, conscious but in severe pain.

1. The paramedics find the woman conscious, with respiratory difficulty, and in great pain. The boy tells you what has happened. List at least three possible blunt chest injuries the woman could have sustained.

2. What is the paramedics' most important concern in chest trauma?

3. As the paramedics begin their assessment, the signs and symptoms lead them to believe that the patient has a flail chest. Define *flail chest*.

4. List at least five signs of a flail chest.

5. David notes paradoxical motion on the right side of the patient's chest. Define *paradoxical motion*.

6. Describe the treatment that should be given and how the patient should be transported.

Handout 25-5

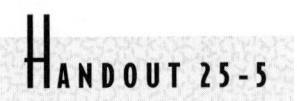

Student's Name _____

CHAPTER 25 REVIEW

Write the word or words that best complete the following sentences in the space provided.

1. The _____ of the blunt trauma victim may affect the trauma received and its seriousness.
2. _____ _____ injuries are by far the most common injuries encountered in blunt chest trauma.
3. Paradoxical chest wall motion seen in a chest injury patient indicates a(n) _____ chest.
4. _____-_____ ventilation of the patient with flail chest reverses the mechanism that causes the paradoxical chest wall movement.
5. The buildup of air under pressure within the thorax is called a(n) _____ _____.
6. Signs and symptoms of a tension pneumothorax include _____ / _____ mismatch, jugular vein _____, _____-tension and _____-volemia.
7. Blood within the pleural space is called a(n) _____.
8. A sign of a hemothorax is _____ percussive sounds over the injury site.
9. _____ is the coughing up of blood that has its origin in the respiratory tract.
10. When the heart impacts the inside of the anterior chest wall and is then compressed between the sternum and the thoracic spine, the condition is known as _____ _____.
11. The restriction to cardiac filling caused by blood or other fluid within the pericardial sac is known as _____ _____.
12. A condition associated with pericardial tamponade, a drop greater than 10 mmHg in the systolic blood pressure during inspiration, is known as _____ _____.
13. _____ _____ occurs when severe compressive force is applied to the thorax and leads to backwards flow of blood from the right heart into the superior vena cava and into the venous vessels of the upper extremities.
14. During the rapid trauma assessment you will examine the patient's chest in detail, carefully _____, _____ about, _____, and auscultating the region.
15. Auscultate _____ lung lobes, both _____ and _____.
16. Penetrating trauma to the heart is likely to cause pericardial _____ and present with jugular vein _____, _____ heart sounds, and systemic _____.
17. The findings in question 16 are known as _____ triad.
18. Rapid fluid administration in the chest injury patient may increase the rate of _____ and dilute the _____ factors.
19. _____ _____ for pain control is contraindicated in chest trauma.
20. A sucking chest wound should be sealed with a(n) _____ dressing, taped on _____ sides to prevent tension pneumothorax.

REINFORCEMENT

638 ESSENTIALS OF PARAMEDIC CARE

HANDOUT 25-6

Student's Name _____

THORACIC TRAUMA PROBLEMS

1. Describe the respiratory system's physiological response to a simple rib fracture. What are the long-term effects?

2. Briefly describe those situations in which morphine sulfate may be indicated and when it is contraindicated for the patient suffering from thoracic trauma. Why may morphine sulfate be beneficial, and why may it be detrimental to a patient?

3. For what condition might needle decompression be necessary? How would you perform this procedure?

4. You are providing positive-pressure ventilation to a patient with a flail chest. Why is this good for the patient, and why might it be bad for the patient?

Handout 25-7

Student's Name _____

SIGNS OF TENSION PNEUMOTHORAX AND HEMOTHORAX

A. *Identify the signs of a tension pneumothorax.*

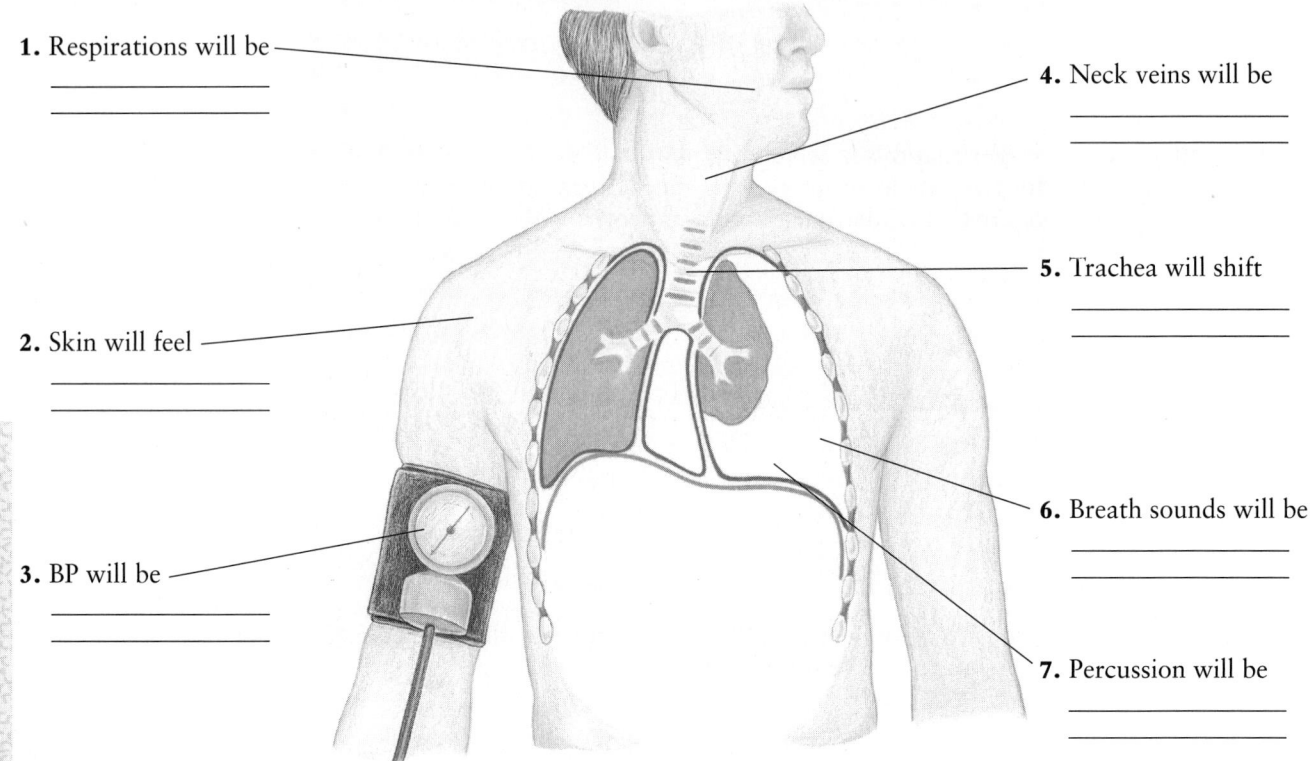

1. Respirations will be
_____
_____

2. Skin will feel
_____
_____

3. BP will be
_____
_____

4. Neck veins will be
_____
_____

5. Trachea will shift
_____

6. Breath sounds will be
_____
_____

7. Percussion will be
_____
_____

REINFORCEMENT

640 ESSENTIALS OF PARAMEDIC CARE

HANDOUT 25-7 Continued

B. *Identify the signs of a hemothorax.*

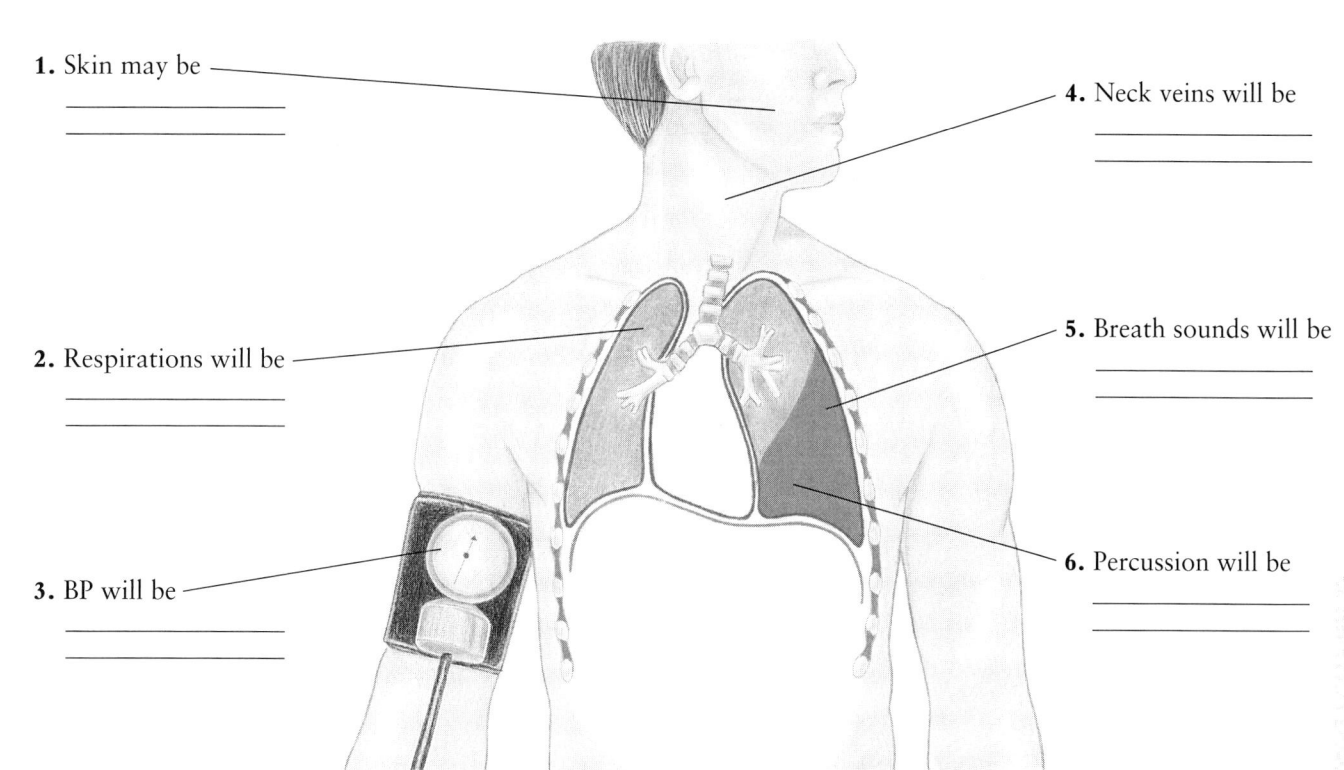

1. Skin may be _____

2. Respirations will be _____

3. BP will be _____

4. Neck veins will be _____

5. Breath sounds will be _____

6. Percussion will be _____

Chapter 25 Answer Key

HANDOUT 25-3: Chapter 25 Quiz

1. B	6. B	11. D	16. A
2. C	7. C	12. B	17. D
3. B	8. D	13. D	18. B
4. B	9. D	14. A	19. D
5. D	10. A	15. B	20. D

Handout 25-4: Chapter 25 Scenario

1. Any of the following are likely: flail chest, pulmonary contusion, tension pneumothorax, or hemothorax.
2. Hypoxia.
3. Three or more adjacent ribs fractured in multiple locations.
4. Signs include severe pain at the injury site, paradoxical chest wall movement, deformity and crepitation over the fractured rib, respiratory difficulty, and cyanosis.
5. Motion of the flail segment that is opposite to the motion of the rest of the chest.
6. Immobilize the spinal cord, administer oxygen via positive-pressure ventilation and a bag-valve device, apply gentle splinting of the flail segment with a pillow or a pad, and transport the patient on long spine board.

Handout 25-5: Chapter 25 Review

1. age
2. Chest wall
3. flail
4. Positive-pressure
5. tension pneumothorax
6. ventilation/perfusion, distention, hypo-, hypo-
7. hemothorax
8. dull
9. Hemoptysis
10. myocardial contusion
11. pericardial tamponade
12. pulsus paradoxus
13. Traumatic asphyxia
14. observing, questioning, palpating
15. all, anteriorly, posteriorly
16. tamponade, distention, distant, hypotension
17. Beck's
18. hemorrhage, clotting
19. Nitrous oxide
20. occlusive, three

Handout 25-6: Thoracic Trauma Problems

1. Because of the painful nature of the rib fracture, the patient will limit chest excursion with each breath. This limits tidal volume and reduces alveolar air. Additionally, the patient is breathing shallowly because chest expansion is painful. This results in alveolar collapse or atelectasis. The long-term effects may include pneumonia or respiratory infection.
2. Morphine sulfate may be appropriate for pain relief in the patient suffering from a simple rib fracture. However, morphine is a respiratory depressant. You should carefully monitor the patient's respiratory rate and depth of respirations if morphine sulfate is administered. Morphine sulfate is contraindicated in patients with possible abdominal injury, since it may hide the signs and symptoms of that injury.
3. Tension pneumothorax. First, locate the second or third intercostal space at the mid-clavicular line. Next, insert a large-bore (10–14 gauge) over-the-needle catheter just above the lower rib at a 90-degree angle. Then advance the needle until you hear air escape. Stop and advance the catheter and remove the needle. Secure the hub of the catheter with tape. Cover the hub with the finger of a latex or rubber glove. Tie or tape the glove finger to the hub, and cut the fingertip to allow air to escape.
4. Good: Positive pressure pushes both the normal chest wall and the flail segment outward. The chest wall and flail segment work in unison, thereby reducing the pain of chest expansion and improving air exchange. Sometimes you may have to ask the patient when he feels the need for a breath. Bad: It may exacerbate injury to the pulmonary tissues, possibly beneath the flail segment.

Handout 25-7: Signs of Tension Pneumothorax and Hemothorax

A. Tension pneumothorax
1. impaired, difficult
2. cool, clammy
3. low, indicative of shock
4. distended
5. toward the normal side
6. diminished or absent
7. hyperresonant

B. Hemothorax
1. cyanotic
2. minimally disturbed, early, difficult, late
3. low, indicative of shock
4. flat
5. absent
6. dull, flat

Chapter 26

Abdominal Trauma

INTRODUCTION

The abdominal cavity is one of the body's largest cavities. It also contains many vital organs. Serious injury to the abdomen may not only damage these organs, but also result in the loss of a great deal of blood before the loss is detected. Many of the outward signs of abdominal injury, such as deformity, swelling, and discoloration of contusions, take time to develop, and are not always seen in the prehospital setting. The anticipation of abdominal injuries, especially based on the mechanism of injury, and careful abdominal assessment are critical for the essential care of the patient. This chapter presents the anatomy and physiology, pathophysiology, assessment, and management of abdominal trauma.

TOTAL TEACHING TIME:
5.19 HOURS
The total teaching time is only a guideline based on the didactic and practical lab averages in the National Standard Curriculum. Instructors should take into consideration such factors as the pace at which students learn, the size of the class, and breaks. The actual time devoted to teaching objectives is the responsibility of the instructor.

CHAPTER OBJECTIVES

After reading this chapter, you should be able to:

1. Describe the epidemiology, including morbidity/mortality, for patients with abdominal trauma as well as prevention strategies to avoid the injuries. (p. 1062)
2. Apply the epidemiologic principles to develop prevention strategies for abdominal injuries. (p. 1062)
3. Describe the anatomy and physiology of the abdominal organs and structures. (see Chapter 3)
4. Predict abdominal injuries based on blunt and penetrating mechanisms of injury. (pp. 1062–1069)
5. Describe open and closed abdominal injuries. (pp. 1062–1065)
6. Identify the need for rapid intervention and transport of the patient with abdominal injuries based on assessment findings. (pp. 1069–1074)
7. Explain the pathophysiology of solid and hollow organ injuries, abdominal vascular injuries, pelvic fractures, and other abdominal injuries. (pp. 1065–1069)
8. Describe the assessment findings associated with and the management of solid and hollow organ injuries, abdominal vascular injuries, pelvic fractures, and other abdominal injuries. (pp. 1069–1077)

9. Differentiate between abdominal injuries based on the assessment and history. (pp. 1069–1075)
10. Given several preprogrammed and moulaged abdominal trauma patients, provide the appropriate scene size-up, initial assessment, rapid trauma or focused physical exam and history, detailed exam, and ongoing assessment and provide appropriate patient care and transportation. (pp. 1062–1077)

FRAMING THE LESSON

Begin by reviewing the important points of Chapter 25, "Thoracic Trauma." Use this time to answer any questions about the previous chapter and discuss any items not completely understood by students. Then begin the discussion of Chapter 26.

Begin with a review of the anatomy of the abdomen. Prepare life-sized cardboard cutouts of each organ found in the abdomen. Distribute them to students. Using a drawing of the human body on either a flip chart or chalkboard, have students tape each organ in its appropriate location. To make this exercise more enjoyable, have a student stand in front of the class in the anatomical position, and tape the abdominal organs to the student. As students attach each organ cutout, have them briefly describe what the function of the organ is, whether it is solid or hollow, and so on. Discuss the lack of skeletal structures in the abdomen and the difficulty sometimes associated with determining injuries. Stress the seriousness of injury and bleeding from solid abdominal organs.

TEACHING STRATEGIES

People learn in a variety of ways. Some do better with the spoken word, whereas others prefer the written. Some prefer to work alone, whereas others profit from working in groups. Recognizing these different ways of acquiring knowledge, the authors of this *Instructor's Resource Manual* have provided a variety of teaching strategies for the different types of learners. These strategies are intended to foster higher-level cognitive skills and encourage creative learning and problem solving. For greatest effectiveness, incorporate these strategies into your class lecture. Symbols in the Lecture Outline indicate the points at which various exercises might be most appropriate. Other strategies can be used to preview the lesson or to summarize it.

The following strategies are keyed to specific sections of the lesson.

1. Autopsy Observation. If possible, arrange through the coroner's office to have students observe an autopsy, paying particular attention to the abdomen. If this is not possible, the coroner's office or law enforcement training facility may have films or videos of autopsies for you to borrow. If you have a choice, attempt to obtain a film or video of an autopsy performed on someone with an abdominal injury.

2. Lamaze Class "Sympathy Belly" Palpation. Borrow a "sympathy belly" from a local Lamaze or parenting class. Use the belly on victims in simulations. Students are often reluctant to touch and palpate a pregnant belly. Frequently, when providers are uncomfortable touching a person or body part, they fail to expose the area and palpate too gingerly to actually observe rigidity or masses. Use the belly often enough that students become comfortable with this part of the female anatomy.

3. Written Assessments Based on Scenario Analysis. Create scenarios on paper for your students. Have students write out the assessment, concentrating on the abdominal trauma assessment specifically. There are many questions to ask and multiple physical findings that will more likely be remembered with this type of critical thinking than with rote memorization.

4. *MVA Victim Simulation.* Be sure to simulate victims in all areas of the vehicle during trauma simulations. Patients placed in different areas of the vehicle will present with different injury patterns. For instance, a patient placed in the back seat of an older vehicle would only have access to a lap belt, with no shoulder harness. For this victim, injuries to the abdomen might be expected from a misplaced lap belt, as well as injuries to the head from forward motion. Victims on the passenger side of a new vehicle will have an airbag and could suffer injuries, such as burns, from the bag itself. Preparing your students for field practice includes broadening the scope of what they see in classroom and laboratory simulations. By providing a wide range of experience, your students are more likely to correctly assess and treat patients in the field.

5. *Scenario Writing and Practice.* Divide students into groups of three or four. Have each group develop a scenario involving abdominal trauma. Make sure that each group chooses a different type of injury, such as motor vehicle trauma, stab, gunshot wound, and so on. Both blunt and penetrating abdominal trauma should be represented. Once scenarios have been written, have the groups develop a patient profile including information obtained by paramedics during scene size-up, initial assessment, focused history and physical or rapid trauma assessment, and ongoing assessment. Once this is completed, have a representative from the group read the scenario to the class. Based on the scenario, have students begin their "assessment" of the scene and the patient, asking questions regarding information they would normally want to know. Information should be given to the class only after the appropriate question has been asked. It will then be up to the class to outline the management of the patient in the scenario, including transport.

The following strategies can be used at various points throughout the lesson or to help summarize and demonstrate what students have learned.

Guest Speakers. Invite a trauma surgeon to class, asking him/her to bring any visual aids of abdominal wound patients he/she has encountered. This could include slides, photos, videos, and so on. Ask the trauma surgeon to present each patient's injuries, signs and symptoms, management, and eventual outcome. You may also consider inviting paramedics or law enforcement personnel to discuss victims of abdominal trauma they have dealt with. You may also invite a physician, RN, or other health care provider to discuss dealing with patients who have a colostomy in place.

Cultural Considerations, Legal Notes, and Patho Pearls. The Student CD-ROM contains this series of informative features to enhance the student's understanding of the material covered in this chapter.

TEACHING OUTLINE

Chapter 26, "Abdominal Trauma," is the eleventh lesson in Division 3, *Trauma Emergencies*. Distribute Handout 26-1 so that students can familiarize themselves with the learning goals for this chapter. If students have any questions about the objectives, answer them at this time.

Then present the chapter. One possible lecture outline follows. In the outline, the parenthetical references in regular type are references to text pages; those in bold type are references to figures, tables, or procedures.

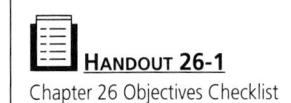

HANDOUT 26-1
Chapter 26 Objectives Checklist

POWERPOINT PRESENTATION
Chapter 26 PowerPoint slides 4–28

TEACHING STRATEGY 1
Autopsy Observation

POWERPOINT PRESENTATION
Chapter 26 PowerPoint slides 29–43

READING/REFERENCE
Criss, E. "Abdominal Gunshot Wounds." *JEMS*, Sept. 2000.

POINT TO EMPHASIZE
Due to the widespread energy transfer and injury pattern, mortality is high from blunt abdominal trauma.

TEACHING STRATEGY 2
Lamaze Class "Sympathy Belly" Palpation

TEACHING STRATEGY 3
Written Assessments Based on Scenario Analysis

POWERPOINT PRESENTATION
Chapter 26 PowerPoint slides 44–49

TEACHING STRATEGY 4
MVA Victim Simulation

POWERPOINT PRESENTATION
Chapter 26 PowerPoint slides 50–54

POINT OF INTEREST
Aortic rupture is the most common cause of sudden death from MVCs or long falls.

TEACHING STRATEGY 5
Scenario Writing and Practice

POWERPOINT PRESENTATION
Chapter 26 PowerPoint slide 55

I. Introduction. Serious direct or secondary injury to the abdominal cavity may damage any one or more of the vital organs contained in the area, including the liver, spleen, stomach, and large and small bowels. Solid organs, especially, may lose large volumes of blood internally without immediate outward signs. It is vital that the paramedic take into account mechanism of injury, as well as other signs and symptoms of abdominal organ damage, bleeding, and shock. Although care for serious abdominal trauma has improved, prevention is the best way to reduce mortality and morbidity. (p. 1062)

II. Pathophysiology of abdominal injury (pp. 1062–1069)

  A. Mechanism of injury (pp. 1062–1064)
   1. Penetrating trauma (**Fig. 26-1, p. 1063**)
   2. Blunt trauma (**Fig. 26-2, p. 1064**)
  B. Injury to the abdominal wall (pp. 1064–1065)
   1. Evisceration
  C. Injury to the hollow organs (p. 1065)
  D. Injury to the solid organs (pp. 1065–1066) (**Fig. 26-3, p. 1065, Fig. 26-4, p. 1066**)
  E. Injury to the vascular structures (p. 1066)
  F. Injury to the mesentery and bowel (pp. 1066–1067)
  G. Injury to the peritoneum (p. 1067)
   1. Peritonitis
   2. Guarding
  H. Injury to the pelvis (p. 1067)
  I. Injury during pregnancy (pp. 1067–1069)
   1. Physiological changes (**Fig. 26-5, p. 1068**)
   2. Abruptio placentae (**Fig. 26-6, p. 1069**)
  J. Injury to pediatric patients (p. 1069)

III. Assessment of the abdominal injury patient (pp. 1069–1074)

  A. Scene size-up (pp. 1069–1071) (**Figs. 26-7, p. 1070; Fig. 26-8, p. 1071**)
  B. Initial assessment (p. 1071)
  C. Rapid trauma assessment (pp. 1072–1074) (**Fig. 26-9, p. 1072**)
   1. Special assessment considerations with pregnant patients
  D. Ongoing assessment (p. 1074)

IV. Management of the abdominal injury patient (pp. 1074–1077)

  A. Management (pp. 1074–1075)
   1. Position
   2. Oxygenation and ventilation
   3. Control of external hemorrhage
   4. Aggressive fluid therapy
   5. PASG if not contraindicated
   6. Evisceration care (**Proc. 26-1, p. 1076**)
  B. Management of the pregnant patient (pp. 1075–1077)

V. Chapter summary (p. 1077). Blunt or penetrating abdominal trauma can result in serious organ damage and life-threatening hemorrhage. Concurrently, the signs of injury are limited, nonspecific, and do not reflect the seriousness of abdominal pathology. It is thus very important for your assessment to carefully determine the mechanism of injury and the region of the abdomen it affects. This information must be communicated to the emergency department to assure its personnel acknowledge the significance of your first-hand knowledge of the mechanism of injury.

Care for significant abdominal injury is provided by rapid transport to the trauma center. Most significant abdominal injury results in serious internal bleeding or organ injury that can neither be cared for nor stabilized in the prehospital setting. Further, the definitive care for the patient with serious abdominal injury is provided via surgery. The patient must be transported to a facility capable of providing immediate surgical intervention when needed. This is a trauma center. Prehospital care is supportive of the airway and breathing, and preventive for shock.

The pregnant patient with abdominal injury deserves special attention because her vascular volume is increased and she will likely not show the signs of shock until the fetus is at risk. Careful observation while preparing for rapid transport to the trauma center is in order. If any of the slightest signs of hypoperfusion is noted, initiate fluid resuscitation.

ASSIGNMENTS

Assign students to complete Chapter 26, "Abdominal Trauma," of the workbook. Also assign them to read Chapter 27, "Pulmonology," before the next class.

EVALUATION

Chapter Quiz and Scenario Distribute copies of the Chapter Quiz provided in Handout 26-2 to evaluate student understanding of this chapter. Make sure each student reads the scenario to reinforce critical thinking on the scene. Remind students not to use their notes or textbooks while taking the quiz.

Student CD Quizzes for every chapter are contained on the dynamic and highly visual in-text student CD.

Companion Website Additional quizzes for every chapter are contained on this exciting website.

TestGen You may wish to create a custom-tailored test using *Prentice Hall TestGen for Essentials of Paramedic Care*, 2nd Edition to evaluate student understanding of this chapter.

On-line Test Preparation (for students and instructors) Additional test preparation is available through Brady's new on-line product, *EMT Achieve: Paramedic Test Preparation* at http://www.prenhall.com/emtachieve/. Instructors can also monitor student mastery on-line.

Review Manual for the EMT-Paramedic This comprehensive exam review contains hundreds of test questions and rationales, including scenarios, along with two 180-question practice tests on CD.

REINFORCEMENT

Handouts If classroom discussion or performance on the quiz indicates that some students have not fully mastered the chapter content, you may wish to assign the Reinforcement Handout for this chapter.

Student CD (for students) A wide variety of material on this CD-ROM will reinforce and also expand student knowledge and skills.

POINT TO EMPHASIZE
The primary factor in assessing and managing abdominal trauma is not the accurate diagnosis of a specific type of injury but rather the recognition that an intraabdominal injury exists and surgery is required. Translation: Rapid transport to a surgical facility is the key to successful handling of abdominal trauma.

WORKBOOK
Chapter 26 Activities

READING/REFERENCE
Textbook, pp. 1080–1120

HANDOUT 26-2
Chapter 26 Quiz

HANDOUT 26-3
Chapter 26 Scenario

PARAMEDIC STUDENT CD
Student Activities

COMPANION WEBSITE
http://www.prenhall.com/bledsoe

TESTGEN
Chapter 26

EMT ACHIEVE: PARAMEDIC TEST PREPARATION
Mistovich & Beasley. *EMT Achieve: Paramedic Test Preparation.*
www.prenhall.com/emtachieve/

REVIEW MANUAL FOR THE EMT-PARAMEDIC
Cherry & Mistovich. *Review Manual for the EMT-Paramedic,* 3rd edition.

HANDOUT 26-4
Reinforcement Activities

PARAMEDIC STUDENT CD
Student Activities

POWERPOINT PRESENTATION
Chapter 26

COMPANION WEBSITE
http://www.prenhall.com/bledsoe

ONEKEY
Chapter 26

ADVANCED LIFE SUPPORT SKILLS
Larmon & Davis. *Advanced Life Support Skills.*

ADVANCED LIFE SKILLS REVIEW
Larmon & Davis. *Advanced Life Skills Review.*

BRADY SKILLS SERIES: ALS
Larmon & Davis. *Brady Skills Series: ALS.*

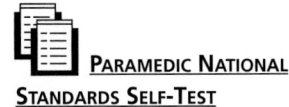

PARAMEDIC NATIONAL STANDARDS SELF-TEST
Miller. *Paramedic National Standards Self-Test*, 4th edition

PowerPoint Presentation (for instructors) The PowerPoint material developed for this chapter offers useful reinforcement of chapter content.

Companion Website (for students) Additional review quizzes and links to EMS resources will contribute to further reinforcement of the chapter.

OneKey On-line support is offered for this course on one of three platforms: CourseCompass, Blackboard, or Web CT. Includes the IRM, PowerPoints, TestGen, and Companion Website for instruction. Ask your local sales representative for more information.

Brady Skills Series: Advanced Life Skills (Video or CD) Have your students watch the skills come to life on VHS or CD-ROM, or they can purchase the highly visual, full-color text with step-by-step procedures and rationales.

HANDOUT 26-1

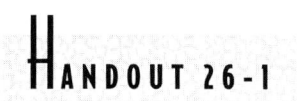

Student's Name _____

CHAPTER 26 OBJECTIVES CHECKLIST

Knowledge	Date Mastered
1. Describe the epidemiology, including morbidity/mortality, for patients with abdominal trauma as well as prevention strategies to avoid the injuries.	
2. Apply the epidemiologic principles to develop prevention strategies for abdominal injuries.	
3. Describe the anatomy and physiology of the abdominal organs and structures.	
4. Predict abdominal injuries based on blunt and penetrating mechanisms of injury.	
5. Describe open and closed abdominal injuries.	
6. Identify the need for rapid intervention and transport of the patient with abdominal injuries based on assessment findings.	
7. Explain the pathophysiology of solid and hollow organ injuries, abdominal vascular injuries, pelvic fractures, and other abdominal injuries.	
8. Describe the assessment findings associated with and the management of solid and hollow organ injuries, abdominal vascular injuries, pelvic fractures, and other abdominal injuries.	
9. Differentiate between abdominal injuries based on the assessment and history.	
10. Given several preprogrammed and moulaged abdominal trauma patients, provide the appropriate scene size-up, initial assessment, rapid trauma or focused physical exam and history, detailed exam, and ongoing assessment and provide appropriate patient care and transportation.	

HANDOUT 26-2

Student's Name _____

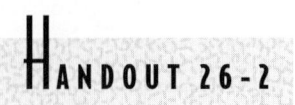

CHAPTER 26 QUIZ

Write the letter of the best answer in the space provided.

_____ 1. When considering the pathophysiology of abdominal injury, remember that:
   A. the abdomen is bound by muscles rather than skeletal structures.
   B. the majority of penetrating abdominal injuries affect the large bowel.
   C. blunt trauma to the abdomen produces the most visible signs of injury.
   D. blast injuries involve only blunt trauma caused by the pressure wave generated by the explosion.

_____ 2. Solid organs may rupture, causing unrestricted hemorrhage. Solid organs include the:
   A. stomach.
   B. rectum.
   C. pregnant uterus.
   D. kidneys.

_____ 3. Which of the following is TRUE regarding the liver?
   A. It is a retroperitoneal organ.
   B. The liver is not as firm as the spleen and pancreas.
   C. It is restrained from forward motion by the ligamentum teres.
   D. The liver is the second largest single organ within the abdomen, being smaller than the stomach.

_____ 4. Peritonitis is:
   A. the release of bowel contents into the abdomen.
   B. inflammation of the peritoneum.
   C. evisceration of the peritoneum.
   D. protective tensing of abdominal muscles due to pain.

_____ 5. The number one killer of pregnant females is:
   A. toxicity.
   B. trauma.
   C. complications of pregnancy.
   D. infection.

_____ 6. Separation of the placenta from the uterine wall during pregnancy is called:
   A. abruptio placentae.
   B. placenta previa.
   C. placenta prolapse.
   D. placenta premature.

_____ 7. Possibly the most important element of the assessment of a patient with abdominal trauma is:
   A. hemorrhage control.
   B. mechanism of injury.
   C. splinting of possible fractures/dislocations.
   D. skin color and condition.

_____ 8. During your initial assessment of a patient with abdominal injury, remember:
   A. that level of consciousness and orientation are not reliable indicators of the patient's condition.
   B. to ask the patient to move from a supine position to a seated or standing position to assess for dizziness or lightheadedness.
   C. that limited chest movement may be due to the pain of peritonitis or blood irritating the diaphragm.
   D. that rapid, shallow respirations, diminished pulse pressure, and a rapid pulse are all late signs of shock not often seen in the prehospital setting.

HANDOUT 26-2 Continued

_____ 9. The principles of managing the abdominal injury patient include:
   A. placing the patient in the prone position for relief of pain.
   B. anticipation of shock based only on the mechanism of injury.
   C. control of all external bleeding prior to transport.
   D. initiation of a large-bore IV line with 5 percent dextrose in water.

_____ 10. Place the late-term pregnant patient in the:
   A. right lateral recumbent position
   B. Trendelenburg position.
   C. Fowler's position.
   D. left lateral recumbent position.

Handout 26-3

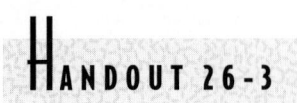

Student's Name _____

CHAPTER 26 SCENARIO

Review the following real-life situation. Then answer the questions that follow.

"My boyfriend's been cut in his stomach by a knife! We need an ambulance!" The dispatcher attempts to calm the excited caller, then dispatches law enforcement and Medic 12, with paramedics Rachel and Damon, to the parking lot of a local tavern known as a "bikers' bar." The ambulance is advised to proceed with caution and not to stage until the scene is secured by law enforcement. As the paramedics arrive, they see three police cars on scene. An officer motions for the ambulance to proceed in and directs the paramedics to a large motorcycle. Lying across the seat of the motorcycle is an adult male, in obvious distress, holding a bloody leather jacket over his abdomen.

1. What should Rachel and Damon do next?

The patient removes his jacket. The paramedics see a protruding bowel.

2. What is the name of this kind of penetrating injury? What are the paramedics' immediate concerns? What is the most common protruding viscera?

3. How should Rachel and Damon conduct an assessment of this patient?

During the assessment, the patient tries to push the bowel back through the wound.

4. How should the paramedics manage this patient? Should they replace the bowel? Should they use the PASG?

HANDOUT 26-4

Student's Name _____

CHAPTER 26 REVIEW

Write the word or words that best complete the following sentences in the space provided.

1. The abdomen is bound by _____ rather than _____ structures.
2. Forty percent of penetrating abdominal trauma affects the _____.
3. _____ trauma to the abdomen produces the least visible signs of injury.
4. Blunt trauma causes trauma through three mechanisms: _____, _____, and _____.
5. With trauma to the abdomen, the discoloration of _____ and noticeable _____ require several hours to develop.
6. The liver, spleen, pancreas, and kidneys are considered _____ organs, while the stomach and bowels are considered _____ organs.
7. Liver injury often presents with pain in the upper right _____ as blood accumulates against the diaphragm.
8. Inflammation of the peritoneum is called _____.
9. _____ is the protective tensing of the abdominal muscles due to pain.
10. Trauma is the number one killer of _____ females.
11. Premature separation of the placenta from the uterine wall is known as _____ _____.
12. Children compensate well for blood loss and may not show any signs or symptoms until they have lost over _____ of their blood volume.
13. For the patient who has sustained abdominal injury, the analysis of the _____ _____ _____ is the most important element of the scene size-up.
14. With a patient who has experienced penetrating trauma you should _____ (remove/not remove) the impaled object.
15. Abnormal _____ in the abdomen suggest arterial injury.
16. The major emphasis of the management of the abdominal injury patient is bringing the patient to _____ as quickly as possible.
17. The use of the PASG is contraindicated for _____ _____ _____ females.
18. Titrate your administration rate of IV fluids to maintain a systolic blood pressure of _____.
19. Assure that you do not exceed _____ of fluid during field care and transport.
20. Place the late-term mother, when possible, in the _____ _____ _____ position.

REINFORCEMENT

©2007 Pearson Education, Inc.
Essentials of Paramedic Care, 2nd ed.

CHAPTER 26 *Abdominal Trauma* 653

Chapter 26 Answer Key

Handout 26-2: Chapter 26 Quiz

1. A
2. D
3. C
4. B
5. B
6. A
7. B
8. C
9. B
10. D

Handout 26-3: Chapter 26 Scenario

1. Determine the mechanism of injury and extent of injury by asking the patient to remove the jacket. (Depending on the circumstances, it may still be a good idea to have the police stay close by to ensure that the scene remains safe.)
2. This type of injury is an evisceration. The paramedics should be concerned about shock, occluded blood supply to the bowel, and bowel contamination. The small bowel is the most common protruding viscera.
3. Though the mechanism of injury may appear obvious, Rachel or Damon should confirm the mechanism of injury by questioning the patient and bystanders. However, this patient needs surgery. The patient should be prepared for immediate transport. With any abdominal trauma, paramedics should suspect cervical spine injury. The patient should be immobilized, and the paramedics should perform a rapid initial assessment. A rapid trauma assessment should then be performed.
4. As mentioned previously, this patient needs definitive surgical care. The paramedics should administer 100 percent oxygen via nonrebreather mask. The bowel should not be replaced. The open wound should be covered with a wet sterile dressing, then an occlusive dressing. The patient's hands may need to be restrained to prevent them from manipulating the bowel. While en route, the paramedics should insert two large-bore IVs. The use of the PASG is controversial for eviscerations. The paramedics should consult their Medical Control, which may advise them to inflate only the leg sections.

Handout 26-4: Chapter 26 Review

1. muscles, skeletal
2. liver
3. Blunt
4. deceleration, compression, shear
5. ecchymosis, swelling
6. solid, hollow
7. shoulder
8. peritonitis
9. Guarding
10. pregnant
11. abruptio placentae
12. half
13. mechanism of injury
14. not remove
15. pulsations
16. surgery
17. late term pregnant
18. 88 mmHg
19. 3,000 mL
20. left lateral recumbent

Essentials of Paramedic Care

Division 4

Medical Emergencies

Chapter 27

Pulmonology

INTRODUCTION

Respiratory emergencies are among some of the most common conditions EMS personnel encounter. Paramedics must promptly recognize respiratory problems and treat them appropriately. This chapter discusses pathophysiology, assessment, and management of the most frequently encountered respiratory emergencies.

CHAPTER OBJECTIVES

After reading this chapter, you should be able to:

1. Discuss the epidemiology of pulmonary diseases and pulmonary conditions. (p. 1081)
2. Identify and describe the function of the structures located in the upper and lower airway. (see Chapter 3)
3. Discuss the physiology of ventilation and respiration. (pp. 1081–1084; also see Chapter 3)
4. Identify common pathological events that affect the pulmonary system. (pp. 1084–1086)
5. Compare various airway and ventilation techniques used in the management of pulmonary diseases. (pp. 1098–1118)
6. Review the use of equipment utilized during the physical examination of patients with complaints associated with respiratory diseases and conditions. (pp. 1091–1092, 1093–1098)
7. Identify the epidemiology, anatomy, physiology, pathophysiology, assessment findings, and management (including prehospital medications) for the following respiratory diseases and conditions:

    - Adult respiratory distress syndrome (pp. 1100–1101)
    - Bronchial asthma (pp. 1101–1102, 1105–1108)
    - Chronic bronchitis (pp. 1101–1102, 1104–1105)
    - Emphysema (pp. 1101–1104)
    - Pneumonia (pp. 1109–1110)
    - Pulmonary edema (pp. 1100–1101)
    - Pulmonary thromboembolism (pp. 1114–1116)
    - Neoplasms of the lung (pp. 1112–1113)
    - Upper respiratory infections (pp. 1108–1109)
    - Spontaneous pneumothorax (p. 1116)
    - Hyperventilation syndrome (pp. 1116–1117)

TOTAL TEACHING TIME:
17.25 HOURS
The total teaching time is only a guideline based on the didactic and practical lab averages in the National Standard Curriculum. Instructors should take into consideration such factors as the pace at which students learn, the size of the class, and breaks. The actual time devoted to teaching objectives is the responsibility of the instructor.

©2007 Pearson Education, Inc.
Essentials of Paramedic Care, 2nd ed.

8. Given several preprogrammed patients with nontraumatic pulmonary problems, provide the appropriate assessment, prehospital care, and transport. (pp. 1081–1118)

FRAMING THE LESSON

Begin the class by taking an informal survey of students, asking if any of them or their family members have experienced any type of respiratory disease or problem. These may include temporary conditions (such as respiratory infections and pneumonia) and chronic conditions (such as asthma or emphysema). Encourage them to describe the signs and symptoms they observed and the treatment that was provided for the condition. Continue by asking: How does it feel to be short of breath? How might patients feel about having to continually be on medication or supplemental oxygen for the rest of their lives? How might patients react to suddenly being unable to breathe normally? Conclude by discussing how organs in the body, especially the brain, react to a decrease in the oxygen level of the blood.

TEACHING STRATEGIES

People learn in a variety of ways. Some do better with the spoken word, whereas others prefer the written. Some prefer to work alone, whereas others profit from working in groups. Recognizing these different ways of acquiring knowledge, the authors of this *Instructor's Resource Manual* have provided a variety of teaching strategies for the different types of learners. These strategies are intended to foster higher-level cognitive skills and encourage creative learning and problem solving. For greatest effectiveness, incorporate these strategies into your class lecture. Symbols in the Lecture Outline indicate the points at which various exercises might be most appropriate. Other strategies can be used to preview the lesson or to summarize it.

The following strategies are keyed to specific sections of the lesson.

1. Filtering the Air. The respiratory system functions much like air filters in your car or shop-vac. Bring in a clean filter and shop-vac the carpet in class. Remove the filter to demonstrate the enormous amount of particulates filtered by the system every day. The filter will likely be visibly changed in color with noticeable hairs, dirt, dust, and other particles attached. This is a very visual activity that will stay with the students for a long time to come.

2. Exploring the Diseased Respiratory System. Divide the pathologies of the respiratory system and have students become "mini-explorers" of a respiratory system that is afflicted by a disease to which they have been assigned. Have students write about what the diseased respiratory system would look like, feel like, and smell like inside a smoker, asthmatic, or victim of an airway obstruction. How would things move in and out? How does breathing occur? For larger classes, include other pathologies such as ALS or MS. Get creative and your students will, too. This will make learning about anatomy and pathophysiology fun and memorable.

3. Replicating Ventilatory Rates and Patterns. Toss a ball or beanbag to the rate and pattern of the respiratory patterns discussed on pages 1084–1085 of the textbook. The graphic representation in Figure 27-2 is good, but a ball or beanbag will get students actively reacting and thinking. For instance, normal respiration should be tossed about 12–20 times per minute in a regular rhythm and pattern. Cheyne-Stokes respirations will get increasingly faster and farther, then slower and closer until someone holds the ball for a minute, and then repeats the patterns.

4. Recognizing Lung Sounds. Lung sounds are challenging for seasoned paramedics, let alone students. So consider using an audio recording of a variety of lung sounds to help students become familiar with them. (Students should apply their stethoscopes directly to the speaker.) To ensure that adequate time has been spent practicing lung sound recognition prior to sending students to clinicals, you may wish to set up an audio quiz using the recording.

The following strategies can be used at various points throughout the lesson or to help summarize and demonstrate what students have learned.

Reviewing Terminology. To help students review terminology related to respiratory anatomy and conditions, play a word game based on the popular game Jeopardy! Use the new terms in Chapter 27 as the "answers" (e.g., "pleuritic"). Have students provide the definitions of those terms as the "questions" (e.g., "What term describes a sharp or tearing pain?"). Each contestant (or team) starts the game with 0 points. Add 10 points for each correct response; subtract 10 points for each incorrect response.

Guest Lecturer. Consider inviting a speaker from the local chapter of the Lung Association. Most chapters have access to teaching aids and support materials on lung diseases. Such community networking is beneficial to all parties involved.

Learning about Drugs. To help them learn the key information about the drugs used in respiratory emergencies, have your students create a flash card for each drug mentioned in the chapter. Though many drug cards are commercially available, nothing helps students retain data like writing up their own cards.

Practice in the Field. Have students consider assisting their local Lung Association with "Asthma Camps," its annual summer camp program. Because of the availability of paramedics and respiratory therapists on site, children who would otherwise be unable to go to summer camp finally can. In addition to serving a greater purpose while advancing the principles of EMS, students will gain valuable insight and experience.

Practice in the Field. Point out to students that they can obtain some of their clinical observation time while assisting respiratory therapists at local hospitals.

Cultural Considerations, Legal Notes, and Patho Pearls. The Student CD-ROM contains this series of informative features to enhance the student's understanding of the material covered in this chapter.

TEACHING OUTLINE

Chapter 27 is the first lesson in Division 4, *Medical Emergencies*. Distribute Handout 27-1 so that students can familiarize themselves with the learning goals for this chapter. If students have any questions about the objectives, answer them at this time.

Then present the chapter. One possible lecture outline follows. In the outline, the parenthetical references in regular type are references to text pages; those in bold type are reference to figures, tables, and procedures.

I. Introduction (pp. 1081–1084)

A. The respiratory system is a vital body system responsible for providing oxygen to the tissues and removing carbon dioxide. (p. 1081)
B. Respiratory emergencies are among the most common emergencies EMS personnel are called upon to treat. (p. 1081)

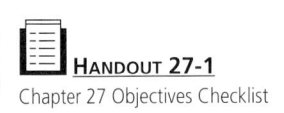

HANDOUT 27-1
Chapter 27 Objectives Checklist

POWERPOINT PRESENTATION
Chapter 27 PowerPoint slides 4–14

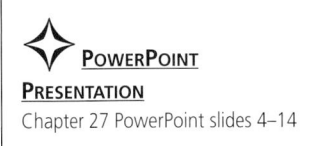

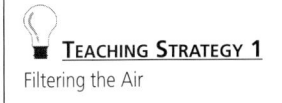

TEACHING STRATEGY 1
Filtering the Air

TEACHING STRATEGY 2
Exploring the Diseased Respiratory System

TEACHING STRATEGY 3
Replicating Ventilatory Rates and Patterns

POWERPOINT PRESENTATION
Chapter 27 PowerPoint slides 15–17

READING/REFERENCE
Frailey, G. "Twenty Respiratory Challenges." *JEMS*, May 2000.

POWERPOINT PRESENTATION
Chapter 27 PowerPoint slides 18–31

TEACHING STRATEGY 4
Recognizing Lung Sounds

POINT TO EMPHASIZE
Common errors in lung auscultation include trying to listen through clothing, listening in a noisy environment, and misinterpreting the stethoscope tube rubbing against objects and chest hair as adventitious sounds.

POINT OF INTEREST
A useful mnemonic for recalling the major causes for acute dyspnea is PPOPPA:
Pulmonary embolism
Pulmonary edema
Obstruction
Pneumothorax
Pneumonia
Asthma (COPD)

READING/REFERENCE
Krauss, B. "Capnography in EMS." *JEMS*, Jan. 2003.
Whitehead, S. "The Coming Capnography Wave." *EMS*, March. 2003.

   C. Risk factors (p. 1081)
      1. Intrinsic risk factors
      2. Extrinsic risk factors
   D. Physiological processes (pp. 1081–1084)
      1. Ventilation
         a. Inspiration and expiration
         b. Airway resistance and lung compliance
         c. Lung volumes
         d. Regulation of ventilation
      2. Diffusion
      3. Perfusion (**Fig. 27-1, p. 1083**)

II. **Pathophysiology** (pp. 1084–1086)
   A. Disruption in ventilation (pp. 1084–1085)
      1. Upper and lower respiratory tracts
      2. Chest wall and diaphragm
      3. Nervous system (**Fig. 27-2, p. 1085**)
         a. Cheyne-Stokes respirations
         b. Kussmaul's respirations
         c. Central neurogenic hyperventilation
         d. Ataxic (Biot's) respirations
         e. Apneustic respiration
   B. Disruption in diffusion (p. 1086)
   C. Disruption in perfusion (p. 1086)

III. **Assessment of the respiratory system** (pp. 1086–1098)
   A. Scene size-up (pp. 1086–1087)
   B. Initial assessment (pp. 1087–1089)
      1. General impression
         a. Position (**Fig. 27-3, p. 1087**)
         b. Color
         c. Mental status
         d. Ability to speak
         e. Respiratory effort
         f. Signs of respiratory distress
      2. Airway
         a. Obstructions
      3. Breathing
         a. Rate
         b. Quality
         c. Effort
   C. Focused history and physical examination (pp. 1089–1098)
      1. History
      2. Physical examination
         a. Inspection (**Fig. 27-4, p. 1091; Fig. 27-5, p. 1092**)
         b. Palpation
         c. Percussion
         d. Auscultation
         e. Normal breath sounds
         f. Abnormal breath sounds
      3. Vital signs
      4. Diagnostic testing
         a. Pulse oximetry (**Fig. 27-6, p. 1093**)
         b. Peak flow (**Fig. 27-7, p. 1094**) (**Table 27-1, p. 1094**)

        c. Capnometry (**Table 27-2**, p. 1095)
           i. Colorimetric devices (**Fig. 27-8**, p. 1096)
           ii. Electronic devices (**Fig. 27-9**, p. 1096; **Fig. 27-10**, p. 1097)
           iii. Capnogram (**Fig. 27-11**, p. 1097)
           iv. Clinical applications (**Fig. 27-12**, p. 1098)

IV. Management of respiratory disorders (p. 1098)

A. Airway is always first priority (p. 1098)
B. Correct hypoxia (p. 1098)
    1. Establish and maintain an airway.
    2. Assist ventilations if needed.
    3. Administer oxygen.
        a. To any patient with respiratory distress
        b. To any patient with an illness or injury that suggests the possibility of hypoxia
        c. When in doubt
    4. Pharmacological agents may also be required.

V. Specific respiratory diseases (pp. 1098–1118)

A. Upper airway obstruction (pp. 1098–1099)
    1. Assessment
        a. Capnography
    2. Management
        a. Conscious adult
        b. Unconscious adult
B. Noncardiogenic pulmonary edema/adult respiratory distress syndrome (ARDS) (pp. 1100–1101)
    1. Pathophysiology
    2. Assessment
    3. Management
C. Obstructive lung diseases (pp. 1101–1108), (**Fig. 27-13**, p. 1102)
    1. Emphysema (**Fig. 27-14**, p. 1103)
        a. Pathophysiology
        b. Assessment
        c. Management
    2. Chronic bronchitis (**Fig. 27-15**, p. 1104)
        a. Pathophysiology
        b. Assessment
        c. Management
    3. Asthma
        a. Pathophysiology
        b. Assessment (**Table 27-3**, p. 1107)
           i. Continuous waveform capnography (**Fig. 27-16**, p. 1107)
        c. Management
        d. Special cases
           i. Status asthmaticus
           ii. Asthma in children
D. Upper respiratory infection (URI) (pp. 1108–1109) (**Table 27-4**, p. 1109)
    1. Pathophysiology
    2. Assessment
    3. Management
E. Pneumonia (pp. 1109–1110)
    1. Pathophysiology
    2. Assessment
    3. Management

POWERPOINT PRESENTATION
Chapter 27 PowerPoint slide 32

POWERPOINT PRESENTATION
Chapter 27 PowerPoint slides 33–86

READING/REFERENCE
Criss, E. "Out-of-Hospital Care of Acute Asthma." *JEMS*, July 2000.
Istvan, D. "Pulmonary Embolism." *JEMS*, Feb. 2000.

READING/REFERENCE
Criss, E. "Out-of-Hospital Care of Acute Asthma." *JEMS*, July 2000.
Istvan, D. "Pulmonary Embolism." *JEMS*, Feb. 2000.

POINT OF INTEREST
Some 5 percent of all hospitalized patients form pulmonary emboli; 66 percent will be undiagnosed.

WORKBOOK
Chapter 27 Activities

READING/REFERENCE
Textbook, pp. 1121–1242

POWERPOINT PRESENTATION
Chapter 27 PowerPoint slide 87

HANDOUT 27-2
Chapter 27 Quiz

HANDOUT 27-3
Chapter 27 Scenario

PARAMEDIC STUDENT CD
Student Activities

F. Severe Acute Respiratory Syndrome (SARS) (pp. 1111–1112) (**Fig. 27-17, p. 1111**)
  1. Pathophysiology
  2. Assessment
  3. Management
G. Lung cancer (pp. 1112–1113)
  1. Pathophysiology
  2. Assessment
  3. Management
H. Toxic inhalation (pp. 1113–1114)
  1. Pathophysiology
  2. Assessment
  3. Management
I. Carbon monoxide inhalation (p. 1114)
  1. Pathophysiology
  2. Assessment
  3. Management
J. Pulmonary embolism (pp. 1114–1116)
  1. Pathophysiology
  2. Assessment
  3. Management
K. Spontaneous pneumothorax (p. 1116)
  1. Pathophysiology
  2. Assessment
  3. Management
L. Hyperventilation syndrome (pp. 1116–1117) (**Table 27-5, p. 1117**)
  1. Pathophysiology
  2. Assessment
  3. Management
M. Central nervous system dysfunction (pp. 1117–1118)
  1. Pathophysiology
  2. Assessment
  3. Management
N. Dysfunction of the spinal cord, nerves, or respiratory muscles (p. 1118)
  1. Pathophysiology
  2. Assessment
  3. Management

VI. Chapter summary (p. 1119). Respiratory emergencies are commonly encountered in prehospital care. It is important to recognize that all respiratory disorders may produce derangements in ventilation, perfusion, or diffusion. Recognition and treatment must be prompt. Understanding the underlying cause of the respiratory disorder can guide therapy. The primary treatment is to correct hypoxia. Necessary steps include establishing and maintaining the airway, assisting ventilations as required, and administering supplemental oxygen. Appropriate pharmacological agents may be subsequently ordered by medical direction.

ASSIGNMENTS

Assign students to complete Chapter 27, "Pulmonology," of the workbook. Also assign them to read Chapter 28, "Cardiology," before the next class.

EVALUATION

Chapter Quiz and Scenario   Distribute copies of the Chapter Quiz provided in Handout 27-2 to evaluate student understanding of this chapter. Make sure each student reads the scenario to reinforce critical thinking on the scene. Remind students not to use their notes or textbooks while taking the quiz.

Student CD   Quizzes for every chapter are contained on the dynamic and highly visual in-text student CD.

Companion Website   Additional quizzes for every chapter are contained on this exciting website.

TestGen   You may wish to create a custom-tailored test using *Prentice Hall TestGen for Essentials of Paramedic Care*, 2nd Edition to evaluate student understanding of this chapter.

On-line Test Preparation (for students and instructors)   Additional test preparation is available through Brady's new on-line product, *EMT Achieve: Paramedic Test Preparation* at *http://www.prenhall.com/emtachieve/*. Instructors can also monitor student mastery on-line.

Review Manual for the EMT-Paramedic   This comprehensive exam review contains hundreds of test questions and rationales, including scenarios, along with two 180-question practice tests on CD

REINFORCEMENT

Handouts   If classroom discussion or performance on the quiz indicates that some students have not fully mastered the chapter content, you may wish to assign some or all of the Reinforcement Handouts for this chapter.

Student CD (for students)   A wide variety of material on this CD-ROM will reinforce and also expand student knowledge and skills.

PowerPoint Presentation (for instructors)   The PowerPoint material developed for this chapter offers useful reinforcement of chapter content.

Companion Website (for students)   Additional review quizzes and links to EMS resources will contribute to further reinforcement of the chapter.

OneKey   On-line support is offered for this course on one of three platforms: CourseCompass, Blackboard, or Web CT. Includes the IRM, PowerPoints, TestGen, and Companion Website for instruction. Ask your local sales representative for more information.

Brady Skills Series: Advanced Life Skills (Video or CD)   Have your students watch the skills come to life on VHS or CD-ROM, or they can purchase the highly visual, full-color text with step-by-step procedures and rationales.

COMPANION WEBSITE
http://www.prenhall.com/bledsoe

TESTGEN
Chapter 27

EMT ACHIEVE: PARAMEDIC TEST PREPARATION
Mistovich &Beasley. *EMT Achieve: Paramedic Test Preparation.*
www.prenhall.com/emtachieve/

REVIEW MANUAL FOR THE EMT-PARAMEDIC
Cherry &Mistovich. *Review Manual for the EMT-Paramedic*, 3rd edition.

HANDOUTS 27-4 AND 27-5
Reinforcement Activities

PARAMEDIC STUDENT CD
Student Activities

POWERPOINT PRESENTATION
Chapter 27

COMPANION WEBSITE
http://www.prenhall.com/bledsoe

ONEKEY
Chapter 27

ADVANCED LIFE SUPPORT SKILLS
Larmon & Davis. *Advanced Life Support Skills.*

ADVANCED LIFE SKILLS REVIEW
Larmon & Davis. *Advanced Life Skills Review.*

BRADY SKILLS SERIES: ALS
Larmon & Davis. *Brady Skills Series: ALS.*

PARAMEDIC NATIONAL STANDARDS SELF-TEST
Miller. *Paramedic National Standards Self-Test*, 4th edition.

Handout 27-1

Student's Name _____

CHAPTER 27 OBJECTIVES CHECKLIST

Knowledge	Date Mastered
1. Discuss the epidemiology of pulmonary diseases and pulmonary conditions.	
2. Identify and describe the function of the structures located in the upper and lower airway.	
3. Discuss the physiology of ventilation and respiration.	
4. Identify common pathological events that affect the pulmonary system.	
5. Compare various airway and ventilation techniques used in the management of pulmonary diseases.	
6. Review the use of equipment utilized during the physical examination of patients with complaints associated with respiratory diseases and conditions.	
7. Identify the epidemiology, anatomy, physiology, pathophysiology, assessment findings, and management (including prehospital medications) for the following respiratory diseases and conditions: • Adult respiratory distress syndrome • Bronchial asthma • Chronic bronchitis • Emphysema • Pneumonia • Pulmonary edema • Pulmonary thromboembolism • Neoplasms of the lung • Upper respiratory infections • Spontaneous pneumothorax • Hyperventilation syndrome	
8. Given several preprogrammed patients with nontraumatic pulmonary problems, provide the appropriate assessment, prehospital care, and transport.	

HANDOUT 27-2

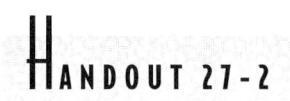

Student's Name _____

CHAPTER 27 QUIZ

Write the letter of the best answer in the space provided.

_____ 1. Lung perfusion is dependent on three conditions, one of which is:
   A. adequate blood volume.
   B. controlled body temperature.
   C. adequate humidity of the air.
   D. adequate atmospheric pressure.

_____ 2. The greatest portion of CO_2 produced during metabolism in cells is converted into:
   A. bicarbonate ions.
   B. hemoglobin.
   C. plasma.
   D. enzymes.

_____ 3. Which one of the following is NOT a common specific finding in patients with breathing difficulty?
   A. They tend to prefer a supine position.
   B. They display peripheral cyanosis.
   C. They may assume the "tripod" position.
   D. They become restless and agitated.

_____ 4. Retraction of the tissues of the neck due to airway obstruction or dyspnea is called:
   A. asphyxia.
   B. hemoptysis.
   C. nasal flaring.
   D. tracheal tugging.

_____ 5. You should suspect a life-threatening respiratory problem in an adult patient if you note:
   A. audible wheezing.
   B. tachycardia ≥ 130 beats per minute.
   C. pursed lips.
   D. 6- to 7-word dyspnea.

_____ 6. Which one of the following is NOT a normal breath sound?
   A. loud and high-pitched over the trachea
   B. soft and medium-pitched over mainstem bronchi
   C. harsh and high-pitched upon inspiration
   D. soft and low-pitched in the lung periphery

_____ 7. Pulsus paradoxus is a:
   A. rise in the systolic blood pressure of 10 mmHg or more with each respiratory cycle.
   B. drop in the systolic blood pressure of 10 mmHg or more with each respiratory cycle.
   C. rise in the systolic blood pressure of 20 mmHg or more with each respiratory cycle.
   D. drop in the systolic blood pressure of 20 mmHg or more with each respiratory cycle.

_____ 8. A form of pulmonary edema that is caused by fluid accumulation in the interstitial space within the lungs is called:
   A. adult respiratory distress syndrome.
   B. positive end-expiratory pressure.
   C. cor pulmonale.
   D. polycythemia.

_____ 9. Common obstructive lung diseases include all of the following EXCEPT:
   A. asthma.
   B. emphysema.
   C. pneumonia.
   D. chronic bronchitis.

_____ 10. COPD is known to be directly caused by:
   A. allergies.
   B. genetic predisposition.
   C. cigarette smoking.
   D. ineffective cardiac output.

HANDOUT 27-2 Continued

_____ 11. Destruction of the alveolar walls distal to the terminal bronchioles is the cause of:
  A. asthma.
  B. emphysema.
  C. pulmonary embolism.
  D. pulmonary edema.

_____ 12. Your assessment of a patient with emphysema may reveal:
  A. a frequent, productive cough.
  B. recent weight gain.
  C. clubbing of the fingers.
  D. Cheyne-Stokes respirations.

_____ 13. With asthma, a common sign is:
  A. persistent cough.
  B. snoring respirations.
  C. narrowing pulse pressure.
  D. gradually decreasing respiratory rate.

_____ 14. Which one of the following is TRUE about carbon monoxide poisoning?
  A. An early sign is cherry red skin.
  B. Carbon monoxide has a distinctive odor.
  C. Anything that produces heat can give off carbon monoxide.
  D. Carbon monoxide easily binds to the hemoglobin molecule.

_____ 15. Which one of the following is TRUE about hyperventilation syndrome?
  A. There is no underlying medical cause for it.
  B. Patients suffering from it require oxygen.
  C. Care includes rebreathing into a paper bag.
  D. Patients often exhibit ataxic respirations.

_____ 16. The measurement of expired CO_2 is known as
  A. capnography.
  B. capnometry.
  C. capnograph.
  D. Capnogram.

_____ 17. Normal $ETCO_2$ is _____ than the partial pressure of carbon dioxide ($PaCO_2$).
  A. 5 percent greater
  B. 7.5 percent greater
  C. 5 percent less
  D. 7.5 percent less

_____ 18. Decreased $ETCO_2$ levels can be found in:
  A. hypoventilation.
  B. bronchospasm.
  C. respiratory depression.
  D. hyperthermia.

_____ 19. During effective CPR, $ETCO_2$ levels have been found to correlate with:
  A. the effectiveness of chest compressions.
  B. cardiac output.
  C. coronary perfusion pressure.
  D. all of these

_____ 20. A patient with SARS is considered contagious:
  A. until the patient is asymptomatic.
  B. for 2–7 days after the onset of symptoms.
  C. for 10–14 days after the onset of symptoms.
  D. for 10 days after the patient is asymptomatic.

HANDOUT 27-3

Student's Name _____

CHAPTER 27 SCENARIO

Review the following real-life situation. Then answer the questions that follow.

The school nurse, frustrated by the apparent lack of progress in treating a child's asthma attack, calls 911. The child has a long-standing history of asthma. He makes numerous visits to her office for his inhaler, especially in the spring. But today's visit is different. The child looks exhausted.

You arrive and immediately assess the patient's airway while auscultating his lungs. You look at your partner quizzically and report, "I don't hear any wheezing." Without hesitation, you open the endotracheal roll and put it at the patient's head. You then start an IV of normal saline. The patient is simultaneously given 100 percent oxygen via a nonrebreather mask. Vital signs are obtained, and the ECG is monitored.

The patient is started on an albuterol treatment via small-volume nebulizer and transported immediately to the closest emergency department. While en route, the patient is not able to hold the nebulizer in his mouth. You elect to nasally intubate the patient and ventilate him prior to arrival at the hospital.

1. This child did not respond well to the nebulized treatments. Why?

2. What would be the next course of action in the emergency department?

3. How could you detect an improvement in this patient's status?

Handout 27-4

Student's Name _____

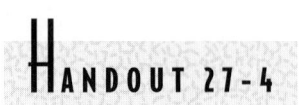

CHAPTER 27 REVIEW

Write the word or words that best complete each sentence in the space(s) provided.

1. The disease characterized by a decreased ability of the lungs to perform the function of ventilation is called _____ _____ _____ _____.
2. _____ is the mechanical process of moving air in and out of the lungs.
3. _____ is the movement of molecules through a membrane from an area of greater concentration to an area of lesser concentration.
4. The circulation of blood through the capillaries is called _____.
5. _____ is the transport protein that carries oxygen in the blood.
6. Lung perfusion is dependent on three conditions: adequate _____ volume, intact pulmonary _____, and efficient pumping of the blood by the _____.
7. The exchange of gases between a living organism and its environment is called _____.
8. A(n) _____ is a collection of air in the pleural space, causing a loss of the negative pressure that binds the lung to the chest wall.
9. A collection of blood in the pleural space is called a(n) _____.
10. A(n) _____ _____ occurs when one or more ribs are fractured in two or more places, creating an unattached rib segment.
11. A state in which insufficient oxygen is available to meet the oxygen requirements of the cells is called _____.
12. The term _____ refers to the absence of breathing.
13. Sweatiness is also called _____.
14. The bluish discoloration of the skin due to an increase in reduced hemoglobin in the blood is called _____, a condition directly related to poor ventilation.
15. Difficult or labored breathing, or a sensation of "shortness of breath," is called _____.
16. A result of interference with respiration, _____ is a decrease in the amount of oxygen and an increase in the amount of carbon dioxide in the blood.
17. Dyspnea while in a supine position is called _____.
18. The short attacks of dyspnea that occur at night and interrupt sleep are called _____ _____ _____.
19. _____ is the expectoration of blood from the respiratory tree.
20. Rapid respiration is called _____, while slow respiration is called _____.
21. A form of pulmonary edema caused by fluid accumulation in the interstitial space within the lungs is known as _____ _____ _____ _____.
22. _____ _____ is hypertrophy of the right ventricle resulting from disorders of the lung.
23. An excess of red blood cells is called _____.
24. The term _____ means sharp or tearing, as a description of pain.
25. A collection of air in the pleural space that occurs in the absence of blunt or penetrating trauma is called a(n) _____ _____.

668 ESSENTIALS OF PARAMEDIC CARE

HANDOUT 27-5

Student's Name _____

RECOGNIZING RESPIRATORY PROBLEMS

Match the terms with the statements that best describe them.

A. Emphysema
B. Chronic bronchitis
C. Asthma
D. Pulmonary embolism
E. Hyperventilation syndrome
F. Carbon monoxide poisoning
G. Cor pulmonale
H. Pneumonia
I. Status asthmaticus
J. Central nervous system dysfunction

_____ 1. Results from an increase in the number of mucus-secreting cells in the respiratory tree; usually associated with a productive cough and copious sputum production.

_____ 2. An infection of the lungs that causes fluid and inflammatory cells to collect in the alveoli.

_____ 3. Chronic inflammatory disorder of the airway, causing symptoms usually associated with widespread but variable air flow obstruction and airway hyperresponsiveness.

_____ 4. Exposure to a gas that has an affinity for hemoglobin 200 times that of oxygen; results in hypoxia at the cellular level and, ultimately, metabolic acidosis.

_____ 5. A blood clot (thrombus) or some other particle that lodges in a pulmonary artery, effectively blocking blood flow.

_____ 6. Hypertrophy of the right ventricle resulting from disorders of the lung.

_____ 7. Results from continued exposure to noxious substances that gradually destroy the alveolar walls.

_____ 8. Characterized by rapid breathing, chest pains, numbness, and other symptoms usually associated with anxiety or a situational reaction; must be considered indicative of a serious medical problem until proven otherwise.

_____ 9. Except in the cases of drug overdose and massive stroke, this condition is rarely the cause of a respiratory emergency, but must always be considered.

_____ 10. Signs include a greatly distended chest from continued air trapping, severe acidosis, exhaustion, and dehydration.

CHAPTER 27 Answer Key

Handout 27-2: Chapter 27 Quiz

1. A	6. C	11. B	16. B
2. A	7. B	12. C	17. C
3. B	8. A	13. A	18. B
4. D	9. C	14. D	19. D
5. B	10. C	15. B	20. A

Handout 27-3: Chapter 27 Scenario

1. The child may be experiencing status asthmaticus. He has progressed past the initial phase of an asthma attack and is in the second phase. The second phase typically will not respond to inhaled beta-agonist drugs.
2. The emergency department would continue the same course and add an antiinflammatory drug such as a corticosteroid. Therefore, the prehospital establishment of an IV access will expedite the patient's care.
3. An increase in wheezing would actually indicate an improvement in aeration and ventilation. A higher oxygen saturation as observed through pulse oximetry also would be an indication of improvement.

Handout 27-4: Chapter 27 Review

1. chronic obstructive pulmonary disease (COPD)
2. Ventilation
3. Diffusion
4. perfusion
5. Hemoglobin
6. blood, capillaries, heart
7. respiration
8. pneumothorax
9. hemothorax
10. flail chest
11. hypoxia
12. apnea
13. diaphoresis
14. cyanosis
15. dyspnea
16. asphyxia
17. orthopnea
18. paroxysmal nocturnal dyspnea
19. Hemoptysis
20. tachypnea, bradypnea
21. adult respiratory distress syndrome (ARDS)
22. Cor pulmonale
23. polycythemia
24. pleuritic
25. spontaneous pneumothorax

Handout 27-5: Recognizing Respiratory Problems

1. B	4. F	7. A	10. I
2. H	5. D	8. E	
3. C	6. G	9. J	

Chapter 28

Cardiology

INTRODUCTION

Cardiovascular disease is a major cause of death and disability in the United States. It is estimated that more than 60 million Americans have some form of it. Each year, on average, 466,000 people die of coronary heart disease. Most cardiac arrests occur outside the hospital setting. Paramedics confront emergencies involving the cardiovascular system on a daily basis.

Due to the size of this chapter, it has been divided into two parts. Part 1 covers cardiovascular anatomy and physiology, ECG monitoring, and dysrhythmia analysis. Part 2 discusses the assessment and management of the cardiovascular patient.

TOTAL TEACHING TIME: 86.20 HOURS
The total teaching time is only a guideline based on the didactic and practical lab averages in the National Standard Curriculum. Instructors should take into consideration such factors as the pace at which students learn, the size of the class, and breaks. The actual time devoted to teaching objectives is the responsibility of the instructor.

CHAPTER OBJECTIVES

Part 1: Cardiovascular Anatomy and Physiology, ECG Monitoring, and Dysrhythmia Analysis (p. 1127)

After reading Part 1 of this chapter, you should be able to:

1. Describe the incidence, morbidity, and mortality of cardiovascular disease. (p. 1126)
2. Discuss prevention strategies that may reduce the morbidity and mortality of cardiovascular disease. (p. 1126)
3. Identify the risk factors most predisposing to coronary artery disease. (p. 1126)
4. Describe the anatomy of the heart, including the position in the thoracic cavity, layers of the heart, chambers of the heart, and location and function of cardiac valves. (pp. 1127–1128; also see Chapter 3)
5. Identify the major structures of the vascular system, the factors affecting venous return, the components of cardiac output, and the phases of the cardiac cycle. (pp. 1128–1130; also see Chapter 3)
6. Define preload, afterload, and left ventricular end-diastolic pressure and relate each to the pathophysiology of heart failure. (see Chapter 3)
7. Identify the arterial blood supply to any given area of the myocardium. (p. 1128; also see Chapter 3)
8. Compare and contrast the coronary arterial distribution to the major portions of the cardiac conduction system. (p. 1128; also see Chapter 3)
9. Identify the structure and course of all divisions and subdivisions of the cardiac conduction system. (pp. 1129–1130; also see Chapter 3)

©2007 Pearson Education, Inc.
Essentials of Paramedic Care, 2nd ed.

10. Identify and describe how the heart's pacemaking control, rate, and rhythm are determined. (p. 1130; also see Chapter 3)
11. Explain the physiological basis of conduction delay in the AV node. (see Chapter 3)
12. Define the functional properties of cardiac muscle. (see Chapter 3)
13. Define the events comprising electrical potential. (see Chapter 3)
14. List the most important ions involved in myocardial action potential and their primary function in this process. (see Chapter 3)
15. Describe the events involved in the steps from excitation to contraction of cardiac muscle fibers. (p. 1130; also see Chapter 3)
16. Describe the clinical significance of Starling's law. (see Chapter 3)
17. Identify the structures of the autonomic nervous system and their effect on heart rate, rhythm, and contractility. (see Chapter 3)
18. Define and give examples of positive and negative inotropism, chronotropism, and dromotropism. (see Chapter 3)
19. Discuss the pathophysiology of cardiac disease and injury. (pp. 1142–1185)
20. Explain the purpose of ECG monitoring and its limitations. (p. 1130)
21. Correlate the electrophysiological and hemodynamic events occurring throughout the entire cardiac cycle with the various ECG waveforms, segments, and intervals. (pp. 1134–1141)
22. Identify how heart rates, durations, and amplitudes may be determined from ECG recordings. (pp. 1134–1141)
23. Relate the cardiac surfaces or areas represented by the ECG leads. (pp. 1131–1132, 1140)
24. Differentiate among the primary mechanisms responsible for producing cardiac dysrhythmias. (pp. 1140, 1142–1185)
25. Describe a systematic approach to the analysis and interpretation of cardiac dysrhythmias. (pp. 1141–1185)
26. Describe the dysrhythmias originating in the sinus node, the AV junction, the atria, and the ventricles. (pp. 1144–1185)
27. Describe the process and pitfalls of differentiating wide QRS complex tachycardias. (pp. 1174–1176)
28. Describe the conditions of pulseless electrical activity. (pp. 1182–1183)
29. Describe the phenomena of reentry, aberration, and accessory pathways. (pp. 1143–1144, 1153, 1184–1185)
30. Identify the ECG changes characteristically produced by electrolyte imbalances and specify their clinical implications. (p. 1185)
31. Identify patient situations where ECG rhythm analysis is indicated. (pp. 1142–1185)
32. Recognize the ECG changes that may reflect evidence of myocardial ischemia and injury and their limitations. (p. 1140)
33. Correlate abnormal ECG findings with clinical interpretation. (pp. 1142–1185)
34. Identify the major mechanical, pharmacological, and electrical therapeutic objectives in the treatment of the patient with any dysrhythmia. (pp. 1142–1185)
35. Describe artifacts that may cause confusion when evaluating the ECG of a patient with a pacemaker. (pp. 1131, 1179, 1181–1182)
36. List the possible complications of pacing. (pp. 1181–1182)
37. List the causes and implications of pacemaker failure. (pp. 1181–1182)
38. Identify additional hazards that interfere with artificial pacemaker function. (pp. 1181–1182)
39. Recognize the complications of artificial pacemakers as evidenced on an ECG. (pp. 1181–1182)

Part 2: Assessment and Management of the Cardiovascular Patient (p. 1186)

After reading Part 2 of this chapter, you should be able to:

1. Identify and describe the components of the focused history as it relates to the patient with cardiovascular compromise. (pp. 1187–1191)
2. Identify and describe the details of inspection, auscultation, and palpation specific to the cardiovascular system. (pp. 1191–1194)
3. Identify and define the heart sounds and relate them to hemodynamic events in the cardiac cycle. (pp. 1192–1193)
4. Describe the differences between normal and abnormal heart sounds. (pp. 1192–1193)
5. Define pulse deficit, pulsus paradoxus, and pulsus alternans. (pp. 1194, 1222)
6. Identify the normal characteristics of the point of maximum impulse (PMI). (p. 1193)
7. Based on field impressions, identify the need for rapid intervention for the patient in cardiovascular compromise. (pp. 1186–1194)
8. Describe the incidence, morbidity, and mortality associated with myocardial conduction defects. (p. 1216)
9. Identify the clinical indications, components, and the function of transcutaneous and permanent artificial cardiac pacing. (pp. 1179, 1181–1182, 1206, 1207–1208)
10. Explain what each setting and indicator on a transcutaneous pacing system represents and how the settings may be adjusted. (pp. 1207–1208)
11. Describe the techniques of applying a transcutaneous pacing system. (pp. 1206, 1207)
12. Describe the characteristics of an implanted pacemaking system. (pp. 1179, 1181–1182)
13. Describe the epidemiology, morbidity, mortality, and pathophysiology of angina pectoris. (pp. 1211–1212)
14. Describe the assessment and management of a patient with angina pectoris. (pp. 1213–1214)
15. Identify what is meant by the OPQRST of chest pain assessment. (pp. 1187–1188)
16. List other clinical conditions that may mimic signs and symptoms of coronary artery disease and angina pectoris. (p. 1212)
17. Identify the ECG findings in patients with angina pectoris. (p. 1213)
18. Based on the pathophysiology and clinical evaluation of the patient with chest pain, list the anticipated clinical problems according to their life-threatening potential. (p. 1212)
19. Describe the epidemiology, morbidity, mortality, and pathophysiology of myocardial infarction. (pp. 1214–1215)
20. List the mechanisms by which a myocardial infarction may be produced from traumatic and nontraumatic events. (p. 1214)
21. Identify the primary hemodynamic changes produced in myocardial infarction. (pp. 1214–1215)
22. List and describe the assessment parameters to be evaluated in a patient with a suspected myocardial infarction. (pp. 1215–1216)
23. Identify the anticipated clinical presentation of a patient with a suspected acute myocardial infarction. (pp. 1215–1216)

24. Differentiate the characteristics of the pain/discomfort occurring in angina pectoris and acute myocardial infarction. (p. 1215)
25. Identify the ECG changes characteristically seen during evolution of an acute myocardial infarction. (p. 1216)
26. Identify the most common complications of an acute myocardial infarction. (pp. 1214–1216)
27. List the characteristics of a patient eligible for fibrinolytic therapy. (pp. 1218–1220)
28. Describe the "window of opportunity" as it pertains to reperfusion of a myocardial injury or infarction. (p. 1218)
29. Based on the pathophysiology and clinical evaluation of the patient with a suspected acute myocardial infarction, list the anticipated clinical problems according to their life-threatening potential. (pp. 1214–1220)
30. Specify the measures that may be taken to prevent or minimize complications in the patient suspected of myocardial infarction. (pp. 1216–1220)
31. Describe the most commonly used cardiac drugs in terms of therapeutic effect and dosages, routes of administration, side effects, and toxic effects. (pp. 1199, 1200, 1218; also see Chapter 6)
32. Describe the epidemiology, morbidity, mortality, and physiology associated with heart failure. (pp. 1220–1221)
33. Identify the factors that may precipitate or aggravate heart failure. (pp. 1220–1221)
34. Define acute pulmonary edema and describe its relationship to left ventricular failure. (pp. 1220–1221)
35. Differentiate between early and late signs and symptoms of left ventricular failure and those of right ventricular failure. (pp. 1220–1221)
36. Define and explain the clinical significance of paroxysmal nocturnal dyspnea, pulmonary edema, and dependent edema. (pp. 1221–1222)
37. List the interventions prescribed for the patient in acute congestive heart failure. (pp. 1223–1224)
38. Describe the most commonly used pharmacological agents in the management of congestive heart failure in terms of therapeutic effect, dosages, routes of administration, side effects, and toxic effects. (pp. 1999, 1200, 1223; also see Chapter 6)
39. Define and describe the incidence, mortality, morbidity, pathophysiology, assessment, and management of the following cardiac-related problems:

    - Cardiac tamponade (pp. 1224–1225)
    - Hypertensive emergency (pp. 1225–1226)
    - Cardiogenic shock (pp. 1226–1229)
    - Cardiac arrest (pp. 1229–1233)

40. Identify the limiting factor of pericardial anatomy that determines intrapericardiac pressure. (p. 1224)
41. Describe how to determine if pulsus paradoxus, pulsus alternans, or electrical alternans is present. (pp. 1222, 1224)
42. Explain the essential pathophysiological defect of hypertension in terms of Starling's law of the heart. (pp. 1221, 1226)
43. Rank the clinical problems of patients in hypertensive emergencies according to their sense of urgency. (pp. 1225–1226)

44. Identify the drugs of choice for hypertensive emergencies, cardiogenic shock, and cardiac arrest, including their indications, contraindications, side effects, route of administration, and dosages. (pp. 1999, 1200, 1226, 1227–1229, 1230; also see Chapter 6)
45. Describe the major systemic effects of reduced tissue perfusion caused by cardiogenic shock. (pp. 1226–1227)
46. Explain the primary mechanisms by which the heart may compensate for a diminished cardiac output and describe their efficiency in cardiogenic shock. (pp. 1226–1227)
47. Identify the clinical criteria and progressive stages of cardiogenic shock. (pp. 1226–1227)
48. Describe the dysrhythmias seen in cardiac arrest. (p. 1229)
49. Explain how to confirm asystole using the 3-lead ECG. (p. 1229)
50. Define the terms *defibrillation* and *synchronized cardioversion*. (pp. 1999, 1204)
51. Specify the methods of supporting the patient with a suspected ineffective implanted defibrillation device. (p. 1201)
52. Describe resuscitation and identify circumstances and situations where resuscitation efforts would not be initiated. (pp. 1229–1233)
53. Identify communication and documentation protocols with medical direction and law enforcement used for termination of resuscitation efforts. (pp. 1232–1233)
54. Describe the incidence, morbidity, mortality, pathophysiology, assessment, and management of vascular disorders including occlusive disease, phlebitis, aortic aneurysm, and peripheral artery occlusion. (pp. 1233–1237)
55. Identify the clinical significance of claudication and presence of arterial bruits in a patient with peripheral vascular disorders. (pp. 1233–1237)
56. Describe the clinical significance of unequal arterial blood pressure readings in the arms. (p. 1236)
57. Recognize and describe the signs and symptoms of dissecting thoracic or abdominal aneurysm. (pp. 1233–1234)
58. Differentiate between signs and symptoms of cardiac tamponade, hypertensive emergencies, cardiogenic shock, and cardiac arrest. (pp. 1224–1229)
59. Utilize the results of the patient history, assessment findings, and ECG analysis to differentiate between, and provide treatment for, patients with the following conditions (pp. 1186–1237):

    - Cardiovascular disease
    - Chest pain
    - In need of a pacemaker
    - Angina pectoris
    - A suspected myocardial infarction
    - Heart failure
    - Cardiac tamponade
    - A hypertensive emergency
    - Cardiogenic shock
    - Cardiac arrest

60. Based on the pathophysiology and clinical evaluation of the patient with chest pain, characterize the clinical problems according to their life-threatening potential. (p. 1212)
61. Given several preprogrammed patients with cardiac complaints, provide the appropriate assessment, treatment, and transport. (pp. 1186–1237)

FRAMING THE LESSON

Begin the lesson by reviewing important points from Chapter 27, "Pulmonology." Review as needed to be sure students understand the chapter material before moving on to Chapter 28. Begin Chapter 28 by discussing the prevalence of cardiovascular disease in the United States. Discuss the role of EMS in prevention and public education, as well as in the care and treatment of patients. Consider inviting a guest lecturer from your local Heart Association office to discuss local statistics and prevention programs. Have students name and discuss risk factors of cardiovascular disease and how these risk factors may be eliminated or minimized. Also, discuss the importance of good cardiovascular health in paramedics.

TEACHING STRATEGIES

People learn in a variety of ways. Some do better with the spoken word, whereas others prefer the written. Some prefer to work alone, whereas others profit from working in groups. Recognizing these different ways of acquiring knowledge, the authors of this *Instructor's Resource Manual* have provided a variety of teaching strategies for the different types of learners. These strategies are intended to foster higher-level cognitive skills and encourage creative learning and problem solving. For greatest effectiveness, incorporate these strategies into your class lecture. Symbols in the Lecture Outline indicate the points at which various exercises might be most appropriate. Other strategies can be used to preview the lesson or to summarize it.

The following strategies are keyed to specific sections of the lesson.

1. Dissecting a Heart. Visit your butcher for beef hearts. They are usually readily available and will provide the best possible anatomy lesson for the heart itself. The thickness of the chamber walls, the size of the aorta, and the pericardium will all be "larger than life" when the student holds a heart in his or her hand. Additionally, beef hearts are quite large, so a group of four to eight students can easily share one heart. Allow dissection of the heart and labeling of the important structures. A photocopy from this text or a lab manual illustrating a cross-section would likely be useful as well.

2. Inspecting Diseased Human Hearts. Human hearts can be borrowed from your hospital pathology lab or medical school cadaver laboratory. Hearts affected by left ventricular hypertrophy, atrial fibrillation, mitral valve prolapse, and other pathologies will be collected there. Sometimes, they are preserved in jars, but frequently they are kept in buckets so that students can actually hold and examine the heart. You might also invite the pathologist to discuss the specimens. This activity illustrates both normal and abnormal anatomy and pathology.

3. Viewing Coronary Vessels. Your hospital lab will have photographs of normal coronary circulation, occluded vessels, vessels recently opened by catheterization, and vessels in spasm. In fact, they may have videotapes of procedures during which reperfusion took place. Coronary vessels are often difficult for students to memorize, yet important to the understanding of myocardial infarction. The chances of them remembering this information are greater if they can see the perfusion in action.

4. Using a Memory Aid. Help students remember which electrolytes are inside the cells by telling them about "Circle K," which in many states is the name of a convenience store chain. Potassium exists inside the cell at rest and is illustrated by a K with a circle around it, thus the "Circle K." From there, students can usually remember the sodium-potassium pump and the concept of polarization of the cell.

5. Interpreting Rhythm Strips. Cardiology is like math in that it takes practice to be good at it. To instill good habits, require your students to list rate, rhythm, P waves, PRI, QRS complexes, and interpretations. When students are successful 90 percent of the time, allow them to transition to "interpretation only" as a reward. Remember, if you don't require enough practice now, later students will still be struggling with interpretation as they also attempt to learn pharmacology and ACLS algorithms. Photocopy hundreds of rhythms for practice, and leave time in class to correct the homework and answer questions.

The following strategies can be used at various points throughout the lesson or to help summarize and demonstrate what students have learned.

Practice with ECGs. Just as you may have students perform vital sign checks on each other at the beginning of each class session, have students perform ECGs on each other. This will help them become familiar with the device and the procedure. Ask for volunteers and connect leads to them to create rhythm strips illustrating the basic components of the ECG. Run several rhythm strips and save them for continuing practice in recognizing the basic components of the ECG.

Clinical Observation. Arrange for students to complete a portion of their clinical observation requirements with the ECG team (or whichever staff or department performs ECGs) of the local hospital. This will give students an opportunity to observe how 12-lead ECGs are conducted and interpreted. If possible, have students bring copies of ECGs to class.

Guest Lecturer. Invite a cardiologist to visit the class and discuss the pathophysiology of certain abnormal ECG findings. What electrical events are occurring in the heart with abnormal findings such as a wide QRS or prolonged PR interval? What clinical significance do rhythms such as atrial fibrillation or tachycardia have? Encourage students to think of questions prior to the physician's visit. Ask the cardiologist to bring in examples of ECGs in which the rhythm interpretation is not initially obvious. Invite students to interpret these rhythms and justify to the physician why they believe their interpretation is correct.

Signs and Symptoms. Distribute several different ECGs to student groups or individuals. Given a specific ECG, have students make up a patient scenario, outlining the signs and symptoms the patient may be having with the specific rhythm. Include normal ECGs as well as abnormal ones. Stress that patients may be having cardiac events while showing no initial ECG changes.

What's My ECG? Have students take turns reading descriptions of ECG patterns to the class. Based on the description, have students name the ECG rhythm. Then have the student who correctly named the rhythm draw the rhythm on the blackboard or flip chart.

Risk Factors. Have students determine their own risk. This will require some delving into family history, as well as some physical and social assessment scales. Publications assisting in this assessment are available from Hope Health Publications and range from stress-level indices to exercise plans and diet programs. Tests for blood sugar and hypertension can be done right in the classroom. Be sure to provide follow-up information for any student who receives an abnormal reading on any of these assessments. Emphasize the importance of provider health as you conduct your risk factor assessments.

Cultural Considerations, Legal Notes, and Patho Pearls. The Student CD-ROM contains this series of informative features to enhance the student's understanding of the material covered in this chapter.

HANDOUTS 28-1 AND 28-2
Chapter 28 Objectives Checklists

TEACHING STRATEGY 1
Dissecting a Heart

TEACHING STRATEGY 2
Inspecting Diseased Human Hearts

TEACHING STRATEGY 3
Viewing Coronary Vessels

POWERPOINT PRESENTATION
Chapter 28 PowerPoint slides 5–16 (Part 1)

TEACHING TIP
Compare the pericardium with the pleura, which both have visceral and parietal layers with a lubricating middle layer.

POINT OF INTEREST
The main reason artificial hearts cause complications is that their makers still haven't been able to duplicate surfaces as smooth as the endocardium. Everything they have tried still won't prevent clots from forming.

POINT OF INTEREST
Blood leaves the left heart at a rate of 3 feet per second. It takes about 1 minute for this blood to return from the toes to the right heart.

TEACHING TIP
Have students be drops of blood. Set up the room to depict the heart and lungs. Then have them line up as in a long train and travel through the various chambers, blood vessels, valves, and so on. Let them experience, firsthand, what happens when an obstruction occurs.

TEACHING TIP
Use an analogy everyone understands all too well: "Detour, road under construction." As one road shuts down, another opens up to nourish the heart.

TEACHING OUTLINE

Chapter 28 is the second lesson in Division 4, *Medical Emergencies*. Distribute Handouts 28-1 and 28-2 so that students can familiarize themselves with the learning goals for this chapter. If students have any questions about the objectives, answer them at this time.

Then present the chapter. One possible lecture outline follows. In the outline, the parenthetical references in regular type are references to text pages; those in bold type are references to figures, tables, and procedures.

Introduction. According to current estimates, more than 60 million Americans have some form of cardiovascular disease (CVD). Coronary heart disease (CHD), a type of CVD, is the single largest killer of Americans. Each year, on average, 466,000 people die of CHD. Approximately 225,000 of them, a little more than half, die before ever reaching the hospital. Another way of looking at the impact of coronary heart disease is this: An American will suffer a non-fatal heart attack every 29 seconds. About once every minute, an American will die from CHD. (p. 1126)

PART 1: CARDIOVASCULAR ANATOMY AND PHYSIOLOGY, ECG MONITORING, AND DYSRHYTHMIA ANALYSIS (pp. 1127–1185)

I. Review of cardiovascular anatomy and physiology (pp. 1127–1130)

A. Cardiovascular anatomy (pp. 1127–1128)
   1. Tissue layers
      a. Endocardium
      b. Myocardium
      c. Pericardium
   2. Chambers
      a. Atria
      b. Ventricles
   3. Valves
      a. Tricuspid
      b. Pulmonary
      c. Mitral
      d. Aortic
   4. Blood flow (**Fig. 28-1, p. 1127**)
      a. Venae cavae
      b. Pulmonary arteries
      c. Pulmonary veins
      d. Aorta
   5. Coronary circulation (**Fig. 28-2, p. 1128**)
      a. Left coronary artery
         i. Anterior descending artery
         ii. Circumflex artery
      b. Right coronary artery
         i. Posterior descending artery
         ii. Marginal artery
   6. Anatomy of the peripheral circulation
      a. Arterial system
      b. Venous system

B. Cardiac physiology (pp. 1128–1129)
   1. Cardiac cycle
      a. Diastole
      b. Systole

678 ESSENTIALS OF PARAMEDIC CARE

    c. Ejection fraction
    d. Stroke volume
    e. Preload
    f. Starling's law of the heart
    g. Afterload
    h. Cardiac output
   2. Heart function
    a. Sympathetic components
    b. Parasympathetic components
    c. Chronotropy
    d. Inotropy
    e. Dromotropy
    f. Role of electrolytes
     i. Sodium (Na^+)
     ii. Calcium (Ca^{++})
     iii. Potassium (K^+)
     iv. Chloride (Cl^-)
     v. Magnesium (Mg^{++})
 C. Electrophysiology (pp. 1129–1130)
   1. Cardiac depolarization
    a. Resting potential
    b. Action potential
   2. Repolarization
   3. Cardiac conductive system (**Fig. 28-3, p. 1130**)
    a. Excitability
    b. Conductivity
    c. Automaticity
    d. Contractility

II. Electrocardiographic monitoring (pp. 1130–1142)
 A. Electrocardiogram (pp. 1131–1134)
   1. Artifacts
   2. ECG leads (**Table 28-1, p. 1231**) (**Fig. 28-4, p. 1232**)
    a. Bipolar leads
    b. Unipolar (augmented) leads
    c. Precordial leads
   3. Routine ECG monitoring
   4. ECG graph paper (**Fig. 28-5, p. 1133; Fig. 28-6, p. 1134**)
 B. Relationship of the ECG to electrical events in the heart (pp. 1134–1141)
   1. ECG tracing components (**Fig. 28-7, p. 1135**)
    a. P wave (**Figs. 28-8 through 28-12, pp. 1136–1138**)
    b. QRS complex (**Fig. 28-13, p. 1138**)
    c. T wave (**Fig. 28-14, p. 1139**)
    d. U wave
   2. Important time intervals (**Fig. 28-15, p. 1139**)
    a. PR interval
    b. QRS interval
    c. ST segment
    d. Refractory period (**Fig. 28-16, p. 1140**)
     i. Absolute refractory period
     ii. Relative refractory period
   3. ST segment changes
    a. Ischemia
    b. Injury
    c. Necrosis
   4. Lead systems and heart surfaces (**Table 28-2, p. 1141**)

TEACHING TIP
Liken the parasympathetic and sympathetic systems to a car's accelerator and brake pedals. Both systems work in opposition to one another.

TEACHING STRATEGY 4
Using a Memory Aid

TEACHING TIP
Use the domino principle to illustrate the syncytium of cardiac depolarization. Set up some dominos and watch them knock each other down in whatever direction you set the rows. Later, you can demonstrate how ectopic beats can cause depolarization from different directions, just like knocking down some middle dominos in both directions.

POWERPOINT PRESENTATION
Chapter 28 PowerPoint slides 17–38 (Part 1)

TEACHING TIP
Take things slowly when discussing the relationship of the ECG to electrical events. The more students understand what they are looking at and what is happening when they see the ECG waves, the easier it will be for them to learn the dysrhythmias later. Time spent here is well worth it.

TEACHING TIP
Liken the refractory period to a toilet flushing. After the flush, it is impossible to flush again until the tank is about half full. A half-tank flush, however, does not provide the powerful flush of a full tank. The same is true of the heart and its refractory periods.

TEACHING STRATEGY 5
Interpreting Rhythm Strips

TEACHING TIP
Liken the PR interval to a border checkpoint where you must show credentials before crossing. There is always some delay, even if your credentials are in order. When they are not in order, there is a greater delay, or even a refusal to allow the crossing.

POWERPOINT PRESENTATION
Chapter 28 PowerPoint slides 39–121 (Part 1)

POINT TO EMPHASIZE
Repeat this often: Always correlate the monitor with the patient's pulse.

   C. Interpretation of rhythm strips (pp. 1141–1142)
   1. Analyzing rate
      a. Six-second method
      b. Heart rate calculator rulers
      c. R-R interval
      d. Triplicate method
   2. Analyzing rhythm
      a. Fairly regular
      b. Occasionally irregular
      c. Regularly irregular
      d. Irregularly irregular
   3. Analyzing P waves
   4. Analyzing PR interval
   5. Analyzing QRS complex

III. Dysrhythmias (pp. 1142–1185) (**Fig. 28-17, p. 1143**)
   A. Mechanism of impulse formation (pp. 1143–1144)
   1. Ectopic foci
   2. Reentry
   B. Classification of dysrhythmias (p. 1144)
   1. Nature of origin
   2. Magnitude
   3. Severity
   4. Site of origin
      a. SA node
      b. Atria
      c. AV junction
      d. Ventricles
      e. Disorders of conduction
   C. Dysrhythmias originating in the SA node (pp. 1144–1149)
   1. Sinus bradycardia (**Fig. 28-18, p. 1145; Fig. 28-19, p. 1146**)
      a. Description
      b. Etiology
      c. Rules of interpretation
      d. Clinical significance
      e. Treatment
   2. Sinus tachycardia (**Fig. 28-20, p. 1147**)
      a. Description
      b. Etiology
      c. Rules of interpretation
      d. Clinical significance
      e. Treatment
   3. Sinus dysrhythmia (**Fig. 28-21, p. 1148**)
      a. Description
      b. Etiology
      c. Rules of interpretation
      d. Clinical significance
      e. Treatment
   4. Sinus arrest (**Fig. 28-22, p. 1149**)
      a. Description
      b. Etiology
      c. Rules of interpretation
      d. Clinical significance
      e. Treatment
   D. Dysrhythmias originating in the atria (pp. 1150–1159)

1. Wandering atrial pacemaker (**Fig. 28-23, p. 1151**)
   a. Description
   b. Etiology
   c. Rules of interpretation
   d. Clinical significance
   e. Treatment
2. Multifocal atrial tachycardia (**Fig. 28-24, p. 1152**)
   a. Description
   b. Etiology
   c. Rules of interpretation
   d. Clinical significance
   e. Treatment
3. Premature atrial contractions (**Fig. 28-25, p. 1153**)
   a. Description
   b. Etiology
   c. Rules of interpretation
   d. Clinical significance
   e. Treatment
4. Paroxysmal supraventricular tachycardia (**Fig. 28-26, p. 1154; Fig. 28-27, p. 1156**)
   a. Description
   b. Etiology
   c. Rules of interpretation
   d. Clinical significance
   e. Treatment
5. Atrial flutter (**Fig. 28-28, p. 1157**)
   a. Description
   b. Etiology
   c. Rules of interpretation
   d. Clinical significance
   e. Treatment
6. Atrial fibrillation (**Fig. 28-29, p. 1158**)
   a. Description
   b. Etiology
   c. Rules of interpretation
   d. Clinical significance
   e. Treatment

E. Dysrhythmias originating within the AV junction (AV blocks) (pp. 1159–1165) (**Fig. 28-30, p. 1160**)
   1. Atrioventricular blocks
   2. First-degree AV block (**Fig. 28-31, p. 1161**)
      a. Description
      b. Etiology
      c. Rules of interpretation
      d. Clinical significance
      e. Treatment
   3. Type I second-degree AV block (**Fig. 28-32, p. 1162**)
      a. Description
      b. Etiology
      c. Rules of interpretation
      d. Clinical significance
      e. Treatment
   4. Type II second-degree AV block (**Fig. 28-33, p. 1163**)
      a. Description
      b. Etiology
      c. Rules of interpretation

- **d.** Clinical significance
- **e.** Treatment
  5. Third-degree AV block (**Fig. 28-34, p. 1165**)
     - **a.** Description
     - **b.** Etiology
     - **c.** Rules of interpretation
     - **d.** Clinical significance
     - **e.** Treatment
- **F.** Dysrhythmias sustained or originating in the AV junction (pp. 1165–1170)
  1. Premature junctional contractions (**Fig. 28-35, p. 1166**)
     - **a.** Description
     - **b.** Etiology
     - **c.** Rules of interpretation
     - **d.** Clinical significance
     - **e.** Treatment
  2. Junctional escape complexes and rhythms (**Fig. 28-36, p. 1167**)
     - **a.** Description
     - **b.** Etiology
     - **c.** Rules of interpretation
     - **d.** Clinical significance
     - **e.** Treatment
  3. Accelerated junctional rhythm (**Fig. 28-37, p. 1169**)
     - **a.** Description
     - **b.** Etiology
     - **c.** Rules of interpretation
     - **d.** Clinical significance
     - **e.** Treatment
  4. Paroxysmal junctional tachycardia (**Fig. 28-38, p. 1170**)
     - **a.** Description
     - **b.** Etiology
     - **c.** Rules of interpretation
     - **d.** Clinical significance
     - **e.** Treatment
- **G.** Dysrhythmias originating in the ventricles (pp. 1171–1182)
  1. Ventricular escape complexes and rhythms (**Fig. 28-39, p. 1172**)
     - **a.** Description
     - **b.** Etiology
     - **c.** Rules of interpretation
     - **d.** Clinical significance
     - **e.** Treatment
  2. Accelerated idioventricular rhythm
  3. Premature ventricular contractions (**Fig. 28-40, p. 1174**)
     - **a.** Description
       - **i.** Bigeminy
       - **ii.** Trigeminy
       - **iii.** Quadrigeminy
       - **iv.** Repetitive PVCs
     - **b.** Etiology
     - **c.** Rules of interpretation
     - **d.** Clinical significance
       - **i.** More than six PVCs per minute
       - **ii.** R-on-T phenomenon
       - **iii.** Couplets or runs
       - **iv.** Multifocal
       - **v.** Associated chest pain
       - **vi.** Lown grading system
         - **a)** Grade 0: No premature beats

- **b)** Grade 1: Occasional (< 30/hr) PVCs
- **c)** Grade 2: Frequent (> 30/hr) PVCs
- **d)** Grade 3: Multiform (multifocal)
- **e)** Grade 4: Repetitive (couplets, salvos of 3 consecutive) PVCs
- **f)** Grade 5: R-on-T phenomenon
            - **e.** Treatment
        - **4.** Ventricular tachycardia (**Fig. 28-41, p. 1175**)
            - **a.** Description
            - **b.** Etiology
            - **c.** Rules of interpretation
            - **d.** Clinical significance
            - **e.** Treatment
            - **f.** Torsades de Pointes (**Fig. 28-42, p. 1177**)
                - **i.** "Twisting on a point"
        - **5.** Ventricular fibrillation (**Fig. 28-43, p. 1178**)
            - **a.** Description
            - **b.** Etiology
            - **c.** Rules of interpretation
            - **d.** Clinical significance
            - **e.** Treatment
        - **6.** Asystole (**Fig. 28-44, p. 1179; Fig. 28-45, p. 1180**)
            - **a.** Description
            - **b.** Etiology
            - **c.** Rules of interpretation
            - **d.** Clinical significance
            - **e.** Treatment
        - **7.** Artificial pacemaker rhythm (**Fig. 28-46, p. 1181**)
            - **a.** Description
            - **b.** Etiology
            - **c.** Rules of interpretation
            - **d.** Problems with pacemakers
            - **e.** Considerations for management
            - **f.** Use of a magnet
- **H.** Pulseless electrical activity (pp. 1182–1183) (**Table 28-3, p. 1182**) (**Fig. 28-47, p. 1183**)
    - **1.** Causes of PEA include:
        - **a.** Hypovolemia
        - **b.** Cardiac tamponade
        - **c.** Tension pneumothorax
        - **d.** Hypoxemia
        - **e.** Acidosis
        - **f.** Massive pulmonary embolism
        - **g.** Ventricular wall rupture
- **I.** Dysrhythmias resulting from disorders of conduction (pp. 1184–1185)
    - **1.** Atrioventricular blocks
    - **2.** Disturbances of ventricular conduction
        - **a.** Aberrant conduction
        - **b.** Bundle branch block
    - **3.** Preexcitation syndromes (**Fig. 28-48, p. 1185**)
        - **a.** Wolff-Parkinson-White (WPW) syndrome
- **J.** ECG changes due to electrolyte abnormalities and hypothermia (p. 1185)
    - **1.** Hyperkalemia
    - **2.** Hypokalemia
    - **3.** Hypothermia (**Fig. 28-49, p. 1185**)

POWERPOINT PRESENTATION
Chapter 28 PowerPoint slides 5–14 (Part 2)

PART 2: ASSESSMENT AND MANAGEMENT OF THE CARDIOVASCULAR PATIENT (pp. 1186–1240)

I. **Assessment of the cardiovascular patient** (pp. 1186–1194)
   A. Scene size-up and initial assessment (pp. 1186–1187)
   B. Focused history (pp. 1187–1191)
      1. Common symptoms
         a. Chest pain or discomfort
         b. Dyspnea
         c. Cough
         d. Syncope
         e. Palpitation
         f. Other related signs and symptoms
      2. Allergies
      3. Medications
      4. Past medical history
      5. Last oral intake
      6. Events preceding the incident
   C. Physical examination (pp. 1191–1194)
      1. Inspection (**Fig. 28-50, p. 1191; Fig. 28-51, p. 1192**)
      2. Auscultation (**Figs. 28-52 and 28-53, p. 1193**)
      3. Palpation (**Fig. 28-54, p. 1194**)

II. **Management of cardiovascular emergencies** (pp. 1194–1211)
   A. Basic life support (p. 1194)
   B. Advanced life support (p. 1195)
   C. Monitoring ECG in the field (pp. 1195–1198) (**Proc. 28-1, pp. 1196–1197**)
   D. Vagal maneuvers (p. 1198)
   E. Precordial thump (pp. 1198–1199) (**Fig. 28-55, p. 1199**)
   F. Pharmacological management (pp. 1199, 1200) (**Table 28-4, p. 1200**)
      1. Antidysrhythmics
         a. Atropine sulfate
         b. Lidocaine
         c. Procainamide
         d. Bretylium
         e. Adenosine
         f. Amiodarone
         g. Verapamil
      2. Sympathomimetic agents
         a. Epinephrine
         b. Norepinephrine
         c. Isoproterenol
         d. Dopamine
         e. Dobutamine
         f. Vasopressin
      3. Drugs used for myocardial ischemia
         a. Oxygen
         b. Nitrous oxide
         c. Nitroglycerin
         d. Morphine sulfate
         e. Fentanyl
         f. Nalbuphine
      4. Fibrinolytic agents
         a. Aspirin
         b. Alteplase (Activase) (tPA)
         c. Relteplase (Retavase)
         d. Tenecteplase (TNKase)

POWERPOINT PRESENTATION
Chapter 28 PowerPoint slides 15–24 (Part 2)

5. Other prehospital drugs
      a. Furosemide
      b. Diazepam
      c. Promethazine
      d. Sodium nitroprusside
   6. Drugs infrequently used in the prehospital setting
      a. Digitalis
      b. Beta blockers
      c. Calcium channel blockers
      d. Alkalinizing agents
G. Defibrillation (pp. 1199–1204) (Proc. 28-2, pp. 1202–1203)
H. Emergency synchronized cardioversion (pp. 1204–1205) (Fig. 28-56, p. 1204; Fig. 28-57, p. 1205)
I. Transcutaneous cardiac pacing (pp. 1206–1208) (Proc. 28-3, pp. 1207–1208)
J. Carotid sinus massage (pp. 1206, 1209–1210) (Proc. 28-4, pp. 1209–1210)
K. Support and communication (p. 1211)

III. **Managing specific cardiovascular emergencies** (pp. 1211–1237)
A. Acute coronary syndrome (ACS) (p. 1211)
   1. Angina pectoris
      a. Prinzmeta's (vasospastic angina)
      b. Stable angina
      c. Unstable angina
   2. Myocardial infarction
      a. Subendocardial myocardial infarction
      b. Transmural myocardial infarction
B. Angina pectoris (pp. 1211–1214)
   1. Introduction
   2. Field assessment
   3. Management
C. Myocardial infarction (pp. 1214–1220) (Fig. 28-58, p. 1215)
   1. Introduction
   2. Field assessment
   3. Management (Fig. 28-59, p. 1217)
   4. Cardiac enzymes (Fig. 28-60, p. 1220)
   5. In-hospital management of MI
D. Heart failure (pp. 1220–1224)
   1. Introduction
      a. Left ventricular failure
      b. Right ventricular failure
      c. Pulmonary embolism
      d. Congestive heart failure
   2. Field assessment
   3. Management
E. Cardiac tamponade (pp. 1224–1225)
   1. Introduction
   2. Field assessment
   3. Management
F. Hypertensive emergencies (pp. 1225–1226)
   1. Introduction
   2. Field assessment
   3. Management
G. Cardiogenic shock (pp. 1226–1229)
   1. Introduction
   2. Field assessment
   3. Management (Fig. 28-61, p. 1228)

POWERPOINT PRESENTATION
Chapter 28 PowerPoint slides 25–113 (Part 2)

READING/REFERENCE
Mattera, C. "Heart Failure and Pulmonary Edema." *JEMS*, May 2000.

- **H.** Cardiac arrest (pp. 1229–1233)
    1. Introduction
    2. Field assessment
    3. Management (**Fig. 28-62, p. 1231**)
        a. Resuscitation
        b. Return of spontaneous circulation
        c. Survival
    4. Withholding or terminating resuscitation
- **I.** Peripheral vascular and other cardiovascular emergencies (pp. 1233–1237)
    1. Atherosclerosis
    2. Aneurysm
        a. Abdominal aortic aneurysm (**Fig. 28-63, p. 1234**)
        b. Dissecting aortic aneurysm
    3. Acute pulmonary embolism
    4. Acute arterial occlusion
    5. Vasculitis
    6. Noncritical peripheral vascular conditions
        a. Peripheral arterial atherosclerotic disease
        b. Deep venous thrombosis
        c. Varicose veins
    7. General assessment and management of vascular disorders
        a. Assessment
        b. Management

IV. Prehospital ECG monitoring (pp. 1237–1240)

A. Prehospital 12-lead ECG monitoring (pp. 1237–1240) (**Proc. 28-5, pp. 1238–1239**)

V. Chapter summary (p. 1240). Cardiovascular disease is the leading cause of death in the United States and Canada. Many deaths from heart attack occur within the first 24 hours—frequently within the first hour. With the advent of fibrinolytic therapy, time is of the essence when managing the patient with suspected ischemic heart disease. EMS plays an ever-increasing role in the early recognition of patients suffering coronary ischemia. In certain areas, EMS provides definitive care by initiating fibrinolytic therapy in the field. This is especially important in cases where transport times can be long. With cardiovascular disease, EMS can truly mean the difference between life and death.

SKILLS DEMONSTRATION AND PRACTICE

Students can practice skills discussed in this chapter in the following settings.

Skills Lab: Divide the class into as many groups as appropriate. Have the groups circulate through the stations. Monitor the groups to be sure all students have a chance to practice each of the skills. You may wish to have other instructors or qualified paramedics assist students in these activities.

POWERPOINT PRESENTATION
Chapter 28 PowerPoint slide 114 (Part 2)

Station	Equipment and Personnel Needed	Activities
ECG Monitoring	ECG monitor 1 instructor	Have students practice hooking each other to the ECG monitor and running a strip.
Defibrillation	Monitor/defibrillator ECG simulator ALS trainer 1 instructor	Have students practice defibrillating on the mannequin.
Synchronized Cardioversion	Monitor/defibrillator ECG simulator ALS trainer 1 instructor	Have students practice synchronized cardioversion on the mannequin.
External Cardiac Pacing	Monitor/defibrillator with pacer Pacing simulator ALS trainer 1 instructor	Have students practice pacing on the mannequin.
Basic Life Support	Adult CPR mannequin AHA skill sheets 1 instructor	Have students practice CPR on adult mannequin.
Carotid Sinus Massage	Monitor/defibrillator ECG simulator ALS trainer 1 instructor	Have students practice locating the carotid sinus on each other and practice carotid sinus massage on the mannequin.

HANDOUT 28-3
ECG Monitoring

HANDOUT 28-4
Defibrillation

HANDOUT 28-5
External Cardiac Pacing

HANDOUT 28-6
Carotid Sinus Massage

HANDOUT 28-7
12-Lead Prehospital ECG Monitoring

ADVANCED LIFE SUPPORT SKILLS
Larmon & Davis. *Advanced Life Support Skills.*

ADVANCED LIFE SKILLS REVIEW
Larmon & Davis. *Advanced Life Skills Review.*

BRADY SKILLS SERIES: ALS
Larmon & Davis. *Brady Skills Series: ALS.*

Scenario Lab: Divide the class into teams. Have the teams circulate through the stations. Monitor the groups to be sure all groups have a chance to manage each of the cases and so that every student has the opportunity to be team leader. You may wish to have other instructors or qualified paramedics assist students in these activities.

Station	Equipment and Personnel Needed	Activities
Acute MI	Medications box Airway management kit Monitor/defibrillator ALS trainer 1 patient 1 instructor	Have students practice assessing and managing patients in acute MI.
Acute Pulmonary Edema	Medications box Airway management kit Monitor/defibrillator ALS trainer 1 patient 1 instructor	Have students practice assessing and managing patients in acute pulmonary edema.
Cardiogenic Shock	Medications box Airway management kit	Have students practice assessing and managing

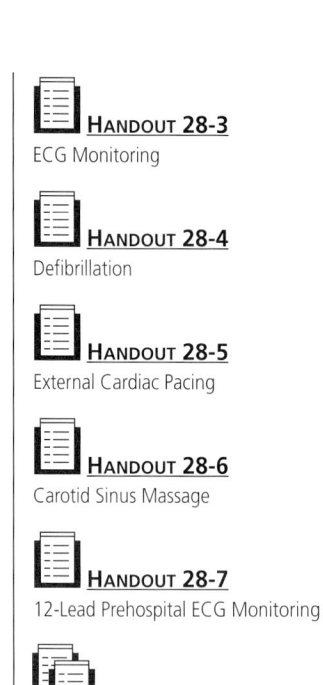

	Monitor/defibrillator ALS trainer 1 patient 1 instructor	patients in cardiogenic shock.
Asystole	Medications box Airway management kit Monitor/defibrillator ALS trainer 1 patient 1 instructor	Have students practice assessing and managing patients in asystole.
Pulseless Electrical Activity	Medications box Airway management kit Monitor/defibrillator ALS trainer 1 patient 1 instructor	Have students practice assessing and managing patients in pulseless electrical activity.
Bradycardia	Medications box Airway management kit Monitor/defibrillator ALS trainer 1 patient 1 instructor	Have students practice assessing and managing patients in bradycardia.
Stable Tachycardia	Medications box Airway management kit Monitor/defibrillator ALS trainer 1 patient 1 instructor	Have students practice assessing and managing patients in stable tachycardia.
Unstable Tachycardia	Medications box Airway management kit Monitor/defibrillator ALS trainer 1 patient 1 instructor	Have students practice assessing and managing patients in unstable tachycardia.
Ventricular Fibrillation and Pulseless Ventricular Tachycardia	Medications box Airway management kit Monitor/defibrillator ALS trainer 1 patient 1 instructor	Have students practice assessing and managing patients in ventricular fibrillation and pulseless ventricular tachycardia.

WORKBOOK
Chapter 28 Activities

READING/REFERENCE
Textbook, pp. 1243–1279

HANDOUTS 28-8 AND 28-9
Chapter 28 Quizzes

HANDOUTS 28-10 AND 28-11
Chapter 28 Scenarios

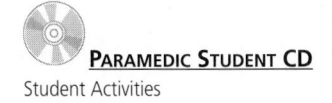

PARAMEDIC STUDENT CD
Student Activities

Hospital: Practice reading ECGs in the coronary care unit (CCU). Chart reviews, assessment, and management of cardiac patients in the CCU. Observe cardiac diagnostic procedures in a cardiologist's office. Assess and manage cardiac emergencies in the emergency department.

Field Internship: Assess and manage cardiac patients in the field.

ASSIGNMENTS

Assign students to complete Chapter 28, "Cardiology," of the workbook. Also assign them to read Chapter 29, "Neurology," before the next class.

EVALUATION

Chapter Quiz and Scenario Distribute copies of the Chapter Quizzes provided in Handouts 28-8 and 28-9 to evaluate student understanding of this chapter. Make sure each student reads the scenario to reinforce critical thinking on the scene. Remind students not to use their notes or textbooks while taking the quiz.

Student CD Quizzes for every chapter are contained on the dynamic and highly visual in-text student CD.

Companion Website Additional quizzes for every chapter are contained on this exciting website.

TestGen You may wish to create a custom-tailored test using *Prentice Hall TestGen for Essentials of Paramedic Care*, 2nd Edition to evaluate student understanding of this chapter.

On-line Test Preparation (for students and instructors) Additional test preparation is available through Brady's new on-line product, *EMT Achieve: Paramedic Test Preparation* at *http://www.prenhall.com/emtachieve/*. Instructors can also monitor student mastery on-line.

Review Manual for the EMT-Paramedic This comprehensive exam review contains hundreds of test questions and rationales, including scenarios, along with two 180-question practice tests on CD.

REINFORCEMENT

Handouts If classroom discussion or performance on the quiz indicates that some students have not fully mastered the chapter content, you may wish to assign some or all of the Reinforcement Handouts for this chapter.

Student CD (for students) A wide variety of material on this CD-ROM will reinforce and also expand student knowledge and skills.

PowerPoint Presentation (for instructors) The PowerPoint material developed for this chapter offers useful reinforcement of chapter content.

Companion Website (for students) Additional review quizzes and links to EMS resources will contribute to further reinforcement of the chapter.

OneKey On-line support is offered for this course on one of three platforms: Course Compass, Blackboard, or Web CT. Includes the IRM, PowerPoints, TestGen, and Companion Website for instruction. Ask your local sales representative for more information.

Brady Skills Series: Advanced Life Skills (Video or CD) Have your students watch the skills come to life on VHS or CD-ROM, or they can purchase the highly visual, full-color text with step-by-step procedures and rationales.

COMPANION WEBSITE
http://www.prenhall.com/bledsoe

TESTGEN
Chapter 28

EMT ACHIEVE: PARAMEDIC TEST PREPARATION
Mistovich & Beasley. *EMT Achieve: Paramedic Test Preparation.*
www.prenhall.com/emtachieve/

REVIEW MANUAL FOR THE EMT-PARAMEDIC
Cherry & Mistovich. *Review Manual for the EMT-Paramedic*, 3rd edition.

HANDOUTS 28-12 TO 28-14
Reinforcement Activities

PARAMEDIC STUDENT CD
Student Activities

POWERPOINT PRESENTATION
Chapter 28

COMPANION WEBSITE
http://www.prenhall.com/bledsoe

ONEKEY
Chapter 28

ADVANCED LIFE SUPPORT SKILLS
Larmon & Davis. *Advanced Life Support Skills.*

ADVANCED LIFE SKILLS REVIEW
Larmon & Davis. *Advanced Life Skills Review.*

BRADY SKILLS SERIES: ALS
Larmon & Davis. *Brady Skills Series: ALS.*

PARAMEDIC NATIONAL STANDARDS SELF-TEST
Miller. *Paramedic National Standards Self-Test*, 4th edition.

HANDOUT 28-1

Student's Name _____

CHAPTER 28 OBJECTIVES CHECKLIST

PART 1: CARDIOVASCULAR ANATOMY AND PHYSIOLOGY, ECG MONITORING, AND DYSRHYTHMIA ANALYSIS

Knowledge	Date Mastered
1. Describe the incidence, morbidity, and mortality of cardiovascular disease.	
2. Discuss prevention strategies that may reduce the morbidity and mortality of cardiovascular disease.	
3. Identify the risk factors most predisposing to coronary artery disease.	
4. Describe the anatomy of the heart, including the position in the thoracic cavity, layers of the heart, chambers of the heart, and location and function of cardiac valves.	
5. Identify the major structures of the vascular system, the factors affecting venous return, the components of cardiac output, and the phases of the cardiac cycle.	
6. Define preload, afterload, and left ventricular end-diastolic pressure and relate each to the pathophysiology of heart failure.	
7. Identify the arterial blood supply to any given area of the myocardium.	
8. Compare and contrast the coronary arterial distribution to the major portions of the cardiac conduction system.	
9. Identify the structure and course of all divisions and subdivisions of the cardiac conduction system.	
10. Identify and describe how the heart's pacemaking control, rate, and rhythm are determined.	
11. Explain the physiological basis of conduction delay in the AV node.	
12. Define the functional properties of cardiac muscle.	
13. Define the events comprising electrical potential.	
14. List the most important ions involved in myocardial action potential and their primary function in this process.	
15. Describe the events involved in the steps from excitation to contraction of cardiac muscle fibers.	
16. Describe the clinical significance of Starling's law.	

HANDOUT 28-1 Continued

Knowledge	Date Mastered
17. Identify the structures of the autonomic nervous system and their effect on heart rate, rhythm, and contractility.	
18. Define and give examples of positive and negative inotropism, chronotropism, and dromotropism.	
19. Discuss the pathophysiology of cardiac disease and injury.	
20. Explain the purpose of ECG monitoring and its limitations.	
21. Correlate the electrophysiological and hemodynamic events occurring throughout the entire cardiac cycle with the various ECG waveforms, segments, and intervals.	
22. Identify how heart rates, durations, and amplitudes may be determined from ECG recordings.	
23. Relate the cardiac surfaces or areas represented by the ECG leads.	
24. Differentiate among the primary mechanisms responsible for producing cardiac dysrhythmias.	
25. Describe a systematic approach to the analysis and interpretation of cardiac dysrhythmias.	
26. Describe the dysrhythmias originating in the sinus node, the AV junction, the atria, and the ventricles.	
27. Describe the process and pitfalls of differentiating wide QRS complex tachycardias.	
28. Describe the conditions of pulseless electrical activity.	
29. Describe the phenomena of reentry, aberration, and accessory pathways.	
30. Identify the ECG changes characteristically produced by electrolyte imbalances and specify their clinical implications.	
31. Identify patient situations where ECG rhythm analysis is indicated.	
32. Recognize the ECG changes that may reflect evidence of myocardial ischemia and injury and their limitations.	
33. Correlate abnormal ECG findings with clinical interpretation.	
34. Identify the major mechanical, pharmacological, and electrical therapeutic objectives in the treatment of the patient with any dysrhythmia.	
35. Describe artifacts that may cause confusion when evaluating the ECG of a patient with a pacemaker.	
36. List the possible complications of pacing.	

©2007 Pearson Education, Inc.
Essentials of Paramedic Care, 2nd ed.

HANDOUT 28-1 Continued

Knowledge	Date Mastered
37. List the causes and implications of pacemaker failure.	
38. Identify additional hazards that interfere with artificial pacemaker function.	
39. Recognize the complications of artificial pacemakers as evidenced on an ECG.	

OBJECTIVES

HANDOUT 28-2

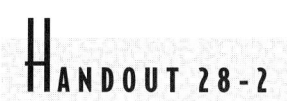

Student's Name _____

CHAPTER 28 OBJECTIVES CHECKLIST

PART 2: ASSESSMENT AND MANAGEMENT OF THE CARDIOVASCULAR PATIENT

Knowledge	Date Mastered
1. Identify and describe the components of the focused history as it relates to the patient with cardiovascular compromise.	
2. Identify and describe the details of inspection, auscultation, and palpation specific to the cardiovascular system.	
3. Identify and define the heart sounds and relate them to hemodynamic events in the cardiac cycle.	
4. Describe the differences between normal and abnormal heart sounds.	
5. Define pulse deficit, pulsus paradoxus, and pulsus alternans.	
6. Identify the normal characteristics of the point of maximum impulse (PMI).	
7. Based on field impressions, identify the need for rapid intervention for the patient in cardiovascular compromise.	
8. Describe the incidence, morbidity, and mortality associated with myocardial conduction defects.	
9. Identify the clinical indications, components, and the function of transcutaneous and permanent artificial cardiac pacing.	
10. Explain what each setting and indicator on a transcutaneous pacing system represents and how the settings may be adjusted.	
11. Describe the techniques of applying a transcutaneous pacing system.	
12. Describe the characteristics of an implanted pacemaking system.	
13. Describe the epidemiology, morbidity, mortality, and pathophysiology of angina pectoris.	
14. Describe the assessment and management of a patient with angina pectoris.	
15. Identify what is meant by the OPQRST of chest pain assessment.	
16. List other clinical conditions that may mimic signs and symptoms of coronary artery disease and angina pectoris.	
17. Identify the ECG findings in patients with angina pectoris.	

OBJECTIVES

HANDOUT 28-2 Continued

Knowledge	Date Mastered
18. Based on the pathophysiology and clinical evaluation of the patient with chest pain, list the anticipated clinical problems according to their life-threatening potential.	
19. Describe the epidemiology, morbidity, mortality, and pathophysiology of myocardial infarction.	
20. List the mechanisms by which a myocardial infarction may be produced from traumatic and nontraumatic events.	
21. Identify the primary hemodynamic changes produced in myocardial infarction.	
22. List and describe the assessment parameters to be evaluated in a patient with a suspected myocardial infarction.	
23. Identify the anticipated clinical presentation of a patient with a suspected acute myocardial infarction.	
24. Differentiate the characteristics of the pain/discomfort occurring in angina pectoris and acute myocardial infarction.	
25. Identify the ECG changes characteristically seen during evolution of an acute myocardial infarction.	
26. Identify the most common complications of an acute myocardial infarction.	
27. List the characteristics of a patient eligible for fibrinolytic therapy.	
28. Describe the "window of opportunity" as it pertains to reperfusion of a myocardial injury or infarction.	
29. Based on the pathophysiology and clinical evaluation of the patient with a suspected acute myocardial infarction, list the anticipated clinical problems according to their life-threatening potential.	
30. Specify the measures that may be taken to prevent or minimize complications in the patient with suspected myocardial infarction.	
31. Describe the most commonly used cardiac drugs in terms of therapeutic effect and dosages, routes of administration, side effects, and toxic effects.	
32. Describe the epidemiology, morbidity, mortality, and physiology associated with heart failure.	
33. Identify the factors that may precipitate or aggravate heart failure.	
34. Define acute pulmonary edema and describe its relationship to left ventricular failure.	

OBJECTIVES

694 ESSENTIALS OF PARAMEDIC CARE

©2007 Pearson Education, Inc.
Essentials of Paramedic Care, 2nd ed.

HANDOUT 28-2 Continued

Knowledge	Date Mastered
35. Differentiate between early and late signs and symptoms of left ventricular failure and those of right ventricular failure.	
36. Define and explain the clinical significance of paroxysmal nocturnal dyspnea, pulmonary edema, and dependent edema.	
37. List the interventions prescribed for the patient in acute congestive heart failure.	
38. Describe the most commonly used pharmacological agents in the management of congestive heart failure in terms of therapeutic effect, dosages, routes of administration, side effects, and toxic effects.	
39. Define and describe the incidence, mortality, morbidity, pathophysiology, assessment, and management of the following cardiac-related problems: • Cardiac tamponade • Hypertensive emergency • Cardiogenic shock • Cardiac arrest	
40. Identify the limiting factor of pericardial anatomy that determines intrapericardiac pressure.	
41. Describe how to determine if pulsus paradoxus, pulsus alternans, or electrical alternans is present.	
42. Explain the essential pathophysiological defect of hypertension in terms of Starling's law of the heart.	
43. Rank the clinical problems of patients in hypertensive emergencies according to their sense of urgency.	
44. Identify the drugs of choice for hypertensive emergencies, cardiogenic shock, and cardiac arrest, including their indications, contraindications, side effects, route of administration, and dosages.	
45. Describe the major systemic effects of reduced tissue perfusion caused by cardiogenic shock.	
46. Explain the primary mechanisms by which the heart may compensate for a diminished cardiac output and describe their efficiency in cardiogenic shock.	
47. Identify the clinical criteria and progressive stages of cardiogenic shock.	
48. Describe the dysrhythmias seen in cardiac arrest.	
49. Explain how to confirm asystole using the 3-lead ECG.	
50. Define the terms *defibrillation* and *synchronized cardioversion*.	

HANDOUT 28-2 Continued

Knowledge	Date Mastered
51. Specify the methods of supporting the patient with a suspected ineffective implanted defibrillation device.	
52. Describe resuscitation and identify circumstances and situations where resuscitation efforts would not be initiated.	
53. Identify communication and documentation protocols with medical direction and law enforcement used for termination of resuscitation efforts.	
54. Describe the incidence, morbidity, mortality, pathophysiology, assessment, and management of vascular disorders including occlusive disease, phlebitis, aortic aneurysm, and peripheral artery occlusion.	
55. Identify the clinical significance of claudication and presence of arterial bruits in a patient with peripheral vascular disorders.	
56. Describe the clinical significance of unequal arterial blood pressure readings in the arms.	
57. Recognize and describe the signs and symptoms of dissecting thoracic or abdominal aneurysm.	
58. Differentiate between signs and symptoms of cardiac tamponade, hypertensive emergencies, cardiogenic shock, and cardiac arrest.	
59. Utilize the results of the patient history, assessment findings, and ECG analysis to differentiate between, and provide treatment for, patients with the following conditions: • Cardiovascular disease • Chest pain • In need of a pacemaker • Angina pectoris • A suspected myocardial infarction • Heart failure • Cardiac tamponade • A hypertensive emergency • Cardiogenic shock • Cardiac arrest	
60. Based on the pathophysiology and clinical evaluation of the patient with chest pain, characterize the clinical problems according to their life-threatening potential.	
61. Given several preprogrammed patients with cardiac complaints, provide the appropriate assessment, treatment, and transport.	

Handout 28-3

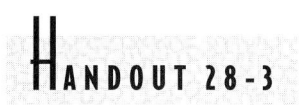

Student's Name _____

ECG MONITORING

Charting Student Progress:
1. *Learning skill*
2. *Performs skill with direction*
3. *Performs skill independently*

Procedure	1	2	3
1. Turn on the machine.			
2. Prepare the skin.			
3. Apply the electrodes.			
4. Check the ECG.			
5. Obtain a tracing.			
6. Continue ALS care.			

Comments:

Handout 28-4

Student's Name _____

DEFIBRILLATION

Charting Student Progress:
1. *Learning skill*
2. *Performs skill with direction*
3. *Performs skill independently*

Procedure	1	2	3
1. Identify rhythm on the cardiac monitor.			
2. Apply electrode gel to the paddles or place commercial defibrillation pads on the patient's exposed thorax.			
3. Charge the defibrillation paddles.			
4. Reconfirm the rhythm on the cardiac monitor.			
5. Verbally and visually clear everybody, including yourself, from the cardiac patient.			
6. Deliver a shock by pressing both buttons simultaneously.			
7. Reconfirm the rhythm on the cardiac monitor.			

Comments:

HANDOUT 28-5

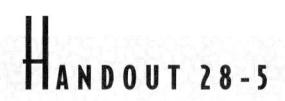

Student's Name _____

EXTERNAL CARDIAC PACING

Charting Student Progress:
1. *Learning skill*
2. *Performs skill with direction*
3. *Performs skill independently*

Procedure	1	2	3
1. Establish an IV line.			
2. Place ECG electrodes.			
3. Carefully assess vital signs and contact medical direction.			
4. If external pacing is ordered, apply the pacing electrodes according to the manufacturer's recommendations.			
5. Connect the electrodes.			
6. Select the desired pacing rate and current.			
7. Monitor the patient's response to treatment.			

Comments:

Handout 28-6

Student's Name _____

CAROTID SINUS MASSAGE

Charting Student Progress:
1. *Learning skill*
2. *Performs skill with direction*
3. *Performs skill independently*

Procedure	1	2	3
1. Assess the patient.			
2. Turn on the monitor.			
3. Listen to both carotids for the presence of bruits.			
4. Start an IV line.			
5. Rub either carotid. Wait.			
6. Check the rhythm.			
7. If unsuccessful, rub the other carotid.			
8. Reevaluate the patient.			

Comments:

Handout 28-7

Student's Name _____

12-LEAD PREHOSPITAL ECG MONITORING

Charting Student Progress:
1. *Learning skill*
2. *Performs skill with direction*
3. *Performs skill independently*

Procedure	1	2	3
1. Prep the skin.			
2. Place the four limb leads according to the manufacturer's recommendations.			
3. Place lead V1.			
4. Place lead V2.			
5. Place lead V3.			
6. Place lead V4.			
7. Place lead V5.			
8. Place lead V6.			
9. Ensure that all leads are attached.			
10. Turn on the machine.			
11. Check the quality of the tracing being received from each channel.			
12. Record the tracing.			
13. Examine the tracing.			
14. Transmit the tracing to the receiving hospital.			

Comments:

Handout 28-8

Student's Name _____

CHAPTER 28 QUIZ, PART 1

Write the letter of the best answer in the space provided.

_____ 1. The heart consists of three tissue layers, including the:
  A. epithelium.
  B. endocardium.
  C. subcardium.
  D. parathelium.

_____ 2. After blood circulates through the lungs and becomes oxygenated, it returns to the heart by way of the:
  A. pulmonary arteries.
  B. myocardial arteries.
  C. pulmonary veins.
  D. superior and inferior vena cava.

_____ 3. Which one of the following statements about the circulation of blood is TRUE?
  A. Intracardiac pressures are higher on the left of the heart.
  B. The left atrium sends oxygenated blood into the left ventricle.
  C. Pulmonary arteries are the only arteries that carry oxygenated blood.
  D. The right myocardium is thicker than the left myocardium.

_____ 4. The heart receives its nutrients from the:
  A. anterior great cardiac vein.
  B. blood within its chambers.
  C. coronary arteries.
  D. aorta.

_____ 5. The term *collateral circulation* refers to:
  A. both sides of the heart receiving blood at the same time.
  B. blood being sent from the atria into the ventricles.
  C. an alternate path for blood flow in case of blockage.
  D. blood flow to the lungs and heart at the same time.

_____ 6. The connection points between the arterial and venous systems are called:
  A. lumens.
  B. capillaries.
  C. venules.
  D. tunica.

_____ 7. Which one of the following statements about arteries is TRUE?
  A. They carry oxygenated blood.
  B. They carry blood away from the heart.
  C. They carry blood under low pressure.
  D. They cannot change the size of their lumen.

_____ 8. The period of time from the end of one cardiac contraction to the end of the next is called the cardiac:
  A. fraction.
  B. diastole.
  C. systole.
  D. cycle.

_____ 9. Pressure in the filled ventricle at the end of diastole is called:
  A. afterload.
  B. preload.
  C. cardiac output.
  D. stroke volume.

_____ 10. The equation used to determine cardiac output is:
  A. stroke volume × heart rate.
  B. systolic pressure × heart rate.
  C. preload × stroke volume.
  D. preload × afterload.

HANDOUT 28-8 Continued

_____ 11. Which one of the following statements about the nervous system's control of the heart is TRUE?
   A. In the heart's normal state, the sympathetic system is dominant.
   B. During sleep, the parasympathetic and sympathetic systems balance.
   C. In stressful situations, the sympathetic system becomes dominant.
   D. In the heart's normal state, the parasympathetic system is dominant.

_____ 12. A positive chronotropic agent will:
   A. increase heart rate.
   B. increase respiratory rate.
   C. strengthen cardiac contraction.
   D. speed impulse conduction.

_____ 13. Cardiac depolarization may be defined as:
   A. a negative charge on the outside of a cell.
   B. similar to the resting potential of cardiac cells.
   C. the opposite of the cell's resting state.
   D. the release of sodium and calcium from a cell.

_____ 14. The return of a cardiac muscle cell to its preexcitation resting state is called:
   A. resting potential.
   B. depolarization.
   C. action potential.
   D. repolarization.

_____ 15. The term *automaticity* refers to a cell's capability of:
   A. responding to electrical stimuli.
   B. propagating an electrical impulse from one cell to another.
   C. self-depolarization.
   D. contraction or shortening.

_____ 16. Muscle tremors, shivering, and loose electrodes can cause deflections on the ECG called:
   A. anomalies.
   B. artifacts.
   C. aberrant conduction.
   D. FLBs.

_____ 17. The AV node has an intrinsic rate of self-excitation, which is _____ beats per minute.
   A. 20–40
   B. 40–60
   C. 60–80
   D. 80–100

_____ 18. The three types of ECG leads include:
   A. augmented.
   B. quadripolar.
   C. triangle.
   D. paradoxical.

_____ 19. Leads designated aVR, aVL, and aVF are known as _____ leads.
   A. unipolar
   B. bipolar
   C. precordial
   D. anterior

_____ 20. Leads I, II, and III are considered _____ leads.
   A. unipolar
   B. bipolar
   C. precordial
   D. anterior

_____ 21. Leads I, II, and III form:
   A. Starling's triad.
   B. Cushing's quadrant.
   C. Einthoven's triangle.
   D. the circle of Willis.

_____ 22. A single monitoring lead can indicate:
   A. presence or location of an infarct.
   B. axis deviation or chamber enlargement.
   C. right-to-left differences in impulse formation.
   D. the time it takes to conduct an impulse through the heart.

_____ 23. One small box on ECG graph paper equals:
   A. 0.20 sec.
   B. 0.02 sec.
   C. 0.04 sec.
   D. 0.40 sec.

HANDOUT 28-8 Continued

_____ 24. Time interval markings on ECG paper are placed at _____-second intervals.
  A. 1
  B. 2
  C. 3
  D. 6

_____ 25. The QRS complex reflects:
  A. atrial depolarization.
  B. ventricular depolarization.
  C. ventricular repolarization.
  D. atrial repolarization.

_____ 26. Waves associated with electrolyte abnormalities, but that may be a normal finding, are the _____ waves.
  A. P
  B. U
  C. T
  D. P, U, and T

_____ 27. Which one of the following statements about the P wave is TRUE?
  A. It is a negative deflection in Lead II.
  B. It is a rounded wave appearing after the QRS complex.
  C. It corresponds to atrial depolarization.
  D. It follows the T wave on normal ECGs.

_____ 28. A prolonged PR interval:
  A. is 0.12 to 0.20 seconds.
  B. indicates a delay in the AV node.
  C. may indicate a bundle branch block.
  D. is related to an increased risk of sudden death.

_____ 29. The interval of time in the cardiac cycle when a sufficiently strong stimulus may produce depolarization is called the _____ refractory period.
  A. absolute
  B. comparative
  C. relative
  D. prolonged

_____ 30. The ST segment may be:
  A. affected by myocardial infarction.
  B. positive and rounded.
  C. invisible in the normal ECG.
  D. isoelectric in the presence of ischemia.

_____ 31. The five-step procedure for interpreting ECG rhythm strips includes analyzing all of the following EXCEPT:
  A. QRS complex.
  B. rhythm.
  C. PR interval.
  D. ST segment.

_____ 32. A nonpacemaker heart cell that automatically depolarizes is called a(n) _____ focus.
  A. ectopic
  B. irritable
  C. ischemic
  D. reentry

_____ 33. Dysrhythmias are classified by all of the following EXCEPT:
  A. nature of origin.
  B. magnitude.
  C. severity.
  D. amplitude.

_____ 34. Dysrhythmias that originate in the SA node include:
  A. asystole.
  B. accelerated junctional rhythm.
  C. sinus tachycardia.
  D. atrial fibrillation.

_____ 35. An ectopic focus in the atrium resulting in an early P wave is called:
  A. atrial fibrillation.
  B. premature atrial contractions (PACs).
  C. atrial tachycardia.
  D. atrial flutter.

HANDOUT 28-8 Continued

_____ 36. Which of the following may be used in the treatment of symptomatic paroxysmal supraventricular tachycardia (PSVT)?
　　A. lidocaine
　　B. epinephrine
　　C. defibrillation
　　D. vagal maneuvers

_____ 37. Which one of the following statements about first-degree AV blocks is TRUE?
　　A. The rhythm is irregularly irregular.
　　B. The pacemaker site is the AV node.
　　C. The PR interval is greater than 0.20 sec.
　　D. It is usually a life-threatening dysrhythmia.

_____ 38. The absence of conduction between the atria and the ventricles is called _____ AV block.
　　A. first-degree
　　B. type I second-degree
　　C. type II second-degree
　　D. third-degree

_____ 39. Ventricular escape rhythms:
　　A. should be treated with lidocaine.
　　B. serve as safety mechanisms to prevent cardiac standstill.
　　C. look identical to a normal QRS complex.
　　D. cause an ST segment elevation.

_____ 40. Since PVCs do not usually depolarize the SA node:
　　A. the pause following the PVC is fully compensatory.
　　B. the PVCs will appear as inverted QRS complexes.
　　C. each PVC will appear to be from a different focus.
　　D. increasing the heart rate will eliminate them.

_____ 41. PVCs are considered malignant when more than _____ occur(s) per minute.
　　A. one
　　B. two
　　C. four
　　D. six

_____ 42. Ventricular fibrillation should be treated with immediate:
　　A. intubation.
　　B. IV lidocaine.
　　C. synchronized cardioversion.
　　D. defibrillation.

_____ 43. Defibrillation is used to treat:
　　A. nonperfusing ventricular tachycardia.
　　B. atrial fibrillation.
　　C. complete AV block.
　　D. malignant PVCs.

_____ 44. The "P" in PEA stands for:
　　A. pneumothorax.
　　B. postdefibrillation.
　　C. pericardiocentesis.
　　D. pulseless.

_____ 45. A kind of interventricular heart block in which conduction through either the right or left bundle branches is blocked or delayed is called a:
　　A. third-degree AV block.
　　B. bundle branch block.
　　C. type II second-degree AV block.
　　D. junctional block.

CHAPTER 28 QUIZ, PART 2

Write the letter of the best answer in the space provided.

_____ 1. All of the following statements about chest pain are true EXCEPT:
   A. Diabetic patients may have a myocardial infarction with no chest pain.
   B. Chest pain associated with pain in the jaw is benign.
   C. Differentiating between benign and life-threatening chest pain is not difficult in the field.
   D. Follow OPQRST to obtain the patient's description of the pain.

_____ 2. The letter "P" in SAMPLE stands for:
   A. pain.
   B. provocation.
   C. past medical history.
   D. provocation/palliation.

_____ 3. When monitoring your patient's ECG, a point to remember is:
   A. thick chest hair should be shaved before placing electrodes.
   B. paddles should be cleaned with alcohol before use.
   C. the negative electrode should be placed on the left lower chest.
   D. diaphoresis improves skin contact and useful ECG signals.

_____ 4. Which one of the following statements about a precordial thump is TRUE?
   A. There is little risk of causing rib fractures or other problems.
   B. It is most effective immediately after the onset of ventricular fibrillation.
   C. Strike the midsternum from a distance of no more than 6 inches.
   D. It stimulates polarization of ventricular cells, causing a resumption of an organized rhythm.

_____ 5. The parasympatholytic agent used to treat symptomatic bradycardias is:
   A. adenosine.
   B. verapamil.
   C. atropine sulfate.
   D. amiodarone.

_____ 6. Supraventricular tachydysrhythmia is managed by:
   A. amiodarone.
   B. adenosine.
   C. lidocaine.
   D. bretylium.

_____ 7. Sympathomimetic agents are similar to naturally occurring hormones, one of which is:
   A. atropine sulfate.
   B. lidocaine.
   C. verapamil.
   D. epinephrine.

_____ 8. The drug used in cardiac arrest resuscitation that acts on both alpha and beta adrenergic receptors is:
   A. dopamine.
   B. epinephrine.
   C. isoproterenol.
   D. atropine sulfate.

_____ 9. A potent beta agonist that increases heart rate and cardiac contractile force, but is rarely used with the advent of transcutaneous pacing, is:
   A. isoproterenol.
   B. dopamine.
   C. norepinephrine.
   D. dobutamine.

_____ 10. Morphine sulfate is important in managing MI because it:
   A. increases myocardial oxygen demand.
   B. has few side effects, none of which are toxic.
   C. increases sympathetic nervous system discharge.
   D. acts directly on the central nervous system.

HANDOUT 28-9 Continued

_____ 11. Which one of the following statements about nitrous oxide is TRUE?
   A. It is used to treat MI because of its hemodynamic effects.
   B. It can be used to increase myocardial oxygen supply.
   C. Its effects subside within 10–15 hours.
   D. You may give it to intoxicated patients.

_____ 12. Aspirin is used in the treatment of myocardial ischemia because it:
   A. is a thrombolytic.
   B. has analgesic effects.
   C. inhibits the aggregation of platelets.
   D. can cause gastric upset and bleeding.

_____ 13. When using alteplase, a potent thrombolytic, an important point to remember is:
   A. it must be administered within 3 hours after the onset of coronary ischemia.
   B. the typical dose is a single 10-unit bolus given IV push over 2 minutes.
   C. complications include potentially life-threatening dysrhythmias.
   D. unlike other fibrinolytics, hemorrhage is not a complication.

_____ 14. The purpose of defibrillation is to:
   A. deliver an electric shock to jump-start the heart.
   B. depolarize the cells and allow them to repolarize uniformly.
   C. deliver a regular impulse to pace a bradycardic heart.
   D. suppress ectopic beats, such as PVCs.

_____ 15. Several factors influence the success of defibrillation, including:
   A. duration of ventricular fibrillation.
   B. age of the patient.
   C. antidysrhythmic drugs.
   D. previous medical history.

_____ 16. Steps in performing defibrillation include:
   A. making sure the defibrillator paddles are clean and dry.
   B. using firm downward pressure on the paddles to decrease transthoracic resistance.
   C. verifying that the synchronizer is turned on.
   D. charging the defibrillator to 360 joules for all three shocks.

_____ 17. Indications for emergency synchronized cardioversion of an unstable patient include:
   A. pulseless ventricular tachycardia.
   B. ventricular fibrillation.
   C. rapid atrial fibrillation.
   D. pulseless electrical activity.

_____ 18. The procedure for synchronized cardioversion is the same as for defibrillation EXCEPT:
   A. the button on only one paddle is pressed.
   B. the energy used is much less.
   C. the electrodes are placed in different positions.
   D. clearing the patient before delivery is unnecessary.

_____ 19. Symptomatic patients in atrial fibrillation with a slow ventricular response may be treated with:
   A. defibrillation.
   B. synchronized cardioversion.
   C. external cardiac pacing.
   D. none of these

_____ 20. Chest pain that results when the blood supply's oxygen demand exceeds the heart's is called:
   A. myocardial infarction.
   B. heart failure.
   C. Prinzmetal's angina.
   D. angina pectoris.

_____ 21. The major difference between stable and unstable angina is that unstable angina:
   A. occurs at rest.
   B. responds more readily to treatment.
   C. indicates the patient's condition is improving.
   D. causes cardiac muscle cell death.

©2007 Pearson Education, Inc.
Essentials of Paramedic Care, 2nd ed.

HANDOUT 28-9 Continued

_____ 22. Which one of the following statements about angina pectoris is TRUE?
  A. It results from underlying coronary artery disease.
  B. For relief, angina pain requires morphine.
  C. With angina, peripheral pulses are typically unequal.
  D. Blood pressure will lower during the episode.

_____ 23. Myocardial infarction:
  A. is the death of a portion of the heart muscle.
  B. can result from coronary artery spasm.
  C. may be caused by hypotension.
  D. is all of these.

_____ 24. The most common complication of myocardial infarction is:
  A. heart failure.
  B. dysrhythmias.
  C. ventricular aneurysm.
  D. pulmonary edema.

_____ 25. To determine specifics about chest pain, use _____ to help you.
  A. SAMPLE
  B. AVPU
  C. DCAP-BTLS
  D. OPQRST

_____ 26. Rapid transport of a patient with chest pain is indicated if:
  A. the patient has a cardiac history.
  B. pathological Q waves are present on the 12-lead.
  C. the ST segment has no changes.
  D. the patient is over 35 years of age.

_____ 27. The clinical syndrome in which the heart's mechanical performance is compromised so that cardiac output cannot meet the body's needs is called:
  A. angina pectoris.
  B. pneumothorax.
  C. heart failure.
  D. cardiac tamponade.

_____ 28. The condition in which the heart's reduced stroke volume causes an overload of fluid in the body's other tissues is called:
  A. congestive heart failure.
  B. myocardial infarction.
  C. Prinzmetal's angina.
  D. angina pectoris.

_____ 29. Management of the patient with congestive heart failure includes placing the patient in a:
  A. supine position with legs slightly raised.
  B. standing position to ease anxiety.
  C. seated position with feet dangling.
  D. left lateral recumbent position.

_____ 30. Your patient is extremely hypertensive with a diastolic reading of over 130 mmHg. He complains of a severe headache, vomiting, and dizziness. You should suspect:
  A. noncardiogenic pulmonary edema.
  B. hypertensive encephalopathy.
  C. dissecting aortic aneurysm.
  D. meningitis.

_____ 31. Sudden death is defined as death:
  A. immediately after the onset of symptoms.
  B. without any signs or symptoms.
  C. within 1 hour after the onset of symptoms.
  D. that is unexpected for any reason.

_____ 32. Return of spontaneous circulation (ROSC) occurs when resuscitation results in:
  A. survival.
  B. sudden death.
  C. a spontaneous pulse and respirations.
  D. a spontaneous pulse, with or without breathing.

HANDOUT 28-9 Continued

_____ 33. When resuscitation is indicated, the mainstay of treatment for cardiac arrest is:
   A. intubation.
   B. IV medications.
   C. basic life support.
   D. NSAIDs.

_____ 34. The thickening, loss of elasticity, and hardening of the walls of the arteries from calcium deposits is called:
   A. arteriosclerosis.
   B. atherosclerosis.
   C. claudication.
   D. an aneurysm.

_____ 35. Which one of the following statements about an abdominal aortic aneurysm is TRUE?
   A. It is more common in women than in men.
   B. It is most prevalent between the ages of 60 and 70.
   C. It occurs most frequently above the renal arteries.
   D. Signs and symptoms include pain in the calf muscles.

HANDOUT 28-10

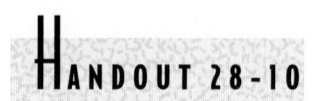

Student's Name _____

CHAPTER 28 SCENARIO 1

Review the following real-life situation. Then answer the questions that follow.

You are called to the local shopping center where a 70-year-old woman has collapsed while shopping. Her daughter called the ambulance. The daughter states that the patient weighs approximately 110 pounds and that she had been experiencing substernal chest pains for approximately 20 minutes when she suddenly "passed out." The patient has not responded to verbal stimuli in the past 5 minutes. Bystanders inform you that the patient was breathing on her own until a few minutes prior to your arrival.

The store manager, who has recently been trained in CPR, has initiated rescue breathing but has not begun chest compressions because he "thought he felt a pulse." You immediately connect the patient to the cardiac monitor and note the rhythm to be sinus tachycardia, with frequent PVCs. You note at this time that the patient has resumed spontaneous respirations.

1. What steps would you take in the management of this patient?

HANDOUT 28-11

Student's Name _____

CHAPTER 28 SCENARIO 2

Review the following real-life situation. Then answer the questions that follow.

You and your partner are called to the scene of a rural residence where you find a 57-year-old male who is complaining of chest pain. The patient reports a history of recent surgery, which was performed to repair a fractured pelvis. Approximately 2 hours ago he began to experience "tightening in his chest," chest discomfort, and shortness of breath. He now reports that he feels nauseated.

1. What would be your initial assessment considerations with this patient?

Your partner records the patient's vital signs as follows: BP, 180/120; heart rate, 140; and respirations, 32. When you connect the patient to the ECG, you see a wide-complex tachycardia (uncertain type). When you contact the base hospital, your medical direction physician instructs you to follow the ACLS algorithm for wide-complex tachycardia and to keep him informed of the patient's status.

2. Prior to initiating drug therapy, what questions would you ask the patient?

3. What is the most important step in the initial management of this patient?

4. Five minutes into your management of this patient, his BP drops to 130/74 and he exhibits a decreased level of consciousness. What should you do next?

EVALUATION

HANDOUT 28-12

Student's Name _____

CHAPTER 28 REVIEW

Write the word or words that best complete each sentence in the space(s) provided.

1. The heart consists of three tissue layers: the _____, _____, and _____.
2. The two superior chambers of the heart are the _____. The larger, inferior chambers are the _____.
3. The heart contains two pairs of valves, the _____ valves and the _____ valves.
4. The _____ _____ _____ receives deoxygenated blood from the head and upper extremities. The _____ _____ _____ receives blood from the areas below the heart.
5. The only veins in the body that carry oxygenated blood are the _____ veins.
6. The term _____ refers to communication between two or more blood vessels.
7. _____ Law states that blood flow through a vessel is directly proportional to the radius of the vessel to the fourth power.
8. The period of time from the end of one cardiac contraction to the end of the next is called the _____ _____.
9. The period of time when the myocardium is relaxed and cardiac filling and coronary perfusion occur is called _____.
10. _____ is the period of the cardiac cycle when the myocardium is contracting.
11. The ratio of blood pumped from the ventricle to the amount of blood remaining at the end of diastole is called the _____ _____.
12. The term _____ refers to the pressure within the ventricles at the end of diastole.
13. The term _____ refers to the resistance against which the heart must pump.
14. The amount of blood pumped by the heart in 1 minute is called the _____ _____.
15. The term _____ _____ refers to the amount of blood ejected by the heart in one cardiac contraction.
16. The term *chronotropy* pertains to heart _____.
17. The term *inotropy* pertains to cardiac _____ _____.
18. The term _____ pertains to the speed of impulse transmission.
19. A reversal of charges at a cell membrane so that the inside of the cell becomes positive in relation to the outside is called cardiac _____.
20. The normal electrical state of cells is called _____ _____.
21. The stimulation of myocardial cells that subsequently spreads across the myocardium is called the _____ _____.
22. The return of a muscle cell to its preexcitation resting state is called _____.
23. The term _____ pertains to cells being able to respond to an electrical stimulus.
24. The term _____ pertains to cells being able to propagate the electrical impulse from one cell to another.
25. The pacemaker cells' capability of self-depolarization is called _____.

712 ESSENTIALS OF PARAMEDIC CARE

HANDOUT 28-12 Continued

26. A deflection on the ECG produced by factors other than the heart's electrical activity is called a(n) _____.
27. Leads I, II, and III are known as _____ limb leads.
28. Leads V1 through V6 are called the _____ leads.
29. Unipolar limb leads are also called _____ limb leads.
30. On ECG graph paper, one small box is equal to _____ seconds.
31. On ECG graph paper, one large box is equal to _____ seconds.
32. The P wave corresponds to _____ depolarization.
33. The QRS complex reflects _____ depolarization.
34. _____ waves may be associated with electrolyte abnormalities.
35. The normal duration of the PR interval is _____ to _____ seconds.
36. The normal QRS complex is _____ to _____ seconds.
37. The period of time when myocardial cells have not yet completely repolarized and cannot be stimulated again is called the _____ _____ period.
38. The _____ _____ _____ is the period of the cardiac cycle when a sufficiently strong stimulus may reproduce depolarization.
39. A heart rate greater than _____ beats per minute is called tachycardia.
40. A heart rate less than 60 beats per minute is called _____.
41. Any deviation from the normal electrical rhythm of the heat is called _____.
42. The absence of cardiac electrical activity is called _____.
43. A nonpacemaker cell that automatically depolarizes is called a(n) _____ focus.
44. Forced expiration against a closed glottis is called a _____ maneuver.
45. The sound of turbulent blood flow through a vessel is called a(n) _____.
46. A delay in conduction at the level of the AV node is called a(n) _____ -degree AV block.
47. An intermittent block at the level of the AV node is called a(n) _____ -degree AV block.
48. The absence of conduction between the atria and the ventricles resulting from complete electrical block at or below the AV node is called a(n) _____ -degree AV block.
49. A single ectopic impulse arising from an irritable focus in either ventricle that occurs earlier than the next expected beat is called a(n) _____ _____ _____.
50. _____ PVCs are termed as malignant if there are more than _____ per minute.
51. _____ _____ is a chaotic ventricular rhythm usually resulting from the presence of many reentry circuits within the ventricles.
52. The dysrhythmia in which there are electrical complexes but no accompanying mechanical contractions of the heart is called _____ _____ _____.
53. Conduction of the electrical impulse through the heart's conductive system in an abnormal fashion is called _____ conduction.
54. A(n) _____ _____ _____ is a kind of interventricular heart block in which conduction through either the right or left bundle branches is blocked or delayed.
55. _____ _____ is the most common presenting symptom in cases of cardiac disease.

HANDOUT 28-12 Continued

56. Use the _____ acronym to help you obtain the patient's description of pain.
57. Systematic, thorough physical examinations involve three components: _____, _____, and _____.
58. _____ life support is the primary skill for managing serious cardiovascular problems.
59. Having the patient bear down as if attempting to have a bowel movement is called a(n) _____ maneuver.
60. Atropine, lidocaine, procainamide, bretylium, and adenosine are all _____ medications.
61. _____ _____ is a parasympatholytic agent used to treat symptomatic bradycardia.
62. _____ is a medication used to manage supraventricular tachydysrhythmia.
63. _____ is a first-line antidysrhythmic used to treat and prevent life-threatening ventricular dysrhythmia.
64. _____, the mainstay medication of cardiac arrest resuscitation, acts on both alpha and beta adrenergic receptors.
65. _____ _____ is a medication that reduces myocardial oxygen demand by reducing preload and afterload.
66. _____ is a medication that inhibits the aggregation of platelets.
67. The process of passing a current through a fibrillating heart to depolarize the cells is called _____.
68. The term _____ _____ refers to the passage of an electrical current through the heart during a specific part of the cardiac cycle to terminate certain kinds of dysrhythmia.
69. Chest pain that results when the blood supply's oxygen demands exceed the heart's is called _____.
70. A variant of angina pectoris caused by vasospasm of the coronary arteries is called _____ angina.
71. Death and subsequent necrosis of the heart muscle caused by inadequate blood supply is called _____ _____.
72. _____ _____ is the clinical syndrome in which the heart's mechanical performance is compromised so that cardiac output cannot meet the body's needs.
73. A blood clot in one of the pulmonary arteries is called a pulmonary _____.
74. _____ _____ _____ is the heart's reduced stroke volume causing an overload of fluid in the body's other tissues.
75. A sudden episode of difficult breathing that occurs after lying down is called _____ _____.
76. The accumulation of excess fluid inside the pericardium is called _____ _____.
77. A cerebral disorder of hypertension indicated by severe headache, nausea, vomiting, and altered mental status is called _____ _____.
78. The inability of the heart to meet the metabolic needs of the body, resulting in inadequate tissue perfusion, is called _____ shock.
79. The absence of any ventricular contraction is called _____ _____.
80. _____ death is death within 1 hour after the onset of symptoms.
81. _____ time is the duration from the beginning of the cardiac arrest until effective CPR is established.

HANDOUT 28-12 Continued

82. The thickening, loss of elasticity, and hardening of the walls of the arteries from calcium deposits is known as _____.

83. Severe pain in the calf muscle due to inadequate blood supply is called _____.

84. The condition in which the ballooning of an arterial wall results from a defect or weakness in the wall is called a(n) _____.

85. _____ _____ _____ is the death or degeneration of a part of the wall of an artery.

86. _____ _____ _____ is a blockage that occurs when a blood clot or other particle lodges in a pulmonary artery.

87. Sudden occlusion of arterial blood flow is called _____ _____ occlusion.

88. Leads I, II, and III are called _____ limb leads.

89. Leads aVR, aVL, and aVF are called _____ limb leads.

90. Leads V1 through V6 are known as the _____ leads.

91. A force that has both magnitude and direction is called a(n) _____.

92. The reduction of all the heart's electrical forces to a single vector represented by an arrow moving in a single plane is called the _____ axis.

93. A calculated axis of the heart's electrical energy that equals or exceeds +105° is known as _____ _____ _____.

94. A calculated axis of the heart's electrical energy that equals or exceeds −30° is known as _____ _____ _____.

95. Deprivation of oxygen and other nutrients to the myocardium is called _____ _____.

96. _____ _____ is the death of myocardial tissue.

97. Myocardial infarction that affects only the deeper levels of the myocardium is called _____ infarction.

98. Myocardial infarction that affects the full thickness of the myocardium is called _____ infarction.

99. A mirror image seen typically on the opposite wall of the injured area is said to be _____.

100. _____ is stretching, enlargement without any additional cells.

Handout 28-13

Student's Name _____

ECG BASICS

Write the names of the indicated components of the ECG tracing in the spaces provided.

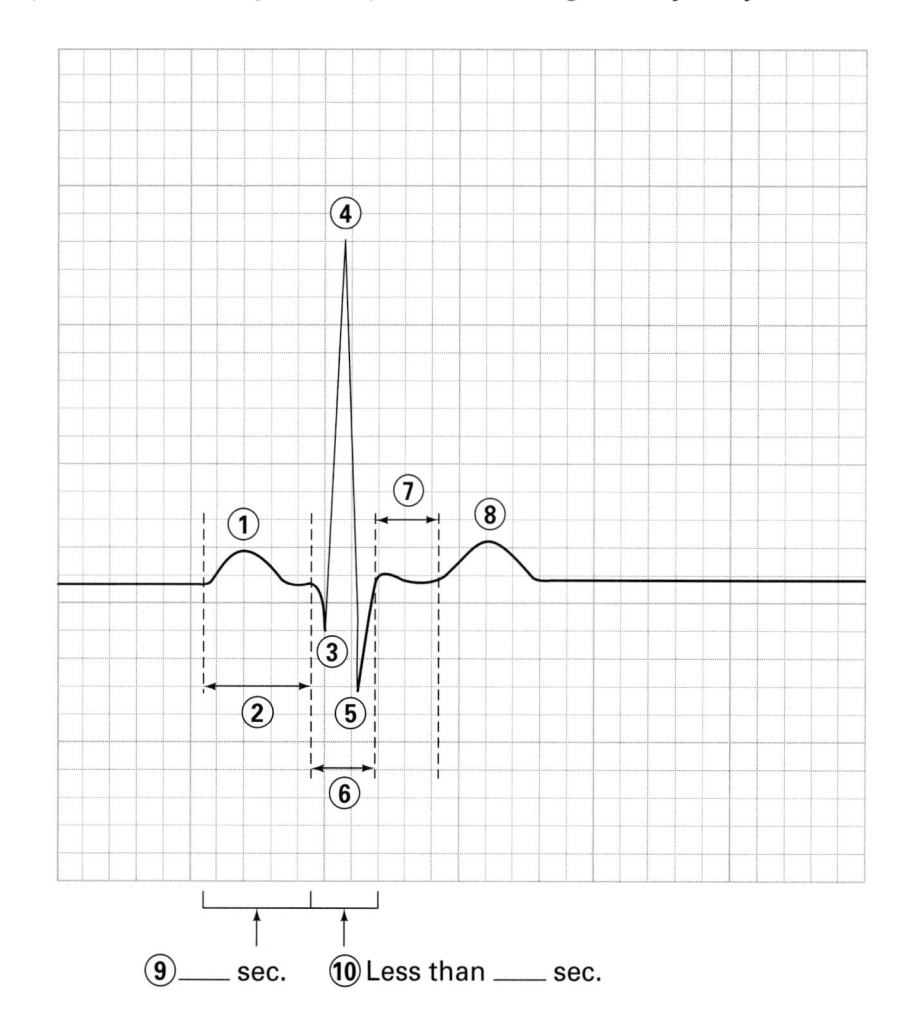

⑨ ___ sec.   ⑩ Less than ___ sec.

1. _____
2. _____
3. _____
4. _____
5. _____
6. _____
7. _____
8. _____
9. _____
10. _____

716 ESSENTIALS OF PARAMEDIC CARE

©2007 Pearson Education, Inc.
Essentials of Paramedic Care, 2nd ed.

HANDOUT 28-14

Student's Name _____

DYSRHYTHMIA MATCHING

Write the letter of the term in the space provided next to the appropriate definition.

A. asystole
B. atrial fibrillation
C. Mobitz II
D. third-degree AV block
E. atrial flutter
F. first-degree AV block
G. PSVT
H. sinus tachycardia
I. PAC
J. PVC
K. sinus arrest
L. ventricular escape
M. sinus bradycardia
N. PJC
O. V-fib
P. V-tach

_____ 1. Result of single electrical impulse originating in the atria outside the SA node; results in premature depolarization.

_____ 2. No electrical activity; no P waves; no PR interval; no QRS complex.

_____ 3. Atrial rate 150–250; ventricular rate varies; rhythm regular; pacemaker in atria; PR interval and QRS normal.

_____ 4. Complete block; absence of conduction between atria and ventricles; atrial and ventricular rhythms regular.

_____ 5. Rate greater than 100; regular rhythm; SA node is pacemaker; P waves, PR interval, QRS normal.

_____ 6. Rhythm regular; pacemaker in SA node or atria; P waves normal, PR interval greater than 0.2 sec, QRS normal.

_____ 7. Atrial rate unaffected, ventricular rate bradycardic; P waves normal, not all followed by QRS; PR interval constant.

_____ 8. Atrial rate 350–750; irregularly irregular rhythm; pacemaker sites are numerous ectopic foci in atria.

_____ 9. Rapid atrial reentry circuit; atrial rate 250–350; rhythm usually regular; pacemaker site in atria outside SA node.

_____ 10. Single ectopic impulse arising from an irritable focus in ventricle; occurring earlier than next expected beat.

_____ 11. Rate 15–40; rhythm irregular in single complex; pacemaker site in ventricle; no P wave; QRS greater than 0.12 sec.

_____ 12. Episode of failure of sinus node to discharge, resulting in short periods of cardiac standstill.

_____ 13. Rate less than 60; regular rhythm; SA node is pacemaker; P waves, PR interval, QRS complex normal.

HANDOUT 28-14 Continued

_____ **14.** Result from single electrical impulse originating in AV node before next expected sinus beat.

_____ **15.** Rate 100–250; regular rhythm; pacemaker site is ventricle; no PR interval; QRS greater than 0.12 sec.

_____ **16.** No organized rhythm; pacemaker sites are numerous ectopic foci in ventricles; P wave, PR interval, QRS complex are absent.

Chapter 28 Answer Key

Handout 28-8: Chapter 28 Quiz, Part 1

1. B	13. C	25. B	37. C
2. C	14. D	26. B	38. D
3. B	15. C	27. C	39. B
4. C	16. B	28. B	40. A
5. C	17. B	29. C	41. D
6. B	18. A	30. A	42. D
7. B	19. A	31. D	43. A
8. D	20. B	32. A	44. D
9. B	21. C	33. D	45. B
10. A	22. D	34. C	
11. C	23. C	35. B	
12. A	24. C	36. D	

Handout 28-9: Chapter 28 Quiz, Part 2

1. D	10. D	19. C	28. A
2. C	11. B	20. D	29. C
3. A	12. C	21. A	30. B
4. B	13. C	22. A	31. C
5. C	14. B	23. D	32. D
6. B	15. A	24. B	33. C
7. D	16. B	25. D	34. A
8. B	17. C	26. B	35. B
9. A	18. B	27. C	

Handout 28-10: Chapter 28 Scenario 1

1. Steps in the management of this patient would include:

   A. Immediately reassess the patient's level of consciousness and ABCs.
   B. Place the patient on 100 percent oxygen via nonrebreather mask.
   C. Obtain baseline vital signs and contact medical direction.
   D. Establish an IV per protocols/medical direction.
   E. Consider IV bolus of lidocaine per protocols/medical direction.

Handout 28-11: Chapter 28 Scenario 2

1. As with all patients who are ill or injured, the initial assessment considerations include immediate assessment of the patient's level of consciousness, airway, breathing, and circulatory status.
2. Do you have any allergies? Have you ever experienced this type of pain before? What medications are you currently taking?
3. Administration of high-flow oxygen (100 percent at 15 liters per minute) via nonrebreather mask.
4. An IV NS would have been established. Administer lidocaine 1–1.5 mg/kg IV push. The lidocaine can be repeated until 3 mg/kg has been given. If the rhythm has not changed, administer adenosine, 6 mg rapid IV push; repeat the adenosine 12 mg rapid IV push over 1–23 sec (may repeat once in 1–2 minutes). Carefully monitor the patient en route to the hospital, maintaining contact with medical direction.

Handout 28-12: Chapter 28 Review

1. endocardium, myocardium, pericardium
2. atria, ventricles
3. atrioventricular, semilunar
4. superior vena cava, inferior vena cava
5. pulmonary
6. anastomosis
7. Poiseuille's
8. cardiac cycle
9. diastole
10. Systole
11. ejection fraction
12. preload
13. afterload
14. cardiac output
15. stroke volume
16. rate
17. contractile force
18. dromotropy
19. depolarization
20. resting potential
21. action potential
22. repolarization
23. excitability
24. conductivity
25. automaticity
26. artifact
27. bipolar
28. precordial
29. augmented
30. 0.04
31. 0.20
32. atrial
33. ventricular
34. Q
35. 0.12 to 0.20
36. 0.08 to 0.12
37. absolute refractory
38. relative refractory period
39. 100
40. bradycardia
41. dysrhythmia
42. arrhythmia
43. ectopic
44. vagal (or Valsalva)
45. bruit
46. first
47. second
48. third
49. premature ventricular contraction (PVC)
50. Six
51. Ventricular fibrillation
52. pulseless electrical activity
53. aberrant
54. bundle branch block
55. Chest pain
56. OPQRST
57. inspection, auscultation, palpation
58. Basic

59. vagal (or Valsalva)
60. antidysrhythmic
61. Atropine sulfate
62. Adenosine
63. Lidocaine
64. Epinephrine
65. Morphine sulfate
66. Aspirin
67. defibrillation
68. synchronized cardioversion
69. angina pectoris
70. Prinzmetal's
71. myocardial infarction
72. Heart failure
73. embolism
74. Congestive heart failure
75. paroxysmal nocturnal dyspnea
76. cardiac tamponade
77. hypertensive encephalopathy
78. cardiogenic
79. cardiac arrest
80. Sudden
81. Down
82. arteriosclerosis
83. claudication
84. aneurysm
85. Cystic medial necrosis
86. Acute pulmonary edema
87. acute arterial
88. bipolar
89. unipolar
90. precordial
91. vector
92. QRS
93. right axis deviation
94. left axis deviation
95. myocardial ischemia
96. Myocardial infarction
97. subendocardial
98. transmural
99. reciprocal
100. Hypertrophy

Handout 28-13: ECG Basics

1. P wave
2. PR interval
3. Q wave
4. R wave
5. S wave
6. QRS interval
7. ST segment
8. T wave
9. 0.12–0.20 sec
10. 0.12 sec

Handout 28-14: Dysrhythmia Matching

1. I
2. A
3. G
4. D
5. H
6. F
7. C
8. B
9. E
10. J
11. L
12. K
13. M
14. N
15. P
16. O

Chapter 29

Neurology

INTRODUCTION

Emergencies involving the nervous system affect millions of lives in the United States and are often difficult to recognize and to treat. These disorders include stroke, epilepsy, Parkinson's disease, and many others. This chapter presents an overview of the common neurological conditions the paramedic may encounter in the prehospital setting, including the relevant anatomy and physiology of the nervous system, patient assessment, and patient management.

TOTAL TEACHING TIME:
13.17 HOURS
The total teaching time is only a guideline based on the didactic and practical lab averages in the National Standard Curriculum. Instructors should take into consideration such factors as the pace at which students learn, the size of the class, and breaks. The actual time devoted to teaching objectives is the responsibility of the instructor.

CHAPTER OBJECTIVES

After reading this chapter, you should be able to:

1. Describe the incidence, morbidity, and mortality of neurological emergencies. (p. 1244)
2. Identify the risk factors most predisposing to diseases of the nervous system. (pp. 1258–1259, 1263–1264, 1267, 1268, 1276)
3. Discuss the anatomy and physiology of the nervous system. (see Chapter 3)
4. Define and discuss the epidemiology (including the morbidity/mortality and preventative strategies), pathophysiology, assessment findings, and management for the following neurologic problems:

   - Coma and altered mental status (pp. 1256–1257)
   - Seizures (pp. 1264–1267)
   - Syncope (pp. 1267–1268)
   - Headache (pp. 1268–1270)
   - Neoplasms (pp. 1270–1272)
   - Abscess (p. 1272)
   - Stroke (pp. 1257–1263)
   - Intracranial hemorrhage (pp. 1259–1263)
   - Transient ischemic attack (pp. 1260–1261)
   - Degenerative neurological diseases (pp. 1272–1275)

5. Describe and differentiate the major types of seizures. (pp. 1264–1265)
6. Describe the phases of a generalized seizure. (pp. 1264–1265)
7. Define the following:

   - Muscular dystrophy (p. 1272)
   - Multiple sclerosis (pp. 1272–1273)
   - Dystonia (p. 1273)
   - Parkinson's disease (p. 1273)
   - Trigeminal neuralgia (pp. 1273–1274)
   - Bell's palsy (p. 1274)

©2007 Pearson Education, Inc.
Essentials of Paramedic Care, 2nd ed.

- Amyotrophic lateral sclerosis (p. 1274)
- Peripheral neuropathy (pp. 1246–1247)
- Myoclonus (p. 1274)
- Spina bifida (p. 1274)
- Poliomyelitis (p. 1274)

8. Define and discuss the pathophysiology, assessment findings, and management for nontraumatic spinal injury, including:

- Low back pain (pp. 1275–1276)
- Herniated intervertebral disk (p. 1276)
- Spinal cord tumors (p. 1276)

9. Differentiate between neurologic emergencies based on assessment findings. (pp. 1247–1277)

10. Given several preprogrammed, nontraumatic neurological emergency patients, provide the appropriate assessment, management, and transport. (pp. 1244–1277)

FRAMING THE LESSON

Begin the lesson by reviewing the important points from Chapter 28, "Cardiology." Discuss any aspects of the chapter not fully understood by students. Then go on to the Chapter 29 material. As a class exercise, discuss the various causes of altered mental status. First have students identify the things that the brain needs to function normally, such as chemicals, oxygen, and space. As each item is identified, list it on the board. After all items are identified, have students describe a condition that could cause alteration in function and the central nervous system signs and symptoms that might result. Students need to understand that there are a variety of conditions that may present as altered mental status. It is important that all of them be carefully considered before dismissing a patient as "intoxicated."

TEACHING STRATEGIES

People learn in a variety of ways. Some do better with the spoken word, whereas others prefer the written. Some prefer to work alone, whereas others profit from working in groups. Recognizing these different ways of acquiring knowledge, the authors of this *Instructor's Resource Manual* have provided a variety of teaching strategies for the different types of learners. These strategies are intended to foster higher-level cognitive skills and encourage creative learning and problem solving. For greatest effectiveness, incorporate these strategies into your class lecture. Symbols in the Lecture Outline indicate the points at which various exercises might be most appropriate. Other strategies can be used to preview the lesson or to summarize it.

The following strategies are keyed to specific sections of the lesson.

1. ***Recognizing Respiratory Patterns.*** Prepare index cards with the name and description of a respiratory pattern seen with central nervous system (CNS) dysfunction, such as Cheyne-Stokes, ataxic, and so on. Distribute the cards to small groups of students. Instruct students, one at a time, to demonstrate the breathing pattern on the card they hold. Have other students in the group decide which pattern is being demonstrated.

2. ***Practice Using the Glasgow Coma Scale.*** Give students practice using the Glasgow Coma Scale by presenting case studies of patients and asking students to

assign a GCS to each. This will assist students in memorizing the tool and also allows them time to ask you questions about how to use it. Though the GCS is intended to be objective, some subjective assessment is required. To reinforce the importance of using the GCS correctly, discuss how different hospitals and EMS systems allocate resources or make treatment decisions based on the GCS score.

The following strategies can be used at various points throughout the lesson or to help summarize and demonstrate what students have learned.

Guest Lecturer. A move toward "stroke center designation" is being made among hospitals in the United States. These are hospitals that conduct stroke research, participate in aggressive stroke therapy, or actually have a "stroke team" much like a code team or trauma team. Have students identify which hospitals in your region are participating in such stroke care. Invite a member of a stroke team to discuss what his or her hospital does differently, or how stroke care today is different than 5 years ago. It is important that students recognize the advancements in stroke care in order for them to make good transport decisions for their patients.

Practice in the Field. No single activity will accomplish as much understanding of, interest in, and empathy for the victims and families of Alzheimer's disease than a clinical rotation at an Alzheimer's treatment center. Special centers with highly trained staff exist for patients because there are so many facets of caring for this type of patient. A 4-or 8-hour rotation will not only allow students to assist with daily activities, assessments, and medication therapy, but also will allow them to hear from families who are dealing with the patient's emotional outbursts, regressive behavior, and the cost of care.

Nerve Game. Draw or obtain a diagram of the spinal cord and its branches. (You may prefer to use Figure 3-69, page 168, on an opaque projector.) In either case, cover up the labels identifying the names of the nerves branching off from the spinal cord. Then divide the class into teams. Equip each team with a buzzer, horn, or some noise-making device. Then use a pointer to indicate the branch to be identified. The first team to signal gets first crack at naming the nerve. If the team identifies the nerve correctly, it gets 3 points. If the team fails to identify it correctly, it loses 2 points and the other teams signal again for the chance to name the nerve. Continue with the game until all nerves have been identified. Members of the team with the highest total points could be awarded simple prizes such as key chains or pens.

Mnemonic Review. Up to this point in the course, students have been exposed to a number of mnemonics to use in helping them remember various causes of problems, assessments, and so on. Either have students recall the mnemonics themselves, or write them on the board. Then have students take turns naming one finding and matching it to one letter of any of the mnemonics. Include the following: AEIOU-TIPS, AVPU, OPQRST, and SAMPLE.

Cultural Considerations, Legal Notes, and Patho Pearls. The Student CD-ROM contains this series of informative features to enhance the student's understanding of the material covered in this chapter.

TEACHING OUTLINE

HANDOUT 29-1
Chapter 29 Objectives Checklist

Chapter 29 is the third lesson in Division 4, *Medical Emergencies*. Distribute Handout 29-1 so that students can familiarize themselves with the learning goals for this chapter. If students have any questions about the objectives, answer them at this time.

Then present the chapter. One possible lecture outline follows. In the outline, the parenthetical references in regular type are references to text pages; those in bold type are references to figures, tables, and procedures.

I. Introduction (pp. 1244–1245)

A. Nervous system conditions and diseases affect millions of U.S. lives. (p. 1244), **(Fig. 29-1, p. 1245)**

B. Common conditions and diseases (p. 1244)
1. Strokes
2. Epilepsy
3. Parkinson's disease
4. Multiple sclerosis
5. Syncope
6. Headache

II. Pathophysiology (pp. 1245–1247)

A. Alteration in cognitive systems (p. 1245)

B. Central nervous system disorders (pp. 1245–1246)
1. Structural lesions
2. Toxic-metabolic states
3. Common causes of altered mental status
    a. Drugs
    b. Cardiovascular
    c. Respiratory
    d. Infectious

C. Cerebral homeostasis (p. 1246)

D. Peripheral nervous system disorders (pp. 1246–1247)
1. Mononeuropathy
2. Polyneuropathy
3. Autonomic nervous system disorders

III. General assessment findings (pp. 1247–1255)

A. Scene size-up and initial assessment (pp. 1247–1249)
1. General appearance
2. Speech
3. Skin
4. Facial drooping
5. Posture/gait
6. AVPU method
7. Mood
8. Thought
9. Perception
10. Judgment
11. Memory and attention

B. Focused history and exam (pp. 1249–1255)
1. History (trauma)
    a. When?
    b. How?
    c. Loss of consciousness?
    d. Evidence of incontinence?
    e. Chief complaint?
    f. Any change in symptoms?
    g. Any complicating factors?
2. History (no trauma)
    a. Chief complaint?

POWERPOINT PRESENTATION
Chapter 29 PowerPoint slides 4–14

POINT OF INTEREST
One beer permanently destroys 10,000 brain cells. (Brain cells do not regenerate.)

POWERPOINT PRESENTATION
Chapter 29 Powerpoint Slides 15–16

POINT OF INTEREST
The brainstem is where we live; the cerebrum is where we play.

POINT TO EMPHASIZE
The brain is a greedy 3-pound organ, demanding 17 percent of cardiac output and 20 percent of all available oxygen.

POWERPOINT PRESENTATION
Chapter 29 PowerPoint slides 17–25

   b. Details of present illness, or nature of illness?
   c. Pertinent underlying medical problems?
   d. Have these symptoms occurred before?
   e. Any environmental clues?
  3. Physical examination
   a. Face
   b. Eyes
   c. Nose/mouth
   d. Respiratory status (**Fig. 29-2, p. 1257**)
    i. Cheyne-Stokes respirations
    ii. Kussmaul's respirations
    iii. Central neurogenic hyperventilation
    iv. Ataxic respirations
    v. Apneustic respirations
   e. Cardiovascular status
    i. Heart rate
    ii. ECG/rhythm
    iii. Bruits
    iv. Jugular venous distention
   f. Nervous system status
    i. Sensorimotor evaluation (**Figs. 29-3 and 29-4, p. 1252**)
     a) Decorticate posturing
     b) Decerebrate posturing
    ii. Motor system status
     a) Muscle tone
     b) Strength
     c) Flexion
     d) Coordination
     e) Balance
    iii. Cranial nerves status
   g. Glasgow Coma Scale (GCS) (**Fig. 29-5, p. 1254**)
   h. Pediatric Glasgow Coma Scale (**Fig. 29-5, p. 1254**)
  4. Vital signs (**Table 29-1, p. 1254**)
   a. Cushing's triad
    i. Increased blood pressure
    ii. Decreased pulse
    iii. Irregular respirations
  5. Additional assessment tools
   a. End-tidal CO_2 detector
   b. Pulse oximeter
   c. Blood glucometer
  6. Geriatric considerations
 C. Ongoing assessment (p. 1255)

IV. Management of nervous system emergencies (pp. 1255–1277)

A. Steps in management (pp. 1255–1256)
 1. Airway and breathing
 2. Circulatory support
 3. Pharmacological interventions
 4. Psychological support
 5. Transport considerations

B. Altered mental status (pp. 1256–1257)
 1. AEIOU-TIPS
 2. Assessment
 3. Management
  a. Establish an IV of normal saline or lactated Ringer's.

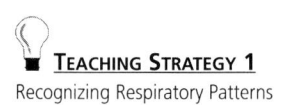

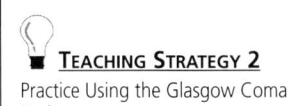

TEACHING STRATEGY 1
Recognizing Respiratory Patterns

TEACHING STRATEGY 2
Practice Using the Glasgow Coma Scale

POWERPOINT PRESENTATION
Chapter 29 PowerPoint slides 26–57

READING/REFERENCE
Benner, R., and C. Soltis. "Neuromuscular Disorders." *JEMS*, Jan. 2000.

POINT OF INTEREST

If the clinical deficit resolves itself within 24 hours, it is a TIA. If it lasts more than 24 hours, it is a stroke.

READING/REFERENCE

Brocato, C. "Twenty Questions about Emergency Stroke and Cardiac Care." *JEMS,* Oct. 2000.
Losavio, K. "Cooling Stroke Victims Reduces Brain Damage and Death." *JEMS,* Oct. 2000.
Nicholl, J. S. "EMD and Acute Stroke Response." *JEMS,* Oct. 2000.

SLIDES/VIDEO

"Stroke," *24-7 EMS,* Spring 2004.

POINT TO EMPHASIZE

Always check an elderly stroke patient's wrists for possible fractures from trying to break the fall.

      b. Determine blood glucose level.
          i. If low, administer 50 percent dextrose.
          ii. It will not harm a hyperglycemic patient.
      c. Administer naloxone if you suspect a narcotic overdose.
      d. Consider administering 100 mg thiamine if patient is suspected alcoholic.
   4. Chronic alcoholism
      a. Wernicke's syndrome
      b. Korsakoff's psychosis
   5. Increased intracranial pressure
C. Stroke and intracranial hemorrhage (pp. 1257–1263) (**Fig. 29-6, p. 1258**)
   1. Two broad categories of stroke
      a. Occlusive
          i. Embolic strokes
          ii. Thrombotic stroke
      b. Hemorrhagic (**Fig. 29-7, p. 1260**)
   2. Assessment
      a. Cincinnati Prehospital Stroke Scale (**Table 29-2, p. 1261**)
      b. Los Angeles Prehospital Stroke Screen (**Table 29-3, p. 1262**)
   3. Transient ischemic attacks (TIAs)
   4. Management (**Fig. 29-8, p. 1263**)
D. Seizures and epilepsy (pp. 1264–1267)
   1. Types of seizures
      a. Generalized seizures
          i. Tonic-clonic
          ii. Absence
          iii. Pseudoseizures
      b. Partial seizures
          i. Simple partial
          ii. Complex partial
   2. Assessment
      a. Signs and symptoms
      b. Syncope versus true seizure (**Table 29-4, p. 1266**)
   3. Management (**Fig. 29-9, p. 1266; Fig. 29-10, p. 1267**)
   4. Status epilepticus
E. Syncope (pp. 1267–1268)
   1. Assessment
      a. Cardiovascular conditions
      b. Noncardiovascular disease
      c. Idiopathic
   2. Management
F. Headache (pp. 1268–1270)
   1. Classification
      a. Vascular
      b. Tension
      c. Organic
   2. Assessment
   3. Management
G. "Weak and dizzy" (p. 1270)
   1. Assessment
   2. Management
H. Neoplasms (pp. 1270–1272)
   1. Assessment
      a. Benign
      b. Malignant
   2. Management
I. Brain abscess (p. 1272)

J. Degenerative neurological disorders (pp. 1272–1275)
  1. Types of degenerative neurological disorders
     a. Alzheimer's disease
     b. Muscular dystrophy (MD)
     c. Multiple sclerosis (MS)
     d. Dystonias
     e. Parkinson's disease
     f. Central pain syndrome
     g. Bell's palsy
     h. Amyotrophic lateral sclerosis
     i. Myoclonus
     j. Spina bifida
        i. Myelomeningocele
        ii. Meningocele
        iii. Occulta
     k. Poliomyelitis
  2. Assessment
  3. Management
K. Back pain and nontraumatic spinal disorders (pp. 1275–1277)
  1. Low back pain
  2. Causes of nontraumatic spinal disorders and back pain
     a. Disk injury
     b. Vertebral injury
     c. Cysts and tumors
     d. Other medical causes
  3. Assessment
  4. Management

V. Summary (p. 1278). Nervous system emergencies include a complex variety of illnesses and injuries. A thorough patient assessment and medical history will help guide your care and will prove invaluable for subsequent hospital management.

Initial field management is directed at ensuring an adequate airway and ventilation. The brain requires a constant supply of oxygen, glucose, and vitamins. After 10 to 20 seconds without blood flow, the patient becomes unconscious. Significant loss of oxygen (anoxia) or low blood sugar (hypoglycemia) can cause coma or seizures. Supply high-flow, high-concentration oxygen to patients with neurological disorders. Administer dextrose to any neurological patient with hypoglycemia.

Neurological injuries and illnesses often require treatment as soon as possible to prevent progressive damage. Patients suffering from an altered level of consciousness, stroke, transient ischemic attack, seizures, and syncope require early intervention and transportation to the closest appropriate facility.

You will also be called to care for patients suffering from a headache, neoplasm, a degenerative neurological disorder, or a complaint of back pain. These conditions may be relatively minor, or indicative of a much more serious underlying condition. They too require a complete patient assessment, medical history, and supportive care.

Care for the neurological patient may simply entail being supportive. In other cases, you should provide drug therapy or other interventions to limit or reduce the presenting symptoms. Airway management remains a priority in caring for any patient with an alteration in neurological function.

POWERPOINT PRESENTATION
Chapter 29 PowerPoint slide 58

WORKBOOK
Chapter 29 Activities

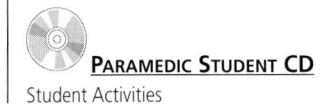

READING/REFERENCE
Textbook, pp. 1280–1294

HANDOUT 29-2
Chapter 29 Quiz

HANDOUT 29-3
Chapter 29 Scenario

PARAMEDIC STUDENT CD
Student Activities

COMPANION WEBSITE
http://www.prenhall.com/bledsoe

TESTGEN
Chapter 29

EMT ACHIEVE: PARAMEDIC TEST PREPARATION
Mistovich & Beasley. *EMT Achieve: Paramedic Test Preparation.*
www.prenhall.com/emtachieve/

REVIEW MANUAL FOR THE EMT-PARAMEDIC
Cherry & Mistovich. *Review Manual for the EMT-Paramedic,* 3rd edition.

HANDOUTS 29-4 AND 29-5
Reinforcement Activities

PARAMEDIC STUDENT CD
Student Activities

POWERPOINT PRESENTATION
Chapter 29

COMPANION WEBSITE
http://www.prenhall.com/bledsoe

ONEKEY
Chapter 29

ADVANCED LIFE SUPPORT SKILLS
Larmon & Davis. *Advanced Life Support Skills.*

ADVANCED LIFE SKILLS REVIEW
Larmon & Davis. *Advanced Life Skills Review.*

BRADY SKILLS SERIES: ALS
Larmon & Davis. *Brady Skills Series: ALS.*

PARAMEDIC NATIONAL STANDARDS SELF-TEST
Miller. *Paramedic National Standards Self-Test,* 4th edition.

ASSIGNMENTS

Assign students to complete Chapter 29, "Neurology," of the workbook. Also assign them to read Chapter 30, "Endocrinology," before the next class.

EVALUATION

Chapter Quiz and Scenario Distribute copies of the Chapter Quiz provided in Handout 29-2 to evaluate student understanding of this chapter. Make sure each student reads the scenario to reinforce critical thinking on the scene. Remind students not to use their notes or textbooks while taking the quiz.

Student CD Quizzes for every chapter are contained on the dynamic and highly visual in-text student CD.

Companion Website Additional quizzes for every chapter are contained on this exciting website.

TestGen You may wish to create a custom-tailored test using *Prentice Hall TestGen for Essentials of Paramedic Care,* 2nd Edition to evaluate student understanding of this chapter.

On-line Test Preparation (for students and instructors) Additional test preparation is available through Brady's new on-line product, *EMT Achieve: Paramedic Test Preparation* at *http://www.prenhall.com/emtachieve/*. Instructors can also monitor student mastery on-line.

Review Manual for the EMT-Paramedic This comprehensive exam review contains hundreds of test questions and rationales, including scenarios, along with two 180-question practice tests on CD.

REINFORCEMENT

Handouts If classroom discussion or performance on the quiz indicates that some students have not fully mastered the chapter content, you may wish to assign some or all of the Reinforcement Handouts for this chapter.

Student CD (for students) A wide variety of material on this CD-ROM will reinforce and also expand student knowledge and skills.

PowerPoint Presentation (for instructors) The PowerPoint material developed for this chapter offers useful reinforcement of chapter content.

Companion Website (for students) Additional review quizzes and links to EMS resources will contribute to further reinforcement of the chapter.

OneKey On-line support is offered for this course on one of three platforms: CourseCompass, Blackboard, or Web CT. Includes the IRM, PowerPoints, TestGen, and Companion Website for instruction. Ask your local sales representative for more information.

Brady Skills Series: Advanced Life Skills (Video or CD) Have your students watch the skills come to life on VHS or CD-ROM, or they can purchase the highly visual, full-color text with step-by-step procedures and rationales.

HANDOUT 29-1

Student's Name _____

CHAPTER 29 OBJECTIVES CHECKLIST

Knowledge	Date Mastered
1. Describe the incidence, morbidity, and mortality of neurological emergencies.	
2. Identify the risk factors most predisposing to diseases of the nervous system.	
3. Discuss the anatomy and physiology of the nervous system.	
4. Define and discuss the epidemiology (including the morbidity/mortality and preventative strategies), pathophysiology, assessment findings, and management for the following neurologic problems: • Coma and altered mental status • Seizures • Syncope • Headache • Neoplasms • Abscess • Stroke • Intracranial hemorrhage • Transient ischemic attack • Degenerative neurological diseases	
5. Describe and differentiate the major types of seizures.	
6. Describe the phases of a generalized seizure.	
7. Define the following: • Muscular dystrophy • Multiple sclerosis • Dystonia • Parkinson's disease • Trigeminal neuralgia • Bell's palsy • Amyotrophic lateral sclerosis • Peripheral neuropathy • Myoclonus • Spina bifida • Poliomyelitis	
8. Define and discuss the pathophysiology, assessment findings, and management for nontraumatic spinal injury, including: • Low back pain • Herniated intervertebral disk • Spinal cord tumors	

HANDOUT 29-1 Continued

Knowledge	Date Mastered
9. Differentiate between neurologic emergencies based on assessment findings.	
10. Given several preprogrammed, nontraumatic neurological emergency patients, provide the appropriate assessment, management, and transport.	

OBJECTIVE

CHAPTER 29 QUIZ

Write the letter of the best answer in the space provided.

_____ 1. A mechanism capable of producing alterations in mental status is a structural lesion. One cause of structural lesions is:
   A. hepatic failure.
   B. hypoglycemia.
   C. brain tumor (neoplasm).
   D. anoxia.

_____ 2. Any malfunction of or damage to the peripheral nerves is called peripheral:
   A. neuropathy.
   B. cyanosis
   C. diaphoresis.
   D. encephalopathy.

_____ 3. You can quickly assess a patient's mental status by using the _____ method.
   A. SAMPLE
   B. AVPU
   C. AEIOU-TIPS
   D. OPQRST

_____ 4. Abnormal pupils can be an early indicator of increasing intracranial pressure that is compressing cranial nerve:
   A. I.
   B. II.
   C. III.
   D. IV.

_____ 5. The breathing pattern characterized by a period of apnea that lasts 10–60 seconds, followed by gradually increasing depth and frequency of respirations, is called:
   A. Kussmaul's respiration.
   B. Guillian-Barré respiration.
   C. apneustic respiration.
   D. Cheyne-Stokes respiration.

_____ 6. Ataxic respirations are:
   A. intercostal muscle dysfunctions.
   B. poor respirations due to CNS damage.
   C. prolonged inspirations unrelieved by expirations.
   D. lesions caused by hyperventilation.

_____ 7. Your patient opens his eyes only when you pinch his shoulder. He has no verbal responses, and withdraws from pain. His Glasgow Coma Score Total is:
   A. 2.
   B. 3.
   C. 4.
   D. 7.

_____ 8. On the Glasgow Coma Scale, a patient with a total score of _____ or better has an estimated 94 percent favorable outcome.
   A. 8
   B. 7
   C. 6
   D. 5

_____ 9. Cushing's reflex is associated with increasing intracranial pressure and:
   A. decreased blood pressure.
   B. increased pulse.
   C. decreased respirations.
   D. decreased temperature.

_____ 10. The words _____ and _____ are assigned to the letter "A" in the mnemonic AEIOU-TIPS.
   A. airway, altered
   B. alert, awake
   C. abdomen, acute
   D. acidosis, alcohol

_____ 11. Stroke is referred to as a "brain attack" because in both a stroke and a heart attack:
   A. overabundance of cerebrospinal fluid is produced.
   B. a sudden, acute onset is reported by the patient.
   C. oxygen deprivation causes damage to affected tissue.
   D. a myocardial infarction may result.

HANDOUT 29-2 Continued

_____ 12. Studies have proven that _____ and other thrombolytic agents used in the treatment of heart attack are also effective in treating certain occlusive strokes.
  A. epinephrine
  B. tPa
  C. morphine sulfate
  D. lidocaine

_____ 13. A stroke caused by the gradual development of a blood clot in a cerebral artery is called a(n):
  A. thrombotic stroke.
  B. embolic stroke.
  C. hemorrhagic stroke.
  D. aneurism.

_____ 14. Symptoms from a transient ischemic attack (TIA) generally resolve within:
  A. 6 hours.
  B. 12 hours.
  C. 24 hours.
  D. 48 hours.

_____ 15. When caring for a patient suffering from a nervous system condition or disease, your first priority in patient care is to:
  A. administer thrombolytic therapy.
  B. assess for any neurological deficits.
  C. establish and maintain an adequate airway.
  D. apply high-concentration oxygen by nonrebreather mask.

_____ 16. A generalized motor seizure that produces a loss of consciousness is known as a(n):
  A. absence seizure.
  B. tonic-clonic seizure.
  C. hysterical seizure.
  D. complex partial seizure.

_____ 17. The phases of a generalized seizure include all of the following EXCEPT:
  A. aura.
  B. loss of consciousness.
  C. postical.
  D. absence.

_____ 18. Management of the seizure patient includes:
  A. inserting an oral airway while the patient is seizing.
  B. protecting the patient from hitting nearby objects.
  C. establishing an IV containing a dextrose solution.
  D. holding a tongue blade in the patient's mouth.

_____ 19. The term *status epilepticus* refers to a:
  A. chronic seizure patient taking anticonvulsant medication regularly.
  B. generalized seizure lasting more than 1 minute.
  C. two or more seizures with no intervening periods of consciousness.
  D. patient experiencing a seizure for the first time.

_____ 20. Management of the adult patient in status epilepticus includes administration of:
  A. 5–10 mg diazepam IV push.
  B. oral glucose if hypoglycemia is present.
  C. dextrose, Narcan, and thiamine IV push.
  D. sumatriptan and prochlorperazine.

_____ 21. A series of one-sided headaches that are sudden, intense, and may continue for 15 minutes to 4 hours is referred to as:
  A. syncope headaches.
  B. migraine headaches.
  C. organic headaches.
  D. cluster headaches.

_____ 22. Consider a headache a potentially serious condition if the patient describes it as:
  A. sudden in onset and "the worst headache of my life."
  B. lasting for more than 24 hours.
  C. being accompanied by nausea and photosensitivity.
  D. dull or achy pain with a feeling of forceful pressure.

HANDOUT 29-2 Continued

_____ 23. The term _____ is used to describe the new growth of a tumor.
   A. malignant
   B. metastasized
   C. benign
   D. neoplasm

_____ 24. The disease that involves inflammation of certain nerve cells followed by demyelination is called:
   A. dystonia.
   B. muscular dystrophy.
   C. multiple sclerosis.
   D. Alzheimer's disease.

_____ 25. A neural defect that results from the failure of one or more of the fetal vertebrae to close properly during the first month of pregnancy is called:
   A. myoclonus.
   B. poliomyelitis.
   C. amyotrophic lateral sclerosis (ALS).
   D. spina bifida.

HANDOUT 29-3

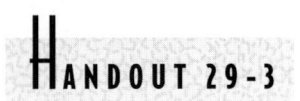

Student's Name _____

CHAPTER 29 SCENARIO

Review the following real-life situation. Then answer the questions that follow.

Your crew has just finished lunch when your pagers go off. It's a call for an unconscious patient at 1324 Amsterdam Avenue. After a relatively short trip, the ambulance pulls up to the address given by the dispatcher. A man meets you at the front door of the house and says that his wife has just had a seizure.

As you enter the residence, you see three small children standing in the spotless living room. The children and the husband are all very upset and concerned about the patient, who is a well-dressed, 32-year-old woman who appears to be sleeping on the couch. You begin to assess the patient while another paramedic obtains a history. The paramedic student, who is riding with your crew today, prepares to hook the patient up to oxygen and the cardiac monitor.

When you speak to the patient, she opens her eyes for a moment, mumbles something unintelligible, and goes back to sleep. She is breathing normally (rate 16 and regular) and her breath sounds are clear bilaterally. The pulse is strong and regular at the wrist, but the rate is slightly elevated at 105. She can move all extremities and responds to pain. Her pupils are equal and reactive (although sluggish) to light. Blood glucose is 100 and the ECG shows a sinus tachycardia.

The husband reports that his wife has a history of epilepsy. She takes Tegretol as directed by her physician (three times a day), but she ran out after last night's dose. They were getting ready to go to the drugstore to pick up the refill when she began to seize. Her epilepsy is fairly well controlled, and she has not had a seizure for a couple of months. The seizure appeared to be typical for the patient—tonic-clonic twitching for about 1 minute followed by a postictal phase. The patient has no other health problems, her recent health has been good, and the only medication she takes is Tegretol. She is allergic to codeine and her last meal was lunch, about 45 minutes ago.

The patient wakes and starts speaking to you. She states that she does not want to go to the hospital. If she gets her medicine, she says, she will be okay, and there is nothing the hospital can do for her. You ask some questions to determine if she is alert and oriented. Not only does she pass all of the tests, she even manages to make a small joke when asked who the president is. The patient and her husband thank you and your crew profusely, but they insist that no further services are required. A refusal form is signed by the patient and witnessed before you return to the station.

1. Why did the crew pay attention to the condition of the house and the dress and appearance of the patient?

2. What are some considerations the crew should raise before allowing this patient to refuse transportation?

HANDOUT 29-3 Continued

3. Was the crew right to let the patient refuse treatment?

4. Who should witness the patient's refusal, and what information should be relayed to the patient?

Handout 29-4

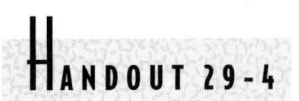

Student's Name _____

CHAPTER 29 REVIEW

Write the word or words that best complete each sentence in the space(s) provided.

1. Anoxia, diabetic ketoacidosis, and renal failure are among the various causes of _____ - _____ states, which can produce diffuse depression of both sides of the cerebrum.

2. Brain tumor, intracranial hemorrhage, parasites, and trauma are among the causes of _____ _____, which are capable of producing alterations in mental status.

3. Any malfunction or damage of the peripheral nerves is called _____ _____.

4. The "A" in the mnemonic _____ means the patient is alert and aware of his surroundings.

5. Breathing characterized by a prolonged inspiration that is unrelieved by expiration attempts is called _____ respiration.

6. Poor respirations due to CNS damage, causing ineffective thoracic muscular coordination, are called _____.

7. A(n) _____ posture is one in which the patient presents with the arms flexed, fists clenched, and legs extended.

8. A(n) _____ posture is one in which the patient presents with stiff and extended extremities and retracted head.

9. A collective change in vital signs associated with increasing intracranial pressure is called the _____ reflex.

10. _____ syndrome is a condition characterized by loss of memory and disorientation, and is associated with chronic alcohol intake and a diet deficient in thiamine.

11. Ischemic or hemorrhagic lesion to a portion of the brain, resulting in damage or destruction of brain tissue, is called a(n) _____.

12. "Brain attacks" are divided into two broad categories: _____ and _____.

13. Seizures that begin as an electrical discharge in a small area of the brain but spread to involve the entire cerebral cortex, causing widespread malfunction, are called _____ seizures.

14. In the _____ phase of a generalized seizure, the patient may awaken confused and fatigued.

15. A type of generalized seizure with sudden onset, characterized by a brief loss of awareness and rapid recovery, is called a(n) _____ seizure.

16. A series of two or more generalized motor seizures without any intervening periods of consciousness is called _____ _____.

17. _____ is a sedative and anticonvulsant medication used in treating seizures.

18. The term _____ is used to describe the new growth of a tumor.

19. Alzheimer's disease, muscular dystrophy, and multiple sclerosis are all examples of _____ _____ disorders.

20. Lou Gehrig's disease, or _____ _____ _____, is a progressive degeneration of specific nerve cells that control voluntary movement.

HANDOUT 29-5

Student's Name _____

TREATMENT IN NERVOUS SYSTEM EMERGENCIES

A number of treatments are performed for the patient with CNS problems. For each one described below, give a brief rationale of why the treatment is beneficial.

1. Administration of oxygen
2. Initiating IV normal saline or lactated Ringer's solution (not 5 percent dextrose)
3. Determining the blood glucose level
4. Protecting the airway
5. Providing assurance to the patient
6. Monitoring cardiac rhythm

CHAPTER 29 Answer Key

HANDOUT 29-2: Chapter 29 Quiz

1. C	6. C	11. C	16. C	21. C
2. A	7. A	12. A	17. A	21. A
3. B	8. B	13. B	18. B	23. B
4. C	9. C	14. C	19. C	24. C
5. D	10. D	15. D	20. D	25. D

Handout 29-3: Chapter 29 Scenario

1. If a patient is taking care of the living environment and personal appearance, he or she may exercise similar care about personal health and adherence to a physician's orders.
2. The patient cannot drive to the drugstore in her condition, and the husband should not leave her alone with three small children. The paramedics have an obligation to ensure that these considerations are brought up and resolved reasonably.
3. The patient was alert and oriented. Additionally, the patient is familiar with her seizure pattern and can make a reasonable assessment of her need for transport.
4. Ideally, the refusal should be witnessed by the woman's husband. As part of the refusal process, the patient should be informed of the risks of refusing treatment (another seizure) and other possible causes of the seizure (hypoxia, diabetes, and so on) that cannot be ruled out by the paramedics. The family should also be informed that if the patient should have another seizure, they are to call 911 without hesitation. Finally, the patient should inform her private physician that she had a seizure.

Handout 29-4: Chapter 29 Review

1. toxic-metabolic
2. structural lesions
3. peripheral neuropathy
4. AVPU
5. apneustic
6. ataxic
7. decorticate
8. decerebrate
9. Cushing's
10. Wernicke's
11. stroke
12. occlusive, hemorrhagic
13. generalized
14. postictal
15. absence
16. status epilepticus
17. Diazepam
18. neoplasm
19. degenerative neurological
20. amyotrophic lateral sclerosis

Handout 29-5: Treatment in Nervous System Emergencies

1. The brain is very sensitive to hypoxia. Administration of oxygen is important to minimizing further CNS damage.
2. An IV is needed for vascular access. Saline or lactated Ringer's solution is used because they are isotonic solutions, which should not contribute significantly to cerebral edema. In addition, the emergency department staff may have to administer phenytoin, which is incompatible with dextrose solutions.
3. Hypoglycemia may be the cause of the CNS problems.
4. The patient cannot protect his airway on his own. Also, in a CNS emergency patient, the risk of vomiting is increased.
5. Often, the patient cannot communicate and may not understand what is happening.
6. Cardiac rhythm disturbances may be causing the CNS problem, or damage to the cardiac and respiratory centers of the brain may result in dysrhythmias.

Chapter 30

Endocrinology

INTRODUCTION

The endocrine system is an important body system. Closely linked to the nervous system, it controls numerous physiological processes. It controls many body functions through the release of hormones. Endocrine system emergencies result from the release of either too much or too little of these hormones. This chapter discusses the endocrine system and some of the more common emergencies seen in the field.

TOTAL TEACHING TIME:
6.47 HOURS
The total teaching time is only a guideline based on the didactic and practical lab averages in the National Standard Curriculum. Instructors should take into consideration such factors as the pace at which students learn, the size of the class, and breaks. The actual time devoted to teaching objectives is the responsibility of the instructor.

CHAPTER OBJECTIVES

After reading this chapter, you should be able to:

1. Describe the incidence, morbidity, and mortality of endocrinologic emergencies. (pp. 1282, 1284–1285, 1289)
2. Identify the risk factors that predispose a person to endocrinologic disease. (pp. 1284–1285, 1289, 1292)
3. Discuss the anatomy and physiology of the endocrine system. (see Chapter 3)
4. Discuss the pathophysiology, assessment findings, need for rapid intervention and transport, and management of endocrinologic emergencies. (pp. 1282–1293)
5. Describe osmotic diuresis and its relationship to diabetes mellitus. (p. 1284)
6. Describe the pathophysiology of adult and juvenile onset diabetes mellitus. (pp. 1284–1285)
7. Differentiate between the pathophysiology of normal glucose metabolism and diabetic glucose metabolism. (pp. 1282–1284)
8. Describe the mechanism of ketone body formation and its relationship to ketoacidosis. (pp. 1283, 1285–1287)
9. Discuss the physiology of the excretion of potassium and ketone bodies by the kidneys. (p. 1284)
10. Describe the relationship of insulin to serum glucose levels. (pp. 1282–1288)
11. Describe the effects of decreased levels of insulin on the body. (pp. 1284–1288)
12. Describe the effects of increased serum glucose levels on the body. (p. 1288)
13. Discuss the pathophysiology, assessment findings, and management of the following endocrine emergencies:
    - Nonketotic hyperosmolar coma (pp. 1285–1286, 1287–1288)
    - Diabetic ketoacidosis (pp. 1285–1287)

©2007 Pearson Education, Inc.
Essentials of Paramedic Care, 2nd ed.

739

- Hypoglycemia (p. 1288)
- Hyperglycemia (pp. 1287–1288)
- Thyrotoxicosis (pp. 1289–1290)
- Myxedema (pp. 1290–1291)
- Cushing's syndrome (pp. 1291–1292)
- Adrenal insufficiency, or Addison's disease (pp. 1292–1293)

14. Describe the actions of epinephrine as it relates to the pathophysiology of hypoglycemia. (p. 1288)

15. Describe the compensatory mechanisms utilized by the body to promote homeostasis when hypoglycemia is present. (pp. 1282, 1288)

16. Differentiate among different endocrine emergencies based on assessment and history. (pp. 1282–1293)

17. Given several scenarios involving endocrine emergency patients, provide the appropriate assessment, management, and transportation. (pp. 1281–1293)

FRAMING THE LESSON

Begin class by reviewing the important points from Chapter 29, "Neurology." Discuss any aspects of the chapter not fully understood by students. Then introduce Chapter 30 material. During the class prior to this session, ask if any students are diabetic. If so and they don't mind sharing information, ask them to speak to the class, relating how they first discovered they had diabetes, what type they have, what is being done to treat it, and how it has changed their everyday lives. Or arrange for someone with the disease to come to class and address students. Often, local hospitals will have a "speakers bureau" that may have either speakers with diabetes or diabetes educators available for such a class.

If possible, have examples of insulin and oral diabetic medications, along with a blood glucometer for demonstration and instruction. If you have students routinely take each other's vital signs before the start of each class session, consider having them check each other's blood glucose levels at the same time. Stress the recent increase in diabetes, especially adult onset, or Type II, and the importance of having one's blood glucose levels checked as part of routine physical exams.

TEACHING STRATEGIES

People learn in a variety of ways. Some do better with the spoken word, whereas others prefer the written. Some prefer to work alone, whereas others profit from working in groups. Recognizing these different ways of acquiring knowledge, the authors of this *Instructor's Resource Manual* have provided a variety of teaching strategies for the different types of learners. These strategies are intended to foster higher-level cognitive skills and encourage creative learning and problem solving. For greatest effectiveness, incorporate these strategies into your class lecture. Symbols in the Lecture Outline indicate the points at which various exercises might be most appropriate. Other strategies can be used to preview the lesson or to summarize it.

The strategies below are keyed to specific sections of the lesson.

1. Researching Endocrine Disorders. Have students research a particular endocrine disorder that interests them. Let them write a page or two on the pathophysiology, presentation, and treatment of the disorder. Then have them present their mini-papers to the class. This activity will broaden their exposure to the discipline of endocrinology and improve their written and oral communication skills.

2. Representing Diabetes Insipidus. Students may wonder how a diagnosis of diabetes insipidus is made. Borrow from your local lab the urine collection jugs used to measure urine output over 24-hour periods—they literally look like brown milk jugs. This will help students capture the magnitude of the volume of urine produced during this condition.

The following strategies can be used at various points throughout the lesson or to help summarize and demonstrate what students have learned.

Guest Lecturer. Invite a diabetes educator from your local hospital, research center, diabetes education office, or diabetes foundation to discuss the disease and its treatment. The expert will be able to answer questions beyond physiology. Because the disease is so common, it is wise to expose students to information on how people live with the disease.

Food Label Watching. Because the body handles carbohydrates and sugars similarly, have students keep track of both—the amount of sugar and the amount of carbohydrates that are in the processed (canned and packaged) foods and drinks they consume. Very likely, they will be surprised at the total amounts. Encourage discussion about why it is important for people with diabetes to monitor both their sugar and carbohydrate intake.

Cultural Considerations, Legal Notes, and Patho Pearls. The Student CD-ROM contains this series of informative features to enhance the student's understanding of the material covered in this chapter.

TEACHING OUTLINE

Chapter 30 is the fourth lesson in Division 4, *Medical Emergencies*. Distribute Handout 30-1 so that students can familiarize themselves with the learning goals for this chapter. If students have any questions about the objectives, answer them at this time.

Then present the chapter. One possible lecture outline follows. In the outline, the parenthetical references in regular type are references to text pages; those in bold type are to figures, tables, and procedures.

I. Introduction (pp. 1281–1282)

A. The endocrine system controls numerous physiological processes by way of specialized chemical messengers called *hormones*. (p. 1281)
B. Fundamental structures are the endocrine glands. (p. 1281) (**Table 30-1, p. 1281**)
C. Unlike exocrine glands, which have a local effect, the endocrine glands secrete hormones directly into the circulatory system. (pp. 1281–1282)

II. Endocrine disorders and emergencies (pp. 1282–1293)

A. Disorders of the pancreas (pp. 1282–1288)
   1. Diabetes mellitus
   2. Glucose metabolism (**Table 30-2, p. 1283**)
   3. Regulation of blood glucose
   4. Type I diabetes mellitus
   5. Type II diabetes mellitus
   6. Diabetic ketoacidosis (diabetic coma) (**Table 30-3, p. 1285; Table 30-4, p. 1286**) (**Fig. 30-1, p. 1287**)

HANDOUT 30-1
Chapter 30 Objectives Checklist

TEACHING TIP
Use the analogy of an elaborate system of thermostats to explain how the glands work.

POWERPOINT PRESENTATION
Chapter 30 PowerPoint slides 4–21

POWERPOINT PRESENTATION
Chapter 30 PowerPoint slides 22–57

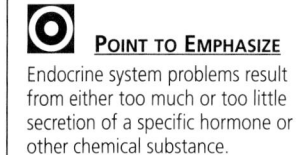

POINT TO EMPHASIZE
Endocrine system problems result from either too much or too little secretion of a specific hormone or other chemical substance.

TEACHING STRATEGY 1
Researching Endocrine Disorders

POINT OF INTEREST

Chen Ch'uan was a Chinese doctor who died in A.D. 643. He was the first person to note the symptoms of diabetes. Frederick Banting and Charles Best were Canadian scientists who discovered insulin in 1921. With the help of J.B. Collip, they purified extracts of insulin and used them to treat diabetic patients.

TEACHING STRATEGY 2

Representing Diabetes Insipidus

POINT TO EMPHASIZE

Emphasize the three polys: polydipsia, polyphagia, and polyuria.

READING/REFERENCE

C. Mattera. Diabetes, Part 1 of 2. *JEMS,* March 2002.
C. Mattera. Glucose Gone Wild: Diabetes, Part 2 of 2. *JEMS,* April 2002.

POINT OF INTEREST

Thyroid disease is common. However, life-threatening extremes (myxedema coma and thyroid storm) are rare (1 percent to 2 percent).

POWERPOINT PRESENTATION

Chapter 30 PowerPoint slide 58

ADVANCED LIFE SUPPORT SKILLS

Larmon & Davis. *Advanced Life Support Skills.*

ADVANCED LIFE SKILLS REVIEW

Larmon & Davis. *Advanced Life Skills Review.*

BRADY SKILLS SERIES: ALS

Larmon & Davis. *Brady Skills Series: ALS.*

      a. Pathophysiology
      b. Signs and symptoms
      c. Assessment and management
   7. Hyperglycemic hyperosmolar nonketotic (HHNK) coma
      a. Pathophysiology
      b. Signs and symptoms
      c. Assessment and management
   8. Hypoglycemia (insulin shock)
      a. Pathophysiology
      b. Signs and symptoms
      c. Assessment and management
  B. Disorders of the thyroid gland (pp. 1289–1291)
   1. Graves' disease (**Fig. 30-2, p. 1290**)
      a. Pathophysiology
      b. Signs and symptoms
      c. Assessment and management
   2. Thyrotoxic crisis ("thyroid storm")
      a. Pathophysiology
      b. Signs and symptoms
      c. Assessment and management
   3. Hypothyroidism and myxedema (**Fig. 30-3, p. 1291**)
      a. Pathophysiology
      b. Signs and symptoms
      c. Assessment and management
  C. Disorders of the adrenal glands (pp. 1291–1293)
   1. Hyperadrenalism (Cushing's syndrome) (**Fig. 30-4, p. 1292**)
      a. Pathophysiology
      b. Signs and symptoms
      c. Assessment and management
   2. Adrenal insufficiency (Addison's disease)
      a. Pathophysiology
      b. Signs and symptoms
      c. Assessment and management

III. Chapter summary (p. 1293). In conjunction with the nervous system, the endocrine system regulates body functions. The vast majority of endocrine emergencies involve complications of diabetes mellitus such as hypoglycemia or ketoacidosis. Other endocrine emergencies tend to be rare and will more likely be part of the history rather than the emergency. In the field, always suspect diabetes when patients present with unexplained changes in mental status. Hypoglycemia, the most urgent diabetic emergency, must be quickly treated to prevent serious nervous system damage. When the exact type of diabetic emergency is undetermined, treat for hypoglycemia. Treatment of diabetic ketoacidosis is primarily a hospital procedure.

SKILLS DEMONSTRATION AND PRACTICE

Students can practice skills discussed in this chapter in the following settings.

Skills Lab: The following stations should be part of a larger medical scenario lab. Divide the class into teams. Have the teams circulate through the stations. Monitor the groups to be sure all groups have a chance to manage each of the cases and to be sure that every student has the opportunity to be team leader. You may wish to have other instructors or qualified paramedics assist students in these activities.

Station	Equipment and Personnel Needed	Activities
Hypoglycemia	Medication box Glucometer 1 patient 1 instructor	Have students practice assessing and managing patients with hypoglycemia.
Diabetic Coma	Medication box Glucometer 1 victim 1 instructor	Have students practice assessing and managing patients with DKA.

Hospital: Begin patient assessment in the emergency department.

Field Internship: Begin patient assessment on simple emergency calls.

ASSIGNMENTS

Assign students to complete Chapter 30, "Endocrinology," of the workbook. Also assign them to read Chapter 31, "Allergies and Anaphylaxis," before the next class.

EVALUATION

Chapter Quiz and Scenario Distribute copies of the Chapter Quiz provided in Handout 30-3 to evaluate student understanding of this chapter. Make sure each student reads the scenario to reinforce critical thinking on the scene. Remind students not to use their notes or textbooks while taking the quiz.

Student CD Quizzes for every chapter are contained on the dynamic and highly visual in-text student CD.

Companion Website Additional quizzes for every chapter are contained on this exciting website.

TestGen You may wish to create a custom-tailored test using *Prentice Hall TestGen for Essentials of Paramedic Care,* 2nd Edition to evaluate student understanding of this chapter.

On-line Test Preparation (for students and instructors) Additional test preparation is available through Brady's new on-line product, *EMT Achieve: Paramedic Test Preparation* at *http://www.prenhall.com/emtachieve/*. Instructors can also monitor student mastery on-line.

Review Manual for the EMT-Paramedic This comprehensive exam review contains hundreds of test questions and rationales, including scenarios, along with two 180-question practice tests on CD.

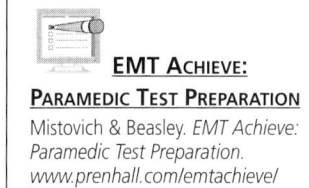

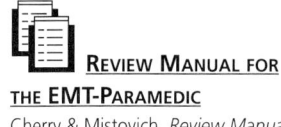

HANDOUT 30-2
Determining Blood Glucose

WORKBOOK
Chapter 30 Activities

READING/REFERENCE
Textbook, pp. 1295–1305

HANDOUT 30-3
Chapter 30 Quiz

HANDOUT 30-4
Chapter 30 Scenario

PARAMEDIC STUDENT CD
Student Activities

COMPANION WEBSITE
http://www.prenhall.com/bledsoe

TESTGEN
Chapter 30

EMT ACHIEVE: PARAMEDIC TEST PREPARATION
Mistovich & Beasley. *EMT Achieve: Paramedic Test Preparation.* www.prenhall.com/emtachieve/

REVIEW MANUAL FOR THE EMT-PARAMEDIC
Cherry & Mistovich. *Review Manual for the EMT-Paramedic,* 3rd edition.

HANDOUTS 30-5 TO 30-7
Reinforcement Activities

PARAMEDIC STUDENT CD
Student Activities

POWERPOINT PRESENTATION
Chapter 30

COMPANION WEBSITE
http://www.prenhall.com/bledsoe

ONEKEY
Chapter 30

ADVANCED LIFE SUPPORT SKILLS
Larmon & Davis. *Advanced Life Support Skills.*

ADVANCED LIFE SKILLS REVIEW
Larmon & Davis. *Advanced Life Skills Review.*

BRADY SKILLS SERIES: ALS
Larmon & Davis. *Brady Skills Series: ALS.*

PARAMEDIC NATIONAL STANDARDS SELF-TEST
Miller. *Paramedic National Standards Self-Test,* 4th edition.

REINFORCEMENT

Handouts   If classroom discussion or performance on the quiz indicates that some students have not fully mastered the chapter content, you may wish to assign some or all of the Reinforcement Handouts for this chapter.

Student CD (for students)   A wide variety of material on this CD-ROM will reinforce and also expand student knowledge and skills.

PowerPoint Presentation (for instructors)   The PowerPoint material developed for this chapter offers useful reinforcement of chapter content.

Companion Website (for students)   Additional review quizzes and links to EMS resources will contribute to further reinforcement of the chapter.

OneKey   On-line support is offered for this course on one of three platforms: Course Compass, Blackboard, or Web CT. Includes the IRM, PowerPoints, TestGen, and Companion Website for instruction. Ask your local sales representative for more information.

Brady Skills Series: Advanced Life Skills (Video or CD)   Have your students watch the skills come to life on VHS or CD-ROM, or they can purchase the highly visual, full-color text with step-by-step procedures and rationales.

HANDOUT 30-1

Student's Name _____

CHAPTER 30 OBJECTIVES CHECKLIST

Knowledge	Date Mastered
1. Describe the incidence, morbidity, and mortality of endocrinologic emergencies.	
2. Identify the risk factors that predispose a person to endocrinologic disease.	
3. Discuss the anatomy and physiology of the endocrine system.	
4. Discuss the pathophysiology, assessment findings, need for rapid intervention and transport, and management of endocrinologic emergencies.	
5. Describe osmotic diuresis and its relationship to diabetes mellitus.	
6. Describe the pathophysiology of adult and juvenile onset diabetes mellitus.	
7. Differentiate between the pathophysiology of normal glucose metabolism and diabetic glucose metabolism.	
8. Describe the mechanism of ketone body formation and its relationship to ketoacidosis.	
9. Discuss the physiology of the excretion of potassium and ketone bodies by the kidneys.	
10. Describe the relationship of insulin to serum glucose levels.	
11. Describe the effects of decreased levels of insulin on the body.	
12. Describe the effects of increased serum glucose levels on the body.	
13. Discuss the pathophysiology, assessment findings, and management of the following endocrine emergencies: • Nonketotic hyperosmolar coma • Diabetic ketoacidosis • Hypoglycemia • Hyperglycemia • Thyrotoxicosis • Myxedema • Cushing's syndrome • Adrenal insufficiency, or Addison's disease	
14. Describe the actions of epinephrine as it relates to the pathophysiology of hypoglycemia.	

OBJECTIVES

©2007 Pearson Education, Inc.
Essentials of Paramedic Care, 2nd ed.

HANDOUT 30-1 Continued

Knowledge	Date Mastered
15. Describe the compensatory mechanisms utilized by the body to promote homeostasis when hypoglycemia is present.	
16. Differentiate among different endocrine emergencies based on assessment and history.	
17. Given several scenarios involving endocrine emergency patients, provide the appropriate assessment, management, and transportation.	

OBJECTIVES

HANDOUT 30-2

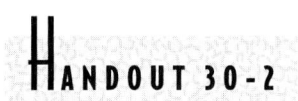

Student's Name _____

DETERMINING BLOOD GLUCOSE

Charting Student Progress:
1. Learning skill
2. Performs skill with direction
3. Performs skill independently

Procedure	1	2	3
1. Choose a vein.			
2. Prep the site.			
3. Perform the venipuncture.			
4. Place a drop of blood on the reagent strip.			
5. Activate the timer.			
6. Wait until the timer sounds.			
7. Wipe the reagent strip.			
8. Place the reagent strip on the glucometer.			
9. Read the blood glucose level.			
10. Administer 50 percent dextrose intravenously, if the blood glucose level is less than 80 mg.			

Comments:

Handout 30-3

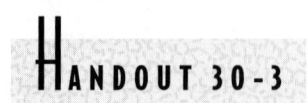

Student's Name _____

CHAPTER 30 QUIZ

Write the letter of the best answer in the space provided.

_____ 1. The disorder marked by inadequate insulin activity in the body is called diabetes:
   A. insipidus.
   B. mellitus.
   C. pectoris.
   D. glycogen.

_____ 2. The constructive or "building up" phase of metabolism is called:
   A. catabolism.
   B. aerobolism.
   C. anabolism.
   D. ionolism.

_____ 3. Physical signs of hypoglycemia may include tachycardia and:
   A. Kussmaul's respirations.
   B. abdominal pain.
   C. diaphoresis.
   D. fruity breath.

_____ 4. The basis of the excessive urination characteristic of untreated diabetes is called:
   A. facilitated elimination.
   B. facilitated diffusion.
   C. osmotic diuresis.
   D. gluconeogenesis.

_____ 5. The compounds produced during the catabolism of fatty acids, including acetoacetic acid and acetone, are called:
   A. ketone bodies.
   B. islets of Langerhans.
   C. T lymphocytes.
   D. peptides.

_____ 6. Which one of the following is a sign or symptom of hypoglycemia?
   A. abdominal pain
   B. cold, clammy skin
   C. increased mental function
   D. polyuria and polydipsia

_____ 7. The hallmark of diabetic ketoacidosis is:
   A. polyuria.
   B. excessive thirst.
   C. sweet, fruity breath odor.
   D. decreased mental function.

_____ 8. Which one of the following is NOT true of Type II diabetes mellitus?
   A. Heredity may play a role in predisposition.
   B. Insulin may not be required for treatment.
   C. It usually begins in early childhood.
   D. Patients can develop nonketotic hyperosmolar coma.

_____ 9. With both diabetic ketoacidosis and hypoglycemia, emergency intervention may call for the IV administration of:
   A. naloxone.
   B. dexamethasone.
   C. 50 percent dextrose.
   D. diazepam.

_____ 10. All of the following signs and symptoms are characteristic of a thyrotoxic crisis EXCEPT:
   A. tachycardia and hypotension.
   B. vomiting and diarrhea.
   C. delirium or coma.
   D. profound hypothermia.

HANDOUT 30-4

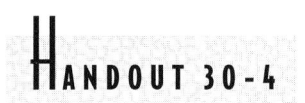

Student's Name _____

CHAPTER 30 SCENARIO

Review the following real-life situation. Then answer the questions that follow.

You have just gone to the bunkroom to get some much needed sleep. As you finish making up your bunk, you get a dispatch for an unconscious patient. When you arrive on scene, a middle-aged man meets you at the curb. He tells you that he tried to call his mother on the phone and was unable to reach her. He drove 45 miles to her house and found her unconscious on the floor of the upstairs bathroom.

You and your partner enter through the front door and are overwhelmed at the sight and stench of a house strewn with garbage. It also appears that the electricity to the house has been shut off. The patient, a 63-year-old woman, is lying unconscious on the floor of the bathroom. She was incontinent of both feces and urine and appears to have been lying there for some time.

1. What are your initial priorities in this situation?

Your partner takes cervical-spine control and places her on a nonrebreather face mask at 15 liters per minute. You notice that she has a rapid, weak pulse and that her breathing is rapid and deep. Her skin is warm and dry. Upon auscultation, some rales are detected in all lung fields. The abdomen, pelvis, and extremities are normal. She is unresponsive to pain, and her pupils are dilated and slow to react. You ask the EMTs to get a set of vitals, place the patient on a long backboard, and place the backboard on a stretcher to move her to the paramedic unit for treatment.

While they are performing these tasks under the direction of your partner, you ask the son to accompany you to the unit and provide you with the patient's history while you set up an IV and the ECG monitor.

2. With the information available to this point, what are the possible diagnoses?

While you set up the IV, you ask the son what happened. He says that he hadn't seen or heard from his mother for about 3 weeks, so he decided to give her a call this evening. When she did not answer the phone, he became concerned and drove over to see if she was okay. He adds that his mother has a severe alcohol problem. She sometimes forgets to pay her bills and that is probably why the electrical power has been shut off. You inquire about any other health problems. He says that she has been diagnosed with emphysema, high blood pressure, and "some type of blood sugar problem." When you ask about medications, he replies that she has not seen a doctor in years so there is little likelihood that she is taking medicine. He is unable to provide any further useful information. Your partner and the EMTs come out of the house with the patient and load her into the ambulance.

3. What do you want to do at this time?

©2007 Pearson Education, Inc.
Essentials of Paramedic Care, 2nd ed.

CHAPTER 30 *Endocrinology* 749

HANDOUT 30-4 Continued

You complete your assessment and find BP is 90/50, pulse is 126, respirations are 42 and labored (with a strong, sweet odor on her breath), breath sounds reveal slight diffuse rales, pulse oximetry is 98 percent; and the ECG shows a sinus tachycardia, without ectopy. Her blood sugar is at the maximum of your ability to determine it (999 on the glucometer).

4. What does this information tell you about the patient?

You start two large-bore (16-gauge) IVs of 0.9 percent normal saline, running them wide open. (Before hooking up the IV tubing on the first IV, you draw 20 mL of blood to fill two red-top tubes.) Per your service's protocols, you administer 100 mg thiamine IV, 50 ml of 50 percent dextrose in water, and 1 mg of naloxone.

There is no change in the patient's condition following these treatments. Medical direction is contacted, and you give your report. You are told that there are no further orders and the patient will be placed in Bed 5 on your arrival.

5. What information should be included in the report to medical direction?

6. Why would your protocols require administration of dextrose when her blood sugar is so high?

On your arrival at the hospital, you transfer your patient to the hospital stretcher and give a report to the nurse. While you fill out the run sheet, your partner cleans and restocks the ambulance. A couple days later, you call the emergency department to follow up on the patient's status. You are informed that she was diagnosed with diabetic ketoacidosis, pneumonia, and malnutrition. She has been admitted to ICU, is currently on a respirator, and has a poor prognosis.

HANDOUT 30-5

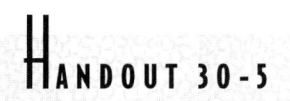

Student's Name _____

CHAPTER 30 REVIEW

Write the word or words that best complete each sentence in the space(s) provided.

1. The endocrine system includes _____ major body glands.

2. Hormones such as growth hormone and thyroid hormone regulate _____.

3. _____, or insulin shock, is a complication of diabetes characterized by low levels of blood glucose and resulting from too high a dose of insulin or from inadequate food intake following a normal insulin dose.

4. _____, or diabetic coma, is a complication of diabetes characterized by high levels of glucose in the blood, metabolic acidosis and, in advanced stages, coma.

5. An endocrine disorder characterized by inadequate insulin production by the beta cells of the islets of Langerhans is _____ _____.

6. Hyperactivity of the thyroid gland may result in a condition known as _____, which may present with tachycardia, nervous symptoms, and rapid metabolism.

7. The _____ system secretes hormones into the blood.

8. A(n) _____ is a chemical substance released by a gland that controls or affects other glands or body systems.

9. Very deep, rapid respirations, called _____ respirations, represent the body's attempt to compensate for metabolic acidosis.

10. Of the two diabetic emergencies, _____ is considered to be a true medical emergency that requires prompt intervention to prevent permanent brain injury.

REINFORCEMENT

Handout 30-6

Student's Name _____

DIABETIC EMERGENCIES

Write the letter of the diabetic emergency next to the sign or symptom associated with it.

A. Diabetic ketoacidosis
B. Hypoglycemia
C. Either diabetic ketoacidosis or hypoglycemia

_____ 1. The patient has not taken insulin.
_____ 2. The patient has overexerted himself.
_____ 3. Cold and clammy skin.
_____ 4. Altered mental status.
_____ 5. Seizures.
_____ 6. Polyuria.
_____ 7. Rapid, deep respirations.
_____ 8. Headache.
_____ 9. Tachycardia.
_____ 10. The patient has not eaten.
_____ 11. History of recent illness.
_____ 12. Skin that is warm and dry.
_____ 13. Hypotension.
_____ 14. Hand tremor.
_____ 15. Sweet, fruity breath odor.
_____ 16. Intense thirst.
_____ 17. Unconsciousness.
_____ 18. Severe electrolyte imbalance.
_____ 19. True medical emergency.
_____ 20. Dysrhythmias.

HANDOUT 30-7

Student's Name _____

DIAGNOSTIC SIGNS OF DIABETIC EMERGENCIES

Complete the chart by filling in the diagnostic signs and symptoms in the correct column. The first line has been filled in for you.

	DIABETIC KETOACIDOSIS	**HYPOGLYCEMIA**
Pulse	Rapid	Normal (may be rapid)
Blood Pressure		
Respirations		
Breath Odor		
Headache		
Mental State		
Tremors		
Convulsions		
Mouth		
Thirst		
Vomiting		
Abdominal Pain		
Ocular Vision		

REINFORCEMENT

Chapter 30 Answer Key

Handout 30-3: Chapter 30 Quiz

1. B
2. C
3. A
4. C
5. A
6. B
7. C
8. C
9. C
10. D

Handout 30-4: Chapter 30 Scenario

1. Priority assessment is cervical-spine control and supplemental oxygen by nonrebreather face mask.
2. Possibilities include the following: trauma, cerebrovascular accident, diabetic emergency, dehydration, poisoning.
3. Patient care should include: ECG; blood sugar check; blood sample for lab analysis; two IVs with 0.9 percent NS or LR; 100 mg thiamine, 25 g dextrose (D50); 1–2 mg naloxone.
4. The assessment indicates the patient may be suffering from diabetic ketoacidosis/diabetic coma.
5. Your unit call name and names and numbers of crew; description of scene; patient's age, sex, and weight; chief complaint; primary problem; associated symptoms; brief history of present illness; pertinent past medical history; physical exam findings; treatment given; estimated time of arrival.
6. The additional glucose load is negligible compared to the quantity already present in the body.

Handout 30-5: Chapter 30 Review

1. eight
2. metabolism
3. Hypoglycemia
4. Ketoacidosis
5. diabetes mellitus
6. thyrotoxicosis
7. endocrine
8. hormone
9. Kussmaul's
10. hypoglycemia (insulin shock)

Handout 30-6: Diabetic Emergencies

1. A
2. B
3. B
4. C
5. B
6. A
7. A
8. B
9. C
10. B
11. A (or C)
12. A
13. A
14. B
15. A
16. A
17. C
18. A
19. B
20. A

Handout 30-7: Diagnostic Signs of Diabetic Emergencies

	DIABETIC KETOACIDOSIS	HYPOGLYCEMIA
Pulse	Rapid	Normal (may be rapid)
Blood Pressure	Low	Normal
Respirations	Exaggerated air hunger (Kussmaul's respirations)	Normal or shallow
Breath Odor	Acetone (sweet, fruity)	None
Headache	Absentness	Present
Mental State	Restlessness, unconsciousness	Apathy, irritability
Tremors	Absent	Present
Convulsions	None	In late stages
Mouth	Dry	Drooling
Thirst	Intense	Absent
Vomiting	Common	Uncommon
Abdominal Pain	Frequent	Absent
Ocular Vision	Dim	Double vision (diplopia)

Chapter 31

Allergies and Anaphylaxis

INTRODUCTION

An allergic reaction is an exaggerated response by the immune system to a foreign substance. Allergic reactions can range from mild skin rashes to severe, life-threatening reactions that involve virtually every body system. The most severe type of allergic reaction is called anaphylaxis. Anaphylaxis is an acute, generalized, and violent antigen-antibody reaction that may be fatal even with prompt recognition and treatment. It is a true life-threatening emergency requiring appropriate prehospital field intervention. This chapter discusses the pathophysiology of allergy and anaphylaxis, and the assessment and management of anaphylaxis.

TOTAL TEACHING TIME:
4.33 HOURS
The total teaching time is only a guideline based on the didactic and practical lab averages in the National Standard Curriculum. Instructors should take into consideration such factors as the pace at which students learn, the size of the class, and breaks. The actual time devoted to teaching objectives is the responsibility of the instructor.

CHAPTER OBJECTIVES

After reading this chapter, you should be able to:

1. Describe the incidence, morbidity, and mortality of anaphylaxis. (p. 1296)
2. Identify the risk factors most predisposing to anaphylaxis. (p. 1296)
3. Discuss the anatomy and physiology of the organs and structures related to anaphylaxis. (pp. 1296–1298)
4. Discuss the pathophysiology of allergy and anaphylaxis. (pp. 1296–1299)
5. Describe the common routes of substance entry into the body. (p. 1298)
6. Define allergic reaction, anaphylaxis, antigen, antibody, and natural and acquired immunity. (pp. 1296–1299)
7. List the common antigens most frequently associated with anaphylaxis. (p. 1297)
8. Discuss human antibody formation. (pp. 1296–1298)
9. Describe the physical manifestations of anaphylaxis. (pp. 1299–1301, 1303)
10. Identify and differentiate between the signs and symptoms of an allergic reaction and anaphylaxis. (p. 1303)
11. Explain the various treatment and pharmacological interventions used in the management of allergic reactions and anaphylaxis. (pp. 1301–1303)
12. Correlate abnormal findings in assessment with the clinical significance in the patient with an allergic reaction or anaphylaxis. (pp. 1299–1301, 1303)

©2007 Pearson Education, Inc.
Essentials of Paramedic Care, 2nd ed.

13. Given several preprogrammed and moulaged patients, provide the appropriate assessment, care, and transport for the allergic reaction and anaphylaxis patient. (pp. 1296–1303)

FRAMING THE LESSON

Begin class by reviewing the important points from Chapter 30, "Endocrinology." Discuss any aspects of the chapter not fully understood by students. Then begin with Chapter 31 material.

Prior to this class session, assign a few students to take a field trip to a local department store or pharmacy. Instruct students to make a list of all the over-the-counter antihistamine products. This list should include products that are specifically antihistamines, as well as the "shotgun" medications that include antihistamines with other ingredients, such as decongestants, cough suppressants, and so forth.

Discuss the prevalence of these products related to the number of people who have allergies. Poll the class and ask students what allergies they have. Ask them to classify their treatment (e.g., OTC medications, prescription medications, "allergy shots," and so on). If any students have a severe allergy, ask them to relate their symptoms and treatment the last time they were exposed to the allergen. You will find a wide variety of signs and symptoms, ranging from simple airborne allergic reactions (itchy, watery eyes, runny nose, and sneezing) to reactions to ingested or injected allergens (itching, hives) to severe allergic reactions (airway swelling and signs and symptoms of shock) as in anaphylaxis. Stress the number of substances that can cause allergic reactions and the severity of anaphylaxis.

TEACHING STRATEGIES

People learn in a variety of ways. Some do better with the spoken word, whereas others prefer the written. Some prefer to work alone, whereas others profit from working in groups. Recognizing these different ways of acquiring knowledge, the authors of this *Instructor's Resource Manual* have provided a variety of teaching strategies for the different types of learners. These strategies are intended to foster higher-level cognitive skills and encourage creative learning and problem solving. For greatest effectiveness, incorporate these strategies into your class lecture. Symbols in the Lecture Outline indicate the points at which various exercises might be most appropriate. Other strategies can be used to preview the lesson or to summarize it.

The following strategies are keyed to specific sections of the lesson.

1. Creating a Master List of Allergens. To create a master list of allergens, have students each think of 10 items that can cause an allergic reaction. Go around the room, having students read their lists aloud. Write the items on a large sheet of paper or the board. Whenever an item is mentioned that is not already on the list, it gets added, but nothing makes the list twice. Every student is able to participate, creating a great camaraderie in the classroom, as well as a useful and very visual list of allergens.

2. The Signs of Allergic Reaction. Slides illustrating the signs of an allergic reaction are the best way to demonstrate to students signs that they may rarely see—such as urticaria, wheals, and angioedema. Should you not be able to find a prepackaged slide set with these slides, copy and scan photos from an illustrated book of allergies, dermatology, or emergency medicine. Remember to get permission from the publisher when required.

*3. **Removal of Bee Stingers.*** Removing a bee stinger takes practice. Embed the tips of dry pine needles into the soft pads of your practice IV arms. Have students practice removing the "stingers" without sticking themselves or squeezing the poison into the patient's flesh. The pine needles are sharp yet safe and unlikely to injure a student.

*4. **Auto-Injecting Epinephrine.*** Although it is an EMT-B skill, all paramedics should know how to use the EpiPen®. Acquire EpiPen trainers from the manufacturer and have students practice administration of epinephrine with the auto-injector. Be sure students know the dose and concentration of the EpiPen. Emphasize that paramedics can use or assist in the use of the EpiPen if their drugs are not readily available.

*5. **Breathing Difficulty Demonstration.*** Obtain several plastic coffee stir sticks, one for each student. These need to be the hollow, plastic type, with very small openings at the ends. To simulate the feeling of breathing difficulty, such as with anaphylaxis, have students pinch their noses and breathe exclusively through the tiny straws.

The following strategies can be used at various points throughout the lesson or to help summarize and demonstrate what students have learned.

Clinical Decision Making. Be sure to use case studies or simulations of patients in this unit because allergic reactions vary so greatly in severity and clinical presentation. Also, the questions required to obtain a comprehensive history vary far more than other assessments such as those for chest pain or abdominal pain. Students will need practice with the clinical decision making in this chapter. Consider some of the following patient situations to give students a variety of patients and complaints:

- Patient who has a severe allergic reaction to IVP dye at an outpatient radiology clinic
- Mild allergy to cats in a pediatric patient
- Bronchospasm after inhalation of room deodorizer
- Localized reaction to a first-time bee sting
- Unconscious after ingestion of two doses of a new antibiotic

Scenario for Discussion. Baby Joanne is 1 week old. As her mother is getting her out of the car seat, a wasp stings the baby on the head. Mom, who is herself allergic to bee stings, becomes hysterical and immediately calls 911. Baby Joanne has never been stung before and, besides a red welt on her head, she appears to be okay. Does Mom have to worry?

Through student discussion, explore the pathophysiology of the immune response, with particular emphasis on the primary and secondary responses. You can also discuss the genetic link of hypersensitivity, as well as the pathophysiology of an allergic reaction. This is a good time to reinforce the importance of "not playing doctor" and contacting medical control when confronted with a situation such as this.

Ask One Question, or Do One Thing. Tell students to imagine that they have been dispatched for an anaphylaxis call. You may use information from your own records or draw on the textbook case study or Handout 31-3, Chapter 31 Scenario. Tell them what they see when they arrive on the scene.

Now tell students that their goal as a class is to find out what is wrong with this patient and to treat him or her. To do this, you will call on each student in turn. When you do, each will be allowed either to ask one question or to perform one action. They must explain what they are looking for and why they are asking a question. If they are performing an action, they must describe how they propose to perform it and why they want to do it (e.g., "Administer oxygen via nonrebreather face mask at 10–15 liters/minute to help prevent hypoxia."). Students must thus work together to coordinate their questions and their actions. If a student proposes something inappropriate, the rest of the class is obligated to point out that there is a problem with the proposed action and explain what it is. Your task as instructor is to be prepared to give details of the case when asked for them. If a student proposes an inappropriate action and no one else picks up on it, you should let the exercise go on, but state what the consequences of that action would be at an appropriate time.

Work your way around the class, being sure each student is called upon before allowing any student a second question or action. See how long it takes for the class to find out what is wrong and to take appropriate action.

(Note: This exercise may be performed several times during the course, whenever you feel it would be beneficial.)

Allergy Round Robin. Have each student make a list on a sheet of paper of 10 items that can cause an allergic/anaphylactic reaction. For each item on their lists, students should indicate the most probable route the antigen would use to enter the body. They should also indicate what they think the speed and severity of reaction would be. Finally, they might also list the most likely initial signs and symptoms produced by each item on their lists (e.g., drug reaction usually initially presents as a rash, a bee sting as redness and swelling around the sting site, and so on.)

After the students have completed their lists, call on class members in random order and have each present one item on his or her list. As the presentations are made, reinforce the pathophysiology of an allergic reaction, the effects on various body systems, and the management of anaphylaxis. It may be helpful to list items presented by students on the board to help prevent duplication. Keep calling on students until no new items are added to the list.

Allergen Desensitization. The concept of desensitization is similar to tolerance. Liken desensitization to an allergen to pain or alcohol tolerance whereby a person gradually accommodates to a situation or stimuli after repeated exposure. You will likely have a student who has built up a tolerance to alcohol due to repeated exposure to the stimuli. The same may be true for caffeine or tobacco. These are examples that your adult learners can apply directly to their lives, so they are likely to remember the concept represented here.

Cultural Considerations, Legal Notes, and Patho Pearls. The Student CD-ROM contains this series of informative features to enhance the student's understanding of the material covered in this chapter.

TEACHING OUTLINE

Chapter 31 is the fifth lesson in Division 4, *Medical Emergencies*. Distribute Handout 31-1 so that students can familiarize themselves with the learning goals for this chapter. If students have any questions about the objectives, answer them at this time.

Then present the chapter. One possible lecture outline follows. In the outline, the parenthetical references in regular type are references to text pages; those in bold type are references to figures, tables, or procedures.

I. Introduction. An allergic reaction is an exaggerated response by the immune system to a foreign substance. The most severe type of allergic reaction is called anaphylaxis, which can be life-threatening and requires prompt

---

POINT OF INTEREST
In 1992, British doctors at Oxford discovered that there is one "allergy" gene causing hay fever, asthma, and eczema. They also concluded that one in three people carries this gene, showing varying degrees of symptoms.

POINT TO EMPHASIZE
Most fatalities from anaphylaxis occur within the first 30 minutes following exposure. Act quickly!

PATHO PEARLS
Allergic Responses... Some Are Life-Saving, Some Can Kill

HANDOUT 31-1
Chapter 31 Objectives Checklist

POINT TO EMPHASIZE
The immune system is responsible for the 3 Rs: recognizing, reacting to, and removing the dangerous substance.

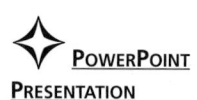

POWERPOINT PRESENTATION
Chapter 31 PowerPoint slide 4

recognition and treatment by paramedics. Anaphylaxis results from exposure to a particular substance that sets off a biochemical chain of events that can ultimately lead to shock and death. (p. 1296)

II. Pathophysiology (pp. 1296–1299)

A. The immune system (pp. 1296–1298)
   1. Pathogens
   2. Toxins
   3. Cellular immunity
   4. Humoral immunity
   5. Antibodies
   6. Immunoglobulins
   7. Antigens (**Table 31-1, p. 1297**)
   8. Primary response
   9. Secondary response
   10. Natural immunity
   11. Acquired immunity
   12. Induced active immunity
   13. Active immunity
   14. Passive immunity

B. Allergies (pp. 1298–1299)
   1. Delayed hypersensitivity
   2. Immediate hypersensitivity

C. Anaphylaxis (p. 1299) (**Table 31-1, p. 1297**)

III. Assessment findings in anaphylaxis (pp. 1299–1301) (**Table 31-2, p. 1303**)

A. Initial assessment (pp. 1299–1300)
B. Skin (p. 1300) (**Fig 31-1, p. 1300**)
C. Respiratory system (p. 1300)
D. Cardiovascular system (p. 1300)
E. Gastrointestinal system (p. 1300)
F. Nervous system (p. 1300)
G. Monitoring devices (pp. 1300–1301)

IV. Management of anaphylaxis (pp. 1301–1303)

A. Protect the airway (p. 1301)
B. Administer medications (pp. 1301–1302)
   1. Oxygen
   2. Epinephrine
   3. Antihistamines
   4. Corticosteroids
   5. Vasopressors
   6. Beta-agonists
   7. Other agents
C. Offer psychological support (p. 1303)

V. Assessment findings in allergic reaction (p. 1303) (**Table 31-2, p. 1303**)

A. Mild allergic reactions (p. 1303)
B. Severe allergic reactions (p. 1303)

VI. Management of allergic reactions (pp. 1303–1304)

A. Mild allergic reactions (p. 1303)
B. Severe allergic reactions (pp. 1303–1304) (**Fig. 31-2, p. 1304**)

TEACHING STRATEGY 1
Creating a Master List of Allergens

POWERPOINT PRESENTATION
Chapter 31 PowerPoint slides 5–11

TEACHING STRATEGY 2
The Signs of Allergic Reaction

TEACHING TIP
Take time to review respiratory pharmacology. Several of these drugs are used in obstructive airway diseases. Ask students to explain why they would help in anaphylaxis.

POWERPOINT PRESENTATION
Chapter 31 PowerPoint slides 12–14

TEACHING STRATEGY 3
Removal of Bee Stingers

POWERPOINT PRESENTATION
Chapter 31 PowerPoint slides 15–17

TEACHING STRATEGY 4
Auto-Injecting Epinephrine

TEACHING STRATEGY 5
Breathing Difficulty Demonstration

POWERPOINT PRESENTATION
Chapter 31 PowerPoint slide 18

POWERPOINT PRESENTATION
Chapter 31 PowerPoint slides 19–20

POWERPOINT PRESENTATION
Chapter 31 PowerPoint slide 21

POINT TO EMPHASIZE
Airway management is the top priority. If ET intubation is indicated, it should be done by the most experienced paramedic. One shot is probably all you will get. Often with a severe attack, peripheral circulation will be shut down. A subcutaneous injection of epinephrine will be of little benefit if it fails to reach central circulation.

ADVANCED LIFE SUPPORT SKILLS
Larmon & Davis. *Advanced Life Support Skills.*

ADVANCED LIFE SKILLS REVIEW
Larmon & Davis. *Advanced Life Skills Review.*

BRADY SKILLS SERIES: ALS
Larmon & Davis. *Brady Skills Series: ALS.*

WORKBOOK
Chapter 31 Activities

READING/REFERENCE
Textbook, pp. 1306–1327

HANDOUT 31-2
Chapter 31 Quiz

HANDOUT 31-3
Chapter 31 Scenario

PARAMEDIC STUDENT CD
Student Activities

COMPANION WEBSITE
http://www.prenhall.com/bledsoe

VII. Chapter summary (p. 1304). Fortunately, severe allergies and anaphylaxis are uncommon. However, when they do occur, they can progress quickly and result in death in minutes. The central physiological action in anaphylaxis is the massive release of histamine and other mediators. Histamine causes bronchospasm, airway edema, peripheral vasodilation, and increased capillary permeability. The prehospital treatment of anaphylaxis is intended to reverse the effects of these agents.

The primary and most important drug used in the treatment of anaphylaxis is epinephrine. Epinephrine helps reverse the effects of histamine. It also supports the blood pressure and reverses detrimental capillary leakage. Following the administration of epinephrine, potent antihistamines should be used to block the adverse effects of the massive histamine release. Inhaled beta-agonists are useful in cases of severe bronchospasm and airway involvement. Intravenous fluid replacement is crucial in preventing hypovolemia and hypotension.

The key to successful prehospital management of anaphylaxis is prompt recognition and treatment.

SKILLS DEMONSTRATION AND PRACTICE

Students can practice the skills discussed in this chapter in the following settings.

Scenario Lab: The following stations will be part of a larger medical scenario lab. Divide the class into teams. Have the teams circulate through the stations. Monitor the teams to be sure that all groups have a chance to manage each of the cases and so that every student has the opportunity to be team leader. You may wish to have other instructors or qualified paramedics assist students in these activities.

Station	Equipment and Personnel Needed	Activities
Anaphylaxis	Airway management kit IV/Med equipment 1 patient 1 instructor	Have students practice managing a patient with anaphylaxis.

Hospital: Assist in assessment and management of anaphylaxis in the ED.

Field Internship: Assist in assessment and management of anaphylaxis in the field.

ASSIGNMENTS

Assign students to complete Chapter 31, "Allergies and Anaphylaxis," of the workbook. Also assign them to read Chapter 32, "Gastroenterology," before the next class.

EVALUATION

Chapter Quiz and Scenario Distribute copies of the Chapter Quiz provided in Handout 31-2 to evaluate student understanding of this chapter. Make sure each student reads the scenario to reinforce critical thinking on the scene. Remind students not to use their notes or textbooks while taking the quiz.

Student CD   Quizzes for every chapter are contained on the dynamic and highly visual in-text student CD.

Companion Website   Additional quizzes for every chapter are contained on this exciting website.

TestGen   You may wish to create a custom-tailored test using *Prentice Hall TestGen for Essentials of Paramedic Care,* 2nd Edition to evaluate student understanding of this chapter.

On-line Test Preparation (for students and instructors)   Additional test preparation is available through Brady's new on-line product, *EMT Achieve: Paramedic Test Preparation* at *http://www.prenhall.com/emtachieve/.* Instructors can also monitor student mastery on-line.

Review Manual for the EMT-Paramedic   This comprehensive exam review contains hundreds of test questions and rationales, including scenarios, along with two 180-question practice tests on CD.

REINFORCEMENT

Handouts   If classroom discussion or performance on the quiz indicates that some students have not fully mastered the chapter content, you may wish to assign some or all of the Reinforcement Handouts for this chapter.

Student CD (for students)   A wide variety of material on this CD-ROM will reinforce and also expand student knowledge and skills.

PowerPoint Presentation (for instructors)   The PowerPoint material developed for this chapter offers useful reinforcement of chapter content.

Companion Website (for students)   Additional review quizzes and links to EMS resources will contribute to further reinforcement of the chapter.

OneKey   On-line support is offered for this course on one of three platforms: CourseCompass, Blackboard, or Web CT. Includes the IRM, PowerPoints, TestGen, and Companion Website for instruction. Ask your local sales representative for more information.

Brady Skills Series: Advanced Life Skills (Video or CD)   Have your students watch the skills come to life on VHS or CD-ROM, or they can purchase the highly visual, full-color text with step-by-step procedures and rationales.

TestGen
Chapter 31

EMT Achieve: Paramedic Test Preparation
Mistovich & Beasley. *EMT Achieve: Paramedic Test Preparation.* www.prenhall.com/emtachieve/

Review Manual for the EMT-Paramedic
Cherry & Mistovich. *Review Manual for the EMT-Paramedic,* 3rd edition.

Handouts 31-4 to 31-6
Reinforcement Activities

Paramedic Student CD
Student Activities

PowerPoint Presentation
Chapter 31

Companion Website
http://www.prenhall.com/bledsoe

OneKey
Chapter 31

Advanced Life Support Skills
Larmon & Davis. *Advanced Life Support Skills.*

Advanced Life Skills Review
Larmon & Davis. *Advanced Life Skills Review.*

Brady Skills Series: ALS
Larmon & Davis. *Brady Skills Series: ALS.*

Paramedic National Standards Self-Test
Miller. *Paramedic National Standards Self-Test,* 4th edition.

HANDOUT 31-1

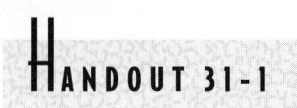

Student's Name _____

CHAPTER 31 OBJECTIVES CHECKLIST

Knowledge	Date Mastered
1. Describe the incidence, morbidity, and mortality of anaphylaxis.	
2. Identify the risk factors most predisposing to anaphylaxis.	
3. Discuss the anatomy and physiology of the organs and structures related to anaphylaxis.	
4. Discuss the pathophysiology of allergy and anaphylaxis.	
5. Describe the common routes of substance entry into the body.	
6. Define allergic reaction, anaphylaxis, antigen, antibody, and natural and acquired immunity.	
7. List the common antigens most frequently associated with anaphylaxis.	
8. Discuss human antibody formation.	
9. Describe the physical manifestations of anaphylaxis.	
10. Identify and differentiate between the signs and symptoms of an allergic reaction and anaphylaxis.	
11. Explain the various treatment and pharmacological interventions used in the management of allergic reactions and anaphylaxis.	
12. Correlate abnormal findings in assessment with the clinical significance in the patient with an allergic reaction or anaphylaxis.	
13. Given several preprogrammed and moulaged patients, provide the appropriate assessment, care, and transport for the allergic reaction and anaphylaxis patient.	

HANDOUT 31-2

Student's Name _____

CHAPTER 31 QUIZ

Write the letter of the best answer in the space provided.

_____ 1. The two most common causes of fatal anaphylaxis are:
   A. injected penicillin and *Hymenoptera* stings.
   B. peanuts and sulfites.
   C. MSG and bee stings.
   D. lidocaine and tetanus vaccine.

_____ 2. Immunity that develops over time and results from exposure to an antigen is called:
   A. natural immunity.
   B. humoral immunity.
   C. cellular immunity.
   D. acquired immunity.

_____ 3. Induced active immunity is immunity that:
   A. is genetically predetermined and is present at birth.
   B. begins to develop after birth and is continually enhanced by exposure to new pathogens and antigens throughout life.
   C. is achieved through a vaccination given to generate an immune response that results in the development of antibodies specific for the injected antigen.
   D. results from a direct attack of a foreign substance by specialized cells of the immune system.

_____ 4. Which of the following is TRUE regarding anaphylaxis?
   A. The signs and symptoms of anaphylaxis begin within 30 to 60 seconds.
   B. Reactions that develop more slowly tend to be much more severe.
   C. Angioneurotic edema is a rare manifestation of anaphylaxis.
   D. The release of histamine causes gastrointestinal motility to decrease.

_____ 5. The primary effect of antihistamines is to:
   A. reverse the action of macrophages.
   B. displace histamine from the receptor sites.
   C. cause bronchodilation.
   D. block the histamine receptor sites.

_____ 6. The primary drug for management of anaphylaxis is:
   A. oxygen.
   B. epinephrine.
   C. diphenhydramine.
   D. methylprednisolone.

_____ 7. Albuterol, Alupent, and Bronkosol are examples of:
   A. vasopressors.
   B. corticosteroids.
   C. antihistamines.
   D. beta-agonists.

_____ 8. A common sign in mild allergic reactions is urticaria, or:
   A. raised areas, or wheals, that occur on the skin.
   B. an itching or tickling sensation in the upper airway.
   C. itchy, watery eyes.
   D. sneezing or a "runny" nose.

HANDOUT 31-2 Continued

_____ 9. Administration of corticosteroids in the patient with anaphylaxis helps to:
   A. block histamine receptors.
   B. suppress the inflammatory response.
   C. cause direct bronchodilation.
   D. increase the blood pressure.

_____ 10. Of the following, which sign would you generally NOT expect to see in the patient with anaphylaxis?
   A. bradycardia
   B. wheezing
   C. facial flushing
   D. hypotension

HANDOUT 31-3

Student's Name _____

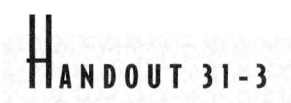

CHAPTER 31 SCENARIO

Review the following real-life situation. Then answer the questions that follow.

Medic 12 and Engine 2 arrive on the scene of an injury on a very hot summer day. The scene, a single-family suburban house on a half-acre plot, appears safe to enter. The crews find an unconscious 42-year-old man wearing nothing but running shorts and sandals, lying in a flower bed next to a ladder. His wife reports that she heard a noise and found him on the ground in that position. As one member of the crew takes c-spine control, the lead paramedic begins an initial assessment. The other firefighters set up the oxygen with a nonrebreather face mask, begin to get the long spine board ready, and take a complete set of vital signs. The second paramedic talks to the wife to obtain a history.

1. What are some of the possibilities that would account for this situation?

2. What should the paramedic look for during the initial assessment and focused physical exam?

3. What information should the second paramedic attempt to obtain from the patient's wife?

    Mr. Wilson's wife reports that her husband has no health problems and takes no medications. Other than indicating that he had lunch about an hour ago and that he is allergic to wasps, she cannot provide any more useful information.
    The paramedic performing the assessment finds that the patient has a contusion on the back of the head, but no other apparent injuries. (Because the patient is wearing only the running shorts, only the sandals are removed.) There are some expiratory wheezes, and Mr. Wilson appears to be working to breathe. His vital signs are as follows: BP 114/78; pulse 120 and weak at the wrist; capillary refill time is more than 2 seconds; respirations 30. The ECG shows sinus tachycardia, without ectopy. The pulse oximeter reading shows SaO_2 to be 95 percent. Mr. Wilson's blood sugar is 120. Assessment of level of consciousness reveals that Mr. Wilson responds to pain by moaning, but is unresponsive otherwise. No other marks or deformity are found.

4. What treatment is indicated at this time?

HANDOUT 31-3 Continued

Mr. Wilson is immobilized and secured to a long spine board and moved to the unit. Total time on the scene was less than 7 minutes. An IV is initiated en route to the hospital and run at a rate of 100 mL/hour. By the time the patient arrives at the ED, he is wheezing loudly and has developed stridor. The ED physician administers 0.5 mg of epinephrine, followed by 25 mg of diphenhydramine. Mr. Wilson's breathing rapidly improves and he wakes up. When he is fully conscious, he reports that he was on the ladder cleaning out the gutters, when he came upon a wasp's nest. One wasp flew up his shorts and stung him on his left hip (there is a large circular welt on his hip that is visible when his shorts are removed). As he tried to swat the wasp, he lost his balance and fell. He does not remember anything further. Mr. Wilson receives a second injection of epinephrine and some oral Benadryl. After a full workup, the head injury is determined to be a concussion, and Mr. Wilson is discharged to home.

5. What are the lessons to be learned from this case?

Handout 31-4

Student's Name _____

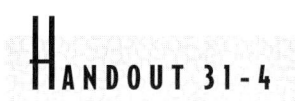

CHAPTER 31 REVIEW

Write the word or words that best complete the following sentences in the space(s) provided.

1. _____ is the most severe form of allergic reaction and is often life-threatening.
2. An exaggerated response by the immune system to a foreign substance is called a(n) _____ _____.
3. _____ are a unique class of chemicals that are manufactured by specialized cells of the immune system called _____.
4. _____ is an order of highly specialized insects such as bees and wasps.
5. The two most common causes of fatal anaphylaxis are _____ _____ and _____ _____.
6. A substance capable of inducing an immune response is called a(n) _____.
7. Immunity achieved through vaccination is called _____ _____ immunity.
8. An unexpected and exaggerated reaction to a particular antigen is called _____. It is used synonymously with the term _____.
9. Allergens can enter the body by _____ ingestion, _____, _____, and through _____ or _____.
10. A(n) _____ is a type of white blood cell that participates in allergic responses. A(n) _____ cell is a specialized cell of the immune system that contains chemicals that assist in the immune response.
11. _____ is a product of mast cells and basophils that causes vasodilation, capillary permeability, bronchoconstriction, and contraction of the gut.
12. A common manifestation of severe allergic reactions is _____ edema of the head, neck, face, and upper airway.
13. _____ are the raised areas, or wheals, that occur on the skin and are associated with vasodilation due to histamine release; they are commonly called _____.
14. The primary drug for the management of anaphylaxis is _____.
15. _____ is probably the most frequently used antihistamine in the treatment of allergic reactions and anaphylaxis. The standard dose is _____ - _____ mg intravenously or intramuscularly.
16. Albuterol is the most commonly used _____ - _____ in prehospital care.
17. Epinephrine 1:1,000 is administered _____ or _____, while epinephrine 1:10,000 is given _____.
18. The severity of an allergic reaction can be diminished in certain cases through a process called _____ or the administering of an extremely small amount of the allergen that causes the patient's anaphylactic reaction.
19. A _____ _____ by the immune system that takes place if the body is exposed to the same antigen again; antibodies specific for the offending antigen are released.
20. _____ _____ _____ begins to develop after birth and is continually enhanced by exposure to new pathogens and antigens throughout life.

REINFORCEMENT

HANDOUT 31-5

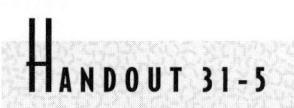

Student's Name _____

CLINICAL PRESENTATIONS OF ALLERGIES AND ANAPHYLAXIS

In the following spaces, list the signs and symptoms that you would expect to see in each specified body system of a patient with anaphylaxis.

1. SKIN
   _____
   _____
   _____
   _____

2. RESPIRATORY SYSTEM
   _____
   _____
   _____
   _____

3. CARDIOVASCULAR SYSTEM
   _____
   _____
   _____
   _____

4. GASTROINTESTINAL SYSTEM
   _____
   _____
   _____
   _____

5. NERVOUS SYSTEM
   _____
   _____
   _____
   _____

REINFORCEMENT

Handout 31-6

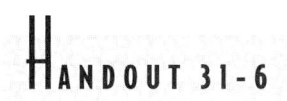

Student's Name _____

ANAPHYLAXIS MEDICATIONS

In the space provided, briefly describe what the following medications are used for and what their actions are when used to treat patients with anaphylaxis.

1. OXYGEN
   _____
   _____
   _____
   _____

2. EPINEPHRINE
   _____
   _____
   _____
   _____

3. ANTIHISTAMINES (Give examples of)
   _____
   _____
   _____
   _____

4. CORTICOSTEROIDS (Give examples of)
   _____
   _____
   _____
   _____

5. VASOPRESSORS (Give examples of)
   _____
   _____
   _____
   _____

6. BETA-AGONISTS (Give examples of)
   _____
   _____
   _____
   _____

REINFORCEMENT

Chapter 31 Answer Key

Handout 31-2: Chapter 31 Quiz

1. A
2. D
3. C
4. A
5. D
6. B
7. D
8. A
9. B
10. A

Handout 31-3: Chapter 31 Scenario

1. Possibilities include heat exhaustion, heatstroke, fall from the ladder, hypoglycemia, allergic reaction, electrocution, cardiac problem.
2. He should perform a standard trauma survey with emphasis on the ABCs. He should look for injuries resulting from the fall as well as for possible causes of the fall (e.g., low blood sugar, signs of dehydration, dysrhythmias, burns, stings).
3. The paramedic should ask questions about the patient's medical history using the SAMPLE mnemonic.
4. The crew should provide oxygen at 10–15 liters/minute via nonrebreather mask, apply a cervical spinal immobilization device, and immobilize the patient to a long spine board. They should establish one or two IVs of NS or LR. They should follow standing orders or contact medical control and consider treatment for allergic reaction.
5. Trauma can frequently accompany an allergic reaction. You should try to determine what caused trauma to occur. There may be an underlying medical cause. Remove all of a patient's clothing when performing an assessment. This scenario also underscores the fact that a well-coordinated effort by all emergency responders can minimize scene time.

Handout 31-4: Chapter 31 Review

1. Anaphylaxis
2. allergic reaction
3. Antibodies, B cells
4. *Hymenoptera*
5. injected penicillin, *Hymenoptera* stings
6. antigen
7. induced active
8. hypersensitivity, allergy
9. oral, inhalation, topically, injection, envenomation
10. basophil, mast
11. Histamine
12. angioneurotic
13. Urticaria, hives
14. epinephrine
15. Diphenhydramine, 25–50
16. beta-agonist
17. intramuscularly, subcutaneously, intravenously
18. desensitization
19. secondary response
20. Naturally acquired immunity

Handout 31-5: Clinical Presentations of Allergies and Anaphylaxis

1. *Skin:* Rash, urticaria (hives), itching, swelling, pallor, diaphoresis
2. *Respiratory System:* Dyspnea, coughing, sneezing, wheezing, stridor, tightness of the neck/throat, pulmonary edema, tracheal/laryngeal edema, tachypnea
3. *Cardiovascular System:* Tachycardia, dysrhythmias, hypotension, pallor, diaphoresis, dryness of the mouth
4. *Gastrointestinal System:* Nausea, vomiting, diarrhea, abdominal cramping, dryness of the mouth
5. *Nervous System:* Anxiety, restlessness, headache, unconsciousness, convulsions

Handout 31-6: Anaphylaxis Medications

1. *Oxygen:* Oxygen is always the first drug to administer to treat hypoxia in a patient with an anaphylactic reaction. Administer high-concentration oxygen with a nonrebreather mask. If the patient is not breathing adequately, administer oxygen via mechanical ventilation device, such as a BVM.
2. *Epinephrine:* Epinephrine is the primary drug for use in treatment of severe allergic reactions and anaphylaxis. It is a sympathetic agonist. It causes an increase in heart rate, increase in the strength of the cardiac contractile force, and peripheral vasoconstriction. It can also reverse some of the bronchospasm associated with anaphylaxis. Epinephrine also reverses much of the capillary permeability caused by histamine. It acts within minutes of administration. In severe anaphylaxis with hypotension and/or severe airway obstruction, administer epinephrine 1:10,000 IV. Standard adult dose is 0.3–0.5 mg. In severe cases of sustained anaphylaxis, medical control may order an epinephrine drip.
3. *Antihistamines:* Antihistamines are second-line agents. They should be given only following the administration of epinephrine. Antihistamines block the effects of histamine by blocking histamine receptors. They do not displace histamine from the receptors. They only block additional histamine from binding. They also help reduce histamine release from mast cells and basophils. Most antihistamines are nonselective and block both H1 and H2 receptors. Diphenhydramine (Benadryl) is the most frequently used antihistamine. Other antihistamines used are hydroxyzine (Atarax, Vistaril) and promethazine (Phenergan). The standard dose of diphenhydramine is 25–50 mg slow IV or IM.
4. *Corticosteroids:* Corticosteroids are of little benefit in the initial stages of treatment of anaphylaxis, but they help suppress the inflammatory response associated with these emergencies. Commonly used corticosteroids include methylprednisolone (Solu-Medrol), hydrocortisone (Solu-Cortef), and dexamethasone (Decadron).
5. *Vasopressors:* Vasopressors are used to treat severe and prolonged anaphylactic reactions to support

blood pressure. Use these medications in conjunction with first-line therapy and adequate fluid resuscitation. Commonly used agents include dopamine, norepinephrine, and epinephrine. These medications are prepared as infusions and are continuously administered to support blood pressure and cardiac output.

6. *Beta-agonists:* Inhaled beta-agonists are used to treat anaphylaxis with bronchospasm, laryngeal edema, or both. The most frequently used is albuterol (Ventolin, Proventil), usually used in the treatment of asthma. Adult dose is 0.5 mL of albuterol in 3 mL of NS via a handheld nebulizer. Other beta-agonists are metaproterenol (Alupent) and isoetharine (Bronkosol).

Chapter 32: Gastroenterology

INTRODUCTION

Gastrointestinal emergencies are a frequent prehospital complaint, accounting for over 500,000 emergency visits and hospitalizations each year. These numbers will rise as the general population ages. An understanding of life-threatening abdominal problems and how to deal with them is essential. This chapter discusses a wide variety of problems that arise within the gastrointestinal system.

CHAPTER OBJECTIVES

After reading this chapter, you should be able to:

1. Describe the incidence, morbidity, and mortality of gastrointestinal emergencies. (p. 1307)
2. Identify the risk factors most predisposing to gastrointestinal emergencies. (p. 1307)
3. Discuss the anatomy and physiology of the gastrointestinal system. (see Chapter 3)
4. Discuss the pathophysiology of abdominal inflammation and its relationship to acute pain. (pp. 1307–1308)
5. Define somatic, visceral, and referred pain as they relate to gastroenterology. (p. 1308)
6. Differentiate between hemorrhagic and nonhemorrhagic abdominal pain. (p. 1310)
7. Discuss the signs and symptoms and differentiate between local, general, and peritoneal inflammation relative to acute abdominal pain. (p. 1308)
8. Describe the questioning technique and specific questions when gathering a focused history in a patient with abdominal pain. (pp. 1309–1310)
9. Describe the technique for performing a comprehensive physical examination on a patient complaining of abdominal pain. (p. 1310)
10. Discuss the pathophysiology, assessment findings, and management of the following gastroenterological problems:
    - Upper gastrointestinal bleeding (pp. 1311–1312)
    - Lower gastrointestinal bleeding (pp. 1317–1318)
    - Acute gastroenteritis (pp. 1314–1315)
    - Colitis (p. 1318)
    - Gastroenteritis (pp. 1314–1315)
    - Diverticulitis (pp. 1319–1320)
    - Appendicitis (pp. 1322–1323)

TOTAL TEACHING TIME:
7.19 HOURS
The total teaching time is only a guideline based on the didactic and practical lab averages in the National Standard Curriculum. Instructors should take into consideration such factors as the pace at which students learn, the size of the class, and breaks. The actual time devoted to teaching objectives is the responsibility of the instructor.

©2007 Pearson Education, Inc.
Essentials of Paramedic Care, 2nd ed.

- Ulcer disease (pp. 1315–1317)
- Bowel obstruction (pp. 1320–1322)
- Crohn's disease (pp. 1318–1319)
- Pancreatitis (p. 1324)
- Esophageal varices (pp. 1313–1314)
- Hemorrhoids (p. 1320)
- Cholecystitis (pp. 1323–1324)
- Acute hepatitis (pp. 1324–1325)

11. Differentiate between gastrointestinal emergencies based on assessment findings. (pp. 1308–1310)

12. Given several preprogrammed patients with abdominal pain and symptoms, provide the appropriate assessment, treatment, and transport. (pp. 1307–1325)

FRAMING THE LESSON

Begin class by reviewing the important points from Chapter 31, "Allergies and Anaphylaxis." Discuss any aspects of the chapter not fully understood by students. Then begin with Chapter 32 material. Begin with a review of the anatomy and physiology of the gastrointestinal system by obtaining a diagram of the system. Either obtain a large, poster-size copy, draw the diagram on the board, or make a copy of the diagram for each student. Starting at either the front or back of the class, have a student identify a structure and label it. Have the next student in line identify the function of the structure. Then have the next student in line identify any problems that may occur with that structure. Repeat for each structure. Stress the seriousness of the life-threatening emergencies that may exist and the need for rapid identification and transport. Discuss the in-hospital treatment, such as surgery, that may be required for serious problems.

TEACHING STRATEGIES

People learn in a variety of ways. Some do better with the spoken word, whereas others prefer the written. Some prefer to work alone, whereas others profit from working in groups. Recognizing these different ways of acquiring knowledge, the authors of this *Instructor's Resource Manual* have provided a variety of teaching strategies for the different types of learners. These strategies are intended to foster higher-level cognitive skills and encourage creative learning and problem solving. For greatest effectiveness, incorporate these strategies into your class lecture. Symbols in the Lecture Outline indicate the points at which various exercises might be most appropriate. Other strategies can be used to preview the lesson or to summarize it.

The following strategies are keyed to specific sections of the lesson.

1. *Abdominal Physical Exam.* Too many paramedics miss obvious abdominal conditions due to poor physical exam techniques. The acute abdomen cannot be properly assessed without visualizing the abdomen or placing the patient supine for palpation. Instill good habits in your students by insisting that they properly position the patient and expose the abdomen EVERY time an abdominal exam is to be performed. Be sure to remind your clinical instructors of this "policy" as well.

2. *Balloon Simulations.* Fill balloons with different substances to simulate the feeling of different abdominal findings. A balloon filled with maximum air will simulate a distended abdomen while a water balloon only partially full feels like ascites. A balloon filled with shaving cream feels a lot like a soft, non-tender abdomen. Use your imagination for pulsating masses, rigidity, and other findings. For added realism, insert your balloons into the abdominal cavity of your infant CPR or OB mannequins, causing the exam to be performed through a layer of skin.

3. Abdominal Organ ID. Place paper cutouts of each of the abdominal organs in a bag. Allow each student to blindly remove one organ from the bag. Have the student identify the retrieved organ by name and function, and pin it onto a large cardboard cutout of the abdominopelvic cavity. This game is like "pin-the-tail-on-the-donkey" for the abdomen. It is not only fun but is a good anatomy and physiology review.

4. Gastrointestinal Structure Anatomy. Using poster board or heavy construction paper, make life-size cutouts of the GI structures. Place a student in front of the class in the anatomical position. Then distribute the cutouts to students, placing a piece of masking tape on the back of each piece. Have students, one at a time, place the structure cutouts on the student standing in front of the class. As each student places the cutout, have them describe the function of the structure.

5. Colonoscopy and Endoscopy Videos. Patients experiencing acute abdominal pain are frequently anxious about the procedures they will undergo once at the hospital. Paramedics become advocates for these patients when they can explain what is to be expected. Borrow videotapes on gastroenterology procedures such as colonoscopy and endoscopy from your internist. Viewing these tapes will allow your students to provide patient education, as well as get a great anatomy lesson.

The following strategies can be used at various points throughout the lesson or to help summarize and demonstrate what students have learned.

GI System Clinical Rotation. During clinical rotations, assign students to one of each of the conditions of the GI system. Have them interview a patient with the assigned diagnosis. They should discover not only the signs, symptoms, and history, but also how the condition affects the patient's lifestyle. As paramedics, we often forget to consider how a condition affects a person's diet, bowel or bladder habits, appetite, or medication therapy. This activity not only improves oral communication and interview skills, but is an excellent way to develop empathy for patients. Students can then present their conditions during a subsequent class session.

Autopsy Observation or Video. Nothing so graphically demonstrates the potential for problems and injuries as observation of an autopsy. If possible, have students observe an autopsy. If this is not possible, obtain a video of an autopsy. Several of these are available. One video is titled "Autopsy" and was produced by *Emergency Medical Update*. Your county coroner's office may also have training videos or films showing autopsies.

Surgical Observation. If possible, have students obtain some of their required clinical hours by observing abdominal surgeries. Local surgeons may be willing to allow one or two students at a time to observe surgeries.

Abdominal Organ Dissection. Sometimes local supermarkets or meat packing companies will have porcine abdominal organs available. If possible, obtain organs such as the stomach, liver, small and large intestine, and so on, and allow students to inspect them. This will give students a good knowledge base of the organs and their structure. (Note: Always use appropriate body substance isolation precautions.)

HANDOUT 32-1
Chapter 32 Objectives Checklist

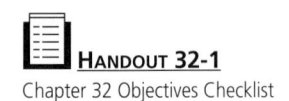

POINT OF INTEREST
It takes about 24 hours to completely digest a typical meal. Food spends about 4 hours in the stomach, 6 hours in the small intestine, 6–7 hours in the colon, and 6–7 hours in the rectum before the waste is expelled as feces.

POINT OF INTEREST
The liver can detoxify approximately one shot of alcohol per hour.

POINT TO EMPHASIZE
The patient's general body language is important. The quieter patients lie, the more ill they are likely to be.

POWERPOINT PRESENTATION
Chapter 32 PowerPoint slides 4–8

POINT OF INTEREST
In 40 to 50 percent of cases, the ED diagnosis is nonspecific abdominal pain.

POWERPOINT PRESENTATION
Chapter 32 PowerPoint slides 9–39

TEACHING STRATEGY 1
Abdominal Physical Exam

TEACHING STRATEGY 2
Balloon Simulations

TEACHING STRATEGY 3
Abdominal Organ ID

TEACHING STRATEGY 4
Gastrointestinal Structure Anatomy

TEACHING STRATEGY 5
Colonoscopy and Endoscopy Videos

POINT OF INTEREST
The most common cause of upper GI bleeding is peptic ulcer. Some 80 percent of upper GI bleeds stop by themselves.

Guest Speaker: Hospital Surgeon. Ask a surgeon from a local hospital to address the class regarding GI problems resolved by surgery. If possible, request that the surgeon bring in any X-rays, photos, and so on, he or she may have of cases handled.

Cultural Considerations, Legal Notes, and Patho Pearls. The Student CD-ROM contains this series of informative features to enhance the student's understanding of the material covered in this chapter.

TEACHING OUTLINE

Chapter 32 is the sixth lesson in Division 4, *Medical Emergencies*. Distribute Handout 32-1 so that students can familiarize themselves with the learning goals for this chapter. If students have any questions about the objectives, answer them at this time.

Then present the chapter. One possible lecture outline follows. In the outline, the parenthetical references in regular type are references to text pages; those in bold type are references to figures, tables, or procedures.

I. Introduction. Gastrointestinal emergencies account for over 500,000 emergency visits and hospitalizations each year. This is approximately 5 percent of all visits to the emergency department. Of that number, more than 300,000 are due to gastrointestinal bleeding. (p. 1307)

II. General pathophysiology, assessment, and treatment (pp. 1307–1311)
  A. General pathophysiology (p. 1308)
  B. General assessment (pp. 1308–1310)
    1. Scene size-up and initial assessment
    2. History and physical exam
    3. Physical exam
      a. Cullen's sign
      b. Grey Turner's sign
  C. General treatment (pp. 1310–1311)

III. Specific injuries and illnesses (pp. 1311–1325)
  A. Upper gastrointestinal diseases (pp. 1311–1317)
    1. Upper gastrointestinal bleeding
    2. Esophageal varices (**Fig. 32-1, p. 1313**)
    3. Acute gastroenteritis
    4. Chronic gastroenteritis
    5. Peptic ulcers (**Fig. 32-2, p. 1316**)
  B. Lower GI diseases (pp. 1317–1322)
    1. Lower GI bleeding
    2. Ulcerative colitis
    3. Crohn's disease
    4. Diverticulitis
    5. Hemorrhoids
    6. Bowel obstruction
      a. Four most frequent causes
        i. Intestinal hernia (**Fig. 32-3a, p. 1321**)
        ii. Intestinal intussusception (**Fig. 32-3b, p. 1321**)
        iii. Intestinal adhesions (**Fig. 32-3c, p. 1321**)
        iv. Intestinal volvulus (**Fig. 32-3d, p. 1321**)

b. Other common causes
   - **i.** Foreign bodies
   - **ii.** Gallstones
   - **iii.** Tumors
   - **iv.** Adhesions from previous abdominal surgery
   - **v.** Bowel infarctions
- **C.** Accessory organ diseases (pp. 1322–1325)
   1. Appendicitis (**Fig. 32-4, p. 1323**)
   2. Cholecystitis
   3. Pancreatitis
   4. Hepatitis

IV. Chapter summary (pp. 1325–1326). Abdominal pain can originate from a wide variety of causes, either from the abdominal organs or from areas outside of the abdominal cavity. The prehospital management priorities for the abdominal patient are to establish and maintain his airway, breathing, and circulation. The differential diagnosis can include a multitude of causes that usually cannot be identified without laboratory and radiographic analysis. Airway management is of paramount importance, as patients frequently suffer from severe bouts of nausea and vomiting. Be prepared to turn the patient onto his side if necessary to clear large amounts of vomitus from the airway. Oxygenation usually can be adequately stabilized by placing the patient on high-flow, high-concentration oxygen via a nonrebreather mask. Fluid loss, hemorrhage, or sepsis may compromise the circulatory status. Initiate fluid resuscitation for the hemodynamically unstable patient in the field, but never delay transport. Patients who have abdominal pain lasting over 6 hours should always be evaluated by a physician.

SKILLS DEMONSTRATION AND PRACTICE

Students can practice skills discussed in this chapter in the following settings.

Scenario Lab. The following station will be part of a larger medical scenario lab. Divide the class into teams. Have the teams circulate through the station. Monitor the groups to be sure all groups have a chance to manage each of the cases and so that every student has the opportunity to be team leader. You may wish to have other instructors or qualified paramedics assist students in these activities.

Station	Equipment Needed	Activities
Acute Abdomen	Medication box 1 patient 1 instructor	Students assess and manage patients with an acute abdomen.

Hospital: Assist in assessment and management of the acute abdomen in the ED.

Field Internship: Assist in assessment and management of the acute abdomen in the field.

POINT OF INTEREST
The most common cause of acute abdomen is appendicitis. The two most commonly missed diagnoses among patients who are wrongfully discharged from EDs are acute appendicitis and acute intestinal obstruction.

POWERPOINT PRESENTATION
Chapter 32 PowerPoint slide 40

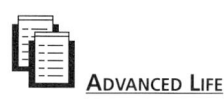

ADVANCED LIFE SUPPORT SKILLS
Larmon & Davis. *Advanced Life Support Skills*.

ADVANCED LIFE SKILLS REVIEW
Larmon & Davis. *Advanced Life Skills Review*.

BRADY SKILLS SERIES: ALS
Larmon & Davis. *Brady Skills Series: ALS*.

WORKBOOK
Chapter 32 Activities

READING/REFERENCE
Textbook, pp. 1328–1348

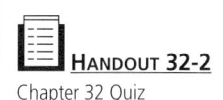

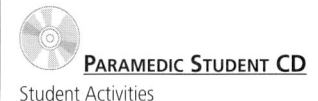

HANDOUT 32-2
Chapter 32 Quiz

HANDOUT 32-3
Chapter 32 Scenario

PARAMEDIC STUDENT CD
Student Activities

ASSIGNMENTS

Assign students to complete Chapter 32, "Gastroenterology," of the workbook. Also assign them to read Chapter 33, "Urology and Nephrology," before the next class.

EVALUATION

Chapter Quiz and Scenario Distribute copies of the Chapter Quiz provided in Handout 32-2 to evaluate student understanding of this chapter. Make sure each student reads the scenario to reinforce critical thinking on the scene. Remind students not to use their notes or textbooks while taking the quiz.

Student CD Quizzes for every chapter are contained on the dynamic and highly visual in-text student CD.

Companion Website Additional quizzes for every chapter are contained on this exciting website.

TestGen You may wish to create a custom-tailored test using *Prentice Hall TestGen for Essentials of Paramedic Care*, 2nd Edition to evaluate student understanding of this chapter.

On-line Test Preparation (for students and instructors) Additional test preparation is available through Brady's new on-line product, *EMT Achieve: Paramedic Test Preparation* at *http://www.prenhall.com/emtachieve/*. Instructors can also monitor student mastery on-line.

Review Manual for the EMT-Paramedic This comprehensive exam review contains hundreds of test questions and rationales, including scenarios, along with two 180-question practice tests on CD.

REINFORCEMENT

Handouts If classroom discussion or performance on the quiz indicates that some students have not fully mastered the chapter content, you may wish to assign some or all of the Reinforcement Handouts for this chapter.

Student CD (for students) A wide variety of material on this CD-ROM will reinforce and also expand student knowledge and skills.

PowerPoint Presentation (for instructors) The PowerPoint material developed for this chapter offers useful reinforcement of chapter content.

Companion Website (for students) Additional review quizzes and links to EMS resources will contribute to further reinforcement of the chapter.

OneKey On-line support is offered for this course on one of three platforms: CourseCompass, Blackboard, or Web CT. Includes the IRM, PowerPoints, TestGen, and Companion Website for instruction. Ask your local sales representative for more information.

Brady Skills Series: Advanced Life Skills (Video or CD) Have your students watch the skills come to life on VHS or CD-ROM, or they can purchase the highly visual, full-color text with step-by-step procedures and rationales.

Handout 32-1

Student's Name _____

CHAPTER 32 OBJECTIVES CHECKLIST

Knowledge	Date Mastered
1. Describe the incidence, morbidity, and mortality of gastrointestinal emergencies.	
2. Identify the risk factors most predisposing to gastrointestinal emergencies.	
3. Discuss the anatomy and physiology of the gastrointestinal system.	
4. Discuss the pathophysiology of abdominal inflammation and its relationship to acute pain.	
5. Define somatic, visceral, and referred pain as they relate to gastroenterology.	
6. Differentiate between hemorrhagic and nonhemorrhagic abdominal pain.	
7. Discuss the signs and symptoms and differentiate between local, general, and peritoneal inflammation relative to acute abdominal pain.	
8. Describe the questioning technique and specific questions when gathering a focused history in a patient with abdominal pain.	
9. Describe the technique for performing a comprehensive physical examination on a patient complaining of abdominal pain.	
10. Discuss the pathophysiology, assessment findings, and management of the following gastroenterological problems: • Upper gastrointestinal bleeding • Lower gastrointestinal bleeding • Acute gastroenteritis • Colitis • Gastroenteritis • Diverticulitis • Appendicitis • Ulcer disease • Bowel obstruction • Crohn's disease • Pancreatitis • Esophageal varices • Hemorrhoids • Cholecystitis • Acute hepatitis	
11. Differentiate between gastrointestinal emergencies based on assessment findings.	
12. Given several preprogrammed patients with abdominal pain and symptoms, provide the appropriate assessment, treatment, and transport.	

OBJECTIVES

CHAPTER 32 QUIZ

Write the letter of the best answer in the space provided.

_____ 1. All of the following are gastrointestinal emergency risk factors EXCEPT:
   A. excessive smoking.
   B. poor bowel habits.
   C. excessive fat consumption.
   D. increased stress.

_____ 2. Pain that originates in the walls of hollow organs is called:
   A. visceral pain.
   B. peritoneal pain.
   C. somatic pain.
   D. referred pain.

_____ 3. Somatic pain is described as:
   A. a dull, achy pain that is vague in nature and difficult to localize.
   B. a sharp pain that travels along definite neural routes to the spinal column.
   C. pain that originates in a region other than where it is felt.
   D. pain originating in the walls of hollow organs, in the capsules of solid organs, or in the visceral peritoneum.

_____ 4. The mnemonic used to help remember questions to ask regarding the history of the present illness for gastrointestinal patients is:
   A. SAMPLE.
   B. DCAP-BTLS.
   C. OPQRST-ASPN.
   D. AVPU.

_____ 5. Usually patients with severe abdominal pathology will:
   A. be moving around as they cannot get comfortable.
   B. want to lie supine with legs straight out.
   C. be seated, leaning forward in an attempt to relieve the pain.
   D. lie as still as possible in the fetal position.

_____ 6. The highest priority when treating a patient with abdominal pain is to:
   A. transport the patient in the most comfortable position.
   B. treat the patient for shock.
   C. maintain the airway, breathing, and circulation.
   D. palpate the abdomen for a pulsating mass.

_____ 7. Always transport a patient with abdominal pain if the:
   A. patient is tachycardic.
   B. pain has lasted longer than 6 hours.
   C. patient is diaphoretic.
   D. pain radiates.

_____ 8. A Mallory-Weiss tear is a(n):
   A. separation of the small and large intestine.
   B. rupture of the abdominal aorta.
   C. esophageal laceration, usually secondary to vomiting.
   D. laceration within the rectum, resulting in bloody stool.

_____ 9. A swollen vein in the esophagus is called a(n):
   A. portal.
   B. esophageal aneurysm.
   C. diverticulitis.
   D. esophageal varix.

_____ 10. A sudden onset of diarrhea associated with mucosal inflammation is called:
   A. gastroenteritis.
   B. acute gastroenteritis.
   C. peptic ulcer.
   D. Zollinger-Ellison syndrome.

HANDOUT 32-2 Continued

_____ 11. Which of the following statements is TRUE regarding lower GI bleeding?
   A. Lower GI bleeding originates distal to the duodenum.
   B. Major causes of lower GI bleeding include varix rupture and gastritis.
   C. Lower GI bleeding is usually chronic and rarely results in exsanguinating hemorrhage.
   D. Patients with lower GI bleeding will often present with hematemesis.

_____ 12. Crohn's disease is:
   A. acute pain associated with cramping or spasms in the abdominal organs.
   B. ulcerative colitis that has spread throughout the entire colon.
   C. a condition that causes the stomach to secrete excessive amounts of hydrochloric acid and pepsin.
   D. a bowel disorder that can affect any portion of the GI tract.

_____ 13. Zollinger-Ellison syndrome is associated with:
   A. esophageal varices.   C. duodenal ulcers.
   B. hemorrhoids.   D. bowel obstruction.

_____ 14. Your patient presents with colicky pain, low-grade fever, nausea and vomiting, and tenderness to the lower left side of the abdomen. He is most likely suffering from:
   A. hemorrhoids.   C. hernia.
   B. peptic ulcer.   D. diverticulitis.

_____ 15. Hernias, intussusception, volvulus, and adhesions are the four most frequent causes of:
   A. abdominal pain.   C. inflammatory bowel disorder.
   B. gastroenteritis.   D. bowel obstruction.

_____ 16. Ninety percent of cholecystitis cases are caused by:
   A. bowel obstruction.   C. gallstones.
   B. hepatitis.   D. colon lesions.

_____ 17. Which of the following is TRUE regarding hepatitis B?
   A. It is commonly referred to as "infectious hepatitis."
   B. It is spread through the oral-fecal route.
   C. It is marked by chronic and often debilitating damage to the liver.
   D. It can stay active in body fluids outside the body for days.

_____ 18. Hemorrhoids are:
   A. small masses of swollen veins in the anus.
   B. ulcerations of the anus.
   C. infected mucosal tissue in the anus.
   D. outpouching of the lining of the anus.

_____ 19. A common site of pain in cases of appendicitis is:
   A. Hey's ligament.   C. Charcot's joint.
   B. Schultze's tract.   D. McBurney's point.

_____ 20. The most common form of hepatitis is:
   A. hepatitis A.   C. hepatitis C.
   B. hepatitis B.   D. hepatitis E.

HANDOUT 32-3

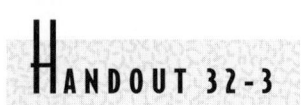

Student's Name _____

CHAPTER 32 SCENARIO

Review the following real-life situation. Then answer the questions that follow.

Community One Ambulance is dispatched for a sickness call. On arrival, they find a 42-year-old female complaining of nausea, vomiting, and abdominal pain. The lead paramedic begins performing his physical assessment and begins to obtain a history.

1. What are important aspects of the assessment?

2. What are important aspects of the history?

The patient had dinner about 7:00 P.M. (It is now 1:00 A.M.) and began feeling nauseous at 9:30. She thought that perhaps her problem was related to some "bad salad dressing." At 10:15 she began vomiting and continued until 911 was called at 12:45 A.M. Abdominal pain, described as "achy," began about the time the vomiting started. The patient says that the pain started around her belly button and has moved down into her right lower quadrant.

The patient has no significant medical history. Her last menstrual period was 10 days ago and she had a tubal ligation 7 years ago. She takes no medications and the only surgery is two c-sections.

On physical examination, her abdomen is tender, with some guarding. There is some rebound tenderness in the right lower quadrant. Vital signs are: BP 105/66; pulse 78 (negative tilt test); respirations are 20 and regular, unlabored, breath sounds equal, clear bilaterally; ECG is NSR, without ectopy; pulse oximeter is 99 percent on room air. Her skin is warm, dry, and flushed. All other physical examination findings are normal.

3. What is this patient's problem, and what leads to that conclusion?

4. What treatment is indicated for this patient?

5. What would be the best way to transport the patient?

HANDOUT 32-4

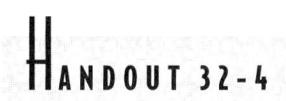

Student's Name _____

CHAPTER 32 REVIEW

Write the word or words that best complete the following sentences in the space(s) provided.

1. The three types of gastrointestinal pain are _____, _____, and _____.
2. Gastrointestinal disease risk factors include excessive _____ consumption, excessive _____, increased _____, ingestion of _____ substances, and poor _____ habits.
3. _____ is the inflammation of the peritoneum, which lines the abdominal cavity.
4. Pain that originates in walls of the body such as skeletal muscles is called _____ pain.
5. Pain that originates in a region other than where it is felt is known as _____ pain.
6. When using the mnemonic OPQRST-ASPN to gain the history of the present illness of your gastrointestinal patient, the AS stands for _____ _____, and the PN stands for _____ _____.
7. _____ of the abdomen is usually an ominous sign.
8. If you _____ the abdomen, you must do so before _____ it.
9. Persistent abdominal pain lasting longer than _____ hours always requires transport.
10. Upper gastrointestinal bleeding is within the GI tract proximal to the _____ _____ _____.
11. A Mallory-Weiss tear is a(n) _____ laceration, usually secondary to _____.
12. Bloody vomitus is known as _____, and dark, tarry, foul smelling stool is known as _____.
13. A swollen vein in the esophagus is called an esophageal _____.
14. A degenerative disease of the liver is called _____.
15. Sudden onset of diarrhea associated with mucosal inflammation is called _____ _____.
16. The condition in which the stomach secretes excessive amounts of hydrochloric acid and pepsin is called _____-_____ _____.
17. Lower GI bleeding is usually _____ and rarely results in _____ hemorrhage.
18. Acute pain associated with cramping or spasms in the abdominal organs is called _____.
19. Prehospital diagnosis of _____ disease is next to impossible because the patient's clinical presentations can vary drastically as the disease progresses.
20. _____ are small outpouchings in the mucosal lining of the intestinal tract.
21. The four most frequent causes of bowel obstruction are _____, _____, _____, and _____.
22. A common site of pain is 1 to 2 inches above the anterior iliac crest in a direct line with the umbilicus. This site is known as _____ _____.
23. Hepatitis _____ is transmitted as a blood-borne pathogen and can stay active in bodily fluids outside the body for days.
24. In patients with hepatitis, the stool is often a(n) _____ color, while the skin is _____.
25. The key to successful treatment of GI ailments is prompt _____, _____, and _____ transport to the hospital.

GASTROINTESTINAL STRUCTURE/FUNCTION/PROBLEMS

Structure	Substructures/Action	Function	Problems
Mouth	Lips Cheeks Gums Teeth Tongue Secretes saliva	Breaking down food into smaller particles Saliva begins digestion of starches Saliva lubricates Saliva important for oral hygiene Taste buds in tongue cause GI secretions	Dental disease
Esophagus	Secretes mucus	Pathway from mouth to the stomach Mucus lubricates food passage and protects esophagus from reflux of gastric juice	Esophageal varices Esophageal ulcers Reflux
Stomach	Secretes hydrochloric acid Secretes enzymes	Chemical food breakdown Digestion of protein Protection of stomach lining Storage of food until it can be accommodated by duodenum Mixing of food with acid	Gastritis Gastric ulcers GI hemorrhage
Pancreas	Secretes pancreatic juice Secretes bicarbonate ion	Digestion of carbohydrates, proteins, fats Neutralize gastric acid upon entering duodenum	Pancreatitis
Liver	Secretes bile Secretes bile salts	Digestion of fat Help with absorption of lipids	Hepatitis
Gall bladder	Stores bile and bile salts	Store up to 12 hours of bile secretion	Cholecystitis
Small intestine	Receives bile and pancreatic juice Secretes mucus Secretes enzymes	Completion of digestion Mixing of chyme with juices Propulsion of chyme Absorption of nutrients Absorption of water Absorption of electrolytes Protection of intestinal wall Lubrication	Duodenal ulcers GI hemorrhage Perforated viscus
Large intestine	Secretes mucus Produces feces Stores feces	Protect intestinal wall Lubricate Absorption of water Absorption of electrolytes	Diverticulosis Carcinoma Appendicitis Bowel obstruction GI hemorrhage Perforated viscus

Chapter 33

Urology and Nephrology

INTRODUCTION

The urinary system performs a number of vital functions, including maintaining blood volume and the proper balance of water, electrolytes, and pH. It also ensures that key substances such as glucose remain in the bloodstream. In addition, it removes a variety of toxic wastes from the blood, plays a major role in arterial blood-pressure regulation, and controls the development of red blood cells.

The most significant medical disorders involving the urinary system affect the kidneys and kidney function. Renal and urologic disorders affect more than 20 million Americans, with more than 50,000 dying annually from kidney disease. This chapter presents a number of the common disorders of the urinary system.

CHAPTER OBJECTIVES

After reading this chapter, you should be able to:

1. Describe the incidence, morbidity, mortality, and risk factors predisposing to urologic and nephrologic emergencies. (pp. 1329–1330, 1335, 1338–1339, 1343–1344, 1345–1346)
2. Discuss the anatomy and physiology of the organs and structures related to the urinary system. (see Chapter 3)
3. Define referred pain and visceral pain as they relate to urology. (p. 1331)
4. Describe the questioning technique and specific questions the paramedic should use when gathering a focused history in a patient with abdominal pain. (pp. 1323–1333)
5. Describe the technique for performing a comprehensive physical examination of a patient complaining of abdominal pain. (pp. 1333–1334)
6. Define acute renal failure. (p. 1335)
7. Discuss the pathophysiology of acute renal failure. (pp. 1335–1337)
8. Recognize the signs and symptoms related to acute renal failure. (pp. 1337–1338)
9. Describe the management of acute renal failure. (p. 1338)

TOTAL TEACHING TIME: 4.22 HOURS
The total teaching time is only a guideline based on the didactic and practical lab averages in the National Standard Curriculum. Instructors should take into consideration such factors as the pace at which students learn, the size of the class, and breaks. The actual time devoted to teaching objectives is the responsibility of the instructor.

10. Integrate pathophysiological principles and assessment findings to formulate a field impression and implement a treatment plan for the patient with acute renal failure. (pp. 1335–1338)
11. Define chronic renal failure. (pp. 1338–1339)
12. Discuss the pathophysiology of chronic renal failure. (pp. 1339–1340)
13. Recognize the signs and symptoms related to chronic renal failure. (pp. 1340–1341)
14. Describe the management of chronic renal failure. (pp. 1341–1343)
15. Integrate pathophysiological principles and assessment findings to formulate a field impression and implement a treatment plan for the patient with chronic renal failure. (pp. 1339–1343)
16. Define renal dialysis. (pp. 1342–1343)
17. Discuss the common complications of renal dialysis. (pp. 1342–1343)
18. Define renal calculi. (pp. 1343–1344)
19. Discuss the pathophysiology of renal calculi. (p. 1344)
20. Recognize the signs and symptoms related to renal calculi. (p. 1345)
21. Describe the management of renal calculi. (p. 1345)
22. Integrate pathophysiological principles and assessment findings to formulate a field impression and implement a treatment plan for the patient with renal calculi. (pp. 1343–1345)
23. Define urinary tract infection. (pp. 1345–1346)
24. Discuss the pathophysiology of urinary tract infection. (pp. 1346–1347)
25. Recognize the signs and symptoms related to urinary tract infection. (p. 1347)
26. Describe the management of a urinary tract infection. (p. 1347)
27. Integrate pathophysiological principles and assessment findings to formulate a field impression and implement a treatment plan for the patient with a urinary tract infection. (pp. 1345–1347)
28. Apply epidemiology to develop prevention strategies for urologic and nephrologic emergencies. (p. 1330)
29. Integrate pathophysiological principles to the assessment of a patient with abdominal pain. (pp. 1331–1334)
30. Synthesize assessment findings and patient history information to accurately differentiate between pain of a urologic or nephrologic emergency and that of another origin. (pp. 1331–1334)
31. Develop, execute, and evaluate a treatment plan based on the field impression made in the assessment. (pp. 1329–1347)

FRAMING THE LESSON

Begin class by reviewing the important points from Chapter 32, "Gastroenterology." Discuss any aspects of the chapter not fully understood by students. Then begin with Chapter 33 material by discussing the anatomy of the kidney. Using a diagram of the kidney, point out the major structures. Provide students with a number of colored pencils or markers and have students color or label the various structures found in the kidney and the nephron at one time or as they are discussed throughout the lesson. Ask students to name as many functions of the kidney as they can think of. Stress that there are many more functions of the kidney besides the formation and elimination of urine. Improperly functioning kidneys affect the entire body.

TEACHING STRATEGIES

People learn in a variety of ways. Some do better with the spoken word, whereas others prefer the written. Some prefer to work alone, whereas others profit from working in groups. Recognizing these different ways of acquiring knowledge, the authors of this *Instructor's Resource Manual* have provided a variety of teaching strategies for the different types of learners. These strategies are intended to foster higher-level cognitive skills and encourage creative learning and problem solving. For greatest effectiveness, incorporate these strategies into your class lecture. Symbols in the Lecture Outline indicate the points at which various exercises might be most appropriate. Other strategies can be used to preview the lesson or to summarize it.

The following strategies are keyed to specific sections of the lesson.

1. Word Cube. Make a word cube to help students with the gross amount of foreign terminology in this section. Wrap a square gift box in wrapping paper that is either fun or relevant to this chapter. Place stickers on all six sides that will indicate the type of term the student is going to get. For instance, anatomy, physiology, treatments, conditions, medications, and hodgepodge. Students take turns tossing the cube to each other, and whatever side the cube lands on, the student is responsible for that type of term. You read the term, and the student gives the definition. All of the key words in the text's margins could be used in this game.

2. Kidney Stone Display. To properly appreciate the pain associated with renal calculi or kidney stones, borrow some stones from your hospital pathologist. When students observe stones the size of peas and marbles with their sharp, jagged edges, they are likely to have instant empathy for their patients suffering this condition.

The following strategies can be used at various points throughout the lesson or to help summarize and demonstrate what students have learned.

Guest Speaker: Member of Kidney Transplant Team. There would be no better person to discuss kidney physiology than a member of the kidney transplant team. Invite a team member to discuss the anatomy and physiology of the kidney, as well as pathologies of the kidney, process for nephrectomy, and complications of living with one kidney. This is likely to be an exciting guest lecture.

Research Project. Assign students to prepare a report on a specific genitourinary or kidney dysfunction using local public or college medical libraries for sources. Prior to students writing the report, have each student submit the name of the condition for your approval, making sure that each student chooses a different condition or dysfunction. After the reports have been turned in, select a few to be presented to the class by the writers.

Laboratory Visit. Arrange for students to tour a medical laboratory either in a clinic or area hospital. Have them observe how specimens are obtained, handled, and tested.

Clinical Rotation in a Dialysis Center. To properly appreciate the pathophysiology of the dialysis patient, students must do clinical time, even solely observation time, in a dialysis center. Establish a relationship with staff members who are willing to educate students on shunts and grafts, the dialysis process, common dialysis candidates, risks and complications of dialysis, and even patient interviews in the unit. Paramedics are frequently called upon to transport patients to and from dialysis appointments,

HANDOUT 33-1
Chapter 33 Objectives Checklist

TEACHING STRATEGY 1
Word Cube

TEACHING TIP
Compare the kidneys to a coffee filter. As a graphic demonstration, mix some sand in water. Then pour the water through the coffee filter and note the water after it is filtered.

POINT OF INTEREST
The kidney has the highest blood supply/gm of any tissue in the body.

POWERPOINT PRESENTATION
Chapter 33 PowerPoint slides 4–10

POWERPOINT PRESENTATION
Chapter 33 PowerPoint slide 11

POINT TO EMPHASIZE
You may have difficulty determining the source of an abdominal problem when pain is the sole complaint because many emergencies have similar presentations.

POWERPOINT PRESENTATION
Chapter 33 PowerPoint slides 12–16

POINT TO EMPHASIZE
Once you have palpated an area of the abdomen that is painful, there is no need to palpate it again, causing additional pain to the patient.

POINT TO EMPHASIZE
As with all patients, monitoring and supporting the ABCs is the key to good patient management.

POINT TO EMPHASIZE
Remember body substance isolation precautions when handling blood or body fluid samples.

---

during complications of peritoneal dialysis at home, and during complications during hemodialysis in outpatient settings. Being familiar with the process, equipment, and pathology will be imperative for proper management of this patient population at a later date.

Cultural Considerations, Legal Notes, and Patho Pearls. The student CD-ROM contains this series of informative features to enhance the student's understanding of the material covered in this chapter.

TEACHING OUTLINE

Chapter 33 is the seventh lesson in Division 4, *Medical Emergencies*. Distribute Handout 33-1 so that students can familiarize themselves with the learning goals for this chapter. If students have any questions about the objectives, answer them at this time.

Then present the chapter. One possible lecture outline follows. In the outline, the parenthetical references in regular type are references to text pages; those in bold type are references to figures, tables, or procedures.

I. Introduction. A properly functioning urinary system is vital to all systems of the body. The kidney's regulation of water and other important substances in blood is an example of homeostasis. The most significant medical disorders involving the urinary system affect the kidneys and kidney function. Dysfunctions of the urinary system and the kidneys are sufficiently common, and you will often see them in the field. (pp. 1329–1330)

II. General mechanisms of nontraumatic tissue problems (p. 1330)
   A. Traumatic (p. 1330)
   B. Nontraumatic (p. 1330)
      1. Inflammatory or immune-mediated disease
      2. Infectious disease
      3. Physical obstruction
      4. Hemorrhage

III. General pathophysiology, assessment, and management (pp. 1331–1335)
   A. Pathophysiologic basis of pain (p. 1331)
      1. Causes of pain
      2. Types of pain
   B. Assessment and management (pp. 1331–1335)
      1. Scene size-up
      2. Initial assessment
      3. Focused history
         a. OPQRST
         b. Previous history of similar event
         c. Nausea/vomiting
         d. Changes in bowel habit or stool
         e. Weight loss
         f. Last oral intake
         g. Chest pain
      4. Focused physical examination
         a. Appearance
         b. Posture
         c. Level of consciousness

        d. Apparent state of health
        e. Skin color
        f. Examination of the abdomen
        g. Assessment tools
        h. Vital signs
    5. Management and treatment plans
        a. ABCs
        b. Pharmacological interventions
        c. Nonpharmacological interventions
        d. Transport considerations

IV. Renal and urological emergencies (pp. 1335–1347)

A. Acute renal failure (ARF) (pp. 1335–1338)
    1. Pathophysiology (**Table 33-1, p. 1336**)
        a. ARF prerenal
        b. Renal ARF
            i. Microangiopathy
            ii. Acute tubular necrosis
            iii. Interstitial nephritis
        c. Postrenal ARF
    2. Assessment (**Figs. 33-1 and 33-2, p. 1338**)
    3. Management

B. Chronic renal failure (pp. 1338–1343)
    1. End-stage renal failure
    2. Pathophysiology
        a. Reduction in nephron mass (**Table 33-2, p. 1339**)
    3. Assessment (**Table 33-3, p. 1340**)
    4. Management
        a. Immediate management
        b. Long-term management
            i. Hemodialysis (**Fig. 33-3, p. 1342**)
            ii. Peritoneal dialysis (**Fig. 33-4, p. 1343**)

C. Renal calculi (pp. 1343–1345) (**Fig. 33-5, p. 1344**)
    1. Pathophysiology
    2. Assessment
    3. Management

D. Priapism (p. 1345)

E. Urinary tract infection (pp. 1345–1347)
    1. Pathophysiology
        a. Urethritis
        b. Cystitis
        c. Prostatitis
        d. Pyelonephritis
        e. Intrarenal abscesses
        f. Perinephric abscesses
        g. Community-acquired infections
        h. Nosocomial infections
    2. Assessment
    3. Management

V. Chapter summary (pp. 1347–1348). The urinary system (1) maintains blood volume and the proper balance of water, electrolytes, and pH; (2) enables the blood to retain key substances such as glucose and removes a variety of toxic wastes from the blood; (3) plays a major role in regulation of arterial blood pressure; and (4) controls maturation of red blood cells. Kidney nephrons produce urine. Homeostasis through urine production is responsible for the first

---

POINT TO EMPHASIZE
A decrease in the level of consciousness in a patient with previously good mental function suggests severe ARF and a potential threat to life.

POINT OF INTEREST
Causes of prerenal ARF (inadequate renal perfusion) include heatstroke and burns.

POWERPOINT PRESENTATION
Chapter 33 PowerPoint slides 17–39

POINT OF INTEREST
In some unusual circumstances, dialysis has been used to treat specific poisonings.

POINT TO EMPHASIZE
Use care and caution when caring for hemodialysis patients. Two of the most common complications are bleeding from the needle puncture site and local infection.

POINT TO EMPHASIZE
In cases of abdominal pain, use analgesics as sparingly as possible. They may mask the signs and symptoms of the problem.

PATHO PEARLS
About Kidney Stones

TEACHING STRATEGY 2
Kidney Stone Display

POINT TO EMPHASIZE
Personal and family history play an important part in the diagnosis of kidney stones.

POINT OF INTEREST
One way of treating or preventing urinary tract infections is the regular ingestion of cranberry juice, which makes urine more acidic. Bacteria cannot live in acidic conditions.

POWERPOINT PRESENTATION
Chapter 33 PowerPoint slide 40

two functions and assists in the third, regulating blood pressure, by producing renin, the enzyme through which blood pressure is controlled. Other kidney cells produce erythropoietin, the hormone that stimulates red blood cell maturation. Renal and urologic emergencies typically present as an acute abdomen. The most common are acute renal failure (ARF), chronic renal failure (CRF, with the subset of end-stage renal disease), and renal calculi. Both ARF and CRF may present with life-threatening complications and impaired function of other systems. Be prepared for apparently stable patients to acutely develop destabilizing complications (often, cardiovascular). Urinary tract infections (UTIs) are divided into those of the lower urinary tract (urethra, bladder, and prostate in men) and those of the upper urinary tract (kidney). Both types of infection can present with considerable pain, but pyelonephritis is the more serious, with fever likely and complications including abscesses possible. Because renal function is often lowered in the elderly and in persons with hypertension or diabetes, consider it potentially impaired in all of these patients. The best prevention strategies are to minimize the likelihood of prerenal failure by protecting blood volume and blood pressure and to investigate possible postrenal urinary tract obstruction.

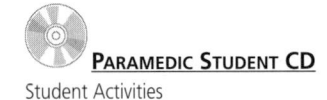

ASSIGNMENTS

Assign students to complete Chapter 33, "Urology and Nephrology," of the workbook. Also assign them to read Chapter 34, "Toxicology and Substance Abuse," before the next class.

EVALUATION

Chapter Quiz and Scenario Distribute copies of the Chapter Quiz provided in Handout 33-2 to evaluate student understanding of this chapter. Make sure each student reads the scenario to reinforce critical thinking on the scene. Remind students not to use their notes or textbooks while taking the quiz.

Student CD Quizzes for every chapter are contained on the dynamic and highly visual in-text student CD.

Companion Website Additional quizzes for every chapter are contained on this exciting website.

TestGen You may wish to create a custom-tailored test using *Prentice Hall TestGen for Essentials of Paramedic Care*, 2nd Edition to evaluate student understanding of this chapter.

On-line Test Preparation (for students and instructors) Additional test preparation is available through Brady's new on-line product, *EMT Achieve: Paramedic Test Preparation* at *http://www.prenhall.com/emtachieve/*. Instructors can also monitor student mastery on-line.

Review Manual for the EMT-Paramedic This comprehensive exam review contains hundreds of test questions and rationales, including scenarios, along with two 180-question practice tests on CD.

REINFORCEMENT

Handouts If classroom discussion or performance on the quiz indicates that some students have not fully mastered the chapter content, you may wish to assign some or all of the Reinforcement Handouts for this chapter.

Student CD (for students) A wide variety of material on this CD-ROM will reinforce and also expand student knowledge and skills.

PowerPoint Presentation (for instructors) The PowerPoint material developed for this chapter offers useful reinforcement of chapter content.

Companion Website (for students) Additional review quizzes and links to EMS resources will contribute to further reinforcement of the chapter.

OneKey On-line support is offered for this course on one of three platforms: CourseCompass, Blackboard, or Web CT. Includes the IRM, PowerPoints, TestGen, and Companion Website for instruction. Ask your local sales representative for more information.

Brady Skills Series: Advanced Life Skills (Video or CD) Have your students watch the skills come to life on VHS or CD-ROM, or they can purchase the highly visual, full-color text with step-by-step procedures and rationales.

HANDOUT 33-4
Reinforcement Activity

PARAMEDIC STUDENT CD
Student Activities

POWERPOINT PRESENTATION
Chapter 33

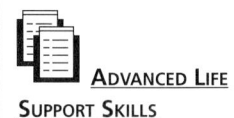

COMPANION WEBSITE
http://www.prenhall.com/bledsoe

ONEKEY
Chapter 33

ADVANCED LIFE SUPPORT SKILLS
Larmon & Davis. *Advanced Life Support Skills.*

ADVANCED LIFE SKILLS REVIEW
Larmon & Davis. *Advanced Life Skills Review.*

BRADY SKILLS SERIES: ALS
Larmon & Davis. *Brady Skills Series: ALS.*

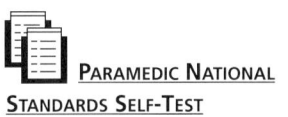

PARAMEDIC NATIONAL STANDARDS SELF-TEST
Miller. *Paramedic National Standards Self-Test,* 4th edition.

Handout 33-1

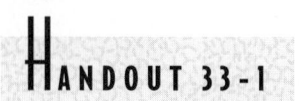

Student's Name _____

CHAPTER 33 OBJECTIVES CHECKLIST

Knowledge	Date Mastered
1. Describe the incidence, morbidity, mortality, and risk factors predisposing to urologic and nephrologic emergencies.	
2. Discuss the anatomy and physiology of the organs and structures related to the urinary system.	
3. Define referred pain and visceral pain as they relate to urology.	
4. Describe the questioning technique and specific questions the paramedic should use when gathering a focused history in a patient with abdominal pain.	
5. Describe the technique for performing a comprehensive physical examination of a patient complaining of abdominal pain.	
6. Define acute renal failure.	
7. Discuss the pathophysiology of acute renal failure.	
8. Recognize the signs and symptoms related to acute renal failure.	
9. Describe the management of acute renal failure.	
10. Integrate pathophysiological principles and assessment findings to formulate a field impression and implement a treatment plan for the patient with acute renal failure.	
11. Define chronic renal failure.	
12. Discuss the pathophysiology of chronic renal failure.	
13. Recognize the signs and symptoms related to chronic renal failure.	
14. Describe the management of chronic renal failure.	
15. Integrate pathophysiological principles and assessment findings to formulate a field impression and implement a treatment plan for the patient with chronic renal failure.	
16. Define renal dialysis.	
17. Discuss the common complications of renal dialysis.	
18. Define renal calculi.	
19. Discuss the pathophysiology of renal calculi.	

HANDOUT 33-1 Continued

Knowledge	Date Mastered
20. Recognize the signs and symptoms related to renal calculi.	
21. Describe the management of renal calculi.	
22. Integrate pathophysiological principles and assessment findings to formulate a field impression and implement a treatment plan for the patient with renal calculi.	
23. Define urinary tract infection.	
24. Discuss the pathophysiology of urinary tract infection.	
25. Recognize the signs and symptoms related to urinary tract infection.	
26. Describe the management of a urinary tract infection.	
27. Integrate pathophysiological principles and assessment findings to formulate a field impression and implement a treatment plan for the patient with a urinary tract infection.	
28. Apply epidemiology to develop prevention strategies for urologic and nephrologic emergencies.	
29. Integrate pathophysiological principles to the assessment of a patient with abdominal pain.	
30. Synthesize assessment findings and patient history information to accurately differentiate between pain of a urologic or nephrologic emergency and that of another origin.	
31. Develop, execute, and evaluate a treatment plan based on the field impression made in the assessment.	

Handout 33-2

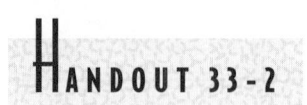

Student's Name _____

CHAPTER 33 QUIZ

Write the letter of the best answer in the space provided.

_____ 1. An extreme failure of kidney function due to nephron loss is called:
  A. acute polynephritis.
  B. chronic renal failure.
  C. chronic nephritis.
  D. end-stage renal failure.

_____ 2. Benign prostatic hypertrophy is:
  A. a noncancerous enlargement of the prostate associated with aging.
  B. a noncancerous enlargement of the prostate due to fluid/blood engorgement.
  C. tissue necrosis of the prostate due to decreased perfusion.
  D. infection caused by swelling of the prostate gland, which eventually compresses the urethra.

_____ 3. Pain arising in hollow organs such as the ureter and bladder is called:
  A. referred pain.
  B. visceral pain.
  C. rebound pain.
  D. inflammatory pain.

_____ 4. Besides the OPQRST mnemonic used to obtain information about a patient's pain, also ask about:
  A. changes in bowel habits or stool.
  B. weight loss.
  C. chest pain.
  D. all of these

_____ 5. If your patient is suffering from peritonitis, his position of comfort will most likely be:
  A. standing erect.
  B. lying prone.
  C. seated, leaning forward.
  D. lying with knees drawn to the chest.

_____ 6. Pain induced by percussion of the flanks indicates:
  A. ureter blockage.
  B. kidney infection.
  C. bladder infection.
  D. prostatic enlargement.

_____ 7. Patients are considered surgical emergencies if their abdominal pain has lasted longer than:
  A. 24 hours.
  B. 12 hours.
  C. 6 hours.
  D. 4 hours.

_____ 8. A sudden drop in urine output to less than 400–500 ml per day, or no urine output, is an indication of:
  A. renal calculi.
  B. acute renal failure.
  C. chronic renal failure.
  D. acute urinary tract infection.

_____ 9. Acute renal failure due to decreased blood perfusion to the kidneys is called:
  A. postrenal ARF.
  B. renal ARF.
  C. prerenal ARF.
  D. anurimic ARF.

_____ 10. Common causes of the condition described in question 19 include:
  A. hemorrhage.
  B. heart failure.
  C. shock.
  D. all of these

_____ 11. More than half of all cases of end-stage renal failure are caused by hypertension and:
  A. heart failure.
  B. infections.
  C. diabetes mellitus.
  D. alcoholism.

_____ 12. The dialysis procedure relying on vascular access to the blood and on an artificial membrane is known as:
  A. dialysate.
  B. hemodialysis.
  C. peritoneal dialysis.
  D. semipermeable dialysis.

HANDOUT 33-2 (Continued)

_____ 13. Benign prostatic hypertrophy is a:
  A. cancerous shrinkage of the prostate.
  B. noncancerous shrinkage of the prostate.
  C. cancerous enlargement of the prostate.
  D. noncancerous enlargement of the prostate.

_____ 14. Priapism is a painful and prolonged erection of the penis affecting:
  A. only the corpora cavernosa.
  B. only the corpora spongiosum.
  C. both the corpora cavernosa and the corpora spongiosum.
  D. neither the corpora cavernosa and the corpora spongiosum.

_____ 15. Possible causes of priapism include:
  A. MDMA (ecstasy).   C. carbon monoxide poisoning.
  B. sickle cell disease.   D. all of these

Handout 33-3

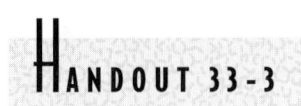

Student's Name _____

CHAPTER 33 SCENARIO

Review the following real-life situation. Then answer the questions that follow.

Highland Medic 6 is dispatched for a sickness at the rest area on U.S. Highway 41. On arrival, they find a 48-year-old male complaining of excruciating pain in his back. He was driving to a vacation site in the woods when the pain suddenly came upon him. No longer able to drive, he pulled into the rest area, and his wife used the pay phone to call 911.

Mr. Clark is a slightly overweight man with a history of gout (for which he takes Zyloprim) and high blood pressure. Other than the chronic problems, he has been in excellent health until today.

As the crew attempts to obtain a history on Mr. Clark, he is very restless and will not sit still. He keeps asking for something for the pain, but the crew tells him that they have nothing to give him. After some effort, they find that the patient is having difficulty urinating and there is some blood in his urine. The patient also reports that he has felt very nauseous since the pain started.

Except for the patient's obvious distress and slightly elevated vital signs (BP is 150/100 and pulse 105), the crew can find nothing abnormal on their physical exam. The patient is placed in the ambulance and an IV of normal saline is started and run at 100 mL/hour. The patient is transported to the hospital without incident.

1. What is Mr. Clark's problem and what leads you to that conclusion?

2. What prehospital treatment is indicated for this condition?

3. How will this treatment help alleviate the problem?

4. What will be Mr. Clark's hospital course and what is his prognosis?

HANDOUT 33-4

Student's Name _____

CHAPTER 33 REVIEW

Write the word or words that best complete the following sentences in the space(s) provided.

1. _____ is the medical specialty dealing with the kidneys.
2. An extreme failure of the kidneys due to the loss of nephrons is _____-_____ _____ _____.
3. The common term for renal calculi is _____ _____.
4. The noncancerous enlargement of the prostate associated with aging is called _____ _____ _____.
5. _____ pain is pain arising in hollow organs such as the ureter and bladder.
6. Pain felt in a location other than that of its origin is called _____ pain.
7. Management of the patient with abdominal pain includes the administration of fluids or medication only by _____ or _____ routes. Give nothing by _____.
8. _____ _____ _____ is indicated by the sudden onset of severely decreased urine production, or _____; urine output falling to zero is a condition called _____.
9. Permanently inadequate renal function due to nephron loss is called _____ _____ _____.
10. _____ dialysis is a dialysis procedure that relies on the peritoneal membrane as the semipermeable membrane.
11. _____ is an infection and inflammation of the urinary bladder.
12. UTI management should center on the _____ and _____ _____.
13. Priapism affects only the _____ _____. The _____ _____ remains flaccid.
14. A _____ is a medical emergency and requires prompt intervention by a urologist to prevent permanent damage and penile dysfunction.
15. The _____ _____ maintains blood volume and the proper balance of water, electrolytes, and pH; enables the blood to retain key substances such as glucose and removes a variety of toxic wastes from the blood; plays a major role in regulation of arterial blood pressure; and controls maturation of red blood cells.

REINFORCEMENT

Chapter 33 Answer Key

Handout 33-2: Chapter 33 Quiz

1. D	6. B	11. C
2. A	7. C	12. B
3. B	8. B	13. D
4. D	9. C	14. A
5. D	10. D	15. D

Handout 33-3: Chapter 33 Scenario

1. The problem is a kidney stone, indicated by excruciating back pain of sudden onset, history of gout, difficulty urinating, hematuria, nausea, and anxiousness/restlessness.
2. Treatment is to make the patient as comfortable as possible, provide pain relief as directed by medical control, and provide IV fluids.
3. The IV fluids will cause dilation of the ureter and help facilitate passage of the stone.
4. The hospital will provide pain relief and fluids to help pass the stone. If it doesn't pass, they will use lithotripsy to break up the stone or surgery to remove the stone. Prognosis is good, but possible complications include inflammation, infection, and partial or total urinary obstruction.

Handout 33-4: Chapter 33 Review

1. Nephrology
2. end-stage renal failure
3. kidney stones
4. benign prostatic hypertrophy
5. Visceral
6. referred
7. IV, IM, mouth
8. Acute renal failure, oliguria, anuria
9. chronic renal failure
10. Peritoneal
11. Cystitis
12. ABCs, circulatory support
13. corpora cavernosa, corpora spongiosum
14. priapism
15. urinary system

Chapter 34
Toxicology and Substance Abuse

INTRODUCTION

Toxicological emergencies have become more prevalent in recent years. These emergencies can be challenging to the paramedic because there are so many substances that can cause accidental or intentional overdoses. This chapter discusses the various aspects of toxicological emergencies as they apply to prehospital care.

CHAPTER OBJECTIVES

After reading this chapter, you should be able to:

1. Describe the incidence, morbidity, and mortality of toxic and drug abuse emergencies. (p. 1351)
2. Identify the risk factors most predisposing to toxic emergencies. (p. 1351)
3. Discuss the anatomy and physiology of the organs and structures related to toxic emergencies. (pp. 1352–1353)
4. Describe the routes of entry of toxic substances into the body. (pp. 1352–1353)
5. Discuss the role of poison control centers in the United States. (p. 1351)
6. Discuss the pathophysiology, assessment findings, need for rapid intervention and transport, and management of toxic emergencies. (pp. 1350–1386)
7. List the most common poisonings, pathophysiology, assessment findings, and management of poisoning by ingestion, inhalation, absorption, injection, and overdose. (pp. 1352–1386)
8. Define the following terms:
   - Substance or drug abuse (p. 1380)
   - Substance or drug dependence (p. 1380)
   - Tolerance (p. 1380)
   - Withdrawal (p. 1380)
   - Addiction (p. 1380)

TOTAL TEACHING TIME:
9.03 HOURS
The total teaching time is only a guideline based on the didactic and practical lab averages in the National Standard Curriculum. Instructors should take into consideration such factors as the pace at which students learn, the size of the class, and breaks. The actual time devoted to teaching objectives is the responsibility of the instructor.

©2007 Pearson Education, Inc.
Essentials of Paramedic Care, 2nd ed.

9. List the most commonly abused drugs (both by chemical name and by street names). (pp. 1381, 1382–1383)
10. Describe the pathophysiology, assessment findings, and management of commonly used drugs. (pp. 1380–1386)
11. List the clinical uses, street names, pharmacology, assessment findings, and management for patients who have taken the following drugs or been exposed to the following substances:

    - Cocaine (pp. 1361, 1381, 1382)
    - Marijuana and cannabis compounds (p. 1383)
    - Amphetamines and amphetamine-like drugs (pp. 1381, 1383)
    - Barbiturates (pp. 1381, 1382)
    - Sedative-hypnotics (p. 1383)
    - Cyanide (pp. 1359, 1362)
    - Narcotics/opiates (pp. 1361, 1381, 1382)
    - Cardiac medications (p. 1363)
    - Caustics (pp. 1363–1364)
    - Common household substances (pp. 1363–1364)
    - Drugs abused for sexual purposes/sexual gratification (p. 1381)
    - Carbon monoxide (pp. 1359, 1361, 1362–1363)
    - Alcohols (pp. 1361, 1381, 1382, 1383–1386)
    - Hydrocarbons (p. 1365)
    - Psychiatric medications (pp. 1365–1367)
    - Newer antidepressants and serotonin syndromes (pp. 1366–1367)
    - Lithium (p. 1367)
    - MAO inhibitors (p. 1366)
    - Nonprescription pain medications: (1) nonsteroidal antiinflammatory agents, (2) salicylates, (3) acetaminophen (pp. 1368–1369)
    - Theophylline (p. 1369)
    - Metals (pp. 1361, 1369–1370)
    - Plants and mushrooms (pp. 1371–1372)

12. Discuss common causative agents or offending organisms, pharmacology, assessment findings, and management for a patient with food poisoning, a bite, or a sting. (pp. 1370–1371, 1373–1380)
13. Given several scenarios of poisoning or overdose, provide the appropriate assessment, treatment, and transport. (pp. 1350–1386)

FRAMING THE LESSON

Begin class by reviewing the important points from Chapter 33, "Urology and Nephrology." Discuss any aspects of the chapter that students do not fully understand. Then begin with Chapter 34 material. You may wish to begin the lesson with a review of the anatomy and physiology of the organs affected by toxic substances and substance abuse, including the liver and kidneys. Ask students to name some of the substances that can be toxic or poisonous. These should include household cleaners, medications, agricultural products, and so on. Prior to the class, obtain information and reports from the area poison prevention agency, often part of state or district health departments. These agencies will often have annual poisoning reports listed by substance, age range, and geographic area. Stress that the number of incidents involving young children ages 1–5 account for half of all poisonings. Obtain pamphlets, phone stickers, and other materials from the Poison Control Center (PCC) that covers your geographic area, and distribute them to students. Obtain standing orders from your area EMS units on poisoning calls and discuss them now and during other classes. Ask any students who have had an occasion to call the

PCC for any type of poisoning or ingestion to briefly tell the class about the situation.

TEACHING STRATEGIES

People learn in a variety of ways. Some do better with the spoken word, whereas others prefer the written. Some prefer to work alone, whereas others profit from working in groups. Recognizing these different ways of acquiring knowledge, the authors of this *Instructor's Resource Manual* have provided a variety of teaching strategies for the different types of learners. These strategies are intended to foster higher-level cognitive skills and encourage creative learning and problem solving. For greatest effectiveness, incorporate these strategies into your class lecture. Symbols in the Lecture Outline indicate the points at which various exercises might be most appropriate. Other strategies can be used to preview the lesson or to summarize it.

The following strategies are keyed to specific sections of the lesson.

1. Flash Cards. This is an excellent chapter for the use of flash cards. You could divide students into two groups. One group is to make cards with names of poisons on one side and signs and symptoms of poisoning by that substance on the other. The second group should make cards with the names of the poisons on one side and the field treatment for poisoning by that substance on the other. When all cards are done you can have the class as a whole try identifying poisons by signs and symptoms or treatments or matching treatments with signs and symptoms.

2. Poison Control Center Stickers. Print or obtain stickers with the number to the Poison Control Centers in your area. Give students several of these to place in their ambulance and home. Encourage the use of the centers for both emergencies and consultations during potential emergencies.

3. Household Poison Look-Alike Kit. Create a look-alike kit for household poisons. Many poisons look like other benign products, and having them next to each other can be a powerful visual tool for your students. Examples include: Comet and parmesan cheese, toothpaste and nitroglycerine paste, Pine-Sol and apple juice, medicines and candy.

4. Antidote Pocket Reference. Make and distribute a pocket reference card for the antidotes of toxicological emergencies listed in Table 33-1. This will encourage students to use the proper treatment when one exists.

5. Simulation Props. Enhance your simulations with props that will facilitate a history or exam centered around a toxin exposure. Use paint on the fingertips of a patient who has been "huffing"; place a patient in the bathroom who has succumbed to cleaning vapors in a confined space; place a patient outside who has been fertilizing the lawn; or place patients in the backseat of a vehicle that has a leaky exhaust system, poisoning the occupants with carbon monoxide. Scenarios like these will require critical thinking skills and clinical decision making on behalf of your students because they are outside the normal overdoses and exposures commonly encountered, yet are still very plausible.

6. Carbon Monoxide Detector Demonstration. Bring in a carbon monoxide detector to demonstrate its use and limitations. The devices are now as common in households as smoke detectors. You might even ask a fire prevention officer to explain how it is supposed to be used.

7. Zoo-Toxicity. If you live in an area in which snake bites are rare, have an expert from your local zoo come in and talk about them. No one is more familiar or experienced in handling these situations. Request that the speaker bring in examples of various snakes and insects that cause toxicological emergencies. If it is not possible for someone from a local zoo to come to class, organize a field trip to the zoo for students.

The following strategies can be used at various points throughout the lesson or to help summarize and demonstrate what students have learned.

Poison Control Center Visit. If there is one close by, arrange for students to visit a regional/local Poison Control Center for a clinical rotation. Have students listen in on calls received by the PCC. You may also consider having someone from the PCC come and visit the class to discuss the types of calls they receive and how they are handled.

Clinical Rotation in Chemical Dependency Unit of Hospital. Clinical time in the chemical dependency or dual-diagnosis unit of your hospital is useful for students in the understanding of substance abuse patients. They will likely be able to participate in group therapy and recreational activities of the patients. The time spent with patients, talking and understanding their weaknesses, fears, addictions, and pathologies, will probably teach students more than time spent with the staff. However, a staff member with excellent verbal management skills can be priceless in teaching students to use words instead of touching to manage potentially violent or disruptive patients.

Toxi-Bingo. Make up several sets of cards four squares wide by four squares high. Randomly distribute 16 numbers chosen from 1 through 25 in the squares. Write the numbers 1 to 25 on separate slips of paper and place them in a container. Prepare a list of 25 questions about toxicology and substance abuse and number the questions.

Distribute the "toxi-bingo" cards to students. Explain that you'll draw numbers from the container and read the question from your list that corresponds to that number. Students who have the number on their cards should write in what they think is the correct answer. The first student to complete a row of correct answers across the card—horizontally, vertically, or diagonally—wins. Be sure, however, to check winning cards to ensure that answers are correct.

Cultural Considerations, Legal Notes, and Patho Pearls. The student CD-ROM contains this series of informative features to enhance the student's understanding of the material covered in this chapter.

HANDOUT 34-1
Chapter 34 Objectives Checklist

TEACHING STRATEGY 1
Flash Cards

READING/REFERENCE
Schaeffer, J. "CDC Funds Exclusive Hotline for Poison Control." *JEMS*, March 2000.

TEACHING TIP
What are the medical control or Poison Control Center procedures in your system? Can the PCC give orders to administer activated charcoal or other treatments?

TEACHING OUTLINE

Chapter 34 is the eighth lesson in Division 4, *Medical Emergencies*. Distribute Handout 34-1 so that students can familiarize themselves with the learning goals for this chapter. If students have any questions about the objectives, answer them at this time.

Then present the chapter. One possible lecture outline follows. In the outline, the parenthetical references in regular type are references to text pages; those in bold type are references to figures, tables, or procedures.

I. Introduction. Toxicological emergencies result from the ingestion, inhalation, surface absorption, or injection of toxic substances that exert their adverse effects on the body. This chapter discusses various aspects of toxicological emergencies as they apply to prehospital care, including general treatment guidelines and specific issues surrounding the more common substances involved. (pp. 1350–1351)

II. Epidemiology (p. 1351)

A. Over 4 million poisonings occur annually. (p. 1351)
B. Ten percent of all ED and EMS responses involve toxic exposures. (p. 1351)
C. Seventy percent of accidental poisonings occur in children < 6 years of age. (p. 1351)
D. Eighty percent of all attempted suicides involve a drug overdose. (p. 1351)

III. Poison Control Centers (p. 1351)

IV. Routes of toxic exposure (pp. 1351–1353)

A. Ingestion (p. 1352)
B. Inhalation (p. 1352)
C. Surface absorption (p. 1352)
D. Injection (p. 1353)

V. General principles of toxicologic assessment and management (pp. 1353–1355)

A. Scene size-up (p. 1353)
B. Initial assessment (p. 1353)
C. History, physical exam, and ongoing assessment (pp. 1353–1354)
D. Treatment (pp. 1354–1355)
   1. Decontamination
   2. Antidotes (**Table 34-1, p. 1355**)
E. Suicidal patients and protective custody (p. 1355)

VI. Ingested toxins (pp. 1356–1357)

A. Assessment (pp. 1356–1357)
   1. History
   2. Physical examination
      a. Skin
      b. Eyes
      c. Mouth
      d. Chest
      e. Circulation
      f. Abdomen
B. Management (p. 1357)
   1. Prevent aspiration
   2. Administer fluids and drugs
   3. Do not induce vomiting

VII. Inhaled toxins (pp. 1357–1358)

A. Assessment (pp. 1357–1358)
   1. Central nervous system
   2. Respiratory
   3. Cardiac
B. Management (p. 1358)
   1. Safely remove patient from poisonous environment.
      a. Wear protective clothing.
      b. Use appropriate respiratory protection.
      c. Remove patient's contaminated clothing.
   2. Perform the initial assessment, history, and physical exam.
   3. Initiate supportive measures.
   4. Contact the Poison Control Center and medical direction, per local protocols.

POWERPOINT PRESENTATION
Chapter 34 PowerPoint slide 4

POWERPOINT PRESENTATION
Chapter 34 PowerPoint slide 5

POWERPOINT PRESENTATION
Chapter 34 PowerPoint slides 6–9

POWERPOINT PRESENTATION
Chapter 34 PowerPoint slides 10–16

TEACHING STRATEGY 2
Poison Control Center Stickers

POWERPOINT PRESENTATION
Chapter 34 PowerPoint slides 17–19

POINT OF INTEREST
To remember the signs and symptoms of acute cholinergic poisoning, students can use the mnemonic DUMBELS: Diarrhea, Urination, Meiosis, Bronchospasm, Emesis, Lacrimation, Salivation.

TEACHING STRATEGY 3
Household Poison Look-Alike Kit

POINT TO EMPHASIZE
Like an astute detective, the paramedic must use all senses (except taste) to gather information from the scene.

POWERPOINT PRESENTATION
Chapter 34 PowerPoint slides 20–21

TEACHING STRATEGY 4
Antidote Pocket Reference

POINT TO EMPHASIZE
Where is there freon in every home?

POWERPOINT PRESENTATION
Chapter 34 PowerPoint slide 22

TEACHING TIP
Have students come up with commonly encountered examples of toxic gases.

TEACHING STRATEGY 5
Simulation Props

POWERPOINT PRESENTATION
Chapter 34 PowerPoint slides 23–51

TEACHING TIP
During the discussion of surface-absorbed poisons, review the effects of parasympathetic nervous system stimulation.

TEACHING STRATEGY 6
Carbon Monoxide Detector Demonstration

VIII. **Surface-absorbed toxins** (pp. 1358–1359)
   A. Assessment (p. 1358)
   B. Management (pp. 1358–1359)
      1. Safely remove patient from poisonous environment.
         a. Wear protective clothing.
         b. Use appropriate respiratory protection.
         c. Remove patient's contaminated clothing.
      2. Perform the initial assessment, history, and physical exam.
      3. Initiate supportive measures.
      4. Contact the Poison Control Center and medical direction, per local protocols.

IX. **Specific toxins** (pp. 1359–1372) (Table 34-2, pp. 1360–1361)
   A. Cyanide (p. 1359) (Fig. 34-1, p. 1362)
      1. Signs and symptoms
      2. Management
   B. Carbon monoxide (pp. 1359, 1362–1363) (Fig. 34-2, p. 1362)
      1. Signs and symptoms
      2. Management
   C. Cardiac medications (p. 1363)
      1. Signs and symptoms
      2. Management
   D. Caustic substances (pp. 1363–1364)
      1. Signs and symptoms
      2. Management
   E. Hydrofluoric acid (p. 1364)
      1. Signs and symptoms
      2. Management
   F. Hydrocarbons (p. 1365)
      1. Signs and symptoms
      2. Management
   G. Tricyclic antidepressants (pp. 1365–1366)
      1. Signs and symptoms
      2. Management
   H. MAO inhibitors (p. 1366)
      1. Signs and symptoms
      2. Management
   I. Newer antidepressants (pp. 1366–1367)
      1. Signs and symptoms
      2. Management
   J. Lithium (p. 1367)
      1. Signs and symptoms
      2. Management
   K. Salicylates (p. 1368)
      1. Signs and symptoms
      2. Management
   L. Acetaminophen (p. 1368)
      1. Signs and symptoms
      2. Management
   M. Other nonprescription pain medications (p. 1369)
      1. Signs and symptoms
      2. Management
   N. Theophylline (p. 1369)
      1. Signs and symptoms
      2. Management

- **O.** Metals (pp. 1369–1370)
    1. Iron
        a. Signs and symptoms
        b. Management
    2. Lead and mercury
        a. Signs and symptoms
        b. Management
- **P.** Contaminated food (pp. 1370–1371)
    1. Signs and symptoms
    2. Management
- **Q.** Poisonous plants and mushrooms (pp. 1371–1372) (**Fig. 34-3, p. 1372**)
    1. Signs and symptoms
    2. Management

X. Injected toxins (pp. 1372–1380)

- **A.** General principles of management (pp. 1372–1373)
- **B.** Insect bites and stings (pp. 1372–1379)
    1. Insect stings
        a. Signs and symptoms
        b. Management
    2. Brown recluse spider bite (**Figs. 34-4 and 34-5, p. 1374; Fig 34-6, p. 1375**)
        a. Signs and symptoms
        b. Management
    3. Black widow spider bites (**Fig. 34-7, p. 1375**)
        a. Signs and symptoms
        b. Management
    4. Scorpion stings (**Fig. 34-8, p. 1376**)
        a. Signs and symptoms
        b. Management
    5. Snakebites (**Fig. 34-9, p. 1377**)
        a. Pit viper bites
            i. Signs and symptoms
            ii. Management
        b. Coral snakebites
            i. Signs and symptoms
            ii. Management
- **C.** Marine animal injection (pp. 1379–1380) (**Fig. 34-10, p. 1379**)
    1. Signs and symptoms
    2. Management

XI. Substance abuse and overdose (pp. 1380–1381)

- **A.** Drugs of abuse (p. 1381)
    1. Drugs commonly abused (**Table 34-3, pp. 1382–1383**)
        a. Alcohol
        b. Cocaine
        c. Narcotics/opiates
        d. Amphetamines
        e. Hallucinogens
        f. Benzodiazepines
        g. Barbiturates
    2. Drugs used for sexual purposes
        a. Ecstasy/MDMA
        b. Rohypnol

XII. Alcohol abuse (pp. 1381–1386)

- **A.** Psychological effects (pp. 1381, 1384)

POINT OF INTEREST
There are 2,600 black widow spider bites reported each year, over one-half of them with severe reactions. The black widow is the leading cause of spider-related death in the United States.

POINT TO EMPHASIZE
To distinguish the poisonous coral snake from nonpoisonous snakes, refer to the snake's color rings and this poem: Red on black, venom lack; red on yellow, kills a fellow.

POWERPOINT PRESENTATION
Chapter 34 PowerPoint slides 52–65

TEACHING STRATEGY 7
Zoo-Toxicity

TEACHING TIP
Have someone from the local aquarium come to your class and teach about marine animals and injection poisoning.

TEACHING TIP
Contact local law enforcement agencies and invite a street drug expert to talk about this topic. Ask the expert to bring in samples of paraphernalia associated with drug use.

READING/REFERENCE
Gross, J. "Clinical Clues to Illicit Drug Use." *JEMS*, March 1999.
Newman, E. "Drug Abuse Trends." *EMS*, Nov. 1999.

POWERPOINT PRESENTATION
Chapter 34 PowerPoint slides 66–71

POINT TO EMPHASIZE
Many health-care workers are "turned-off" by the intoxicated or suicidal patient. Don't be judgmental. Instead, meet the challenge your patient presents, and you will be rewarded.

POWERPOINT PRESENTATION
Chapter 34 PowerPoint slides 72–75

> **PowerPoint Presentation**
> Chapter 34 PowerPoint slide 76

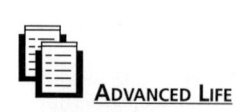

B. General alcoholic profile (p. 1384) (Fig. 34-11, p. 1385)
   1. Drinks early in the day
   2. Prone to drink alone and secretly
   3. Periodic binges (may last for several days)
   4. Partial or total loss of memory ("blackouts") during period of drinking
   5. Unexplained history of gastrointestinal problems (especially bleeding)
   6. "Green tongue syndrome" (using chlorophyll-containing substances to disguise the odor of alcohol on the breath)
   7. Cigarette burns on clothing
   8. Chronically flushed face and palms
   9. Tremulousness
   10. Odor of alcohol on breath under inappropriate conditions
C. Consequences of chronic alcohol ingestion: withdrawal syndrome (pp. 1384–1386)
   1. Signs and symptoms
      a. Delirium tremens (DTs)
   2. Management

XIII. **Chapter summary** (p. 1386). Clearly, there is much to remember when dealing with toxicological emergencies. To effectively manage these situations you must focus on three things:

- Recognize the poisoning promptly. In other words, you must have a high index of suspicion when circumstances suggest a toxin may be involved.
- Be thorough in your initial assessment and evaluation of the patient. This will facilitate your efforts to identify the toxin and the measures needed to control the situation.
- Initiate the standard treatment procedures required for all toxicological emergencies. Beyond the usual concern for rescuer safety and rapid implementation of ABCs and supportive measures, consider the methods needed to minimize any further exposure to the toxin, decontaminate the patient from the toxins already involved, and finally administer any useful antidote if one exists for the particular toxin.

If you remember these three steps, you will be equipped to handle most toxicological emergencies promptly and efficiently.

SKILLS DEMONSTRATION AND PRACTICE

> **Advanced Life Support Skills**
> Larmon & Davis. *Advanced Life Support Skills.*
>
> **Advanced Life Skills Review**
> Larmon & Davis. *Advanced Life Skills Review.*
>
> **Brady Skills Series: ALS**
> Larmon & Davis. *Brady Skills Series: ALS.*

Students can practice skills discussed in this chapter in the following settings.

Scenario Lab: The following stations will be part of a larger medical scenario lab. Divide the class into teams. Have the teams circulate through the stations. Monitor the groups to be sure that all groups have a chance to manage each of the cases and so that every student has the opportunity to be team leader. You may wish to have other instructors or qualified paramedics assist students in these activities.

Station	Equipment Needed	Activities
Ingested Poisoning	Medication box 1 instructor 1 patient	Have students practice assessing and managing patients who have ingested poison.
Inhaled Poisoning	Medication box 1 patient 1 instructor	Have students practice assessing and managing patients who have inhaled poison.

Injected Poisoning	Medication box 1 patient 1 instructor	Have students practice assessing and managing patients who have injected poison.
Surface-Absorbed Poisoning	Medication box 1 patient 1 instructor	Have students practice assessing and managing patients who have absorbed a surface poison.

Hospital:

- Observe the management of poisonings at the regional poison center.
- Assist in the assessment and management of all types of toxicological emergencies in the ED.

Field Internship: Assist in the assessment and management of all types of toxicological emergencies in the field.

ASSIGNMENTS

Assign students to complete Chapter 34, "Toxicology and Substance Abuse," of the workbook. Also assign them to read Chapter 35, "Hematology," before the next class.

EVALUATION

Chapter Quiz and Scenario Distribute copies of the Chapter Quiz provided in Handout 34-2 to evaluate student understanding of this chapter. Make sure each student reads the scenario to reinforce critical thinking on the scene. Remind students not to use their notes or textbooks while taking the quiz.

Student CD Quizzes for every chapter are contained on the dynamic and highly visual in-text student CD.

Companion Website Additional quizzes for every chapter are contained on this exciting website.

TestGen You may wish to create a custom-tailored test using *Prentice Hall TestGen for Essentials of Paramedic Care*, 2nd Edition to evaluate student understanding of this chapter.

On-line Test Preparation (for students and instructors) Additional test preparation is available through Brady's new on-line product, *EMT Achieve: Paramedic Test Preparation* at *http://www.prenhall.com/emtachieve/*. Instructors can also monitor student mastery on-line.

Review Manual for the EMT-Paramedic This comprehensive exam review contains hundreds of test questions and rationales, including scenarios, along with two 180-question practice tests on CD.

REINFORCEMENT

Handouts If classroom discussion or performance on the quiz indicates that some students have not fully mastered the chapter content, you may wish to assign some or all of the Reinforcement Handouts for this chapter.

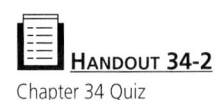

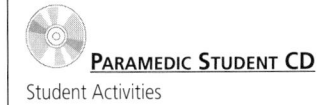

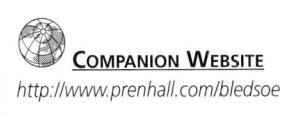

WORKBOOK
Chapter 34 Activities

READING/REFERENCE
Textbook, pp. 1389–1404

HANDOUT 34-2
Chapter 34 Quiz

HANDOUT 34-3
Chapter 34 Scenario

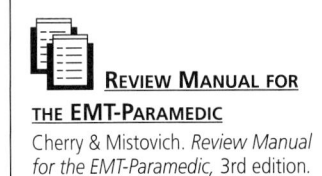

PARAMEDIC STUDENT CD
Student Activities

COMPANION WEBSITE
http://www.prenhall.com/bledsoe

TESTGEN
Chapter 34

EMT ACHIEVE:
PARAMEDIC TEST PREPARATION
Mistovich & Beasley. *EMT Achieve: Paramedic Test Preparation.*
www.prenhall.com/emtachieve/

REVIEW MANUAL FOR THE EMT-PARAMEDIC
Cherry & Mistovich. *Review Manual for the EMT-Paramedic*, 3rd edition.

HANDOUTS 34-4 TO 34-7
Reinforcement Activities

PARAMEDIC STUDENT CD
Student Activities

POWERPOINT PRESENTATION
Chapter 34

COMPANION WEBSITE
http://www.prenhall.com/bledsoe

ONEKEY
Chapter 34

ADVANCED LIFE SUPPORT SKILLS
Larmon & Davis. *Advanced Life Support Skills.*

ADVANCED LIFE SKILLS REVIEW
Larmon & Davis. *Advanced Life Skills Review.*

BRADY SKILLS SERIES: ALS
Larmon & Davis. *Brady Skills Series: ALS.*

PARAMEDIC NATIONAL STANDARDS SELF-TEST
Miller. *Paramedic National Standards Self-Test*, 4th edition.

Student CD (for students)   A wide variety of material on this CD-ROM will reinforce and also expand student knowledge and skills.

PowerPoint Presentation (for instructors)   The PowerPoint material developed for this chapter offers useful reinforcement of chapter content.

Companion Website (for students)   Additional review quizzes and links to EMS resources will contribute to further reinforcement of the chapter.

OneKey   On-line support is offered for this course on one of three platforms: CourseCompass, Blackboard, or Web CT. Includes the IRM, PowerPoints, TestGen, and Companion Website for instruction. Ask your local sales representative for more information.

Brady Skills Series: Advanced Life Skills (Video or CD)   Have your students watch the skills come to life on VHS or CD-ROM, or they can purchase the highly visual, full-color text with step-by-step procedures and rationales.

HANDOUT 34-1

Student's Name _____

CHAPTER 34 OBJECTIVES CHECKLIST

Knowledge	Date Mastered
1. Describe the incidence, morbidity, and mortality of toxic and drug abuse emergencies.	
2. Identify the risk factors most predisposing to toxic emergencies.	
3. Discuss the anatomy and physiology of the organs and structures related to toxic emergencies.	
4. Describe the routes of entry of toxic substances into the body.	
5. Discuss the role of poison control centers in the United States.	
6. Discuss the pathophysiology, assessment findings, need for rapid intervention and transport, and management of toxic emergencies.	
7. List the most common poisonings, pathophysiology, assessment findings, and management of poisoning by ingestion, inhalation, absorption, injection, and overdose.	
8. Define the following terms: • Substance or drug abuse • Substance or drug dependence • Tolerance • Withdrawal • Addiction	
9. List the most commonly abused drugs (both by chemical name and by street names).	
10. Describe the pathophysiology, assessment findings, and management of commonly used drugs.	
11. List the clinical uses, street names, pharmacology, assessment findings, and management for patients who have taken the following drugs or been exposed to the following substances: • Cocaine • Marijuana and cannabis compounds • Amphetamines and amphetamine-like drugs • Barbiturates • Sedative-hypnotics • Cyanide • Narcotics/opiates • Cardiac medications • Caustics	

OBJECTIVES

©2007 Pearson Education, Inc.
Essentials of Paramedic Care, 2nd ed.

HANDOUT 34-1 Continued

Knowledge	Date Mastered
• Common household substances • Drugs abused for sexual purposes/sexual gratification • Carbon monoxide • Alcohols • Hydrocarbons • Psychiatric medications • Newer antidepressants and serotonin syndromes • Lithium • MAO inhibitors • Nonprescription pain medications: (1) nonsteroidal antiinflammatory agents, (2) salicylates, (3) acetaminophen • Theophylline • Metals • Plants and mushrooms	
12. Discuss common causative agents or offending organisms, pharmacology, assessment findings, and management for a patient with food poisoning, a bite, or a sting.	
13. Given several scenarios of poisoning or overdose, provide the appropriate assessment, treatment, and transport.	

HANDOUT 34-2

Student's Name _____

CHAPTER 34 QUIZ

Write the letter of the best answer in the space provided.

_____ 1. Which of the following statistics is TRUE regarding toxicological emergencies in the United States?
   A. Less than 1 percent of all emergency department visits and EMS responses involve toxic exposures.
   B. A child who has experienced an accidental ingestion has a 75 percent chance of another, similar ingestion within 1 year.
   C. Some 80 percent of all attempted suicides involve a drug overdose.
   D. Some 25 percent of accidental poisonings occur in children under the age of 6 years.

_____ 2. Ingestion is the most common route of entry for toxic exposure. Other routes of entry include all of the following EXCEPT:
   A. inhalation.
   B. surface absorption.
   C. tertiary.
   D. injection.

_____ 3. Many toxic substances can pass through the skin without puncturing it. An example of this type of substance is:
   A. snakebite venom.
   B. carbon tetrachloride.
   C. gasoline.
   D. organophosphates.

_____ 4. General principles of toxicologic assessment and management include:
   A. reducing absorption of ingested toxins with administration of syrup of ipecac.
   B. enhancing the elimination of ingested toxins by administering activated charcoal.
   C. reducing intake of a surface-absorbed toxin by removing clothing and cleaning the skin with soap and water.
   D. all of these

_____ 5. Benzodiazepine overdoses are treated with the antidote:
   A. diazepam.
   B. amyl nitrite.
   C. flumazenil.
   D. naloxone.

_____ 6. One of your major objectives in treating a poisoning patient is:
   A. the administration of an antidote.
   B. prevention of aspiration.
   C. administration of IV fluids.
   D. induction of vomiting.

_____ 7. Cyanide enters the body by:
   A. ingestion.
   B. absorption.
   C. inhalation.
   D. all of these

_____ 8. You are caring for a patient with carbon monoxide poisoning. An important point to remember is which of the following?
   A. Carbon monoxide has a distinctive, "rotten egg" odor.
   B. Oxygen has more than 200 times the affinity of carbon monoxide to bind with hemoglobin.
   C. Once the carbon monoxide molecule binds with hemoglobin, it is very resistant to removal.
   D. Because carbon monoxide binds with red blood cells, internal hemorrhage is a serious complication of exposure.

HANDOUT 34-2 Continued

_____ 9. Your patient has been working in the fields of his farm for several hours. When you arrive, he presents with sweating, constricted pupils, lacrimation, excessive salivation, wheezing, cramps, vomiting, diarrhea, and urinary incontinence. You suspect his problem is:
   A. a snake bite.
   B. a spider bite.
   C. carbon monoxide poisoning.
   D. organophosphate poisoning.

_____ 10. Once airway and breathing have been managed, treatment for the patient in question 9 would include what medication?
   A. lidocaine
   B. atropine
   C. epinephrine
   D. flumazenil

_____ 11. Activated charcoal does not bind with caustic substances, so it should not be given in cases of:
   A. lithium overdose.
   B. hydrocarbon ingestion.
   C. alkali or acid ingestion.
   D. all of these

_____ 12. The range between curative and toxic doses of medications is called the:
   A. therapeutic index.
   B. toxic window.
   C. cumulative dosage.
   D. curative level.

_____ 13. A young man tells you he believes his wife has overdosed on some medication she is on for obsessive-compulsive disorder. She is complaining of a headache, nausea, and palpitations. She is very agitated, restless, and you note tremors. You suspect she may have overdosed on:
   A. lithium.
   B. an MAO inhibitor.
   C. Prozac.
   D. a tricyclic antidepressant.

_____ 14. Your patient has deliberately ingested a large dose of aspirin. Which of the following is TRUE regarding salicylate overdoses?
   A. Signs and symptoms associated with the overdose are likely to include hyperthermia, confusion, and rapid respirations.
   B. About 150 mg/kg is the dose required to cause toxicity.
   C. Aspirin overdose can result in metabolic alkalosis, further injuring organ systems.
   D. The antidote for aspirin overdose, N-acetylcysteine, is most effective when given rapidly in the prehospital setting.

_____ 15. Signs and symptoms of poisonous mushroom ingestion include:
   A. hallucinations.
   B. dry mouth.
   C. diaphoresis.
   D. constipation.

_____ 16. You are caring for a patient who is complaining of chills, fever, and nausea developed since he awoke this morning. He discovered a small, painful, erythematous macule surrounded by a white ring on his arm. You suspect a:
   A. brown recluse spider bite.
   B. black widow spider bite.
   C. scorpion sting.
   D. _Hymenoptera_ sting.

_____ 17. Management of the patient who has been bitten by a pit viper includes:
   A. application of constricting bands above and below the bite.
   B. application of a cold pack to reduce swelling and pain.
   C. maintaining the extremity in a neutral position.
   D. application of electrical stimulation to retard venom spread.

_____ 18. To relieve the pain and inactivate the venom of a marine animal injection, you should:
   A. administer acetaminophen orally.
   B. apply constricting bands above and below the site.
   C. apply ice or cold pack to relieve pain and reduce swelling.
   D. apply heat or hot water (110–113°F).

_____ 19. The condition in which the body reacts severely when deprived of an abused substance is called:
   A. withdrawal.
   B. addiction.
   C. tolerance.
   D. dependence.

HANDOUT 34-2 Continued

_____ **20.** An absolute contraindication in the treatment of cocaine overdose is:
    A. benzodiazepines.
    B. naloxone.
    C. flumazenil.
    D. beta-blockers.

_____ **21.** Alcohol abuse may be indicated by a number of warning signs, including "green tongue syndrome" resulting from:
    A. an adverse reaction of the taste buds in the tongue to excessive exposure to alcohol.
    B. decreased oxygen perfusion to tissues caused by chronic lung diseases often experienced by alcoholics.
    C. the use of chlorophyll-containing substances to disguise alcohol odor on the breath.
    D. toxins in the blood caused by liver disease.

_____ **22.** Chronic alcoholics may exhibit or experience which of the following?
    A. death resulting from delirium tremens
    B. decreased xyphoid-umbilical distance
    C. distended external jugular veins
    D. testicular enlargement

_____ **23.** The drug commonly referred to as the "date rape drug" is:
    A. Restoril.
    B. Halcion.
    C. Rohypnol.
    D. PCP.

_____ **24.** The drugs for which flumazenil is used to counteract adverse effects are:
    A. hallucinogens.
    B. benzodiazepines.
    C. marijuana derivatives.
    D. barbiturates.

_____ **25.** Delirium tremens usually develop in habitual alcoholics within how long after cessation of drinking?
    A. 10 to 12 hours
    B. 24 to 36 hours
    C. 48 to 72 hours
    D. 72 to 96 hours

HANDOUT 34-3

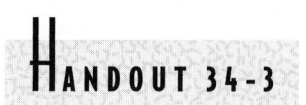

Student's Name _____

CHAPTER 34 SCENARIO

Review the following real-life situation. Then answer the questions that follow.

A woman returns home after work and finds her 14-year-old son unconscious in the empty bathtub. When she is unable to waken him, she calls 911 and returns to the bathroom, where the boy is having a generalized tonic-clonic seizure. Shortly thereafter, both police and paramedic units arrive on the scene.

The police indicate that the scene is secure, and the paramedics enter the house. They find the boy still in the bathtub. A quick assessment of the scene reveals a syringe lying beside the patient in the bathtub. A tie is secured around the boy's upper arm, and a fresh puncture wound is noted just below the tie. The initial assessment reveals that the patient is unresponsive, breathing at a rate of 4 per minute with a weak radial pulse of 132. Blood pressure is palpated at 94. Pupils are dilated and slow to react. Several needle tracks are noticed on both arms. As the assessment is completed, the patient begins another generalized tonic-clonic seizure. After paramedics manage the patient's airway, they place him on the ECG monitor, initiate an IV, and obtain a blood glucose reading of 88. The monitor shows a sinus tachycardia with frequent unifocal PVCs.

Per protocol, the paramedics administer 1 mg/kg of lidocaine IV push, and a lidocaine drip at 2 mg/min. They contact the hospital, report their findings and treatment to the emergency room physician, and request an order to administer 5 mg of Valium. The physician gives the order for the Valium, and it is administered. The patient is packaged and transported rapidly to the hospital. En route, the patient goes into respiratory arrest and is intubated. The patient remains unresponsive with a slight twitching to the right arm. Another set of vital signs taken after medication administration show a radial pulse of 100, blood pressure of 98/60, and respirations of 0. The monitor shows a sinus tachycardia with an occasional PVC. The paramedics turn the patient over to the emergency department staff with an update on his condition.

1. What type of drug would you suspect that the patient overdosed on?

2. Why do you suspect this drug?

3. Was administration of lidocaine indicated? Why or why not?

4. What information was necessary to convey to the emergency department physician?

HANDOUT 34-4

Student's Name _____

CHAPTER 34 REVIEW

Write the word or words that best complete the following sentences in the space(s) provided.

1. Any chemical that causes adverse effects on an organism that is exposed to it is called a(n) _____.
2. The term _____ is used to describe exposure to nonpharmacological substances, while _____ is used to describe exposure to pharmacological substances.
3. Some _____ percent of accidental poisonings occur in children under the age of 6.
4. Some 80 percent of all attempted suicides involve _____ _____.
5. _____ is the most common route of entry to toxic exposure.
6. The entry of a substance into the body through the respiratory tract is called _____.
7. The process of minimizing toxicity by reducing the amount of toxin absorbed into the body is called _____.
8. Principles of decontamination include reducing _____, reducing _____, and enhancing _____.
9. N-Acetylcysteine is the antidote for _____ overdose.
10. Ethyl alcohol is considered the antidote for _____ _____.
11. Preventing _____ must be one of the major objectives in treating a poisoning patient.
12. _____ _____ _____ is no longer an accepted routine intervention for patients who have ingested toxins.
13. Your first priority in any inhalation emergency is _____ _____.
14. A group of typical signs and symptoms consistently associated with exposure to a particular type of toxin is called a(n) _____.
15. Once cyanide enters the body, it acts as a cellular _____.
16. _____ _____ is an odorless, tasteless gas that is often the byproduct of incomplete combustion.
17. A cyanide antidote kit contains _____ _____ ampules.
18. _____ overdose is characterized by CNS depression, pinpoint pupils, and slowed respirations.
19. A(n) _____ is a substance that liberates hydrogen ions when in solution.
20. A(n) _____ is a substance that liberates hydroxyl ions when in solution.
21. _____ _____ penetrates deeply into tissues and is inactivated only when it comes in contact with cations such as calcium.
22. The range between curative and toxic dosages of a medication is called the _____ _____.
23. To reverse an overdose of benzodiazepines, administer _____.
24. _____ _____ have recently been used, on a limited basis, to treat obsessive-compulsive disorders.
25. Activated charcoal does not bind with _____, _____, and _____ substances.
26. In toxic amounts, _____ inhibit normal energy production and acid buffering in the body, resulting in metabolic _____.

REINFORCEMENT

©2007 Pearson Education, Inc.
Essentials of Paramedic Care, 2nd ed.

CHAPTER 34 *Toxicology and Substance Abuse* 817

HANDOUT 34-4 Continued

27. Aspirin overdose patients may require urine alkalinization with _____ _____.
28. A soluble poisonous substance secreted during growth of a bacterium is called a(n) _____.
29. Gastrointestinal symptoms and diseases such as food poisoning are produced by _____.
30. Except for _____, food poisoning is rarely life-threatening.
31. _____ account for over 90 percent of all mushroom poisoning deaths.
32. Signs and symptoms of _____ _____ _____ bites start as immediate localized pain, redness, and swelling, progressing to spasms of large muscle groups with severe pain.
33. Severe muscle spasms due to certain insect bites may be treated with either IV _____ or IV _____ _____.
34. When caring for a patient who has been bitten by a pit viper, three "don'ts" include: DO NOT apply _____ or a _____ pack or _____ spray to the wound; DO NOT apply an arterial _____ ; and DO NOT apply _____ stimulation from any device.
35. Treat marine animal injection by applying _____ or _____ water.
36. Use of a pharmacological substance for purposes other than medically defined reasons is known as _____ _____.
37. A compulsive and overwhelming dependence on a drug is called a(n) _____.
38. The need to progressively increase the dose of a drug to reproduce the effect originally achieved by smaller doses is called _____.
39. The term _____ refers to the patient's body reacting severely when deprived of the abused substance.
40. A disorder found in habitual and excessive users of alcoholic beverages after cessation of drinking for 48 to 72 hours is known as _____ _____.

REINFORCEMENT

HANDOUT 34-5

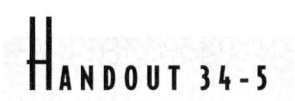

Student's Name _____

POISON TREATMENT TRUE OR FALSE

Indicate if the following statements are true or false by writing T or F in the space provided.

_____ 1. Syrup of ipecac is widely used in both the prehospital and hospital phases of decontamination in poisoning cases.

_____ 2. Cyanide poisoning should initially be treated by inhaling a crushed pearl of amyl nitrite for 30 seconds, then oxygen for 30 seconds.

_____ 3. Naloxone has been found to be beneficial in the treatment of benzodiazepine overdose.

_____ 4. Treatment of comatose patients should always include a "coma cocktail" consisting of $D_{50}W$, Narcan, and thiamine.

_____ 5. Induction of vomiting is a routine intervention for patients who have ingested a toxin or overdose of medication.

_____ 6. Severe cases of carbon monoxide poisoning may require treatment in a hyperbaric chamber to remove CO from hemoglobin.

_____ 7. Ingestion of caustic substances (acids, alkalis) may be treated by the administration of activated charcoal to absorb the substances.

_____ 8. Since activated charcoal does not bind with lithium, administration of it is unnecessary.

_____ 9. A dose of 100 mg/kg is usually sufficient to cause toxicity in an adult patient.

_____ 10. Acetaminophen overdose is effectively treated with N-acetylcysteine.

_____ 11. Activated charcoal binds well with heavy metals such as lead and mercury.

_____ 12. Except for botulism, food poisoning is rarely life-threatening.

_____ 13. Management of patients with *Hymenoptera* stings should include applying hot water or a hot pack to the injection site.

_____ 14. Patients experiencing severe muscle spasms resulting from a black widow spider bite may be treated with calcium gluconate.

_____ 15. Constricting bands should be placed above and below the injection site of either a scorpion sting or pit viper bite.

_____ 16. Treatment for a marine animal injection includes applying a constricting band between the wound and the heart, and application of heat or hot water to the site.

_____ 17. Naloxone is effective in reversing the effects of benzodiazepine overdose.

_____ 18. Forced diuresis and alkalinization of the urine improve elimination of barbiturates from the body.

_____ 19. Mixed overdoses that include benzodiazepines should be treated with Flumazenil to prevent seizures.

_____ 20. Beta-blockers may be beneficial in the treatment of cocaine abuse.

HANDOUT 34-6

Student's Name _____

TOXICOLOGY MATCHING

Write the letter of each term below in the space provided next to the appropriate description.

A. Absorption
B. Acid
C. Alkali
D. Antidote
E. Benzodiazepine
F. Activated charcoal
G. DTs
H. Ingestion
I. Inhalation
J. Injection
K. Overdose
L. Poison control
M. Toxin
N. Toxicology
O. Toxidrome

_____ 1. The entrance of a substance into the body through the gastrointestinal tract.

_____ 2. The entrance of a substance into the body through a break in the skin.

_____ 3. A substance used to absorb toxins by chemically binding to its surface area.

_____ 4. The entrance of a substance into the body directly through the skin or mucous membrane.

_____ 5. Medical or biological science that studies poisons.

_____ 6. General term to describe one of a group of tranquilizing drugs with similar chemical structures.

_____ 7. A substance that neutralizes a poison or the effects of a poison.

_____ 8. Any chemical that causes adverse effects on an organism that is exposed to it.

_____ 9. Disorder found in habitual and excessive users of alcoholic beverages after cessation of drinking.

_____ 10. Information center staffed by trained personnel that provides up-to-date toxicologic information.

_____ 11. Dose of a drug in excess of that usually prescribed.

_____ 12. The entrance of a substance into the body through the respiratory tract.

_____ 13. A group of typical signs and symptoms consistently associated with exposure to a particular type of toxin.

_____ 14. A substance that liberates hydroxyl ions when in solution.

_____ 15. A substance that liberates hydrogen ions when in solution.

HANDOUT 34-7

Student's Name _____

TOXICOLOGY SIGNS AND SYMPTOMS

For each of the following sources of poisoning pictured, describe the route of entry and the signs and symptoms it commonly produces in a victim.

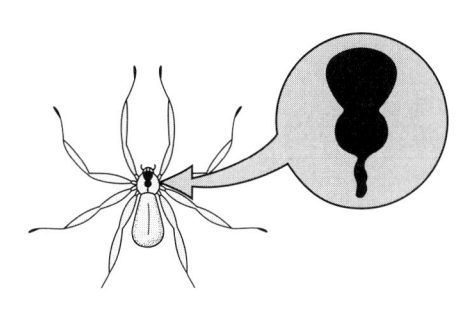

1. Route: _____
   Signs and Symptoms:

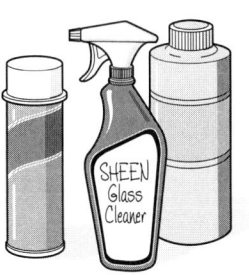

Household cleaners

2. Route: _____
   Signs and Symptoms:

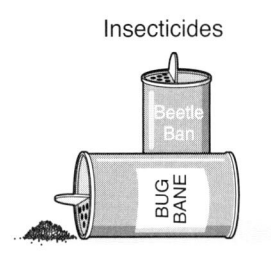

Insecticides

3. Route: _____
   Signs and Symptoms:

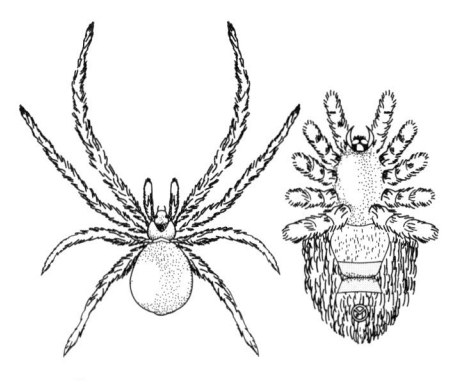

4. Route: _____
   Signs and Symptoms:

REINFORCEMENT

©2007 Pearson Education, Inc.
Essentials of Paramedic Care, 2nd ed.

CHAPTER 34 *Toxicology and Substance Abuse* 821

Chapter 34 Answer Key

Handout 34-2: Chapter 34 Quiz

1. C	8. C	15. C	22. A
2. C	9. D	16. A	23. C
3. D	10. B	17. C	24. B
4. C	11. C	18. D	25. C
5. C	12. A	19. A	
6. B	13. B	20. D	
7. D	14. A	21. C	

Handout 34-3: Chapter 34 Scenario

1. Cocaine.
2. It is the prime suspect because of method of administration, seizure activity, dysrhythmias, dilated pupils, and tachycardia.
3. Administration of lidocaine was indicated for the frequent PVCs. A cocaine overdose may cause life-threatening dysrhythmias that should be treated according to protocol.
4. The report to the ER physician should include how the patient was found, initial vital signs, heart rhythm, treatment administered, results of the treatment, and current patient condition.

Handout 34-4: Chapter 34 Review

1. toxin
2. poisoning, overdose
3. 70
4. drug overdose
5. Ingestion
6. inhalation
7. decontamination
8. intake, absorption, elimination
9. acetaminophen
10. methyl alcohol
11. aspiration
12. Syrup of ipecac
13. personal safety
14. toxidrome
15. asphyxiant
16. Carbon monoxide
17. amyl nitrite
18. Narcotic
19. acid
20. alkali
21. Hydrofluoric acid
22. therapeutic index
23. flumazenil
24. MAO inhibitors
25. lithium, hydrocarbons, caustic
26. salicylates, acidosis
27. sodium bicarbonate
28. exotoxin
29. enterotoxins
30. botulism
31. Amanita
32. black widow spider
33. diazepam, calcium gluconate
34. ice, cold, freon, tourniquet, electrical
35. heat, hot
36. substance abuse
37. addiction
38. tolerance
39. withdrawal
40. delirium tremens

Handout 34-5: Poison Treatment True or False

1. F	6. T	11. F	16. T
2. T	7. F	12. T	17. F
3. F	8. T	13. F	18. T
4. F	9. F	14. T	19. F
5. F	10. T	15. F	20. F

Handout 34-6: Toxicology Matching

1. H	5. N	9. G	13. O
2. J	6. E	10. L	14. C
3. F	7. D	11. K	15. B
4. A	8. M	12. I	

Handout 34-7: Toxicology Signs and Symptoms

1. *Route:* Injection (brown recluse spider).
   Signs and symptoms include: small bleb surrounded by white ring; localized pain, redness, swelling; localized tissue necrosis; chills; fever; nausea and vomiting; joint pain; bleeding disorders.
2. *Route:* Inhalation.
   Signs and symptoms include: coughing, choking, and respiratory collapse; irritation of the eyes; nausea, vomiting, and abdominal pain; seizures.
3. *Route:* Surface absorption.
   Signs and symptoms include: excessive salivation; lacrimation; urination; diarrhea; gastrointestinal distress; emesis; constricted pupils.
4. *Route:* Injection (black widow spider).
   Signs and symptoms include: immediate localized pain, redness, and swelling; progressive muscle spasms; severe back, shoulder, or chest pain—upper extremity bite; severe abdominal pain—lower extremity bite; nausea and vomiting; sweating; seizures; paralysis; hypertension; diminished level of consciousness.

Chapter 35

Hematology

INTRODUCTION

Hematology is the study of the blood and the blood-forming organs. Although hematological disorders are common, they rarely are the primary cause of a medical emergency. They usually accompany other ongoing disease processes. Often, laboratory findings are needed to confirm the diagnosis. It is essential that paramedics have a good understanding of the basic pathophysiological processes of their patients' diseases, including hematological disorders. This chapter will discuss the pathology and clinical manifestations and prognoses associated with many of the common hematological diseases and abnormalities.

CHAPTER OBJECTIVES

After reading this chapter, you should be able to:

1. Identify the anatomy and physiology of the hematopoietic system. (see Chapter 3)
2. Discuss the following: (see Chapter 3)
    - Plasma
    - Red blood cells (erythrocytes)
    - Hemoglobin
    - Hematocrit
    - White blood cells (leukocytes)
    - Platelets, clotting, and fibrinolysis
    - Hemostasis
3. Identify the following (see Chapter 4):
    - Inflammatory process
    - Cellular and humoral immunity
    - Alterations in immunological response
4. Identify blood groups. (pp. 1390–1391)
5. List erythrocyte disorders. (pp. 1397–1399)
6. List leukocyte disorders. (pp. 1399–1401)
7. List platelet and clotting disorders. (pp. 1401–1402)
8. Describe how acquired factor deficiencies may occur. (pp. 1401–1402)
9. Identify the components of the physical assessment as they relate to the hematology system. (pp. 1392–1396)

TOTAL TEACHING TIME: 4.66 HOURS

The total teaching time is only a guideline based on the didactic and practical lab averages in the National Standard Curriculum. Instructors should take into consideration such factors as the pace at which students learn, the size of the class, and breaks. The actual time devoted to teaching objectives is the responsibility of the instructor.

©2007 Pearson Education, Inc.
Essentials of Paramedic Care, 2nd ed.

10. Describe the pathology and clinical manifestations and prognoses associated with:
    - Anemia (pp. 1397–1398)
    - Leukemia (p. 1400)
    - Lymphomas (pp. 1400–1401)
    - Polycythemia (p. 1399)
    - Disseminated intravascular coagulopathy (p. 1402)
    - Hemophilia (pp. 1401–1402)
    - Sickle cell disease (pp. 1398–1399)
    - Multiple myeloma (pp. 1401–1403)

11. Given several preprogrammed patients with hematological problems, provide the appropriate assessment, management, and transport. (pp. 1390–1403)

FRAMING THE LESSON

Begin class by reviewing the important points from Chapter 34, "Toxicology and Substance Abuse." Discuss any aspects of the chapter not fully understood by students. Then begin with Chapter 35 material. You may wish to begin the lesson with a review of the anatomy and physiology of the organs involved in the formation of blood, including the liver, spleen, kidneys, and bone marrow. If possible, obtain from the local Red Cross or blood bank examples of various blood products, such as whole blood, packed red cells, and so on, in IV bags to show students. Ask students to name all of the functions of blood and its components that they can think of. These should include the transportation of oxygen and nutrients, clotting factors, dealing with infections, and so on. Discuss how disorders of the blood or its components affect every system of the body and can be devastating in severe cases. You may also ask students if any of them, or someone they know, has any type of blood disorder that they would be willing to discuss. Stress that blood disorders are not often the cause of an EMS call, but that they may exacerbate any other medical or traumatic problems the patient is having. As an example, explain that for the hemophiliac patient with a relatively minor traumatic injury, bleeding, both internal and external, may be excessive, resulting in shock.

TEACHING STRATEGIES

People learn in a variety of ways. Some do better with the spoken word, whereas others prefer the written. Some prefer to work alone, whereas others profit from working in groups. Recognizing these different ways of acquiring knowledge, the authors of this *Instructor's Resource Manual* have provided a variety of teaching strategies for the different types of learners. These strategies are intended to foster higher-level cognitive skills and encourage creative learning and problem solving. For greatest effectiveness, incorporate these strategies into your class lecture. Symbols in the Lecture Outline indicate the points at which various exercises might be most appropriate. Other strategies can be used to preview the lesson or to summarize it.

The following strategies are keyed to specific sections of the lesson.

1. ***Working with Lab Reports.*** During the discussion of white blood cells, bring in several laboratory reports of CBCs with differentials. After taking precautions to ensure patient confidentiality, have students look for reports from patients with various disorders, such as a bacterial infection, viral infection,

anemia, or leukemia. Having the report to look at, as well as a clinical presentation, will lend validity to the discussion.

2. Researching Hematological Diseases. To increase interest and participation during discussion of each of the hematological diseases, make students responsible for researching and presenting one disease each. Either bring books into the classroom or release the students into your medical library for 30 minutes during this session. Have students determine the pathophysiology, signs and symptoms, and treatment, including pharmacology, for the disease. Have students take turns presenting their reports aloud. This activity improves research and verbal presentation skills.

The following strategies can be used at various points throughout the lesson or to help summarize and demonstrate what students have learned.

Organizing a Blood Drive. To emphasize the importance of adequate blood supply in health care, offer extra credit for students who donate blood during your field trip. Alternately, have students organize a blood drive for the hospital or Red Cross. Give students credit for working the blood drive or donating blood. This activity works to create class spirit, community activism, and volunteerism.

Field Trip. Few will be able to explain hematology better than the experts in the blood bank of your hospital or Red Cross blood donation center. Take a field trip to the blood bank so that students can not only speak with an expert, but also see the equipment used for donation, typing and cross-matching, storage, and so on.

Guest Speaker: Blood Lab Tests. Invite someone from a local clinic or hospital laboratory to come to class and discuss the various lab tests performed on blood, how they are done, and the normal and abnormal findings. Have the guest speaker stress body substance isolation precautions taken while obtaining and testing the specimens.

Laboratory Observation Time. Arrange for students to obtain part of their required clinical observation time at a local clinic or hospital laboratory to observe and, if possible, assist in the obtaining and testing of blood specimens. Request the lab technician(s) to discuss the purpose of various blood tests, and what abnormal findings may mean clinically.

Guest Speaker: Hematologist. Invite a hematologist from an area medical center to discuss the pathophysiology and clinical manifestations of disorders of the blood. Request that the hematologist bring slides, overheads, or other AV material with examples of microscopic blood samples, both normal and abnormal. Obtain microscopes, if possible, to view samples.

Playing "The Memory Game." Write each of the new terms in this chapter on a piece of construction paper and the term's meaning on a separate piece. Turn the pieces of paper over and number each. Students then request number pairs in attempt to match up the term and the correct meaning. When they have successfully remembered a term and meaning, pull the pair off and hand them to the student. The student with the most cards at the end of the game wins a small prize of your choosing. This game is fun, improves student vocabulary, and encourages healthy competition.

Cultural Considerations, Legal Notes, and Patho Pearls. The Student CD-ROM contains this series of informative features to enhance the student's understanding of the material covered in this chapter.

TEACHING OUTLINE

HANDOUT 35-1
Chapter 35 Objectives Checklist

READING/REFERENCE
Martini, F. *Fundamentals of Anatomy and Physiology*, Englewood Cliffs, NJ: Prentice Hall, 2001.

POWERPOINT PRESENTATION
Chapter 35 PowerPoint slides 4–20

TEACHING STRATEGY 1
Working with Lab Reports

POINT TO EMPHASIZE
About 2.5 million red blood cells die every second, but they are replaced just as quickly.

TEACHING TIP
Liken the process of clot formation to a beaver building a dam.

TEACHING TIP
To illustrate the hematocrit, bring in a tube of blood from the emergency department or lab and allow the red cells to settle.

POWERPOINT PRESENTATION
Chapter 35 PowerPoint slides 21–23

POINT OF INTEREST
Blood products are good only for 21 days, while fresh frozen plasma is good for 6 months.

POWERPOINT PRESENTATION
Chapter 35 PowerPoint slides 24–35

TEACHING TIP
Have students perform a search on the Internet using phrases such as "blood diseases" or "blood disorders" and list some of the sites found relating to various hematological problems.

TEACHING STRATEGY 2
Researching Hematological Diseases

Chapter 35 is the ninth lesson in Division 4, *Medical Emergencies*. Distribute Handout 35-1 so that students can familiarize themselves with the learning goals for this chapter. If students have any questions about the objectives, answer them at this time.

Then present the chapter. One possible lecture outline follows. In the outline, the parenthetical references in regular type are references to text pages; those in bold type are references to figures, tables, or procedures.

I. Introduction. Hematology is the study of blood and blood-forming organs. Although blood disorders are common, they are rarely the primary cause of the medical emergency. Some hematological diseases are genetic in nature, and others are more common in certain ethnic groups. Paramedics must use all their assessment skills to recognize and treat injuries, pain, and instabilities. It is essential to have a good understanding of the basic pathophysiological processes of patients' diseases, including hematological disorders. (pp. 1390–1392)

   A. Blood products and blood typing (pp. 1390–1391)
   1. Blood types
      a. A
      b. B
      c. AB
      d. O
   2. Types of transfusions (**Fig. 35-1, p. 1391**)(**Table 35-1, p. 1391**)
      a. Whole blood
      b. Packed red cells
      c. Platelets
      d. Fresh frozen plasma
      e. Clotting factors
   B. Transfusion reactions (p. 1392)

II. General assessment and management (pp. 1392–1397)

   A. Scene size-up (p. 1393)
   B. Initial assessment (p. 1393)
   C. Focused history and physical exam (pp. 1393–1396)
   1. SAMPLE history
   2. Physical exam (**Fig. 35-2, p. 1395**)
      a. Nervous system
      b. Skin
      c. Lymphatic
      d. Gastrointestinal
      e. Musculoskeletal
   D. General management of hematopoietic emergencies (pp. 1396–1397)

III. Managing specific patient problems (pp. 1397–1403)

   A. Diseases of the red blood cells (pp. 1397–1399)
   1. Anemias (**Table 35-2, p. 1398**)
   2. Sickle cell disease (**Fig. 35-3, p. 1398**)
   3. Polycythemia
   B. Diseases of the white blood cells (pp. 1399–1401)
   1. Leukopenia/neutropenia
   2. Leukocytosis
   3. Leukemia
   4. Lymphomas

C. Diseases of the platelets/blood-clotting abnormalities (pp. 1401–1402)
  1. Thrombocytosis
  2. Thrombocytopenia
  3. Hemophilia
  4. Von Willebrand's disease
D. Other hematopoietic disorders (pp. 1402–1403)
  1. Disseminated intravascular coagulation
  2. Multiple myeloma

IV. Chapter summary (p. 1403). Hematology is the study of the blood and blood-forming organs. Hematological disorders include red blood cell disorders, white blood cell disorders, platelet disorders, and coagulation problems. Problems can also be caused when the body has an immunological response to antigens present on red blood cells from a foreign donor. Although hematological disorders are common, they are seldom the primary reason for an emergency call. Rather, they are likely to accompany another ongoing disease process.

The signs and symptoms that accompany hematological problems seldom point directly to the underlying disease. Generally, lab findings are necessary to clarify the diagnosis. However, an understanding of hematological pathophysiology is important to understanding the disease process your patient may be undergoing and to helping you to form a field impression and make appropriate decisions about emergency care.

ASSIGNMENTS

Assign students to complete Chapter 35, "Hematology," of the workbook. Also assign them to read Chapter 36, "Environmental Emergencies," before the next class.

EVALUATION

Chapter Quiz and Scenario Distribute copies of the Chapter Quiz provided in Handout 35-2 to evaluate student understanding of this chapter. Make sure each student reads the scenario to reinforce critical thinking on the scene. Remind students not to use their notes or textbooks while taking the quiz.

Student CD Quizzes for every chapter are contained on the dynamic and highly visual in-text student CD.

Companion Website Additional quizzes for every chapter are contained on this exciting website.

TestGen You may wish to create a custom-tailored test using *Prentice Hall TestGen for Essentials of Paramedic Care,* 2nd Edition to evaluate student understanding of this chapter.

On-line Test Preparation (for students and instructors) Additional test preparation is available through Brady's new on-line product, *EMT Achieve: Paramedic Test Preparation* at *http://www.prenhall.com/emtachieve/*. Instructors can also monitor student mastery on-line.

Review Manual for the EMT-Paramedic This comprehensive exam review contains hundreds of test questions and rationales, including scenarios, along with two 180-question practice tests on CD.

POWERPOINT PRESENTATION
Chapter 35 PowerPoint slide 36

WORKBOOK
Chapter 35 Activities

READING/REFERENCE
Textbook, pp. 1405–1438

HANDOUT 35-2
Chapter 35 Quiz

HANDOUT 35-3
Chapter 35 Scenario

PARAMEDIC STUDENT CD
Student Activities

COMPANION WEBSITE
http://www.prenhall.com/bledsoe

TESTGEN
Chapter 35

EMT ACHIEVE: PARAMEDIC TEST PREPARATION
Mistovich & Beasley. *EMT Achieve: Paramedic Test Preparation.*
www.prenhall.com/emtachieve/

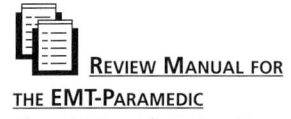

REVIEW MANUAL FOR THE EMT-PARAMEDIC
Cherry & Mistovich. *Review Manual for the EMT-Paramedic,* 3rd edition.

HANDOUTS 35-4 AND 35-5
Reinforcement Activities

PARAMEDIC STUDENT CD
Student Activities

POWERPOINT PRESENTATION
Chapter 35

COMPANION WEBSITE
http://www.prenhall.com/bledsoe

ONEKEY
Chapter 35

ADVANCED LIFE SUPPORT SKILLS
Larmon & Davis. *Advanced Life Support Skills.*

ADVANCED LIFE SKILLS REVIEW
Larmon & Davis. *Advanced Life Skills Review.*

BRADY SKILLS SERIES: ALS
Larmon & Davis. *Brady Skills Series: ALS.*

PARAMEDIC NATIONAL STANDARDS SELF-TEST
Miller. *Paramedic National Standards Self-Test,* 4th edition.

REINFORCEMENT

Handouts   If classroom discussion or performance on the quiz indicates that some students have not fully mastered the chapter content, you may wish to assign some or all of the Reinforcement Handouts for this chapter.

Student CD (for students)   A wide variety of material on this CD-ROM will reinforce and also expand student knowledge and skills.

PowerPoint Presentation (for instructors)   The PowerPoint material developed for this chapter offers useful reinforcement of chapter content.

Companion Website (for students)   Additional review quizzes and links to EMS resources will contribute to further reinforcement of the chapter.

OneKey   On-line support is offered for this course on one of three platforms: CourseCompass, Blackboard, or Web CT. Includes the IRM, PowerPoints, TestGen, and Companion Website for instruction. Ask your local sales representative for more information.

Brady Skills Series: Advanced Life Skills (Video or CD)   Have your students watch the skills come to life on VHS or CD-ROM, or they can purchase the highly visual, full-color text with step-by-step procedures and rationales.

HANDOUT 35-1

Student's Name_____

CHAPTER 35 OBJECTIVES CHECKLIST

Knowledge	Date Mastered
1. Identify the anatomy and physiology of the hematopoietic system.	
2. Discuss the following: • Plasma • Red blood cells (erythrocytes) • Hemoglobin • Hematocrit • White blood cells (leukocytes) • Platelets, clotting, and fibrinolysis • Hemostasis	
3. Identify the following: • Inflammatory process • Cellular and humoral immunity • Alterations in immunological response	
4. Identify blood groups.	
5. List erythrocyte disorders.	
6. List leukocyte disorders.	
7. List platelet and clotting disorders.	
8. Describe how acquired factor deficiencies may occur.	
9. Identify the components of the physical assessment as they relate to the hematology system.	
10. Describe the pathology and clinical manifestations and prognoses associated with: • Anemia • Leukemia • Lymphomas • Polycythemia • Disseminated intravascular coagulopathy • Hemophilia • Sickle cell disease • Multiple myeloma	
11. Given several preprogrammed patients with hematological problems, provide the appropriate assessment, management, and transport.	

OBJECTIVES

©2007 Pearson Education, Inc.
Essentials of Paramedic Care, 2nd ed.

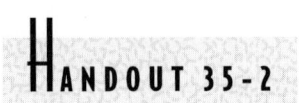

CHAPTER 35 QUIZ

Write the letter of the best answer in the space provided.

_____ 1. A person with which blood type is considered the "universal donor?"
   A. A
   B. AB
   C. B
   D. O

_____ 2. Fresh frozen plasma is often used for replacing:
   A. red blood cells in anemic patients.
   B. blood loss from hemorrhage.
   C. volume in hypovolemia secondary to low oncotic pressure.
   D. factors missing due to inadequate production as in hemophilia.

_____ 3. Erythroblastosis fetalis is caused by:
   A. sensitization to antigens on the white blood cells, platelets, or plasma proteins.
   B. a recipient of a blood transfusion receiving an incompatible blood type.
   C. erythrocytes being damaged during the transfusion process.
   D. an Rh$^-$ mother previously sensitized by pregnancy with an Rh$^+$ child becoming pregnant with an Rh$^+$ child.

_____ 4. During your physical exam of a patient, you note jaundice, or yellow skin. This could be caused by:
   A. decreased perfusion to vital organs.
   B. hemolysis of red blood cells.
   C. kidney disease.
   D. anemia.

_____ 5. The most common cause of priapism in the emergency setting is:
   A. spinal cord injuries.
   B. polycythemia.
   C. sickle cell disease.
   D. hemophilia.

_____ 6. Employing proper isolation techniques is extremely important when caring for patients with leukemia and lymphoma because:
   A. these patients are at an increased risk of developing infection.
   B. both diseases are transmitted by airborne pathogens.
   C. these patients will typically have open lesions.
   D. both diseases are highly infectious in the early stages.

_____ 7. Hemophilia A is a blood disorder caused by a deficiency of:
   A. erythrocytes.
   B. factor VIII.
   C. leukocytes.
   D. factor IX.

_____ 8. An abnormal decrease in the number of platelets is known as:
   A. thrombocytosis.
   B. DIC.
   C. thrombocytopenia.
   D. factor IX disease.

_____ 9. A disorder of coagulation caused by systemic activation of the coagulation cascade is:
   A. thrombocytosis.
   B. DIC.
   C. thrombocytopenia.
   D. factor IX disease.

_____ 10. A cancerous disorder of plasma cells is:
   A. von Willebrand's disease.
   B. DIC.
   C. thrombocytopenia.
   D. multiple myeloma.

HANDOUT 35-3

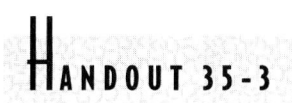

Student's Name _____

CHAPTER 35 SCENARIO

Review the following real-life situation. Then answer the questions that follow.

Placerville Rescue 2 has been called to a nearby mobile home park for a patient with weakness and shortness of breath. The paramedics arrive to find a 72-year-old male seated in a chair. They immediately note that the patient is conscious and breathing, but appears pale and fatigued. His wife relates that her husband (your patient), George, had made reservations for a whitewater rafting trip next month and, in order to prepare himself physically, had purchased a treadmill to use in the house for exercise. But every time he used it, he quickly became tired. In fact, lately, he has become very tired and short of breath with even small amounts of activity, such as getting out of his chair and walking from the living room to other rooms in the house. He had a recent appointment with his doctor and had an ECG, which was normal. He is scheduled for other tests but has not had them yet. His weakness and shortness of breath with exertion has gotten worse over the past several weeks. George's wife tells the paramedics that he has also been very irritable lately. When asked about bleeding disorders, George admits that he has had some rectal bleeding for a few weeks, but he hasn't told his doctor about it.

Upon performing a physical exam, the paramedics find clear lungs, pale but warm skin, and a slightly tachycardic heart rate. George's heart rhythm is regular and the ECG shows a sinus tachycardia. Postural vitals are basically unchanged. The paramedics apply high-flow, high-concentration oxygen via nonrebreather mask and start an IV of normal saline at a keep-open rate. George is placed in the semi-Fowler position on the stretcher and moved to the ambulance. Another set of vital signs is taken and George is transported to the hospital a few miles away without incident.

1. What do you believe George's problem is, and what might be causing it?

2. What signs and symptoms lead you to the conclusion in question 1?

3. What might the hospital treatment for this condition be?

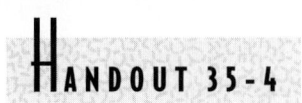

CHAPTER 35 REVIEW

Write the word or words that best complete the following sentences in the space(s) provided.

1. _____ is the study of blood and the blood-forming organs.
2. Blood type _____ is considered the universal donor, and blood type _____ is considered the universal recipient.
3. Yellow skin is known as _____; reddish-purple spots are known as _____; reddish-purple blotches are known as _____.
4. Bleeding gums are often associated with a decreased _____ count.
5. An oral yeast infection in an adult is commonly associated with _____.
6. _____ _____ disease is a common cause of priapism in the emergency setting.
7. _____ is an excess of red blood cells.
8. _____ is an inadequate number of red blood cells.
9. A cancer of the hematopoietic cells is known as _____.
10. Too few white cells is known as _____, and too many white blood cells is known as _____.

HANDOUT 35-5

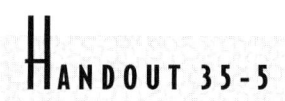

Student's Name _____

TRANSFUSION TABLE

Complete the table below by filling in the missing information about transfusions.

Type of Transfusion	Contents of Transfusion	Use
Whole blood	All blood cells, platelets, clotting factors, and plasma	
Packed red blood cells (PRBCs)		
Platelets	Thrombocytes and some plasma	
Fresh frozen plasma (FFP)		
Clotting factors	Specific clotting factors needed for coagulation	

Chapter 35 Answer Key

Handout 35-2: Chapter 35 Quiz

1. D
2. C
3. D
4. B
5. C
6. A
7. B
8. C
9. B
10. D

Handout 35-3: Chapter 35 Scenario

1. George's problem is anemia, possibly caused by internal bleeding as evidenced by his reporting rectal bleeding for a few weeks. Remember that anemia is a sign, and not a disease in itself.
2. George is showing several signs and symptoms of anemia. These include dyspnea and fatigue during exercise or physical activity, irritability, and tachycardia.
3. For mild anemia, treatment may begin with oral iron supplements. More severe cases may be treated by administration of packed red cells, as the problem is a decrease in the number of red cells in the blood. The most definitive treatment is to find the cause of the anemia and correct it. In George's case, it may be a lower GI bleed, based on his admission of having rectal bleeding. Control of the bleeding would be the final, definitive treatment.

Handout 35-4: Chapter 35 Review

1. Hematology
2. O, AB
3. jaundice, petechiae, purpura
4. platelet
5. AIDS
6. Sickle cell
7. Polycythemia
8. Anemia
9. leukemia
10. leukopenia, leukocytosis

Handout 35-5: Transfusion Table

Whole blood. Use: Replace blood loss from hemorrhage.
Packed red blood cells. Contents: Red blood cells and some plasma. *Use:* Replace blood cells in anemic patients.
Platelets. Use: Replace platelets in a patient with thrombocytopenia.
Fresh frozen plasma. Contents: Plasma, a combination of fluids, clotting factors, and proteins. *Use:* Replace volume in a burn patient or in hypovolemia secondary to low oncotic pressure.
Clotting factors. Use: Replace factors missing due to inadequate production, as in hemophilia.

Chapter 36

Environmental Emergencies

INTRODUCTION

The environment is defined as all of the surrounding external factors that affect the development and functioning of a living organism. Paramedics frequently encounter medical and traumatic emergencies related to environmental conditions. Temperature, weather, terrain, and atmospheric pressure can create stresses for which the unprotected body is unable to compensate. A good understanding of the causes and underlying pathophysiologies of the body can help the paramedic recognize these emergencies promptly and manage them effectively. This chapter will focus on problems related to temperature extremes, drowning and near-drowning, diving emergencies, high-altitude illness, and nuclear radiation.

CHAPTER OBJECTIVES

After reading this chapter, you should be able to:

1. Define "environmental emergency." (p. 1407)
2. Describe the incidence, morbidity, and mortality associated with environmental emergencies. (p. 1423)
3. Identify risk factors most predisposing to environmental emergencies. (p. 1407)
4. Identify environmental factors that may cause illness or exacerbate a preexisting illness or complicate treatment or transport decisions. (p. 1407)
5. Define "homeostasis" and relate the concept to environmental influences. (p. 1407)
6. Identify normal, critically high, and critically low body temperatures. (pp. 1408–1410)
7. Describe several methods of temperature monitoring. (p. 1409)
8. Describe human thermal regulation, including system components, substances used, and wastes generated. (pp. 1407–1411, 1416)
9. List the common forms of heat and cold disorders. (pp. 1411–1423)
10. List the common predisposing factors and preventive measures associated with heat and cold disorders. (pp. 1411–1412, 1416–1417)
11. Define heat illness, hypothermia, frostbite, near-drowning, decompression illness, and altitude illness. (pp. 1411, 1416, 1422, 1423, 1428, 1433)

TOTAL TEACHING TIME: 6.64 HOURS
The total teaching time is only a guideline based on the didactic and practical lab averages in the National Standard Curriculum. Instructors should take into consideration such factors as the pace at which students learn, the size of the class, and breaks. The actual time devoted to teaching objectives is the responsibility of the instructor.

©2007 Pearson Education, Inc.
Essentials of Paramedic Care, 2nd ed.

12. Describe the pathophysiology, signs and symptoms, and predisposing factors, preventive actions, and treatment for heat cramps, heat exhaustion, heatstroke, and fever. (pp. 1411–1416)
13. Describe the contribution of dehydration to the development of heat disorders. (p. 1415)
14. Describe the differences between classical and exertional heatstroke. (p. 1414)
15. Identify the fundamental thermoregulatory difference between fever and heatstroke. (p. 1415)
16. Discuss the role of fluid therapy in the treatment of heat disorders. (pp. 1412, 1413, 1414)
17. Describe the pathophysiology, predisposing factors, signs, symptoms, and management of the following:
    - Hypothermia (pp. 1416–1422)
    - Superficial and deep frostbite (pp. 1422–1423)
    - Near-drowning (pp. 1423–1426)
    - Decompression illness (pp. 1428, 1429–1431)
    - Diving emergency (pp. 1427–1433)
    - Altitude illness (pp. 1433–1436)
18. Identify differences between mild, severe, chronic, and acute hypothermia. (p. 1417)
19. Discuss the impact of severe hypothermia on standard BCLS and ACLS algorithms and transport considerations. (pp. 1419–1422)
20. Differentiate between freshwater and saltwater immersion as they relate to near-drowning. (p. 1424)
21. Discuss the incidence of "wet" versus "dry" drownings and the differences in their management. (p. 1424)
22. Discuss the complications and protective role of hypothermia in the context of near-drowning. (pp. 1423, 1424)
23. Define self-contained underwater breathing apparatus (scuba). (p. 1426)
24. Describe the laws of gases and relate them to diving emergencies and altitude illness. (pp. 1426–1427)
25. Differentiate between the various diving emergencies. (pp. 1427–1428)
26. Identify the various conditions that may result from pulmonary overpressure accidents. (pp. 1428, 1431)
27. Describe the function of the Divers Alert Network (DAN) and how its members may aid in the management of diving-related illnesses. (p. 1433)
28. Describe the specific function and benefit of hyperbaric oxygen therapy for the management of diving accidents. (pp. 1429–1430)
29. Define acute mountain sickness (AMS), high-altitude pulmonary edema (HAPE), and high-altitude cerebral edema (HACE). (pp. 1434–1436)
30. Discuss the symptomatic variations presented in progressive altitude illnesses. (pp. 1434–1436)
31. Discuss the pharmacology appropriate for the treatment of altitude illnesses. (pp. 1435–1436)
32. Given several preprogrammed simulated environmental emergency patients, provide the appropriate assessment, management, and transportation. (pp. 1407–1436)

FRAMING THE LESSON

Begin class by reviewing the important points from Chapter 35, "Hematology." Discuss any aspects of the chapter not fully understood by students. Then go on to Chapter 36. Begin by discussing the normal temperature ranges in your geographical area. What are the normal high temperatures in the summer? What are the normal low temperatures in the winter? Discuss the need for protection from temperature extremes. What do we do to protect ourselves from excessive heat? Excessive cold? How do we protect ourselves from temperature extremes when we are out in the environment? At what temperatures do we feel "comfortable" when outside? What are the body's reactions to hot weather? To cold weather? During the discussions, introduce the information that age, pre-existing medical conditions, and general health influence the body's reaction to temperature.

TEACHING STRATEGIES

People learn in a variety of ways. Some do better with the spoken word, whereas others prefer the written. Some prefer to work alone, whereas others profit from working in groups. Recognizing these different ways of acquiring knowledge, the authors of this *Instructor's Resource Manual* have provided a variety of teaching strategies for the different types of learners. These strategies are intended to foster higher-level cognitive skills and encourage creative learning and problem solving. For greatest effectiveness, incorporate these strategies into your class lecture. Symbols in the Lecture Outline indicate the points at which various exercises might be most appropriate. Other strategies can be used to preview the lesson or to summarize it.

The strategies below are keyed to specific sections of the lesson.

1. Demonstrating Convection. Try the "warm cookie" trick. Pass out cookies that are too warm to eat without first blowing on them to cool them off. Have half of the class blow on theirs, and have the other half just let their cookies cool at room temperature without intervention. The blowers will get to eat their cookies much faster than the their classmates, thus illustrating the principles of convection.

2. Demonstrating Conduction and Radiation. A good example of conduction is an ice cube or a snowball melting in one's hand. A good example of radiation is body heat raising the temperature of a small room. The ice gains the heat of one's hand, causing cold fingers and a melted ice cube, and most people can relate to feeling overheated in a small room or elevator that gets packed with people. Using common, realistic examples will help students to remember these concepts.

3. Demonstrating Evaporation. A desktop water fountain, the kind that seems to be popular because of its supposedly soothing effects, will easily demonstrate evaporation. Fill the fountain in the morning at the beginning of class, mark the waterline, and go about your business of the day. By the end of class, the fountain will have evaporated appreciably, changing the waterline.

4. Using Case Studies. Because the treatment for specific heat disorders is not the same, do case presentations of each type in class. Create a likely location and situation, and add the patient's clinical information including vitals and history. Allow students to work through and apply the correct assessment and management on paper. Discuss the cases to be sure all students came to the correct prehospital diagnosis and treatment. Such an activity requires clinical decision making, yet fosters discussion and use of verbal reasoning skills as well.

5. Creating a Safety Campaign. Have students work in groups to create a drowning education and prevention campaign. Allow the class to choose the best presentation, and work with your local fire department or EMS agency to implement the idea prior to summer session. This activity promotes community service, patient education, injury prevention, and teamwork.

The following strategies can be used at various points throughout the lesson or to help summarize and demonstrate what students have learned.

Purchasing the Proper Equipment. Teach students that "cotton is rotten" in the back country because it traps moisture and promotes heat loss. You may wish to assist students in purchasing proper outdoor gear by establishing a *pro forma* deal with outdoor clothing and gear companies such as Patagonia, Sierra Designs, and Marmot. Such companies offer discounts to instructors and students of rescue programs. Contact the customer service or corporate sales department.

Adjusting the Environment. Depending on the season in which you teach this lesson, you might try turning the heat or air conditioning in your classroom either up or down to allow your students to feel the effects of thermoregulation as you teach about it. You may consider adjusting the temperature without telling students and watch for their reactions.

Field Experience. An additional activity that may enhance the didactic presentation of environmental emergencies is to have students participate as medical personnel in a local foot race or marathon. This enables them to experience heat illnesses firsthand.

Guest Speaker. Inviting a certified rescue diver or instructor to class brings experience and expertise to the material on diving injuries. Such a guest can provide a demonstration of proper use of diving equipment, which is an added benefit. This can familiarize students with situations they may encounter only rarely during their EMS careers. A short water rescue familiarization course with hands-on practicals is equally beneficial.

Clinical Observation. If there is one in your area, have students obtain part of their required clinical observation time at a U.S. Navy or Coast Guard facility that has a clinic or hospital. Such a facility would have a high probability of receiving and treating patients with water-related hypothermia or diving emergencies.

Guest Speaker. Invite an employee of your hospital's hyperbaric chamber to class to discuss the pathophysiology of hyperbaric medicine. He or she will likely be able to explain dive injuries and other injuries and conditions currently being treated with hyperbaric pressure, such as carbon monoxide poisoning and extremity wounds.

Cultural Considerations, Legal Notes, and Patho Pearls. The Student CD-ROM contains this series of informative features to enhance the student's understanding of the material covered in this chapter.

TEACHING OUTLINE

Chapter 36 is the tenth lesson in Division 4, *Medical Emergencies*. Distribute Handout 36-1 so that students can familiarize themselves with the learning goals for this chapter. If students have any questions about the objectives, answer them at this time.

Then present the chapter. One possible lecture outline follows. In the outline, the parenthetical references in regular type are references to text pages; those in bold type are references to figures, tables, and procedures.

I. Introduction (p. 1407)

A. Human beings depend on the environment for life but must also be protected from its extremes. (p. 1407)
B. The environment acts on the body and can create stresses for which the body is unable to compensate. (p. 1407)
  1. Temperature
  2. Weather
  3. Terrain
  4. Atmospheric pressure
C. Risk factors for environmental illnesses (p. 1407)
  1. Age
  2. Poor general health
  3. Fatigue
  4. Medical conditions
  5. Certain medications

II. Pathophysiology of heat and cold disorders (pp. 1407–1411)

A. Mechanisms of heat gain and loss (pp. 1407–1408)
B. Thermogenesis (heat generation) (p. 1408)
  1. Work-induced
  2. Thermoregulatory
  3. Diet-induced
C. Thermolysis (heat loss) (p. 1408) (**Fig. 36-1, p. 1409**)
  1. Conduction
  2. Convection
  3. Radiation
  4. Evaporation
  5. Respiration
D. Thermoregulation (pp. 1408–1411) (**Fig. 36-2, p. 1410**)
  1. Thermoreceptors
  2. Metabolic rate
     a. Basal
     b. Exertional

III. Heat disorders (pp. 1411–1416)

A. Hyperthermia (p. 1411)
B. Predisposing factors (pp. 1411–1412)
  1. Age
  2. Health
  3. Medications
  4. Level of acclimatization
  5. Length of exposure
  6. Intensity of exposure
  7. Environmental factors

HANDOUT 36-1
Chapter 36 Objectives Checklist

POWERPOINT PRESENTATION
Chapter 36 PowerPoint slide 4

POWERPOINT PRESENTATION
Chapter 36 PowerPoint slides 5–8

TEACHING STRATEGY 1
Demonstrating Convection

TEACHING STRATEGY 2
Demonstrating Conduction and Radiation

TEACHING STRATEGY 3
Demonstrating Evaporation

POINT TO EMPHASIZE
At over 90 percent relative humidity, evaporation theoretically stops.

POWERPOINT PRESENTATION
Chapter 36 PowerPoint slides 9–17

TEACHING STRATEGY 4
Using Case Studies

C. Preventative measures (p. 1412)
1. Adequate fluid intake
2. Gradual acclimatization
3. Limited exposure
D. Specific heat disorders (pp. 1412–1415)
1. Heat (muscle) cramps
   a. Signs and symptoms
   b. Treatment
2. Heat exhaustion
   a. Signs and symptoms
   b. Treatment
3. Heatstroke
   a. Signs and symptoms
   b. Treatment
E. Role of dehydration in heat disorders (p. 1415)
F. Fever (pyrexia) (pp. 1415–1416)

IV. **Cold disorders** (pp. 1416–1423)
A. Hypothermia (p. 1416)
B. Mechanisms of heat conservation and loss (p. 1416)
C. Predisposing factors (pp. 1416–1417)
1. Age
2. Health
3. Medications
4. Prolonged or intense exposure
5. Coexisting weather conditions
D. Preventative measures (p. 1417)
1. Warm clothing
2. Rest
3. Regular, appropriate meals
4. Limited exposure
E. Degrees of hypothermia (p. 1417)
F. Assessment and management of hypothermia (pp. 1417–1422)
1. Signs and symptoms (**Table 36-1, p. 1418; Table 36-2, p. 1418**) (**Fig. 36-3, p. 1419**)
2. Treatment of hypothermia (**Fig. 36-4, p. 1420**)
   a. Passive rewarming
   b. Active rewarming
   c. Rewarming shock
   d. Cold diuresis
3. Resuscitation
   a. BCLS
   b. ACLS
4. Transportation
G. Frostbite (pp. 1422–1423) (**Fig. 36-5, p. 1422**)
1. Superficial and deep frostbite
2. Treatment for frostbite
H. Trench foot (p. 1423)

V. **Near-drowning and drowning** (pp. 1423–1426)
A. Pathophysiology of drowning and near-drowning (pp. 1423–1425) (**Fig. 36-6, p. 1425**)
1. Dry versus wet drowning
2. Freshwater versus saltwater drowning
3. Factors affecting survival

B. Treatment for near-drowning (pp. 1425–1426)
    1. Adult respiratory distress syndrome

VI. Diving emergencies (pp. 1426–1433)
  A. Effects of air pressure on gases (pp. 1426–1427)
    1. Boyle's law
    2. Dalton's law
    3. Henry's law
  B. Pathophysiology of diving emergencies (p. 1427)
  C. Classification of diving injuries (pp. 1427–1428)
    1. Injuries on the surface
    2. Injuries during descent
    3. Injuries on the bottom
    4. Injuries during ascent
  D. General assessment of diving emergencies (pp. 1428–1429)
  E. Pressure disorders (pp. 1429–1432)
    1. Decompression illness (**Table 36-3**, p. 1430)
      a. Signs and symptoms
      b. Treatment (**Fig. 36-7**, p. 1430)
    2. Pulmonary overpressure accidents
      a. Signs and symptoms
      b. Treatment
    3. Arterial gas embolism (AGE)
      a. Signs and symptoms
      b. Treatment
    4. Pneumomediastinum
      a. Signs and symptoms
      b. Treatment
    5. Nitrogen narcosis
      a. Signs and symptoms
      b. Treatment
  F. Other diving-related illnesses (p. 1432)
  G. Divers Alert Network (DAN) (p. 1433)

VII. High-altitude illness (pp. 1433–1436)
  A. Prevention (pp. 1433–1434)
    1. Gradual ascent
    2. Limited exertion
    3. Sleeping altitude
    4. High-carbohydrate diet
    5. Medications
  B. Types of high-altitude illness (pp. 1434–1436)
    1. Acute mountain sickness (AMS)
      a. Signs and symptoms
      b. Treatment
    2. High-altitude pulmonary edema (HAPE)
      a. Signs and symptoms
      b. Treatment
    3. High altitude cerebral edema (HACE)
      a. Signs and symptoms
      b. Treatment

VIII. Chapter summary (p. 1436). Our environment provides us with all that we need to survive and prosper. The extremes of our environment, however, can have significant impact on human metabolism. Our bodies will, of course, compensate for these extremes, but sometimes it is not enough. Sometimes the heat

---

POINT OF INTEREST
It takes approximately 25 seconds for the mammalian diving reflex to work in adults and 45 seconds in children under 5 years old.

POWERPOINT PRESENTATION
Chapter 36 PowerPoint slides 34–45

POWERPOINT PRESENTATION
Chapter 36 PowerPoint slides 46–49

POWERPOINT PRESENTATION
Chapter 36 PowerPoint slide 50

gain or loss is too much. Sometimes the pressure change is too much. As a result, medical illnesses and emergencies arise. These can range from abnormal core body temperatures to decompensation, shock, and even death.

Basic knowledge of common environmental, recreational, and exposure emergencies is necessary in order for you to administer prompt and proper treatment in the prehospital setting. It is not easy to remember this type of information because these problems are not usually encountered on a daily basis. Remember the general principles involved. Remove the environmental influence causing the problem. Support the patient's own attempt to compensate. Finally, select a definitive care location and transport the patient as rapidly as possible.

In every case, remember that you must maintain your own safety. There are too many cases in which paramedics have lost their lives as a result of attempting a rescue for which they were not properly trained. Rapid action is always necessary when performing an environmental rescue; however, common sense must prevail.

SKILLS DEMONSTRATION AND PRACTICE

Students can practice skills discussed in this chapter in the following settings.

Skills Lab: The following stations should be part of a larger medical scenario lab. Divide the class into teams. Have the teams circulate through the stations. Monitor the groups to be sure all groups have a chance to manage each of the cases and so that every student has the opportunity to be team leader. You may wish to have other instructors or qualified paramedics assist students in these activities.

Station	Equipment and Personnel Needed	Activities
Hypothermia	Immobilization set Medication box Resuscitation gear 1 patient 1 instructor	Have students practice assessing and managing patients with hypothermia.
Heat Illness	1 patient 1 instructor	Have students practice assessing and managing patients with a heat-related illness

Hospital: Visit a hyperbaric chamber. Assist in assessing and managing environmental emergencies in the emergency department.

Field Internship: Assist in assessing and managing environmental emergencies in the field.

ASSIGNMENTS

Assign students to complete Chapter 36, "Environmental Emergencies," of the workbook. Also assign them to read Chapter 37, "Infectious Disease," before the next class.

EVALUATION

Chapter Quiz and Scenario Distribute copies of the Chapter Quiz provided in Handout 36-3 to evaluate student understanding of this chapter. Make sure each student reads the scenario to reinforce critical thinking on the scene. Remind students not to use their notes or textbooks while taking the quiz.

Student CD Quizzes for every chapter are contained on the dynamic and highly visual in-text student CD.

Companion Website Additional quizzes for every chapter are contained on this exciting website.

TestGen You may wish to create a custom-tailored test using *Prentice Hall TestGen for Essentials of Paramedic Care*, 2nd Edition to evaluate student understanding of this chapter.

On-line Test Preparation (for students and instructors) Additional test preparation is available through Brady's new on-line product, *EMT Achieve: Paramedic Test Preparation* at *http://www.prenhall.com/emtachieve/*. Instructors can also monitor student mastery on-line.

Review Manual for the EMT-Paramedic This comprehensive exam review contains hundreds of test questions and rationales, including scenarios, along with two 180-question practice tests on CD.

REINFORCEMENT

Handouts If classroom discussion or performance on the quiz indicates that some students have not fully mastered the chapter content, you may wish to assign some or all of the Reinforcement Handouts for this chapter.

Student CD (for students) A wide variety of material on this CD-ROM will reinforce and also expand student knowledge and skills.

PowerPoint Presentation (for instructors) The PowerPoint material developed for this chapter offers useful reinforcement of chapter content.

Companion Website (for students) Additional review quizzes and links to EMS resources will contribute to further reinforcement of the chapter.

OneKey On-line support is offered for this course on one of three platforms: CourseCompass, Blackboard, or Web CT. Includes the IRM, PowerPoints, TestGen, and Companion Website for instruction. Ask your local sales representative for more information.

Brady Skills Series: Advanced Life Skills (Video or CD) Have your students watch the skills come to life on VHS or CD-ROM, or they can purchase the highly visual, full-color text with step-by-step procedures and rationales.

EMT ACHIEVE: PARAMEDIC TEST PREPARATION
Mistovich & Beasley. *EMT Achieve: Paramedic Test Preparation.*
www.prenhall.com/emtachieve/

REVIEW MANUAL FOR THE EMT-PARAMEDIC
Cherry & Mistovich. *Review Manual for the EMT-Paramedic,* 3rd edition.

HANDOUTS 36-5 TO 35-7
Reinforcement Activities

PARAMEDIC STUDENT CD
Student Activities

POWERPOINT PRESENTATION
Chapter 36

COMPANION WEBSITE
http://www.prenhall.com/bledsoe

ONEKEY
Chapter 36

ADVANCED LIFE SUPPORT SKILLS
Larmon & Davis. *Advanced Life Support Skills.*

ADVANCED LIFE SKILLS REVIEW
Larmon & Davis. *Advanced Life Skills Review.*

BRADY SKILLS SERIES: ALS
Larmon & Davis. *Brady Skills Series: ALS.*

PARAMEDIC NATIONAL STANDARDS SELF-TEST
Miller. *Paramedic National Standards Self-Test,* 4th edition.

HANDOUT 36-1 Student's Name _____

CHAPTER 36 OBJECTIVES CHECKLIST

Knowledge	Date Mastered
1. Define "environmental emergency."	
2. Describe the incidence, morbidity, and mortality associated with environmental emergencies.	
3. Identify risk factors most predisposing to environmental emergencies.	
4. Identify environmental factors that may cause illness or exacerbate a preexisting illness or complicate treatment or transport decisions.	
5. Define "homeostasis" and relate the concept to environmental influences.	
6. Identify normal, critically high, and critically low body temperatures.	
7. Describe several methods of temperature monitoring.	
8. Describe human thermal regulation, including system components, substances used, and wastes generated.	
9. List the common forms of heat and cold disorders.	
10. List the common predisposing factors and preventive measures associated with heat and cold disorders.	
11. Define heat illness, hypothermia, frostbite, near-drowning, decompression illness, and altitude illness.	
12. Describe the pathophysiology, signs and symptoms, and predisposing factors, preventive actions, and treatment for heat cramps, heat exhaustion, heatstroke, and fever.	
13. Describe the contribution of dehydration to the development of heat disorders.	
14. Describe the differences between classical and exertional heatstroke.	
15. Identify the fundamental thermoregulatory difference between fever and heatstroke.	
16. Discuss the role of fluid therapy in the treatment of heat disorders.	
17. Describe the pathophysiology, predisposing factors, signs, symptoms, and management of the following: • Hypothermia • Superficial and deep frostbite • Near-drowning	

844 ESSENTIALS OF PARAMEDIC CARE

HANDOUT 36-1 Continued

Knowledge	Date Mastered
• Decompression illness • Diving emergency • Altitude illness	
18. Identify differences between mild, severe, chronic, and acute hypothermia.	
19. Discuss the impact of severe hypothermia on standard BCLS and ACLS algorithms and transport considerations.	
20. Differentiate between freshwater and saltwater immersion as they relate to near-drowning.	
21. Discuss the incidence of "wet" versus "dry" drownings and the differences in their management.	
22. Discuss the complications and protective role of hypothermia in the context of near-drowning.	
23. Define self-contained underwater breathing apparatus (scuba).	
24. Describe the laws of gases and relate them to diving emergencies and altitude illness.	
25. Differentiate between the various diving emergencies.	
26. Identify the various conditions that may result from pulmonary overpressure accidents.	
27. Describe the function of the Divers Alert Network (DAN) and how its members may aid in the management of diving-related illnesses.	
28. Describe the specific function and benefit of hyperbaric oxygen therapy for the management of diving accidents.	
29. Define acute mountain sickness (AMS), high-altitude pulmonary edema (HAPE), and high-altitude cerebral edema (HACE).	
30. Discuss the symptomatic variations presented in progressive altitude illnesses.	
31. Discuss the pharmacology appropriate for the treatment of altitude illnesses.	
32. Given several preprogrammed simulated environmental emergency patients, provide the appropriate assessment, management, and transportation.	

OBJECTIVES

Handout 36-2

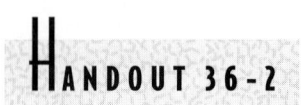

Student's Name _____

EMERGENCY CARE FOR HEAT DISORDERS

Charting Student Progress:
1. *Learning skill*
2. *Performs skill with direction*
3. *Performs skill independently*

HEAT CRAMPS

Procedure	1	2	3
1. Remove patient from hot environment.			
2. Place patient in a cool, shaded, or air-conditioned area.			
3. Administer oral fluids, if patient is alert and able to swallow, or an IV of normal saline.			

HEAT EXHAUSTION

Procedure	1	2	3
1. Remove patient from hot environment.			
2. Place patient in a cool, shaded, or air-conditioned area.			
3. Administer oral fluids, if patient is alert and able to swallow, or an IV of normal saline.			
4. Place patient in a supine position.			
5. Remove some clothing and fan the patient, but do not chill the patient.			
6. Treat for shock, if shock is suspected, but do not overheat the patient.			

HEATSTROKE

Procedure	1	2	3
1. Remove patient from hot environment.			
2. Place patient in a cool, shaded, or air-conditioned area.			

HANDOUT 36-2 Continued

Procedure	1	2	3

3. Initiate rapid active cooling en route to hospital by:
   a. Removing patient's clothing.
   b. Covering the patient with sheets soaked in tepid water.
   c. Cooling body temperature to no lower than 102°F/30°C.			

4. Administer high-flow oxygen by nonrebreather mask.			
5. Administer oral fluids if patient is alert and able to swallow.			
6. Begin one or two IVs of normal saline, wide open.			
7. Monitor the ECG.			
8. Monitor body temperature.			

HANDOUT 36-3

Student's Name _____

CHAPTER 36 QUIZ

Write the letter of the best answer in the space provided.

_____ 1. A medical condition caused or exacerbated by the weather, terrain, atmospheric pressure, or other local factors is called a(n):
  A. homeostatic emergency.
  B. external emergency.
  C. environmental emergency.
  D. localized emergency.

_____ 2. All of the following factors can predispose certain individuals to developing environmental illnesses EXCEPT:
  A. age.
  B. complexion.
  C. fatigue.
  D. medications.

_____ 3. The natural tendency of the body to maintain a steady and normal internal environment is called:
  A. homeostasis.
  B. stability.
  C. homeopathy.
  D. normostasis.

_____ 4. Thermal gradient is the difference in temperature between the:
  A. highest and lowest normal body temperature.
  B. lowest and highest tolerable temperatures.
  C. hypothermia and hyperthermia.
  D. environment and the body.

_____ 5. Thermoregulatory thermogenesis is the production of heat resulting from the:
  A. high environmental temperatures.
  B. increase in the rate of cellular metabolism.
  C. exercise of muscles working effectively.
  D. processing of food and nutrients.

_____ 6. Heat loss from direct contact of the body's surfaces with another, cooler object is called:
  A. convection.
  B. conduction.
  C. radiation.
  D. evaporation.

_____ 7. An unclothed person will lose approximately 60 percent of total body heat at room temperature by the mechanism of:
  A. convection.
  B. conduction.
  C. radiation.
  D. evaporation.

_____ 8. The portion of the brain responsible for temperature regulation is the:
  A. pituitary gland.
  B. sternomastoid.
  C. hypothalamus.
  D. pineal gland.

_____ 9. The rate at which the body consumes energy just to maintain stability is called the:
  A. basal metabolic rate.
  B. homeostatic rate.
  C. normostatic rate.
  D. thermoregulatory rate.

_____ 10. The lowest body temperature at which cardiac resuscitation is possible and the recovery prognosis favorable is at least:
  A. 80°F.
  B. 82°F.
  C. 84°F.
  D. 86°F.

_____ 11. The general signs of heat loss include all of the following EXCEPT:
  A. diaphoresis.
  B. increased skin temperature.
  C. flushing.
  D. cyanosis.

HANDOUT 36-3 (Continued)

_____ 12. For heatstroke, you should lower the patient's body temperature to no lower than:
  A. 94°F.
  B. 98°F.
  C. 102°F.
  D. 106°F.

_____ 13. Your patient has been working in his garden on a very hot, humid day and has not been drinking fluids. His body temperature is about 101°F, his skin is cool and clammy with heavy perspiration, his breathing is rapid and shallow, and his pulse is weak. He is conscious and tells you he feels weak. You suspect:
  A. heat cramps.
  B. heat exhaustion.
  C. heatstroke.
  D. heat shock.

_____ 14. Signs and symptoms of heatstroke may include:
  A. bradycardia initially, tachycardia later.
  B. cool, clammy skin.
  C. hot, dry skin.
  D. hypertension.

_____ 15. The first essential step in the treatment of a patient with heatstroke is to:
  A. initiate rapid active cooling.
  B. remove him from the hot environment.
  C. administer high-flow oxygen.
  D. administer fluid therapy.

_____ 16. Efforts to cool the body temperature of a pediatric patient with a fever should include:
  A. immersion in cool water.
  B. rubbing-alcohol sponge bath.
  C. cold packs in the armpits and groin.
  D. administration of an antipyretic medication.

_____ 17. When the core temperature of the body drops to below _____, an individual is considered to be hypothermic.
  A. 99°F
  B. 98.6°F
  C. 97°F
  D. 95°F

_____ 18. The ECG deflection associated with hypothermia and seen at a core temperature below 32°C is a(n):
  A. elevated ST segment.
  B. U wave.
  C. first degree AV block.
  D. J wave.

_____ 19. Guidelines for handling cardiac arrest patients whose core temperature is below 30°C include:
  A. checking for pulse and respirations for longer periods.
  B. administrating up to six defibrillation shocks.
  C. avoiding orotracheal intubation.
  D. increasing doses of epinephrine.

_____ 20. Your patient has been skiing all day and has developed frostbite to both of his feet. Your treatment may include:
  A. massaging the feet to restore circulation.
  B. providing analgesia prior to thawing.
  C. thawing the feet because refreezing is possible.
  D. rewarming the feet so the patient can walk away.

_____ 21. Which one of the following statements is TRUE?
  A. Drowning is the leading cause of death in children under the age of 5.
  B. Drowning is the third most common cause of accidental death in the United States.
  C. Approximately 85 percent of near-drowning victims are female.
  D. Two-thirds of the males who are near-drowning victims know how to swim.

HANDOUT 36-3 Continued

_____ 22. The term "dry drowning" refers to death:
   A. more than 24 hours after a submersion.
   B. from submersion in small containers such as buckets.
   C. from submersion if water does not enter the lungs.
   D. from long-term exposure to pulmonary irritants.

_____ 23. Although the physiology of freshwater and saltwater drownings differs, there is _____ difference in the end metabolic result or in prehospital management.
   A. no
   B. only a slight
   C. somewhat of a
   D. considerable

_____ 24. The mammalian diving reflex _____ blood flow everywhere except to the brain.
   A. increases
   B. constricts
   C. ceases
   D. dilates

_____ 25. If rescue personnel must go into the water to rescue a patient, they should wear protective clothing if water temperature is less than:
   A. 90°F.
   B. 87°F.
   C. 83°F.
   D. 70°F.

_____ 26. One emergency a diver may experience is "nitrogen narcosis." Which of the following is true regarding this condition?
   A. It is commonly called "the bends" and causes severe pain.
   B. It is caused by the development of nitrogen bubbles within body tissues.
   C. It is a state of stupor due to nitrogen's effect on cerebral function.
   D. The most serious effect is pulmonary overpressure.

_____ 27. Patients who complain of joint and abdominal pain, fatigue, paresthesia, and CNS disturbances within 24 hours after a dive are most likely suffering from:
   A. "the squeeze."
   B. decompression illness.
   C. nitrogen narcosis.
   D. arterial gas embolism.

_____ 28. High-altitude illnesses usually becomes manifest at altitudes greater than:
   A. 4,000 feet.
   B. 6,000 feet.
   C. 8,000 feet.
   D. 10,000 feet.

_____ 29. Signs and symptoms of high-altitude pulmonary edema include:
   A. coughing producing frothy sputum.
   B. decreased urine output.
   C. abdominal pain
   D. severe vomiting.

_____ 30. High-altitude cerebral edema (HACE) will cause a(n):
   A. decrease in intracranial pressure.
   B. increase in intracranial pressure.
   C. initial decrease in intracranial pressure following by a marked increase.
   D. initial increase in intracranial pressure following by a marked decrease.

HANDOUT 36-4

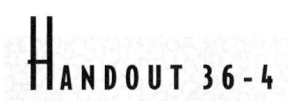

Student's Name _____

CHAPTER 36 SCENARIO

Review the following real-life situation. Then answer the questions that follow.

Your Medic 6 team is dispatched to a track and field event. Dispatch informs you that athletic trainers are currently working on a female athlete who collapsed during a 5K run. It is late in the afternoon and the temperature and humidity are high.

When you arrive, the patient is in the trainer's tent. She is unconscious and unresponsive, her skin hot and dry, her pupils dilated and fixed, and alternating deep and shallow breathing is evident. The athletic training staff has packed the patient in wet towels with ice located at the armpits, knees, groin, wrists, ankles, and neck. A brief history finds that the athlete has recently had the flu. Her fluid intake during the race was minimal. Following the race, the patient sat down to stretch and became unconscious.

The patient is loaded into the ambulance where cooling is continued. Vitals are: pulse 130 and weak, BP 80/30, respirations 26. Oxygen is administered via nonrebreather mask at 15 liters/minute. Two large-bore IVs are initiated and run wide open with lactated Ringer's. The ECG monitor shows a sinus tachycardia without ectopy. The patient is transported in emergency status and the hospital is notified of the patient's condition en route.

1. What is the athlete's problem?

2. Describe the physiological events that have led to the athlete's condition.

3. Why do you think the athlete experienced this episode?

4. How should the paramedics alter treatment if the patient begins to have seizure activity?

Handout 36-5

Student's Name _____

CHAPTER 36 REVIEW

Write the word or words that best completes each sentence in the space(s) provided.

1. _____ is the natural tendency of the body to maintain a steady and normal internal environment.
2. An _____ emergency is a medical condition caused or exacerbated by the weather, terrain, atmospheric pressure, or other local factors.
3. The difference in temperature between the environment and the body is called the _____ _____.
4. _____ is the production of heat, especially within the body.
5. Loss of body heat by direct contact with a cooler object or surface is called heat loss by _____.
6. Heat loss to air currents passing over the body is called _____.
7. The body temperature of the deep tissues is called the _____ temperature.
8. _____ is the maintenance or regulation of a particular temperature of the body.
9. The _____, which is in the brain, is the body's thermostat.
10. The rate at which the body consumes energy just to maintain stability is called the _____ _____ _____.
11. The rate at which the body consumes energy during activity is called the _____ metabolic rate.
12. _____ is an unusually high core body temperature, while _____ is an unusually low core body temperature.
13. The condition characterized by acute painful spasms of the voluntary muscles following strenuous activity in a hot environment without adequate fluid or salt intake is called _____ _____.
14. An acute, dangerous reaction to heat exposure characterized by central nervous system disturbances and a body temperature above 105°F is called _____.
15. When caring for a child with a fever, consider administering an _____ primarily for patient comfort.
16. A core temperature less than _____ with signs and symptoms of hypothermia is considered severe hypothermia.
17. Hypothermia patients who experience body temperatures above _____ will usually have a favorable prognosis.
18. Treatment of the hypothermic patient includes avoiding rough handling, which can trigger _____.
19. The use of warm blankets and heat packs to treat a hypothermic patient is known as _____ _____.
20. The ECG deflection associated with hypothermia is called the _____ _____.
21. The return of cool blood and acids from extremities to the core of a hypothermic patient being rewarmed by the application of heat packs may result in _____ _____.
22. The environmentally induced freezing of body tissues causing destruction of cells is called _____.
23. Freezing involving epidermal and subcutaneous tissues, resulting in a white appearance, hard feeling on palpation, and loss of sensation is called _____ _____.

HANDOUT 36-5 Continued

24. An incident of potentially fatal submersion in liquid that did not result in death is called _____-_____.

25. In a near-drowning or drowning situation, freshwater washes away _____, causing alveoli to collapse.

26. A complex cardiovascular reflex resulting from the submersion of the face and nose in cold water is called the _____ _____ reflex.

27. The cold-water drowning victim is not dead until he or she is _____ and dead.

28. _____ Law states that the amount of gas dissolved in a given volume of fluid is proportional to the pressure of the gas above it.

29. _____ _____ is a state of stupor that develops during deep dives due to nitrogen's effect on cerebral functions; another term for the condition is "_____ _____ _____ _____."

30. The development of nitrogen bubbles within the tissues due to a rapid reduction of air pressure is called _____ illness, or "_____ _____."

31. Patients suffering from severe barotrauma may require treatment in a _____ oxygen chamber.

32. Signs and symptoms such as a rapid, dramatic onset of sharp, tearing pain within 2 to 10 minutes of ascent from a deep dive indicate blocked blood flow caused by an _____ _____ _____.

33. Increased pulmonary pressure and hypertension caused by changes in blood flow at high altitude is called high-altitude _____ _____.

34. Increased fluid in the brain causing a rise in intracranial pressure at high altitudes is known as high-altitude _____ _____.

35. _____ occurs from increasing pressure during a diving descent and is commonly called "the squeeze."

Handout 36-6

Student's Name _____

WATER EMERGENCIES

Describe the physiological processes affecting patients and treatment in each of the following situations.

1. Freshwater Drowning
   Processes: _____
   _____
   _____
   _____

   Treatment: _____
   _____

2. Saltwater Drowning
   Processes: _____
   _____
   _____
   _____

   Treatment: _____
   _____

3. Barotrauma
   Processes: _____
   _____
   _____
   _____

   Treatment: _____
   _____

4. Nitrogen Narcosis
   Processes: _____
   _____
   _____
   _____

   Treatment: _____
   _____

5. Decompression Illness
   Processes: _____
   _____
   _____
   _____

   Treatment: _____
   _____

HANDOUT 36-6 Continued

6. Arterial Gas Embolism
   Processes: _____
   _____
   _____
   _____

   Treatment: _____
   _____

7. Pulmonary Overpressure Accidents
   Processes: _____
   _____
   _____
   _____

   Treatment: _____
   _____

8. Pneumomediastinum
   Processes: _____
   _____
   _____
   _____

   Treatment: _____
   _____

REINFORCEMENT

HANDOUT 36-7

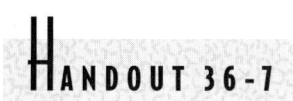

Student's Name _____

THERMAL DISORDERS

Describe the physiological processes affecting patients and treatment in each of the following situations.

1. Heat Cramps
   Processes: _____
   _____
   _____
   _____

   Treatment: _____
   _____

2. Heat Exhaustion
   Processes: _____
   _____
   _____
   _____

   Treatment: _____
   _____

3. Heatstroke
   Processes: _____
   _____
   _____
   _____

   Treatment: _____
   _____

4. Mild Hypothermia
   Processes: _____
   _____
   _____
   _____

   Treatment: _____
   _____

5. Severe Hypothermia
   Processes: _____
   _____
   _____
   _____

   Treatment: _____
   _____

HANDOUT 36-7 Continued

6. Frostbite
Processes: _____
_____
_____
_____

Treatment: _____
_____

Chapter 36 Answer Key

Handout 36-3: Chapter 36 Quiz

1. C	9. A	17. D	25. D
2. B	10. D	18. D	26. C
3. A	11. D	19. A	27. B
4. D	12. C	20. B	28. C
5. B	13. B	21. B	29. A
6. B	14. C	22. C	30. B
7. C	15. B	23. A	
8. C	16. D	24. B	

Handout 36-4: Chapter 36 Scenario

1. Heatstroke.
2. Temperature regulation has been lost, probably from insufficient water replacement during exertion in the high temperature. This loss of thermoregulation can lead to cell death and physiologic collapse.
3. Because the athlete recently was ill with the flu, she probably did not have an ideal fluid/electrolyte balance prior to beginning the race. During the race, she failed to adequately replace fluids that were being lost, which resulted in a loss of temperature regulation.
4. Treatment with diazepam would be appropriate.

Handout 36-5: Chapter 36 Review

1. Homeostasis
2. environmental
3. thermal gradient
4. Thermogenesis
5. conduction
6. convection
7. core
8. Thermoregulation
9. hypothalamus
10. basal metabolic rate
11. exertional
12. Hyperthermia, hypothermia
13. heat cramps
14. heatstroke
15. antipyretic
16. 90°F
17. 86°F
18. dysrhythmias
19. active rewarming
20. J wave
21. rewarming shock
22. frostbite
23. deep frostbite
24. near-drowning
25. surfactant
26. mammalian diving
27. warm
28. Henry's
29. Nitrogen narcosis, raptures of the deep
30. decompression, the bends
31. hyperbaric
32. arterial gas embolism
33. pulmonary edema
34. cerebral edema
35. Barotrauma

Handout 36-6: Water Emergencies

1. Freshwater drowning
   Processes: due to the large surface area of the lungs, a large amount of water is allowed to enter the vascular space. Hemodilution results. Surfactant is washed away causing alveoli to collapse.
   Treatment: symptomatic and should, in the case of cardiac arrest, follow ACLS protocols, unless the patient is hypothermic.
2. Saltwater drowning
   Processes: the hypertonic nature of the solution causes fluid to be drawn from the vascular space into the lungs, causing pulmonary edema.
   Treatment: should be the same as for freshwater drowning.
3. Barotrauma
   Processes: caused by inability of a diver to equalize the pressure between the nasopharynx and middle ear.
   Treatment: includes decreasing the amount of nitrogen present in the blood.
4. Nitrogen narcosis
   Processes: caused by nitrogen's effect on cerebral function. Diver appears intoxicated.
   Treatment: includes decreasing the amount of nitrogen present in the blood.
5. Decompression illness
   Processes: caused by air bubbles forming in the blood and joints due to a rapid ascent to the surface.
   Treatment: should be symptomatic with transport to a hyperbaric oxygen chamber facility. Transport patient in Trendelenburg position.
6. Arterial gas embolism
   Processes: air bubbles enter the circulatory system during a rapid ascent because of rupture of small pulmonary vessels.
   Treatment: same as for decompression sickness.
7. Pulmonary overpressure accidents
   Processes: lung overinflation due to rapid ascent. Air trapped in the lungs by mucous plugs, bronchospasm, or simple breath-holding. With rapid ascent, ambient pressure drops quickly, causing the trapped air to expand.
   Treatment: the same as for pneumothorax caused by any other mechanism. Rest and supplemental oxygen are important, but hyperbaric oxygen is not usually necessary.
8. Pneumomediastinum
   Processes: a release of air through the visceral pleura into the mediastinum and pericardial sac.
   Treatment: includes high-flow oxygen, IV, and rapid transport.

Handout 36-7: Thermal Disorders

1. Heat cramps
   Processes: intermittent, painful contractions of various skeletal muscles caused by a rapid change in extracellular fluid osmolarity resulting from sodium and water losses.
   Treatment: includes removing patient from the environment with an increase of fluid and sodium intake. Severe cases may need IV fluid replacement.

2. Heat exhaustion
   Processes: caused by dehydration and salt loss from exposure to a hot environment. History is important to determine appropriate assessment.
   Treatment: includes removing patient from the environment and replacing fluids with IV normal saline solution. If untreated, may progress to heatstroke.
3. Heatstroke
   Processes: hypothalamic temperature regulation is lost.
   Treatment: includes rapid patient cooling, oxygen, two large-bore IVs wide open initially, monitoring of core temperature.
4. Mild hypothermia
   Processes: lowing of body core temperature to between 86°F and 97°F, leading to a lowered metabolic rate and lowered cardiac output and a shift in fluids from the vascular to the extravascular compartment.
   Treatment: includes removing all wet clothing and protecting against heat loss, avoiding rough handling, monitoring core temperature and cardiac rhythm, rewarming patient as able, giving warm fluids if patient has stopped uncontrolled shivering.
5. Severe hypothermia
   Processes: core temperature below 86°F, processes described for mild hypothermia continue, leading to cell ischemia and necrosis eventually resulting in death.
   Treatment: includes everything for mild hypothermia as well as warm IV fluids and warmed oxygen. Avoid medication administration. If vital signs are absent and core temperature is less than 86°F, cardiac arrest medications should be avoided.
6. Frostbite
   Processes: caused by environmentally induced freezing of body tissues, resulting in ice crystals forming within and water being drawn out of the cells into the extracellular space. Ice crystals expand, causing the destruction of cells.
   Treatment: do not thaw if there is any possibility of refreezing. Do not massage or rub with snow. Administer analgesia prior to thawing. Transport for rewarming by immersion. Cover thawed part with loosely applied, dry, sterile dressings. Elevate and immobilize thawed part. Do not puncture or drain blisters. Do not rewarm frozen feet if they are required for walking out of a hazardous situation.

Chapter 37

Infectious Disease

INTRODUCTION

Infectious diseases are illnesses caused by infection or infestation of the human body by various biological agents. All health care professionals must maintain a strong working knowledge of public health principles and infectious diseases. This chapter discusses infectious diseases, including the types of disease-causing organisms, functions of the immune system, and general pathophysiology of infectious diseases. It also emphasizes the specific diseases, discussing those most likely encountered by the paramedic in the field, as well as during interhospital transports or out-of-hospital care.

CHAPTER OBJECTIVES

After reading this chapter, you should be able to:

1. Describe the specific anatomy and physiology pertinent to infectious and communicable diseases. (pp. 1443–1446; also see Chapter 4)
2. Define specific terminology identified with infectious/communicable diseases. (pp. 1441–1482)
3. Discuss public health principles relevant to infectious/communicable diseases. (pp. 1441–1442)
4. Identify public health agencies involved in the prevention and management of disease outbreaks. (p. 1442)
5. List and describe the steps of an infectious process. (pp. 1446–1449)
6. Discuss the risks associated with infection. (pp. 1441, 1446–1449)
7. List and describe the stages of infectious diseases. (pp. 1446–1449)
8. List and describe infectious agents, including bacteria, viruses, fungi, protozoans, and helminths (worms). (pp. 1443–1446)
9. Describe characteristics of the immune system. (see Chapters 4 and 31)
10. Describe the processes of the immune system defenses, including humoral and cell-mediated immunity. (see Chapters 4 and 31)
11. In specific diseases, identify and discuss the issues of personal isolation. (pp. 1449–1484)
12. Describe and discuss the rationale for the various types of personal protection equipment. (pp. 1449–1453)

TOTAL TEACHING TIME: 7.67 HOURS

The total teaching time is only a guideline based on the didactic and practical lab averages in the National Standard Curriculum. Instructors should take into consideration such factors as the pace at which students learn, the size of the class, and breaks. The actual time devoted to teaching objectives is the responsibility of the instructor.

©2007 Pearson Education, Inc.
Essentials of Paramedic Care, 2nd ed.

13. Discuss what constitutes a significant exposure to an infectious agent. (pp. 1453–1454)
14. Describe the assessment of a patient suspected of, or identified as having, an infectious/communicable disease. (pp. 1454–1455)
15. Discuss the proper disposal of contaminated supplies such as sharps, gauze, sponges, and tourniquets. (pp. 1451–1452)
16. Discuss disinfection of patient care equipment and areas where patient care occurred. (pp. 1452–1453)
17. Discuss the seroconversion rate after direct significant HIV exposure. (pp. 1448–1449)
18. Discuss the causative agent, body systems affected, and potential secondary complications, routes of transmission, susceptibility and resistance, signs and symptoms, patient management and protective measures, and immunization for each of the following:
    - HIV (pp. 1447, 1451, 1456–1458)
    - Hepatitis A (pp. 1447, 1459)
    - Hepatitis B (pp. 1447, 1459–1460)
    - Hepatitis C (pp. 1447, 1460)
    - Hepatitis D (p. 1460)
    - Hepatitis E (pp. 1460–1461)
    - Tuberculosis (pp. 1461–1463)
    - Meningococcal meningitis (pp. 1466–1468)
    - Pneumonia (pp. 1447, 1463–1464)
    - Tetanus (pp. 1476–1477)
    - Rabies (pp. 1475–1476)
    - Hantavirus (p. 1473)
    - Chickenpox (pp. 1465–1466)
    - Mumps (pp. 1447, 1469)
    - Rubella (p. 1470)
    - Measles (pp. 1447, 1469–1470)
    - Pertussis (whooping cough) (pp. 1470–1471)
    - Influenza (pp. 1447, 1468–1469)
    - Mononucleosis (p. 1471)
    - Herpes simplex 1 and 2 (pp. 1447, 1471–1472, 1480)
    - Syphilis (pp. 1447, 1478–1479)
    - Gonorrhea (pp. 1447, 1478)
    - Chlamydia (p. 1480)
    - Scabies (p. 1482)
    - Lice (pp. 1481–1482)
    - Lyme disease (pp. 1447, 1477–1478)
    - Gastroenteritis (pp. 1473–1474)
19. Discuss other infectious agents known to cause meningitis, including streptococcus pneumonia, haemophilus influenza type B, and various varieties of viruses. (pp. 1466–1468)
20. Identify common pediatric viral diseases. (pp. 1465–1466, 1469–1471, 1472)
21. Discuss the characteristics of and organisms associated with febrile and afebrile diseases including bronchiolitis, bronchitis, laryngitis, croup, epiglottitis, and the common cold. (pp. 1468–1473)
22. Articulate the pathophysiological principles of an infectious process given a case study of a patient with an infectious/communicable disease. (pp. 1441–1484)
23. Given several preprogrammed infectious disease patients, provide the appropriate body substance isolation procedure, assessment, management, and transport. (pp. 1441–1484)

FRAMING THE LESSON

Begin class by reviewing the important points from Chapter 36, "Environmental Emergencies."; Discuss any aspects of the chapter not fully understood by students. Then begin with Chapter 37 material. Review the importance of and the procedures for body substance isolation (BSI) when handling specific types of patients. Review which specific diseases may require special precautions or equipment. Have each piece of personal protective equipment (PPE) available for students to practice with during scenarios. Discuss the importance of students having their own personal protective equipment, such as a "pocket mask." Because many EMTs and paramedics have their own personal "jump kit" in their car or at home, ask students to bring theirs to class and inventory what PPE they may have or need. You may approach your school about allowing you to place a bulk order of gloves, masks, and so on for students to purchase at a reduced price. Stress that if students are going to make patient contacts when they are not on duty or equipment from an emergency service is not available, they must have the proper personal protective equipment.

TEACHING STRATEGIES

People learn in a variety of ways. Some do better with the spoken word, whereas others prefer the written. Some prefer to work alone, whereas others profit from working in groups. Recognizing these different ways of acquiring knowledge, the authors of this *Instructor's Resource Manual* have provided a variety of teaching strategies for the different types of learners. These strategies are intended to foster higher-level cognitive skills and encourage creative learning and problem solving. For greatest effectiveness, incorporate these strategies into your class lecture. Symbols in the Lecture Outline indicate the points at which various exercises might be most appropriate. Other strategies can be used to preview the lesson or to summarize it.

The following strategies are keyed to specific sections of the lesson.

1. Review of the Immune System. This is an excellent time to review the immune system response from Chapter 4. Make these associations as often as you can throughout your course. Attaching new information to old information helps students learn.

2. Immunization Inventory. Have students bring in documentation of the various vaccinations and immunizations required for health care workers, including the normal "childhood" immunizations: HBV, chickenpox, measles, mumps, and so on. If any students are deficient in any of the necessary immunizations, now is the time to discover that and correct it.

3. Revealing Contaminants with Luminol. Body fluids are a major carrier of infectious disease. Use Luminol (available from law enforcement, used at crime scene investigations) in your classroom and lavatory to "illuminate" the contaminants lurking about.

4. Pharmacology of a Disease. Because students have likely already had pharmacology at this point in the program, liken the factors affecting infection to some pharmacology terms they already know. The concepts are remarkably similar:

Mode = Route

Virulence = Potency

Dose = Dose

Resistance = Tolerance

5. Job Exposure Brainstorming. Give students 5 minutes each to think of a situation in which they could be exposed to a communicable disease on the job. Share the stories aloud. Too often, health care workers think a dirty needle is their biggest enemy. However, this exercise will bring to light 20 to 30 different situations in which an exposure could occur, from being coughed on to spat upon to exposure due to faulty personal protective equipment.

The following strategies can be used at various points throughout the lesson or to help summarize and demonstrate what students have learned.

Infection Simulations. During lab, run students through simulations of infected patients. Insist that students use the appropriate personal protective equipment, even in class. This way, students will get used to recognizing signs and symptoms of various infectious diseases and selecting and wearing the appropriate PPE.

Interviewing Hospital Personnel. Have students interview hospital personnel to determine the emergency department's procedures for receiving patients with infectious diseases. This activity will lend additional information to the practical care of an infected patient, as well as improving provider relationships the next time a communicable patient is brought to that receiving facility. Additionally, check with your hospital's exposure control department for their next drill on receiving contaminated patients. It may be possible for your class to participate.

Guest Speaker: EMS Disease Control Officer. Invite the infectious disease control officer from a local EMS agency to address the class on how potential infectious disease exposures are handled within their system. What is the reporting procedure? What forms are used? How are results and information passed on to those potentially exposed? What are the responsibilities of the EMS agency in the testing and treatment, if needed, for those exposed?

Infection Control Scenarios. Divide the class into small groups. Have each group create a scenario that would pose a variety of infection risks to responding EMS personnel and have them list the precautions that the personnel should take. Then have the groups take turns presenting just their scenarios to the class as a whole. What precautions does the class as a whole come up with? Discuss and debate any differences in responses.

Guest Speaker: Hospital Infection Control Specialist. Hospitals usually have infection control specialists within their system as well as physicians specializing in infectious diseases. Invite such individuals to address the class.

Cultural Considerations, Legal Notes, and Patho Pearls. The Student CD-ROM contains this series of informative features to enhance the student's understanding of the material covered in this chapter.

TEACHING OUTLINE

Chapter 37 is the eleventh lesson in Division 4, *Medical Emergencies*. Distribute Handout 37-1 so that students can familiarize themselves with the learning goals for this chapter. If students have any questions about the objectives, answer them at this time.

HANDOUT 37-1
Chapter 37 Objectives Checklist

Then present the chapter. One possible lecture outline follows. In the outline the parenthetical references in regular type are references to text pages; those in bold type are references to figure, tables, or procedures.

I. Introduction. Infectious diseases are illnesses caused by infestation of the body by biological organisms such as bacteria, viruses, fungi, protozoans, and helminths. Though most infectious disease states are not life-threatening, some types of infection, such as HIV, HBV, and acute bacterial meningitis, are particularly dangerous and may result in death or permanent disability. Early recognition and management of patients with these diseases may make a difference in the patient's outcome as well as prevent exposure to providers. (p. 1441)

II. Public health principles (pp. 1441–1442)

  A. Epidemiologists (p. 1442)
  B. Population identification (p. 1442)
  C. Tracking progress of infection (p. 1442)
  D. Index case (p. 1442)

III. Public health agencies (p. 1442)

  A. Local agencies (p. 1442)
  B. State agencies (p. 1442)
  C. Federal agencies (p. 1442)
   1. U.S. Department of Health and Human Services (DHHS)
   2. Centers for Disease Control and Prevention (CDC)
   3. National Institute for Occupational Safety and Health (NIOSH)
   4. Occupational Safety and Health Administration (OSHA)
   5. Federal Emergency Management Agency (FEMA)
   6. National Fire Protection Association (NFPA)
   7. United States Fire Protection Administration (USFPA)
   8. International Association of Fire Fighters (IAFF)

IV. Microorganisms (pp. 1442–1446)

  A. Types (p. 1443)
   1. Normal flora
   2. Pathogen
   3. Opportunistic pathogen
  B. Bacteria (pp. 1443–1444) (**Fig. 37-1, p. 1443**)
   1. Gram staining
    a. Blue = positive
    b. Red = negative
   2. General appearance
    a. Spheres
    b. Rods
    c. Spirals
   3. Endotoxins
   4. Bactericidal
   5. Bacteriostatic
  C. Viruses (pp. 1444–1445) (**Fig. 37-2, p. 1445**)
   1. Obligate intraclluealr parasites
  D. Other microorganisms (pp. 1445–1446)
   1. Prions
   2. Fungi
   3. Protozoa
   4. Parasites
   5. Pinworms

POWERPOINT
PRESENTATION
Chapter 37 PowerPoint slide 4

POINT TO EMPHASIZE
Ask whether any of your students have seen the movie *City of Joy*. It is a story of medical care in the third world that will lead to increased appreciation for sanitation and universal precautions.

POWERPOINT
PRESENTATION
Chapter 37 PowerPoint slide 4

POWERPOINT
PRESENTATION
Chapter 37 PowerPoint slides 5–7

POINT OF INTEREST
Viruses were discovered by Dmitry Ivanovsky, a Russian scientist, in 1892.

TEACHING STRATEGY 1
Review of the Immune System

TEACHING STRATEGY 2
Immunization Inventory

POINT TO EMPHASIZE
Despite the abundance of antibiotics available, infectious diseases are still common and often serious illnesses.

TEACHING STRATEGY 3
Revealing Contaminants with Luminol

POWERPOINT PRESENTATION
Chapter 37 PowerPoint slides 8–15

TEACHING STRATEGY 4
Pharmacology of a Disease

TEACHING STRATEGY 5
Job Exposure Brainstorming

HANDOUT 37-6
Categorization of Infectious Diseases and Precautions

POWERPOINT PRESENTATION
Chapter 37 PowerPoint slides 16–26

TEACHING TIP
Ask students how many of their agencies have infection control policies in place and adhere to them.

HANDOUT 37-7
Decontamination of Vehicles and Equipment

POINT TO EMPHASIZE
AIDS has become a worldwide epidemic. Regardless of where you work or travel, you will encounter people with this disease.

POWERPOINT PRESENTATION
Chapter 37 PowerPoint slides 27–29

POWERPOINT PRESENTATION
Chapter 37 PowerPoint slides 30–78

READING/REFERENCE
Coughlin, C., and A. Craft. "Hepatitis C: The Silent Epidemic." *JEMS*, March 2000.

    6. Hookworms
    7. Trichinosis

V. Contraction, transmission, and stages of disease (pp. 1446–1449)
  A. Bloodborne (p. 1447)
  B. Airborne (p. 1447)
  C. Fecal-oral route (p. 1447)
  D. Factors affecting disease transmission (p. 1447)
    1. Mode of entry (**Table 37-1, p. 1447**)
    2. Virulence
    3. Number of organisms transmitted
    4. Host resistance
    5. Other host factors
  E. Phases of the infectious process (pp. 1448–1449)
    1. Latent period
    2. Communicable period
    3. Incubation period
    4. Antigens
    5. Antibodies
    6. Seroconversion
    7. Window phase
    8. Disease period

VI. Infection control in prehospital care (pp. 1449–1454) (**Fig. 37-3, p. 1449**)
  A. Preparation for response (pp. 1449–1450)
  B. Response (p. 1450)
  C. Patient contact (pp. 1450–1451) (**Table 37-2, p. 1451**)
  D. Recovery (pp. 1451–1452) (**Fig. 37-4, p. 1452**)
  E. Decontamination methods and procedures (pp. 1451–1453)
    1. Low-level disinfection
    2. Intermediate-level disinfection
    3. High-level disinfection
    4. Sterilization
  F. Infectious disease exposures (pp. 1453–1454)
    1. Reporting an infectious disease exposure
    2. The Ryan White Act
    3. Postexposure
    4. Confidentiality

VII. Assessment of the patient with infectious disease (pp. 1454–1455)
  A. Past medical history (p. 1454)
  B. Physical examination (p. 1455)

VIII. Selected infectious diseases (pp. 1455–1483)
  A. Diseases of immediate concern to EMS providers (pp. 1455–1472)
    1. HIV
      a. Pathogenesis
      b. Risk to the general public
      c. Risk to health care workers
      d. Clinical presentation
      e. Postexposure prophylaxis
      f. Summary of HIV
      g. Universal precautions
    2. Hepatitis

    a. Hepatitis A (infectious or viral hepatitis)
    b. Hepatitis B (serum hepatitis)
    c. Hepatitis C
    d. Hepatitis D
    e. Hepatitis E
  3. Tuberculosis
    a. Skin testing
    b. Pathogenesis
    c. Clinical presentation
    d. EMS response (**Figs. 37-5a and 37-5b, p. 1463**)
    e. Masks
    f. Postexposure identification and management
  4. Pneumonia
    a. History and assessment
    b. Patient management and PPE
    c. Immunization and postexposure management
  5. Severe Acute Respiratory Syndrome (SARS) (**Fig. 36-7, p. 1465**)
    a. Pathophysiology
    b. Assessment
    c. Management
  6. Chickenpox
    a. Clinical presentation
    b. Assessing immunity
    c. Immunization
    d. EMS response and postexposure
  7. Meningitis
    a. Transmission factors
    b. Clinical presentation
    c. Immunization
    d. EMS response and postexposure
  8. Other job-related airborne diseases
    a. Influenza and the common cold
    b. Measles
    c. Mumps
    d. Rubella
    e. Respiratory syncytial virus (RSV)
    f. Pertussis
  9. Viral diseases transmitted by contact
    a. Mononucleosis
    b. Herpes simplex virus type 1
B. Other infectious conditions of the respiratory system (pp. 1472–1473)
  1. Epiglottitis
  2. Croup
  3. Pharyngitis
  4. Sinusitis
  5. Hantavirus
C. GI system infections (pp. 1473–1475)
  1. Gastroenteritis
  2. Food poisoning
D. Nervous system infections (pp. 1475–1478)
  1. Encephalitis
  2. Rabies
  3. Tetanus
  4. Lyme disease
    a. Early localized stage

POINT TO EMPHASIZE
Any child under the age of 2 with a high-grade fever has meningitis until proven otherwise.

POINT TO EMPHASIZE
Infection control begins long before an emergency call.

READING/REFERENCE
Murphy, P., and S. Alfaro. "Meningitis." *JEMS,* May 2000.

POINT OF INTEREST
Influenza was first recorded in Paris in 1414, but there may have been cases even before this date.

POINT OF INTEREST
People born before 1957 are probably immune to measles. If a pregnant woman contracts rubella during the first trimester, fetal infection occurs in up to 80 percent of cases.

POINT OF INTEREST
Once thought to be a disease of the past, over 25,000 cases of measles occurred in the United States in 1991.

POINT OF INTEREST

As early as 1930, Dr. Benjamin Washburn wrote regarding sexually transmitted diseases, "No matter how exemplary one's conduct may be, there is always a chance, which is not so remote as many people imagine, for an accidental infection. Many women are infected by their husbands, who had the disease and thought they were cured before they were married."

POINT OF INTEREST

About 12 million people in the United States contract a sexually transmitted disease each year.

POWERPOINT PRESENTATION

Chapter 37 PowerPoint slides 79–80

POWERPOINT PRESENTATION

Chapter 37 PowerPoint slide 81

ADVANCED LIFE SUPPORT SKILLS

Larmon & Davis. *Advanced Life Support Skills.*

ADVANCED LIFE SKILLS REVIEW

Larmon & Davis. *Advanced Life Skills Review.*

BRADY SKILLS SERIES: ALS

Larmon & Davis. *Brady Skills Series: ALS.*

      b. Early disseminated stage
      c. Late stage
  E. Sexually transmitted diseases (pp. 1478–1481)
    1. Gonorrhea
    2. Syphilis
      a. Primary syphilis (first stage)
      b. Secondary syphilis (second stage)
      c. Latent syphilis (third stage)
      d. Tertiary syphilis (fourth stage)
    3. Genital warts
    4. Herpes simplex type 2
    5. Chlamydia
    6. Trichomoniasis
    7. Chancroid
  F. Diseases of the skin (pp. 1481–1482)
    1. Impetigo
    2. Lice
    3. Scabies
  G. Nosocomial infections (pp. 1482–1483)
    1. Vancomycin-resistant enterococcus (VRE)
    2. Methicillin-resistant *Staphylococcus aureus* (MRSA)
    3. Resistant strains of tuberculosis

IX. Preventing disease transmission (pp. 1483–1484)

X. Chapter summary (p. 1484). Over the past 30 years, medical science has made tremendous progress in diagnosing and treating infectious diseases. New vaccines and antibiotics are continually being developed. Advances in laboratory technology, notably the polymerase chain reaction (PCR), have made the presence and identification of microorganisms easier, quicker, and more accurate. Despite these tremendous advances, many infectious diseases cannot be effectively treated. Specific treatments for most viral diseases remain elusive, and each year countless people die from AIDS, hepatitis, pneumonia, sexually transmitted diseases, and other infectious diseases.

    EMS can have a significant impact on the incidence of infectious disease if providers remain knowledgeable, are leaders in public education, and are consistently alert in protecting themselves and their patients. The title of the International Association of Fire Fighters (IAFF) hepatitis B curriculum, *The Silent War*, provides a metaphor for the dilemma of infectious diseases in EMS: EMS personnel deal with few infectious disease emergencies; however, when we do respond to such emergencies, we often are unaware of the disease's presence until after the call. Standard (universal) precautions, often written for clinical and research facilities with more predictable hazards and risks, are increased to body substance isolation (BSI) for emergency health care providers because of the uncertainties of our profession. Constant vigilance and personal accountability are the keys to reducing those risks.

SKILLS DEMONSTRATION AND PRACTICE

Students can practice skills discussed in this chapter in the following settings.

Scenario Lab: The following station will be part of a larger medical scenario lab. Divide the class into teams. Have the teams circulate through the station. Monitor the groups to be sure all groups have a chance to manage each of the cases and so that every student has the opportunity to be team leader. You may wish to have other instructors or qualified paramedics assist students in these activities.

Station	Equipment and Personnel Needed	Activities
Universal precautions and masks	Set of gowns, goggles, gloves, 1 instructor	Students practice taking universal precautions.

Hospital: Assist in assessment and management of infectious diseases in the ED.

Field Internship: Assist in assessment and management of infectious diseases in the field.

ASSIGNMENTS

Assign students to complete Chapter 37, "Infectious Disease," of the workbook. Also assign them to read Chapter 38, "Psychiatric and Behavioral Disorders," before the next class.

EVALUATION

Chapter Quiz and Scenario Distribute copies of the Chapter Quiz provided in Handout 37-2 to evaluate student understanding of this chapter. Make sure each student reads the scenario to reinforce critical thinking on the scene. Remind students not to use their notes or textbooks while taking the quiz.

Student CD Quizzes for every chapter are contained on the dynamic and highly visual in-text student CD.

Companion Website Additional quizzes for every chapter are contained on this exciting website.

TestGen You may wish to create a custom-tailored test using *Prentice Hall TestGen for Essentials of Paramedic Care*, 2nd Edition to evaluate student understanding of this chapter.

On-line Test Preparation (for students and instructors) Additional test preparation is available through Brady's new on-line product, *EMT Achieve: Paramedic Test Preparation* at *http://www.prenhall.com/emtachieve/*. Instructors can also monitor student mastery on-line.

Review Manual for the EMT-Paramedic This comprehensive exam review contains hundreds of test questions and rationales, including scenarios, along with two 180-question practice tests on CD.

REINFORCEMENT

Handouts If classroom discussion or performance on the quiz indicates that some students have not fully mastered the chapter content, you may wish to assign some or all of the Reinforcement Handouts for this chapter.

Student CD (for students) A wide variety of material on this CD-ROM will reinforce and also expand student knowledge and skills.

WORKBOOK
Chapter 37 Activities

READING/REFERENCE
Textbook, pp. 1486–1508

HANDOUT 37-2
Chapter 37 Quiz

HANDOUT 37-3
Chapter 37 Scenario

PARAMEDIC STUDENT CD
Student Activities

COMPANION WEBSITE
http://www.prenhall.com/bledsoe

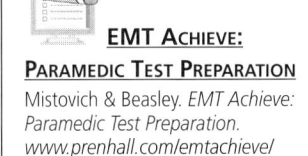

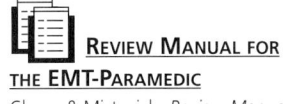

TESTGEN
Chapter 37

EMT ACHIEVE:
PARAMEDIC TEST PREPARATION
Mistovich & Beasley. *EMT Achieve: Paramedic Test Preparation.*
www.prenhall.com/emtachieve/

REVIEW MANUAL FOR THE EMT-PARAMEDIC
Cherry & Mistovich. *Review Manual for the EMT-Paramedic,* 3rd edition.

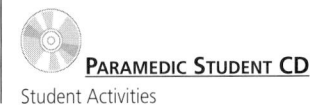

HANDOUTS 37-4 TO 37-7
Reinforcement Activities

PARAMEDIC STUDENT CD
Student Activities

POWERPOINT PRESENTATION
Chapter 37

COMPANION WEBSITE
http://www.prenhall.com/bledsoe

ONEKEY
Chapter 37

ADVANCED LIFE SUPPORT SKILLS
Larmon & Davis. *Advanced Life Support Skills.*

ADVANCED LIFE SKILLS REVIEW
Larmon & Davis. *Advanced Life Skills Review.*

BRADY SKILLS SERIES: ALS
Larmon & Davis. *Brady Skills Series: ALS.*

PARAMEDIC NATIONAL STANDARDS SELF-TEST
Miller. *Paramedic National Standards Self-Test,* 4th edition.

PowerPoint Presentation (for instructors) The PowerPoint material developed for this chapter offers useful reinforcement of chapter content.

Companion Website (for students) Additional review quizzes and links to EMS resources will contribute to further reinforcement of the chapter.

OneKey On-line support is offered for this course on one of three platforms: CourseCompass, Blackboard, or Web CT. Includes the IRM, PowerPoints, TestGen, and Companion Website for instruction. Ask your local sales representative for more information.

Brady Skills Series: Advanced Life Skills (Video or CD) Have your students watch the skills come to life on VHS or CD-ROM, or they can purchase the highly visual, full-color text with step-by-step procedures and rationales.

HANDOUT 37-1

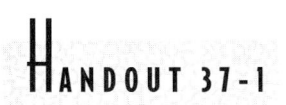

Student's Name _____

CHAPTER 37 OBJECTIVES CHECKLIST

Knowledge	Date Mastered
1. Describe the specific anatomy and physiology pertinent to infectious and communicable diseases.	
2. Define specific terminology identified with infectious/communicable diseases.	
3. Discuss public health principles relevant to infectious/communicable diseases.	
4. Identify public health agencies involved in the prevention and management of disease outbreaks.	
5. List and describe the steps of an infectious process.	
6. Discuss the risks associated with infection.	
7. List and describe the stages of infectious diseases.	
8. List and describe infectious agents, including bacteria, viruses, fungi, protozoans, and helminths (worms).	
9. Describe characteristics of the immune system.	
10. Describe the processes of the immune system defenses, including humoral and cell-mediated immunity.	
11. In specific diseases, identify and discuss the issues of personal isolation.	
12. Describe and discuss the rationale for the various types of personal protection equipment.	
13. Discuss what constitutes a significant exposure to an infectious agent.	
14. Describe the assessment of a patient suspected of, or identified as having, an infectious/communicable disease.	
15. Discuss the proper disposal of contaminated supplies such as sharps, gauze, sponges, and tourniquets.	
16. Discuss disinfection of patient care equipment and areas where patient care occurred.	
17. Discuss the seroconversion rate after direct significant HIV exposure.	

HANDOUT 37-1 Continued

Knowledge	Date Mastered
18. Discuss the causative agent, body systems affected, and potential secondary complications, routes of transmission, susceptibility and resistance, signs and symptoms, patient management and protective measures, and immunization for each of the following: • HIV • Hepatitis A • Hepatitis B • Hepatitis C • Hepatitis D • Hepatitis E • Tuberculosis • Meningococcal meningitis • Pneumonia • Tetanus • Rabies • Hantavirus • Chickenpox • Mumps • Rubella • Measles • Pertussis (whooping cough) • Influenza • Mononucleosis • Herpes simplex 1 and 2 • Syphilis • Gonorrhea • Chlamydia • Scabies • Lice • Lyme disease • Gastroenteritis	
19. Discuss other infectious agents known to cause meningitis, including streptococcus pneumonia, haemophilus influenza type B, and various varieties of viruses.	
20. Identify common pediatric viral diseases.	
21. Discuss the characteristics of and organisms associated with febrile and afebrile diseases including bronchiolitis, bronchitis, laryngitis, croup, epiglottitis, and the common cold.	
22. Articulate the pathophysiological principles of an infectious process given a case study of a patient with an infectious/communicable disease.	
23. Given several preprogrammed infectious disease patients, provide the appropriate body substance isolation procedure, assessment, management, and transport.	

OBJECTIVES

HANDOUT 37-2

Student's Name _____

CHAPTER 37 QUIZ

Write the letter of the best answer in the space provided.

_____ 1. The individual who first introduces an infectious agent to a population is called the:
   A. initial infection.
   B. index case.
   C. index carrier.
   D. pathogen introduction.

_____ 2. Organisms that live inside our bodies without ordinarily causing disease are known as:
   A. benign pathogens.
   B. host flora.
   C. normal flora.
   D. harmless flora.

_____ 3. An ordinarily harmless bacterium that may cause disease if a patient has a weakened immune system or is under unusual stress is called a(n):
   A. advantageous bacteria.
   B. immune deficient pathogen.
   C. susceptible bacteria.
   D. opportunistic pathogen.

_____ 4. Microscopic single-celled organisms that range in length from 1 to 20 micrometers are called:
   A. bacteria.
   B. exotoxins.
   C. viruses.
   D. fungi.

_____ 5. Living pathogenic bacteria may harm their human hosts by releasing toxic waste products called:
   A. endotoxins.
   B. bactericides.
   C. spheres.
   D. exotoxins.

_____ 6. It is necessary to use an electron microscope to see:
   A. bacteria.
   B. viruses.
   C. fungi.
   D. protozoa.

_____ 7. Viruses are known as obligate intracellular parasites because they:
   A. can only grow and reproduce within a host cell.
   B. are folded in such a way that protease enzymes cannot act upon them.
   C. can remain active for several days in fluid outside of the body.
   D. can reproduce quickly in any body fluid.

_____ 8. Yeasts, molds, and mushrooms are all types of:
   A. bacteria.
   B. viruses.
   C. fungi.
   D. spores.

_____ 9. Protozoa cause diseases such as:
   A. pneumonia.
   B. malaria.
   C. Lyme disease.
   D. meningitis.

_____ 10. Hookworms and pinworms are called parasites because they:
   A. cause disease.
   B. live within cells.
   C. live in or on another organism.
   D. reproduce in body fluids.

_____ 11. An example of a disease transmitted by contact with blood or body fluid is:
   A. hepatitis B.
   B. tuberculosis.
   C. measles.
   D. meningitis.

_____ 12. An example of a disease that may be transmitted by bloodborne, sexual, and indirect contact is:
   A. pneumonia.
   B. hepatitis A.
   C. mumps.
   D. herpes virus.

HANDOUT 37-2 Continued

_____ 13. Agents and diseases that are capable of being transmitted to another host are called:
  A. contaminant.
  B. virile.
  C. communicable.
  D. virulent.

_____ 14. The period of time when a host cannot transmit an infectious agent to someone else is called the:
  A. incubation period.
  B. latent period.
  C. noncommunicable period.
  D. window period.

_____ 15. Seroconversion is said to have occurred when:
  A. a person begins to show signs and symptoms of the disease.
  B. signs and symptoms of a disease disappear.
  C. the host is now able to transmit the disease to someone else.
  D. the person develops antibodies after exposure to a disease.

_____ 16. The duration from the onset of signs and symptoms of disease until the resolution of symptoms or death is called the:
  A. disease period.
  B. communicable period.
  C. window phase.
  D. latent period.

_____ 17. Neutrophils and macrophages are both types of:
  A. antigens.
  B. immunoglobulins.
  C. leukocytes.
  D. antibodies.

_____ 18. There are five classes of human antibodies. The class that attaches to mast cells and plays a major role in allergic reactions is:
  A. IgG.
  B. IgA.
  C. IgD.
  D. IgE.

_____ 19. The overflow circulatory fluid in spaces between tissues is called:
  A. plasma.
  B. lymph.
  C. serum.
  D. synovial.

_____ 20. Cells that line the lymph nodes and attach to and destroy particulate matter are called:
  A. reticuloendothelial cells.
  B. T lymphocytes
  C. macrophages.
  D. retroendothelial cells.

_____ 21. An immunity provided by antibodies that the patient did not manufacture is called:
  A. active immunity.
  B. acquired immunity.
  C. passive immunity.
  D. artificial immunity.

_____ 22. There are four phases of prehospital infection control. Putting on gloves and donning eye and face protection are part of which phase?
  A. preparation for response
  B. response
  C. patient contact
  D. recovery

_____ 23. Guidelines for prehospital infection control during patient contact include:
  A. wearing gloves, goggles, and gowns on all calls.
  B. allowing only necessary personnel to make patient contact.
  C. carefully recapping IV needles after use.
  D. eating or drinking in the patient compartment only after it has been cleaned.

_____ 24. Any reusable item that comes in contact with the patient's mucous membranes should receive:
  A. low-level disinfection.
  B. high-level disinfection.
  C. intermediate-level disinfection.
  D. sterilization.

HANDOUT 37-2 Continued

_____ 25. Which of the following is TRUE regarding the human immunodeficiency virus?
  A. HIV causes a cellular immune system response and then remains in a dormant phase.
  B. HIV specifically targets T-lymphocytes with the CD4 marker.
  C. Reports of the transmission rate from mother to infant range from 60 to 70 percent.
  D. HIV is much more contagious than hepatitis B.

_____ 26. When caring for a patient with hepatitis B, which of the following is an important point to remember?
  A. Transmission has been known to occur with tattooing, acupuncture, and communally used razors and toothbrushes.
  B. Infection of health care workers from HBV-infected patients is extremely rare.
  C. The virus is unstable and quickly dies on surfaces with dried, visible blood.
  D. Sexual transmission of HBV is not common in the general populace.

_____ 27. The most common preventable adult infectious disease in the world is:
  A. pneumonia.   C. measles.
  B. hepatitis A.   D. tuberculosis.

_____ 28. Positive Brudzinski's sign is suggestive of meningitis. Brudzinski's sign is the:
  A. inability to fully extend the knees with hips flexed.
  B. inability to form a fist with one or both hands.
  C. physical exam finding in which flexion of the neck causes flexion of the hips and knees.
  D. inability to flex one's head forward and touch the chin to the chest.

_____ 29. A very contagious infection of the skin caused by staphylococci or streptococci is:
  A. scabies.   C. impetigo.
  B. warts.   D. herpes.

_____ 30. An example of a viral disease transmitted by contact is:
  A. mononucleosis.   C. measles.
  B. pertussis.   D. mumps.

_____ 31. A patient with SARS is considered contagious:
  A. until the patient is asymptomatic.
  B. for 2 to 7 days after the onset of symptoms.
  C. for 10 to 14 days after the onset of symptoms.
  D. for 10 days after the patient is asymptomatic.

_____ 32. Signs and symptoms associated with SARS include:
  A. rhinorrhea.   C. diarrhea.
  B. rigors.   D. all of these

_____ 33. All of the following are treatment steps for a patient with suspected SARS, EXCEPT:
  A. ventilatory assistance, as needed.
  B. low-flow, low-concentration oxygen.
  C. place the patient in a position of comfort.
  D. IV fluids if patient is dehydrated.

_____ 34. SARS stands for:
  A. Secondary Acute Respiratory Syndrome.
  B. Secondary Adult Respiratory Syndrome.
  C. Severe Acute Respiratory Syndrome.
  D. Severe Adult Respiratory Syndrome.

_____ 35. The paramedic's primary concern when dealing with a suspected SARS patient is:
  A. notifying the receiving facility.
  B. donning personal protective equipment.
  C. assuring a patent airway.
  D. none of these

Handout 37-3

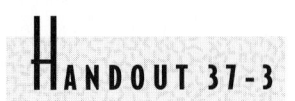

Student's Name _____

CHAPTER 37 SCENARIO

Review the following real-life situation. Then answer the questions that follow.

Medic 1 is dispatched to assist another ambulance at the scene of a multiple-vehicle crash. Upon arrival on the scene, Medic 1's crew is directed to an inverted vehicle some 25 feet off the edge of the road. The vehicle's driver has been ejected from the vehicle and is supine on the ground. Fire department personnel are performing CPR.

The paramedics' assessment confirms the pulseless and apneic patient. CPR is continued as the patient is prepared for intubation. Due to the massive facial injuries, intubation is impossible. It is impossible to maintain an airway for adequate ventilation, so the senior paramedic prepares to perform a cricothyrotomy, while her partner secures the heart monitor and intravenous access to the patient.

The first round of medications are administered, and the cricothyrotomy is performed, producing good ventilations. The patient is packaged and loaded into the unit for a short trip to an improvised landing zone. There a helicopter awaits to transport the patient to a trauma center. Patient care is transferred to the helicopter medical personnel. At transfer, the patient has two large-bore IVs and is in an idioventricular rhythm. Ventilations through the cricothyrotomy are continuing. Medic 1 confirms this information in a verbal report to the air transport personnel and the patient is transported to the trauma center.

1. What precautions against infectious diseases should have been followed by the paramedics in this scenario?

2. What infectious diseases might the crew of Medic 1 have been exposed to from this patient?

HANDOUT 37-4

Student's Name _____

CHAPTER 37 REVIEW

Write the word or words that best complete the following sentences in the space(s) provided.

1. The individual who first introduced an infectious agent to a population is called the _____ _____.
2. An illness caused by an infestation of the body by biological organisms is called a(n) _____ _____.
3. _____ _____ are organisms that live inside our bodies without ordinarily causing disease.
4. An organism capable of causing disease is called a(n) _____.
5. An ordinarily harmless bacterium that causes disease only under unusual circumstances is called a(n) _____ _____.
6. _____ are microscopic single-celled organisms that range in length from 1 to 20 micrometers.
7. Three types of bacteria are _____, _____, and _____.
8. _____ are toxic waste products released by living bacteria, while _____ are toxic products released when bacteria die and decompose.
9. _____ means a substance is capable of inhibiting bacterial growth or reproduction, while _____ means capable of killing bacteria.
10. A(n) _____ is a disease-causing organism that can be seen only with an electron microscope.
11. A(n) _____ _____ _____ is an organism that can grow and reproduce only within a host cell.
12. Plant-like microorganisms are called _____.
13. An organism that lives in or on another organism is called a(n) _____.
14. Any living creature or environment that can harbor an infectious agent is called a(n) _____.
15. The presence of an agent only on the surface of the host without penetrating it is called _____. The presence of an agent within the host, without necessarily causing disease, is called _____.
16. _____ is an organism's strength or ability to infect or overcome the body's defenses.
17. The _____ period is when a host cannot transmit an infectious agent to someone else, while the _____ period is when a host can transmit an infectious agent to someone else.
18. Phases of prehospital infection control include _____ for _____, _____, _____, _____, and _____.
19. To destroy certain forms of microorganisms, but not all, is to _____. To destroy all microorganisms is to _____.
20. _____ is the inflammation of the liver characterized by diffuse or patchy tissue necrosis.
21. Hepatitis D seems only to coexist with _____ infection.
22. _____ is the most common preventable adult infectious disease in the world.
23. _____ is inflammation of the membranes protecting the brain and spinal cord, and cerebrospinal fluid.
24. _____ is an acute viral disease characterized by painful enlargement of the salivary glands.

HANDOUT 37-4 Continued

25. _____ is a highly contagious, acute viral disease characterized by a reddish rash that appears on the fourth or fifth day of illness.

26. The three phases of pertussis are _____, _____, and _____.

27. The viral disease known as the "kissing disease" is _____.

28. _____ is an inflammation caused by infection of the brain and its structures.

29. The three stages of Lyme disease are _____ _____, _____ _____, and _____.

30. Infections that are acquired while in the hospital are called _____.

HANDOUT 37-5

Student's Name _____

INFECTIOUS DISEASE MATCHING

Write the letter of the disease in the space next to the appropriate description.

A. Tetanus
B. Herpes simplex, type 1
C. Meningitis
D. Hepatitis B
E. Tuberculosis
F. Hepatitis D
G. Scabies
H. Syphilis
I. Lice
J. Gonorrhea
K. Measles
L. Herpes simplex, type 2
M. Mumps
N. AIDS
O. Varicella

_____ 1. Bloodborne virus that requires a helper virus to replicate.

_____ 2. Infestation characterized by severe itching and small white specks in the hair.

_____ 3. Foodborne viral disease characterized by malaise, weakness, loss of appetite, and jaundice.

_____ 4. Infection of the lining of the brain and spinal cord.

_____ 5. Viral disease in which the patient may develop skin tumors known as Kaposi's sarcoma.

_____ 6. Bacterial disease in which patients develop coughs, chills, fever, fatigue, weight loss, and night sweats.

_____ 7. Viral disease characterized by swelling of the salivary glands under the jaw and around the cheeks.

_____ 8. Sexually transmitted bacterial disease characterized in males by burning urination and yellowish penile discharge.

_____ 9. Disease in which toxin travels through the blood to skeletal muscles, causing spastic rigidity.

_____ 10. Sexually transmitted viral disease that results in thin-walled vesicles on the genitalia.

_____ 11. Bloodborne viral disease characterized by malaise, weakness, loss of appetite, and pronounced jaundice.

_____ 12. Disease commonly called the "seven-year itch."

_____ 13. Sexually transmitted bacterial disease whose early presentation is characterized by a painless chancre in the genital area.

_____ 14. Viral disease that begins with fever and a reddish rash that appears first on the face and spreads to the rest of the body.

_____ 15. Viral disease characterized by a rash of fluid-filled vesicles that rupture, forming small ulcers that eventually scab.

REINFORCEMENT

HANDOUT 37-6

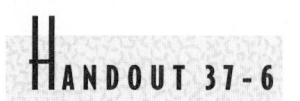

Student's Name _____

CATEGORIZATION OF INFECTIOUS DISEASES AND PRECAUTIONS

INFECTIONS OF THE NERVOUS SYSTEM

Meningitis **Precautions:** gloves, mask; bag and label linen; intermediate-level disinfection; medical surveillance for health care personnel.

Encephalitis

Brain abscess

INFECTIONS OF THE RESPIRATORY SYSTEM

Tuberculosis **Precautions:** gloves and mask; patient mask; avoid prolonged confined-space contact; avoid sputum contact; bag and label linen; intermediate or high-level disinfection; medical surveillance for health care personnel.

INFECTIONS OF THE SKIN

Scabies **Precautions:** gloves; hand washing following patient contact; sterilization or disposal of all instruments used; bag and label linen; notification of ED personnel.

Lice

CHILDHOOD DISEASES

Measles **Precautions:** masks for respiratory isolation, gloves; hand washing following contact with body secretions; sterilization or disposal of instruments used; bag and label linen; notification of ED personnel; follow up with emergency department for confirmation of type of infection, medical surveillance if needed.

Mumps

Chickenpox

INFECTIONS OF THE GASTROINTESTINAL SYSTEM

Gastroenteritis **Precautions:** gloves at all times; gowns, goggles, gloves, and mask when exposed to secretions or cleaning instruments or equipment; hand washing following contact with any body secretions; sterilization or disposal of instruments or equipment; bag and label linen, follow up with ED for type of infection, medical surveillance if needed.

Hepatitis A, B, C, D, E

HANDOUT 37-6 Continued

SEXUALLY TRANSMITTED DISEASES

Syphilis **Precautions:** gloves; hand washing following contact with any secretions; sterilization or disposal of instruments and equipment; bag and label linen; notification of ED personnel.

Gonorrhea

Chlamydia

Herpes simplex, 1 and 2

HIV INFECTION

HIV **Precautions:** gloves at all times—changed and discarded after each patient contact; glasses or face shields with procedures likely to generate blood or body fluids; gowns or aprons if splashing of blood or body fluids is likely; hand washing following contact with blood or body fluids; use of mouthpieces, resuscitation bags, or ventilation devices during resuscitation; proper disposal of sharps; sterilization or disposal of instruments and equipment; bag and label linen; notification of ED personnel.

AIDS

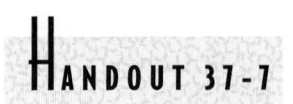

DECONTAMINATION OF VEHICLES AND EQUIPMENT

Low-Level
Used for routine housekeeping, cleaning, and removing visible body fluids. Should be used after every patient encounter.
Procedure: Use any EPA-registered disinfectant.

Intermediate-Level
Used to kill most viruses, fungi, and *Mycobacterium tuberculosis*. Does not destroy bacterial spores. Should be used on stethoscopes, splints, blood pressure cuffs, and other equipment that has come into contact with intact skin.
Procedure: Use 1:10 to 1:100 dilution of water and chlorine bleach solution or hard-surface germicides or EPA-registered disinfectants/chemical germicides.

High-Level
Used to destroy all forms of microorganisms except certain bacterial spores. Should be used on all reusable devices that have come into contact with mucous membranes.
Procedure: Immerse in an EPA-approved chemical sterilizing agent for short periods (10–45 seconds, usually) or immersion in hot water (176–212°F) for 30 minutes.

Sterilization
Used to destroy all microorganisms and is required for all contaminated invasive instruments.
Procedure: Use an autoclave with steam under pressure or with ethylene-oxide gas. Alternatively, use extended immersion in an EPA-approved chemical sterilizing agent for 6 to 10 hours.

Chapter 37 Answer Key

Handout 37-2: Chapter 37 Quiz

1. B	10. C	19. B	28. C
2. C	11. A	20. B	29. C
3. D	12. D	21. A	30. A
4. A	13. C	22. B	31. A
5. D	14. B	23. B	32. D
6. B	15. D	24. C	33. B
7. A	16. A	25. B	34. C
8. C	17. C	26. A	35. B
9. B	18. D	27. D	

Handout 37-3: Chapter 37 Scenario

1. Precautions should have included gloves, goggles, mask or shield (because of large amount of blood), bagging and labeling of linens, intermediate- and high-level disinfections of vehicle and instruments, and medical follow-up.
2. Possibilities include tuberculosis, hepatitis, HIV.

Handout 37-4: Chapter 37 Review

1. index case
2. infectious disease
3. Normal flora
4. pathogen
5. opportunistic pathogen
6. Bacteria
7. spheres, rods, spirals
8. Exotoxins, endotoxins
9. Bacteriostatic, bactericidal
10. virus
11. obligate intracellular parasite
12. fungi
13. parasite
14. reservoir
15. contamination, infection
16. Virulence
17. latent, communicable
18. preparation, response, response, patient contact, recovery
19. disinfect, sterilize
20. Hepatitis
21. hepatitis B
22. Tuberculosis
23. Meningitis
24. Mumps
25. Measles
26. catarrhal, paroxysmal, convalescent
27. mononucleosis
28. Encephalitis
29. early localized, early disseminated, late
30. nosocomial

Handout 37-5: Infectious Disease Matching

1. K	6. C	11. J
2. E	7. G	12. D
3. H	8. M	13. L
4. B	9. A	14. F
5. O	10. N	15. I

Chapter 38

Psychiatric and Behavioral Disorders

INTRODUCTION

Behavioral emergencies pose a special challenge to the paramedic. Up until now, most of the topics studied have had objective diagnostic criteria. ECGs are interpreted, blood pressure and pulse rates are counted, bleeding is controlled, and so on. Caring for patients with psychiatric or behavioral emergencies, however, depends more on communication skills than on treatment of physical illnesses or injuries. Your care includes support, calming reassurance, and occasionally restraint. This chapter discusses the physical and psychological aspects of behavioral problems.

TOTAL TEACHING TIME: 8.45 HOURS
The total teaching time is only a guideline based on the didactic and practical lab averages in the National Standard Curriculum. Instructors should take into consideration such factors as the pace at which students learn, the size of the class, and breaks. The actual time devoted to teaching objectives is the responsibility of the instructor.

CHAPTER OBJECTIVES

After reading this chapter, you should be able to:

1. Define behavior and distinguish among normal behavior, abnormal behavior, and the behavioral emergency. (pp. 1487–1488)
2. Discuss the prevalence of behavioral and psychiatric disorders. (pp. 1487–1488)
3. Discuss the pathophysiology of behavioral and psychiatric disorders. (pp. 1448–1489)
4. Discuss the factors that may alter the behavioral or emotional status of an ill or injured individual. (pp. 1488–1489)
5. Describe the medical legal considerations for management of emotionally disturbed patients. (p. 1504)
6. Describe the overt behaviors associated with behavioral and psychiatric disorders. (pp. 1492–1502)
7. Define the following terms:
   - Affect (p. 1490)
   - Anger (p. 1495)
   - Anxiety (p. 1494)
   - Confusion (p. 1490)
   - Depression (p. 1495)
   - Fear (p. 1490)
   - Mental status (p. 1490)
   - Open-ended question (p. 1490)
   - Posture (p. 1489)

©2007 Pearson Education, Inc.
Essentials of Paramedic Care, 2nd ed.

8. Describe verbal techniques useful in managing the emotionally disturbed patient. (pp. 1490–1491)
9. List the appropriate measures to ensure the safety of the paramedic, the patient, and others. (pp. 1489, 1504)
10. Describe the circumstances when relatives, bystanders, and others should be removed from the scene. (p. 1490)
11. Describe techniques to systematically gather information from the disturbed patient. (pp. 1490–1491, 1503–1504)
12. Identify techniques for physical assessment in a patient with behavioral problems. (pp. 1489–1491, 1502–1507)
13. List situations in which you are expected to transport a patient forcibly and against his will. (p. 1504)
14. Describe restraint methods necessary in managing the emotionally disturbed patient. (pp. 1504–1507)
15. List the risk factors and behaviors that indicate a patient is at risk for suicide. (p. 1501)
16. Use the assessment and patient history to differentiate between the various behavioral and psychiatric disorders. (pp. 1489–1502)
17. Given several preprogrammed behavioral emergency patients, provide the appropriate scene size-up, initial assessment, focused assessment, and detailed assessment, then provide the appropriate care and patient transport. (pp. 1487–1507)

FRAMING THE LESSON

Begin the lesson with a brief review of the important points from Chapter 37, "Infectious Diseases." Discuss any aspects of the chapter not fully understood by students. Then begin with Chapter 38 material. Begin by asking students to describe their idea of how a psychiatric or behavioral emergency patient might act. Have them think about what might cause some of these behaviors. Stress the point that any patient may exhibit what appear to be behavioral problems. Ill or injured patients may present with psychological problems due to the stress they are under. Medical conditions may cause signs and symptoms of what appear to be behavioral problems. These include stroke, head injury, shock, and diabetic problems. Stress that, along with true psychological and behavior problems, any condition that affects blood, oxygen, or glucose flow to the brain may cause the patient to act inappropriately. This would be an excellent time to review diabetic problems, stroke, and shock as they affect the brain.

During this time, also stress the importance of personal safety. Discuss the policies of local EMS agencies in handling potentially violent patients, and the use of restraints. Who can use them? Is EMS involved in the restraining process, or is that strictly a law enforcement function?

TEACHING STRATEGIES

People learn in a variety of ways. Some do better with the spoken word, whereas others prefer the written. Some prefer to work alone, whereas others profit from working in groups. Recognizing these different ways of acquiring knowledge, the authors of this *Instructor's Resource Manual* have provided a variety of teaching strategies for the different types of learners. These strategies are intended to foster higher-level cognitive skills and encourage creative learning and problem solving. For greatest effectiveness, incorporate these strategies into

your class lecture. Symbols in the Lecture Outline indicate the points at which various exercises might be most appropriate. Other strategies can be used to preview the lesson or to summarize it.

The following strategies are keyed to specific sections of the lesson.

1. Determining Reasons for Behavioral Emergencies. To open this lecture, have students brainstorm a list of reasons why one could be experiencing a "breakdown" or "hard time coping" or "excessive stress." Then, point out to students that all of those reasons are triggers for a behavioral emergency. This should help them see that behavioral emergencies are quite common and affect all types of people, regardless of previous psychiatric diagnosis.

2. Categorizing Behavioral Emergencies. Use the previous exercise as a springboard for this one. Have students put the items from their brainstormed list of behavioral emergencies into categories of biological, psychosocial, and sociocultural. Though these are not difficult concepts, they are likely to be new to students and require a bit of practical application before they mean much to students.

3. Role-Playing a Mental Status Exam. Students will need practice with the mental status exam because it is much more complex and complete than most will have ever used before. Have each student think of a psychiatric patient situation that they could role-play. Then, have half of the class act to carry out the MSE of their "patient" partners, while the other half of the class role-plays the patients. Then switch. Do this three or four times to give all students ample practice with the new examination tool. Done en masse like this, each student should be able to complete several assessments in 30 to 60 minutes of class time.

4. Illustrating Psychiatric Behaviors. Show movie video clips to illustrate behaviors associated with certain psychiatric conditions. Some examples are:

Rain Man, Autism
Patch Adams, Schizophrenia
Girl, Interrupted, Eating disorders, depression
As Good As It Gets, Anxiety disorders (OCD)

This use of visual aids assists the visual learner, while appealing to a broad audience of popular culture.

5. Contrasting Delusions and Hallucinations. To explain the difference between delusions and hallucinations, use a crown and a lava lamp. Crown the most unlikely student "King for a Day" and allow this student to make requests of the other students. Thought disorders such as thinking you are the president of the United States, an alien, or the king are examples of delusions. In contrast, hallucinations involve sensory perceptions. Plug in the lava lamp while giving this explanation, and allow it to work its magic throughout this lecture. Not only were the 1970s, when lava lamps were popular, full of psychedelic images, but the bright colors and eye teasers the lamp projects are similar to the sound and visual hallucinations experienced by some patients.

6. Guest Speaker: Patient Restraint. Invite a representative from local law enforcement to discuss methods of restraint and methods of self-protection when dealing with violent individuals.

The following strategies can be used at various points throughout the lesson or to help summarize and demonstrate what students have learned:

HANDOUTS 38-5 TO 38-7
Role-Playing Sheets

Role-Playing Behavioral Emergencies. Role-play the following scenarios in class. Provide students with copies of Handouts 38-5 and 38-6 for instructions and

Handout 38-7 for evaluation. Use the scenarios laid out in Handout 38-6 as the bases for the role-plays. Discuss each scenario with the students who will be role-playing it, but do not reveal the "subject" of the scenario to other class members prior to its start. You may find it helpful to videotape the scenarios for review during the postscenario discussions.

Scenarios include:

- Depression
- Suicide
- Anxiety disorder
- Manic disorder
- Schizophrenia
- Geriatric crisis
- Domestic violence

Allow sufficient time for the scenario to be played out to its logical conclusion. Then ask observers to complete evaluation sheets prior to class discussion. In addition to going over the evaluation sheets, use discussion questions that might include: How did you feel? Which techniques worked? Why? What techniques did not work as well? Why?

In the Field. Arrange for students to do a "clinical rotation" at the local suicide-prevention hotline or mental health facility.

Guest Speaker: Crisis Intervention. Invite a member of the local crisis intervention team or psychiatric care facility to attend your class as a guest speaker.

Cultural Considerations, Legal Notes, and Patho Pearls. The Student CD-ROM contains this series of informative features to enhance the student's understanding of the material covered in this chapter.

TEACHING OUTLINE

Chapter 38 is the twelfth lesson in Division 4, *Medical Emergencies*. Distribute Handout 38-1 so that students can familiarize themselves with the learning goals for this chapter. If students have any questions about the objectives, answer them at this time.

Then present the chapter. One possible lecture outline follows. In the outline the parenthetical references in regular type are references to text pages; those in bold type are references to figures, tables, or procedures.

I. Introduction. Behavioral and psychiatric emergencies are not as clear-cut as other topics studied up to this point. Those other topics have had objective diagnostic criteria. Most of your assessment and care of psychiatric and behavioral patients will depend on your people skills and communication. Reducing anxiety and offering emotional support may be your primary treatment. Care for patients with psychiatric and behavioral emergencies will include calming reassurance, support, and occasionally restraint, and requires interpersonal skills more than diagnostic equipment. (p. 1487)

II. Behavioral emergencies (pp. 1487–1488)

A. Behavior (p. 1487)
B. Behavioral emergency (pp. 1487–1488)

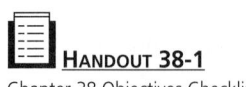

III. Pathophysiology of psychiatric disorders (pp. 1488–1489)

A. Biological (p. 1488)
B. Psychosocial (personal) (pp. 1488–1489)
C. Sociocultural (situational) (p. 1489)

IV. Assessment of behavioral emergency patients (pp. 1489–1492)

A. Scene size-up (p. 1489) (**Fig. 38-1, p. 1490**)
B. Initial assessment (pp. 1489–1490)
C. Focused history and physical examination (pp. 1490–1491) (**Fig. 38-2, p. 1491**)
   1. Listen.
   2. Spend time.
   3. Be assured.
   4. Do not threaten.
   5. Do not fear silence.
   6. Place yourself at the patient's level.
   7. Keep a safe and proper distance.
   8. Appear comfortable.
   9. Avoid appearing judgmental.
   10. Never lie to the patient.
D. Mental status examination (pp. 1491–1492)
   1. General appearance
   2. Behavioral observations
   3. Orientation
   4. Memory
   5. Sensorium
   6. Perceptual processes
   7. Mood and affect
   8. Intelligence
   9. Thought processes
   10. Insight
   11. Judgment
   12. Psychomotor
E. Psychiatric medications (p.1492)

V. Specific psychiatric disorders (pp. 1492–1502)

A. Cognitive disorders (p. 1493)
   1. Delirium
   2. Dementia
B. Schizophrenia (pp. 1493–1494)
   1. Paranoid
   2. Disorganized
   3. Catatonic
   4. Undifferentiated
C. Anxiety and related disorders (pp. 1494–1495)
   1. Panic attack
   2. Phobias
   3. Posttraumatic stress syndrome
D. Mood disorders (pp. 1495–1497)
   1. Depression
   2. Bipolar disorder
E. Substance-related disorders (p. 1497)
F. Somatoform disorders (pp. 1497–1498)
   1. Somatization disorder
   2. Conversion disorder

POWERPOINT PRESENTATION
Chapter 38 PowerPoint slide 5

POWERPOINT PRESENTATION
Chapter 38 PowerPoint slides 6–9

TEACHING STRATEGY 2
Categorizing Behavioral Emergencies

READING/REFERENCE
Doyle, T. J., and R. J. Vissers. "An EMS Approach to Psychiatric Emergencies." *EMS,* June 1999.

TEACHING STRATEGY 3
Role-Playing Mental Status Exam

TEACHING STRATEGY 4
Illustrating Psychiatric Behaviors

TEACHING STRATEGY 5
Contrasting Delusions and Hallucinations

POWERPOINT PRESENTATION
Chapter 38 PowerPoint slides 10–26

TEACHING TIP
Ask students how many of them have experienced anxiety attacks during the course. Ask them to describe their symptoms.

POINT OF INTEREST
Depression is the most common mental illness in the United States.

3. Hypochondriasis
4. Body dysmorphic disorder
5. Pain disorder
G. Factitious disorders (p. 1498)
1. Munchausen syndrome
H. Dissociative disorders (p. 1498)
1. Psychogenic amnesia
2. Fugue state
3. Multiple personality disorder
4. Depersonalization
I. Eating disorders (pp. 1498–1499)
1. Anorexia nervosa
2. Bulimia nervosa
J. Personality disorders (pp. 1499–1500)
1. Cluster A personality disorders
   a. Paranoid
   b. Schizoid
   c. Schizotypal
2. Cluster B personality disorders
   a. Antisocial
   b. Borderline
   c. Histrionic
   d. Narcissistic
3. Cluster C personality disorders
   a. Avoidant
   b. Dependent
   c. Obsessive-compulsive
K. Impulse control disorders (p. 1500)
1. Kleptomania
2. Pyromania
3. Pathological gambling
4. Trichotillomania
5. Intermittent explosive disorder
L. Suicide (pp. 1500–1501)
1. Assessing potentially suicidal patients
2. Risk factors for suicide
M. Age-related conditions (pp. 1591–1592)
1. Crisis in the geriatric patient
2. Crisis in the pediatric patient

VI. **Management of behavioral emergencies** (pp. 1502–1504)

A. General (p. 1502)
1. Assure scene safety and BSI precautions.
2. Provide a supportive and calm environment.
3. Treat any existing medical conditions.
4. Do not allow the suicidal patient to be alone.
5. Do not confront or argue with the patient.
6. Provide realistic reassurance.
7. Respond to the patient in a direct, simple manner.
8. Transport to an appropriate receiving facility.
B. Medical (p. 1502)
C. Psychological (pp. 1503–1504) (**Fig. 38-3, p. 1503**)

POINT TO EMPHASIZE

Don't think that you can accurately predict who will commit suicide. We are, more often than not, absolutely shocked and devastated by the news of a suicide, especially when it happens to an EMS colleague.

POWERPOINT PRESENTATION

Chapter 38 PowerPoint slides 27–29

TEACHING TIP

Gather information regarding the committal laws in your state. Paramedics should be thoroughly versed in these laws.

TEACHING STRATEGY 6

Guest Speaker: Patient Restraint

TEACHING TIP

Obtain information from local law enforcement regarding the legality of restraining a patient. Who can do it? What are the justifications for it?

VII. Violent patients and restraint (pp. 1504–1507)

  A. Methods of restraint (pp. 1504–1507)

    1. Verbal deescalation

    2. Physical restraint (**Proc. 38-1, p. 1506**)

    3. Chemical restraint

VIII. Chapter summary (p. 1507). Calls involving psychiatric and behavioral emergencies will challenge your skills as a paramedic. Differentiating physiological and psychological conditions will try your diagnostic skills, and developing the interview abilities that form the basis of psychiatric assessment and care will test your people skills. Ultimately, you will be called on to help patients in a time of great need—the time of crisis. Once you determine that the patient is experiencing a purely behavioral emergency your compassion and communication skills rather than medications and procedures will benefit him most.

    Emergency medical services providers routinely encounter patients who are violent or combative as a result of behavioral illness or a medical condition or trauma. Verbal, physical, and chemical restraint techniques provide effective ways of restraining patients who are a threat to themselves or others or who require medical assessment and treatment for a condition associated with combative or agitated behavior. Life-threatening adverse events have occurred in restrained individuals, but adherence to the principles of restraint presented in this chapter will minimize the occurrence of such adverse events. EMS personnel and their medical directors should ensure that their systems are prepared to treat violent or combative patients responsibly by providing appropriate training, policies, and protocols to deal with these situations.

    Situations involving crisis can drain your emotions. Observing a suicide or attempted suicide or struggling with or restraining a patient can take its toll. Take care of yourself before, during, and after these calls.

POWERPOINT PRESENTATION
Chapter 38 PowerPoint slides 30–36

POWERPOINT PRESENTATION
Chapter 38 PowerPoint slide 37

SKILLS DEMONSTRATION AND PRACTICE

Students can practice skills discussed in this chapter in the following settings.

Skills Lab: Divide the class into teams with a minimum of three students each. Have teams take turns practicing the following activity. Students within the teams should take turns acting as the "violent" patient until all students have had the chance to apply restraints. You may wish to have other instructors or qualified paramedics or law enforcement officers assist and monitor students in this activity.

Station	Equipment and Personnel Needed	Activities
Violent Patient Restraint	Commercial restraint systems or small towels, cravats, triangular bandages, webbed straps, or other materials for improvised restraints 1 patient 1 instructor	After you have demonstrated the techniques, student teams will practice taking down and restraining an unarmed, violent patient. Caution students to be extremely careful in applying the restraints. Remind them to use minimum reasonable force. Monitor this exercise closely.

TEACHING TIP
Use the Skills Demonstration and Practice exercise to allow students to experience how it feels to be restrained. Ask students how they felt about being restrained after the exercise.

ADVANCED LIFE SUPPORT SKILLS
Larmon & Davis. *Advanced Life Support Skills.*

ADVANCED LIFE SKILLS REVIEW
Larmon & Davis. *Advanced Life Skills Review.*

BRADY SKILLS SERIES: ALS
Larmon & Davis. *Brady Skills Series: ALS.*

Hospital:

- Observe interviewing techniques of social caseworkers in the psychiatric unit.
- Assist in assessment and management of behavioral emergencies in the ED.

Field Internship: Assist in assessment and management of behavioral emergencies in the field.

ASSIGNMENTS

Assign students to complete Chapter 38, "Psychiatric and Behavioral Disorders," of the workbook. Also assign them to read Chapter 39, "Gynecology," before the next class.

EVALUATION

Chapter Quiz and Scenario   Distribute copies of the Chapter Quiz provided in Handout 38-2 to evaluate student understanding of this chapter. Make sure each student reads the scenario to reinforce critical thinking on the scene. Remind students not to use their notes or textbooks while taking the quiz.

Student CD   Quizzes for every chapter are contained on the dynamic and highly visual in-text student CD.

Companion Website   Additional quizzes for every chapter are contained on this exciting website.

TestGen   You may wish to create a custom-tailored test using *Prentice Hall TestGen for Essentials of Paramedic Care*, 2nd Edition to evaluate student understanding of this chapter.

On-line Test Preparation (for students and instructors)   Additional test preparation is available through Brady's new on-line product, *EMT Achieve: Paramedic Test Preparation* at *http://www.prenhall.com/emtachieve/*. Instructors can also monitor student mastery on-line.

Review Manual for the EMT-Paramedic   This comprehensive exam review contains hundreds of test questions and rationales, including scenarios, along with two 180-question practice tests on CD.

REINFORCEMENT

Handouts   If classroom discussion or performance on the quiz indicates that some students have not fully mastered the chapter content, you may wish to assign some or all of the Reinforcement Handouts for this chapter.

Student CD (for students)   A wide variety of material on this CD-ROM will reinforce and also expand student knowledge and skills.

PowerPoint Presentation (for instructors)   The PowerPoint material developed for this chapter offers useful reinforcement of chapter content.

Companion Website (for students)   Additional review quizzes and links to EMS resources will contribute to further reinforcement of the chapter.

OneKey On-line support is offered for this course on one of three platforms: CourseCompass, Blackboard, or Web CT. Includes the IRM, PowerPoints, TestGen, and Companion Website for instruction. Ask your local sales representative for more information.

Brady Skills Series: Advanced Life Skills (Video or CD) Have your students watch the skills come to life on VHS or CD-ROM, or they can purchase the highly visual, full-color text with step-by-step procedures and rationales.

ONEKEY
Chapter 38

ADVANCED LIFE SUPPORT SKILLS
Larmon & Davis. *Advanced Life Support Skills.*

ADVANCED LIFE SKILLS REVIEW
Larmon & Davis. *Advanced Life Skills Review.*

BRADY SKILLS SERIES: ALS
Larmon & Davis. *Brady Skills Series: ALS.*

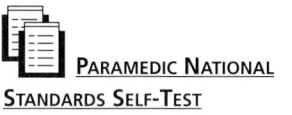

PARAMEDIC NATIONAL STANDARDS SELF-TEST
Miller. *Paramedic National Standards Self-Test,* 4th edition.

Handout 38-1

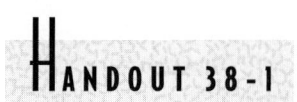

Student's Name _____

CHAPTER 38 OBJECTIVES CHECKLIST

Knowledge	Date Mastered
1. Define behavior and distinguish among normal behavior, abnormal behavior, and the behavioral emergency.	
2. Discuss the prevalence of behavioral and psychiatric disorders.	
3. Discuss the pathophysiology of behavioral and psychiatric disorders.	
4. Discuss the factors that may alter the behavioral or emotional status of an ill or injured individual.	
5. Describe the medical legal considerations for management of emotionally disturbed patients.	
6. Describe the overt behaviors associated with behavioral and psychiatric disorders.	
7. Define the following terms: • Affect • Anger • Anxiety • Confusion • Depression • Fear • Mental status • Open-ended question • Posture	
8. Describe verbal techniques useful in managing the emotionally disturbed patient.	
9. List the appropriate measures to ensure the safety of the paramedic, the patient, and others.	
10. Describe the circumstances when relatives, bystanders, and others should be removed from the scene.	
11. Describe techniques to systematically gather information from the disturbed patient.	
12. Identify techniques for physical assessment in a patient with behavioral problems.	
13. List situations in which you are expected to transport a patient forcibly and against his will.	
14. Describe restraint methods necessary in managing the emotionally disturbed patient.	

HANDOUT 38-1 Continued

Knowledge	Date Mastered
15. List the risk factors and behaviors that indicate a patient is at risk for suicide.	
16. Use the assessment and patient history to differentiate between the various behavioral and psychiatric disorders.	
17. Given several preprogrammed behavioral emergency patients, provide the appropriate scene size-up, initial assessment, focused assessment, and detailed assessment, then provide the appropriate care and patient transport.	

Handout 38-2

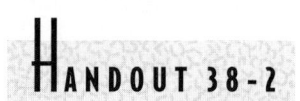

Student's Name _____

CHAPTER 38 QUIZ

Write the letter of the best answer in the space provided.

_____ 1. A person's observable conduct and activity is known as his or her:
  A. makeup.
  B. affect.
  C. behavior.
  D. socialization.

_____ 2. Which of the following is NOT one of the general causes of behavioral emergencies?
  A. social (situational)
  B. psychosocial (personal)
  C. genetic (physical)
  D. biological (organic)

_____ 3. Conditions related to a patient's personality style, dynamics of unresolved conflict, or crisis management methods are called:
  A. psychosocial.
  B. sociocultural.
  C. biological/organic.
  D. sociobehavioral.

_____ 4. In behavioral emergencies, as with any other emergency calls, it is of utmost importance to determine:
  A. the number of patients.
  B. the chief complaint.
  C. scene safety.
  D. the patient's level of consciousness.

_____ 5. When faced with a violent patient with a weapon, you should:
  A. immediately take the weapon from the patient.
  B. have your partner assist you in "taking down" the patient.
  C. ask a family member to take the weapon from the patient.
  D. request law enforcement assistance.

_____ 6. A patient who has a feeling of alarm and discontentment in the expectation of danger is said to be:
  A. confused.
  D. fearful.
  C. in a rage.
  D. anxious.

_____ 7. When assessing a patient with a behavioral emergency, guidelines include:
  A. standing close to the patient so he must focus on you.
  B. positioning yourself at a higher level than the patient, so he must look up at you.
  C. realizing that silence is nothing to fear and can be appropriate.
  D. spending as little time on-scene as possible; proper treatment will only begin at the care facility.

_____ 8. A structured exam designed to quickly evaluate a patient's level of mental functioning is called the:
  A. focused mental examination (FME).
  B. focused mental evaluation (FME).
  C. mental status examination (MSE).
  D. field psychiatric evaluation (FPE).

_____ 9. Psychiatric disorders with organic causes are known as cognitive disorders, one example of which is:
  A. delirium.
  B. delusions.
  C. anxiety disorder.
  D. posttraumatic stress.

_____ 10. Common symptoms of schizophrenia include:
  A. gradual impairment of memory.
  B. extreme periods of anxiety resulting in emotional stress.
  C. excessive fear that interferes with functioning.
  D. sensory perceptions with no basis in reality.

HANDOUT 38-2 Continued

_____ 11. The appearance of being disinterested, often lacking facial expression, is called:
   A. catatonia.
   B. flat affect.
   C. delirium.
   D. depression.

_____ 12. One of the cognitive disturbances seen in dementia is:
   A. aphasia.
   B. delusions.
   C. hallucinations.
   D. anxiety.

_____ 13. One of the major types of schizophrenia is "catatonic." This means that the patient:
   A. displays grossly disorganized behavior.
   B. does not readily fit into one of the defined categories.
   C. is preoccupied with a feeling of persecution.
   D. exhibits rigidity, immobility, stupor, or peculiar movements.

_____ 14. A pervasive and sustained emotion that colors a person's perception of the world is:
   A. a mood disorder.
   B. an anxiety disorder
   C. schizophrenia.
   D. a cognitive disorder.

_____ 15. Symptoms of a major depressive disorder include:
   A. loss of any feelings of guilt.
   B. hyperactivity, increased agitation.
   C. recurrent thoughts of death.
   D. the impaired ability to deal with reality.

_____ 16. A screening acronym for major depression is:
   A. *BAD NEWS.*
   B. *In SAD CAGES.*
   C. *BEREAVE.*
   D. *A DOWN DAY.*

_____ 17. Bipolar disorder is characterized by one or more manic episodes. The term *manic* refers to:
   A. excessive excitement or activity.
   B. profound sadness or feeling of melancholy.
   C. excessive fear that interferes with functioning.
   D. hostility or rage.

_____ 18. Somatoform disorders are characterized by:
   A. a state of constant sleepiness or drowsiness.
   B. physical symptoms that have no apparent physiological cause.
   C. the relatively rapid onset of widespread disorganized thought.
   D. failure to recall, as opposed to inability to recall.

_____ 19. Similar personality disorders are grouped into three broad types, or clusters. Which of the following is NOT a disorder in Cluster A?
   A. obsessive-compulsive
   B. paranoid
   C. schizoid
   D. schizotypal

_____ 20. A condition characterized by the patient's failure to control recurrent impulses is called:
   A. obsessive-compulsive disorder.
   B. personality disorder.
   C. impulse control disorder.
   D. somatoform disorder.

_____ 21. Which of the following statements is TRUE regarding suicide?
   A. Men attempt suicide more than women.
   B. The most common method of suicide is poisoning.
   C. Suicide is the third leading cause of death in the 15–24 age group.
   D. Suicide rates for younger age groups and the elderly are decreasing.

_____ 22. A patient with Munchausen syndrome is suffering from a(n):
   A. somatoform disorder.
   B. factitious disorder.
   C. dissociative disorder.
   D. eating disorder.

HANDOUT 38-2 Continued

_____ 23. A patient in a fugue state is suffering from a(n):
  A. somatoform disorder.
  B. factitious disorder.
  C. dissociative disorder.
  D. eating disorder.

_____ 24. A patient with bulimia nervosa is suffering from a(n):
  A. somatoform disorder.
  B. factitious disorder.
  C. dissociative disorder.
  D. eating disorder.

_____ 25. When considering the need for restraining a patient, it is important to remember:
  A. patients who are physically restrained must receive frequent and close monitoring.
  B. never use "hog-tie" or hobble restraints.
  C. restrain one arm at the patient's side and the other above his head.
  D. all of these

_____ 26. Methods of restraint include:
  A. physical restraint.
  B. chemical restraint.
  C. verbal deescalation.
  D. all of these

_____ 27. Verbal deescalation involves all the following EXCEPT:
  A. avoid entering the patient's personal space.
  B. look the patient directly in the eyes.
  C. be honest.
  D. use a friendly tone of voice.

_____ 28. All of the following are examples of soft restraints EXCEPT:
  A. leathers.
  B. chest Posey.
  C. sheets.
  D. wristlets.

_____ 29. Which of the following is NOT a benzodiazepine commonly used for chemical restraint?
  A. midazolam (Versed).
  B. diazepam (Valium).
  C. haloperidol (Haldol).
  D. lorazepam (Ativan).

_____ 30. Positional asphyxia is most commonly a result of a patient restrained in the:
  A. supine position.
  B. prone position.
  C. right lateral recumbent position.
  D. left lateral recumbent position.

HANDOUT 38-3

Student's Name _____

CHAPTER 38 SCENARIO

Review the following real-life situation. Then answer the questions that follow.

It is early evening in late spring. You have been dispatched to a home in an upper-middle-class neighborhood for an "unknown medical" call. The dispatcher tells you that police will meet you at the scene, as the caller reported that she could hear things being thrown against the walls and lots of shouting.

The police car is in the driveway when you arrive. A middle-aged woman comes out of the house next door and joins the officer on the front sidewalk as you and your partner grab your jump kit and approach. As you get closer to the front door you can hear the sounds from inside the house. Dispatch was right; it does sound like things are being thrown. But you only hear a single voice shouting. The neighbor, Mrs. Rozenman, reports that the family who lives at this address is fairly new to the neighborhood. She says that she knows they have a teenage son and thinks that both parents are attorneys.

The police officer goes to the front door, knocks, and identifies himself. There is no answer. So he knocks again. Still no answer. He then tries the doorknob and finds the door unlocked. He motions for you to join him as he enters the house. You and your partner enter the house behind the officer.

The noise seems to be coming from the room with the open door just to the right of the front door. You all turn in the direction of the noise, with the police officer, again, identifying himself. Inside is a slightly built adolescent male who is standing in the center of the room amidst overturned furniture. His clothes are disheveled and it appears that he is sweating profusely. Although he is looking at you, your impression is that he is not aware that you are there, but he does stop yelling.

1. What are at least three possible causes for the young man's condition?

The police officer again identifies himself and identifies you and your partner as paramedics. The patient acknowledges this by shouting, "Go to hell!" Your partner goes to check the medicine cabinets for a clue about what's going on, while you and the police officer prepare to "take down" the patient.

2. How should this "takedown" be handled?

Just as you get the patient into a prone position, a well-dressed middle-aged woman enters the room with your partner. She identifies herself as Mrs. Spencer, the patient's mother, and tells you that her son, Bob, is diabetic and that they recently changed his insulin dosage.

3. What should you do now?

After your intervention, Bob is alert and oriented, quiet and cooperative. He apologizes for giving you such a hard time. Mrs. Spencer thanks you for coming and tells you that she will contact Bob's doctor immediately. You contact medical control and are cleared to return to quarters.

HANDOUT 38-4

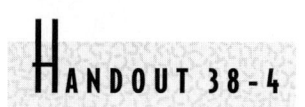

Student's Name _____

CHAPTER 38 REVIEW

Write the word or words that best complete each sentence in the space(s) provided.

1. A person's observable conduct and activity is called _____.
2. A(n) _____ _____ is a situation in which a patient's behavior becomes so unusual that it alarms the patient or another person and requires intervention.
3. _____ / _____ causes of behavioral emergencies are related to disease processes or structural changes.
4. _____ conditions are related to a patient's personality style, dynamics of unresolved conflict, or crisis management methods.
5. _____ causes of behavioral disorders are related to the patient's actions and interactions within society.
6. Position, attitude, or bearing of the body is called _____.
7. _____ is the feeling of alarm and discontentment in the expectation of danger.
8. _____ is the state of being unclear or unable to make a decision easily.
9. _____ _____ is the state of the patient's cerebral functioning.
10. _____ is the visible indicator of mood, and _____ _____ is the appearance of being disinterested, often lacking facial expression.
11. The initials MSE stand for _____ _____ _____.
12. Components of an MSE include general _____ and behavioral _____.
13. Cognitive disorders include _____ and _____.
14. Symptoms of schizophrenia include _____, _____, disorganized speech, grossly _____ behavior, and _____ symptoms.
15. Types of schizophrenia are _____, _____, _____, and _____.
16. A(n) _____ disorder is a condition characterized by dominating apprehension and fear.
17. A(n) _____ _____ is an extreme period of anxiety resulting in great emotional stress.
18. An excessive fear that interferes with functioning is called a(n) _____.
19. Hostility or rage to compensate for an underlying feeling of anxiety is called _____.
20. A pervasive and sustained emotion that colors a person's perception of the world is called a(n) _____ _____.
21. _____ is profound sadness or feeling of melancholy.
22. The acronym _____ provides a screening mnemonic for major depression.
23. The condition characterized by one or more manic episodes, with or without periods of depression, is called a(n) _____ disorder.
24. A drug used to treat bipolar disorder is _____, which has a very narrow therapeutic index.
25. If a patient has a somatization disorder, he is preoccupied with _____ symptoms.
26. A(n) _____ disorder is the condition in which the patient feigns illness in order to assume the sick role.

HANDOUT 38-4 Continued

27. _____ nervosa is characterized by voluntary refusal to eat, and _____ nervosa is recurrent episodes of binge eating.

28. Kleptomania and pyromania are examples of _____ _____ disorders.

29. An extreme response to stress characterized by impaired ability to deal with reality is called a(n) _____.

30. The main object in restraint is to restrict the patient's _____ in order to stop _____ behaviors and prevent him from _____ himself.

HANDOUT 38-5

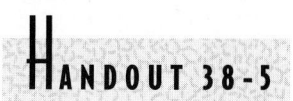

Student's Name _____

BEHAVIORAL EMERGENCY ROLE-PLAY INSTRUCTIONS

Instructions: This activity will be a role-play for dealing with behavioral emergencies. You may not hurt any of your fellow students. Take the role assigned to you and use your education and experience to fill in the blanks. If there are any medical questions, first verbalize the actions you would take, and then ask the instructor for the results. Make no assumptions. Act as you would in a similar situation in the real world.

At the conclusion of each scenario, you will be asked to evaluate the performance of the caregivers in the following areas, using the sheets provided.

- *Scene size-up*
- *Assessment*
- *Interview techniques*
- *General management and intervention techniques*

HANDOUT 38-6

Student's Name _____

BEHAVIORAL EMERGENCY ROLE-PLAYS

Scenario #1

Caregivers: You have been dispatched to a rest stop on the interstate for an "unknown emergency."
Patient: DEPRESSION You are a young college student who has just failed out of school and are found crying at the rest stop phone booth. You are very depressed and do not know how you can face your parents. You are on your way home and are at a loss as to what to do.
Engine Company: Arrive with the paramedics. Crew to take no action unless ordered to by the paramedics.

Scenario #2

Caregivers: You have been dispatched to a townhouse for an "illness." Dispatch reports that this was a third-party call from the adult child (who lives in another state) of this patient. The caller reported that the patient "sounded very sick on the phone."
Patient: SUICIDE You are a 54-year-old who has been very sick for the past several months. You are divorced, living alone, and very depressed. You are planning to take an overdose due to your recent diagnosis of cancer. Although you have not told your 30-year-old daughter anything about your illness, you did tell her that you were sending her a revised copy of your will.
Engine Company: Arrive with the paramedics. Crew to take no action unless ordered to by the paramedics.

Scenario #3

Caregivers: You have been dispatched to assist another paramedic unit at a multiple-fatality auto collision. They are transporting one of two survivors, a pregnant adult female who is critically injured. You are assigned to the other survivor who was just extricated from the wreckage.
Patient: ANXIETY DISORDER You were just involved in a multiple-vehicle auto collision in which two people were killed and one was seriously injured. You were alone in your car and were unhurt from the accident, but were trapped in the wreckage. You were saved by your seat belt and the air bag. You are unable to function. You are overwhelmed by having had to look at the two dead people in the other vehicle while extrication was taking place. You are hyperventilating, and have chest pain (non–cardiac-related). You are trembling all over. You doubt that you'll ever be able to drive again. You were not at fault; the other driver ran the red light.
Engine Company: Arrive with the paramedics. Crew to take no action unless ordered to by the paramedics.

Scenario #4

Caregivers: You are dispatched to a local high school for an "illness."
Patient: MANIC DISORDER You are a high school student using cocaine. You are experiencing mood swings. You alternate between depression and elation. You have greatly increased activity levels and have been sleeping a lot less lately. You are restless and talkative. You can't concentrate but don't think there is a problem you can't handle.
Teacher: You report that this kid has really changed over the past several weeks. Grades have fallen dramatically and truancy has increased. You called 911 because, from your viewpoint, the student is really acting crazy today and was very restless and talkative in class. You are very concerned about the student's health and think that the student is "whacked out" on drugs.

Scenario #5

Caregivers: You are dispatched to assist the police for a "mental patient" at a local homeless shelter.
Patient: SCHIZOPHRENIA You are a young adult who has withdrawn from society. You are dirty, dull-witted, and have difficulty communicating. You can communicate that you are a close personal

HANDOUT 38-6 Continued

friend of television character Beavis and Butthead and have been asked to attend the next Black Sabbath concert as their reviewer. You have accepted the assignment and now need to go get your tickets and press pass. You are quite excited about the opportunity and are anxious to leave, but you are worried that everyone is going to try to steal your tickets and backstage pass. You are nonviolent, but not cooperative.

Shelter Manager: You are concerned that the agitation of the patient will set off a chain reaction among your clientele, many of whom are deinstitutionalized psychiatric patients. You want the patient out of your facility, but are concerned about his safety on the street in his present condition.

Scenario #6

Caregivers: You are dispatched to a residential neighborhood for an "elderly patient with an illness." This is the fourth time this month that you have gone to this address for an 82-year-old who seems to be trying to test your assessment skills. On the first trip, the patient was in heart block and had experienced a syncopal episode. The second and third trips were to deal with an "injury from a fall." Your last trip was again for a syncopal episode.

Patient: GERIATRIC CRISIS You are an 82-year-old who is failing fast, but you have all of your mental faculties and want to stay in your own home until the end if at all possible. All you did was refuse breakfast, but your daughter got angry and called 911 because she wants you to go to a "home." You want to stay in your own house. After all, you've lived here since you got married 62 years ago. Your spouse died 10 years ago, and you have lived alone ever since. You still think you can manage your own affairs. It seems to you that the doctor solved your "palpitation" problem just fine. You weren't in any mood to eat after fighting with your child about her wanting you to go to the "raisin farm," so you refused breakfast.

Daughter: You are the 54-year-old only child of this patient. You want the paramedics to convince your parent to go to the "home." Your parent has been getting sicker and has refused to eat today. When further probed, you can identify your own problems (financial since your husband got "pink-slipped" last week) and your inability to deal with caring for your parent because you need to work full-time.

Scenario #7

Caregivers: You are dispatched for an "injury" at a home in a middle-class residential neighborhood.
Patient: DOMESTIC VIOLENCE You are a husband and wife who have been fighting. The husband has been hitting the wife in the face and she is holding her head but does not appear to be seriously injured. Both are quite agitated.
Engine Company: Arrive with the paramedics. Crew to take no action unless ordered to by the paramedics. If asked, acknowledge that the police are en route and should arrive in the next 10 minutes.

HANDOUT 38-7

Student's Name _____

BEHAVIORAL EMERGENCIES ROLE-PLAY EVALUATION SHEET

Using the following scale, rank the "performance" of the caregivers in the scenario you have just observed.

1 = Well done
2 = Not bad
3 = Needs improvement
4 = Don't come to my house

Component	Score
Scene Size-up Comments:	
Assessment Comments:	
Interview Techniques Comments:	
General Management and Intervention Techniques Comments:	

Total = _____

Handout 38-8

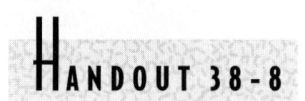

Student's Name _____

TABLE OF BEHAVIORAL EMERGENCIES

Complete the following table.

Behavioral Emergency	Characteristics, Signs/Symptoms	Prescribed Medications	EMS Management
Depression			
Schizophrenia			
Anxiety Disorder			
Manic Disorders			
Suicide	Risk Factors:		

Chapter 38 Answer Key

Handout 38-2: Chapter 38 Quiz

1.	C	9.	A	17.	A	25.	D
2.	C	10.	D	18.	B	26.	D
3.	A	11.	B	19.	A	27.	B
4.	C	12.	A	20.	C	28.	A
5.	D	13.	D	21.	C	29.	C
6.	B	14.	A	22.	B	30.	B
7.	C	15.	C	23.	C		
8.	C	16.	B	24.	D		

Handout 38-3: Chapter 38 Scenario

1. Possible causes include alcohol abuse, drug abuse, trauma, and medical illness (e.g., diabetes).
2. Make sure you have enough assistance. Offer the patient one final opportunity to cooperate. If there is no response to this request, at least two persons should move swiftly toward the patient at the same time while one paramedic continues talking to the patient. The two persons should cautiously move closer toward the patient. If the patient calms down, you may elect to transport without restraints. Continue to reassure the patient. Have the patient lie down and position yourself between him and the door. If the patient continues to resist, position your inside leg in front of the patient's leg and force the patient forward into a prone position. Continue to reassure the patient. Once subdued, the patient should be positioned prone or on his side, then secure the arms and legs. Transport.
3. Follow local protocols for management of a diabetic emergency. Get baseline vital signs and draw a blood sample to check his blood sugar. Establish an IV and administer 50% dextrose IV.

Handout 38-4: Chapter 38 Review

1. behavior
2. behavioral emergency
3. Biological/organic
4. Psychosocial
5. Sociocultural
6. posture
7. Fear
8. Confusion
9. Mental status
10. Affect, flat affect
11. mental status examination
12. appearance, observations
13. delirium, dementia
14. delusions, hallucinations, disorganized, negative
15. paranoid, disorganized, catatonic, undifferentiated
16. anxiety
17. panic attack
18. phobia
19. anger
20. mood disorder
21. Depression
22. In SAD CAGES
23. bipolar
24. lithium
25. physical
26. factitious
27. Anorexia, bulimia
28. impulse control
29. psychosis
30. movement, dangerous, harming

Handout 38-8: Table of Behavioral Emergencies

Behavioral Emergency	Characteristics, Signs/Symptoms	Prescribed Medications	EMS Management
Depression Consider: organic cause or part of bipolar disorder?	Feels helpless or hopeless Lack of interest Changing appetite Malaise Feelings of guilt or worthlessness	*Antidepressants* Amitriptyline Imipramine Phenelzine Buproprion Fluoxetine	Provide supportive care. Encourage patient to talk. Ask about suicidal thoughts. Transport.
Schizophrenia Several forms: • Catatonic • Paranoia • Undifferentiated • Disorganized	Hallucinations Delusions Altered thought Inappropriate affect Disorganization in thought or dress	*Antipsychotics:* Haloperidol Chlorpromazine Fluphenazine Thioridazine Thiothixene	Depends upon the situation. If violent, consider meds. If EPS symptoms, consider diphenhydramine. Transport.
Anxiety Disorder Also known as panic attack	Acute onset Chest pain Palpitations Dyspnea Syncope Vertigo Diarrhea Choking sensation	*Antianxiety:* Diazepam Alprazolam Lorazepam Buspirone	Provide supportive care. Consider possible physical causes. Calm and reassure. Transport.

Handout 38-8: Table of Behavioral Emergencies (continued)

Manic Disorders May be part of a bipolar disorder or induced by street drugs such as PCP, cocaine, or amphetamines.	Appears "high" Elevated mood Get details of history Increased activity use restraints Decreased need for sleep Poor concentration Sense of inflated self-esteem	Lithium or *antipsychotics*: Haloperidol Chlorpromazine	Management is variable. If nonviolent, "talk down." If violent, you may need to transport.
Suicide Likely in severe depression	*Risk Factors:* Previous attempts Age Alcohol/drug abuse Major separation trauma or physical stresses Loss of independence Mechanism for suicide available	May be taking antidepressants	Protect from harm. Ask about intent. Ask about prior attempts. Evaluate lethality of suicide plan.

Chapter 39

Gynecology

INTRODUCTION

Gynecology is the branch of medicine that deals with the health maintenance and the diseases of women, primarily of their reproductive organs. Paramedics are often called to handle emergencies involving the female reproductive anatomy. Patients often present with either abdominal pain or vaginal bleeding. This chapter focuses on the assessment and care of nonpregnant patients.

CHAPTER OBJECTIVES

After reading this chapter, you should be able to:

1. Review the anatomic structures and physiology of the female reproductive system. (see Chapter 3)
2. Identify the normal events of the menstrual cycle. (see Chapter 3)
3. Describe how to assess a patient with a gynecological complaint. (pp. 1510–1511)
4. Explain how to recognize a gynecological emergency. (pp. 1510–1511)
5. Describe the general care for any patient experiencing a gynecological emergency. (pp. 1512, 1514, 1515)
6. Describe the pathophysiology, assessment, and management of the following gynecological emergencies.
   - Pelvic inflammatory disease (pp. 1512–1513)
   - Ruptured ovarian cyst (p. 1513)
   - Cystitis (p. 1513)
   - Mittelschmertz (p. 1513)
   - Endometritis (p. 1513)
   - Endometriosis (pp. 1513–1514)
   - Ectopic pregnancy (p. 1514)
   - Vaginal hemorrhage (p. 1514)
7. Describe the assessment, care, and emotional support of the sexual assault patient. (pp. 1515–1516)
8. Given several preprogrammed gynecological patients, provide the appropriate assessment, management, and transportation. (pp. 1510–1516)

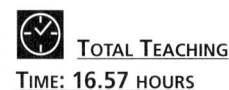

TOTAL TEACHING TIME: 16.57 HOURS
The total teaching time is only a guideline based on the didactic and practical lab averages in the National Standard Curriculum. Instructors should take into consideration such factors as the pace at which students learn, the size of the class, and breaks. The actual time devoted to teaching objectives is the responsibility of the instructor.

FRAMING THE LESSON

Begin the class session by reviewing the important points from Chapter 38, "Psychiatric and Behavioral Disorders." Discuss any aspects of the chapter not fully understood by students. Then begin with Chapter 39 material. This is an excellent opportunity to review the anatomy and physiology of the female reproductive system. Briefly review the structures and functions of the organs and the system. Encourage students to ask any questions about the system at this time, because a good understanding of the female reproductive system anatomy and physiology will enhance their understanding of the various problems associated with the system. As this topic may be embarrassing for some students, stress that as EMS professionals, they may be dealing with these types of patients frequently, and must present themselves in a calm, caring, professional manner.

TEACHING STRATEGIES

People learn in a variety of ways. Some do better with the spoken word, whereas others prefer the written. Some prefer to work alone, whereas others profit from working in groups. Recognizing these different ways of acquiring knowledge, the authors of this *Instructor's Resource Manual* have provided a variety of teaching strategies for the different types of learners. These strategies are intended to foster higher-level cognitive skills and encourage creative learning and problem solving. For greatest effectiveness, incorporate these strategies into your class lecture. Symbols in the Lecture Outline indicate the points at which various exercises might be most appropriate. Other strategies can be used to preview the lesson or to summarize it.

The following strategies are keyed to specific sections of the lesson.

1. ***Learning Technical Terms.*** Chapters 39 and 40 use numerous new terms. Play a word game such as Pictionary® to help students understand their meanings. Write one new term on a scrap of paper, a different one for each student. Have students use their books or a medical dictionary to look up the meaning of the term. Students then volunteer to come to the board to "draw their word." The other students guess the term and meaning based on the drawing. Give treats for correct answers, and for having the courage to be the "artist"! This right-brain activity has been shown to improve memory of new language terms. Additionally, it is fun and builds a sense of community among classmates.

2. ***Assessing the OB/GYN Patient.*** The gynecological assessment uses a good number of questions not asked of every patient. Create a flow sheet for students to use during assessment of the OB/GYN patient, and encourage its use during simulations. The flow sheet should prompt students to ask the pertinent questions exclusive to the assessment of the OB/GYN patient.

3. ***Taking the OB/GYN Patient's History.*** The history and exam of gynecological patients requires the gathering of sensitive information that can make both patient and provider uncomfortable. Do not allow the first real patient your students see to become their guinea pig. Instead, create scenarios in class that *require* the difficult questions, such as questions about PID, abortion, and STDs. The more students ask the questions, the more comfortable and thorough they will be with real patients in need of quality prehospital care.

The following strategies can be used at various points throughout the lesson or to help summarize and demonstrate what students have learned.

Guest Speaker: Sexually Transmitted Disease. The issues of sexually transmitted diseases and female abdominal pain can be closely linked. You might want to consider having a local infection control nurse speak to the class about the prevalence of such diseases, modes of transmission, and especially symptom patterns of the diseases.

Working a Shift at an STD Clinic or Public Health Clinic. Many STD clinics or public health clinics are staffed by volunteers who can both use your students' help as well as teach them a great deal about assessment and treatment of gynecological disorders. During clinical rotations, arrange for students to do a shift at one of these clinics. They can help take vitals as well as observe the history and physical exam of the clinic patients. The professionals at the clinic will not be uncomfortable with the sensitive nature of these questions, and can help lend some comfort to students who may still be shy with this line of questioning.

Observing at a Rape Crisis or Hotline Center. Arrange for students to observe at a rape crisis or hotline center. While they will not be able to provide care, or even do the history, they can gain a good deal of skill in dealing with human beings in crisis from the professionals who work these centers. A short 4-hour session will be a huge advantage to students in their practice.

Guest Speaker: Crime Scene Preservation after Sexual Assault. Invite a speaker from the Special Victims Unit to come to class and instruct students on crime scene preservation after a sexual assault. They will have innumerable cases to draw from when discussing possible scenarios and situations in which your students may encounter a survivor of a sex crime.

Guest Speaker: Sexual Assault and Rape. The issue of sexual assault and rape is a complex and sensitive one. It can be difficult to know the right information to pass along to your students without encouraging them to become "junior detectives" or "psychologists in training." Inviting a speaker from the local rape crisis hotline or center can be invaluable when discussing this topic. These highly trained individuals can encourage your students to "do the right thing" without harming the patient or endangering a police investigation.

Simulations: Gynecological Emergencies. Create a variety of gynecological scenarios for students to practice assessing. Make the patterns of signs and symptoms in these scenarios purposely confusing, pointing to multiple possible diagnoses. This is a great way to reinforce the priorities of prehospital care and to underscore the danger and urgency of a situation involving a possible ectopic pregnancy.

Cultural Considerations, Legal Notes, and Patho Pearls. The Student CD-ROM contains this series of informative features to enhance the student's understanding of the material covered in this chapter.

TEACHING OUTLINE

Chapter 39 is the thirteenth lesson in Division 4, *Medical Emergencies*. Distribute Handout 39-1 so that students can familiarize themselves with the learning goals for this chapter. If students have any questions about the objectives, answer them at this time.

Then present the chapter. One possible lecture outline follows. In the outline, the parenthetical references in regular type are references to text pages; those in bold type are references to figures, tables, or procedures.

HANDOUT 39-1
Chapter 39 Objectives Checklist

TEACHING STRATEGY 1
Learning Technical Terms

POINT TO EMPHASIZE
The uterus is normally the size of a small pear, but it stretches during pregnancy to about 12 inches in length.

POINT TO EMPHASIZE
Most women release one ripe egg every month for about 35 years. That adds up to over 400 eggs. A woman's ovaries contain thousands of unripe eggs that never develop.

PowerPoint Presentation
Chapter 39 PowerPoint slides 4–14

PowerPoint Presentation
Chapter 39 PowerPoint slides 15–18

? What Would You Do
Your 24-year-old patient swears there is no way she could be pregnant, yet she presents with lower abdominal pain and vaginal bleeding. What would you do?

Teaching Strategy 2
Assessing the OB/GYN Patient

PowerPoint Presentation
Chapter 39 PowerPoint slide 19

PowerPoint Presentation
Chapter 39 PowerPoint slides 20–30

Teaching Strategy 3
Taking the OB/GYN Patient's History

Point of Interest
The classic "Chandelier Sign" is consistent for PID. Jiggling the stretcher jiggles the cervix, causing pain.

Point to Emphasize
Ectopic pregnancy kills women. Consider it as a possibility in every woman with abdominal pain and vaginal bleeding.

Point to Emphasize
Rape is a crime of violence, degradation, and dominance, not a sexual act.

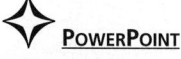

PowerPoint Presentation
Chapter 39 PowerPoint slide 31

I. Introduction. The term *gynecology* is derived from Greek, *gynaik*, meaning "woman." Gynecology is the branch of medicine that deals with the health maintenance and the diseases of women, primarily of their reproductive organs. *Obstetrics*, on the other hand, is the branch of medicine that deals with the care of women throughout pregnancy. Most gynecological emergencies paramedics encounter will be patients experiencing abdominal pain or vaginal bleeding. (p. 1510)

II. Assessment of the gynecological patient (pp. 1510–1511)

  A. Most common complaints (p. 1510)
      1. Abdominal pain
      2. Vaginal bleeding
  B. History (pp. 1510–1511)
      1. Dysmenorrhea
      2. Dyspareunia
      3. Previous pregnancies
      4. Last menstrual period
      5. Contraception
  C. Physical exam (p. 1511)

III. Management of gynecological emergencies (p. 1512)

  A. Generally focused on supportive care (p. 1512)
  B. Do not pack dressings in the vagina. (p. 1512)
  C. Do not perform an internal vaginal exam in the field. (p. 1512)

IV. Specific gynecological emergencies (pp. 1512–1516)

  A. Medical gynecological emergencies (pp. 1512–1514)
      1. Gynecological abdominal pain
          a. Pelvic inflammatory disease
          b. Ruptured ovarian cyst
          c. Cystitis
          d. Mittelschmerz
          e. Endometritis
          f. Endometriosis
          g. Ectopic pregnancy
      2. Management of gynecological abdominal pain
          a. Make the patient comfortable.
          b. Transport.
      3. Nontraumatic vaginal bleeding
      4. Management of nontraumatic vaginal bleeding
          a. Absorb blood flow, but do not pack vagina.
          b. Transport.
          c. Initiate oxygen therapy and IV access based on patient's condition.
  B. Traumatic gynecological emergencies (pp. 1514–1516)
      1. Causes of gynecological trauma
      2. Management of gynecological trauma
      3. Sexual assault (**Fig. 39-1**, p. 1516)
          a. Assessment
          b. Management
          c. Documentation

V. Chapter summary (pp. 1516–1517). Most gynecological emergency patients have either abdominal pain or vaginal bleeding. The patient with abdominal pain should be made comfortable and transported to the emergency department. The management of vaginal bleeding depends on the severity. Minor bleeding should be simply monitored. Severe bleeding should be treated with IV fluids, if indicated.

In the case of sexual assault, first determine if any life-threatening physical injuries exist. Second, respect the patient's wishes and offer emotional support. Third, in treating victims of sexual assault, make every effort to preserve physical evidence. As with any type of emergency care, the primary concern is the patient.

SKILLS DEMONSTRATION AND PRACTICE

Students can practice skills discussed in this chapter in the following settings.

Scenario Lab: Divide the class into teams. Have the teams circulate through the stations and practice the skill. Monitor the groups to be sure that every student is involved. You may wish to have other instructors or qualified paramedics assist students in these activities.

Station	Equipment Needed	Activities
Ruptured Ectopic Pregnancy	Medication boxes 1 patient 1 instructor	Have students practice assessing and managing a patient with a ruptured ectopic pregnancy.

Hospital: Assist in assessment and management of gynecological emergencies in the ED.

Field Internship: Assist in assessment and management of gynecological emergencies in the field.

ASSIGNMENTS

Assign students to complete Chapter 39, "Gynecology," of the workbook. Also assign them to read Chapter 40, "Obstetrics," before the next class.

EVALUATION

Chapter Quiz and Scenario Distribute copies of the Chapter Quiz provided in Handout 39-2 to evaluate student understanding of this chapter. Make sure each student reads the scenario to reinforce critical thinking on the scene. Remind students not to use their notes or textbooks while taking the quiz.

Student CD Quizzes for every chapter are contained on the dynamic and highly visual in-text student CD.

Companion Website Additional quizzes for every chapter are contained on this exciting website.

TestGen You may wish to create a custom-tailored test using *Prentice Hall TestGen for Essentials of Paramedic Care*, 2nd Edition to evaluate student understanding of this chapter.

On-line Test Preparation (for students and instructors) Additional test preparation is available through Brady's new on-line product, *EMT Achieve: Paramedic Test Preparation* at *http://www.prenhall.com/emtachieve/*. Instructors can also monitor student mastery on-line.

ADVANCED LIFE SUPPORT SKILLS
Larmon & Davis. *Advanced Life Support Skills.*

ADVANCED LIFE SKILLS REVIEW
Larmon & Davis. *Advanced Life Skills Review.*

BRADY SKILLS SERIES: ALS
Larmon & Davis. *Brady Skills Series: ALS.*

WORKBOOK
Chapter 39 Activities

READING/REFERENCE
Textbook, pp. 1518–1552

HANDOUT 39-2
Chapter 39 Quiz

HANDOUT 39-3
Chapter 39 Scenario

PARAMEDIC STUDENT CD
Student Activities

COMPANION WEBSITE
http://www.prenhall.com/bledsoe

TESTGEN
Chapter 39

EMT ACHIEVE: PARAMEDIC TEST PREPARATION
Mistovich & Beasley. *EMT Achieve: Paramedic Test Preparation.*
www.prenhall.com/emtachieve/

Review Manual for the EMT-Paramedic This comprehensive exam review contains hundreds of test questions and rationales, including scenarios, along with two 180-question practice tests on CD.

REINFORCEMENT

Handouts If classroom discussion or performance on the quiz indicates that some students have not fully mastered the chapter content, you may wish to assign some or all of the Reinforcement Handouts for this chapter.

Student CD (for students) A wide variety of material on this CD-ROM will reinforce and also expand student knowledge and skills.

PowerPoint Presentation (for instructors) The PowerPoint material developed for this chapter offers useful reinforcement of chapter content.

Companion Website (for students) Additional review quizzes and links to EMS resources will contribute to further reinforcement of the chapter.

OneKey On-line support is offered for this course on one of three platforms: CourseCompass, Blackboard, or Web CT. Includes the IRM, PowerPoints, Test-Gen, and Companion Website for instruction. Ask your local sales representative for more information.

Brady Skills Series: Advanced Life Skills (Video or CD) Have your students watch the skills come to life on VHS or CD-ROM, or they can purchase the highly visual, full-color text with step-by-step procedures and rationales.

REVIEW MANUAL FOR THE EMT-PARAMEDIC
Cherry & Mistovich. *Review Manual for the EMT-Paramedic*, 3rd edition.

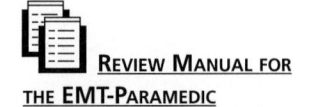

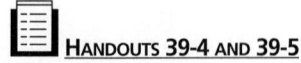

HANDOUTS 39-4 AND 39-5
Reinforcement Activities

PARAMEDIC STUDENT CD
Student Activities

POWERPOINT PRESENTATION
Chapter 39

COMPANION WEBSITE
http://www.prenhall.com/bledsoe

ONEKEY
Chapter 39

ADVANCED LIFE SUPPORT SKILLS
Larmon & Davis. *Advanced Life Support Skills.*

ADVANCED LIFE SKILLS REVIEW
Larmon & Davis. *Advanced Life Skills Review.*

BRADY SKILLS SERIES: ALS
Larmon & Davis. *Brady Skills Series: ALS.*

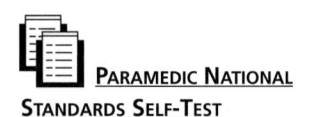

PARAMEDIC NATIONAL STANDARDS SELF-TEST
Miller. *Paramedic National Standards Self-Test*, 4th edition.

HANDOUT 39-1

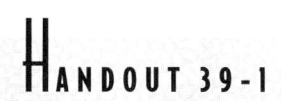

Student's Name _____

CHAPTER 39 OBJECTIVES CHECKLIST

Knowledge	Date Mastered
1. Review the anatomic structures and physiology of the female reproductive system.	
2. Identify the normal events of the menstrual cycle.	
3. Describe how to assess a patient with a gynecological complaint.	
4. Explain how to recognize a gynecological emergency.	
5. Describe the general care for any patient experiencing a gynecological emergency.	
6. Describe the pathophysiology, assessment, and management of the following gynecological emergencies. • Pelvic inflammatory disease • Ruptured ovarian cyst • Cystitis • Mittelschmertz • Endometritis • Endometriosis • Ectopic pregnancy • Vaginal hemorrhage	
7. Describe the assessment, care, and emotional support of the sexual assault patient.	
8. Given several preprogrammed gynecological patients, provide the appropriate assessment, management, and transportation.	

HANDOUT 39-2

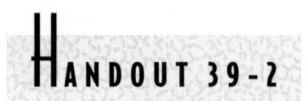

Student's Name _____

CHAPTER 39 QUIZ

Write the letter of the best answer in the space provided.

_____ 1. The branch of medicine that deals with health maintenance and the diseases of women, primarily of the reproductive organs, is called:
   A. obstetrics.
   B. gynecology.
   C. endocrinology.
   D. perinatalistics.

_____ 2. The female external genitalia are known collectively as the:
   A. vagina.
   B. vulva.
   C. perineum.
   D. labia.

_____ 3. The _____ drains the urinary bladder.
   A. vagina
   B. mons pubis
   C. prepuce
   D. urethra

_____ 4. The part of the female internal genitalia that provides an outlet for menstrual blood and tissue leaving the body is called the:
   A. vagina.
   B. uterus.
   C. fallopian tube.
   D. urethra.

_____ 5. The normal site for fetal development is (are) the:
   A. ovaries.
   B. uterus.
   C. urethra.
   D. fallopian tubes.

_____ 6. The fundus is the:
   A. uppermost portion of the uterus, above where the fallopian tubes connect.
   B. lower portion of the uterus, also called the cervix.
   C. upper two-thirds of the uterus, comprised of smooth muscle.
   D. body, or corpus, of the uterus.

_____ 7. The sloughing of the uterine lining is referred to as:
   A. endometriosis.
   B. pelvic inflammatory disease.
   C. the menstrual cycle.
   D. menopause.

_____ 8. During the proliferative phase of a menstrual cycle:
   A. the uterine lining thickens and becomes engorged with blood.
   B. uterine vascularity increases in anticipation of implantation of a fertilized egg.
   C. vascular changes cause the endometrium to become pale, and small blood vessels rupture.
   D. the ischemic endometrium is shed.

_____ 9. Fertilization of the egg takes place during the:
   A. proliferative phase.
   B. secretory phase.
   C. ischemic phase.
   D. menstrual phase.

_____ 10. One of the two most common emergency gynecological complaints is:
   A. vomiting.
   B. fever.
   C. abdominal pain.
   D. back pain.

_____ 11. Severe discomfort during a woman's menstrual period is known as:
   A. PID
   B. dysmenorrhea
   C. dyspareunia
   D. LMP

HANDOUT 39-2 Continued

_____ 12. General guidelines in assessing and caring for a gynecological emergency patient include:
   A. packing the vagina with sterile dressings to control excessive hemorrhage.
   B. performing a thorough internal vaginal exam in the field.
   C. realizing that psychological support may be more important than emergency medical care.
   D. application of direct pressure, over the uterus, to control vaginal hemorrhage.

_____ 13. Your patient is complaining of abdominal pain, which increases when she walks. To avoid this, she walks with a shuffling gate. She also complains of fever, chills, nausea, and vomiting. She is most likely experiencing:
   A. an ectopic pregnancy.
   B. a ruptured ovarian cyst.
   C. pelvic inflammatory disease.
   D. endometritis.

_____ 14. An ectopic pregnancy is a pregnancy in which the:
   A. baby is delivered prematurely.
   B. developing fetus implants outside of the uterus.
   C. fetus develops in an abnormal position, such as buttocks superior.
   D. fetus is spontaneously expelled during the first trimester.

_____ 15. During your assessment of the victim of a sexual assault, you should:
   A. ask specific questions about the assault to report to law enforcement.
   B. perform a brief vaginal exam to verify penetration.
   C. place bloody articles in a brown paper bag.
   D. allow the patient to clean up before the medical examination.

HANDOUT 39-3

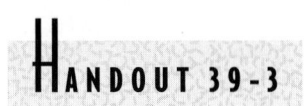

Student's Name _____

CHAPTER 39 SCENARIO

Review the following real-life situation. Then answer the questions at the end of the scenario.

As a working paramedic in the Emergency Department, you start the assessment of patients off with a battery of routine procedures—vital signs, weight, IV as needed. Today you encounter a 29-year-old female who has a complaint of severe abdominal pain. Unwilling to have her walk to the department, you place her in a wheelchair where she draws her knees up into the seat. Peculiar behavior, you think, for a woman wearing a dress.

After the patient disrobes in private and puts on the hospital gown, you reenter the room. The patient complains of diffuse abdominal pain that she characterizes as 8 on a scale of 0 to 10. She is presently having her menstrual period. She also relates she has had a light yellow discharge from the vagina lately.

On physical examination, she is pale and diaphoretic. Her pulse is a sustained 120 beats per minute. Her blood pressure is 140/76, elevated according to the patient. Palpation elicits severe pain and rebound tenderness. Your medical director has indicated that you are to follow your prehospital protocols and then report your patient to either the charge nurse or the attending physician, depending on the severity of the patient's condition.

1. What would be some of your leading working diagnoses for this patient?

2. How would you treat this patient?

HANDOUT 39-4

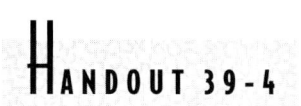

Student's Name _____

CHAPTER 39 REVIEW

Write the word or words that best complete the following sentences in the space(s) provided.

1. _____ is the branch of medicine that deals with the health maintenance and the diseases of women, primarily of the reproductive organs. _____ is the branch of medicine that deals with the care of women throughout pregnancy.

2. The female external genitalia are known collectively as the _____, or the _____.

3. The _____ is a roughly diamond-shaped, skin-covered muscular tissue that separates the vagina from the anus.

4. The structures that protect the vagina and the urethra are the _____.

5. Although not truly a part of the female reproductive system, the _____ drains the urinary bladder.

6. The _____ is the female organ of copulation, forms the final passageway for the infant during childbirth, and provides an outlet for menstrual blood to leave the body.

7. The primary function of the _____ is to provide a site for fetal development.

8. The _____ is the uppermost portion of the uterus.

9. The fundal _____, measured in centimeters, is generally comparable to the _____ of gestation.

10. The inner layer of the uterine wall where the fertilized egg implants is called the _____.

11. The term _____ refers to the onset of menses, usually occurring between ages 10 and 14 years.

12. The _____ are the primary female gonads, or sex organs.

13. The function of the _____ _____ is to conduct the egg from the space around the ovaries into the uterine cavity.

14. The female sex hormones _____ and _____ control the ovarian-menstrual cycle, pregnancy, and lactation.

15. During the _____ phase of the menstrual cycle, the uterine lining thickens and becomes engorged with blood.

16. Fertilization of the egg may take place during the _____ phase of the menstrual cycle.

17. During the _____ phase, the ischemic endometrium is shed, along with a discharge of blood, mucus, and cellular debris.

18. The cessation of menses and ovarian function due to decreased secretion of estrogen is called _____.

19. The two most common emergency gynecological complaints are _____ _____ and _____ _____.

20. When obtaining the history of any female patient of childbearing age, the paramedic should always document the patient's last _____ _____.

21. Do not perform a(n) _____ vaginal exam in the field.

22. General management of gynecological emergencies is focused on _____ care.

23. While caring for the female patient with vaginal bleeding, do not pack _____ in the _____.

REINFORCEMENT

©2007 Pearson Education, Inc.
Essentials of Paramedic Care, 2nd ed.

CHAPTER 39 *Gynecology* 919

HANDOUT 39-4 Continued

24. An acute infection of the reproductive organs is called _____ _____ _____.
25. _____ is an infection of the urinary bladder.
26. Painful urination often associated with cystitis is called _____.
27. The commonly used term to describe a pregnancy which ends before 20 weeks gestation is called a(n) _____, or spontaneous _____.
28. Treatment for vaginal bleeding includes _____ blood flow, _____, and initiating _____ therapy and _____ access based on the patient's condition.
29. When caring for a victim of sexual assault, consider the patient a _____ scene.
30. _____ and _____ support are the most important elements of care for the sexual assault victim.

HANDOUT 39-5

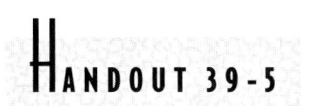

Student's Name _____

GYNECOLOGICAL TRUE OR FALSE

Indicate if the following statements are true or false by writing T or F in the space provided.

_____ 1. Most gynecological emergency patients experience either abdominal pain or vaginal bleeding.

_____ 2. The uterus produces LH and FSH.

_____ 3. The ovaries produce eggs for reproduction.

_____ 4. The perineum is the lining of the uterus that sloughs off during the menstrual period.

_____ 5. Women are more susceptible to bladder disease than men because they have longer urethras.

_____ 6. Actual menstruation occurs during the secretory phase of the menstrual cycle.

_____ 7. The number of times a woman has been pregnant is referred to as her gravidity.

_____ 8. The number of a woman's pregnancies that have resulted in a viable infant are referred to as her parity.

_____ 9. The use of IUDs can cause hypertension, stroke, and pulmonary embolism.

_____ 10. The internal vaginal exam should be performed immediately after history taking.

_____ 11. Probably the most common cause of nontraumatic abdominal pain in women is PID.

_____ 12. PID may be difficult to distinguish from appendicitis in the field.

_____ 13. Patients with PID often draw their knees up to the chest as a way of decreasing tension on the peritoneum.

_____ 14. In an ectopic pregnancy, the egg implants in the uterus.

_____ 15. Ectopic pregnancy is a life-threatening condition.

_____ 16. Endometritis is caused by the rupture of an ovarian cyst.

_____ 17. The condition known as mittelschmerz is associated with the release of an egg from the ovary.

_____ 18. Any woman with significant abdominal pain should be transported to the hospital.

_____ 19. Never pack the vagina with any material or dressing to control bleeding.

_____ 20. If you are the first person to reach a rape victim, question her to establish details of the incident while they are fresh in her mind.

Chapter 39 Answer Key

Handout 39-2: Chapter 39 Quiz

1. B	5. B	9. A	13. C
2. B	6. A	10. C	14. B
3. D	7. C	11. B	15. C
4. A	8. A	12. C	

Handout 39-3: Chapter 39 Scenario

1. The symptom pattern is similar to that of either pelvic inflammatory disease or acute appendicitis. However, the possibility of an ectopic pregnancy cannot be ruled out.
2. The question of an ectopic pregnancy is pressing. According to the ectopic pregnancy/abdominal pain protocols, the patient should have a large-bore IV line established with a fluid bolus of 500 to 1000 cc of NS or LR. The patient should be prepared for the possibility of imminent shock as well. It is imperative that blood be drawn and sent to the lab to confirm or deny the presence of pregnancy.

Handout 39-4: Chapter 39 Review

1. Gynecology, Obstetrics
2. vulva, pudendum
3. perineum
4. labia
5. urethra
6. vagina
7. uterus
8. fundus
9. height, weeks
10. endometrium
11. menarche
12. ovaries
13. fallopian tubes
14. estrogen, progesterone
15. proliferative
16. proliferative
17. menstrual
18. menopause
19. abdominal pain, vaginal bleeding
20. menstrual period
21. internal
22. supportive
23. dressings, vagina
24. pelvic inflammatory disease
25. Cystitis
26. dysuria
27. miscarriage, abortion
28. absorbing, transport, oxygen, IV
29. crime
30. Psychological, emotional

Handout 39-5: Gynecological True or False

1. T	6. F	11. T	16. F
2. F	7. T	12. T	17. T
3. T	8. T	13. T	18. T
4. F	9. F	14. F	19. T
5. F	10. F	15. T	20. F

Chapter 40

Obstetrics

INTRODUCTION

Pregnancy and childbirth are natural processes, but sometimes complications do occur. Though complications of pregnancy are uncommon, paramedics must be able to recognize these complications, which may be life-threatening to the mother or baby, and manage them effectively. This chapter deals with the pregnancy and childbirth process and its complications.

CHAPTER OBJECTIVES

After reading this chapter, you should be able to:

1. Describe the anatomic structures and physiology of the reproductive system during pregnancy. (pp. 1519–1522)
2. Identify the normal events of pregnancy. (pp. 1522–1525)
3. Describe how to assess an obstetrical patient. (pp. 1525–1527)
4. Identify the stages of labor and the paramedic's role in each stage. (pp. 1537–1539)
5. Differentiate between normal and abnormal delivery. (pp. 1544–1549)
6. Identify and describe complications associated with pregnancy and delivery. (pp. 1527–1537, 1549–1550)
7. Identify predelivery emergencies. (pp. 1527–1537)
8. State indications of an imminent delivery. (pp. 1538–1539)
9. Identify the contents of an obstetrical kit and explain the use of each item. (pp. 1539–1542)
10. Differentiate the management of a patient with predelivery emergencies from a normal delivery. (p. 1527)
11. State the steps in the predelivery preparation of the mother. (pp. 1538–1539)
12. Establish the relationship between body substance isolation and childbirth. (p. 1539)
13. State the steps to assist in the delivery of a newborn. (pp. 1539–1542)
14. Describe how to care for the newborn. (pp. 1542–1544)
15. Describe how and when to cut the umbilical cord. (p. 1542)
16. Discuss the steps in the delivery of the placenta. (pp. 1541, 1542)
17. Describe the management of the mother postdelivery. (pp. 1542, 1549–1550)
18. Summarize neonatal resuscitation procedures. (pp. 1543–1544)

TOTAL TEACHING TIME:
12.00 HOURS
The total teaching time is only a guideline based on the didactic and practical lab averages in the National Standard Curriculum. Instructors should take into consideration such factors as the pace at which students learn, the size of the class, and breaks. The actual time devoted to teaching objectives is the responsibility of the instructor.

19. Describe the procedures for handling abnormal deliveries, complications of pregnancy, and maternal complications of labor. (pp. 1527–1537, 1544–1550)
20. Describe special considerations when meconium is present in amniotic fluid or during delivery. (p. 1549)
21. Describe special considerations of a premature baby. (pp. 1536–1537)
22. Given several simulated delivery situations, provide the appropriate assessment, management, and transport for the mother and child. (pp. 1519–1550)

FRAMING THE LESSON

Begin class by reviewing the important points from Chapter 39, "Gynecology." Discuss any aspects of the chapter not fully understood by students. Then begin with Chapter 40 material. Start by asking if any of the students have ever witnessed or assisted at a childbirth. If any students have, ask them to briefly describe the situation. You may also wish to begin the class with a film or videotape of an actual delivery. Stress that most pregnancies and deliveries are normal, but that problems that do occur during the pregnancy and the delivery of the baby are often serious and life-threatening for the baby, the mother, or both. Emphasize that childbirth has been occurring for thousands of years—and until the past few hundred years without the aid of medical care professionals. Though EMTs and paramedics may tell about the number of babies they have "delivered," in fact, it is the mothers who have delivered. Prehospital care providers have assisted these mothers with what is in most cases a natural process.

TEACHING STRATEGIES

People learn in a variety of ways. Some do better with the spoken word, whereas others prefer the written. Some prefer to work alone, whereas others profit from working in groups. Recognizing these different ways of acquiring knowledge, the authors of this *Instructor's Resource Manual* have provided a variety of teaching strategies for the different types of learners. These strategies are intended to foster higher-level cognitive skills and encourage creative learning and problem solving. For greatest effectiveness, incorporate these strategies into your class lecture. Symbols in the Lecture Outline indicate the points at which various exercises might be most appropriate. Other strategies can be used to preview the lesson or to summarize it.

The following strategies are keyed to specific sections of the lesson.

1. ***Using the Affective Domain.*** To use an activity in the affective domain, view *A Baby Story* from the Lifetime cable channel. Touching stories of families having or trying to have babies are played daily on the channel.

2. ***Flash Cards.*** Suggest that students create flash cards with the names of complications of pregnancy, labor, and delivery on one side and the signs and symptoms for assessment of the conditions on the other. Students can take turns quizzing each other with the cards.

3. ***Placing a Pregnant Patient on a Stretcher.*** Positioning of the pregnant patient, especially backboarding, can be difficult. Moulage a patient as pregnant, and have students practice placing the patient on the stretcher and in various immobilization devices. You may be able to borrow a weighted abdomen,

lending additional realism to the scenario, from your high school's parenting class or from a costume shop.

4. Creating APGAR Blankets. For use during the neonatal resuscitation portion of class, make (or have the students make) an APGAR blanket. Use iron-on transfers illustrating the mnemonic for APGAR, so that the students have a visual reminder after delivering the infant. For example, use a clock for pulse rate or Grimace, the purple character from McDonald's, for irritability. If you have the students create these blankets, consider donating them to your local EMS agency after class.

5. Using Neonatal Equipment. The equipment used for preemies and neonates is *tiny*. Most paramedics have only used pediatric equipment, which, though it looks small compared to adult equipment, is actually much bigger than preemie or neonate equipment. Be sure to have at least one full set of neonatal resuscitation equipment for students to use in class. If money is tight, contact the special care nursery in your area to solicit a donation. Most have education funds and would likely provide oxygen masks, BVM face masks, IV catheters, EKG patches, diapers, and other commonly used equipment.

6. Viewing Birthing Videotapes. "Delivery Room" from The Learning Channel shows all types of birthing situations, including some challenging deliveries such as precipitous labor, breech birth, and placenta previa. In addition to the special programming, most TLC programs are available to purchase, with three shows per tape for under $30. The web address is *www.TLC.com*.

The following strategies can be used at various points throughout the lesson or to help summarize and demonstrate what students have learned.

Field Trip. Some health care centers and birthing centers will allow students to come to classes and visit with expectant mothers. The students can then practice history gathering and physical exams (to practice measuring fundal height and listening for fetal heart tones).

Clinical Observation Time. If your community has a clinic or care center operated by a nurse-midwife, arrange for clinical observation time for students at the center or at a home delivery. Ask if students would be allowed to assist the midwife in the assessment, care, and eventual delivery by the patients.

Guest Speaker: Pregnant Woman. If you are unable to arrange a field trip or clinical observation time, invite to the class a pregnant woman willing to allow students to inspect, palpate, and auscultate her baby. She can also answer a lot of questions about the pregnancy for your class.

Clinical Time in Labor and Delivery. Few conditions are the same as being present during a birth and neonatal resuscitation. Be sure to secure clinical time in labor and delivery. Hospitals may be reluctant, as obstetrics is a major area of litigation in health care. However, most hospitals will at least allow observation. Generally, clinical time should be hands-on and interactive. This is one area in which even a single observation will be valuable when the paramedic is called upon to deliver a baby.

Guest Speaker: Nurse from NICU or Neonatal Transport. A nurse from the NICU or Neonatal Transport Team would make an excellent guest speaker in class.

Cultural Considerations, Legal Notes, and Patho Pearls. The Student CD-ROM contains this series of informative features to enhance the student's understanding of the material covered in this chapter.

TEACHING OUTLINE

Chapter 40 is the fourteenth lesson in Division 4, *Medical Emergencies*. Distribute Handout 40-1 so that students can familiarize themselves with the learning goals for this chapter. If students have any questions about the objectives, answer them at this time.

Then present the chapter. One possible lecture outline follows. In the outline, the parenthetical references in regular type are references to text pages; those in bold type are references to figures, tables, or procedures.

I. Introduction. Pregnancy is a normal, natural process of life. Complications of pregnancy are uncommon but can be life-threatening. It is therefore important that the paramedic be prepared to recognize them quickly and manage them appropriately. Childbirth occurs every day, usually requiring only the most basic assistance. However, childbirth complications do occur. This chapter will prepare students to assess and care for the female patient throughout her pregnancy and the delivery of her child. (p. 1519)

II. The prenatal period (pp. 1519–1525)

    A. Anatomy and physiology of the obstetric patient (pp. 1519–1521) (**Figs. 40-1 and 40-2, p. 1520**)
        1. Ovulation
        2. Placenta
        3. Afterbirth
        4. Umbilical cord
        5. Amniotic sac
        6. Amniotic fluid

    B. Physiologic changes of pregnancy (pp. 1521–1522) (**Fig. 40-3, p. 1521**)
        1. Reproductive system
        2. Respiratory system
        3. Cardiovascular system
        4. Gastrointestinal system
        5. Urinary system
        6. Musculoskeletal system

    C. Fetal development (pp. 1522–1523) (**Table 40-1, p. 1523**)
        1. Estimated date of confinement (EDC)
        2. Trimesters
        3. Stages of development
            a. Preembryonic stage
            b. Embryonic stage
            c. Fetal stage
            d. Obstetric terminology

    D. Fetal circulation (pp. 1523–1525) (**Fig. 40-4, p. 1524**)

III. General assessment of the obstetric patient (pp. 1525–1527)

    A. Initial assessment (p. 1525)
    B. History (pp. 1525–1526)
        1. General information
        2. Preexisting or aggravated medical conditions

HANDOUT 40-1
Chapter 40 Objectives Checklist

TEACHING STRATEGY 1
Using the Affective Domain

POWERPOINT PRESENTATION
Chapter 40 PowerPoint slides 4–12

POINT TO EMPHASIZE
At 12 to 13 weeks, you should need a Doppler device to detect fetal heart tones; at 18 to 20 weeks you should need only a stethoscope. Expect a rate of 140 to 200.

POINT OF INTEREST
A mother's pregnancy history is normally described as follow: G4P2-2022. Translated, this is Gravida 4 (4 times pregnant), Para 2 (2 viable deliveries) – 2 ful-term pregnancies, 0 preemies, 2 abortions, 2 viable children.

POWERPOINT PRESENTATION
Chapter 40 PowerPoint slides 13–14

a. Diabetes
  b. Heart disease
  c. Hypertension
  d. Seizure disorders
  e. Neuromuscular disorders
 3. Pain
 4. Vaginal bleeding
 5. Active labor
C. Physical examination (pp. 1526–1527)
 1. Fundal height
 2. Vitals
 3. Crowning
 4. Prolapsed cord

IV. **General management of the obstetric patient** (p. 1527)

A. Focus on ABCs. (p. 1527)
B. Monitor for shock. (p. 1527)
C. Administer oxygen. (p. 1527)
D. Initiate IV. (p. 1527)
E. Consider fluid resuscitation. (p. 1527)
F. Monitor heart. (p. 1527)
G. Place patient in position of comfort. (p. 1527)

V. **Complications of pregnancy** (pp. 1527–1537)

A. Trauma (pp. 1527–1528)
 1. Application of c-collar, backboard
 2. High-flow, high-concentration oxygen
 3. Two large-bore IVs
 4. Transport tilted to the left.
 5. Reassess frequently.
 6. Monitor the fetus.
B. Medical conditions (p. 1528)
C. Bleeding during pregnancy (pp. 1528–1532)
 1. Abortion
  a. Classifications
  b. Assessment
  c. Management
 2. Ectopic pregnancy
  a. Assessment
  b. Management
 3. Placenta previa (**Fig. 40-5, p. 1531**)
  a. Assessment
  b. Management
 4. Abruptio placentae (**Fig 40-6, p. 1532**)
  a. Assessment
  b. Management
D. Medical complications of pregnancy (pp. 1532–1535)
 1. Hypertensive disorders
  a. Preeclampsia and eclampsia
  b. Chronic hypertension
  c. Chronic hypertension superimposed with preeclampsia
  d. Transient hypertension
  e. Assessment
  f. Management
   i. Hypertension
   ii. Preeclampsia

POINT TO EMPHASIZE

When the mother is in shock, the body's compensatory mechanism considers the fetus an unnecessary appendage and shunts blood from it to the heart, brain, and lungs. This means that the baby may be in distress long before the mother shows signs of trouble. Life-threatening vaginal bleeding occurs with a ruptured ectopic pregnancy, placenta previa, and abruptio placentae.

POWERPOINT PRESENTATION

Chapter 40 PowerPoint slide 15

TEACHING STRATEGY 3

Placing a Pregnant Patient on a Stretcher

POWERPOINT PRESENTATION

Chapter 40 PowerPoint slides 16–34

TEACHING STRATEGY 2

Flash Cards

POINT OF INTEREST

Some 99 percent of bleedings in pregnancy occur in the first or third trimesters. The vast majority of these (20:1) occur in the first trimester.

READING/REFERENCE

Mattera, C. "Obstetrical Complications." *JEMS*, March 1999.

POINT OF INTEREST

About 10 percent of abortions are spontaneous. Patients usually complain of crampy lower abdominal or back pain.

READING/REFERENCE

Dominguez, O. J. "Ruptured Ectopic Pregnancy," *EMS*, Nov. 1999.

POINT TO EMPHASIZE

What differentiates eclampsia from preeclampsia are the accompanying seizures.

            iii. Eclampsia
        2. Supine-hypotensive syndrome (**Fig. 40-7, p. 1535**)
            a. Assessment
            b. Management
        3. Gestational diabetes
            a. Assessment
            b. Management
    E. Braxton-Hicks contractions (p. 1536)
    F. Preterm labor (pp. 1536–1537)
        1. Maternal factors
        2. Placental factors
        3. Fetal factors
        4. Assessment
        5. Management

VI. **The puerperium** (pp. 1537–1544)
    A. Labor (pp. 1537–1538)
        1. Stage one (Dilation stage)
        2. Stage two (Expulsion stage)
        3. Stage three (Placental stage)
    B. Management of the patient in labor (pp. 1538–1539)
    C. Field delivery (pp. 1539–1542) (**Proc. 40-1, p. 1540**) (**Figs. 40-8 through 40-16, p. 1541**)
    D. Neonatal care (pp. 1542–1544) (**Fig. 40-17, p. 1542; Fig. 40-18, p. 1543**)
        1. Routine care of the neonate
        2. APGAR scoring (**Table 40-2, p. 1544**)
        3. Neonatal resuscitation

VII. **Abnormal delivery situations** (pp. 1544–1547)
    A. Breech presentation (pp. 1544–1545) (**Figs. 40-19 and 40-20, p. 1545**)
    B. Prolapsed cord (pp. 1546–1547) (**Fig. 40-21, p. 1546; Fig. 40-22, p. 1547**)
    C. Limb presentation (p. 1547)
    D. Other abnormal presentations (p. 1547)

VIII. **Other delivery complications** (pp. 1548–1549)
    A. Multiple births (p. 1548)
    B. Cephalopelvic disproportion (p. 1548)
    C. Precipitous delivery (p. 1548)
    D. Shoulder dystocia (p. 1548)
    E. Meconium staining (p. 1549)

IX. **Maternal complications of labor and delivery** (pp. 1549–1550)
    A. Postpartum hemorrhage (p. 1549)
    B. Uterine rupture (p. 1550)
    C. Uterine inversion (p. 1550)
    D. Pulmonary embolism (p. 1550)

X. **Chapter summary** (p. 1551). Childbirth is a normal process and obstetrical emergencies are fairly uncommon. However, all pregnant patients are at risk for developing complications, and it is impossible to predict which ones will actually occur. It is therefore important to recognize these complications and act accordingly. Keep in mind that you are caring for two patients, and as long as you remember the priorities of patient care, the situation should go smoothly. Relax and enjoy the opportunity to help bring a new life into the world.

POWERPOINT PRESENTATION
Chapter 40 PowerPoint slides 35–42

TEACHING STRATEGY 4
Creating APGAR Blankets

TEACHING STRATEGY 5
Using Neonate Equipment

TEACHING STRATEGY 6
Viewing Birthing Videotapes

POWERPOINT PRESENTATION
Chapter 40 PowerPoint slides 43–49

POWERPOINT PRESENTATION
Chapter 40 PowerPoint slides 50–55

POINT TO EMPHASIZE
The highest number of children ever produced from a multiple birth is 10!

POWERPOINT PRESENTATION
Chapter 40 PowerPoint slides 56–60

POWERPOINT PRESENTATION
Chapter 40 PowerPoint slide 61

SKILLS DEMONSTRATION AND PRACTICE

Students can practice skills discussed in this chapter in the following settings.

Scenario Lab: The following stations will be part of a larger trauma scenario lab. Divide the class into teams. Have teams circulate through the stations. Monitor the groups to be sure all groups have a chance to manage each of the cases and so that every student has the opportunity to be team leader. You may wish to have other instructors or qualified paramedics assist students in these activities.

Station	Equipment Needed	Activities
Normal Delivery	OB mannequin OB kit Instructor	Have students practice normal deliveries on the OB model.
Abnormal Delivery	OB mannequin OB kit Instructor	Have students practice abnormal deliveries on the OB model

Hospital:

- Observe and assist in normal and abnormal deliveries in the labor and delivery suite.
- Observe and assist in perinatal care of the mother and baby.
- Observe and assist in postpartum hemorrhage control.

Field Internship:

- Assist in normal and abnormal deliveries in the field.
- Assist in perinatal care of the mother and baby.
- Assist in postpartum hemorrhage control.

ASSIGNMENTS

Assign students to complete Chapter 40, "Obstetrics," of the workbook. Also assign them to read Chapter 41, "Neonatology," before the next class.

EVALUATION

Chapter Quiz and Scenario Distribute copies of the Chapter Quiz provided in Handout 40-2 to evaluate student understanding of this chapter. Make sure each student reads the scenario to reinforce critical thinking on the scene. Remind students not to use their notes or textbooks while taking the quiz.

Student CD Quizzes for every chapter are contained on the dynamic and highly visual in-text student CD.

Companion Website Additional quizzes for every chapter are contained on this exciting website.

TestGen You may wish to create a custom-tailored test using *Prentice Hall TestGen for Essentials of Paramedic Care*, 2nd Edition to evaluate student understanding of this chapter.

On-line Test Preparation (for students and instructors) Additional test preparation is available through Brady's new on-line product, *EMT Achieve: Paramedic Test Preparation* at *http://www.prenhall.com/emtachieve/*. Instructors can also monitor student mastery on-line.

ADVANCED LIFE SUPPORT SKILLS
Larmon & Davis. *Advanced Life Support Skills.*

ADVANCED LIFE SKILLS REVIEW
Larmon & Davis. *Advanced Life Skills Review.*

BRADY SKILLS SERIES: ALS
Larmon & Davis. *Brady Skills Series: ALS.*

WORKBOOK
Chapter 40 Activities

READING/REFERENCE
Textbook, pp. 1554–1584

HANDOUT 40-2
Chapter 40 Quiz

HANDOUT 40-3
Chapter 40 Scenario

PARAMEDIC STUDENT CD
Student Activities

COMPANION WEBSITE
http://www.prenhall.com/bledsoe

TESTGEN
Chapter 40

EMT ACHIEVE: PARAMEDIC TEST PREPARATION
Mistovich & Beasley. *EMT Achieve: Paramedic Test Preparation*, www.prenhall.com/emtachieve/

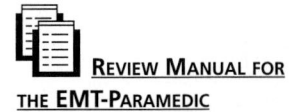

REVIEW MANUAL FOR THE EMT-PARAMEDIC
Cherry & Mistovich. *Review Manual for the EMT-Paramedic*, 3rd edition.

HANDOUTS 40-4 TO 40-6
Reinforcement Activities

PARAMEDIC STUDENT CD
Student Activities

POWERPOINT PRESENTATION
Chapter 40

COMPANION WEBSITE
http://www.prenhall.com/bledsoe

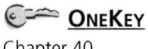

ONEKEY
Chapter 40

ADVANCED LIFE SUPPORT SKILLS
Larmon & Davis. *Advanced Life Support Skills.*

ADVANCED LIFE SKILLS REVIEW
Larmon & Davis. *Advanced Life Skills Review.*

BRADY SKILLS SERIES: ALS
Larmon & Davis. *Brady Skills Series: ALS.*

PARAMEDIC NATIONAL STANDARDS SELF-TEST
Miller. *Paramedic National Standards Self-Test*, 4th edition.

Review Manual for the EMT-Paramedic   This comprehensive exam review contains hundreds of test questions and rationales, including scenarios, along with two 180-question practice tests on CD.

REINFORCEMENT

Handouts   If classroom discussion or performance on the quiz indicates that some students have not fully mastered the chapter content, you may wish to assign some or all of the Reinforcement Handouts for this chapter.

Student CD (for students)   A wide variety of material on this CD-ROM will reinforce and also expand student knowledge and skills.

PowerPoint Presentation (for instructors)   The PowerPoint material developed for this chapter offers useful reinforcement of chapter content.

Companion Website (for students)   Additional review quizzes and links to EMS resources will contribute to further reinforcement of the chapter.

OneKey   On-line support is offered for this course on one of three platforms: CourseCompass, Blackboard, or Web CT. Includes the IRM, PowerPoints, TestGen, and Companion Website for instruction. Ask your local sales representative for more information.

Brady Skills Series: Advanced Life Skills (Video or CD)   Have your students watch the skills come to life on VHS or CD-ROM, or they can purchase the highly visual, full-color text with step-by-step procedures and rationales.

HANDOUT 40-1

Student's Name _____

CHAPTER 40 OBJECTIVES CHECKLIST

Knowledge	Date Mastered
1. Describe the anatomic structures and physiology of the reproductive system during pregnancy.	
2. Identify the normal events of pregnancy.	
3. Describe how to assess an obstetrical patient.	
4. Identify the stages of labor and the paramedic's role in each stage.	
5. Differentiate between normal and abnormal delivery.	
6. Identify and describe complications associated with pregnancy and delivery.	
7. Identify predelivery emergencies.	
8. State indications of an imminent delivery.	
9. Identify the contents of an obstetrical kit and explain the use of each item.	
10. Differentiate the management of a patient with predelivery emergencies from a normal delivery.	
11. State the steps in the predelivery preparation of the mother.	
12. Establish the relationship between body substance isolation and childbirth.	
13. State the steps to assist in the delivery of a newborn.	
14. Describe how to care for the newborn.	
15. Describe how and when to cut the umbilical cord.	
16. Discuss the steps in the delivery of the placenta.	
17. Describe the management of the mother postdelivery.	
18. Summarize neonatal resuscitation procedures.	
19. Describe the procedures for handling abnormal deliveries, complications of pregnancy, and maternal complications of labor.	

HANDOUT 40-1 Continued

Knowledge	Date Mastered
20. Describe special considerations when meconium is present in amniotic fluid or during delivery.	
21. Describe special considerations of a premature baby.	
22. Given several simulated delivery situations, provide the appropriate assessment, management, and transport for the mother and child.	

OBJECTIVES

HANDOUT 40-2

Student's Name _____

CHAPTER 40 QUIZ

Write the letter of the best answer in the space provided.

_____ 1. The release of an egg from the ovary is called:
   A. the preembryonic stage.
   B. ovulation.
   C. menstruation.
   D. gestation.

_____ 2. Fertilization of the egg takes place in the:
   A. uterus.
   B. vagina.
   C. fallopian tube.
   D. cervix.

_____ 3. The placenta, or "organ of pregnancy,":
   A. is an organ always present in the female uterus.
   B. is the organ in which the fetus will develop.
   C. secretes hormones necessary for fetal survival.
   D. becomes thick and engorged with blood at the time of fertilization.

_____ 4. Which of the following statements is TRUE regarding the umbilical cord?
   A. If it is found to be around the baby's neck at the time of delivery, it must immediately be clamped and cut.
   B. It is a flexible, rope-like structure, usually several feet in length.
   C. It circulates amniotic fluid through the uterus.
   D. It contains two arteries and one vein.

_____ 5. When a pregnant patient advises you that her "water has broken," she means:
   A. contractions have begun.
   B. the mucus plug has been expelled.
   C. the membranes have ruptured.
   D. she is experiencing vaginal bleeding.

_____ 6. The most significant pregnancy-related changes occur in the uterus. These changes include:
   A. an increase in weight of the uterus to approximately 2 pounds.
   B. an increase in the vascular system of the uterus to about one-fourth of the mother's total blood volume.
   C. the development of a layer of mucus on the lining of the uterus.
   D. an increase in the capacity of the uterus to nearly a liter of fluid.

_____ 7. When maternal blood volume increases, pregnant women receive supplemental iron to prevent anemia. This is because:
   A. the mother's red blood cells do not carry as much oxygen as they did prior to the pregnancy.
   B. there is a decrease in the number of the mother's red blood cells because they are now shared with the fetus.
   C. although both red blood cells and plasma increase, there is slightly more plasma.
   D. there is only an increase in plasma, not in red blood cells.

_____ 8. Hemodynamic changes of pregnancy include:
   A. the stroke volume progressively declining to term following a rise early in the pregnancy.
   B. cardiac output increasing 2.5–3 L/min during the first trimester.
   C. blood volume decreasing slightly, by 1–5 percent.
   D. heart rate remaining about the same.

HANDOUT 40-2 Continued

_____ 9. Supine-hypotensive syndrome occurs when the:
   A. heart is compressed by the gravid uterus when the mother lies supine.
   B. gravid uterus compresses the inferior vena cava when the mother lies in the supine position.
   C. body reacts to the mother lying in the supine position by dilation of the major blood vessels.
   D. fetus, lying at the same level as the mother when she is lying in the supine position, now requires more blood.

_____ 10. Which of the following statements is TRUE regarding fetal development?
   A. Fetal heart tones may be detected with a stethoscope by the 16th week.
   B. The baby may be able to survive if born before the 20th week.
   C. By the 38th week, the baby is considered fully developed.
   D. The sex of the infant can usually be determined by 8 weeks' gestation.

_____ 11. The fetus receives its blood from the placenta by means of the:
   A. umbilical arteries.   C. pulmonary arteries.
   B. umbilical vein.   D. pulmonary veins.

_____ 12. A pregnant woman may develop diabetes during the pregnancy. This is called:
   A. gravid diabetes.   C. gestational diabetes.
   B. obstetrical diabetes.   D. uterine diabetes.

_____ 13. Because cardiac output increases up to 30 percent during pregnancy, patients who have serious preexisting heart disease may develop:
   A. pulmonary embolism.   C. palpitations.
   B. congestive heart failure.   D. angina pectoris.

_____ 14. When caring for a pregnant patient who is experiencing vaginal bleeding, you should:
   A. gain information about the color, amount, and duration.
   B. assess the amount of bleeding by counting the number of sanitary pads used.
   C. save any passed clots or tissue for evaluation.
   D. all of these

_____ 15. Indications of imminent delivery include:
   A. contractions less than 5 minutes apart for a patient who is pregnant for the first time.
   B. the bulging of the fetal head past the opening of the vagina during a contraction.
   C. pain in the lower back.
   D. all of these

_____ 16. When caring for a pregnant patient who has experienced a major trauma, remember that:
   A. the later in the pregnancy, the less the likelihood of injury to the uterus.
   B. the fetus may be in danger even though the mother is showing no signs or symptoms of shock.
   C. the primary cause of fetal mortality is direct injury to the fetus, while the mother survives.
   D. the amniotic fluid provides little protection to the fetus from blunt trauma.

_____ 17. Spontaneous abortion is the term used to describe:
   A. an elective termination of pregnancy.
   B. the expulsion of the fetus prior to 8 weeks' gestation.
   C. the loss of a fetus by natural means.
   D. the loss of a fetus due to a traumatic injury to the mother.

_____ 18. An ectopic pregnancy refers to a pregnancy in which:
   A. delivery occurs within the first 24 weeks of the pregnancy.
   B. the egg has split in two, resulting in maternal twins.
   C. any aspect of it is abnormal.
   D. the fetus is implanted abnormally outside of the uterus.

HANDOUT 40-2 Continued

_____ 19. The abnormal implantation of the placenta on the lower half of the uterine wall, resulting in partial or complete coverage of the cervical opening, is called:
   A. placenta previa.
   B. abruptio placentae.
   C. prolapsed placenta.
   D. nucal placenta.

_____ 20. The hallmark of the condition described in question 19 is:
   A. severe abdominal pain and vaginal bleeding.
   B. increased blood pressure and seizures.
   C. painless, bright red vaginal bleeding.
   D. abdominal pain accompanied by fever.

_____ 21. Sharp, tearing pain and a stiff, boardlike abdomen without vaginal bleeding in a pregnant patient indicate:
   A. a central abruption of the placenta.
   B. placenta previa.
   C. an ectopic pregnancy.
   D. spontaneous abortion.

_____ 22. Care for the preeclamptic patient includes:
   A. administration of IV diazepam.
   B. transport of the patient in the left lateral recumbent position.
   C. administration of IV Lasix to reduce edema.
   D. two large-bore IVs of lactated Ringer's, initiating a 250-ml fluid challenge.

_____ 23. Labor consists of uterine contractions that cause the dilation and effacement of the cervix. The term *effacement* means that the uterus is:
   A. thinning and shortening.
   B. thinning and lengthening.
   C. releasing the placenta.
   D. returning to its normal, prepregnancy size.

_____ 24. The term *tocolysis* refers to:
   A. the acceleration of labor by administration of Pitocin.
   B. an infection acquired by the mother, passed on to the fetus.
   C. the process of stopping labor.
   D. the disruption of blood flow from the placenta to the fetus.

_____ 25. During the second stage of labor:
   A. contractions are usually mild, occurring every 10 to 20 minutes.
   B. the patient feels the urge to push or "bear down."
   C. the placenta (afterbirth) is delivered.
   D. the cervix dilates to 10 centimeters.

_____ 26. If you note crowning prior to transporting the patient to the hospital:
   A. have the mother cross her legs and transport immediately.
   B. place the mother in the knee-chest position and transport.
   C. prepare to deliver the baby, as the birth is imminent.
   D. place the mother in the Trendelenburg position and transport.

_____ 27. During the delivery of the baby, you should:
   A. pull gently on the umbilical cord to encourage the placenta to deliver.
   B. "milk" the cord, toward the baby.
   C. suction the baby's mouth first, then the nose.
   D. administer high-flow, high-concentration oxygen to the baby.

HANDOUT 40-2 Continued

_____ 28. Guidelines of neonatal resuscitation include:
  A. initiating chest compressions if the infant's heart rate is below 100, and it does not respond to ventilations.
  B. assisting ventilations if the infant's respiratory rate is below 30, and tactile stimulation does not increase the rate.
  C. intubating the infant and initiating ACLS procedures if the heart rate falls below 80.
  D. administering 25 percent dextrose IV if the infant's respiratory rate is less than 15.

_____ 29. If the umbilical cord is seen in the vagina (prolapsed cord), you should:
  A. insert a gloved hand to gently push the fetus back up the birth canal.
  B. immediately clamp and cut the cord.
  C. place the mother in the knee-chest position.
  D. encourage the mother to continue to push to speed up the delivery.

_____ 30. If your patient complains of excruciating abdominal pain with the onset of labor, and shows signs and symptoms of shock without external hemorrhage, consider:
  A. uterine inversion.   C. uterine rupture.
  B. placenta previa.   D. abruptio placentae.

HANDOUT 40-3

Student's Name _____

CHAPTER 40 SCENARIO

Review the following real-life situation. Then answer the questions that follow.

You respond to a call to find a 19-year-old female complaining of vaginal bleeding and abdominal pain. The patient is lying in the fetal position in obvious distress when you arrive. Her vital signs are pulse, 140; BP, 84/50; respirations, 24 normal; lungs clear; skin cool, pale, and moist. While obtaining her history, you discover that she has been having irregular bleeding for approximately 2 weeks. She says her last menstrual period was almost 2 months ago. She denies pregnancy because she uses a protective device. Her abdomen is warm and tender to palpation to the right lower quadrant, causing severe pain. She denies any further medical problems.

1. Based on this evidence, what problem do you believe this patient is having? Why?

2. What other problems might she be having?

3. What other questions might help you in your diagnosis?

4. What treatment should be given to this patient?

5. Is there a need for a visual exam? Why or why not?

HANDOUT 40-4

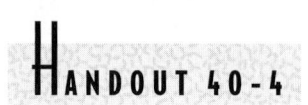

Student's Name _____

CHAPTER 40 REVIEW

Write the word or words that best complete the following sentences in the space(s) provided.

1. The release of an egg from the ovary is called _____.
2. The organ that serves as a lifeline for the developing fetus is the _____.
3. The structure that connects the placenta and the fetus is the _____ _____, which has _____ artery(ies) and _____ vein(s).
4. The clear, watery fluid that surrounds and protects the developing fetus is called _____ fluid.
5. The membranes that surround and protect the developing fetus throughout the period of intrauterine development are the _____ _____.
6. The normal duration of pregnancy is _____ weeks, or _____ days, or _____ calendar months.
7. Generally, pregnancy is divided into _____, each being 13 weeks long.
8. The approximate date the infant will be born is called the _____ _____ of _____.
9. A woman who has given birth to her first child is called _____, while a woman who has delivered more than one baby is called _____.
10. The bulging of the fetal head past the opening of the vagina during a contraction is called _____, which is an indication of _____ delivery.
11. Transport all trauma patients at _____ weeks or more gestation.
12. Termination of pregnancy before the 20th week of gestation is called a(n) _____.
13. Another term for miscarriage is _____ _____.
14. Assume that any female of childbearing age with lower abdominal pain is experiencing a(n) _____ _____.
15. _____ _____ occurs as a result of abnormal implantation of the placenta on the lower half of the uterine wall.
16. The premature separation of a normally implanted placenta from the uterine wall is called _____ _____.
17. The difference between preeclampsia and eclampsia is the onset of _____.
18. _____-_____ _____ occurs when the gravid uterus compresses the inferior vena cava when the mother lies in a supine position.
19. The thinning and shortening of the cervix during labor is called _____.
20. The process of stopping labor is called _____.
21. After the delivery of the infant, place the first clamp on the umbilical cord _____ cm from the baby, and the second clamp _____ cm above the first clamp.
22. A(n) _____ _____ occurs when the umbilical cord precedes the fetal presenting part.
23. With limb presentation, place the mother in the _____-_____ position.
24. A delivery that occurs after less than 3 hours of labor is called a(n) _____ delivery.
25. _____ _____ occurs when the fetus passes feces into the amniotic fluid.

REINFORCEMENT

938 ESSENTIALS OF PARAMEDIC CARE

©2007 Pearson Education, Inc.
Essentials of Paramedic Care, 2nd ed.

HANDOUT 40-4 Continued

26. _____ _____ is the loss of more than 500 cc of blood immediately following delivery.
27. The actual tearing of the uterus is called _____ _____.
28. _____ _____ occurs when the uterus turns inside out after delivery.
29. _____ _____ is a clear, watery liquid that surrounds and protects the developing fetus.
30. _____ _____ is the presence of a blood clot in the pulmonary vascular system.

Handout 40-5

Student's Name _____

OBSTETRICAL TERMINOLOGY MATCHING

Write the letter of the appropriate term in the space provided next to the description.

A. Primigravida
B. Nulligravida
C. Multigravida
D. Primipara
E. Multipara
F. Nullipara
G. Ectopic pregnancy
H. Abruptio placenta
I. Placenta previa
J. Preeclampsia
K. Eclampsia
L. Supine-hypotensive syndrome
M. Cephalopelvic disproportion
N. Prolapsed cord
O. Shoulder dystocia

_____ 1. Woman who has not yet delivered her first child.

_____ 2. Pregnancy toxemia resulting in hypertension, edema, headache, and vision disturbances.

_____ 3. Woman who is pregnant for the first time.

_____ 4. Woman who has delivered her first child.

_____ 5. When the umbilical cord is the presenting part and is compressed in the birth canal.

_____ 6. When the baby's head is too large for the birth canal.

_____ 7. Implantation of an egg other than in the uterus.

_____ 8. Woman who has delivered more than one baby.

_____ 9. Compression of the major vessels by the uterus.

_____ 10. Separation of the placenta from the uterine wall.

_____ 11. Woman who has not been pregnant.

_____ 12. When the baby's shoulders are larger than the head.

_____ 13. Woman who has been pregnant more than once.

_____ 14. Low attachment of the placenta interfering with the cervix.

_____ 15. Pregnancy toxemia resulting in seizures.

HANDOUT 40-6

Student's Name _____

OBSTETRICAL PROBLEMS TRUE OR FALSE

Indicate if the following statements are true or false by writing T or F in the space provided.

_____ 1. Pregnant diabetics should generally be managed with oral drugs.

_____ 2. Women who were borderline hypertensive before becoming pregnant may become dangerously hypertensive when pregnant.

_____ 3. In cases involving abortions, the physical exam should include orthostatic vital signs, if possible.

_____ 4. In cases of ectopic pregnancy, start an IV of D_5W.

_____ 5. Patients suffering abruptio placenta most often report heavy bleeding with no pain.

_____ 6. The definitive treatment for placenta previa is cesarean section.

_____ 7. The most common sign of placenta previa is brownish vaginal discharge.

_____ 8. Eclampsia is characterized by seizures.

_____ 9. Medical control may order the administration of Valium and/or magnesium sulfate to eclampsia patients.

_____ 10. Supine-hypotensive syndrome is most common in the first trimester.

_____ 11. Tocolysis is the recommended procedure in cases of preeclampsia.

_____ 12. Braxton-Hicks contractions are a true medical emergency requiring rapid transport.

_____ 13. The presence of crowning indicates that delivery is imminent.

_____ 14. "Milk" the umbilical cord after delivery to lessen the possibility of vaginal bleeding.

_____ 15. Cephalopelvic disproportion tends to develop most frequently in the primigravida.

_____ 16. It may be necessary to insert a gloved hand into the vagina and use the fingers to form an airway for the infant in cases of breech birth.

_____ 17. With a prolapsed cord, use a dressing moistened with sterile saline to push the cord back.

_____ 18. Pulmonary embolism is one of the most common causes of maternal death.

_____ 19. In cases of postpartum hemorrhage, administer oxygen and begin fundal massage.

_____ 20. In cases of uterine inversion, initiate IVs of NS or LR immediately after pulling the placenta free.

REINFORCEMENT

Chapter 40 Answer Key

Handout 40-2: Chapter 40 Quiz

1. B	9. B	17. C	25. B
2. C	10. C	18. D	26. C
3. C	11. B	19. A	27. C
4. D	12. C	20. C	28. B
5. C	13. B	21. A	29. C
6. A	14. D	22. B	30. C
7. C	15. B	23. A	
8. A	16. B	24. C	

Handout 40-3: Chapter 40 Scenario

1. There is a strong likelihood of an ectopic pregnancy, based on the irregular bleeding, missed period, tender lower right quadrant, and vital sign findings.
2. Acute abdomen and appendicitis are possibilities.
3. What type of birth control protection does she use (IUD)? Were there any previous pelvic infections? Abdominal surgery? Tubal ligations? Any other pregnancy-related symptoms?
4. She should receive high-flow oxygen and an IV of LR or NS, with rapid transport.
5. No. If this is a delivery of a pregnancy, the dates would indicate a nonviable fetus.

Handout 40-4: Chapter 40 Review

1. ovulation
2. placenta
3. umbilical cord, two, one
4. amniotic
5. amniotic sac
6. 40, 280, 9
7. trimesters
8. estimated date, confinement
9. primipara, multipara
10. crowning, imminent
11. 20
12. abortion
13. spontaneous abortion
14. ectopic pregnancy
15. Placenta previa
16. abruptio placentae
17. seizures
18. Supine-hypotensive syndrome
19. effacement
20. tocolysis
21. 10, 5
22. prolapsed cord
23. knee-chest
24. precipitous
25. Meconium staining
26. Postpartum hemorrhage
27. uterine rupture
28. Uterine inversion
29. Amniotic fluid
30. Pulmonary embolism

Handout 40-5: Obstetrical Terminology Matching

1. F	5. N	9. L	13. C
2. J	6. M	10. H	14. I
3. A	7. G	11. B	15. K
4. D	8. E	12. O	

Handout 40-6: Obstetrical Problems True or False

1. F	6. T	11. F	16. T
2. T	7. F	12. F	17. F
3. T	8. T	13. T	18. T
4. F	9. T	14. F	19. T
5. F	10. F	15. T	20. F

Essentials of Paramedic Care

Division 5

Special Considerations/Operations

Chapter 41

Neonatology

INTRODUCTION

Most deliveries in the pre-hospital setting occur without complications. However, emergency deliveries can present a number of challenges to the paramedic. The risk of death or serious neurological injury is much greater when a child is born after a spontaneous, pre-hospital delivery compared to a controlled, in-hospital delivery. Care given in the first few minutes after birth may have a significant impact on future quality of life. A child born in the pre-hospital setting also is more likely to be preterm, increasing the risk of complications. Finally, the presence of two patients—the mother and the newborn—adds to the challenges. This chapter discusses the assessment and management of the normal newborn, resuscitation of distressed neonates, and management of common problems encountered in infants during the first month of their lives.

TOTAL TEACHING TIME: 10.23 HOURS
The total teaching time is only a guideline based on the didactic and practical lab averages in the National Standard Curriculum. Instructors should take into consideration such factors as the pace at which students learn, the size of the class, and breaks. The actual time devoted to teaching objectives is the responsibility of the instructor.

CHAPTER OBJECTIVES

After reading this chapter, you should be able to:

1. Define newborn and neonate. (p. 1555)
2. Identify important antepartum factors that can affect childbirth. (p. 1556)
3. Identify important intrapartum factors that can determine high-risk newborn patients. (p. 1556)
4. Identify the factors that lead to premature birth and low-birth-weight newborns. (pp. 1556, 1573, 1576–1577)
5. Distinguish between primary and secondary apnea. (p. 1557)
6. Discuss pulmonary perfusion and asphyxia. (p. 1557)
7. Identify the primary signs utilized for evaluating a newborn during resuscitation. (pp. 1559–1560)
8. Identify the appropriate use of the APGAR scale. (pp. 1559–1560)
9. Calculate the APGAR score given various newborn situations. (pp. 1559–1560; see also Chapter 40)
10. Formulate an appropriate treatment plan for providing initial care to a newborn. (pp. 1560–1563)
11. Describe the indications, equipment needed, application, and evaluation of the following management techniques for the newborn in distress:
    - Blow-by oxygen (pp. 1565, 1567)
    - Ventilatory assistance (pp. 1565, 1567–1568)
    - Endotracheal intubation (pp. 1564, 1566–1567, 1568)
    - Orogastric tube (p. 1570)
    - Chest compressions (pp. 1570, 1571)
    - Vascular access (pp. 1570, 1571)

©2007 Pearson Education, Inc.
Essentials of Paramedic Care, 2nd ed.

12. Discuss the routes of medication administration for a newborn. (pp. 1570, 1571, 1572)
13. Discuss the signs of hypovolemia in a newborn. (p. 1578)
14. Discuss the initial steps in resuscitation of a newborn. (pp. 1564–1573)
15. Discuss the effects of maternal narcotic usage on the newborn. (p. 1573)
16. Determine the appropriate treatment for the newborn with narcotic depression. (p. 1573)
17. Discuss appropriate transport guidelines for a newborn. (p. 1573)
18. Determine appropriate receiving facilities for low- and high-risk newborns. (p. 1573)
19. Describe the epidemiology, including the incidence, morbidity/mortality, risk factors and prevention strategies, pathophysiology, assessment findings, and management for the following neonatal problems:
    - Meconium aspiration (pp. 1574–1575)
    - Apnea (p. 1575)
    - Diaphragmatic hernia (pp. 1575–1576)
    - Bradycardia (p. 1576)
    - Prematurity (pp. 1576–1577)
    - Respiratory distress/cyanosis (pp. 1577–1578)
    - Seizures (pp. 1578–1579)
    - Fever (p. 1579)
    - Hypothermia (pp. 1579–1580)
    - Hypoglycemia (p. 1580)
    - Vomiting (pp. 1580–1581)
    - Diarrhea (p. 1581)
    - Common birth injuries (pp. 1581–1582)
    - Cardiac arrest (p. 1582)
    - Post-arrest management (p. 1582)
20. Given several neonatal emergencies, provide the appropriate procedures for assessment, management, and transport. (pp. 1555–1582)

FRAMING THE LESSON

Begin with a brief review of the important points from Chapter 40, "Obstetrics." Discuss any material or information that students have not completely understood. Then proceed to the neonatology material in Chapter 41. Stress that though most pre-hospital deliveries occur without complications, in situations where there are problems immediate intervention can make a significant difference in a newborn's survival and future quality of life. Ask the class if anyone would be willing to share experiences they have had with their children or children of friends or relatives having to spend time in a neonatal intensive care unit. Ask the students to describe how they think they might feel in this situation.

TEACHING STRATEGIES

People learn in a variety of ways. Some do better with the spoken word, whereas others prefer the written. Some prefer to work alone, whereas others profit from working in groups. Recognizing these different ways of acquiring knowledge, the authors of this *Instructor's Resource Manual* have provided a variety of teaching strategies for the different types of learners. These strategies are intended to foster higher-level cognitive skills and encourage creative learning and problem solving. For greatest effectiveness, incorporate these strategies into

your class lecture. Symbols in the Lecture Outline indicate the points at which various exercises might be most appropriate. Other strategies can be used to preview the lesson or to summarize it.

The following strategies are keyed to specific sections of the lesson.

1. *In-the-Field Deliveries.* Delivering a baby in the field is both frightening and exciting. Add meaning and interest to this lecture by inviting paramedics who have had the privilege of delivering a baby to speak to your class. Ask them to share their experiences, challenges, and feelings. If you cannot get them to come to class, at least interview these folks and videotape, audiotape, or write down what they have to share. This activity is not only interesting but also covers objectives in the affective domain.

2. *Identifying Risk Factors.* Help students identify risk factors for delivery complications by placing the conditions in Table 41-1 and others discussed in the text on index cards. Have them sort by antepartum, intrapartum, and non-risk factors for newborn complications. The students can do this in groups and compare piles when they are finished. Ask groups to justify or defend their decisions if any piles are different than the other groups' piles. This activity promotes critical thinking by forcing students to discuss or defend their choices for placement of the cards. Additionally, students practice oral communication skills, cooperative learning skills, and acceptance of opinions and decisions different than their own.

3. *NICU Field Trip.* Neonatal resuscitation seems overwhelming because students often lack experience with this type of patient, situation, and even equipment. Improve the students' ability and desire to care for neonates by ensuring that they are very comfortable with the equipment involved in neonatal resuscitation. A field trip to the NICU or invitation for the neonatal transport team to visit your class would be beneficial here. Have the special care nursery staff cover the equipment used, noting the tiny sizes and differences in concentrations of medications and the like. This activity gets students out of the traditional classroom environment, provides a preview to the clinical experience, and can improve relations with the nursery staff and transport nurses whom your students will likely work with as practicing professionals.

4. *Realistic Neonate Mannequin.* When practicing childbirth in class and lab situations, coat the neonate mannequin in realistic material like K-Y jelly mixed with powdered blood. Delivering a baby for the first time is often challenging because paramedics have never felt how slippery a newborn is and are surprised by the mess of fluids and blood. Give your students this experience in the classroom to improve their performance during the real thing. Adding realism to scenarios is a key element of problem-based learning.

5. *Practice Determining APGAR.* Use neonatal resuscitation case studies either in class as overheads, as a PowerPoint® presentation, or as a written assignment. Students need a great deal of practice determining APGAR scores and using the inverted triangle. Because this information is new and foreign, the amount of time available in classroom labs and simulations is not enough to reach mastery level, and this information will likely always seem frightening to your students. Give them the extra preparation needed by assigning case studies first, reinforcing with laboratory simulations, and, when possible, following up with clinical time in the NICU or with the neonatal transport team.

6. *Mnemonic Memory Aid.* Students often forget which should be suctioned first, the mouth or nose of a newborn. Help them remember to do this in alphabetical order: mouth first, then nose. Infants are obligate nose breathers, so as soon as the nostrils are stimulated, they will inhale everything in the upper airway, which includes the mouth and nose. Therefore, it is important to clear the mouth of any fluid or obstructions.

7. *Resuscitation Reference Card*. Make a pocket card of the resuscitation information in Table 41-4. Allow use of the reference card in simulations and classroom case studies. Following the American Heart Association's approach to PALS, encourage familiarity and understanding of equipment, drugs, and procedures rather than simple memorization. This improves the comfort level of most students and therefore their ability to learn.

The following strategies can be used at various points throughout the lesson or to help summarize and demonstrate what students have learned.

Guest Speaker. Consider inviting a neonatologist from the local or regional hospital to the class.

Clinical Rotations. During labor and delivery rotations, encourage students to seek out opportunities to observe the management of patients with high-risk pregnancies. Students should observe and, if possible, assist with the management of distressed newborns in the delivery room. If possible, students should do clinical rotations in a neonatal intensive care unit.

Cultural Considerations, Legal Notes, and Patho Pearls. The Student CD-ROM contains this series of informative features to enhance the student's understanding of the material covered in this chapter.

TEACHING OUTLINE

Chapter 41 is the first lesson in Division 5, *Special Considerations/Operations*. Distribute Handout 41-1 so that students can familiarize themselves with the learning goals for this chapter. If students have any questions about the objectives, answer them at this time.

Then present the chapter. One possible lecture outline follow. In the outline, the parenthetical references in regular type are references to text pages; those in bold type are references to figures, tables, or procedures.

I. Introduction. This chapter concerns itself with babies 1 month old or younger. (pp. 1555–1556)

  A. Definitions (p. 1555)
      1. Neonate
          a. Infant from birth to 1 month of age
      2. Newborn
          a. Baby in the first few hours of life (**Fig. 41-1, p. 1556**)
      3. Newborns also called *newly born infants*
  B. Considerations in unscheduled field deliveries (p. 1555)
      1. Two patients: mother and infant
      2. Care of mother was discussed in the obstetrics module.

II. General pathophysiology, assessment, and management (pp. 1556–1563)

  A. Epidemiology (p. 1556)
      1. Risk of complications
          a. Approximately 6 percent of field deliveries require life support.
          b. About 80 percent of newborns weighing less than 1,500 grams (3 pounds, 5 ounces) at birth require resuscitation.

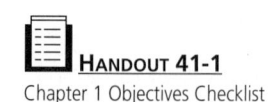

HANDOUT 41-1
Chapter 1 Objectives Checklist

TEACHING STRATEGY 1
In-the-Field Deliveries

POWERPOINT PRESENTATION
Chapter 41 PowerPoint slides 4–5

POINT TO EMPHASIZE
For newborns who require additional care, your quick actions can make the difference between life and death.

TEACHING STRATEGY 2
Identifying Risk Factors

POWERPOINT PRESENTATION
Chapter 41 PowerPoint slides 6–27

TEACHING STRATEGY 3
NICU Field Trip

2. Risk factors (Table 41-1, p. 1556)
    a. Antepartum factors
        i. Multiple gestation
        ii. Inadequate prenatal care
        iii. Mother's age <16 or >35
        iv. History of perinatal morbidity or mortality
        v. Postterm gestation
        vi. Drugs/medications
        vii. Toxemia, hypertension, diabetes
    b. Intrapartum factors
        i. Premature labor
        ii. Meconium-stained amniotic fluid
        iii. Rupture of membranes greater than 24 hours prior to delivery
        iv. Use of narcotics within 4 hours of delivery
        v. Abnormal presentation
        vi. Prolonged labor or precipitous delivery
        vii. Prolapsed cord
        viii. Bleeding
3. Factors affecting successful resuscitation
    a. Training
    b. Practice
    c. Proper equipment
4. Transport considerations

B. Pathophysiology (pp. 1557–1559)
    1. Dramatic changes at birth prepare newborn for extrauterine life.
    2. Respiratory system must initiate, maintain oxygenation. (Fig. 41-2, p. 1558)
    3. Transition from fetal to neonatal circulation
        a. Closure of foramen ovale between right and left atria
        b. Closure of ductus arteriosus between pulmonary artery and aorta, forming the ligamentum arteriosum
        c. Diversion of blood flow to lungs
    4. Remain alert to signs of respiratory distress.
    5. Congenital anomalies
        a. May affect a single organ/structure or many organs/structures
        b. Recognized patterns or syndromes
        c. A few make resuscitation more difficult
        d. Causes are largely unknown
        e. Patent ductus arteriosus (also called a persistent ductus arteriosus)
            i. Ductus arteriosus fails to close
            ii. Increases pulmonary blood flow
        f. Septal defects
            i. Hole in the wall between the atria or the ventricles
            ii. Increases pulmonary blood flow
            iii. Atrial septal defect
                a) Hole between the two atria
            iv. Ventricular septal defect
                a) Hole between the two ventricles
        g. Tetralogy of Fallot
            i. Is a combination of four congenital conditions
            ii. Decreases pulmonary blood flow
        h. Transposition of the great vessels
            i. Normal outflow tracts of the right and left ventricles are switched
            ii. Decreases pulmonary blood flow

POINT TO EMPHASIZE
Your success in treating at-risk newborns increases with training, ongoing practice, and proper stocking of equipment on board the ambulance.

READING/REFERENCE
Jaimovich, D. G., and D. Vidyasagar. *Handbook of Pediatric and Neonatal Transport Medicine*, 2nd ed. Philadelphia, PA: Hanley & Belfus, Inc., 2002.

POINT TO EMPHASIZE
Upon birth, dramatic changes take place within the newborn to prepare it for extrauterine life.

POINT TO EMPHASIZE
The time of a newborn's first breath is unrelated to the cutting of the umbilical cord.

POINT TO EMPHASIZE
Newborns may have congenital anomalies that make resuscitation more difficult.

POINT TO EMPHASIZE
Always assume that apnea in the newborn is secondary apnea and rapidly treat it with ventilatory assistance.

i. Coarctation of the aorta
  i. Narrowing in the arch of the aorta
  ii. Obstructs blood flow
j. Aortic or mitral stenosis
  i. Problems with either the mitral or the aortic valve
  ii. Can cause blood flow obstruction
k. Hypoplastic left heart syndrome
  i. The left side of the heart is underdeveloped.
  ii. Usually fatal by 1 month of age if untreated
l. Diaphragmatic hernia
  i. Defect that allows some of the abdominal contents to enter the chest cavity
  ii. If you suspect a diaphragmatic hernia, do not treat the infant with bag-valve-mask ventilation.
    a) Bag-valve-mask or other positive-pressure ventilation will cause the stomach to distend and protrude into the chest cavity, thus decreasing ventilation capacity.
    b) Immediately intubate the infant.
m. Meningomyelocele
  i. Defect in the area of the spine
  ii. In some cases, spinal canal contents may protrude.
  iii. Place infant in prone or laterally recumbent position and cover spinal defect with sterile gauze pads soaked in warm sterile saline and covered with an occlusive dressing.
n. Omphalocele
  i. Defect in the area of the umbilicus
  ii. In some cases, the abdominal contents will fill this defect.
  iii. If you encounter a newborn with an omphalocele, cover the defect with an occlusive dressing.
o. Choanal atresia
  i. Most common birth defect involving the nose
  ii. Presence of a bony or membranous septum between the nasal cavity and the pharynx
  iii. Suspect this condition if you are unable to pass a catheter through either nare into the oropharynx.
  iv. An oral airway will usually bypass the obstruction.
p. Cleft palate
  i. Fairly common congenital anomaly
  ii. Failure of the palate to completely close during fetal development
  iii. Requires endotracheal intubation if prolonged ventilation needed
q. Cleft lip
  i. Failure of the upper lip to close
  ii. Requires endotracheal intubation if prolonged ventilation is needed
r. Pierre Robin syndrome
  i. Small jaw and large tongue in conjunction with a cleft palate
  ii. Use nasal or oral airway to bypass obstruction; if bypass is unsuccessful, endotracheal intubation may be necessary.

C. Assessment (pp. 1556–1560)
  1. General considerations
    a. Note time of birth.
    b. Remember that newborns are slippery.
    c. Someone needs to be caring for and watching the mother.
  2. Respirations
    a. Should be 40 to 60 per minute
    b. Ventilate if inadequate.

■ **TEACHING STRATEGY 4**
Realistic Neonate Mannequin

3. Heart rate
    a. Should be 150 to 180 per minute at birth, soon slowing to 130 to 140
    b. Less than 100 requires emergency intervention.
4. Skin color
    a. Cyanosis of extremities is common immediately after birth, but central cyanosis or persistent peripheral cyanosis is abnormal.
    b. Give 100 percent oxygen until cause determined or condition corrected.
5. The APGAR Scale (**Table 41-2, p. 1560**)
    a. Appearance (skin color)
        i. Completely pink—2
        ii. Body pink, extremities blue—1
        iii. Blue, pale—0
    b. Pulse rate
        i. Above 100—2
        ii. Below 100—1
        iii. Absent—0
    c. Grimace (irritability)
        i. Cries—2
        ii. Grimaces—1
        iii. No response—0
    d. Activity (muscle tone)
        i. Active motion—2
        ii. Some flexion of extremities—1
        iii. Limp—0
    e. Respiratory effort
        i. Strong cry—2
        ii. Slow and irregular—1
        iii. Absent—0
    f. Significance of scores
        i. 7–10
            a) Active
            b) Vigorous newborn requiring only routine care
        ii. 4–6
            a) Moderately distressed newborn requiring oxygenation and ventilation
        iii. 0–4
            a) Severely distressed newborn requiring immediate resuscitation
        iv. If infant not breathing or otherwise obviously distressed, do not delay resuscitation to obtain APGAR scores.
D. Treatment (pp. 1560–1563)
    1. Establishing the airway (**Fig. 41-3, p. 1561**)
        a. One of the most critical steps in newborn care
        b. As soon as the head delivers, suction mouth then nose so there is nothing to aspirate if infant gasps when nose is suctioned.
        c. After delivery, position infant at level of vagina with head 15 degrees below torso.
        d. If large amount of secretions present, use DeLee suction trap attached to suction source.
    2. Breathing
        a. Stimulate by drying and suctioning.
        b. If additional stimulation needed, flick the soles of feet or rub the infant's back. (**Fig. 41-4, p. 1562**)

TEACHING STRATEGY 5
Practice Determining APGAR

POINT TO EMPHASIZE
If a newborn is not breathing, DO NOT withhold resuscitation to determine the APGAR score.

POINT TO EMPHASIZE
Severely distressed newborns, those with APGAR scores of less than 4, require immediate resuscitation.

TEACHING STRATEGY 6
Mnemonic Memory Aid

POINT TO EMPHASIZE
Airway management is one of the most critical steps in caring for the newborn.

POINT TO EMPHASIZE
Always suction the mouth first so that there is nothing for the infant to aspirate if he or she gasps when the nose is suctioned.

POINT TO EMPHASIZE
If the newborn does not cry immediately, stimulate it by gently rubbing its back or flicking the soles of its feet. Do not spank or vigorously rub a newborn baby.

POINT TO EMPHASIZE
Cold infants quickly become distressed infants.

POINT TO EMPHASIZE
Do not "milk" or strip the umbilical cord.

POINT TO EMPHASIZE
Of the vital signs, fetal heart rate is the most important indicator of neonatal distress.

TEACHING TIP
Problems caused by overextension and underextension of the neck can be illustrated with plastic soda straws simulating the flexible neonatal trachea. Students can see how over- or underextension of a small, flexible tube can result in obstruction and decrease air entry.

POWERPOINT PRESENTATION
Chapter 41 PowerPoint slides 28–62

POINT TO EMPHASIZE
Suctioning of the newborn should take no longer than 10 seconds.

POINT TO EMPHASIZE
Never deprive a newborn of oxygen in the prehospital setting for fear of oxygen toxicity.

---

   c. Do NOT vigorously rub newborn.
   d. Do NOT slap newborn on buttocks.
 3. Prevention of heat loss
   a. Cold infants quickly become distressed infants.
   b. Heat loss
      i. Evaporation
      ii. Convection
      iii. Conduction
      iv. Radiation
   c. To prevent heat loss (**Fig. 41-5, p. 1562**)
      i. Dry the infant.
      ii. Maintain ambient temperature at 23 to 24°C (74 to 76°F).
      iii. Close all windows and doors.
      iv. Swaddle infant in warm, dry receiving blanket or other suitable material.
      v. Cover infant's head.
      vi. Place well-insulated containers of warm water (40°C/104°F) around (but not against) infant.
 4. Cutting the umbilical cord
   a. After airway is stabilized and heat loss minimized
   b. Maintain infant at same level as vagina to prevent under- or overtransfusion.
   c. Do not "milk" or strip the cord.
      i. Causes polycythemia and increased blood viscosity
      ii. Polycythemia can lead to excess red cell destruction and to hyperbilirubinemia.
   d. Clamp cord within 30 to 45 seconds of birth.
   e. Place first clamp about 10 cm (4 inches) from newborn.
   f. Place second clamp about 4 cm (2 inches) away from first.
   g. Cut cord between clamps.
   h. Inspect cord periodically for additional bleeding.

III. The distressed newborn (pp. 1563–1573)

A. Resuscitation (pp. 1563–1564) (**Proc. 41-1, p. 1565**)
 1. The vast majority of newborns require no resuscitation beyond stimulation, airway maintenance, and body temperature maintenance.
 2. Predicting which newborns will require resuscitation is difficult.
 3. Neonatal resuscitation kit should be available in unit.
B. Inverted pyramid for resuscitation (pp. 1564–1572) (**Fig. 41-6, p. 1564; Fig. 41-7, p. 1566**)
 1. Drying, warming, positioning, suctioning, tactile stimulation
   a. Dry newborn to minimize heat loss.
   b. Place in warm, dry blanket.
   c. Position on back with head slightly lower than body, neck slightly extended. (**Fig. 41-8, p. 1567**)
   d. Place small blanket folded to 2 cm (3/4 inch) thickness under shoulders.
   e. Suction using bulb syringe or DeLee suction trap.
   f. Stimulate by flicking soles of feet or rubbing the infant's back.
   g. Assess the infant.
 2. Supplemental oxygen
   a. For central cyanosis or inadequate ventilation, give warmed, humidified supplemental oxygen by blow-by. (**Fig. 41-9, p. 1569**)
   b. Continue oxygen until color has improved.

952 ESSENTIALS OF PARAMEDIC CARE

c. Blow-by oxygen in the prehospital setting will NOT cause oxygen toxicity.
3. Ventilation
   a. Begin positive-pressure ventilation if:
      i. Heart rate is less than 100 beats per minute.
      ii. Apnea is present.
      iii. Central cyanosis is present after oxygen is given.
   b. Ventilate at rate of 40–60 breaths per minute.
   c. Use bag-valve-mask.
   d. Endotracheal intubation (**Proc. 41-2, p. 1568**)
      i. Intubate if:
         a) Bag-valve-mask unit does not work.
         b) Tracheal suctioning is required.
         c) Prolonged ventilation will be required.
         d) Diaphragmatic hernia is suspected.
         e) Inadequate respiratory effort is found.
      ii. Use uncuffed endotracheal tubes because of narrowness of airway at cricoid ring.
4. Chest compressions (**Fig. 41-10, p. 1571**)
   a. Begin chest compressions if the heart rate is
      i. Less than 60 beats per minute, or
      ii. Between 60 and 80 beats per minute and does not increase with 30 seconds of oxygenation and ventilation.
   b. Compress sternum 1.5–2.0 cm (1/2 to 1/3 inch) at 120 compressions per minute.
   c. Ventilate in a ratio of 3 compressions to 1 ventilation.
   d. Reassess after 20 cycles of compressions and ventilations or at about 1 minute.
   e. Stop compressions when heart rate exceeds 80 per minute.
5. Medications and fluids (**Table 41-3, p. 1572**)
   a. Most newborn cardiopulmonary arrests result from hypoxia and respond to oxygenation and ventilation.
   b. Vascular access is most readily obtained through the umbilical vein. (**Fig. 41-11, p. 1571**)
   c. If umbilical vein catheter cannot be placed, lidocaine, atropine, naloxone, and epinephrine can be given via the endotracheal tube.
   d. Other options for vascular access include peripheral veins or the intraosseous route.
   e. Fluid therapy should consist of 10 mL/kg of saline or lactated Ringer's solution as a slow IV push.
C. Maternal narcotic use (p.1573)
   1. Naloxone is treatment of choice for respiratory depression caused by maternal narcotic use within 4 hours of delivery.
   2. Naloxone may induce withdrawal reactions in infants born to narcotic-addicted mothers.
D. Neonatal transport (**p. 1573**) (**Fig. 41-12, p. 1573**)
   1. Neonatal intensive care unit (NICU)

IV. **Specific neonatal situations** (pp. 1574–1582)

A. Meconium-stained amniotic fluid (pp. 1574–1575)
   1. Meconium is dark green substance found in digestive tract of full-term newborns indicative of fetal distress.
   2. Hypoxia can cause meconium to be passed into amniotic fluid.
   3. Presence of thick, particulate (pea-soup) meconium requires suctioning of lower airway BEFORE infant is stimulated to breathe. (**Fig. 41-13, p. 1574**)

TEACHING TIP
Students frequently have difficulty understanding why they do chest compressions on bradycardia infants and small children with pulses, but not on adults. Explain the underlying physiology by reviewing the fact that cardiac output equals heart rate times stroke volume. As hearts become smaller they are less able to vary their stroke volume to compensate for a decreased rate. In infants and small children, cardiac output becomes almost entirely rate-dependent. Therefore, chest compressions become necessary to support cardiac output in the presence of a slow heart rate.

POINT TO EMPHASIZE
In an infant, vascular access for the administration of fluids and drugs can most readily be managed by using the umbilical vein.

POINT TO EMPHASIZE
Keep in mind that naloxone may induce a withdrawal reaction in an infant born to a narcotic-addicted mother.

POINT TO EMPHASIZE
Do not discuss "chances of survival" with a newborn's family or caregivers.

TEACHING TIP
Communication with family members is important during care of neonates. However, paramedics (and other health care providers) frequently have trouble explaining disease processes and their management to laypeople. Try having your students develop verbal or written explanations of disease processes or treatments that a person without specialized training can understand.

POWERPOINT PRESENTATION
Chapter 41 PowerPoint slides 63–94

POINT TO EMPHASIZE
Do not use narcotic antagonists if the mother is a drug abuser.

B. Apnea (p. 1575)
  1. Absence of spontaneous ventilation with stimulation or respiratory pauses of greater than 20 seconds
  2. Assessment findings
     a. Failure to breathe spontaneously after stimulation
     b. Respiratory pauses greater than 20 seconds
  3. Management
     a. Stimulate baby by flicking soles of feet or rubbing back.
     b. Ventilate with BVM.
     c. Suction as needed.
     d. Intubate if apnea is prolonged or heart rate is less than 60 with adequate ventilation and chest compressions.
     e. Gain circulatory access.
     f. Monitor heart rate continuously.
     g. If apnea is due to narcotics given in previous 4 hours, consider naloxone.
     h. Prevent hypothermia.

C. Diaphragmatic hernia (pp. 1575–1576)
  1. Abdominal contents displaced into thorax to varying degrees
  2. Can make the lung on affected side compressed and may displace the heart
  3. Assessment findings
     a. Little to severe distress
     b. Dyspnea and cyanosis unresponsive to ventilations
     c. Scaphoid (flat) abdomen
     d. Bowel sounds heard in chest
     e. Heart sounds displaced to right
  4. Management
     a. Position infant with head and thorax higher than abdomen and feet. (Fig. 41-14, p. 1576)
     b. Place nasogastric tube and apply low, intermittent suction.
     c. Do NOT use bag-valve-mask.
     d. Endotracheal intubation may be necessary.
     e. Explain need for possible surgery to parents.

D. Bradycardia (p. 1576)
  1. Management
     a. Follow procedures in inverted pyramid.
     b. Avoid temptation to treat with pharmacological measures alone.
     c. Avoid prolonged suctioning or airway instrumentation.
     d. Keep newborn warm.

E. Prematurity (pp. 1576–1577) (Fig. 41-15, p. 1577)
  1. Epidemiology
     a. Born before 37 weeks gestation or with weight from 0.6 to 2.2 kg (1 pound, 5 ounces to 4 pounds, 13 ounces)
     b. Healthy premature infants weighing greater than 1,700 g (3 pounds, 12 ounces) have survivability and outcomes approximating those of full-term infants.
     c. Mortality decreases weekly with gestation beyond the onset of viability (currently around 23–24 weeks of gestation).
  2. Assessment findings
     a. Degree of immaturity determines the physical characteristics.
     b. Larger head relative to body size
     c. Generally a large trunk and short extremities
     d. Skin transparent with fewer wrinkles
     e. Less subcutaneous fat

POINT TO EMPHASIZE
If you suspect a diaphragmatic hernia, do not use bag-valve-mask ventilation, which can worsen the condition by causing gastric distension.

POINT TO EMPHASIZE
When administering treatment to a newborn, resist the temptation to treat bradycardia with pharmacological measures alone.

POINT TO EMPHASIZE
Prematurity should not be a factor in short-term management. Resuscitation should be attempted if there is any sign of life.

3. Management
    a. Attempt resuscitation if the infant has any sign of life.
    b. Follow same procedures as those for newborns of normal maturity and weight.
    c. Maintain patent airway.
    d. Avoid potential aspiration of gastric contents.
    e. Consider use of epinephrine.
    f. Maintain body temperature.
    g. Transport to facility with services for low-birth-weight newborns.
F. Respiratory distress/cyanosis (pp. 1577–1578)
  1. Prematurity is the single most common determining factor.
  2. Assessment findings
      a. Tachypnea
      b. Paradoxical breathing
      c. Periodic breathing
      d. Intercostal retractions
      e. Nasal flaring
      f. Expiratory grunt
  3. Management
      a. Follow inverted pyramid of treatment, paying particular attention to airway and ventilation.
      b. Suction as needed.
      c. Provide high concentration of oxygen.
      d. Ventilate as needed with bag-valve-mask.
      e. Consider endotracheal intubation if prolonged ventilation needed.
      f. Perform chest compressions if indicated.
      g. Sodium bicarbonate may be helpful in prolonged resuscitation.
      h. Consider dextrose if newborn is hypoglycemic.
      i. Maintain body temperature.
G. Hypovolemia (p. 1578)
  1. Leading cause of shock in newborns: causes include dehydration, hemorrhage, third-spacing of fluids.
  2. Assessment findings
      a. Pale color
      b. Cool skin
      c. Diminished peripheral pulses
      d. Delayed capillary refill, despite normal ambient temperature
      e. Mental status changes
      f. Diminished urination (oliguria)
  3. Management
      a. Provide fluid bolus resuscitation with isotonic crystalloid (LR or NS).
      b. Give 10 mL/kg over 5 to 10 minutes.
      c. Assess response.
      d. If signs of shock continue, give second bolus.
      e. Hypovolemic infants may require 40 to 60 mL/kg in first hour.
H. Seizures (pp. 1578–1579)
  1. Occur in a very small percentage of all newborns, but represent relative medical emergencies as they are usually a sign of an underlying abnormality
  2. Prolonged and frequent multiple seizures may result in metabolic changes and cardiopulmonary difficulties.
  3. Pathophysiology
      a. Generalized tonic-clonic convulsions normally do not occur in first month of life.

POINT TO EMPHASIZE

In treating hypovolemia in a newborn, do not use solutions containing dextrose, as they can produce hypokalemia or worsen ischemic brain injury.

b. Subtle seizure
  i. Chewing motions
  ii. Excessive salivation
  iii. Blinking
  iv. Sucking
  v. Swimming movements of arms
  vi. Pedaling movements of legs
  vii. Apnea
  viii. Color changes
c. Tonic seizure
  i. Rigid posturing of extremities and trunk
  ii. Sometimes fixed deviation of eyes
  iii. More common in premature infants, especially in those with intraventricular hemorrhage
d. Focal clonic seizure
  i. Rhythmic twitching of muscle groups, particularly extremities and face
  ii. Occur in both full-term and premature infants
e. Multifocal seizure
  i. Similar to focal clonic seizures
  ii. Involves multiple muscle groups
  iii. Randomly migrates to another area of the body
  iv. Occurs primarily in full-term infants
f. Myoclonic seizure
  i. Brief jerks of the upper or lower extremities
  ii. May occur singly or in a series of repetitive jerks

4. Assessment findings
  a. Decreased level of consciousness
  b. Seizure activity
5. Management considerations
  a. Manage airway and ventilation.
  b. Maintain oxygen saturation.
  c. Consider $D_{10}W$ for hypoglycemia.
  d. Consider benzodiazepine (lorazepam) for status epilepticus.
  e. Maintain normal body temperature.

I. Fever (p. 1579)
  1. Epidemiology
    a. Average normal newborn's temperature is 99.5°F (37.5°C).
    b. Rectal temperature greater than 100.4°F (38.0°C) is considered fever.
    c. Neonates do not develop fever as easily as older children.
    d. Fever in neonate may indicate life-threatening condition, requires extensive evaluation.
    e. Any neonate with fever should be considered to have meningitis until proven otherwise.
  2. Assessment findings
    a. Mental status changes (irritability/somnolence)
    b. Decreased intake
    c. Caretaker history
    d. Feels warm
    e. Observe patient for rashes, petechiae.
    f. Term newborns will produce beads of sweat on their brow but not over the rest of their body.
    g. Premature infants will have no visible sweat.
  3. Management
    a. Assure adequate oxygenation and ventilation.
    b. Avoid use of cold packs.

POINT TO EMPHASIZE
Any neonate with a fever should be considered to have meningitis until proven otherwise.

POINT TO EMPHASIZE
In assessing a neonate with a fever, remember that infants have a limited ability to control their body temperature. As a result, fever can be a serious condition.

       c. Perform chest compressions if bradycardia develops.
       d. Administration of antipyretic agent is questionable in the prehospital setting.
  J. Hypothermia (pp. 1579–1580)
     1. Pathophysiology
        a. Increased surface-to-volume ratio makes newborns extremely sensitive to environmental conditions, especially when they are wet after delivery.
        b. Hypothermia can be an indicator of sepsis in the neonate.
        c. Increased metabolic demand can cause metabolic acidosis, pulmonary hypertension, and hypoxemia.
     2. Assessment findings
        a. Pale color
        b. Cool to touch, particularly in extremities
        c. Acrocyanosis
        d. Respiratory distress
        e. Apnea
        f. Bradycardia
        g. Central cyanosis
        h. Initial irritability
        i. Lethargy in later stage
        j. Generally do not shiver
     3. Management
        a. Assure adequate oxygenation and ventilation.
        b. Perform chest compressions if indicated.
        c. Warm IV fluids via IV fluid warmer.
        d. Administer $D_{10}W$ or $D_{25}W$ if hypoglycemic.
        e. Environmental conditions should be 24 to 26.5°C (75.2 to 78.8°F).
        f. Warm hands before touching patient.
  K. Hypoglycemia (p. 1580)
     1. Epidemiology
        a. Newborns are the only age group that can develop severe hypoglycemia without having diabetes mellitus.
        b. May be due to inadequate glucose intake or increased utilization of glucose
        c. Persistent low blood glucose levels may have catastrophic effects on the brain.
     2. Pathophysiology
        a. Glycogen stores are sufficient to meet glucose requirements for 8 to 12 hours.
        b. Time frame is decreased in infants with decreased glycogen stores or with problems that increase glucose utilization.
        c. Body responds to hypoglycemia by releasing counterregulatory hormones including glucagon, epinephrine, cortisol, and growth hormone.
        d. Hormones may cause symptoms of hyperglycemia that last for several hours.
        e. Blood glucose concentration should be determined on all sick infants.
        f. A blood glucose screening test below 45 mg/dL indicates hypoglycemia.
     3. Assessment findings
        a. Twitching or seizures
        b. Limpness
        c. Lethargy

POINT TO EMPHASIZE
Remember to warm your hands before touching a neonate.

POINT TO EMPHASIZE
Because hypoglycemia can have a catastrophic effect on a neonate's brain, you should determine the blood sugar on all sick infants.

    d. Eye-rolling
    e. High-pitched cry
    f. Apnea
    g. Irregular respirations
    h. Possible cyanosis
   4. Management
    a. Assure adequate oxygenation and ventilation.
    b. Perform chest compressions if indicated.
    c. Administer dextrose ($D_{10}W$ or $D_{25}W$).
    d. Maintain normal body temperature.
 L. Vomiting (pp. 1580–1581)
   1. Epidemiology
    a. Vomiting mucus, occasionally blood-streaked, in the first few hours of life is not uncommon.
    b. Persistent vomiting is a warning sign.
    c. Vomiting in the first 24 hours of life suggests obstruction in the upper digestive tract or increased intracranial pressure.
    d. Vomitus containing dark blood is usually a sign of a life-threatening illness.
    e. Aspiration of vomitus can cause respiratory insufficiencies or obstruction of the airway.
   2. Assessment findings
    a. Distended stomach
    b. Infection
    c. Increased ICP
    d. Drug withdrawal
   3. Management considerations
    a. Maintain a patent airway.
    b. Suction/clear vomitus from airway.
    c. Assure adequate oxygenation.
    d. Fluid administration may be required.
    e. Bradycardia may be caused by vagal stimulus of vomiting.
 M. Diarrhea (p. 1581)
   1. Five to six stools per day is normal, especially if infant is breast-feeding, but severe diarrhea can cause dehydration and electrolyte imbalance.
   2. Causes
    a. Bacterial or viral infections
    b. Gastroenteritis
    c. Lactose intolerance
    d. Phototherapy
    e. Neonatal abstinence syndrome
    f. Thyrotoxicosis
    g. Cystic fibrosis
   3. Assessment findings
    a. Loose stools
    b. Decreased urinary output
    c. Signs of dehydration
   4. Management
    a. Take proper BSI precautions.
    b. Assure adequate oxygenation and ventilation.
    c. Perform chest compressions if indicated.
    d. Fluid therapy may be indicated.
 N. Common birth injuries (pp. 1581–1582)
   1. Avoidable and unavoidable mechanical and anoxic trauma incurred by the infant during labor and delivery

POINT TO EMPHASIZE

In treating distressed neonates who have birth injuries or other critical conditions, provide professional and compassionate communication to the parents or caregivers.

2. Pathophysiology
   a. Cranial injuries
   b. Intracranial hemorrhage
   c. Spine and spinal cord injury from strong traction exerted when the spine is hyperextended or pull is lateral
   d. Peripheral nerve injury
   e. Liver injury
   f. Rupture of spleen
   g. Adrenal hemorrhage
   h. Clavicle and extremity fractures
   i. Hypoxia-ischemia
3. Assessment findings
   a. Diffuse, sometimes ecchymotic, edematous swelling of the soft tissues of the scalp
   b. Paralysis below the level of spinal cord injury
   c. Paralysis of the upper arm with or without paralysis of the forearm
   d. Diaphragmatic paralysis
   e. Movement on only one side of the face when newborn cries
   f. Inability to move arm freely on side of fractured clavicle
   g. Lack of spontaneous movement of the affected extremity
   h. Hypoxia
   i. Shock
4. Management
   a. Assure adequate oxygenation and ventilation.
   b. Perform chest compressions if indicated.
   c. Transport to facility capable of providing specialized care.
   d. Provide professional, compassionate communication to parents or caregivers.

O. Cardiac resuscitation, postresuscitation, and stabilization (p. 1582)
   1. Risk factors
      a. Bradycardia
      b. Intrauterine asphyxia
      c. Prematurity
      d. Drugs administered to or taken by the mother
      e. Congenital neuromuscular diseases
      f. Congenital malformations
      g. Intrapartum hypoxemia
   2. Pathophysiology
      a. Primary apnea
      b. Secondary apnea
      c. Bradycardia
      d. Persistent fetal circulation
      e. Pulmonary hypertension
   3. Assessment findings
      a. Peripheral cyanosis
      b. Inadequate respiratory effort
      c. Ineffective or absent heart rate
   4. Management
      a. Follow inverted pyramid.
      b. Consult medical direction and follow its instructions.
      c. Maintain normal body temperature.

V. **Chapter summary** (p. 1583). After a woman gives birth, you must care for two patients—the mother and her newborn child. The newborn has several special needs, the most important of which are protection of the

TEACHING TIP

Because caring for a sick neonate includes communicating with and supporting the parents or other caregivers, patient-care simulations should include "parent" role players. Students should be expected to communicate with the "parents" appropriately during the role play.

TEACHING STRATEGY 7

Resuscitation Reference Card

POWERPOINT PRESENTATION

Chapter 41 PowerPoint slide 95

airway and support of ventilations. The newborn must be kept warm at all times. If assessment reveals a distressed newborn, you should initiate ventilatory support, stimulation, and, if required, CPR. If possible, newborns should be transported to a facility with an NICU. Maintain communications with family members or caregivers, explaining all procedures performed on the newborn.

SKILLS DEMONSTRATION AND PRACTICE

Students can practice skills discussed in this chapter in the following Skills Lab activities.

Skills Lab: Provide students with Handouts 41-5 and 41-6. Demonstrate umbilical vein catheterization and infant resuscitation techniques. Note the following key points:

- The majority of newborns can be resuscitated with drying, warming, positioning, suctioning, and stimulating.
- Bradycardia in a newborn is a result of hypoxia.
- Drug therapy is rarely needed in the resuscitation of the newborn.
- Hypothermia in the newborn must be avoided by rapid drying and warming.
- Meconium aspiration is a potentially lethal complication of delivery. Particulate meconium must be suctioned from the oro-/nasopharynx and from the trachea before the baby takes its first breath.

After your demonstration, have students circulate through the stations, making sure that each station is equipped as detailed in the following tests. Monitor the students to be sure each has a chance to practice each of the skills. You may wish to have other instructors or qualified paramedics assist in these activities.

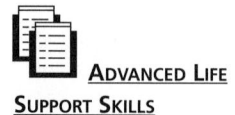

Station	Equipment and Personnel Needed	Activities
Umbilical Vein Catheterization	Disposable gloves, latex and nonlatex Protective eyewear Umbilical cords, kept in sterile saline Baby bottles, 4 oz Nipples Umbilical catheter, 5 French Syringe, 10 mL Umbilical tape Gauze Saline Red food coloring Scalpel blade, #10 1 instructor	Have students cannulate the umbilical vein of a newborn, following the steps in Handout 41-5. Ensure that all participants wear goggles and protective eyewear during this procedure.
Resuscitation of the Normal Newborn	Infant mannequin Infant intubation mannequin Bulb syringe DeLee suction trap Meconium aspirator Endotracheal tubes: 2.5, 3.0, and 3.5	Have students practice resuscitating a normal newborn as described in Handout 41-6, Scenario One. Choose a team leader or allow students to self-select their roles. Follow an interactive format by presenting the initial scenario, and then provide

Station	Equipment and Personnel Needed	Activities
	Suction catheters: 5, 6, and 8 French 20-ml syringe and 8 French feeding tube for gastric suction	additional historical and physical exam information in response to participants' questions.
	Towels Cord clamp Sterile scissors or Scalpel IV catheters: 22- and 24-gauge over-the-needle; 23- and 25-gauge butterfly Tape Bag-valve-mask device with infant-sized mask Stethoscope Blood glucose testing materials Laryngoscope Handle Laryngoscope blades: 0, 1 straight 1 instructor	Advance students to the next case when their actions are acceptable. If a student is having difficulty managing a case, other participants may give suggestions. Continued inappropriate management is better handled by stopping the scenario and discussing key points than by continuing to have the patient's condition deteriorate. When the case is completed, use the suggested steps in the Answer Key to review its management with the students, acknowledging correct treatment decisions and critiquing errors. Any content points not made during the course of the scenario should be addressed in a short didactic session or discussion at this time. Instructor information to be given upon request: 1. What number pregnancy is this? *First* 2. Do you feel like you need to push? *Yes* 3. Baby's head is crowning 4. Meconium present? *No* 5. Twins? *No* 6. Term delivery? *Yes* 7. First ABC assessment: *Beginning to make strong, effective breathing efforts; heart rate is 80 and rising.* 8. Reassessment of ABCs: *Breathing is becoming faster and easier; heart rate is 140.*
Resuscitation of the Distressed Newborn	Infant mannequin Infant intubation mannequin	Have students practice resuscitating a distressed newborn as described in Handout 41-6

Station	Equipment and Personnel Needed	Activities
	Bulb syringe DeLee suction trap Meconium aspirator Endotracheal tubes: 2.5, 3.0, and 3.5 Suction catheters: 5, 6, and 8 French 20-ml syringe and 8 French feeding tube for gastric suction Towels Cord clamp Sterile scissors or Scalpel IV catheters: 22- and 24-gauge over-the-needle; 23- and 25-gauge butterfly Tape Bag-valve-mask device with infant-sized mask Stethoscope	Scenario Two. Choose a team leader or allow students to self-select their roles. Follow an interactive format by presenting the initial scenario, and then provide additional historical and physical exam information in response to participants' questions. Advance students to the next case when their actions are acceptable. If a student is having difficulty managing a case, other participants may give suggestions. Continued inappropriate management is better handled by stopping the scenario and discussing key points than by continuing to have the patient's condition deteriorate. When the case is completed, use the suggested steps in the Answer Key to review its management with the students, acknowledging correct treatment decisions and critiquing errors. Any content points not made during the course of the scenario should be addressed in a short didactic session or discussion at this time. Instructor information given upon request: 1. What number pregnancy is this? *Third* 2. Do you feel like you need to push? *Yes* 3. Baby's head is crowning 4. Meconium present? *Yes* 5. Twins? *No* 6. Term delivery? *Yes* 7. First ABC assessment: *Gasping without air movement; heart rate is 40.* 8. Reassessment of ABCs: *Good chest rise with BMV; heart rate is 55.*

WORKBOOK
Chapter 41 Activities

READING/REFERENCE
Textbook, pp. 1585–1666

HANDOUT 41-2
Chapter 41 Quiz

HANDOUT 41-3
Chapter 41 Scenario

PARAMEDIC STUDENT CD
Student Activities

ASSIGNMENTS

Assign students to complete Chapter 41, "Neonatology" of the workbook. Also assign them to read Chapter 42, "Pediatrics," before the next class.

EVALUATION

Chapter Quiz and Scenario Distribute copies of the Chapter Quiz provided in Handout 41-2 to evaluate student understanding of this chapter. Make sure each student reads the scenario to reinforce critical thinking on the scene. Remind students not to use their notes or textbooks while taking the quiz.

Student CD Quizzes for every chapter are contained on the dynamic and highly visual in-text student CD.

Companion Website Additional quizzes for every chapter are contained on this exciting website.

TestGen You may wish to create a custom-tailored test using *Prentice Hall TestGen for Essentials of Paramedic Care*, 2nd Edition to evaluate student understanding of this chapter.

On-line Test Preparation (for students and instructors) Additional test preparation is available through Brady's new on-line product, *EMT Achieve: Paramedic Test Preparation* at http://www.prenhall.com/emtachieve/. Instructors can also monitor student mastery on-line.

Review Manual for the EMT-Paramedic This comprehensive exam review contains hundreds of test questions and rationales, including scenarios, along with two 180-question practice tests on CD.

REINFORCEMENT

Handouts If classroom discussion or performance on the quiz indicates that some students have not fully mastered the chapter content, you may wish to assign some or all of the Reinforcement Handouts for this chapter.

Student CD (for students) A wide variety of material on this CD-ROM will reinforce and also expand student knowledge and skills.

PowerPoint Presentation (for instructors) The PowerPoint material developed for this chapter offers useful reinforcement of chapter content.

Companion Website (for students) Additional review quizzes and links to EMS resources will contribute to further reinforcement of the chapter.

OneKey On-line support is offered for this course on one of three platforms: Course Compass, Blackboard, or Web CT. Includes the IRM, PowerPoints, TestGen, and Companion Website for instruction. Ask your local sales representative for more information.

Brady Skills Series: Advanced Life Skills (Video or CD) Have your students watch the skills come to life on VHS or CD-ROM, or they can purchase the highly visual, full-color text with step-by-step procedures and rationales.

COMPANION WEBSITE
http://www.prenhall.com/bledsoe

TESTGEN
Chapter 41

EMT ACHIEVE: PARAMEDIC TEST PREPARATION
Mistovich & Beasley. *EMT Achieve: Paramedic Test Preparation*, www.prenhall.com/emtachieve/

REVIEW MANUAL FOR THE EMT-PARAMEDIC
Cherry & Mistovich. *Review Manual for the EMT-Paramedic*, 3rd edition.

HANDOUTS 41-4 TO 41-6
Reinforcement Activities

PARAMEDIC STUDENT CD
Student Activities

POWERPOINT PRESENTATION
Chapter 41

COMPANION WEBSITE
http://www.prenhall.com/bledsoe

ONEKEY
Chapter 41

ADVANCED LIFE SUPPORT SKILLS
Larmon & Davis. *Advanced Life Support Skills*.

ADVANCED LIFE SKILLS REVIEW
Larmon & Davis. *Advanced Life Skills Review*.

BRADY SKILLS SERIES: ALS
Larmon & Davis. *Brady Skills Series: ALS*.

PARAMEDIC NATIONAL STANDARDS SELF-TEST
Miller. *Paramedic National Standards Self-Test*, 4th edition.

HANDOUT 41-1

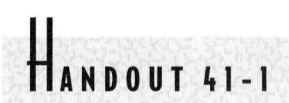

Student's Name _____

CHAPTER 41 OBJECTIVES CHECKLIST

Knowledge	Date Mastered
1. Define newborn and neonate.	
2. Identify important antepartum factors that can affect childbirth.	
3. Identify important intrapartum factors that can determine high-risk newborn patients.	
4. Identify the factors that lead to premature birth and low-birth-weight newborns.	
5. Distinguish between primary and secondary apnea.	
6. Discuss pulmonary perfusion and asphyxia.	
7. Identify the primary signs utilized for evaluating a newborn during resuscitation.	
8. Identify the appropriate use of the APGAR scale.	
9. Calculate the APGAR score given various newborn situations.	
10. Formulate an appropriate treatment plan for providing initial care to a newborn.	
11. Describe the indications, equipment needed, application, and evaluation of the following management techniques for the newborn in distress: • Blow-by oxygen • Ventilatory assistance • Endotracheal intubation • Orogastric tube • Chest compressions • Vascular access	
12. Discuss the routes of medication administration for a newborn.	
13. Discuss the signs of hypovolemia in a newborn.	
14. Discuss the initial steps in resuscitation of a newborn.	
15. Discuss the effects of maternal narcotic usage on the newborn.	
16. Determine the appropriate treatment for the newborn with narcotic depression.	
17. Discuss appropriate transport guidelines for a newborn.	

HANDOUT 41-1 Continued

Knowledge	Date Mastered
18. Determine appropriate receiving facilities for low- and high-risk newborns.	
19. Describe the epidemiology, including the incidence, morbidity/mortality, risk factors and prevention strategies, pathophysiology, assessment findings, and management for the following neonatal problems: • Meconium aspiration • Apnea • Diaphragmatic hernia • Bradycardia • Prematurity • Respiratory distress/cyanosis • Seizures • Fever • Hypothermia • Hypoglycemia • Vomiting • Diarrhea • Common birth injuries • Cardiac arrest • Post-arrest management	
20. Given several neonatal emergencies, provide the appropriate procedures for assessment, management, and transport.	

CHAPTER 41 QUIZ

Write the letter of the best answer in the space provided.

_____ 1. A neonate is an infant from the time of birth to:
   A. 1 week of age.
   B. 2 weeks of age.
   C. 1 month of age.
   D. 3 months of age.

_____ 2. The term *newborn* or *newly born infant* is used to describe a neonate:
   A. until the umbilical cord is cut.
   B. during the time it spends in the delivery room.
   C. until it is discharged from the hospital.
   D. during the first few hours of life.

_____ 3. The difference between primary apnea and secondary apnea in a newborn is that:
   A. infants with primary apnea typically will respond to simple stimulation and oxygen while those in secondary apnea will not.
   B. bradycardia is present in primary apnea but not in secondary apnea.
   C. infants with secondary apnea typically will respond to simple stimulation and oxygen while those in primary apnea will not.
   D. bradycardia is present in secondary apnea but not in primary apnea.

_____ 4. A normal newborn's respiratory rate should average:
   A. 12 to 20 breaths per minute.
   B. 20 to 30 breaths per minute.
   C. 40 to 60 breaths per minute.
   A. 60 to 80 breaths per minute.

_____ 5. A newborn's heart rate should normally be:
   A. 80 to 100 at birth, speeding to 140 to 160 thereafter.
   B. 150 to 180 at birth, slowing to 130 to 140 thereafter.
   C. 170 to 190 at birth, slowing to 80 to 100 thereafter.
   D. 60 to 80 at birth, speeding to 150 to 180 thereafter.

_____ 6. Which of the following statements about skin color in the newborn immediately after birth is correct?
   A. Cyanosis of the extremities is common, but central cyanosis is abnormal.
   B. Central cyanosis is common, but cyanosis of the extremities is abnormal.
   C. Both cyanosis of the extremities and central cyanosis are common and normal.
   D. Both central cyanosis and cyanosis of the extremities are abnormal.

_____ 7. An infant is in distress and requires emergency intervention if its pulse rate is less than:
   A. 60.
   B. 80.
   C. 100.
   D. 120.

_____ 8. Determine the APGAR score for the following infant:

   Appearance—completely pink
   Pulse—over 100
   Grimace—crying
   Activity—some flexion, slowly
   Respiration—strong cry

   A. 5
   B. 7
   C. 9
   D. 10

HANDOUT 41-2 Continued

____ 9. Determine the APGAR score for the following infant:

Appearance—completely cyanotic
Pulse—below 100
Grimace—frowns when stimulated
Activity—limp
Respiration—slow, irregular

  A. 1
  B. 3
  C. 5
  D. 7

____ 10. You have just delivered an infant. The baby is limp with central cyanosis. There is no apparent respiratory effort. You should:
  A. begin resuscitation immediately.
  B. withhold resuscitation for 1 minute so the APGAR score can be used to guide your efforts.
  C. give oxygen by blow-by, but withhold other resuscitative measures until a 1-minute APGAR score can be determined.
  D. position, dry, warm, suction, and stimulate the infant, but withhold other resuscitation until a 1-minute APGAR score can be determined.

____ 11. An infant is considered to be in severe distress and in need of immediate resuscitation if its APGAR score is less than:
  A. 2.
  B. 4.
  C. 6.
  D. 8.

____ 12. When you suction a newborn's airway, you should:
  A. suction the mouth first so there is nothing there to aspirate if the infant gasps when its nose is suctioned.
  B. suction the nose first so there is nothing there to aspirate if the infant gasps when its mouth is suctioned.
  C. suction either the nose or the mouth first depending on which you can reach most easily.
  D. squeeze the suction bulb only after placing it into the infant's mouth.

____ 13. Appropriate methods of stimulating a newborn include:
  A. flicking the soles of its feet; slapping its buttocks.
  B. flicking the soles of its feet; gently rubbing its back.
  C. vigorous rubbing; flicking the soles of the feet.
  D. vigorous rubbing; slapping the buttocks.

____ 14. "Milking" or stripping the umbilical cord is:
  A. contraindicated because it increases blood viscosity and produces polycythemia.
  B. indicated because it increases the newborn's red cell mass and improves oxygenation.
  C. contraindicated because it decreases blood viscosity and causes hypovolemia.
  D. indicated because it helps reverse hypovolemia that may have developed during birth.

____ 15. The first priority following the birth of a baby is to:
  A. clamp and cut the umbilical cord.
  B. deliver the placenta.
  C. ensure that the infant's airway and breathing are adequate.
  D. control maternal blood loss.

____ 16. Acceptable techniques for checking the heart rate of an infant include all of the following EXCEPT:
  A. listening over the cardiac apex with a stethoscope.
  B. lightly grasping the stump of the umbilical cord.
  C. palpating the femoral or brachial pulses.
  D. attaching the infant to an ECG monitor and watching the heart-rate meter.

HANDOUT 41-2 Continued

_____ 17. At 1540 hours you respond to a call in a maternity store at a shopping mall where you find a woman in labor. Exam reveals that the baby's head is crowning, and the mother says she needs to push. When you deliver the infant, it is covered with a greenish-black material. The infant's respirations are gasping and are not moving air. You should:
   A. position the infant head down and rub its back to stimulate breathing.
   B. begin immediate ventilation with oxygen using the bag-valve-mask.
   C. intubate the trachea and apply suction to the ET tube to remove any foreign material from the lower airway.
   D. give blow-by oxygen and transport immediately.

_____ 18. A newborn should receive positive-pressure ventilations with a bag-valve mask if its heart rate is not at least:
   A. 60.
   B. 80.
   C. 100.
   D. 120.

_____ 19. A newborn has a heart rate of 140 and regular, unlabored respirations at 42. Cyanosis of the chest and abdomen are present. You should:
   A. withhold oxygen because central cyanosis is common in the first few minutes after birth.
   B. withhold oxygen because high-concentration oxygen has been linked with blindness in newborn infants.
   C. give oxygen immediately using a bag-valve-mask.
   D. give oxygen by blowing oxygen across the newborn's face.

_____ 20. A newborn has a heart rate of 86 and regular, unlabored respirations at 40. Cyanosis of the extremities is present. You should:
   A. blow oxygen across the newborn's face.
   B. wait for 1 minute, then reassess the pulse to see if it is increasing.
   C. begin chest compressions immediately.
   D. immediately begin positive-pressure ventilation with a bag-valve-mask.

_____ 21. A newborn initially presented with a heart rate of 152 and regular, unlabored respirations at 46. Because central cyanosis was present, oxygen was given by blow-by. After about a minute, the cyanosis was still present. You should:
   A. discontinue the oxygen because the cause is probably not respiratory in nature.
   B. begin positive-pressure ventilation with a bag-valve-mask.
   C. immediately intubate the newborn's trachea, then ventilate with a bag-valve-mask.
   D. begin chest compressions.

_____ 22. Chest compressions should be initiated in a newborn if the heart rate is:
   A. less than 60 beats per minute.
   B. between 60 and 80 beats per minute, but does not increase with 30 seconds of oxygenation and ventilation.
   C. between 80 and 100 beats per minute and central cyanosis is present.
   D. either A or B

_____ 23. Which of the following best describes the correct technique for giving chest compressions and ventilations to a newborn?
   A. rate 120/minute; compression to ventilation ratio 3:1
   B. rate 180/minute; compression to ventilation ratio 5:1
   C. rate 120/minute; compression to ventilation ratio 5:1
   D. rate 100/minute; compression to ventilation ratio 3:1

HANDOUT 41-2 Continued

_____ 24. You are delivering the infant of a 17-year-old female who has been living in a shelter for the homeless. During your assessment of the mother, you notice needle tracks on her arms. Her speech is slurred, and she appears to be drowsy and apathetic. When you question her about drug abuse, she admits to "shooting up with heroin about 2 hours ago to relieve the pain of labor. Which of the following statements best describes your considerations in this situation?
   A. The infant will probably suffer respiratory depression following delivery and should receive naloxone as quickly as possible to reverse this problem.
   B. The infant will probably not suffer significant problems because narcotics do not cross the placental barrier easily.
   C. The infant will probably suffer respiratory depression following delivery but should not be given naloxone because a withdrawal reaction might occur.
   D. Naloxone should be given by IV push to the mother immediately to avoid serious respiratory depression in her newborn.

_____ 25. An infant you have just delivered is in severe respiratory distress. Central cyanosis unresponsive to bag-valve-mask ventilation is present. Physical exam reveals a small, flat abdomen, absent breath sounds over the left lung field, and displacement of the heart sounds to the right. What problem do you suspect?
   A. meconium aspiration   C. diaphragmatic hernia
   B. omphalocele   D. meningomyelocele

_____ 26. Appropriate management of the infant in question 25 would include positioning her head and thorax:
   A. higher than the abdomen and feet; placing a nasogastric or orogastric tube; ventilating with a bag-valve-mask while preparing to intubate.
   B. higher than her abdomen and feet; placing a nasogastric or orogastric tube; withholding further bag-valve-mask ventilation until an endotracheal tube is placed.
   C. lower than her abdomen and feet; placing a nasogastric or orogastric tube; withholding further bag-valve-mask ventilation until an endotracheal tube is placed.
   d. higher than her abdomen and feet; avoiding placement of a nasogastric or orogastric tube; ventilating with a bag-valve-mask while preparing to intubate.

_____ 27. The most common cause of bradycardia in the newborn is:
   A. increased intracranial pressure.   C. hypoxia.
   B. acidosis.   D. hypothyroidism.

_____ 28. The most effective initial treatment for bradycardia in the newborn is to give:
   A. atropine.   C. epinephrine.
   B. oxygen.   D. $D_{10}W$.

_____ 29. A premature newborn is an infant born before:
   A. 40 weeks gestation or with a weight less than 2.2 kg.
   B. 37 weeks gestation or with a weight less than 2.2 kg.
   C. 32 weeks gestation or with a weight less than 0.6 kg.
   D. 28 weeks gestation or with a weight less than 0.6 kg.

_____ 30. Premature infants are susceptible to hypothermia because:
   A. they have a large surface-to-volume ratio.
   B. they have small stores of subcutaneous fat and therefore less insulation.
   C. they are unable to shiver.
   D. all of these

_____ 31. The most common factor causing respiratory distress and cyanosis in the newborn is:
   A. meconium aspiration.
   B. prematurity.
   C. diaphragmatic hernia.
   D. aspiration pneumonitis.

HANDOUT 41-2 Continued

_____ 32. The leading cause of shock in newborns is:
   A. sepsis.
   B. cardiac failure secondary to hypoxia.
   C. hypovolemia.
   D. hypoglycemia.

_____ 33. A newborn suspected of being hypovolemic should be given a bolus of:
   A. 10 mL/kg of Ringer's lactate or normal saline.
   B. 10 mL/kg of D_5LR or D_5NS.
   C. 40 mL/kg of Ringer's lactate or normal saline.
   D. 40 mL/kg of D_5LR or D_5NS.

_____ 34. Fever in a neonate:
   A. is not a cause for concern because their immune systems are immature and they frequently develop mild infections.
   B. is not a cause for concern unless the infant is sweating heavily.
   C. should be treated with application of cold packs to lower the core temperature.
   D. should be considered a sign of meningitis or another life-threatening infection until proven otherwise.

_____ 35. Infants of diabetic mothers should have their blood glucose levels checked about 30 minutes after birth because:
   A. they will frequently develop hypoglycemia.
   B. an elevated blood glucose at this time will help predict whether the infant also will be diabetic.
   C. they will frequently develop hyperglycemia.
   D. a decreased blood glucose at this time will help predict whether the infant also will be diabetic.

HANDOUT 41-3

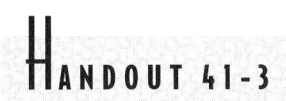

Student's Name _____

CHAPTER 41 SCENARIO

Review the following real-life situation. Then answer the questions that follow.

At 2230 hours on a snowy winter evening, you are dispatched for a woman in preterm labor. Weather and traffic conditions slow your response, and a trip that normally would have taken 5 minutes requires 15. When you finally reach the location of the call, a suburban home, you discover that a 28-year-old female, assisted by her husband, has just delivered a 30-week-gestation boy.

The infant is flaccid with no spontaneous movement. He has no apparent respiratory effort. The pulse, felt at the base of the umbilical cord, is 44 beats/minute and weak. Central cyanosis is present. You estimate the infant's weight at 1 kg. There are no obvious congenital abnormalities.

1. What is this newborn's status and the most likely cause of this situation?

2. What should you do?

3. Thirty seconds after beginning ventilation, the baby's heart rate is still 44 beats/minute. What should you do now?

4. After 30 seconds of CPR, the baby's heart rate rises to 88 beats per minute. What should you do now?

Handout 41-4

Student's Name _____

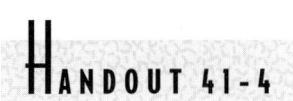

CHAPTER 41 REVIEW

Write the word or words that best complete the following sentences in the space(s) provided.

1. An infant from the time of birth to 1 month of age is a(n) _____.
2. A baby in the first few hours of life is referred to as a(n) _____. These infants also are sometimes called _____ _____ _____.
3. After an unscheduled delivery in the field, you have _____ patients to manage, the _____ and the _____.
4. Factors present before onset of labor that indicate possible complications in newborns are called _____ factors.
5. Factors occurring during childbirth that indicate possible complications in newborns are called _____ factors.
6. The channel between the main pulmonary artery and the aorta in the fetus is the _____ _____.
7. A condition in the newborn in which blood continues to bypass the fetal respiratory system, resulting in ongoing hypoxia, is _____ _____ _____.
8. The initial period of apnea in a hypoxic newborn that can be reversed with simple stimulation and exposure to oxygen is _____ apnea.
9. _____ apnea is a condition characterized by falling heart rate, falling blood pressure, and oxygen saturation that is not responsive to stimulation and that will not spontaneously reverse.
10. Apnea in a newborn should always be assumed to be _____ apnea.
11. Protrusion of abdominal contents into the thoracic cavity through an opening in the diaphragm is a(n) _____ _____.
12. Herniation of the spinal cord and membranes through a defect in the spinal column is a(n) _____.
13. A defect in the area of the umbilicus that results in herniation of the abdominal contents is a(n) _____.
14. The most common birth defect of the nose, which is due to the presence of a bony or membranous septum between the nasal cavity and the pharynx, is _____ _____.
15. A numerical system for distinguishing newborns who need only routine care from those who need greater assistance is the _____ _____, which has five parameters: _____, _____, _____, _____, _____, and _____ _____.
16. As soon as you deliver a newborn's head, suction the _____ first, then the _____.
17. The dark green material that can be expelled from the intestine into the amniotic fluid during periods of distress is _____.
18. Two acceptable methods of stimulating a newborn that does not cry immediately are _____ _____ _____ and _____ _____ _____ _____.
19. Heat loss from the newborn can result from _____, _____, _____, and _____.
20. "Milking" or stripping the umbilical cord can cause _____ _____ _____ and _____.
21. The most important indicator of neonatal distress is the _____ _____.

HANDOUT 41-4 Continued

22. The first steps on the "inverted pyramid" of neonatal resuscitation are _____, _____, _____, _____, and _____ _____.

23. If a newborn has central cyanosis and a heart rate greater than 100, you should administer _____.

24. An infant should receive positive-pressure ventilation if it has a heart rate less than _____, _____, or persistence of _____ _____ after administration of oxygen.

25. An infant who needs positive-pressure ventilation should be ventilated at a rate of _____ to _____ breaths per minute.

26. Chest compressions should be initiated in a newborn if the heart rate is less than _____ or is between _____ and _____ but does not increase with oxygenation and ventilation.

27. Chest compressions in the newborn should be performed at a rate of _____ per minute.

28. Vascular access in the newborn can be most readily obtained by using the _____ _____.

29. If naloxone is given to an infant born to a narcotic-addicted mother, it may induce a _____ _____.

30. If you suspect a diaphragmatic hernia, DO NOT use _____-_____ _____, which can worsen the condition by causing gastric distension.

31. Bradycardia in the newborn is most commonly caused by _____.

32. A premature newborn is an infant born before _____ weeks or who weighs less than _____ kg.

33. The single most common factor causing respiratory distress and cyanosis in the newborn is _____.

34. The most common cause of shock in the newborn is _____.

35. Fluid bolus resuscitation in the newborn consists of _____ ml/kg of isotonic crystalloid.

36. Any neonate with a fever should be considered to have _____ until proven otherwise.

37. Newborns are extremely sensitive to environmental temperatures because of their increased _____ to _____ relationship.

38. Newborns of diabetic mothers have an increased risk of developing _____.

39. Hypoglycemia in the newborn is indicated by a blood glucose of less than _____.

40. Hypoglycemia in the newborn can be corrected by giving _____ or _____.

STEPS FOR UMBILICAL VEIN CATHETERIZATION

1. Fill baby bottle with saline (food coloring may be added to simulate blood).
2. Make two cross-slits in the nipple of the bottle.
3. Pull the umbilical cord through the nipple and attach the nipple to the bottle.
4. Cut the umbilical cord horizontally until the two arteries and the vein are easily seen.
5. Place umbilical tape at the base of the cord.
6. Fill a syringe and the umbilical catheter with saline.
7. Locate the orifice of the umbilical vein and insert the catheter.
8. Advance the catheter slowly until a fluid return is obtained.

    (*Note:* When this procedure is performed on a newborn, the catheter should be advanced only a short distance to avoid entering the hepatic venous system.)

9. When there is good blood return, tighten the tape in a purse string.

    (*Note:* This step should be demonstrated by your instructor but not practiced.)

HANDOUT 41-6

Student's Name _____

NEWBORN RESUSCITATION

SCENARIO ONE: RESUSCITATION OF THE NORMAL NEWBORN

At 2245 hours, you respond to a report of "abdominal pain" in a small community that is about 30 minutes from the closest emergency department. The patient is a 15-year-old female who is screaming as she lies on a couch in the living room of her home. The girl's mother is standing by perplexed. After a quick exam, you determine that the patient is pregnant and is in active labor. What do you do?

HANDOUT 41-6 *Continued*

SCENARIO TWO: RESUSCITATION OF THE DISTRESSED NEWBORN

At 1415 hours, you are dispatched to a report of a "woman in labor" at a shopping mall. When you arrive, mall security quickly escorts you to a maternity store where you find a 28-year-old female in active labor. What do you do?

Chapter 41 Answer Key

Handout 41-2: Chapter 41 Quiz

1. C
2. D
3. A
4. C
5. B
6. A
7. C
8. C
9. B
10. A
11. B
12. A
13. B
14. A
15. C
16. D
17. C
18. C
19. D
20. D
21. B
22. D
23. A
24. C
25. C
26. B
27. C
28. B
29. B
30. D
31. B
32. C
33. A
34. D
35. A

Handout 41-3: Chapter 41 Scenario

1. He is in cardiopulmonary failure, probably as a result of hypoxia.
2. Clamp and cut the umbilical cord. Dry, warm, position, suction, and stimulate the newborn. Reassess for breathing. Then begin bag-valve-mask ventilations at 40 to 60 breaths/min with high-concentration oxygen. After 30 seconds, recheck the heart rate.
3. Check for adequate chest rise and air entry with bag-valve-mask ventilation. Continue to ventilate while your partner begins chest compressions at a rate of 120/minute. Reassess heart rate in 30 seconds.
4. Stop chest compressions. Continue to ventilate with the bag-valve-mask. Reassess heart rate after 30 seconds. Check for spontaneous respirations and for central cyanosis. Make preparations to transport, including maximizing heat in the patient compartment of the ambulance.

Handout 41-4: Chapter 41 Review

1. neonate
2. newborn, newly born infants
3. two, mother, baby
4. antepartum
5. intrapartum
6. ductus arteriosus
7. persistent fetal circulation
8. primary
9. Secondary
10. secondary
11. diaphragmatic hernia
12. meningomyelocele
13. omphalocele
14. choanal atresia
15. APGAR scale, Appearance, Pulse rate, Grimace, Activity, Respiratory effort
16. mouth, nose
17. meconium
18. rubbing its back, flicking its soles
19. conduction, evaporation, convection, radiation
20. increased blood viscosity, polycythemia
21. heart rate
22. drying, warming, positioning, suction, tactile stimulation
23. oxygen
24. 100, apnea, central cyanosis
25. 40, 60
26. 60, 60, 80
27. 120
28. umbilical vein
29. withdrawal reaction
30. bag-mask ventilation
31. hypoxia
32. 37, 2.2
33. prematurity
34. hypovolemia
35. 10
36. meningitis
37. surface, volume
38. hypoglycemia
39. 45 mg/dL
40. $D_{10}W$, $D_{25}W$

Handout 41-6: Newborn Resuscitation

Scenario one: Resuscitation of the Normal Newborn

Expected sequence of interventions

1. Obtained and opened OB kit.
2. Questioned mother about length of gestation and twins.
3. Observed for presence of meconium.
4. Assisted with delivery.
    a. Delivered infant's head.
    b. Suctioned mouth, then nose with bulb syringe.
    c. Allowed mother to push on next contraction to complete delivery.
5. Received baby in sterile towel, warmed if possible.
6. At the perineum, positioned the infant's head in a dependent position.
7. Suctioned mouth, then nose again.
8. Stimulated respirations by drying infant with towel.
9. Assessed ABCs.
10. Continued stimulation/drying.
11. Reassessed breathing and circulation.
12. Applied cord clamps.
13. Cut umbilical cord.
14. Placed infant in new dry towel, dried thoroughly while observing.
15. Wrapped infant to prevent hypothermia.
16. Prepared for transport.

Scenario 2: Resuscitation of the Distressed Newborn

Expected sequence of interventions

1. Obtained and opened OB kit.
2. Prepared suction and intubation equipment.
3. Questioned mother about length of gestation and twins.
4. Assisted with delivery.
    a. Delivered infant's head.
    b. Suctioned mouth, pharynx, nose thoroughly.
    c. Allowed mother to push on next contraction to complete delivery.
5. Received baby in sterile towel, warmed if possible.
6. Clamped and cut the umbilical cord.
7. Positioned infant with head in slightly dependent position.

8. Intubated trachea; observed for presence of meconium on vocal cords during procedure.
9. Withdrew endotracheal tube while applying direct suction to endotracheal tube, using meconium aspiration adaptor.
10. Repeated intubation and suctioning until meconium was no longer returned.
11. Stimulated respirations by drying infant with towel.
12. Assessed ABCs.
13. Administered bag-valve-mask ventilation at 40 to 60 breaths/minute with 100 percent oxygen.
14. Reassessed heart rate after 30 seconds of oxygenation and ventilation.
    a. Breathing (good chest rise with BVM ventilation)
    b. Circulation (heart rate is 140)
15. Began chest compressions, stopping compressions for ventilation after every third compression to deliver 30 breaths and 90 compressions/minute (120 events/minute).
16. Reassessed heart rate after 30 seconds of oxygenation and ventilation.
17. Performed endotracheal intubation.
18. Wrapped infant to prevent hypothermia.
19. Prepared for transport.

Chapter 42 Pediatrics

INTRODUCTION

Management of sick or injured children requires knowledge of common pediatric emergencies, strong patient assessment skills, and a well-organized approach. Children are not little adults. The etiologies that lead to catastrophic events, such as cardiopulmonary arrest, are different from those in adults. Because children typically have healthy cardiovascular and respiratory systems, they tend to compensate well when they are stressed physiologically. Accordingly, the signs and symptoms of distress may be subtle. Paramedics must recognize that although children make up a relatively small portion of the patients cared for by the EMS system, their unique needs require specialized preparation and responses.

TOTAL TEACHING TIME: 27.38 HOURS

The total teaching time is only a guideline based on the didactic and practical lab averages in the National Standard Curriculum. Instructors should take into consideration such factors as the pace at which students learn, the size of the class, and breaks. The actual time devoted to teaching objectives is the responsibility of the instructor.

CHAPTER OBJECTIVES

After reading this chapter, you should be able to:

1. Discuss the paramedic's role in the reduction of infant and childhood morbidity and mortality from acute illness and injury. (pp. 1587–1589)
2. Identify methods/mechanisms that prevent injuries to infants and children. (pp. 1588–1589)
3. Describe Emergency Medical Services for Children (EMSC) and how it can affect patient outcome. (p. 1588)
4. Identify the common family responses to acute illness and injury of an infant or child. (p. 1590)
5. Describe techniques for successful interaction with families of acutely ill or injured infants and children. (p. 1590)
6. Identify key anatomical, physiological, growth, and developmental characteristics of infants and children and their implications. (pp. 1590–1593)
7. Outline differences in adult and childhood anatomy, physiology, and "normal" age-group-related vital signs. (pp. 1593–1597)
8. Describe techniques for successful assessment and treatment of infants and children. (pp. 1597–1623)
9. Discuss the appropriate equipment used to obtain pediatric vital signs. (p. 1605)
10. Determine appropriate airway adjuncts, ventilation devices, and endotracheal intubation equipment; their proper use; and complications of use for infants and children. (pp. 1606–1617)
11. List the indications and methods of gastric decompression for infants and children. (pp. 1617–1619)
12. Define pediatric respiratory distress, failure, and arrest. (pp. 1624–1626)
13. Differentiate between upper airway obstruction and lower airway disease. (pp. 1626–1632)

©2007 Pearson Education, Inc.
Essentials of Paramedic Care, 2nd ed.

14. Describe the general approach to the treatment of children with respiratory distress, failure, or arrest from upper airway obstruction or lower airway disease. (pp. 1626–1632)
15. Discuss the common causes and relative severity of hypoperfusion in infants and children. (pp. 1632–1636)
16. Identify the major classifications of pediatric cardiac rhythms. (pp. 1637–1640)
17. Discuss the primary etiologies of cardiopulmonary arrest in infants and children. (pp. 1624–1625, 1632)
18. Discuss age-appropriate sites, equipment, techniques, and complications of vascular access for infants and children. (pp. 1619–1620)
19. Describe the primary etiologies of altered level of consciousness in infants and children. (pp. 1623–1648, 1653–1654, 1663)
20. Identify common lethal mechanisms of injury in infants and children. (pp. 1649–1651)
21. Discuss anatomical features of children that predispose or protect them from certain injuries. (pp. 1654–1655)
22. Describe aspects of infant and child airway management that are affected by potential cervical spine injury. (pp. 1651–1653)
23. Identify infant and child trauma patients who require spinal immobilization. (pp. 1621, 1623)
24. Discuss fluid management and shock treatment for infant and child trauma patients. (pp. 1632–1636, 1653)
25. Determine when pain management and sedation are appropriate for infants and children. (p. 1653)
26. Define child abuse, child neglect, and sudden infant death syndrome (SIDS). (pp. 1656–1661)
27. Discuss the parent/caregiver responses to the death of an infant or child. (p. 1657)
28. Define children with special health care needs and technology-assisted children. (pp. 1661–1664)
29. Discuss basic cardiac life support (CPR) guidelines for infants and children. (pp. 1599–1602, 1606–1611)
30. Integrate advanced life support skills with basic cardiac life support for infants and children. (pp. 1611–1621, 1637–1640)
31. Discuss the indications, dosage, route of administration, and special considerations for medication administration in infants and children. (pp. 1620–1622)
32. Discuss appropriate transport guidelines for low- and high-risk infants and children. (p. 1623)
33. Describe the epidemiology, including the incidence, morbidity/mortality, risk factors, prevention strategies, pathophysiology, assessment, and treatment of infants and children with:

    - Respiratory distress/failure (pp. 1624–1632)
    - Hypoperfusion (pp. 1632–1636)
    - Cardiac dysrhythmias (pp. 1637–1640)
    - Neurologic emergencies (pp. 1640, 1642–1643)
    - Trauma (pp. 1648–1651)
    - Abuse and neglect (pp. 1657–1661)
    - Special health-care needs, including technology-assisted children (pp. 1661–1664)
    - SIDS (pp. 1656–1657)

34. Given several preprogrammed simulated pediatric patients, provide the appropriate assessment, treatment, and transport. (pp. 1587–1664)

FRAMING THE LESSON

Begin by reviewing the important points from Chapter 41, "Neonatology." Discuss any points that the class does not completely understand. Then move on to Chapter 42. Ask the students to imagine and list the feelings of an acutely ill or injured child entering the emergency health care system. Next ask them to imagine and list the feelings they might experience in the role of the child's parent or other caregiver. Finally, ask the students to imagine and list the feelings they would have if they were the paramedic responding to provide care to this child. List the feelings and emotions of each person involved in a pediatric emergency on a flip chart or board and compare them. Emphasize that pediatric emergencies frequently are emotionally charged, highly stressful situations that require not only knowledge and skill but also a high level of professionalism and mental discipline to manage. Because EMS responses to pediatric patients are relatively infrequent, study, practice, and planning are critical to maintaining the knowledge, skill, and discipline necessary for good outcomes.

TEACHING STRATEGIES

People learn in a variety of ways. Some do better with the spoken word, whereas others prefer the written. Some prefer to work alone, whereas others profit from working in groups. Recognizing these different ways of acquiring knowledge, the authors of this *Instructor's Resource Manual* have provided a variety of teaching strategies for the different types of learners. These strategies are intended to foster higher-level cognitive skills and encourage creative learning and problem solving. For greatest effectiveness, incorporate these strategies into your class lecture. Symbols in the Lecture Outline indicate the points at which various exercises might be most appropriate. Other strategies can be used to preview the lesson or to summarize it.

The following strategies are keyed to specific sections of the lesson:

1. National and Local Agencies. Identify national and local agencies that promote the education of pediatric clinical skills and education, such as the American Heart Association, the American Academy of Pediatrics, the Children's Hospital, and Maternal and Child Health Services. Help students to understand the courses and materials offered by each of these organizations, and their roles in the care and prevention of childhood illness and injuries. Be sure to have brochures and contact information somewhere in your classroom to promote lifelong learning and the importance of continuing education.

2. Pediatric Health Fair. Volunteer your students at a local pediatric health fair. If one does not exist in your area, have students organize such an event. Include blood pressure screening, height and weight measurements, blood sugar checks, and even immunizations if possible. Volunteerism teaches valuable life lessons about being a public servant and giving to others. In addition, this activity can substitute for clinical time in a pediatric health clinic, which is sometimes hard to secure. This event will expose your students to many children of various ages and backgrounds, giving them practice communicating with and assessing children in a noncrisis situation, which is often easier than during an ambulance call.

3. Child Observation Exercise. The differences in development, behavior, and communication abilities of children may seem like a mystery to students, especially those without children of their own. A simple observation exercise can help. Have students, either individually or in small groups, observe children and parents in a public setting, such as the mall, the zoo, a playground, or a park. Have your students record the behaviors and language used by children and their parents, along with an estimation of their age and size. When students come back to class, ask the entire group to share behaviors or characteristics of children in several different developmental stages, such as infant, toddler, preschool, or adolescent. You will likely prepare a list that is remarkably similar to those listed in the text, and the students will have actual behavioral observations to improve their understanding of the material. The skill of observation is important to the paramedic, who often must communicate with and assess a patient while being aware of his or her total environment. This is a social psychology exercise that reaches both the cognitive and affective domains. The assignment should be given prior to the class session on this material to provide a context for discussion.

4. Elementary School Health Clinic. Many elementary schools, especially in urban areas, have health clinics or at least a school nurse's office. Arrange for students to spend time in these clinics, where they are likely to encounter basically healthy children with a single complaint. This allows students to gain comfort communicating with and assessing pediatric patients in the absence of a major crisis that usually accompanies a 911 call. In addition, the staff in these clinics are usually overworked and often appreciate the assistance. This activity improves the quality of clinical time, covers all three educational domains, and improves relationships with community health servants whom your students are likely to encounter as professional paramedics.

5. Researching an EMSC Project. Several years ago, emphasis in EMS was placed on pediatrics. Significant funds were allocated to EMS for Children (EMSC) projects all over the country. Many of these projects were wildly successful, improving the care to children and placing an emphasis on prevention. Have students research an EMSC project and share with the class the project's goals and successes. Have them discuss how their project could be extrapolated to your community, considering and solving any barriers to the project's success. This activity emphasizes research, oral communication, and problem-solving skills. Additionally, it encourages students to look outside their own community or EMS system for solutions to problems.

The following strategies can be used at various points throughout the lesson or to help summarize and demonstrate what students have learned.

Guest Speaker: Developmental or Child Psychologist. Invite a developmental or child psychologist to class to share techniques for interviewing and communicating with children. This person will likely have many tips and tricks to build rapport quickly with children of all ages. He or she should also be able to explain why certain approaches work with children of various ages. Any hospital with a pediatric wing is likely to have a child psychologist on staff. Many even employ psychologists who specialize in working with sick children or those in need of special health care. He or she could be an even greater asset to your classroom. In some cases, use of a subject matter expert is your best bet for an interesting and informative lecture.

Guest Speaker. Consider inviting a pediatrician, pediatric intensivist, pediatric surgeon, or pediatric anesthesiologist from the local or regional hospital to the class to discuss topics related to his or her specialty.

Clinical Rotations. Pediatric clinical rotations should be designed so students can see a wide range of pediatric patients and illnesses. Opportunities include:

- Day care centers, to allow students to see and interact with healthy young children.
- Immunization clinics, to allow students to obtain practice giving IM and SC injections to pediatric patients and interacting with healthy children who are under stress.
- Pediatric clinics and pediatricians' offices, to allow students to interact with children who are presenting with common injuries and illnesses of minor to moderate severity in a primary care setting.
- Pediatric emergency departments, to allow students to interact with children presenting with minor to critical injuries and illnesses.
- Pediatric intensive care units, to allow students to interact with and care for critically ill or injured children.
- Pediatric long-term care facilities, to allow students to interact with and care for chronically ill children, including those who are technology-assisted or technology-dependent.

Cultural Considerations, Legal Notes, and Patho Pearls. The Student CD-ROM contains this series of informative features to enhance the student's understanding of the material covered in this chapter.

TEACHING OUTLINE

Chapter 42 is the second lesson in Division 5, *Special Considerations/Operations*. Distribute Handout 42-1 so that students can familiarize themselves with the learning goals for this chapter. If the students have any questions about the objectives, answer them at this time.

Then present the chapter. One possible lecture outline follows. In the outline, the parenthetical references in regular type are references to text pages; those in bold type are reference to figures,tables, or procedures.

I. Introduction (p. 1587)

A. More than 20,000 pediatric deaths occur each year in the United States. (p. 1587)
B. Top causes of pediatric deaths (p. 1587)
   1. Motor-vehicle collisions
   2. Burns
   3. Drownings
   4. Suicides
   5. Homicides

II. Role of paramedics in pediatric care (pp. 1587–1589)

A. Continuing education and training programs (pp. 1587–1588)
   1. Pediatric Advanced Life Support (PALS)
   2. Pediatric Basic Trauma Life Support (PBTLS)
   3. Advanced Pediatric Life Support (APLS)
   4. Pediatric Emergencies for Prehospital Providers (PEPP)
   5. Regional conferences and seminars
   6. Pediatric education sites on the Internet
   7. Center for Pediatric Medicine (CPEM) at NYU and Bellevue Hospital
   8. Textbooks and journals
   9. Teaching Resource for Instructors of Prehospital Pediatrics (TRIPP)

HANDOUT 42-1
Chapter 42 Objectives Checklist

READING/REFERENCE
Garza, M. A. "Smart Pediatric Transport." *JEMS*, March 2000.
Losavio, K. "EMS for Kids." *JEMS*, Dec. 2000.

READING/REFERENCE
Perkin, R., and D. van Stralen. "20 Things You May Not Know about Pediatrics." *JEMS*, March 2000.

TEACHING STRATEGY 1
National and Local Agencies

POINT TO EMPHASIZE
Tragedies involving children account for some of the most stressful incidents that you will encounter in EMS practice.

POWERPOINT PRESENTATION
Chapter 42 PowerPoint slide 4

TEACHING STRATEGY 2
Pediatric Health Fair

POWERPOINT PRESENTATION
Chapter 42 PowerPoint slides 5–8

POINT TO EMPHASIZE
Because you will encounter pediatric patients less frequently than adult patients, you have a professional responsibility to maintain and improve upon your pediatric knowledge, particularly your clinical skills.

B. Improved health and injury prevention (pp. 1588–1589)
  1. Emergency Medical Services for Children (EMSC)
  2. Coordinated national effort
  3. Identification of specific areas of pediatric health care concern

III. General approach to pediatric emergencies (pp. 1589–1590)

A. Communication and psychological support (p. 1589)
B. Responding to patient needs (p. 1589)
  1. Common fears of children include:
     a. Separation from parents, caregivers
     b. Removal from home and never returning
     c. Injury
     d. Mutilation or disfigurement
     e. The unknown
  2. Be honest with children about what is being done to them and about discomfort and pain associated with procedures.
  3. Use language appropriate for the age of the child.
C. Responding to parents and caregivers (p. 1590)
  1. Caregivers' responses may include
     a. Shock
     b. Grief
     c. Denial
     d. Anger
     e. Guilt
     f. Fear
     g. Complete loss of control
  2. Designate one paramedic to deal with adults on the scene to avoid conflicts in information.
  3. Paramedic confidence and professionalism help parents regain control.

IV. Growth and development (pp. 1590–1593)

A. Newborns (first hours after birth) (p. 1590)
  1. Assessed with APGAR scoring system
  2. Resuscitation follows inverted pyramid and NeoNatal Resuscitation (NNR) guidelines.
B. Neonates (birth to 1 month) (pp. 1590–1591)
  1. Physical development
     a. Initially loses up to 10 percent of birth weight
     b. Lost weight normally recovered within 10 days
     c. Premature neonates not as neurologically or physically developed as their term counterparts
  2. Cognitive and emotional development
     a. Development centers on reflexes.
     b. Personality begins to form.
     c. May stare at faces and smile
     d. Mother, and occasionally father, can comfort and quiet the child.
  3. Common illnesses
     a. Jaundice
     b. Vomiting
     c. Respiratory distress
C. Infants (1 to 5 months) (p. 1591)
  1. Physical development
     a. Should have doubled birth weight
     b. Should be able to follow movements of others with their eyes

---

POWERPOINT PRESENTATION
Chapter 42 PowerPoint slides 9–12

TEACHING STRATEGY 3
Child Observation Exercise

POWERPOINT PRESENTATION
Chapter 42 PowerPoint slides 13–28

POINT TO EMPHASIZE
Examine infants and toddlers in a toe-to-head direction.

- c. Development of muscle tone moves from head to trunk and from trunk to extremities.
- 2. Cognitive and emotional development centers closely on parents and caregivers.
- 3. Common illnesses and accidents
  - a. SIDS
  - b. Vomiting
  - c. Dehydration
  - d. Meningitis
  - e. Child abuse
  - f. Household accidents
- 4. Paramedic considerations

D. Infants (6 to 12 months) (p. 1591)
  1. Physical development
     - a. May stand or walk without assistance
     - b. Active
     - c. Enjoy exploring world with their mouths, causing serious risk for foreign body airway obstruction
  2. Cognitive and emotional development (**Fig. 42-1, p. 1591**)
     - a. Have more fully formed personalities; express themselves readily
     - b. Have anxiety toward strangers
     - c. Don't like lying on backs
     - d. Tend to cling to mother
  3. Common illnesses and accidents
     - a. Febrile seizures
     - b. Vomiting
     - c. Diarrhea
     - d. Dehydration
     - e. Bronchiolitis
     - f. Motor-vehicle collisions
     - g. Croup
     - h. Child abuse
     - i. Poisonings
     - j. Falls
     - k. Airway obstruction
     - l. Meningitis
  4. Paramedic considerations

E. Toddlers (1 to 3 years) (p. 1592)
  1. Physical development
     - a. Great strides in motor development, mobility
     - b. Always on the move
  2. Cognitive and emotional development
     - a. Begin to stray away from parents/caregivers more frequently
     - b. Will cling to parents/caregivers if frightened
     - c. Understand better than they can speak
     - d. Can answer simple, specific questions
  3. Common illnesses and accidents
     - a. Motor-vehicle collisions
     - b. Homicide
     - c. Burn injuries
     - d. Drowning
     - e. Vehicle versus pedestrian collisions
     - f. Vomiting
     - g. Diarrhea
     - h. Febrile seizures
     - i. Poisonings
     - j. Falls

POINT TO EMPHASIZE
Do not trick or lie to the child and always explain what you are going to do.

    k. Child abuse
    l. Croup
    m. Meningitis
    n. Foreign body airway obstruction
   4. Paramedic considerations
  F. Preschoolers (3 to 5 years) (p. 1592)
   1. Physical development
    a. Tremendous increase in fine and gross motor development
    b. Know how to talk, but may refuse to speak, especially to strangers
   2. Cognitive and emotional development
    a. Vivid imaginations
    b. May see monsters as part of their world
    c. Have tempers and will express them
    d. Fear mutilation, may feel threatened by treatment
    e. Often run to a particular parent or caregiver
    f. Are openly affectionate, seek support and comfort from within home
   3. Common illnesses and accidents
    a. Croup
    b. Asthma
    c. Poisonings
    d. Motor-vehicle collisions
    e. Burns
    f. Child abuse
    g. Ingestion of foreign bodies
    h. Drownings
    i. Epiglottitis
    j. Febrile seizures
    k. Meningitis
   4. Paramedic considerations
  G. School-age children (6 to 12 years) (p. 1592) (**Fig. 42-2, p. 1592**)
   1. Physical development
    a. Tend to be active and carefree
    b. Growth spurts may lead to clumsiness.
   2. Cognitive and emotional development
    a. Protective and proud of parents or caregivers
    b. Seek attention of parents/caregivers
    c. Value peers, but also need home support
   3. Common illnesses and accidents
    a. Drownings
    b. Motor-vehicle collisions
    c. Bicycle collisions
    d. Falls
    e. Fractures
    f. Sports injuries
    g. Child abuse
    h. Burns
   4. Paramedic considerations
  H. Adolescents (13 to 18 years) (p. 1593)
   1. Usually defined as end of childhood and beginning of puberty
    a. Highly child-specific
    b. Male, average 13 years
    c. Female, average 11 years
   2. Physical development
    a. Significant variation among children
    b. Tend to be body conscious and concerned about physical image

---

TEACHING STRATEGY 4
Elementary School Health Clinic

POINT TO EMPHASIZE
It may be wise to interview the adolescent patient away from the parents or caregivers.

3. Cognitive and emotional development
      a. Most consider themselves to be grown up.
      b. Take offense at the use of the word "child"
      c. Relationships with peers are very important.
      d. Relationships with parents may be strained by growing need for independence.
   4. Common illnesses and accidents
      a. Mononucleosis
      b. Asthma
      c. Motor-vehicle collisions
      d. Sports injuries
      e. Drug and alcohol problems
      f. Suicide gestures
      g. Sexual abuse
      h. Pregnancy
   5. Paramedic implications

V. **Anatomy and physiology** (pp. 1593–1597) (Table 42-1, p. 1594)

A. Head (pp. 1593–1594) (Fig. 42-3, p. 1595)
   1. Larger size
   2. Larger occipital region
   3. Fontanelles open in infancy
   4. Face small in comparison to size of head
   5. Paramedic implications
      a. Higher proportion of blunt trauma involves the head
      b. Different airway positioning techniques
      c. Examine fontanelles in infants.
         i. Bulging fontanelles suggest increased intracranial pressure.
         ii. Sunken fontanelles suggest dehydration.

B. Airway (pp. 1594–1595)
   1. Narrower at all levels
   2. Infants are obligate nose breathers.
   3. The tongue takes up more space in the mouth.
   4. The jaw is proportionally smaller in young children.
   5. The larynx is higher (C-3 to C-4) and more anterior.
   6. The cricoid ring is narrowest part of airway in young children.
   7. Tracheal cartilage softer
   8. Trachea smaller in both length and diameter and more flexible
   9. Epiglottis
   10. Paramedic implications
       a. Keep nares clear in infants < 6 months.
       b. Keep in mind that narrower upper airways are more easily obstructed.
       c. Differences in intubation technique

C. Chest and lungs (pp. 1595–1596)
   1. Ribs positioned horizontally
   2. Ribs more pliable than adults' and offer less protection to organs
   3. Chest muscles are immature and fatigue easily.
   4. Lung tissue more fragile than adults'
   5. Mediastinum more mobile than adults'
   6. Thin chest wall easily transmits breath sounds.
   7. Paramedic implications
      a. Infants and children are diaphragmatic breathers.
      b. Infants and children are prone to gastric distention.
      c. Rib fractures are less frequent, but not uncommon in child abuse and trauma.

POINT TO EMPHASIZE
In assessing infants, pay special attention to the fontanelles, especially the anterior fontanelle.

POWERPOINT PRESENTATION
Chapter 42 PowerPoint slides 29–32

TEACHING TIP
Ask students to offer explanations as to why infants are nose breathers. Can they figure out that it is related to the fact that infants are designed to breast-feed?

POINT TO EMPHASIZE
Consider use of an oral or nasal airway in a pediatric patient only after other manual maneuvers have failed to keep the airway open.

> **POINT TO EMPHASIZE**
>
> During the early stages of development, injuries to the growth plate by use of an intraosseous needle may disrupt bone growth.

> **POINT TO EMPHASIZE**
>
> Infants and children increase their cardiac output by increasing their heart rate. They have very limited capacity to increase their stroke volume.

> **POINT TO EMPHASIZE**
>
> Bleeding that would not be dangerous in an adult may be life-threatening in an infant or child.

> **TEACHING TIP**
>
> See if students reason from the fact that infants and small children lose heat more rapidly to the fact that they must have higher metabolic rates and, therefore, higher respiratory rates and heart rates.

        d. Following trauma, children can have significant internal injury without external signs.
        e. Pulmonary contusions more common in major trauma
        f. Lungs prone to pneumothorax following barotraumas
        g. Mediastinum has greater shift with tension pneumothorax.
        h. Easy to miss pneumothorax or misplaced intubation due to transmitted breath sounds

D. Abdomen (p. 1596)
    1. Immature abdominal muscles offer less protection.
    2. Abdominal organs closer together
    3. Liver and spleen proportionally larger and more vascular
    4. Paramedic implications
        a. Liver and spleen more frequently injured
        b. Multiple organ injuries more common

E. Extremities (p. 1597)
    1. Bones softer and more porous until adolescence
    2. Growth plate injuries may disrupt bone growth.
    3. Paramedic implications
        a. Immobilize any "sprain" or "strain," as it is likely a fracture.
        b. Avoid piercing growth plate during intraosseous needle insertion.

F. Skin and body surface area (BSA) (p. 1596)
    1. Thinner and more elastic
    2. Thermal exposure results in deeper burn.
    3. Less subcutaneous fat
    4. Larger surface area relative to body mass
    5. Paramedic implications
        a. Children are more easily and deeply burned.
        b. They suffer larger losses of fluid and heat.

G. Respiratory system (infants and children) (p. 1596)
    1. Tidal volume proportionally similar to adolescents' and adults', but children require double metabolic oxygen
    2. Have smaller oxygen reserves
    3. Are susceptible to hypoxia

H. Cardiovascular system (pp. 1596–1597)
    1. Cardiac output is rate-dependent in infants and small children.
    2. Vigorous but limited cardiovascular reserves
    3. Bradycardia in response to hypoxia
    4. Can maintain blood pressure longer than an adult
    5. Circulating blood volume proportionally larger than adults'
    6. Absolute blood volume smaller than adults'
    7. Paramedic implications
        a. Smaller absolute volume of fluid/blood loss needed to cause shock
        b. Larger proportional volume of fluid/blood loss needed to cause shock
        c. Hypotension is a late sign of shock.
        d. A child may be in shock despite normal blood pressure.
        e. Shock assessment is based upon clinical signs of tissue perfusion.
        f. Carefully assess for shock if tachycardia is present.
        g. Monitor carefully for development of hypotension.

I. Nervous system (p. 1597)
    1. Develops throughout childhood
    2. Developing neural tissue is fragile.
    3. Brain and spinal cord less well protected by skull and spinal column
    4. Paramedic implications
        a. Brain injuries more devastating in young children
        b. Greater force transmitted to underlying brain of young children
        c. Spinal cord injury can occur without spinal column injury.

J. Metabolic differences (p. 1597)
  1. Infants and children have limited glycogen and glucose stores.
  2. Significant volume loss can result from vomiting and diarrhea.
  3. Prone to hypothermia due to increased body surface area
  4. Newborns and neonates are unable to shiver to maintain body temperature.
  5. Paramedic implications
     a. Keep child warm during treatment and transport.
     b. Cover the head to minimize heat loss.

VI. General approach to pediatric assessment (pp. 1597–1606)
  A. Basic considerations (p. 1597)
   1. Use "assessment from doorway" patient observation.
   2. Involve parent/caregiver.
   3. Observe parent/caregiver interaction with patient.
  B. Scene size-up (p. 1598)
   1. Observe scene for hazards or potential hazards.
   2. Observe scene for mechanism of injury/illness.
   3. Observe the parent/guardian/caregiver interaction with the child.
  C. Initial assessment (pp. 1598–1603)
   1. General impression
   2. Vital functions (**Table 42-2, p. 1601**)
      a. Level of consciousness
      b. Airway (**Figs. 42-4 and 42-5, p. 1599; Fig. 42-6, p. 1600**)
      c. Breathing (**Fig. 42-7, p. 1600**)
        i. Respiratory rate
        ii. Respiratory effort (**Table 42-3, p. 1602**)
        iii. Color
      d. Circulation
        i. Heart rate
        ii. Peripheral circulation
        iii. End-organ perfusion
   3. Anticipating cardiopulmonary arrest
      a. Respiratory rate greater than 60
      b. Heart rate greater than 180 or less than 80 (under 5 years)
      c. Heart rate greater than 180 or less than 60 (over 5 years)
      d. Respiratory distress
      e. Trauma
      f. Burns
      g. Cyanosis
      h. Altered level of consciousness
      i. Seizures
      j. Fever with petechiae
   4. Transport priority
      a. Urgent
      b. Non-urgent
      c. Pediatric Trauma and Glasgow Coma Scales (**Table 42-4, p. 1603**)
   5. Transitional phase
      a. Allows the infant or child to become familiar with you and your equipment
      b. Use depends on the seriousness of the patient's condition.
      c. Skip transition phase and proceed directly to treatment and transport for unconscious or acutely ill child.
  D. Focused history and physical exam (pp. 1603–1605)
   1. History
      a. For infant, toddler, and preschool-age patient, obtain from parent/guardian.

POINT TO EMPHASIZE
Remember to take appropriate BSI precautions when treating infants and children.

POWERPOINT PRESENTATION
Chapter 42 PowerPoint slides 33–58

POINT TO EMPHASIZE
Airway and respiratory problems are the most common cause of cardiac arrest in infants and young children.

TEACHING STRATEGY 5
Researching an EMSC Project

TEACHING TIP
See if students can explain why younger children require support under the torso to maintain their airways. What is the anatomical difference?

POWERPOINT PRESENTATION
Chapter 42 PowerPoint slides 59–134

POINT TO EMPHASIZE
Never use blind finger sweeps in a pediatric patient.

POINT TO EMPHASIZE
DO NOT use nasal airways on a child with mid-face or head trauma.

TEACHING TIP
Ask students: What is the problem with using these ventilation devices on children?

POINT TO EMPHASIZE
Alternative airways (EOA, PTL, ETC) cannot be used in children. A properly sized laryngeal mask (LMA) can be used in the pediatric patient. However, you should remember that LMAs do not protect the airway from aspiration.

      b. For school-age and adolescent patient, most information may be obtained from patient.
      c. For older adolescent patient, question patient in private regarding sexual activity, pregnancy, and illicit drug and alcohol use.
  2. Physical exam
      a. Head-to-toe in older child
      b. Toe-to-head in younger child
      c. Glasgow Coma Scale (**Table 42-4, p. 1603**)
         i. Mild—GCS 13 to 15
         ii. Moderate—GCS 9 to 12
         iii. Severe—GCS less than or equal to 8
      d. Vital signs
      e. Noninvasive monitoring (**Fig. 42-8, p. 1605**)
         i. Pulse oximeter
         ii. Automated blood pressure devices
         iii. Self-registering thermometers
         iv. ECGs
E. Ongoing assessment (p. 1606)

VII. General management of pediatric patients (pp. 1606–1623)
A. Basic airway management (pp. 1606–1611) (**Table 42-5, p. 1607**)
  1. Manual positioning
  2. Foreign body airway obstruction (FBAO)
      a. Partial obstruction
         i. Place in position of comfort; transport
      b. Complete airway obstruction
         i. Infants
            a) Five back blows, five chest thrusts
         ii. Children
            a) Five abdominal thrusts
  3. Suctioning (**Fig. 42-9, p. 1607**) (**Table 42-6, p. 1607**)
  4. Oxygenation
      a. Nonrebreather mask (**Fig. 42-10, p. 1608**)
      b. Blow-by oxygen if mask is not tolerated
  5. Oropharyngeal airway (**Table 42-7, p. 1609**)
      a. Size by measuring from corner of mouth to front of earlobe.
      b. Use the tongue blade to depress tongue and jaw for insertion. (**Fig. 42-11, p. 1610**)
  6. Nasopharyngeal airway
      a. Use for children who have a gag reflex but require prolonged ventilation.
      b. DO NOT use in patients with head or mid-face trauma.
  7. Ventilation
      a. Avoid excessive bag pressure and volume.
      b. Use properly sized mask. (**Fig. 42-12, p. 1611**)
      c. Obtain chest rise with each breath.
      d. Allow adequate time for exhalation.
      e. Provide 100% oxygen by using BVM reservoir.
      f. Do not use flow-restricted, oxygen-powered ventilation devices in pediatric resuscitation.
      g. Do not use BVMs with pop-off valves unless they can be readily occluded.
      h. Use Sellick maneuver to apply cricoid pressure. (**Fig. 42-13, p. 1611**)
      i. Position to avoid hyperextension of neck.

B. Advanced airway and ventilation management (pp. 1611–1619)
  1. Foreign body clearing methods
  2. Needle cricothyrotomy
  3. Endotracheal intubation
      a. Anatomical and physiological concerns
          i. Creation of a visual plane from mouth to pharynx to glottis is difficult.
          ii. Selection of properly sized tubes is critical.
          iii. Depth of insertion can be estimated based on age. (Table 42-8, p. 1613)
          iv. Narrowing at cricoid cartilage requires use of uncuffed tubes for children less than 8 years old.
          v. Laryngoscopy and passage of an endotracheal tube are likely to cause a vagal response, slowing the heart rate.
      b. Indications
          i. Need for prolonged artificial ventilation
          ii. Inadequate ventilations with a bag-valve mask
          iii. Cardiac or respiratory arrest
          iv. Control of airway in a patient without cough or gag reflex
          v. To obtain a route for drug administration
          vi. Access to the airway for suctioning
      c. Technique (**Fig. 42-14, p. 1616**) (**Proc. 42-1, pp. 1614–1615**)
          i. Tube placement verification, preferably with end-tidal CO_2 detector
          ii. Continuously monitor for tube displacement.
  4. Nasogastric intubation
      a. Indications
          i. Inability to achieve adequate tidal volume during ventilation due to gastric distension
          ii. Presence of gastric distension in unresponsive patient
      b. Contraindicated with head trauma and mid-face trauma
      c. Technique (**Proc. 42-2, p. 1618**)
  5. Rapid sequence intubation
      a. Indications
          i. Advanced airway management required
          ii. Patient has significant level of consciousness or gag reflex.
      b. Medications used are succinylcholine (Anectine) and a sedative agent such as midazolam, diazepam, thiopental, or fentanyl.

C. Circulation (pp. 1619–1621)
  1. Vascular access
      a. Techniques are basically same as in adults.
      b. Additional veins accessible in infants include neck and scalp veins.
  2. Intraosseous infusion (**Fig. 42-15, p. 1620; Fig. 42-16, p. 1621**)
      a. Used for fluids and medications
      b. Indications
          i. Children < 6 years of age
          ii. Existence of shock and cardiac arrest
          iii. Unresponsive patient
          iv. Unsuccessful attempts at peripheral IV insertion
      c. Contraindicated in the presence of fracture in extremity to be used or fracture of pelvis or bone proximal to chosen site
      d. Technique
  3. Fluid therapy
      a. Administer initial dosage of 20 mL/kg of lactated Ringer's or normal saline titrated to perfusion for hypovolemic shock.
      b. Monitor IV infusions closely.

POINT TO EMPHASIZE
NG tube insertion is safest when the airway is protected with an ET tube.

POINT TO EMPHASIZE
There are two problems that lead to cardiopulmonary arrest in children: shock and respiratory failure.

4. Medication objectives
    a. Correction of hypovolemia
    b. Increased perfusion pressure during chest compressions
    c. Stimulation of spontaneous or more forceful cardiac contractions
    d. Acceleration of heart rate
    e. Correction of metabolic acidosis
    f. Suppression of ventricular ectopy
    g. Maintenance of renal perfusion
    h. Dosages (Table 42-9, p. 1622; Table 42-10, p. 1622)
5. Electrical therapy
    a. Used less frequently in pediatric patients than in adults.
    b. Use initial dose of 2 j/kg.
    c. If unsuccessful, increase to 4 j/kg.
    d. If unsuccessful, focus attention on correcting hypoxia and acidosis.
D. C-spine immobilization (pp. 1621–1623)
    1. Special considerations
        a. Spinal injury is less common in children than adults.
        b. The larger head makes cervical spine more vulnerable.
        c. Spinal cord injury can occur without injury to vertebral column.
        d. Children with positive mechanism should be immobilized until evaluated by hospital personnel.
    2. Techniques
E. Transport guidelines (p. 1623) (Fig. 42-17, p. 1623)

VIII. Specific medical emergencies (pp. 1623–1648)

A. Infections (p. 1624)
    1. Account for majority of pediatric illnesses
    2. Varied signs and symptoms, depending on agent and extent of infection
    3. Management
        a. Take all BSI precautions.
        b. Be familiar with common infections in your area.
        c. Be aware of status of your own immunity.
        d. Limit exposure to diseases to which you are not immune.
B. Respiratory emergencies (pp. 1624–1626)
    1. Respiratory distress
        a. Signs and symptoms
            i. Normal mental status deteriorating to irritability and anxiety
            ii. Tachypnea
            iii. Retractions
            iv. Nasal flaring in infants
            v. Good muscle tone
            vi. Tachycardia
            vii. Head bobbing
            viii. Grunting
            ix. Cyanosis that improves with supplemental oxygen
            x. If uncorrected, leads to respiratory failure
    2. Respiratory failure
        a. Assessment
            i. Irritability or anxiety deteriorating to lethargy
            ii. Marked tachypnea later deteriorating to bradypnea
            iii. Poor muscle tone
            iv. Marked tachycardia later deteriorating to bradycardia
            v. Central cyanosis
            vi. Ominous condition; patient is on verge of respiratory arrest

3. Respiratory arrest
    a. Assessment
        i. Unresponsiveness deteriorating to coma
        ii. Bradypnea deteriorating to apnea
        iii. Absent chest wall motion
        iv. Bradycardia deteriorating to asystole
        v. Profound cyanosis
4. Management of respiratory compromise
    a. Use graded approach to treatment based on severity of problem.
    b. Manage upper airway obstructions as needed.
    c. Insert airway adjunct if needed.
    d. Early respiratory failure: administer high-flow oxygen.
    e. Late respiratory failure/respiratory arrest:
        i. Ventilate patient with 100 percent oxygen via age-appropriate sized BVM.
        ii. Intubate patient if positive-pressure ventilation does not rapidly improve condition.
        iii. Consider gastric decompression if abdominal distension is impeding ventilation.
        iv. Consider needle decompression if tension pneumothorax is present.
        v. Consider cricothyrotomy as last resort if complete upper airway obstruction is present.
    f. Obtain venous access.
    g. Transport to appropriate facility.
    h. Provide emotional and psychological support to parents.
C. Specific respiratory emergencies (upper airway obstruction) (pp. 1626–1629)
    1. Croup
        a. Assessment (Table 42-11, p. 1627)
            i. Signs and symptoms of respiratory distress or failure, depending on severity
            ii. Appears sick
            iii. Stridor
            iv. Barking (seal- or dog-like) or brassy cough
            v. Hoarseness
            vi. Low-grade fever
            vii. Usually with history of upper respiratory infection in classic croup (1–2 days)
        b. Management
            i. Maintain airway.
            ii. Administer cool mist oxygen at 4–6 L/min.
            iii. Administer nebulized racemic epinephrine or albuterol.
            iv. Keep child in position of comfort.
            v. Do not agitate patient (no IVs, no BP, etc.).
            vi. Keep parent/caregiver with infant or child if appropriate.
    2. Epiglottitis (Figs. 42-18a and 42-18b, p. 1627)
        a. Assessment (Table 42-11, p. 1627) (Fig. 42-19, p. 1628)
            i. Signs and symptoms of respiratory distress or failure, depending on severity
            ii. Appears agitated, sick
            iii. Stridor
            iv. Muffled voice
            v. Drooling
            vi. Sore throat and pain on swallowing
            vii. High fever
            viii. Usually no previous history but a rapid onset of symptoms (6–8 hours)

TEACHING TIP
Have students compare and contrast croup and epiglottitis.

POINT TO EMPHASIZE
Never attempt to visualize the airway in patients with epiglottitis.

        ix. Can quickly progress to respiratory arrest
    b. Management
        i. Allow parent to administer oxygen. (**Fig. 42-20, p. 1628**)
        ii. Use two-rescuer ventilation with BVM if airway becomes obstructed.
        iii. Attempt intubation with stylet in place if BVM not effective.
        iv. Do not attempt intubation in settings with short transport times.
        v. Know that performing chest compression upon glottic visualization during intubation may produce a bubble at the tracheal opening.
        vi. Consider needle cricothyrotomy per medical direction as a last resort if complete upper airway obstruction is present.
        vii. Allow patient to assume position of comfort.
        viii. Notify hospital of patient status early.
        ix. Do not agitate the patient—no IVs, no BP, do not look in patient's mouth.
        x. Keep the caregiver with the child if appropriate.
3. Bacterial tracheitis
    a. Assessment
        i. Respiratory distress or failure, depending on severity
        ii. Appears agitated, sick
        iii. High-grade fever
        iv. Inspiratory and expiratory stridor
        v. Coughing up pus/mucus
        vi. Hoarse voice
        vii. Pain in throat
        viii. Usually a history of croup in preceding few days
        ix. May progress to respiratory failure or arrest
    b. Management
        i. Assure airway and ventilation.
        ii. Administer oxygen (possibly by blow-by).
        iii. With complete obstruction or respiratory failure/arrest: Use BVM ventilation, intubation, endotracheal suctioning.
        iv. Use high pressure as required to adequately ventilate.
        v. Do not agitate the patient—no IVs, no BP. Do not look in patient's mouth.
        vi. Keep caregiver with child if appropriate.
4. Foreign body aspiration—upper airway
    a. Assessment—partial obstruction
        i. Signs and symptoms of respiratory distress or failure, depending on severity
        ii. Appears irritable or anxious, but not toxic
        iii. Inspiratory stridor
        iv. Muffled or hoarse voice
        v. Drooling
        vi. Pain in throat
        vii. Usually a history of choking if observed by adult
    b. Management—partial obstruction
        i. Place patient in sitting position.
        ii. Deliver oxygen by nonrebreather mask or blow-by.
        iii. Do not attempt to look in mouth.
        iv. Interventions other than oxygen and transport may precipitate complete obstruction.
    c. Assessment—complete obstruction
        i. Signs and symptoms of respiratory failure or arrest, depending on severity

- ii. Appears agitated or lethargic
- iii. No or minimal air movement
- iv. History often lacking
- v. Inability to ventilate despite proper airway positioning
- d. Management—complete obstruction
    - i. Open airway and attempt to visualize the obstruction.
    - ii. Sweep *visible* obstructions with your finger; do NOT perform blind finger sweeps.
    - iii. Perform BLS FBAO maneuvers.
    - iv. Attempt BVM ventilations.
    - v. Perform laryngoscopy if BVM is unsuccessful.
    - vi. Remove object if possible with pediatric Magill forceps.
    - vii. Intubate if possible.
    - viii. Continue BLS FBAO maneuvers if ALS is unsuccessful.
    - ix. Consider needle cricothyrotomy as last resort.
    - x. Notify hospital of patient status.
    - xi. Keep caregiver with child, if appropriate.
- D. Specific respiratory diseases (lower airway distress) (pp. 1629–1632)
    1. Asthma
        a. Assessment
            - i. Respiratory distress or failure, depending on severity
            - ii. Anxiety
            - iii. Wheezing
            - iv. Prolonged expiratory phase
            - v. Symptoms usually began following exposure to known trigger.
        b. Management
            - i. Administer oxygen by tolerated method.
            - ii. Use BVM ventilations for respiratory failure/arrest (progressive lethargy, poor muscle tone, shallow respiratory effort).
            - iii. Use endotracheal intubation for respiratory failure/arrest with prolonged BVM ventilations or inadequate response to BVM.
            - iv. Administer nebulized beta-agonists. (Fig. 42-21, p. 1631)
            - v. Give steroids, particularly if transport times are long.
            - vi. Use subcutaneous epinephrine 1:1000 or terbutaline with severe respiratory distress or failure.
            - vii. Allow patient to assume position of comfort.
            - viii. Keep caregiver with child if appropriate.
    2. Bronchiolitis
        a. Assessment
            - i. Signs and symptoms of respiratory distress or failure, depending on severity
            - ii. Anxiety
            - iii. Wheezing
            - iv. Diffuse crackles (rales)
            - v. Usually history of upper respiratory infection symptoms
            - vi. Bronchiolitis and asthma may present very similarly.
        b. Management
            - i. Administer oxygen by tolerated method.
            - ii. Use BVM ventilations for respiratory failure/arrest (progressive lethargy, poor muscle tone, shallow respiratory effort).
            - iii. Use endotracheal intubation for respiratory failure/arrest with prolonged BVM ventilations or inadequate response to BVM ventilations.

POINT TO EMPHASIZE

Status asthmaticus requires immediate transport with aggressive treatment administered en route.

POINT OF INTEREST
Children with pneumonia in the lower lobes of the lungs frequently present with abdominal pain rather than chest pain. Why?

        iv. Administer nebulized bronchodilators.
        v. Monitor cardiac rhythm and oxygen saturation.
        vi. Keep caregiver with child if appropriate.
    3. Pneumonia
      a. Assessment
        i. Signs and symptoms of respiratory distress or failure, depending on severity
        ii. Anxiety
        iii. Decreased breath sounds
        iv. Crackles (rales)
        v. Rhonchi (diffuse or localized)
        vi. Pain in chest
        vii. Fever
        viii. Usually a history of lower airway respiratory infection
      b. Management
        i. Administer oxygen by tolerated method.
        ii. Use BVM ventilations for respiratory failure/arrest (progressive lethargy, poor muscle tone, shallow respiratory effort).
        iii. Use endotracheal intubation for respiratory failure with prolonged BVM ventilations or inadequate response to BVM ventilations.
        iv. Allow patient to assume position of comfort.
        v. Provide emotional, and psychological support to parents.
        vi. Keep caregiver with child if appropriate.
    4. Foreign body lower airway obstruction—lower airway
      a. Assessment
        i. Signs and symptoms or respiratory distress or failure, depending on severity
        ii. Anxiety
        iii. Decreased breath sounds
        iv. Crackles (rales)
        v. Rhonchi (localized or diffuse)
        vi. Pain in chest
        vii. May be a history of choking if witnessed by an adult
      b. Management
        i. Administer oxygen by tolerated method.
        ii. Use BVM ventilations for respiratory failure/arrest (progressive lethargy, poor muscle tone, shallow respiratory effort).
        iii. Use endotracheal intubation for respiratory failure/arrest with prolonged BVM ventilations or inadequate response to BVM ventilations.
        iv. Do not attempt to retrieve foreign body, as it is beyond the reach of Magill forceps.
        v. Allow patient to assume position of comfort.
E. Shock (hypoperfusion) (pp. 1632–1636)
    1. Severity of shock
      a. Compensated (early) shock—signs and symptoms (**Fig. 42-22**, p. 1633)
        i. Irritability or anxiety
        ii. Tachycardia
        iii. Tachypnea
        iv. Weak peripheral pulses, full central pulses
        v. Delayed capillary refill
        vi. Cool, pale extremities
        vii. Systolic blood pressure within normal limits
        viii. Decreased urinary output

POINT TO EMPHASIZE
A slight increase in the heart rate is one of the earliest signs of shock.

POINT TO EMPHASIZE
The hallmark of decompensated shock is a fall in blood pressure (an ominous sign in children).

b. Decompensated shock—signs and symptoms (**Fig. 42-22, p. 1633**)
      i. Lethargy or coma
      ii. Marked tachycardia or bradycardia
      iii. Marked tachypnea or bradypnea
      iv. Absent peripheral pulses, weak central pulses
      v. Markedly delayed capillary refill
      vi. Cool, pale, dusky, mottled extremities
      vii. Hypotension
      viii. Markedly decreased urinary output
      ix. Absence of tears
   c. Irreversible shock
      i. Occurs when treatment is inadequate or is begun too late to prevent significant tissue damage and death.
2. Categories of shock
   a. Hypovolemic shock
      i. Noncardiogenic shock results from loss of extracellular fluid secondary to vomiting, diarrhea, blood loss, and/or burns.
      ii. Treatment involves giving supplemental oxygen, obtaining vascular access, and giving fluid in 20 mL/kg boluses until perfusion is restored.
3. Distributive shock
   a. Distributive shock (septic shock) is caused by infection of bloodstream by a pathogen (usually bacterial).
   b. Distributive shock (anaphylaxis) is caused by exposure to an antigen to which the patient previously has been sensitized.
   c. Distributive shock (neurogenic shock) is caused by sudden peripheral vasodilation due to interruption of nervous control of the peripheral nervous system.
4. Cardiogenic shock
   a. In children usually occurs secondary to another problem, such as drowning or toxic ingestion.
F. Congenital heart disease (pp. 1636–1640)
   a. Primary cause of heart disease in children
   b. Most cases detected at birth, but some problems not discovered until later in childhood
   c. A common symptom is cyanosis resulting from mixing of oxygenated and unoxygenated blood via openings in cardiac septum or between great vessels.
1. Cardiomyopathy
   a. Disease or dysfunction of the heart muscle
   b. Management
      i. Supplemental oxygen
      ii. Vascular access
      iii. Restriction of IV fluids
      iv. Diuretics
      v. Use of pressor agents
2. Dysrhythmias
   a. Generally uncommon in children
   b. Tachydysrhythmias (**Fig. 42-23a, p. 1638**)
      i. Rate is greater than estimated maximum normal heart rate for child.
      ii. Can result from primary heart disease or secondary causes
      iii. Supraventricular tachycardia
      iv. Ventricular tachycardia with a pulse
   c. Bradydysrhythmias (**Fig. 42-23b, p. 1639**)
      i. Most common type of dysrhythmia

POINT TO EMPHASIZE
Septic shock kills!

> **POINT TO EMPHASIZE**
> The diagnosis of febrile seizure should not be made in the field.

> **POINT TO EMPHASIZE**
> Some medical directors prefer lorazepam (Ativan) as the anticonvulsant of choice for pediatric patients with febrile seizures.

        d. Absent rhythm
           i. Asystole
           ii. Ventricular fibrillation/pulseless ventricular tachycardia
           iii. Pulseless electrical activity (**Fig. 42-24, p. 1641**)
    G. Neurologic emergencies (pp. 1640–1643)
        1. Seizures
           a. Common reason for EMS being summoned for pediatric patients
           b. Results from abnormal firing of neurons in brain
           c. Assessment—generalized seizure
               i. Sudden jerking of both sides of the body followed by tenseness and relaxation of the body
               ii. Loss of consciousness
           d. Assessment—focal seizure
               i. Sudden jerking of a part of the body (arm, leg)
               ii. Lip smacking
               iii. Eye blinking
               iv. Staring
               v. Confusion
               vi. Lethargy
           e. Management
               i. Evaluate
                   a) Adequacy of respirations
                   b) Level of consciousness
                   c) Neurological signs
                   d) Evidence of injury
                   e) Status of hydration
               ii. Maintain patent airway.
               iii. Place patient on side.
               iv. Do not place anything in mouth.
               v. Prevent injury.
               vi. Administer high-flow oxygen.
               vii. If patient is febrile, remove excess clothing but avoid extreme cooling.
               viii. Check blood glucose levels. Give dextrose if hypoglycemic.
               ix. If status epilepticus, give diazepam or lorazepam.
               x. If seizure appears to be due to fever and a long transport time is anticipated, consider acetaminophen elixir or suppositories.
        2. Meningitis
           a. Infection of the meninges, the lining of the brain and spinal cord
           b. Types
               i. Viral
                   a) Aseptic meningitis
               ii. Bacterial
                   a) *Streptococcus pneumoniae*
                   b) *Haemophilus influenzae*
                   c) *Neisseria meningitides*
           c. Assessment
               i. History of recent ear or respiratory tract infection
               ii. High fever
               iii. Lethargy or irritability
               iv. Severe headache
               v. Stiff neck
               vi. Infants may not develop stiff neck, but will become lethargic, will not feed well, and may have a bulging anterior fontanelle.
           d. Management
               i. Supportive care

- ii. Rapid transport to hospital
- iii. 20 mL/kg fluid boluses if shock present
- **H.** Gastrointestinal emergencies (pp. 1643–1644)
  1. Nausea and vomiting
     - **a.** Not diseases in themselves, but symptoms of other diseases
     - **b.** Assessment (Table 42-12, p. 1644)
     - **c.** Management
       - i. Supportive care
       - ii. Vascular access if patient unable to keep fluids down
       - iii. For severe dehydration, 20 mL/kg boluses of LR or NS
  2. Diarrhea
     - **a.** Common occurrence in childhood
     - **b.** Generally considered to be 10 or more stools a day
     - **c.** Usually a result of viral gastroenteritis or secondary to infection elsewhere in body
     - **d.** Management
       - i. Supportive care
       - ii. Vascular access if dehydration present
       - iii. For severe dehydration, 20 mL/kg boluses of LR or NS
- **I.** Metabolic emergencies (pp. 1644–1646)
  1. Hypoglycemia
     - **a.** Usually seen in newborn infants and in children with Type I diabetes
     - **b.** Assessment
       - i. Measure blood glucose. (Fig. 42-25, p. 1645)
     - **d.** Management
       - i. Monitor ABCs.
       - ii. Determine if caregivers have given any glucose-containing material before EMS arrived.
       - iii. Check blood glucose level.
       - iv. If patient is conscious and alert, give oral glucose or glucose-containing fluids.
       - v. If no response or if patient has altered mental status:
         - a) Administer $D_{25}W$ intravenously.
         - b) Administer glucagon IM if IV access is not possible.
         - c) Repeat blood glucose test 10–15 minutes after dextrose infusion.
       - vi. Provide emotional and psychological support to caregivers and patient.
       - vii. Avoid labeling test results as "good" or "bad."
  2. Hyperglycemia
     - **a.** Abnormally high concentration of blood sugar
     - **b.** Most common finding in new-onset diabetics
     - **c.** Early assessment (Table 42-13, p. 1646)
       - i. Increased thirst
       - ii. Increased urination
       - iii. Weight loss
     - **d.** Late assessment (dehydration and early ketoacidosis)
       - i. Weakness
       - ii. Abdominal pain
       - iii. Generalized aches
       - iv. Loss of appetite
       - v. Nausea
       - vi. Vomiting
     - **e.** Measure blood glucose
       - i. > 200 mg/dL indicates hyperglycemia

POINT TO EMPHASIZE
Hypoglycemia is a true medical emergency that must be treated immediately.

POINT TO EMPHASIZE
Diabetic ketoacidosis is a very serious medical emergency that may quickly deteriorate into coma.

f. Management
      i. Monitor ABCs and vital signs.
      ii. Establish vascular access.
      iii. Give 20 mL/kg boluses of IV fluid titrated to vital signs and mental status.
      iv. Be prepared to intubate if patient's respirations decrease.
      v. If patient's blood glucose level cannot be determined reliably and there is uncertainty as to whether patient is hypo- or hyperglycemic, give glucose.
J. Poisoning and toxic exposure (pp. 1646–1648)
   1. Common substances of pediatric poisonings
   2. Assessment (**Fig. 42-26, p. 1648**)
      a. Signs and symptoms vary depending upon both the poisoning/toxic substance and the time since the child was exposed.
      b. Respiratory system depression
      c. Circulatory system depression
      d. Central nervous system stimulation or depression
      e. Alterations of thought or behavior
      f. Gastrointestinal system irritation
   3. Management—responsive patient
      a. Give oxygen.
      b. Contact medical control and/or poison center.
      c. Consider need for activated charcoal.
      d. Transport patient and product.
      e. Monitor patient continuously.
   4. Management—unresponsive patient
      a. Assure patent airway, suction as needed.
      b. Give oxygen.
      c. Be prepared to assist ventilations.
      d. Contact medical control and/or poison center.
      e. Transport.
      f. Monitor patient continuously.
      g. Rule out trauma as cause of altered mental status.

IX. **Trauma emergencies** (pp. 1648–1656)

A. Mechanisms of injury (pp. 1649–1651)
   1. Falls
      a. Single most common cause of injury in children (**Fig. 42-27, p. 1649**)
      b. Serious injury or death resulting from truly accidental falls is relatively uncommon unless from a significant height.
   2. Motor-vehicle collisions (**Fig. 42-28, p. 1650**)
      a. Leading cause of permanent brain injury and new cases of epilepsy
      b. Leading cause of death and serious injury in children
   3. Car versus pedestrian injuries
   4. Drownings and near-drownings
      a. Third leading cause of injury or death in children between birth and 4 years old
   5. Penetrating injuries
   6. Burns
      a. Leading cause of accidental death in the home for children under 14 years old
   7. Physical abuse
      a. Factors influencing
         i. Increased poverty
         ii. Domestic disturbance

POINT TO EMPHASIZE
Trauma is the number one cause of death in children.

POWERPOINT PRESENTATION
Chapter 42 PowerPoint slides 146–153

           iii. Younger-aged parents
           iv. Substance abuse
            v. Community violence
        b. All cases must be thoroughly documented
  B. Special considerations (pp. 1651–1654)
     1. Airway control (**Fig. 42-29, p. 1652**)
        a. Maintain in-line stabilization in neutral, not sniffing, position.
        b. Administer 100% oxygen to all trauma patients.
        c. Maintain patent airway via suctioning and jaw thrust.
        d. Be prepared to assist ineffective respirations.
        e. Perform intubation when airway remains inadequate. (**Fig. 42-30, p. 1652**)
        f. Place gastric tube after intubation.
        g. Know that needle cricothyrotomy is rarely indicated for traumatic upper airway obstruction.
     2. Immobilization
        a. Use appropriate-sized pediatric immobilization equipment.
        b. Maintain supine neutral in-line position for infants, toddlers, and preschoolers by placing padding from shoulders to hips.
     3. Fluid management
        a. Management of the airway and breathing take priority over management of circulation because circulatory compromise is less common in children than adults.
        b. Vascular access
            i. Insert large-bore intravenous catheter into a large peripheral vein.
           ii. Do not delay transport to gain access.
          iii. Use intraosseous access in children < 6 years of age if intravenous access fails.
           iv. Administer initial fluid bolus of 20 mL/kg of LR or NS.
            v. Reassess vital signs and re-bolus with 20 mL/kg if no improvement.
           vi. If improvement does not occur after the second bolus, there is likely to be significant blood loss and the need for rapid surgical intervention.
     4. Pediatric analgesia and sedation
        a. Frequently overlooked aspect of care
        b. Indications for analgesia include burns, long bone fractures, and locations.
        c. Meperidine, morphine, and fentanyl are common choices.
        d. Butorphanol, and nalbuphine have unpredictable effects on children.
        e. Indications for sedation include penetrating eye injuries, prolonged rescues, cardioversion, and painful procedures.
     5. Traumatic brain injury
        a. Early recognition and aggressive management can reduce mortality and morbidity.
        b. Signs of increased intracranial pressure
            i. Elevated blood pressure
           ii. Bradycardia
          iii. Rapid, deep respirations (Kussmaul) progressing to slow, deep respirations alternating with rapid, deep respirations (Cheyne-Stokes)
           iv. Bulging fontanelle (infant)
        c. Specific management
            i. Administer high-concentration oxygen for mild to moderate head injuries (GCS 9–15).

   ii. Intubate and ventilate at normal breathing rate with 100% oxygen for severe head injuries (GCS 3–8).
    a. Use of lidocaine may blunt rise in ICP (controversial).
    b. Consider RSI per medical direction.
 C. Specific injuries (pp. 1654–1656)
  1. Head, face, and neck injury
   a. Larger relative mass of the head and lack of neck muscle strength contribute to increased momentum in acceleration-deceleration injuries and a greater stress to the cervical spine region.
   b. 60 to 70 percent of pediatric fractures occur in C-1 or C-2.
   c. Head injury is the most common cause of death in pediatric trauma victims.
   d. Soft tissues, skull, and brain are more compliant in children than in adults.
   e. Due to open fontanelles and sutures, infants up to an average age of 16 months may be more tolerant of an increase in intracranial pressure and can have delayed signs.
   f. Subdural bleeds in an infant can produce hypotension (extremely rare).
   g. Significant blood loss can occur through scalp lacerations and should be controlled immediately.
   h. The modified Glasgow Coma Scale should be used for infants and young children.
  2. Chest injury
   a. Chest injuries in children under 14 years of age are usually the result of blunt trauma.
   b. Due to the compliance of the chest wall, severe intrathoracic injury can be present without signs of external injury.
   c. Tension pneumothorax is poorly tolerated and is an immediate threat to life.
   d. Flail segment is an uncommon injury in children; when noted without a significant mechanism of injury, suspect child abuse.
   e. Many children with cardiac tamponade will have no physical signs of tamponade other than hypotension.
  3. Abdominal injury
   a. Musculature is minimal and poorly protects the viscera.
   b. The organs most commonly injured are liver, kidney, and spleen.
   c. Onset of symptoms may be rapid or gradual.
   d. Due to the small size of the abdomen, be certain to palpate only one quadrant at a time.
   e. Any child who is hemodynamically unstable without evidence of obvious source of blood loss should be considered as having an abdominal injury until proven otherwise.
  4. Extremity injury
   a. Relatively more common in children than adults
   b. Flexible bones tend to result in incomplete breaks (bend, buckle, and greenstick fractures).
   c. Growth plate injuries are common and may lead to permanent disability.
   d. Compartment syndrome is an emergency in children.
   e. Any sites of active bleeding must be controlled.
   f. Splinting should be performed to prevent further injury and blood loss.
   g. PASG may be useful in unstable pelvic fractures with hypotension.
  5. Burns
   a. Second leading cause of death in children

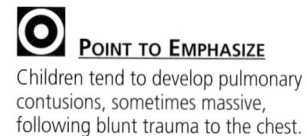

POINT TO EMPHASIZE
Children tend to develop pulmonary contusions, sometimes massive, following blunt trauma to the chest.

POINT TO EMPHASIZE
Burns are the second leading cause of death in children.

- **b.** Leading cause of accidental death in the home in children under age 14
- **c.** Thermal, electrical, and chemical mechanisms
- **d.** Scalding is the most common cause.
- **e.** Rule of nines must be modified to account for child's larger head size. **(Fig. 42-31, p. 1656)**
- **f.** Rule of palm can be used to estimate size of smaller burns.
- **g.** Management priorities
    - **i.** Prompt management of the airway is required, as swelling can develop rapidly.
    - **ii.** If intubation is required, an endotracheal tube up to two sizes smaller than what would normally be used may be required.
    - **iii.** Thermally burned children are very susceptible to hypothermia; maintain normal body temperature.
    - **iv.** Suspect musculoskeletal injuries in electrical burn patients and perform spine immobilization techniques.

X. Sudden infant death syndrome (SIDS) (pp. 1656–1657)

A. Epidemiology (pp. 1656–1657)
1. Sudden death of infant during first year of life from an illness of unknown etiology
2. Leading cause of death from 2 weeks to 1 year old
3. Prevention strategies
    - **a.** Infants should sleep in supine position.
    - **b.** Avoid overwrapping infants.
    - **c.** Avoid smoking before and after pregnancy.
    - **d.** Avoid filling cribs with soft bedding.

B. Assessment (p. 1657)
1. No external signs of injury
2. Lividity
3. Frothy, blood-tinged drainage from nose/mouth
4. Rigor mortis
5. Evidence that the baby was very active just prior to death (rumpled bed clothes, unusual position or location in the bed)

C. Management (p. 1657)
1. Initiate CPR unless the infant is obviously dead (unquestionably dead to a layperson).
2. Perform ALS as indicated.
3. Be prepared for the range of possible family emotional reactions.
4. Parents/caregiver should be allowed to accompany baby in ambulance.
5. Explain that certain information about infant's health is necessary to determine care to be given.
6. Use the baby's name.
7. Phrase questions so that blame is not implied.
8. Critical incident stress debriefing of responders may be needed.

XI. Child abuse and neglect (pp. 1657–1661)

A. Epidemiology (p. 1657)
1. Leading cause of death in infants less than 6 months old
2. Between 2,000 and 5,000 children die each year due to abuse and neglect.

B. Perpetrators of abuse or neglect (pp. 1657–1658)
1. Parent, legal guardian, foster parent; person, institution, agency, or program having custody of the child; person serving as a caretaker (e.g., babysitter)

POWERPOINT PRESENTATION
Chapter 42 PowerPoint slide 154

POINT TO EMPHASIZE
At all points in a SIDS case, use the baby's name when speaking with parents or caregivers.

POINT TO EMPHASIZE
In SIDS, active and aggressive care should continue until delivery to the ER unless the infant is obviously dead.

POWERPOINT PRESENTATION
Chapter 42 PowerPoint slides 155–160

2. Perpetrators can come from any geographic, religious, ethnic, racial, occupational, educational, or social background.
C. Types of abuse (pp. 1658–1659) (**Fig. 42-32, p. 1658; Fig. 42-33, p. 1659**)
 1. Physical
 2. Emotional
 3. Sexual
D. Assessment of potentially abused or neglected child (pp. 1659–1660)
 1. Physical indicators of abuse (**Figs. 42-34 to 42-36, p. 1660**)
    a. Obvious or suspected fractures in child less than 2 years old
    b. Multiple injuries in various stages of healing, especially burns and bruises
    c. More injuries than usually seen in children of same age and size
    d. Injuries scattered on many areas of body
    e. Bruises or burns in patterns that suggest intentional infliction
    f. Increased intracranial pressure in infants
    g. Suspected intraabdominal trauma in a young child
    h. Any injury that does not fit the description given of the cause
 2. Indicators of abuse in the history
    a. History does not match nature or severity of injury.
    b. History is vague or changes during the interview.
    c. Accusations that child injured himself intentionally
    d. Delay in seeking help
    e. Child dressed inappropriately for situation
    f. Revealing comments by bystanders, especially siblings
 3. Indicators of neglect
    a. Extreme malnutrition
    b. Multiple insect bites
    c. Long-standing skin infections
    d. Extreme lack of cleanliness
    e. Verbal or social skills far below those expected of a child of similar age and background
    f. Lack of appropriate medical care
E. Management of the potentially abused or neglected child (p. 1660)
 1. Assess the injuries/neglect and render appropriate care.
 2. Look at the environment for condition and cleanliness.
 3. Look for evidence of anything out of the ordinary.
 4. Look and listen to caregiver/family members.
 5. Assess whether the explanation fits the injury.
 6. Do not "cross-examine" the parents.
 7. Try to be supportive of parents if this will help you to transport the child.
 8. Never leave transport to the alleged abuser.
 9. Document all findings thoroughly.
 10. Report suspicions to appropriate personnel.
F. Resources for abuse and neglect (p. 1661)
 1. State, regional, and local child protection agencies
 2. Hospital social service department

XII. Infants and children with special needs (pp. 1661–1664)

A. Types (p. 1661)
 1. Premature babies
 2. Lung diseases
 3. Heart diseases
 4. Neurological diseases
 5. Chronic diseases

POINT TO EMPHASIZE
Never leave transport of an abused child to an alleged abuser.

POWERPOINT PRESENTATION
Chapter 42 PowerPoint slides 161–162

a. Cystic fibrosis
  b. Asthma
  c. Childhood cancers
  d. Cerebral palsy
 6. Altered functions from birth
  a. Cerebral palsy
  b. Spina bifida
B. Common home care devices (pp. 1661–1663)
 1. Tracheostomy tube (Fig. 42-37, p. 1662)
  a. Complications may include
   i. Obstruction
   ii. Bleeding
   iii. Air leak
   iv. Dislodgement
   v. Infection
  b. Management
   i. Maintain an open airway.
   ii. Suction the tube, as needed.
   iii. Maintain position of comfort.
   iv. Give oxygen if respiratory distress is present.
   v. Intubation orally in absence of upper airway obstruction.
   vi. Intubate via stoma if upper airway obstruction is present.
   vii. Transport.
 2. Apnea monitors
  a. Used to alert parents and caregivers to cessation of breathing in an infant
 3. Home artificial ventilators
  a. Complications include
   i. Mechanical failure
   ii. Power outages
  b. Management
   i. Assure airway.
   ii. Artificially ventilate with BVM and oxygen.
   iii. Transport.
 4. Central venous lines
  a. Intravenous lines that are placed in superior vena cava for long-term use
  b. Uses
   i. Antibiotics
   ii. Chemotherapy
   iii. IV nutrition
  c. Complications
   i. Cracked line
   ii. Infection
   iii. Clots
   iv. Bleeding
   v. Air embolism
  d. Management
   i. If cracked line
    a) Clamp between crack and patient.
   ii. If altered mental status following cracked line
    a) Position on left side with head down.
   iii. If bleeding
    a) Apply pressure.
   iv. Transport.
 5. Gastric feedings and gastrostomy tubes
  a. Tubes placed directly into stomach for feeding

POINT TO EMPHASIZE
Most parents who have infants on apnea monitors have received training in pediatric CPR.

    b. Complications
        i. Bleeding at site
        ii. Dislodged tube
        iii. Respiratory distress secondary to aspiration
        iv. Altered mental status in diabetics due to missed feedings.
    c. Management
        i. Assure adequate airway.
        ii. Administer 100 percent oxygen.
        iii. Suction if needed.
        iv. Consider hypoglycemia in diabetic patient who cannot be fed.
        v. Transport sitting or lying on right side, head elevated.
  6. Shunts
    a. Device running from the brain to abdomen to drain excess cerebrospinal fluid
    b. Complications
        i. Shunt connections may separate due to child's growth.
        ii. Increase in intracranial pressure occurs, producing altered mental status, respiratory distress, posturing.
    c. Management
        i. Manage airway.
        ii. Assure adequate artificial ventilation.
        iii. Transport with head elevated if possible.
C. General assessment and management procedures (pp. 1663–1664)
  1. Patients with special needs require same assessment as other patients.
  2. The child's special need is often an ongoing process.
  3. Concentrate on the acute problem.
  4. Ask the parent or caregiver, "What unusual situation caused you to call an ambulance?"
  5. Most parents or caregivers will be very knowledgeable about the patient's condition.
  6. Avoid using the term "disability."
  7. Never assume the patient cannot understand what you are saying.
  8. Involve the parents or caregivers and the patient.
  9. Treat the patient with a special need with the same respect as any other patient.

XIII. Chapter summary (p. 1664). Pediatric emergencies can be stressful for both you and the adults responsible for the child's well-being. Most pediatric emergencies result from trauma, respiratory distress, ingestion of poisons, or febrile seizure activity. In addition, you must always be on the lookout for signs and symptoms of child abuse or neglect. The approach and management of pediatric emergencies must be modified for the age and size of the child. Certain skills generally considered routine, such as IV administration, become difficult in the pediatric patient because of size and other factors. It is important to remember that children are not "small adults." They have special considerations—both physical and emotional—that must be managed accordingly.

SKILLS DEMONSTRATION AND PRACTICE

Students can practice the skills discussed in this chapter in the following settings.

Skills Lab One: Divide the class into as many groups as appropriate. Have the groups circulate through the stations. Monitor the groups to be sure that all groups have a chance to practice each of the skills.

POINT TO EMPHASIZE
In most cases, concentrate on the acute problem rather than the ongoing special need.

POWERPOINT PRESENTATION
Chapter 42 PowerPoint slide 163

ADVANCED LIFE SUPPORT SKILLS
Larmon & Davis. *Advanced Life Support Skills.*

ADVANCED LIFE SKILLS REVIEW
Larmon & Davis. *Advanced Life Skills Review.*

BRADY SKILLS SERIES: ALS
Larmon & Davis. *Brady Skills Series: ALS.*

Station	Equipment and Personnel Needed	Activities
Station 1-1	Stethoscopes	After demonstrating how to perform a pediatric assessment, have students perform an initial assessment, taking vital signs and identifying IV and IO sites on an infant, toddler, preschooler, grade-school-aged child, and adolescent.
Pediatric Assessment	Blood pressure cuffs	Children of instructors, students, or community members may be recruited to serve as models. They should be accompanied by a parent, and a consent form should be signed by the parent agreeing to the physical exam and accepting responsibility for the child's supervision during the workshop.
	Chairs for parents and children "Exam" table Blankets Pen lights Rewards for children (crayons, books, Legos) Toys/snacks for children to play with/eat during station time 1 instructor 1 infant 1 preschooler 1 grade-school-aged child 1 adolescent	
Station 1-2	Child mannequins	After demonstrating basic life support techniques, have each student practice and demonstrate one-rescuer infant and child CPR, two-rescuer child CPR, infant FBAO management, and child FBAO management. Demonstration should be kept simple to reinforce the priorities and techniques of CPR.
Basic Life Support	Infant mannequins Alcohol wipes Extra lungs CPR skills sheets	

(continued)

Station	Equipment and Personnel Needed	Activities
Station 1-3 Pediatric Airway Adjuncts	Infant mannequins Child mannequins Infant, child, and adult bag-valve-mask devices Oropharyngeal airways: 00, 0, 1, 2, 3, 4 Suction devices: Bulb syringe, DeLee suction, tonsil-tip suction device, meconium aspiration adaptor, and standard suction catheters (5, 6, 8, 10, 14 French) Pediatric and adult oxygen masks Pediatric and adult nasal cannulas Pocket masks	After demonstrating pediatric airway adjuncts, have each student give return demonstrations of the use of oxygen delivery systems, oral airways, bag-valve-mask devices, and suctioning devices.
Station 1-4 Endotracheal Intubation	Infant intubation mannequins Child intubation mannequins Bag-valve-mask device for each mannequin Stethoscopes Tape Laryngoscope handles Laryngoscope blades: Curved 2, 3; Straight 0, 1, 2, 3 Endotracheal tubes: 2.5, 3.0, 3.5, 4.0, 4.5, 5.0, 6.0, 6.5, 7.0 Stylets of appropriate sizes Pediatric and adult Magill forceps	After demonstrating endotracheal intubation, have each student give a return demonstration of proper intubation technique for an infant and child.

Station	Equipment and Personnel Needed	Activities
Station 1-5	Equipment for peripheral IV	After demonstrating peripheral vascular access, have each student give a return demonstration of pediatric vascular access techniques, including:
Peripheral	Over-the-needle catheters: 18-, 20-, 22-, 24-gauge	1. Cannulation of an arm vein
Vascular Access	Butterfly needles: 19-, 21-, 23-, 25-gauge	2. Cannulation of a scalp vein
	Pediatric IV arms Model head for scalp vein IV insertion IV solutions 3-cc syringes Solution administration sets Alcohol prep pads Tourniquets Materials for securing IVs: arm boards, tape Sharps container IV poles Equipment for intraosseous infusion Raw chicken legs Bone marrow needles 5-cc syringes Exam gloves Flush solution (250-cc bag of NS)	3. Placement of an intraosseous line
Station 1-6	Long backboard with attached straps	After demonstrating pediatric immobilization, have students demonstrate effective techniques for adapting adult equipment to immobilizing children.
Pediatric	Short spinal immobilization device (preferably a KED)	
Immobilization	2-inch tape Blankets Pediatric cervical collars: small, medium, and large Towels Pillows Scissors Infant car seat Infant mannequin 1 child, age 4 to 8	

WORKBOOK
Chapter 42 Activities

READING/REFERENCE
Textbook, pp. 1667–1714

HANDOUT 42-2
Chapter 42 Quiz

HANDOUT 42-3
Chapter 42 Scenario

PARAMEDIC STUDENT CD
Student Activities

COMPANION WEBSITE
http://www.prenhall.com/bledsoe

TESTGEN
Chapter 42

EMT ACHIEVE:
PARAMEDIC TEST PREPARATION
Mistovich & Beasley. *EMT Achieve: Paramedic Test Preparation.*
www.prenhall.com/emtachieve/

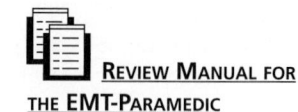

REVIEW MANUAL FOR THE EMT-PARAMEDIC
Cherry & Mistovich. *Review Manual for the EMT-Paramedic,* 3rd edition.

HANDOUTS 42-4 TO 42-7
Reinforcement Activities

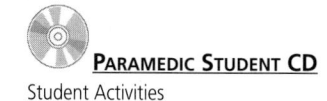

PARAMEDIC STUDENT CD
Student Activities

POWERPOINT PRESENTATION
Chapter 42

COMPANION WEBSITE
http://www.prenhall.com/bledsoe

ONEKEY
Chapter 42

ADVANCED LIFE SUPPORT SKILLS
Larmon & Davis. *Advanced Life Support Skills.*

ADVANCED LIFE SKILLS REVIEW
Larmon & Davis. *Advanced Life Skills Review.*

BRADY SKILLS SERIES: ALS
Larmon & Davis. *Brady Skills Series: ALS.*

PARAMEDIC NATIONAL STANDARDS SELF-TEST
Miller. *Paramedic National Standards Self-Test,* 4th edition.

Hospital: Begin patient assessments in emergency department.

Field Internship: Begin patient assessments on simple emergency calls.

ASSIGNMENTS

Assign students to complete Chapter 42, "Pediatrics," of the workbook. Also assign them to read Chapter 43, "Geriatric Emergencies," before the next class.

EVALUATION

Chapter Quiz and Scenario Distribute copies of the Chapter Quiz provided in Handout 42-2 to evaluate student understanding of this chapter. Make sure each student reads the scenario to reinforce critical thinking on the scene. Remind students not to use their notes or textbooks while taking the quiz.

Student CD Quizzes for every chapter are contained on the dynamic and highly visual in-text student CD.

Companion Website Additional quizzes for every chapter are contained on this exciting website.

TestGen You may wish to create a custom-tailored test using *Prentice Hall TestGen for Essentials of Paramedic Care,* 2nd Edition to evaluate student understanding of this chapter.

On-line Test Preparation (for students and instructors) Additional test preparation is available through Brady's new on-line product, *EMT Achieve: Paramedic Test Preparation* at *http://www.prenhall.com/emtachieve/.* Instructors can also monitor student mastery on-line.

Review Manual for the EMT-Paramedic This comprehensive exam review contains hundreds of test questions and rationales, including scenarios, along with two 180-question practice tests on CD.

REINFORCEMENT

Handouts If classroom discussion or performance on the quiz indicates that some students have not fully mastered the chapter content, you may wish to assign some or all of the Reinforcement Handouts for this chapter.

Student CD (for students) A wide variety of material on this CD-ROM will reinforce and also expand student knowledge and skills.

PowerPoint Presentation (for instructors) The PowerPoint material developed for this chapter offers useful reinforcement of chapter content.

Companion Website (for students) Additional review quizzes and links to EMS resources will contribute to further reinforcement of the chapter.

OneKey On-line support is offered for this course on one of three platforms: CourseCompass, Blackboard, or Web CT. Includes the IRM, PowerPoints, TestGen, and Companion Website for instruction. Ask your local sales representative for more information.

Brady Skills Series: Advanced Life Skills (Video or CD) Have your students watch the skills come to life on VHS or CD-ROM, or they can purchase the highly visual, full-color text with step-by-step procedures and rationales.

HANDOUT 42-1

Student's Name _____

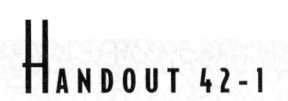

CHAPTER 42 OBJECTIVES CHECKLIST

Knowledge	Date Mastered
1. Discuss the paramedic's role in the reduction of infant and childhood morbidity and mortality from acute illness and injury.	
2. Identify methods/mechanisms that prevent injuries to infants and children.	
3. Describe Emergency Medical Services for Children (EMSC) and how it can affect patient outcome.	
4. Identify the common family responses to acute illness and injury of an infant or child.	
5. Describe techniques for successful interaction with families of acutely ill or injured infants and children.	
6. Identify key anatomical, physiological, growth, and developmental characteristics of infants and children and their implications.	
7. Outline differences in adult and childhood anatomy, physiology, and "normal" age-group-related vital signs.	
8. Describe techniques for successful assessment and treatment of infants and children.	
9. Discuss the appropriate equipment used to obtain pediatric vital signs.	
10. Determine appropriate airway adjuncts, ventilation devices, and endotracheal intubation equipment; their proper use; and complications of use for infants and children.	
11. List the indications and methods of gastric decompression for infants and children.	
12. Define pediatric respiratory distress, failure, and arrest.	
13. Differentiate between upper airway obstruction and lower airway disease.	
14. Describe the general approach to the treatment of children with respiratory distress, failure, or arrest from upper airway obstruction or lower airway disease.	
15. Discuss the common causes and relative severity of hypoperfusion in infants and children.	
16. Identify the major classifications of pediatric cardiac rhythms.	

©2007 Pearson Education, Inc.
Essentials of Paramedic Care, 2nd ed.

HANDOUT 42-1 Continued

Knowledge	Date Mastered
17. Discuss the primary etiologies of cardiopulmonary arrest in infants and children.	
18. Discuss age-appropriate sites, equipment, techniques, and complications of vascular access for infants and children.	
19. Describe the primary etiologies of altered level of consciousness in infants and children.	
20. Identify common lethal mechanisms of injury in infants and children.	
21. Discuss anatomical features of children that predispose or protect them from certain injuries.	
22. Describe aspects of infant and child airway management that are affected by potential cervical spine injury.	
23. Identify infant and child trauma patients who require spinal immobilization.	
24. Discuss fluid management and shock treatment for infant and child trauma patients.	
25. Determine when pain management and sedation are appropriate for infants and children.	
26. Define child abuse, child neglect, and sudden infant death syndrome (SIDS).	
27. Discuss the parent/caregiver responses to the death of an infant or child.	
28. Define children with special health care needs and technology-assisted children.	
29. Discuss basic cardiac life support (CPR) guidelines for infants and children.	
30. Integrate advanced life support skills with basic cardiac life support for infants and children.	
31. Discuss the indications, dosage, route of administration, and special considerations for medication administration in infants and children.	
32. Discuss appropriate transport guidelines for low- and high-risk infants and children.	
33. Describe the epidemiology, including the incidence, morbidity/mortality, risk factors, prevention strategies, pathophysiology, assessment, and treatment of infants and children with: • Respiratory distress/failure • Hypoperfusion • Cardiac dysrhythmias	

HANDOUT 42-1 Continued

Knowledge	Date Mastered
• Neurologic emergencies • Trauma • Abuse and neglect • Special health-care needs, including technology-assisted children • SIDS	
34. Given several preprogrammed simulated pediatric patients, provide the appropriate assessment, treatment, and transport.	

Handout 42-2

Student's Name _____

CHAPTER 42 QUIZ

Write the letter of the best answer in the space provided.

_____ 1. You respond to a private residence to find a 4-month-old infant with a fractured humerus. Your examination also reveals numerous bruises and abrasions in various stages of healing on the child's back and buttocks and what appear to be cigarette burns on the child's palms and soles. The child's mother says the fracture was a result of the infant's rolling off the bed onto the floor. You should:
   A. call the police and have the mother arrested for child abuse.
   B. lecture the mother sternly about her treatment of the child.
   C. transport the child and report your suspicions to the physician at the emergency department.
   D. keep what you suspect to yourself, because you may be liable if you falsely report child abuse.

_____ 2. Headache, seizures, a stiff neck, bulging fontanelles, and a rash consisting of tiny pin-point hemorrhages under the skin indicate:
   A. meningitis.   C. pneumonia.
   B. epiglottitis.   D. laryngotracheobronchitis.

_____ 3. The patient is a 5-year-old female who developed severe respiratory distress with inspiratory stridor about 30 minutes ago. Her mother tells you that the patient "seemed to be perfectly healthy" until about 3 hours earlier when she began to complain of a severe sore throat. The patient is sitting on the side of her bed leaning forward with her neck slightly extended. Respiratory distress with accessory muscle use and intercostal retractions is present. The child is drooling profusely, and when she tries to talk, her voice sounds "muffled." She is suffering from a life-threatening emergency due to potential:
   A. seizures.   C. airway obstruction.
   B. cardiac dysrhythmias.   D. respiratory arrest.

_____ 4. The patient is a 3-year-old male who awakened about 10 minutes ago with respiratory distress and stridor. He is sitting bolt upright in bed. Accessory muscle use and intercostal retractions are present, but drooling is absent. Cyanosis of the lips and nailbeds is present. The patient coughs frequently, producing a sound similar to a seal's bark. When he attempts to talk, he sounds very hoarse. His mother tells you that the patient has had a cold with a low-grade fever for "2 or 3 days." The treatment for this patient would include:
   A. systemic drug therapy with 1:1000 epinephrine.
   B. intubation and high-concentration oxygen.
   C. humidified oxygen and nebulized bronchodilators.
   D. systemic drug therapy with aminophylline.

_____ 5. The patient is a 7-year-old female who experienced a sudden onset of coughing and expiratory wheezing about 20 minutes ago. She has no history of pulmonary or cardiovascular disease. She states that she was eating peanuts immediately prior to the onset of the symptoms and that she "almost choked on one." Auscultation of her chest reveals localized wheezing in the right lung field. She is most likely suffering from:
   A. an acute asthma attack.
   B. anaphylaxis.
   C. aspiration of a foreign body into the lower airways.
   D. pneumonia.

HANDOUT 42-2 Continued

_____ 6. To select the proper size pediatric endotracheal tube, choose one that is:
  A. the same size as the patient's age in months.
  B. the same size as the patient's little finger.
  C. as long as the distance from nose to ear.
  D. the same size as the base of the child's thumb.

_____ 7. The patient is a 3-month-old infant who suddenly developed cyanosis and audible expiratory wheezing. Retractions and nasal flaring with a respiratory rate of 80/minute are present. The patient's mother reports that he has had a mild cold with a cough for 2 or 3 days. The patient has had a low-grade fever. There is no family history of asthma or allergies. The initial treatment of choice for this patient would be:
  A. epinephrine 1:1000 SC.
  B. humidified oxygen.
  C. nebulized racemic epinephrine.
  D. immediate endotracheal intubation.

_____ 8. Before administering epinephrine to a patient who is having an asthma attack, you should always obtain a medication history from the patient because:
  A. the patient may already have severe cardiac irritability from an overdose of bronchodilators from a home inhaler.
  B. medication in inhalers tends to antagonize the effects of epinephrine.
  C. the combination of epinephrine with drugs the patient has already taken may worsen bronchospasm.
  D. the combination of epinephrine with drugs the patient has already taken may slow the patient's heart.

_____ 9. To defibrillate a child, you should use pediatric paddles. If for some reason these special paddles are not available, you would use adult paddles. Which of the following positions best explains how you modify paddle placement in this situation?
  A. below right clavicle; at apex
  B. below right nipple; below left nipple
  C. anterior thorax; posterior thorax
  D. below left clavicle; at apex

_____ 10. Status epilepticus refers to:
  A. a severe seizure that cannot be stopped with diazepam.
  B. two or more seizures without a period of consciousness between them.
  C. a very mild type of seizure that is caused by fever.
  D. a type of grand mal seizure produced by hypoglycemia.

_____ 11. A prolonged asthma attack that cannot be broken with epinephrine is:
  A. status asthmaticus.
  B. beta-resistant primary bronchospasm.
  C. status epilepticus.
  D. sympathorefractory asthma.

_____ 12. The purpose of administering humidified oxygen in the treatment of asthma is to:
  A. dilate the bronchi.
  B. avoid drying of mucus secretions in the airway.
  C. increase the respiratory rate.
  D. correct alveolar dehydration.

_____ 13. Bronchiolitis is best described as a:
  A. viral infection causing inflammation of the larynx, trachea, and bronchi.
  B. bacterial infection causing inflammation of the bronchioles.
  C. bacterial infection causing inflammation of the larynx, trachea, and bronchi.
  D. viral infection causing inflammation of the bronchioles.

EVALUATION

HANDOUT 42-2 Continued

_____ 14. Asthma is best described as an:
   A. obstructive pulmonary disease characterized by distention of the pulmonary air spaces with destructive changes in their walls.
   B. obstructive pulmonary disease characterized by episodes of severe bronchospasm, bronchial edema, and hypersecretion of mucus in the lower airways.
   C. obstructive pulmonary disease characterized by excessive mucus production in the bronchial tree with a chronic productive cough.
   D. inflammation of the bronchioles caused by a viral infection.

_____ 15. Croup is best described as a:
   A. bacterial infection causing inflammation of the larynx.
   B. viral infection causing inflammation of the larynx.
   C. bacterial infection causing inflammation of the oropharynx and epiglottis.
   D. viral infection causing inflammation of the oropharynx and epiglottis.

_____ 16. The initial endotracheal dose of epinephrine for cardiac arrest in children is:
   A. 0.01 mg/kg of 1:10,000 solution.   C. 0.01 mg/kg of 1:1000 solution.
   B. 0.1 mg/kg of 1:10,000 solution.   D. 0.1 mg/kg of 1:1000 solution.

_____ 17. The initial intravenous dose of epinephrine for cardiac arrest in children is:
   A. 0.01 mg/kg of 1:10,000 solution.   C. 0.1 mg/kg of 1:10,000 solution.
   B. 0.01mg/kg of 1:1000 solution.   D. 0.1 mg/kg of 1:1000 solution.

_____ 18. The usual dose of lidocaine for ventricular fibrillation in children is:
   A. 0.01 mg/kg.   C. 0.3 mg/kg.
   B. 0.5 mg/kg.   D. 1.0 mg/kg.

_____ 19. The most common cause of death following seizures is:
   A. hyperthermia.   C. dehydration.
   B. anoxia.   D. head injury.

_____ 20. Which of the following groups of activities best describes the prehospital management of a patient with epiglottitis?
   A. Restrain the patient in a supine position and intubate immediately.
   B. Administer humidified oxygen, allow the patient to assume the most comfortable position, and transport.
   C. Administer humidified oxygen for 5 minutes, and start a TKO IV if doing this does not increase the patient's distress, and attempt to intubate.
   D. Administer humidified oxygen, establish an IV with LR wide open, allow the patient to assume the most comfortable position, and transport.

_____ 21. The least desirable vein to use during CPR is a(n):
   A. scalp vein.   C. femoral vein.
   B. antecubital vein.   D. saphenous vein.

_____ 22. Which of the following combinations of laryngoscope blades and endotracheal tubes should be used when intubating a 2-year-old?
   A. straight blade; uncuffed tube   C. straight blade; cuffed tube
   B. curved blade; uncuffed tube   D. curved blade; cuffed tube

_____ 23. The patient is a 6-month-old infant found unconscious by his mother. The infant has no pulse, no blood pressure, and no respirations. You and another EMT should begin CPR using a rate of at least:
   A. 100/minute; ratio 30:2.   C. 100/minute; ratio 30:2.
   B. 100/minute; ratio 15:2.   D. 80/minute; ratio 30:2.

HANDOUT 42-2 Continued

_____ 24. Cardiac arrest in infants and children usually results from:
   A. heart attack.
   B. respiratory failure or arrest.
   C. electric shock.
   D. drowning.

_____ 25. How many watt-seconds should be used initially to defibrillate a 12-kg infant?
   A. 25 watt-seconds
   B. 50 watt-seconds
   C. 100 watt-seconds
   D. 200 watt-seconds

_____ 26. The initial attempt to defibrillate a 30-kg child is unsuccessful. How many watt-seconds should be used to repeat the defibrillation of the child?
   A. 60 watt-seconds
   B. 120 watt-seconds
   C. 300 watt-seconds
   D. 360 watt-seconds

_____ 27. Which of the following actions is associated with diazepam?
   A. anticonvulsant
   B. antiarrhythmic
   C. bronchodilator
   D. antihistamine

_____ 28. The patient is a 4-year-old female who received an electrical shock. The child has no pulse and no respirations. While your partner prepares equipment, you begin one-rescuer CPR using a rate of:
   A. at least 100/minute; ratio 15:2
   B. 100/minute; ratio 15:2
   C. 100/minute; ratio 5:1
   D. 100/minute; ratio 30:2

_____ 29. If an infant has a complete airway obstruction not relieved by back blows, the rescuer should:
   A. administer five abdominal thrusts.
   B. administer five additional back blows.
   C. administer five chest thrusts.
   D. perform a finger sweep.

_____ 30. Before beginning chest compressions on an infant, you should check for the presence of a pulse at which artery?
   A. temporal
   B. carotid
   C. brachial
   D. femoral

_____ 31. Before beginning chest compressions on a child, you should check for the presence of a pulse at which artery?
   A. temporal
   B. carotid
   C. brachial
   D. femoral

_____ 32. When compressing the chest of a child, use the:
   A. tips of the index and middle fingers of one hand.
   B. heel of one hand.
   C. heels of both hands.
   D. thumbs of both hands.

_____ 33. Which of the following statements best defines sudden infant death syndrome (SIDS)?
   A. The sudden, unexplained, and unexpected death of an infant prior to an autopsy to determine cause of death.
   B. The sudden, unexplained, and unexpected death of an infant where a thorough autopsy fails to reveal the cause of death.
   C. The sudden, unexpected death of an infant where the autopsy reveals the cause of death to be cardiovascular disease.
   D. The sudden, unexpected death of an infant in its sleep caused by suffocation in the bed clothing.

HANDOUT 42-2 Continued

_____ 34. Which of the following statements about asthma and bronchiolitis is correct?
   A. Asthma usually is associated with a family history of the disease, while bronchiolitis is not.
   B. Bronchiolitis is common in infants less than 1 year of age, but asthma is uncommon in that age group.
   C. Asthma produces generalized wheezes, but bronchiolitis produces localized wheezes.
   D. both A and B

_____ 35. Assessment of a patient who is having an asthma attack would include examination for:
   A. state of consciousness, general appearance, vital signs, respiratory movement, skin turgor, dryness of mucous membranes.
   B. state of consciousness, vital signs, general appearance, respiratory movement, pedal edema.
   C. state of consciousness, general appearance, vital signs, respiratory movement, abdominal rebound tenderness.
   D. general appearance, state of consciousness, vital signs, respiratory movement, jugular vein distention.

_____ 36. Differences in the anatomy of the airway that warrant differences in intubation techniques for infants and adults include:
   A. the infant's tongue being larger in relation to other structures in the airway.
   B. the glottis being higher in the infant than in the adult.
   C. the epiglottis being narrower in the infant and its vocal cords slanting upward and backward.
   D. all of these

_____ 37. In which of the following age groups does sudden infant death syndrome (SIDS) most commonly occur?
   A. birth to 2 weeks
   B. 2 months to 4 months
   C. 6 months to 12 months
   D. 12 months to 18 months

_____ 38. What question(s) would be appropriate to ask about a child who has had a seizure?
   A. Does the child have a history of previous seizures, head trauma, diabetes, recent headache, or stiff neck?
   B. Is the child taking any medications?
   C. How many seizures has the child had, and what did they look like?
   D. all of these

_____ 39. Which of the following statements about specific age groups of pediatric patients is correct?
   A. 2- to 3-year-olds are usually cooperative and like to be touched by strangers.
   B. 4- to 5-year-olds are usually cooperative and like to "help out" the paramedic.
   C. School-age children usually do not like to be told what is being done to them.
   D. Adolescents usually are not concerned about lasting effects of injury or illness.

_____ 40. The endotracheal tube used in infant intubation is not cuffed because of anatomical differences in the infant's:
   A. pharynx.
   B. trachea.
   C. glottis.
   D. mandible.

_____ 41. What procedure would be appropriate when examining a toddler?
   A. Decide which parts of the physical exam are essential and get through them as quickly as possible.
   B. Establish ground rules, for example, "It's all right to cry, but not to bite or kick."
   C. Obtain as much information as possible before touching the child.
   D. all of these

HANDOUT 42-2 Continued

_____ 42. The patient is a 5-year-old child who is in respiratory arrest. The child should be ventilated once every:
   A. 3 seconds.
   B. 4 seconds.
   C. 5 seconds.
   D. 6 seconds.

_____ 43. How many times a minute should an infant who is not breathing be ventilated?
   A. 10
   B. 15
   C. 20
   D. 30

_____ 44. A patient with epiglottitis would typically exhibit:
   A. inspiratory stridor, pain on swallowing, high fever, and drooling.
   B. expiratory wheezing, coughing, crackles, and cyanosis.
   C. inspiratory stridor, "seal-bark" cough, low-grade fever, and orthopnea.
   D. expiratory wheezing, rales, coughing, high fever.

_____ 45. A patient with laryngotracheobronchitis would typically exhibit:
   A. inspiratory stridor, pain on swallowing, high fever, drooling.
   B. expiratory wheezing, coughing, crackles, cyanosis.
   C. inspiratory stridor, "seal-bark" cough, low-grade fever, orthopnea.
   D. expiratory wheezing, crackles, coughing, high fever.

_____ 46. Which of the following age groups is usually associated with croup?
   A. 0 to 6 months
   B. 6 months to 4 years
   C. 4 years to 12 years
   D. Over 12 years

_____ 47. The physical exam of a child who has had a seizure should include a check for:
   A. level of consciousness.
   B. evidence of fever or dehydration.
   C. signs of an injury that caused or was caused by the seizures.
   D. all of these

_____ 48. Which group of pediatric patients would generally be expected to be uncooperative?
   A. 2 to 3 years old
   B. 4 to 5 years old
   C. 6 to 10 years old
   D. 10 to 14 years old

_____ 49. A pediatric patient is seen by paramedics for a seizure. The child has a fever of 101°F, was lethargic and irritable before the seizure, and has had no previous seizure activity. The child complained of a headache earlier in the day. What is the most likely problem?
   A. febrile seizure
   B. meningitis
   C. hypoglycemia
   D. hypoxia

_____ 50. You are called to see a 6-month-old infant. The mother's chief complaint is that the child has been irritable for the last few days, is not feeding well, is sweaty, and is "just not acting right." On exam, you find a fussy infant who wants the bottle. Respirations are 40/min. The skin is pink but is cool distally. Capillary refill is 2 seconds. Pulses are very rapid at about 300/min. The ECG shows a narrow complex tachycardia with no P waves visible. You should:
   A. administer oxygen and transport.
   B. cardiovert immediately at 0.5 to 1 j/kg.
   C. administer verapamil.
   D. administer 20 mL/kg lactated Ringer's solution.

HANDOUT 42-2 Continued

51. You respond to a mottled, cyanotic 3-month-old 5-kg infant who responds only to painful stimuli. Proximal pulses are too rapid to count and thready proximally. Distal pulses are absent. The skin is pale and cold distally. Capillary refill is 5 seconds. Respirations are 65/minute, and the patient is working hard to breathe. ECG shows a narrow complex tachycardia with no P waves visible. You should:
    A. administer oxygen and transport.
    B. cardiovert at 0.5 to 1 j/kg.
    C. administer verapamil.
    D. administer 20 mL/kg lactated Ringer's solution.

52. You are called to evaluate an 8-month-old infant with a 5-day history of vomiting and diarrhea. Mom states that the infant is "not acting right." On initial observation, you note a lethargic infant with mottled skin and no spontaneous movement. Respirations are 60, unlabored. Pulse is 170, weak. Capillary refill is 4 seconds. Extremities are cool. The ECG shows a narrow complex tachycardia. P waves are visible and the rhythm is slightly irregular. You should:
    A. administer oxygen and transport.
    B. cardiovert at 0.5 to 1 j/kg.
    C. administer verapamil.
    D. administer 20 mL/kg lactated Ringer's solution.

53. A 2-year-old male fell into a swimming pool and was submersed for about 2 minutes. The child is unresponsive, cyanotic, apneic, and pulseless. A firefighter who first responded on an engine is performing CPR. You are not able to quickly obtain vascular access, but you are able to place an endotracheal tube. EKG shows a sinus bradycardia with a rate of 32. You should:
    A. start an intraosseous line immediately.
    B. administer 0.01 mg/kg epinephrine 1:10,000 down the endotracheal tube.
    C. administer 0.1 mg/kg epinephrine 1:1000 down the endotracheal tube.
    D. administer 0.02 mg/kg atropine down the endotracheal tube.

54. A 5-year-old boy was struck by an automobile when he ran into the street from between two parked cars. He is pale, confused, and sweating heavily. Capillary refill time is 5 seconds. Breath sounds are present bilaterally. The upper left quadrant of the abdomen is bruised and tender. Fluid resuscitation should consist of:
    A. two large-bore IVs with lactated Ringer's infused as rapidly as possible.
    B. a single IV with lactated Ringer's to avoid overhydrating the child.
    C. 20 mL/kg of lactated Ringer's while monitoring him for signs of improved perfusion.
    D. two large-bore IVs of D_5W infused as rapidly as possible, because lactated Ringer's should not be given to small children.

55. Children and infants who are burned are more likely to suffer more significant fluid loss than adults because:
    A. a larger portion of a pediatric patient's body mass consists of water.
    B. IVs cannot be established as easily.
    C. their body surface area is larger in proportion to their body volume.
    D. crying associated with pain and anxiety will add to volume loss.

56. A 3-year-old and his brother were walking along a frozen irrigation ditch. The 3-year-old tried to retrieve a dropped toy and fell through the ice. He is apneic and pulseless with fixed, dilated pupils. No one knows how long he was underwater. ECG shows asystole. You should:
    A. start CPR immediately and transport.
    B. call for the police and the coroner.
    C. attempt to rewarm the patient as rapidly as possible.
    D. transport without doing CPR.

HANDOUT 42-2 Continued

_____ 57. A 4-month-old male infant has been vomiting and having watery diarrhea for two days. His mother says the infant has not urinated at all today. The baby's lips and oral mucosa are dry, and his fontanelles are sunken. The infant's extremities are cold to the elbows and knees. Capillary refill is 5 seconds. Heart rate is 170. ECG shows a narrow complex tachycardia with P waves visible. Management should include:
  A. infusion of 20 mL/kg lactated Ringer's.
  B. cardioversion at 0.5 to 1 j/kg.
  C. checking a dex stik with possible administration of $D_{25}W$ for hypoglycemia.
  D. both A and C

_____ 58. A 3-year-old female ingested six 0.25 mg digoxin tablets about 2 hours ago. She is awake, alert, and taking the bottle. Pulse is 50, strong, regular. Respirations are 30, regular, unlabored. Capillary refill is less than 2 seconds. Skin is pink and warm. BP is 90 by palpation. ECG shows a sinus bradycardia with a first-degree AV block. You should administer:
  A. 0.2 mg/kg atropine IV push.
  B. 0.01 mg/kg epinephrine IV push.
  C. 5 mg/kg calcium chloride IV push.
  D. oxygen by blow-by, then monitor and transport.

_____ 59. Indications that an intraosseous line has been successfully placed include which of the following?
  A. A change in resistance is felt as the marrow cavity is entered.
  B. The needle stands on its own without support.
  C. Bone marrow can be aspirated from the needle.
  D. all of these

_____ 60. You are called to see a 9-month-old baby who has stopped breathing. The mother's boyfriend is babysitting and states that the infant fell off the couch. The baby is lying in the crib. There are no obvious signs of trauma. The child is lethargic and breathing slowly at a rate of 8 per minute. Skin is warm, and capillary refill is normal. Heart rate is 140. The left pupil is dilated and fixed. The right pupil is mid-position and reactive. Linear bruises are present on both upper arms. Management of the infant should include all of the following EXCEPT:
  A. stabilization of the cervical spine.
  B. intubation and hyperventilation with high-concentration oxygen.
  C. infusion of 20 mL/kg of lactated Ringer's solution.
  D. reporting of possible child abuse to the ER physician.

_____ 61. A 15-year-old male has been involved in a swimming accident at a spot that is popular with local teenagers. The boy was reported to have jumped or dove from a rock outcropping into the river. He did not surface immediately and was pulled from the water a few minutes later about 25 yards downstream. The patient is unresponsive. His respiratory rate is 8/minute. His heart rate is 120/minute. His extremities are cold. Management should include all of the following EXCEPT:
  A. opening of the airway with a jaw thrust and stabilization of the cervical spine.
  B. drying and wrapping in warm blankets.
  C. assisted ventilations with a bag-valve mask and oxygen, followed by possible endotracheal intubation.
  D. administration of sodium bicarbonate to correct acidosis.

HANDOUT 42-2 Continued

_____ 62. All of the following statements about the physical assessment of a patient with an acute asthma attack are true EXCEPT:
   A. Sleepiness or stupor indicates severe hypercarbia, hypoxia, and acidosis.
   B. The disappearance of wheezing during a severe asthma attack is a good sign, because it indicates that bronchospasm has stopped.
   C. Tenting of the skin and dryness of the mucous membranes can indicate dehydration due to the asthma attack.
   D. Young children may not show the positional preferences of older children.

_____ 63. You are called to see a 6-year-old child because he has a very high fever. His mother tells you that he became ill about 4 hours ago and has been complaining of a severe sore throat. He will not eat or drink because he says it hurts to swallow. You find the child sitting upright in bed, crying and drooling noticeably. He appears very frightened. His axillary temperature is 104 degrees. His respirations are 30 and shallow, and there is flaring of his nostrils on inhalation. His chest is clear to auscultation. All of the following are part of the management of this child EXCEPT:
   A. administering high-concentration, humidified oxygen.
   B. deferring starting an IV, because this may worsen the patient's distress.
   C. carefully examining the throat to determine whether inflammation is present.
   D. transporting the child in the sitting position.

_____ 64. A call comes in late at night for a sick child. When you arrive, a very distraught mother tells you that her 6-year-old son has been "having fits." He has been ill today with an upper respiratory infection and about half an hour ago began having seizures. He has had three seizures so far. The mother did not notice how the seizures started. You find the child apparently asleep on his bed. He is difficult to arouse. As you examine him, his eyes suddenly open and deviate sharply to the right, and he rapidly develops another generalized tonic-clonic seizure. All of the following should be considered EXCEPT:
   A. administration of high-concentration, humidified oxygen.
   B. placing a bite-block between his teeth to protect his tongue.
   C. checking a blood glucose level and giving glucose if he is hypoglycemic.
   D. administering diazepam to terminate the seizures.

_____ 65. You are called to see a 3-year-old child who is in moderate respiratory distress. His mother says he has appeared well during the day, but for the past two nights he has been waking up around midnight with a high-pitched cough that sounds like a dog barking. You find the child lying in bed, looking very tired and miserable. Axillary temperature is 99.7°F. Respirations are stridorous at 30 per minute, with suprasternal retractions and accessory muscle use. On auscultation of the chest, no wheezing or crackles are heard. All of the following would be included in the management of this patient EXCEPT:
   A. administration of high-concentration, humidified oxygen.
   B. performing direct laryngoscopy to be sure the airway is not obstructed.
   C. administering racemic epinephrine by nebulizer.
   D. transporting to the hospital in the position of comfort.

HANDOUT 42-3

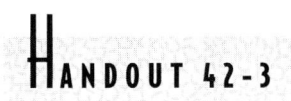

Student's Name _____

CHAPTER 42 SCENARIO

Review the following real-life scenario. Then answer the questions that follow.

At 2330 hours you are called to evaluate a 2-year-old male with a 5-day history of vomiting and diarrhea. The patient's mother says that she called because the child "is not acting right." On initial observation, you note that the child has mottled skin and no spontaneous movement. He is unresponsive to painful stimuli. Respirations are 60/minute, shallow, and regular. Radial pulses are absent. Carotid pulse is 170, weak, and regular. Capillary refill is 5 seconds. The patient's extremities are cool. The ECG shows a narrow complex tachycardia with at rate of 170. P waves are visible.

1. What problem does the patient appear to have?

2. What is the significance of the patient's cool, mottled skin?

3. Why is the patient tachypneic?

4. When you attempt to start an IV on this patient, you cannot find any veins. What alternative route is available for vascular access?

5. How do you know you have achieved vascular access via this route?

6. Once you have achieved vascular access, what method would you use to infuse fluid? Why?

7. You decide to endotracheally intubate the patient. How would you select the proper endotracheal tube size?

Handout 42-4

Student's Name _____

CHAPTER 42 REVIEW

Write the word or words that best complete each sentence in the space(s) provided.

1. In assessing and treating pediatric patients, it is important to keep in mind that they are not simply _____ _____.

2. The federally funded program aimed at improving the health of pediatric patients who suffer from life-threatening illnesses and injuries is _____ _____ _____ for _____.

3. Foremost in approaching any pediatric emergency is consideration of the patient's _____ and _____ development.

4. When assessing or treating a pediatric patient, always use _____ that is appropriate for the age of the child.

5. An infant up to 1 month of age is known as a(n) _____.

6. Infants should have _____ their birth weight by 5 or 6 months of age.

7. _____ are the leading cause of injury deaths in patients aged 1 to 15 years.

8. When examining school-age children, give _____ the responsibility of providing the history.

9. If you must perform a detailed physical exam on an adolescent patient, respect the patient's sense of _____.

10. The pediatric patient's head is proportionally _____ than the adult's, and the occipital region is significantly _____.

11. A child's larynx is _____ than an adult's and extends into the _____.

12. Pediatric patients are prone to _____ because of their greater BSA-to-weight ratio.

13. The three components of the _____ _____ _____ are appearance, breathing, and circulation.

14. _____ and _____ problems are the most common cause of cardiac arrest in infants and children.

15. The normal respiration rate for a preschooler is _____ to _____ breaths per minute.

16. For a patient under 5 years, one of the signs of a risk of cardiopulmonary arrest is a heart rate greater than _____ or less than _____ per minute.

17. A "severe" patient would be one with a Glasgow Coma Scale score of less than or equal to _____.

18. _____ is a late and often sudden sign of cardiovascular decompensation in pediatric patients.

19. For infants less than 1 year old with foreign body airway obstruction, deliver 5 _____ _____, followed by 5 _____ _____.

20. Never do _____ _____ _____ in infant or child FBAO patients.

21. Never use a(n) _____ _____ on a child with mid-face or head trauma.

22. The length of an endotracheal tube for a patient 4 to 6 years old should be _____ cm measured from the teeth to the mid-trachea.

23. When intubating a pediatric patient, you should use a laryngoscope with a(n) _____ blade.

24. If gastric distention is present in a pediatric patient, consider placement of a(n) _____ _____.

1024 ESSENTIALS OF PARAMEDIC CARE

HANDOUT 42-4 Continued

25. One indication for intraosseous infusion is a child patient less than _____ _____ old.
26. The initial dosage of fluid in a pediatric patient suffering from hypovolemia should be _____ of an isotonic fluid.
27. The last stage of respiratory compromise, to which the patient will progress if not treated, is respiratory _____.
28. The viral infection common in children from 6 months to 4 years of age that usually occurs in fall and winter months is _____.
29. If the pediatric patient with epiglottitis is maintaining the airway, do not put anything _____ _____ _____.
30. In severe asthma attacks, an ominous sign is a lack of _____.
31. Common causes of lower airway distress include FBAO, asthma, bronchiolitis, and _____.
32. A slight increase in _____ _____ is one of the earliest signs of shock in the pediatric patient.
33. The child in septic shock may require _____ therapy.
34. _____ _____ _____ is an abnormality or defect in the heart that is present at birth.
35. Most of the pediatric seizures that paramedics encounter are _____.
36. Bacteria and viruses can cause the infection of the GI system known as _____.
37. In the prehospital setting, hypoglycemia in pediatric patients usually results from _____ _____ diabetes.
38. Most poisonings treated by EMS result from accidental _____.
39. _____ are the single most common cause of injury in children.
40. The second leading cause of death in infants less than 6 months of age is _____ _____.

Handout 42-5

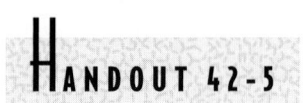

Student's Name _____

CHAPTER 42 SHORT ANSWER A

Answer each of the following questions.

1. Why do infants and small children require special precautions to prevent them from becoming cold?
2. Match the age group with the typical characteristics of that group.

    Adolescents _____

    Toddlers _____

    School-age children _____

    Preschoolers _____

    a. Dislike strange people; strong assertiveness; high mobility, low common sense

    b. Totally subjective worldview; think magically; do not separate fantasy and reality; intense fear of injury, pain, blood loss

    c. Master environment through information; can make compromises, think objectively

    d. Seeking self-determination; fragile self-esteem; very acute body image; high need for modesty

3. What is the most common form of shock in pediatric patients?
4. What are the fontanelles? What change occurs in the fontanelles of a dehydrated infant?
5. What is status asthmaticus?
6. Why should skin turgor be checked in patients who are having an asthma attack?
7. Why is it important to determine the medications taken by an asthmatic prior to beginning any therapy?
8. Why should oxygen be humidified when it is administered to an asthma patient?
9. What is the prehospital treatment for croup?
10. What is the principal danger facing a patient with epiglottitis?

Handout 42-6

Student's Name _____

CHAPTER 42 SHORT ANSWER B

Answer each of the following questions.

1. What is the proper finger position for performing chest compressions on an infant?
2. What are the proper depth and rate for chest compressions on an infant? On a child?
3. How is hypovolemic shock corrected in pediatric patients? Why is this technique used?
4. Should flow-restricted, oxygen-powered breathing devices (demand valves) be used to ventilate children? Why?
5. How is the proper size of endotracheal tube selected for pediatric patients?
6. Why are uncuffed endotracheal tubes used on infants and children less than 8 years old?
7. What is the suggested initial setting for defibrillation of pediatric patients? What energy is used on subsequent shocks?
8. What three routes are available for drug administration to children during cardiopulmonary arrest?
9. What drug is always used FIRST in the management of symptomatic bradycardia in pediatric patients?
10. What is the initial IV dose of epinephrine in pediatric cardiac arrest?

PEDIATRIC CARE SCENARIOS

Answer each of the following questions.

1. A 6-month-old infant was found unconscious and unresponsive. The baby's skin is cool and pale. Capillary refill is greater than 5 seconds. Radial pulses are absent. Carotid and femoral pulses are thready. The ECG shows a narrow complex tachycardia with a rate of 300 and no visible P waves. How would you manage this patient?

2. A 9-month-old infant's mother called you because she says the baby "turns a funny color and sweats" when he feeds and won't take the entire bottle. The infant is awake and alert. His skin is warm and pink. Capillary refill is less than 2 seconds. Radial and pedal pulses are palpable but very fast. How would you manage this patient?

3. A 2-year-old was found floating facedown in a neighbor's swimming pool. He is unconscious and unresponsive. Pulses and respirations are absent. The ECG shows a sinus bradycardia. How would you manage this patient?

4. A 7-month-old infant responds only to painful stimuli. The skin is pale and mottled. Peripheral pulses are weak, and capillary refill is greater than 4 seconds. The infant's respirations are 52 per minute but are unlabored. Rectal temperature is 105°F. What problem do you suspect? How would you manage this patient?

5. An 18-month-old male with a history of nausea, vomiting, and diarrhea for 3 days presents with listlessness and a decreased level of consciousness. Skin and mucous membranes are dry. Skin turgor is decreased. Respirations are rapid and shallow. Peripheral pulses are rapid and weak. Capillary refill is slow. Describe your management of this patient.

Chapter 42 Answer Key

Handout 42-2: Chapter 42 Quiz

1.	C	14.	B	27.	A	40.	B	53.	C
2.	A	15.	B	28.	D	41.	D	54.	C
3.	C	16.	D	29.	C	42.	A	55.	C
4.	C	17.	A	30.	C	43.	C	56.	A
5.	C	18.	D	31.	B	44.	A	57.	D
6.	B	19.	B	32.	B	45.	C	58.	D
7.	B	20.	B	33.	B	46.	B	59.	D
8.	A	21.	A	34.	D	47.	D	60.	C
9.	C	22.	A	35.	A	48.	A	61.	D
10.	B	23.	B	36.	D	49.	B	62.	B
11.	A	24.	B	37.	B	50.	A	63.	C
12.	B	25.	A	38.	D	51.	B	64.	B
13.	D	26.	B	39.	B	52.	D	65.	B

Handout 42-3: Chapter 42 Scenario

1. The patient is suffering from volume depletion (dehydration) and hypovolemic shock.
2. Early in hypovolemic shock, patients vasoconstrict to shunt blood to the body core. As shock persists, compensatory mechanisms begin to fail and dilation begins to occur in localized parts of the periphery. This produces the patchy appearance called mottling. Mottling suggests decompensated shock.
3. Hypoperfusion causes cells to convert to anaerobic metabolism. A byproduct of anaerobic metabolism is lactic acid. This lactic acid is buffered by the carbonate buffer system to produce carbon dioxide. Removal of this carbon dioxide by increased respirations helps compensate for the metabolic acidosis produced by shock.
4. The intraosseous route.
5. Resistance is lost as the needle passes through the cortex of the bone; the needle stands by itself; marrow can be aspirated through the needle; IV fluid will flow freely through the needle.
6. 20 mL/kg boluses of lactated Ringer's or normal saline would be infused. After each bolus, perfusion would be reassessed. This technique restores adequate volume while minimizing the risk of volume overload.
7. Use a device like the Broselow tape; use the formula (age + 16)/4; select a tube the same size as the child's little finger.

Handout 42-4: Chapter 42 Review

1. small adults
2. Emergency Medical Services, Children
3. emotional, psychological
4. language
5. neonate
6. doubled
7. Accidents
8. them (the patients)
9. privacy
10. larger, larger
11. higher, pharynx
12. hypothermia
13. pediatric assessment triangle
14. Airway, respiratory
15. 22, 34
16. 180, 80
17. 8
18. Hypotension
19. back blows, chest thrusts
20. blind finger sweeps
21. nasopharyngeal airway
22. 16
23. straight
24. nasogastric tube
25. 6 years
26. 20 mL/kg
27. arrest
28. croup
29. in the mouth
30. wheezing
31. pneumonia
32. heart rate
33. pressor
34. Congenital heart disease
35. febrile
36. gastroenteritis
37. Type I
38. ingestion
39. Falls
40. child abuse

Handout 42-5: Chapter 42 Short Answer A

1. Infants and small children have a high surface-to-volume ratio; therefore, they tend to lose heat more rapidly than adults.
2. b, d, c, a
3. hypovolemic
4. The fontanelles are areas in the infant's skull that have not yet fused. The fontanelles of a dehydrated infant become sunken.
5. Status asthmaticus is a severe, prolonged asthma attack that cannot be broken by aggressive use of beta adrenergic agonists.
6. Increased respiratory water losses and decreased fluid intake during an asthma attack can lead to dehydration.
7. Asthmatics in distress frequently overuse their inhalers; therefore, an asthmatic may be suffering from increased cardiac irritability from the effects of beta-agonists.
8. If oxygen is not humidified, it will tend to dry the mucus in the asthmatic's airways, worsening the plugging that already is present.
9. Humidified high-concentration oxygen, nebulized racemic epinephrine or albuterol, continuous monitoring of oxygen saturation and ECG, transport. An IV should not be established because it will increase the patient's anxiety.
10. Loss of airway.

Handout 42-6: Chapter 42 Short Answer B

1. One finger-width below the nipple line.
2. Infant: 1/2 to 1 inch at a rate of at least 100 compressions/minute. Child: 1 to 1 1/2 inches at a rate of 100 compressions/minute.

3. With 20 mL/kg fluid boluses, reassessing perfusion between boluses. Because children have smaller cardiovascular systems, they are at increased risk for volume overload.
4. No. Flow-restricted, oxygen-powered breathing devices deliver high pressures and do not allow the operator to feel pulmonary compliance. Therefore, they are more likely to cause pneumothorax in children.
5. Use a length-based resuscitation system such as the Broselow tape; compare the tube to the child's little finger; use the formula (age + 16)/4.
6. The narrowest part of the child's airway is below the glottis at the cricoid ring. This structure forms a functional cuff on the endotracheal tube. If the tube was cuffed, its diameter would have to be so small that resistance to airflow through the tube would be extremely high.
7. 2 j/kg, 4 j/kg
8. endotracheal, intravenous, intraosseous
9. oxygen
10. 0.01 mg/kg of 1:10,000 solution

Handout 42-7: Chapter 42 Pediatric Care Scenarios

1. Give high-concentration oxygen. Perform synchronized cardioversion at 0.5 to 1 j/kg.
2. Give high-concentration oxygen and transport.
3. Begin chest compressions and ventilations with high-concentration oxygen. If child does not respond, place an endotracheal tube. If child still does not respond, establish vascular access and administer epinephrine. Remember that epinephrine also can be given via the endotracheal tube.
4. Septic shock. Give high-concentration oxygen. Establish vascular access. Give 20 mL/kg isotonic crystalloid. Reassess perfusion, respirations, and lung sounds. Repeat fluid boluses until adequate perfusion is restored.
5. Give high-concentration oxygen. Consider assisting ventilations. Establish vascular access. Give 20 mL/kg isotonic crystalloid. Reassess perfusion, respirations, and lung sounds. Repeat fluid boluses until adequate perfusion is restored. Also check blood glucose level. If patient is hypoglycemic secondary to decreased intake, give $D_{25}W$.

Chapter 43

Geriatric Emergencies

INTRODUCTION

Today, approximately one in every eight persons in the United States is over age 65. By the year 2030, one in every four persons will be a member of this age group. The elderly are four times more likely than the nonelderly to use ambulance services. For example, in 1987, 36 percent of ambulance transports to hospital emergency departments were for patients over age 65, and more than 50 percent of all ambulance transports of any kind were for elderly patients. It has been projected that by the year 2030, patients who are 65 or older will represent 70 percent of all ambulance transports. Paramedic students must master the assessment and management of geriatric patients because the practice of paramedics in the twenty-first century will focus heavily on the special problems and needs of the elderly.

CHAPTER OBJECTIVES

After reading this chapter, you should be able to:

1. Discuss the demographics demonstrating the increasing size of the elderly population in the United States. (pp. 1669–1670)
2. Assess the various living environments of elderly patients. (pp. 1670–1671)
3. Discuss society's view of aging and the social, financial, and ethical issues facing the elderly. (pp. 1669–1671)
4. Discuss common emotional and psychological reactions to aging, including causes and manifestations. (pp. 1669–1671)
5. Apply the pathophysiology of multisystem failure to the assessment and management of medical conditions in the elderly patient. (p. 1672)
6. Compare the pharmacokinetics of an elderly patient to that of a young patient, including drug distribution, metabolism, and excretion. (pp. 1672–1673)
7. Discuss the impact of polypharmacy, dosing errors, increased drug sensitivity, and medication noncompliance on assessment and management of the elderly patient. (pp. 1672–1673)
8. Discuss the use and effects of commonly prescribed drugs for the elderly patient. (pp. 1672–1673, 1703–1705)
9. Discuss the problem of mobility in the elderly, and develop strategies to prevent falls. (p. 1673)

TOTAL TEACHING TIME: 9.66 HOURS
The total teaching time is only a guideline based on the didactic and practical lab averages in the National Standard Curriculum. Instructors should take into consideration such factors as the pace at which students learn, the size of the class, and breaks. The actual time devoted to teaching objectives is the responsibility of the instructor.

10. Discuss age-related changes in sensations in the elderly, and describe the implications of these changes for communication and patient assessment. (pp. 1673, 1675–1678)
11. Discuss the problems with continence and elimination in the elderly patient, and develop communication strategies to provide psychological support. (pp. 1674–1675)
12. Discuss factors that may complicate the assessment of the elderly patient. (pp. 1673, 1675–1679)
13. Discuss the principles that should be employed when assessing and communicating with the elderly. (pp. 1673, 1676–1678)
14. Compare the assessment of a young patient with that of an elderly patient. (pp. 1675–1685)
15. Discuss common complaints of elderly patients. (pp. 1672, 1685–1713)
16. Discuss the normal and abnormal changes of age in relation to the:

    - Pulmonary system (pp. 1680–1681)
    - Cardiovascular system (pp. 1681–1682)
    - Nervous system (pp. 1681, 1682–1683)
    - Endocrine system (pp. 1681, 1683)
    - Gastrointestinal system (pp. 1681, 1683–1684)
    - Thermoregulatory system (pp. 1681, 1684)
    - Integumentary system (pp. 1681, 1684)
    - Musculoskeletal system (pp. 1681, 1684)

17. Describe the incidence, morbidity/mortality, risk factors, prevention strategies, pathophysiology, assessment, need for intervention and transport, and management for elderly medical patients with:

    - Pneumonia, chronic obstructive disease, and pulmonary embolism (pp. 1686–1689)
    - Myocardial infarction, heart failure, dysrhythmias, aneurysm, and hypertension (pp. 1689–1692)
    - Cerebral vascular disease, delirium, dementia, Alzheimer's disease, and Parkinson's disease (pp. 1693–1696)
    - Diabetes and thyroid diseases (pp. 1696–1697)
    - Gastrointestinal problems, GI hemorrhage, and bowel obstruction (pp. 1697–1699)
    - Skin diseases and pressure ulcers (pp. 1699–1700)
    - Osteoarthritis and osteoporosis (pp. 1700–1701)
    - Hypothermia and hyperthermia (pp. 1702–1703)
    - Toxicological problems, including drug toxicity, substance abuse, alcohol abuse, and drug abuse (pp. 1703–1706)
    - Psychological disorders, including depression and suicide (pp. 1707–1708)

18. Describe the incidence, morbidity/mortality, risk factors, prevention strategies, pathophysiology, assessment, need for intervention and transport, and management of the elderly trauma patient with:

    - Orthopedic injuries (p. 1712)
    - Burns (pp. 1712–1713)
    - Head injuries (p. 1713)

19. Given several preprogrammed simulated geriatric patients with various complaints, provide the appropriate assessment, management, and transport. (pp. 1669–1713)

FRAMING THE LESSON

Begin by reviewing the important points from Chapter 42, "Pediatrics." Discuss any points that the class does not completely understand. Then move on to Chapter 43. Ask students to describe images that come to mind when they hear the phrases "senior citizen" or "older person." Frequently, EMS students have a very limited range of experience with older people and assume that almost everyone over the age of 65 is confined to a nursing home. Ask students to continue to provide images and impressions until they are describing the entire range of situations in which they are likely to encounter older persons—from the frail, chronically ill patient in the nursing home to the vigorous older adult who has injured himself engaging in a sport normally associated with younger persons. Emphasize to students that providing for the health care needs of the elderly is going to be a critical element of a paramedic's practice in the twenty-first century.

TEACHING STRATEGIES

People learn in a variety of ways. Some do better with the spoken word, whereas others prefer the written. Some prefer to work alone, whereas others profit from working in groups. Recognizing these different ways of acquiring knowledge, the authors of this *Instructor's Resource Manual* have provided a variety of teaching strategies for the different types of learners. These strategies are intended to foster higher-level cognitive skills and encourage creative learning and problem solving. For greatest effectiveness, incorporate these strategies into your class lecture. Symbols in the Lecture Outline indicate the points at which various exercises might be most appropriate. Other strategies can be used to preview the lesson or to summarize it.

The following strategies are keyed to specific sections of the lesson.

1. Interview an Elderly Person. In cooperation with your local senior center or nursing home, have students interview an elderly person. Arm them with a questionnaire that covers such areas as the subject's demographic information, occupations, and education. Be sure to ask additional questions about the person's perspective on issues today such as technology and health care. Discuss the findings of the interviews in class. This activity will lay a foundation of empathy for this unit, broadening each student's perspective on aging.

2. Defining "Old." Ask students to define "when a person becomes old." Many will associate "old" with a number, such as 55 or retirement age. Others will define "old" by the state of mind, such as when a person ceases to socialize or care for him- or herself. Discuss the findings in class. You will likely find that those who have elders close in their lives, such as aging parents or grandparents, respect an elder's knowledge and abilities. In contrast, those with little exposure to the elderly define old by one's illnesses and disabilities.

3. Film Clip: **On Golden Pond.** This movie provides some nice illustrations of changes that take place during the aging process. Show the first 20 minutes, and then ask the students to contrast Henry Fonda's experiences with Katharine Hepburn's.

4. Threats to Elderly. Make a list of threats to the elderly—concerns that plague an aging person. Include topics such as hopelessness, loneliness, loss of independence, lack of choices, institutionalization. Have students create solutions to these concerns in the context of an ambulance call. For example, to combat fear and loneliness, a paramedic could summon a family member to the scene or hospital to sit with the patient during tests and procedures. Or, to empower the patient, allow them to walk to the stretcher if possible, choose which hospital to go to, or gather important belongings prior to leaving the scene. These practices will improve the relationship between patient and provider.

5. Health Care Financing and the Elderly. Paramedics are easily frustrated by patients who do not comply with their medication regime or who fail to seek health care promptly. Help students understand the financial limitations of health care financing and fixed incomes by having each seek health insurance. Give each student a set of demographics and have them use the Internet or an insurance broker to seek health care coverage for their fictitious person. Be sure to compare the cost of coverage and elements covered by their policy. Offer a prize for the most economical and most comprehensive coverage sought. Most likely, everyone will be amazed at the cost and limitations of coverage for older adults.

6. Designing a Safety or Prevention Program. Divide the class into work teams and ask them to design a safety or prevention program that focuses on needs of the elderly. Be sure they address issues of researching the need, identifying the population to be served, financing the project, implementation, data collection and sharing, measuring the impact on the target population, and benefits to EMS providers. These projects should be documented and presented to the class. This activity encourages critical thinking and creative problem solving. Communication skills also are exercised.

7. Explaining the Inconvenience of Aging. Allow students to experience the inconveniences of aging by giving each a disability of aging for the day. Create arthritics by placing Popsicle sticks in the fingers of exam gloves. Imitate cataracts and glaucoma patients by placing clear tape on goggles. The hearing impaired should use disposable earplugs. Emphysema patients can be simulated by wearing a nasal cannula and portable oxygen tank. Be sure to have students do daily activities such as dressing, toileting, eating, and socializing.

The following strategies can be used at various points throughout the lesson or to help summarize and demonstrate what students have learned.

What Might Explain. . .? Encourage students to exercise cause-and-effect thinking by asking them to consider what might explain an event.

Guest Speaker. A number of different options are available for using guest speakers. A gerontologist might discuss the biological and social aspects of the aging process. An internist or family physician with a special interest in geriatrics might be asked to present a program on disease processes affecting a particular organ system. Recognizing elder abuse might be an appropriate topic for a police investigator or adult protective services officer to discuss. Representatives from local or state agencies that provide services to the elderly might be asked to briefly discuss their programs and the resources they have available.

Clinical Rotations. Clinical rotations in nursing homes can provide students with an opportunity to interact with older persons and observe the interplay between normal effects of aging, acute illness, and chronic illness. Rotations with home health services offer students a chance to see older persons living in the community who require varying levels of ongoing health services. A rotation at a community center that serves seniors could give students the chance to interact with older persons who are healthy and living independently and to learn about issues and life changes to which older persons may adapt.

Cultural Considerations, Legal Notes, and Patho Pearls. The Student CD-ROM contains this series of informative features to enhance the student's understanding of the material covered in this chapter.

TEACHING OUTLINE

Chapter 43 is the third lesson in Division 5, *Special Considerations/Operations*. Distribute Handout 43-1 so that the students can familiarize themselves with the learning goals for this chapter. If the students have any questions about the objectives, answer them at this time.

Then present the chapter. One possible lecture outline follows. In the outline, the parenthetical references in regular type are references to text pages; those in bold type are references to figures, tables, or procedures.

I. Introduction. Aging is a complex process that has many implications for EMS, for which it represents a fast-growing number of users. (p. 1669)

II. Epidemiology and demographics (pp. 1669–1671)
  A. Population characteristics (pp. 1669–1670)
    1. Great impact of aging on society
    2. Gerontology
      a. Scientific study of effects of aging and age-related disease on humans
    3. Geriatrics
      a. Study and treatment of diseases of the aged
  B. Societal issues (pp. 1670–1671) (**Fig. 43-1, p. 1670**)
    1. Living environments
      a. Poverty and loneliness
        i. Factors that heavily impact the aged
      b. Social support
        i. Friends and family
          a) Decreasing numbers of each
        ii. Life-care communities
        iii. Congregate care
        iv. Personal-care homes
        v. Independent versus dependent living
    2. Ethics
      a. Advance directives
        i. Applicability to the elderly
      b. Paramedics should follow state laws and local EMS protocols when dealing with the elderly.
  C. Financing and resources for health care (p. 1671)
    1. Government programs
      a. Medicare
      b. Medicaid
      c. Veterans Administration
    2. Health care alternatives
      a. Growing costs of health care need to be contained.
      b. Home care offers possibility of cost cutting.
    3. Prevention and self-help (**Table 43-1, p. 1671**)
      a. Senior centers
        i. Social atmosphere
        ii. Health care endeavors
        iii. Nutrition programs

HANDOUT 43-1
Chapter 43 Objectives Checklist

READING/REFERENCE
Criss, E., and L. Honeycutt. "20 Challenges of Geriatric Care." *JEMS*, April 2000.
Kauder, D. "The Geriatric Puzzle." *JEMS*, July 2000.

POWERPOINT PRESENTATION
Chapter 43 PowerPoint slide 4

POWERPOINT PRESENTATION
Chapter 43 PowerPoint slides 5–17

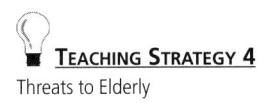

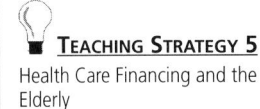

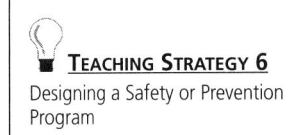

TEACHING STRATEGY 1
Interview an Elderly Person

TEACHING STRATEGY 2
Defining "Old"

TEACHING STRATEGY 3
Film Clip: *On Golden Pond*

TEACHING STRATEGY 4
Threats to Elderly

TEACHING STRATEGY 5
Health Care Financing and the Elderly

TEACHING STRATEGY 6
Designing a Safety or Prevention Program

> **TEACHING STRATEGY 7**
> Explaining the Inconvenience of Aging

> **POWERPOINT PRESENTATION**
> Chapter 43 PowerPoint slides 18–36

> **POINT TO EMPHASIZE**
> The elderly often suffer from more than one illness or disease at a time.

> **POINT TO EMPHASIZE**
> In taking a medical history of an elderly patient, remember to ask if the patient is taking a prescribed medication as directed.

> **POINT TO EMPHASIZE**
> In treating incontinence, remember to respect the patient's modesty and dignity.

> **POINT TO EMPHASIZE**
> Because of the increased risk of tuberculosis in patients who are in nursing homes, consider using a HEPA or N95 respirator.

> **POINT TO EMPHASIZE**
> Try to distinguish the patient's chief complaint from the primary problems.

> **POINT TO EMPHASIZE**
> Be prepared to spend more time obtaining a history from an elderly patient.

  b. Religious organizations
  c. National and state organizations
      i. AARP
      ii. Alzheimer's Association
      iii. Association for Senior Citizens
  d. Government agencies
      i. Local Departments of Health, and so on

III. General pathophysiology, assessment, and management (pp. 1671–1680)

  A. Pathophysiology of the elderly patient (pp. 1672–1675)
    1. Multiple-system failure produces common complaints.
        a. Fatigue/weakness
        b. Dizziness/vertigo/syncope
        c. Falls
        d. Headaches
        e. Insomnia
        f. Dysphagia
        g. Loss of appetite
        h. Inability to void
        i. Constipation/diarrhea
    2. Pharmacology in the elderly
        a. Often use multiple medications for multiple problems
        b. Be alert for problems that may cause lack of compliance with drug programs.
        c. Limited income
        d. Memory loss
        e. Limited mobility
        f. Sensory impairment
        g. Multiple or complicated drug therapies
        h. Fear of toxicity
        i. Childproof containers
        j. Duration of drug therapy
    3. Problems with mobility and falls (contributing factors)
        a. Poor nutrition
        b. Difficulty with elimination
        c. Poor skin integrity
        d. Greater predisposition for falls
        e. Loss of independence and/or confidence
        f. Depression from feeling old
        g. Isolation and lack of social network
    4. Communication difficulties (**Table 43-2, p. 1674**)
    5. Problems with continence and elimination
        a. Incontinence causes
            i. Medical disorders
            ii. Medications
            iii. Age-related physical changes
        b. Elimination (**Table 43-3, p. 1675**)
  B. Assessment considerations (pp. 1675–1679)
    1. Factors in forming general health assessment.
        a. Living situation
        b. Level of activity
        c. Network of social support
        d. Level of independence
        e. Medication history
        f. Sleep patterns

1036   ESSENTIALS OF PARAMEDIC CARE

2. General health assessment
3. Pathophysiology and assessment
   a. Take extra time in gathering a history, which may be difficult but is extremely vital.
4. History-taking can be complicated in several ways.
   a. Communication challenges (**Figs. 43-2 and 43-3, p. 1677; Fig. 43-4, p. 1678**)
      i. Vision difficulties
      ii. Hearing loss
      iii. Trouble speaking
   b. Altered mental status and confusion may be due to (**Fig. 43-5, p. 1679**)
      i. On-scene confusion
      ii. Medical conditions
      iii. Drugs
      iv. Depression
   c. Conclude the history by verifying with a credible source if one is available and the confirmation can be done discreetly.
5. Physical examination
   a. Always respect the needs of the elderly patient when performing a physical exam.
C. Management considerations (pp. 1679–1680)
   1. ABCs
   2. Remain alert for changes in patient's condition.
   3. Provide emotional support.
   4. Treatment based on assessment and history

IV. System pathophysiology in the elderly (pp. 1680–1685) (Table 43-4, p. 1681)

A. Respiratory system (pp. 1680–1681)
   1. Age-related changes
   2. Complications
   3. Management
      a. Positioning
      b. Teach breathing patterns.
      c. Use bronchodilators as needed.
      d. Provide supplemental oxygen as needed.
      e. Monitor patient closely.
B. Cardiovascular system (pp. 1681–1682)
   1. Age-related changes
   2. Complications
   3. Management
      a. Provide high-concentration supplemental oxygen.
      b. Start IV for medication administration.
      c. Inquire about age-related dosages.
      d. Monitor vital signs and rhythm.
      e. Acquire a 12-lead ECG.
      f. Remain calm, professional, and empathetic.
C. Nervous system (pp. 1682–1683)
   1. Age-related changes
   2. Complications
   3. Management
      a. Monitor patient closely.
      b. Assign priority if possible stroke victim.
      c. Provide supplemental oxygen as needed.
      d. Administer medications per protocols and medical direction.

POINT OF INTEREST
Patients who have experienced gradual hearing loss may have compensated by unconsciously learning to read lips.

POINT OF INTEREST
Because initial hearing loss frequently involves high-frequency sounds, some elderly patients may have difficulty hearing higher-pitched voices. This may present a problem for female paramedics when they try to take a history from a geriatric patient.

POINT TO EMPHASIZE
DO NOT assume that a confused, disoriented patient is "just senile." This constitutes failing to assess for a serious underlying problem.

POWERPOINT PRESENTATION
Chapter 43 PowerPoint slides 37–38

POINT TO EMPHASIZE
In treating respiratory disorders in the elderly patient, DO NOT FLUID OVERLOAD.

POINT TO EMPHASIZE
Many endocrine emergencies encountered in the field present as altered mental status, especially with insulin-related disorders.

  D. Endocrine system (p. 1683)
    1. Age-related changes
    2. Complications
       a. Hormonal Replacement Therapy (HRT)
          i. Can increase risk of breast cancer and stroke in menopausal woman.
       b. Thyroid disorders
       c. Marfan's Syndrome
          i. Abnormal growth of distal tissues
    3. Management
       a. Monitor patient carefully.
  E. Gastrointestinal system (pp. 1683–1684)
    1. Age-related changes
    2. Complications
    3. Management
  F. Thermoregulatory system (p. 1684)
    1. Age-related changes
    2. Complications
    3. Management
  G. Integumentary system (p. 1684)
    1. Age-related changes
    2. Complications
    3. Management
  H. Musculoskeletal system (p. 1684)
    1. Age-related changes
    2. Complications
    3. Management
  I. Renal system (p. 1685)
    1. Age-related changes
    2. Complications
    3. Management
       a. Oxygenation
       b. Fluid status
       c. Monitoring
  J. Genitourinary system (p. 1685)
    1. Age-related changes
    2. Complications
    3. Management
  K. Immune system (p. 1685)
    1. Age-related changes
    2. Complications
    3. Management
  L. Hematology system (p. 1685)
    1. Age-related changes
    2. Complications
    3. Management

POWERPOINT PRESENTATION
Chapter 43 PowerPoint slides 39–55

V. **Common medical problems in the elderly** (pp. 1685–1708)
  A. Pulmonary/respiratory disorders (pp. 1686–1689) (**Fig. 43-6, p. 1686**)
    1. Pneumonia
       a. Fourth leading cause of death in elderly
       b. Signs and symptoms
          i. Increasing dyspnea
          ii. Congestion
          iii. Fever/chills
          iv. Tachypnea

POINT TO EMPHASIZE
DO NOT transmit an illness—even a mild cold—to an elderly patient.

        v. Sputum production
        vi. Altered mental status
    c. Treatment
        i. Manage all life threats.
        ii. Maintain adequate oxygenation.
        iii. Transport and monitor.
2. Chronic obstructive pulmonary disease (Fig. 43-7, p. 1688)
    a. Signs and symptoms
        i. Cough
        ii. Increased sputum production
        iii. Dyspnea
        iv. Accessory muscle use
        v. Pursed lip breathing
        vi. Tripod positioning
        vii. Exercise intolerance
        viii. Wheezing
        ix. Pleuritic chest pain
        x. Tachypnea
    b. Treatment
        i. Oxygen
        ii. Drug therapy
3. Pulmonary embolism
    a. Signs and symptoms
        i. Dyspnea
        ii. Pleuritic chest pain
        iii. Right heart failure
        iv. Cardiac dysrhythmias
    b. Treatment
        i. Morphine sulfate for anxiety
        ii. Anticoagulants
        iii. Rapid transport
4. Pulmonary edema
    a. Signs and symptoms
        i. Severe dyspnea
        ii. Congestion
        iii. Rapid labored breathing
        iv. Cough with blood-stained sputum
        v. Cyanosis
        vi. Cold extremities
    b. Treatment is directed toward altering the cause of the condition.
5. Lung cancer
    a. Signs and symptoms
        i. Progressive dyspnea
        ii. Hemotypsis
        iii. Chronic cough
        iv. Weight loss
    b. Treatment is in hospital.
B. Cardiovascular disorders (pp. 1689–1692)
1. Angina pectoris
2. Myocardial infarction
    a. Presentations in elderly
        i. Absence of pain
        ii. Exercise intolerance
        iii. Confusion/dizziness
        iv. Syncope
        v. Dyspnea

TEACHING TIP
Patients with COPD who experience a sudden onset of increased dyspnea often have developed a spontaneous pneumothorax. What changes in the lungs associated with COPD account for this?

POINT TO EMPHASIZE
Keep in mind that heart sounds are generally softer in the elderly, probably because of a thickening of lung tissues between the heart and chest wall.

POINT TO EMPHASIZE
In the elderly patient, exercise intolerance is a key symptom of angina.

POINT TO EMPHASIZE
The elderly patient with myocardial infarction is less likely to present with classic symptoms than a younger counterpart.

TEACHING TIP
Ask students why the elderly are more likely to present with "silent" myocardial infarctions.

> **TEACHING TIP**
> Some older persons who have CHF present with recurring episodes of nocturnal confusion. Why?

           vi. Neck, dental, and/or epigastric pain
          vii. Fatigue/weakness
    3. Heart failure
       a. Signs and symptoms
           i. Fatigue
          ii. Two-pillow orthopnea
         iii. Dyspnea on exertion
         iv. Dry, hacking cough progressing to productive cough
           v. Dependent edema
          vi. Nocturia
         vii. Anoxeria, heptomegaly, ascites
    4. Dysrhythmias
    5. Aortic dissection/aneurysms
       a. Due largely to atherosclerosis combined with hypertension
       b. IV medication and rapid transport
    6. Hypertension
       a. Often no clinically obvious signs or symptoms
       b. Management often with beta-blockers
    7. Syncope
       a. Common presentations
           i. Vasopressor
              a) Common faint
          ii. Orthostatic
              a) On rising from a supine or seated position
         iii. Vasovagal
              a) Result of a valsalva maneuver
         iv. Cardiac
              a) Sudden decrease in cardiac output
           v. Seizures
              a) Syncope may result from a seizure disorder
              b) Syncope may cause seizures
         vi. Transient ischemic attack
              a) May cause syncope
C. Neurological disorders (pp. 1693–1696)
    1. Cerebrovascular disease
       a. Two major categories
           i. Brain ischemia (80 percent of strokes)
          ii. Brain hemorrhage
       b. Be highly suspicious of condition in elderly patient with sudden change in mental status.
       c. Complete Glasgow Coma Scale for later comparison in ER.
    2. Seizures
       a. Easily mistaken for stroke; cause often cannot be determined in field.
    3. Dizziness/vertigo
    4. Delirium (**Table 43-5, p. 1695**)
       a. Signs and symptoms
           i. Acute anxiety
          ii. Inability to focus
         iii. Disordered thinking
         iv. Irritability
           v. Inappropriate behavior
          vi. Fearfulness
         vii. Excessive energy
        viii. Psychotic behavior
         ix. Aphasia/speaking disorders

> **TEACHING TIP**
> Ask students to explain the relationship between major types of antihypertensives and orthostatic syncope.

> **TEACHING TIP**
> Ask students to explain why a syncopal episode could trigger a seizure.

> **TEACHING TIP**
> Strokes caused by thrombus formation frequently occur when older patients are sleeping. Why?

> **POINT TO EMPHASIZE**
> Whenever you suspect stroke, it is essential that you complete the Glasgow Coma Scale for later comparison in the emergency department.

5. Dementia (**Table 43-5, p. 1695**)
   a. Signs and symptoms
      i. More prevalent in elderly than delirium
      ii. Progressive disorientation
      iii. Shortened attention span
      iv. Aphasia/nonsense talking
      v. Hallucinations
6. Alzheimer's disease
   a. Signs and symptoms
      i. Particular type of dementia
      ii. Early stage
         a) Memory loss
         b) Inability to learn new material
         c) Mood swings
         d) Personality changes
         e) Aggression/hostility common
      iii. Intermediate stage
         a) Complete inability to learn new material
         b) Wandering
         c) Increased falls
         d) Loss of ability for self-care
         e) Inability to walk
         f) Regression to infant stage
7. Parkinson's disease
   a. Degenerative disorder characterized by changes in muscle response
   b. Common signs and symptoms
      i. Impossible to distinguish primary and secondary in field setting
      ii. Resting tremor with pill-rolling motion
      iii. Slowed, jerky movements
      iv. Shuffling gait
      v. Kyphotic deformity
      vi. Mask-like face devoid of expression

D. Metabolic and endocrine disorders (pp. 1696–1697)
   1. Diabetes mellitus
      a. Affects 20 percent of older adults
      b. Do not manage the diabetic and hypoglycemic emergencies differently for older patients than for others.
   2. Thyroid disorders
      a. Condition experienced by 2 to 3 percent of older patients
      b. Must be cared for in hospital.

E. Gastrointestinal disorders (pp. 1697–1699)
   1. Common among elderly and require prompt management
   2. Treatment
      a. Airway management
      b. Support of breathing and circulation
      c. High-flow oxygen therapy
      d. IV fluid replacement with crystalloid
      e. PASG if indicated
      f. Rapid transport
   3. Causes of upper GI bleed
      a. Peptic ulcer disease
      b. Gastritis
      c. Esophageal varices
      d. Mallory-Weiss tear
   4. Lower GI bleed
      a. Diverticulosis
      b. Tumors

POINT TO EMPHASIZE
Remember to treat both the Alzheimer's patient and family and/or caregivers with respect and compassion.

POINT TO EMPHASIZE
Patients with gastrointestinal complaints should be aggressively managed, especially the elderly.

          c. Ischemic colitis
          d. Arteriovenous malformations
       5. Bowel obstruction signs and symptoms
          a. Diffuse abdominal pain
          b. Bloating
          c. Nausea
          d. Vomiting
          e. Distended abdomen
          f. Hypoactive/absent bowel sounds
       6. Mesenteric infarct signs and symptoms
          a. Pain out of proportion to physical exam
          b. Bloody diarrhea
          c. Some tachycardia
          d. Abdominal distention
    F. Skin disorders (pp. 1699–1700)
       1. Skin diseases
          a. Itching may camouflage other conditions.
          b. Slower healing and compromised tissue perfusion make the elderly more susceptible to bacterial infection and fungal infections.
          c. Disorders may be drug-induced
             i. e.g., beta-blockers and psoriasis.
       2. Pressure ulcers
          a. Most common in people over 70
          b. Care
             i. Change patient's position frequently.
             ii. Use a pull sheet to move patient.
             iii. Pad skin prior to movement.
             iv. Clean and dry areas of excessive moisture.
             v. Clean ulcers with normal saline and cover with hydrocolloid or hydrogel dressings.
    G. Musculoskeletal disorders (pp. 1700–1701)
       1. Osteoarthritis (Fig. 43-8, p. 1700)
          a. Leading cause of disability of those 65 and older
          b. Initially presents as joint pain, worsened by exercise, improved by rest.
          c. Treatment involves stretching, drug therapy, and, as a last resort, surgery.
       2. Osteoporosis
          a. Softening of bone tissue due to loss of essential minerals
          b. Affects 20 million Americans
          c. Usually asymptomatic until fracture occurs
          d. Management involves prevention through exercise and drug therapy.
    H. Renal disorders (pp. 1701–1702)
       1. Common problems include
          a. Renal failure
          b. Glomerulonephritis
          c. Renal blood clots
       2. Precipitating conditions include
          a. Hypotension
          b. Heart failure
          c. Major surgery
          d. Sepsis
          e. Angiographic procedures
          f. Use of nephrotoxic antibiotics

I. Urinary disorders (p. 1702)
   1. Affects 10 percent of the elderly
   2. Signs and symptoms
      a. Cloudy, foul-smelling urine
      b. Bladder pain
      c. Frequent urination
      d. Signs of septic shock with urosepsis
   3. Treatment
      a. Placement of large-bore IVs for administration of fluids and antibiotics
      b. Prompt transport
J. Environmental emergencies (pp. 1702–1703)
   1. Hypothermia
      a. Elderly may fail to note or report signs/symptoms of hypothermia; may not shiver.
      b. Rewarm as with other patients and provide rapid transport.
   2. Hyperthermia
      a. Nearly half of all heatstroke deaths are to people over 50.
      b. Signs and symptoms may be masked.
      c. Treat as with other patients and provide rapid transport.
K. Toxicological emergencies (pp. 1703–1705)
   1. Aging alters pharmacokinetics and pharmacodynamics in the elderly, while medical conditions lead them to take more medications.
   2. Common drugs that cause problems for elderly patients
      a. Lidocaine
      b. Beta-blockers
      c. Antihypertensives/diurectics
         i. Hydrochlorothiazide
         ii. Furosemide
         iii. Ethacrynic acid
         iv. Bumetanide
         v. Torsemide
      d. Angiotensin-converting enzyme (ACE) inhibitors
      e. Digitalis (digoxin, Lanoxin)
      f. Antipsychotropics/antidepressants
         i. SSRIs:
            a) Prozac
            b) Wellbutrin
         ii. Tricyclic antidepressants
            a) Elavil
            b) Tofranil
         iii. Monamine oxidase inhibitors
            a) Marplan
            b) Nardil
            c) Lithium
         iv. Antipsychotics
            a) Thorazine
            b) Mellaril
            c) Taractan
            d) Navane
            e) Haldol
         v. Benzodiazepines
            a) Flurazepam
            b) Temazepam
            c) Triazolam

POINT TO EMPHASIZE

Remember that the elderly hypothermic patient often does not shiver.

    vi. Antianxiety
     a) Diazepam
     b) Lorazepam
     c) Chlordiazepoxide
   g. Medications for Parkinson's disease
    i. Carbidopa/levadopa
    ii. Bromocriptine
    iii. Benzotropine mesylate
    iv. Amantadine
    v. Tsmar
    vi. Sinemet
   h. Antiseizure medications
   i. Analgesics and antiinflammatory agents
    i. Narcotic analgesics
     a) Codeine
     b) Meperidine
     c) Morphine
     d) Oxycodone
     e) Propoxyphene
    ii. NSAIDs
    iii. Acetaminophen
   j. Corticosteriods
    i. Cortisone
    ii. Hydrocortisone
    iii. Prednisone
 L. Substance abuse (pp. 1705–1706)
  1. Up to 17 percent of the elderly are addicted to substances.
  2. Drug abuse
   a. Polypharmacy
   b. Signs and symptoms
    i. Memory changes
    ii. Drowsiness
    iii. Decreased vision/hearing
    iv. Orthostatic hypotension
    v. Poor dexterity
    vi. Mood changes
    vii. Falling
    viii. Restlessness
    ix. Weight loss
  3. Alcohol abuse
   a. 15 percent of men and 12 percent of women exceed guidelines for use of alcohol.
   b. High risk of toxicity in elderly with abuse of alcohol
   c. Signs and symptoms
    i. Mood swings, denial, hostility
    ii. Confusion
    iii. History of falls
    iv. Anorexia
    v. Insomnia
    vi. Visible anxiety
    vii. Nausea
 M. Behavioral/psychological disorders (pp. 1707–1708)
  1. Common classifications of disorders related to aging include
   a. Organic brain syndrome
   b. Affective disorders
    i. Depression

POINT TO EMPHASIZE

Unless an elderly person is openly intoxicated, discovery of alcohol abuse often depends upon a thorough history.

      c. Personality disorders
          i. Dependent personality
      d. Dissociative disorders
          i. Paranoid
          ii. Schizophrenia
  2. Depression
      a. Up to 15 percent of elderly experience depression
      b. Rising to 30 percent among the institutionalized
  3. Suicide
      a. Highest suicide rates in United States are in those over 65, especially men
      b. Third leading cause of death among the elderly
      c. Warning signs
          i. Loss of interest in once pleasurable activities
          ii. Curtailing of social interaction, grooming, self-care
          iii. Breaking from medical or exercise regimens
          iv. Grieving a personal loss
          v. Feeling useless
          vi. Putting affairs in order, finalizing things
          vii. Stockpiling medications or other means of self-destruction

VI. Trauma in the elderly patient (pp. 1708–1713)

A. Contributing factors (p. 1709)
  1. Osteoporosis
  2. Reduced cardiac reserve
  3. Decreased respiratory function, ARDS
  4. Impaired renal function
  5. Decreased elasticity in blood vessels

B. General assessment (pp. 1709–1710)
  1. Proceed as with other patients, but remember that signs and symptoms in the elderly can be deceptive.
  2. Observe for abuse/neglect; report suspected cases. (**Fig. 43-9, p. 1710**)
  3. Average abused patient
      a. Over 80
      b. Has multiple medical problems
      c. Senile dementia is common

C. General management (pp. 1710–1711)
  1. Cardiovascular considerations
      a. Elderly trauma patients may require higher than usual arterial pressures for perfusion of vital organs
      b. Take care in IV fluid administration because of decreased myocardial reserves.
  2. Respiratory considerations
      a. Remember age-related changes in the respiratory system.
      b. Make necessary adjustments in treatment to provide adequate oxygenation and CO_2 removal.
      c. Use positive-pressure ventilations cautiously.
  3. Renal considerations
      a. Remember age-related changes in the renal system.
      b. Elderly injured are at greater risk for fluid overload and pulmonary edema.
      c. Toxins and medications accumulate more readily in the elderly.
  4. Transport considerations
      a. Remember the frailty of the elderly.
      b. Move gently.

POINT TO EMPHASIZE
All suicidal elderly patients should be transported to the hospital.

POWERPOINT PRESENTATION
Chapter 43 PowerPoint slides 56–67

POINT TO EMPHASIZE
In assessing elderly trauma patients, remember that blood pressure and pulse readings can be deceptive indicators of hypoperfusion.

POINT TO EMPHASIZE
Many states have laws that require prehospital personnel to report suspected cases of geriatric abuse and/or neglect.

READING/REFERENCE
"Geriatric Trauma" and "Abuse in the Elderly and Impaired," in Tintinalli, J. E., et al., eds., *Emergency Medicine: A Comprehensive Study Guide*, 5th ed., New York: McGraw-Hill, 1999.

POINT TO EMPHASIZE
Keep in mind that trauma places an elderly person at increased risk of hypothermia. Ensure that the patient is kept warm at all times.

c. Keep the patient warm.
d. Package appropriately. (**Fig. 43-10a, 43-10b and 43-10c, p. 1711**)
D. Specific injuries (pp. 1712–1713)
1. Orthopedic injuries (**Fig. 43-11, p. 1712**)
a. Elderly suffer the greatest mortality and disability from falls
i. Most commonly a fracture of hip or pelvis
b. When treating orthopedic injuries, remain alert for cardiac emergencies.
2. Burns
a. Elderly more likely to suffer deaths from burns than any other age group except neonates and infants.
b. Factors affecting burns in elderly
i. Slowed reaction time among elderly
ii. Preexisting diseases
iii. Age-related skin changes
iv. Immunological and metabolic changes
v. Reductions in physiologic function and reduced reserve of organ systems
c. Management is the same as for other patients but remember:
i. Elderly are at increased risk for shock.
ii. Fluids are important to prevent renal tubular damage.
3. Head and spinal injuries
a. Remember that elderly are at increased risk of brain injury because of decrease in brain size.
b. Spine is also more subject to injury because of osteoporosis and spondylosis.

VII. Chapter summary (p. 1713). Providing EMS in the twenty-first century means treating a growing elderly population. The "Graying of America" has resulted in a greater number of people age 65 and older, many of whom are in home settings. When treating elderly patients, keep in mind the anatomical, physiological, and emotional changes that occur with age. However, never jump to conclusions based solely on age. Weigh normal age-related changes against abnormal changes, that is, those resulting from a medical condition or trauma. Recall that elderly patients are much more susceptible to medication side effects and toxicity than younger patients. They also are more susceptible to trauma and environmental stressors. Abuse of the elderly occurs, and you should bear this in mind whenever injuries do not match the history. Any suspected abuse or neglect of an elderly patient should be reported to the emergency department and/or the appropriate governmental authorities.

SKILLS DEMONSTRATION AND PRACTICE

Give the students a chance to experience some of the effects of aging by rotating them through the following stations in a skills lab.

Station 1: Vision
Obtain a set of swimmer's goggles or safety goggles and—

- Paste yellow transparent cellophane or lubricating jelly on the lenses to represent yellowing of the lens of the eye and to simulate cataracts.
- Paste strips of black paper on the sides for left and/or right obstruction of peripheral vision.
- Paste black paper in a circle around each eye to depict tunnel vision.

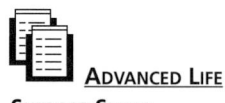

- Paste spots of black paper on the goggles to represent spotted vision commonly experienced by patients with certain forms of retinal disorders.
- Totally blacken the lens to represent blindness.
- Have students wearing the totally blackened goggles take a "blind walk" to illustrate dependence on a companion, the importance of cues and barriers, and the use of handrails.
- Shake a slide in a projector as the slide is shown on a screen to simulate an inability to control ocular motion.
- Have students read or perform other detailed work in a dimly lit room to illustrate effects of reduction in light to the eyes.

Station 2: Hearing
- Obtain a set of swimmer's earplugs, a pair of earmuffs, or a stocking hat to dull the sound of people talking. After the student inserts the earplugs, verbally give him/her directions for accomplishing a task. Time the students to illustrate how hearing loss may even affect how fast a person can accomplish an assignment or process directions.
- Do not forget the interrelation of vision and hearing. Have a blindfolded person listen to instructions given at a fast pace. This will illustrate how often we depend on nonverbal as well as verbal communication cues.

Station 3: Touch
- Have students don plastic or rubber gloves to work in different water temperatures and to pick up small objects, so that they may experience the difficulties the elderly may experience in distinguishing water temperatures and in grasping small objects.
- Ask a person wearing a pair of gloves to tie shoelaces or to perform any other similar task such as buttoning a shirt or buckling a belt.
- Place masking around several fingers and/or joints to simulate a missing finger or stiffened joint. Use elastic bandages to limit the functioning of the hand or wrist.
- Set up some one-handed tasks to demonstrate the difficulty encountered by a person who is missing an arm or who has lost the use of an arm through a stroke.

Station 4: Taste
After blocking out the student's visual and olfactory capacities by use of a blindfold and cotton in the nose—

- Have the student eat and identify raw pieces of apple and potato (foods that have similar textures); a potato chip and a corn chip.
- Ask the student to distinguish between a variety of foods that have been put through a blender so they cannot be recognized by their texture.

Station 5: Smell
The close relationship between smell, taste, and vision makes designing simulation exercises for smell alone difficult.

- As a variation of the exercise suggested for taste, ask students to identify substances by smell. Substances used can range from apples and oranges to peanut butter, mustard, and chocolate, as long as they have distinctive odors. Cotton or swimmer's nose clips can be used to simulate loss of smell.
- Blindfold students and present them with a variety of odors to identify. Be certain to use a range of distinctive odors.
- Use one strong odor, such as musk oil, to mask other odors. Have the blindfolded student try to identify the other odors.

Station 6: Mobility and Gait
- Using a wheelchair and a door, ask the student to maneuver the wheelchair through the door using only one arm or leg, as would a person who had experienced a stroke. While the student is sitting in the wheelchair, have another person come from behind and move the chair without telling the student where they are going.
- Have students attempt to carry packages in their hands while using a walker or cane.
- Have a student sit in a desk chair. After spinning the chair around rapidly a few times, ask the student to walk a straight line. The dizziness experienced is similar to that of a person who has a mobility or balance problem.
- Paste thick sponge rubber on the bottom of a pair of shoes and have the person walk in them. This simulates dizziness or a lack of stability.
- Use elastic bandages on the knees and other joints to simulate stiffness. Then have the student attempt to walk across the room or rise from a low chair.
- Use a combination of these activities and those recommended for vision and touch training to demonstrate the effect of the interrelationship among the senses on mobility and balance.

ASSIGNMENTS

Assign students to complete Chapter 43, "Geriatric Emergencies," of the workbook. Also assign them to read Chapter 44, "Abuse and Assault," before the next class.

EVALUATION

Chapter Quiz and Scenarios   Distribute copies of the Chapter Quiz provided in Handout 43-2 to evaluate student understanding of this chapter. Make sure each student reads the scenarios to reinforce critical thinking on the scene. Remind students not to use their notes or textbooks while taking the quiz.

Student CD   Quizzes for every chapter are contained on the dynamic and highly visual in-text student CD.

Companion Website   Additional quizzes for every chapter are contained on this exciting website.

TestGen   You may wish to create a custom-tailored test using *Prentice Hall TestGen for Essentials of Paramedic Care*, 2nd Edition to evaluate student understanding of this chapter.

On-line Test Preparation (for students and instructors)   Additional test preparation is available through Brady's new on-line product, *EMT Achieve: Paramedic Test Preparation* at *http://www.prenhall.com/emtachieve/*. Instructors can also monitor student mastery on-line.

Review Manual for the EMT-Paramedic   This comprehensive exam review contains hundreds of test questions and rationales, including scenarios, along with two 180-question practice tests on CD.

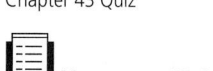

WORKBOOK
Chapter 43 Activities

READING/REFERENCE
Textbook, pp. 1715–1728

HANDOUT 43-2
Chapter 43 Quiz

HANDOUTS 43-3 AND 43-4
Chapter 43 Scenarios

PARAMEDIC STUDENT CD
Student Activities

COMPANION WEBSITE
http://www.prenhall.com/bledsoe

TESTGEN
Chapter 43

EMT ACHIEVE: PARAMEDIC TEST PREPARATION
Mistovich & Beasley. *EMT Achieve: Paramedic Test Preparation*, www.prenhall.com/emtachieve/

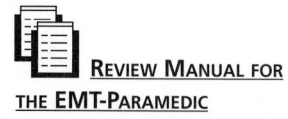

REVIEW MANUAL FOR THE EMT-PARAMEDIC
Cherry & Mistovich. *Review Manual for the EMT-Paramedic*, 3rd edition.

REINFORCEMENT

Handouts If classroom discussion or performance on the quiz indicates that some students have not fully mastered the chapter content, you may wish to assign some or all of the Reinforcement Handouts for this chapter.

Student CD (for students) A wide variety of material on this CD-ROM will reinforce and also expand student knowledge and skills.

PowerPoint Presentation (for instructors) The PowerPoint material developed for this chapter offers useful reinforcement of chapter content.

Companion Website (for students) Additional review quizzes and links to EMS resources will contribute to further reinforcement of the chapter.

OneKey On-line support is offered for this course on one of three platforms: CourseCompass, Blackboard, or Web CT. Includes the IRM, PowerPoints, TestGen, and Companion Website for instruction. Ask your local sales representative for more information.

Brady Skills Series: Advanced Life Skills (Video or CD) Have your students watch the skills come to life on VHS or CD-ROM, or they can purchase the highly visual, full-color text with step-by-step procedures and rationales.

HANDOUTS 43-5 AND 43-6
Reinforcement Activities

PARAMEDIC STUDENT CD
Student Activities

POWERPOINT PRESENTATION
Chapter 43

COMPANION WEBSITE
www.prenhall.com/bledsoe

ONEKEY
Chapter 43

ADVANCED LIFE SUPPORT SKILLS
Larmon & Davis. *Advanced Life Support Skills.*

ADVANCED LIFE SKILLS REVIEW
Larmon & Davis. *Advanced Life Skills Review.*

BRADY SKILLS SERIES: ALS.
Larmon & Davis. *Brady Skills Series: ALS.*

PARAMEDIC NATIONAL STANDARDS SELF-TEST
Miller. *Paramedic National Standards Self-Test,* 4th edition.

Handout 43-1

Student's Name _____

CHAPTER 43 OBJECTIVES CHECKLIST

Knowledge	Date Mastered
1. Discuss the demographics demonstrating the increasing size of the elderly population in the United States.	
2. Assess the various living environments of elderly patients.	
3. Discuss society's view of aging and the social, financial, and ethical issues facing the elderly.	
4. Discuss common emotional and psychological reactions to aging, including causes and manifestations.	
5. Apply the pathophysiology of multisystem failure to the assessment and management of medical conditions in the elderly patient.	
6. Compare the pharmacokinetics of an elderly patient to that of a young patient, including drug distribution, metabolism, and excretion.	
7. Discuss the impact of polypharmacy, dosing errors, increased drug sensitivity, and medication noncompliance on assessment and management of the elderly patient.	
8. Discuss the use and effects of commonly prescribed drugs for the elderly patient.	
9. Discuss the problem of mobility in the elderly, and develop strategies to prevent falls.	
10. Discuss age-related changes in sensations in the elderly, and describe the implications of these changes for communication and patient assessment.	
11. Discuss the problems with continence and elimination in the elderly patient, and develop communication strategies to provide psychological support.	
12. Discuss factors that may complicate the assessment of the elderly patient.	
13. Discuss the principles that should be employed when assessing and communicating with the elderly.	
14. Compare the assessment of a young patient with that of an elderly patient.	
15. Discuss common complaints of elderly patients.	
16. Discuss the normal and abnormal changes of age in relation to the: • Pulmonary system • Cardiovascular system • Nervous system • Endocrine system	

1050 Essentials of Paramedic Care

©2007 Pearson Education, Inc.
Essentials of Paramedic Care, 2nd ed.

HANDOUT 43-1 Continued

Knowledge	Date Mastered
• Gastrointestinal system • Thermoregulatory system • Integumentary system • Musculoskeletal system	
17. Describe the incidence, morbidity/mortality, risk factors, prevention strategies, pathophysiology, assessment, need for intervention and transport, and management for elderly medical patients with: • Pneumonia, chronic obstructive disease, and pulmonary embolism • Myocardial infarction, heart failure, dysrhythmias, aneurysm, and hypertension • Cerebral vascular disease, delirium, dementia, Alzheimer's disease, and Parkinson's disease • Diabetes and thyroid diseases • Gastrointestinal problems, GI hemorrhage, and bowel obstruction • Skin diseases and pressure ulcers • Osteoarthritis and osteoporosis • Hypothermia and hyperthermia • Toxicological problems, including drug toxicity, substance abuse, alcohol abuse, and drug abuse • Psychological disorders, including depression and suicide	
18. Describe the incidence, morbidity/mortality, risk factors, prevention strategies, pathophysiology, assessment, need for intervention and transport, and management of the elderly trauma patient with: • Orthopedic injuries • Burns • Head injuries	
19. Given several preprogrammed simulated geriatric patients with various complaints, provide the appropriate assessment, management, and transport.	

CHAPTER 43 QUIZ

Student's Name _____

Write the letter of the best answer in the space provided.

_____ 1. A 78-year-old nursing home patient is found to have severe pedal edema. His neck veins are flat. No adventitious sounds are present in the lung fields. There is no abdominal distension. The patient reportedly spends 12 to 14 hours a day sitting in front of the TV with his feet in a dependent position. The edema of his ankles and feet probably results from:
   A. right-sided heart failure.
   B. immobility and the dependent position of his feet.
   C. liver disease.
   D. left-sided heart failure.

_____ 2. Kyphosis in a geriatric patient will most likely result in the paramedic having to modify:
   A. interviewing techniques because kyphosis causes hearing loss.
   B. methods for spinal stabilization because kyphosis results in excessive curvature of the upper back and neck.
   C. drug dosages because kyphosis is a result of liver damage.
   D. sedation because kyphosis is associated with manic-depressive disorder.

_____ 3. In the United States, the most common cause of dementia among older persons is:
   A. psychosis.
   B. Alzheimer's disease.
   C. drug and alcohol abuse.
   D. depression.

_____ 4. Which of the following medications poses the greatest risk of adverse effects in the geriatric patient if given at normal adult doses?
   A. lidocaine
   B. adenosine
   C. midazolam
   D. Narcan

_____ 5. The most common psychiatric disorder among geriatric patients is:
   A. schizophrenia.
   B. paranoia.
   C. depression.
   D. posttraumatic stress disorder.

_____ 6. A 90-year-old female has been experiencing episodes of nocturnal confusion for several weeks. Her lower extremities are swollen, with large, translucent fluid-filled areas resembling blisters on the skin. These areas probably are caused by:
   A. an allergic reaction to medication.
   B. toxicity from an antidepressant medication the patient is taking.
   C. increased hydrostatic pressure caused by right-sided CHF and sleeping sitting up.
   D. degenerative effects of old age on the skin of the lower extremities.

_____ 7. A 77-year-old male has been experiencing dizziness and weakness when he attempts to stand quickly. Causes that should be considered include:
   A. beta-blocker use.
   B. use of vasodilators for treatment of hypertension.
   C. hypovolemia secondary to diuretic use or depressed thirst mechanisms.
   D. all of these

HANDOUT 43-2 Continued

_____ 8. An 89-year-old female presents with multiple bruises on her face and upper extremities. She lives with her son, who tells you that the patient is always falling down and is just generally clumsy. The patient appears malnourished and frightened. She cowers when you approach and is reluctant to allow you to examine her. Her son seems to be hostile toward you and your partner and nervously attempts to explain each bruise. In this case you should do all of following EXCEPT:
  A. obtain a complete patient and family history.
  B. report suspicions of elder abuse to the emergency department staff.
  C. be honest and open with the patient's son about your concerns.
  D. listen carefully for inconsistencies in stories.

_____ 9. When you are assessing or managing an older patient, you should:
  A. use physical contact to compensate for loss of sight or hearing.
  B. talk louder than normal because most of the elderly have hearing loss.
  C. separate the patient from friends or family as quickly as possible to reduce anxiety.
  D. call the patient "dear" or "honey" to make the patient feel cared for.

_____ 10. Patients taking diuretics such as furosemide are at special risk for developing which of the following electrolyte imbalances?
  A. hypocalcemia   C. hypercalcemia
  B. hypokalemia   D. hyperkalemia

_____ 11. Which of the following combinations of signs and symptoms would be most suggestive of acute myocardial infarction in a geriatric patient?
  A. extreme weakness, malaise, syncope, jaundice
  B. extreme weakness, syncope, loss of bowel and bladder control, malaise
  C. syncope, loss of bowel and bladder control, confusion, stiff neck and headache
  D. extreme weakness, confusion, syncope, stiff neck and headache

_____ 12. Which of the following statements about medical emergencies in geriatric patients is NOT true?
  A. Dyspnea may be the only symptom with which acute myocardial infarction presents.
  B. Syncope in the elderly is rarely significant.
  C. Congestive heart failure may present with episodes of nocturnal restlessness and confusion.
  D. Occlusive strokes (thrombus formation) tend to be more common in the elderly.

_____ 13. What effect will hypokalemia have if a patient is taking digitalis?
  A. It will enhance the effects of digitalis, possibly resulting in digitalis toxicity.
  B. It will antagonize the action of digitalis, making the digitalis ineffective.
  C. It will not produce any significant effects.
  D. It will antagonize the effects of digitalis if the patient is digitalis toxic, but will enhance the effects if the patient is not digitalis toxic.

_____ 14. Which of the following statements about the care of geriatric trauma patients is NOT true?
  A. The heart's ability to increase its rate and stroke volume to compensate for hypovolemia may be decreased.
  B. The patient may require a greater amount of IV fluid to support the higher arterial pressures needed to perfuse the vital organs.
  C. In the geriatric patient, tissues and organs have less tolerance of hypoxia and hypoperfusion.
  D. Physical deformities may require modification of packaging procedures.

_____ 15. A 73-year-old female has been experiencing episodes of weakness and dizziness. You have placed her on oxygen by nonrebreather mask and attached an ECG monitor. As you continue to take her history, she suddenly complains of feeling light-headed and weak. You look at the monitor and notice that the patient has gone into complete AV block with no escape rhythm. After about 15 seconds of generating only P waves, the patient returns to a sinus rhythm, and her symptoms quickly resolve. The patient has experienced a problem called:
  A. Stokes-Adams syndrome.   C. sick sinus syndrome.
  B. transient ischemic attack.   D. autonomic dysreflexia.

HANDOUT 43-2 Continued

_____ 16. Which of the following statements about elder abuse is NOT true?
   A. Elder abuse generally is limited to low socioeconomic situations.
   B. Injuries that cannot be explained are the primary finding.
   C. The victim frequently is no longer able to be independent, and the family has difficulty upholding commitments to provide care.
   D. It may be important to note inconsistencies between the histories obtained from the patient and from family members.

_____ 17. A 67-year-old male fell while trying to get up from a chair. He had begun to experience pain in his lower back about 15 minutes before. When he tried to get up, he discovered that his legs were weak and numb. The patient has a history of hypertension for about 15 years. He smokes two packs of cigarettes a day. Vital signs are BP 102/60; pulse 120 weak, regular; respirations 18 shallow, regular. He is awake, alert, and responds appropriately to questions. Breath sounds are present and equal bilaterally with no adventitious sounds. Abdomen is very obese and nontender. The lower abdomen is mottled. The lower extremities are mottled and have no spontaneous movement and no response to pain. There are no pedal pulses. The back is nontender to palpation. Upper extremities move spontaneously with equal grip strengths and normal sensation. What problem do you suspect?
   A. cerebrovascular accident   C. abdominal aortic aneurysm
   B. lumbar spine fracture   D. silent acute myocardial infarction

_____ 18. A 76-year-old male called 911 because he could not breathe. He pants as he speaks and must take several breaths between each word. He is diaphoretic, and his lips and nailbeds are cyanotic. The problem has been worsening for about 4 days. When he breathes, he has a sharp pain in his left lower chest that is not constant and lasts only a few seconds at a time. He has a chronic cough and smokes three packs of cigarettes a day. He says he has no history of cardiovascular disease. Vital signs are BP 130/88; pulse 130 strong, regular; respirations 42 labored. The patient's temperature is 102°F. Crackles (rales) and wheezes are present in the left lower chest. The most appropriate medications to use in managing this patient would be:
   A. oxygen, nitroglycerin, morphine.
   B. oxygen, nitroglycerin, morphine, furosemide.
   C. oxygen, morphine.
   D. oxygen, albuterol.

_____ 19. In distinguishing between delirium and dementia, you should recall that delirium:
   A. is a chronic, slowly progressive process; dementia is rapid in onset and has a fluctuating course.
   B. tends not to affect memory; dementia tends to impair memory.
   C. may be reversed if treated early; dementia is an irreversible disorder.
   D. causes global cognitive deficits; dementia causes focal cognitive deficits.

_____ 20. Special problems that may be encountered in geriatric patients may include:
   A. increased susceptibility to general deterioration as a result of illness.
   B. depressed pain and temperature-regulating mechanisms.
   C. increased susceptibility to confusion and depression.
   D. all of these

_____ 21. The key symptom in patients with bowel infarction is:
   A. vomiting of fecal material.
   B. pain out of proportion to physical findings.
   C. uncontrollable diarrhea.
   D. melena.

HANDOUT 43-2 Continued

_____ 22. Which of the following findings is NOT typical of a patient with Parkinson's disease?
   A. tremor combined with pill-rolling motion of the hands
   B. shuffling gait with short steps
   C. mask-like face with no expression
   D. tendency to speak rapidly and loudly

_____ 23. You respond to a report of a "person seizing." The patient is a 74-year-old female who is experiencing uncontrollable movements of the skeletal muscles in her extremities and face. She is awake, alert, and extremely agitated and restless. The patient has no history of cerebrovascular accident, seizures, or other neurological disease. You discover that the patient's physician recently placed her on a new medication, but neither she nor her family can remember what the name of the drug is. Which of the following drugs would be most likely to produce these effects?
   A. Elavil
   B. Thorazine
   C. Librium
   D. Lithium carbonate

_____ 24. Which of the following statements about suicide and suicide risk in the elderly is TRUE?
   A. The elderly have the lowest suicide rate of any age group in the United States.
   B. The elderly are less likely to seek help for depression and suicidal ideation than younger people.
   C. Elderly women are more likely to commit suicide than elderly men.
   D. The elderly are less likely to turn anger and sorrow inward rather than expressing these emotions outward.

_____ 25. An 82-year-old female presents with vague complaints about feeling weak and fatigued. She denies chest pain, dizziness, nausea, or shortness of breath. She has a long history of cardiovascular and respiratory problems. She takes numerous medications but cannot recall their names or which ones she has taken today. During the physical exam, you note pedal edema, weak pedal pulses, and fine bibasilar crackles (rales). Which of the following statements about this patient is true?
   A. Absence of chest pain excludes myocardial infarction as a possible problem.
   B. Her crackles and peripheral edema may be normal findings for her.
   C. Her risk of death is highest during the first few hours following the onset of symptoms.
   D. all of these

HANDOUT 43-3

Student's Name _____

CHAPTER 43 SCENARIO 1

Review the following real-life situation. Then answer the questions that follow.

On a Saturday morning at 0930, you respond to a report of "difficulty breathing" in a residential neighborhood. The patient is a 68-year-old female who complains of weakness and shortness of breath that have increased gradually over the previous 3 days. She denies any history of heart or lung disease. Her only past history has been severe osteoarthritis for which she has been taking "a lot of aspirin." The patient is awake and alert, and she responds to questions appropriately. Vital signs are pulse 114 strong, regular; respirations 22 regular, unlabored; BP 116/86. Her skin is pale, warm, and dry. Pupils are equal and react briskly to light. Breath sounds are present and equal bilaterally with no adventitious sounds. The abdomen is soft and nontender.

1. What problem should you suspect?

2. What questions might you ask?

3. What other problem should you consider as a possible cause for her weakness and dizziness?

HANDOUT 43-4

Student's Name _____

CHAPTER 43 SCENARIO 2

Review the following real-life situation. Then answer the questions that follow.

At 1030 on a Tuesday morning, you respond to a report of a motor vehicle collision. The patient is an 82-year-old male who appears to have lost control of his vehicle, which struck a utility pole. The patient is awake, alert, restless, and anxious. Respirations are rapid and shallow at 24 breaths/minute. Radial pulses are weak at 80 beats/minute. The patient's blood pressure is 128/86. The left lower chest is bruised and is tender to palpation. The left upper abdominal quadrant is tender. Breath sounds are present and equal bilaterally. The patient also complains of pain in his left shoulder. However, there is no bruising, tenderness, or deformity of this area. The patient takes a "blood pressure pill," but he cannot remember its name and does not have the bottle with him.

1. Based on the mechanism of injury and your physical findings, what problem do you suspect?

2. Is the patient's heart rate consistent with this problem? Why or why not?

3. If the patient's heart rate is not consistent with the problem you suspect, how do you explain your findings?

4. Is the patient's blood pressure consistent with the suspected problem? If not, how do you explain your findings?

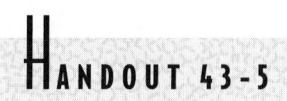

CHAPTER 43 REVIEW

Write the word or words that best complete the following sentences in the space(s) provided.

1. The elderly who are 80 or older are referred to as the _____ - _____.
2. The scientific study of the effects of aging and age-related diseases on humans is known as _____.
3. Discrimination against old people is termed _____.
4. A living arrangement in which the elderly live in, but do not own, individual apartments or rooms and receive select services is _____ _____.
5. A legal document prepared when a person is alive, competent, and able to make informed decisions about health care is a(n) _____ _____.
6. When a paramedic is presented with a DNR, he or she should follow state laws and local EMS system _____.
7. The program under which federal and state governments share responsibility for providing health care to the aged poor, the blind, the disabled, and low-income families with dependent children is _____.
8. In treating the elderly, the best intervention is _____.
9. A person with a decreased ability to meet daily needs on an independent basis suffers from a(n) _____ _____.
10. A complicating factor in the assessment of the elderly is having more than one disease at a time, a condition known as _____ - _____.
11. Another complicating factor in the assessment and care of the elderly is _____, in which there is concurrent use of a number of drugs.
12. _____ - _____ injuries represent the leading cause of accidental death among the elderly.
13. The inability to retain urine or feces because of loss of sphincter control or cerebral or spinal lesions is _____.
14. In the elderly, efforts to force a bowel movement can lead to _____ _____ _____ or _____.
15. Elderly patients are more likely to suffer from _____, a ringing in the ears, or from _____ _____, a condition characterized by vertigo, nerve deafness, and a roar or buzzing in the ears.
16. The condition that can mimic senility and organic brain syndrome and can inhibit patient cooperation with the paramedic is _____.
17. By the time people reach age 65, vital capacity may be reduced by as much as _____ percent.
18. Overall there is an average _____ percent reduction in brain weight from age 20 to age 90.
19. _____ _____, in which a portion of the stomach protrudes upward into the mediastinal cavity, while not age-related per se, can have severe consequences for the elderly.
20. The softening of bone tissue due to loss of essential minerals, which can cause loss of 2 to 3 inches in height in the elderly, is _____.
21. The diminished vigor of the immune response to the challenge and rechallenge by pathogens is referred to as _____ _____.
22. The fourth leading cause of death among those 65 and older is _____.

HANDOUT 43-5 Continued

23. The leading cause of death in the elderly is _____ _____.

24. Unlike younger cardiac patients, the elderly are more apt to suffer a(n) _____ _____ _____.

25. The best-known form of dementia is _____ _____.

26. The most common initial sign of _____ _____ is a resting tremor combined with a pill-rolling motion.

27. The paramedic should not rule out _____ as a complicating factor in cases of hypoglycemia.

28. Gastritis and esophageal varices are likely causes of _____ GI bleeding.

29. Elderly patients are more likely to develop the ischemic damage and subsequent necrosis affecting the skin that is known as a(n) _____ _____.

30. The leading cause of disability among those 65 and older is _____.

31. The drugs that are widely used to treat hypertension, angina pectoris, and dysrhythmias and that are commonly associated with toxicity in the elderly are _____-_____.

32. An exaggerated feeling of depression or unrest, characterized by a mood of general dissatisfaction, restlessness, discomfort, and unhappiness is _____.

33. The syndrome in which an elderly person is physically or psychologically injured by another is _____ _____.

34. The most common fall-related fracture is of the _____ or _____.

35. _____, a degeneration of the vertebral body, is common in the elderly.

Handout 43-6

Student's Name _____

THE PHYSIOLOGY OF AGING

Answer each of the following questions in the space provided.

1. What effect does aging have on dermal blood supply and thickness? How does this affect wound healing? How does this affect severity of burn injuries in the elderly?

2. What effect does aging have on bone resorption? Which gender is particularly affected? What effect does this have in victims of sudden deceleration trauma?

3. What effect does aging have on respiratory reserve capacity? What effect does this have on the ability of older patients to compensate for chest trauma or acute respiratory disease such as pulmonary embolism, spontaneous pneumothorax, or pneumonia?

4. What effect does aging have on myocardial reserve capacity? What effect does this have on volume resuscitation of the older trauma patient?

5. What effect does aging have on the peripheral blood vessels? What effect does this have on the older patient's ability to compensate for volume loss? What effect does this have on the older patient's ability to tolerate hot or cold environments?

6. What effect does aging have on the kidneys? What effect does this have on the response of the patient to drugs? What effect does this have on the response of the patient to fluid therapy for hypovolemia?

HANDOUT 43-6 Continued

7. What effect does aging have on the conduction velocity of the nerves? What effect does this have on the ability of the older patient to feel pain?

8. What effect does aging have on the thirst mechanisms? What effect does this have on patients?

9. What effect does aging have on the size of the brain relative to the size of the cranial cavity? What effect does this produce regarding the onset of signs and symptoms from a subdural hematoma?

10. If a patient is on beta-blocker therapy, what effect does this have on your ability to detect the early signs of shock? Why?

11. What effect does aging have on the cervical spine and spinal canal? What effect do these changes have on the risk of an older person sustaining a cervical spinal cord injury?

12. What effect does aging have on hepatic blood flow and on the ability of the liver to metabolize drugs? What change does this effect dictate for the dosing of most drugs?

Chapter 43 Answer Key

Handout 43-2: Chapter 43 Quiz

1. B	8. C	15. A	22. D
2. B	9. A	16. A	23. B
3. B	10. B	17. C	24. B
4. A	11. B	18. D	25. D
5. C	12. B	19. C	
6. C	13. A	20. D	
7. D	14. B	21. B	

Handout 43-3: Chapter 43 Scenario 1

1. Anemia caused by gastrointestinal hemorrhage caused by excessive aspirin use.
2. Ask the patient about changes in her stool. A dark, tarry consistency helps confirm your suspicions.
3. Silent myocardial infarction.

Handout 43-4: Chapter 43 Scenario 2

1. Intraabdominal hemorrhage and hypovolemic shock, probably from an injury to the spleen.
2. No. If the patient is compensating for volume loss secondary to hemorrhage, the heart rate should be increased.
3. If the "blood pressure pill" is a beta-blocker, the patient may be unable to accelerate his heart rate adequately in response to hypovolemia.
4. It does not appear to be until the history of hypertension is considered. Even with treatment, a hypertensive patient may have a blood pressure significantly above "normal." Therefore, this patient may be hypotensive relative to his "normal" blood pressure.

Handout 43-5: Chapter 43 Review

1. old-old
2. gerontology
3. ageism
4. congregate care
5. advance directive
6. protocols
7. Medicaid
8. prevention
9. functional impairment
10. co-morbidity
11. polypharmacy
12. Fall-related
13. incontinence
14. transient ischemic attack, syncope
15. tinnitus, Meniere's disease
16. depression
17. 50
18. 10
19. Hiatal hernia
20. osteoporosis
21. immune senescence
22. pneumonia
23. cardiovascular disease
24. silent myocardial infarction
25. Alzheimer's disease
26. Parkinson's disease
27. alcohol
28. upper
29. pressure ulcer
30. osteoarthritis
31. beta-blockers
32. dysphoria
33. geriatric abuse
34. hip, pelvis
35. Spondylosis

Handout 43-6: The Physiology of Aging

1. The dermal blood supply decreases, and the dermis thins. Wound healing takes longer. The elderly burn more quickly and more severely at lower temperatures.
2. The rate of bone resorption increases, resulting in a decrease in bone mass and density. Females tend to be affected more frequently. Fractures can occur with less force and at lower velocities than in younger patients.
3. Respiratory reserve capacity in the elderly decreases. This diminishes the ability to compensate for chest trauma or acute respiratory disease.
4. Myocardial reserve capacity decreases. The elderly develop volume overload more easily than younger patients. Volume resuscitation must be carried out cautiously with careful monitoring for signs of overload, particularly pulmonary edema.
5. Peripheral vessel walls become sclerotic and less able to vary the diameter of the vessel. Older patients cannot vasoconstrict as efficiently in response to volume loss. Because the elderly cannot vary the diameter of their peripheral blood vessels effectively, they cannot thermoregulate as well as younger patients.
6. Reductions in the number of nephrons and in renal blood flow occur. Drugs are excreted less effectively via the renal route, so drug action is prolonged. Excess fluid is excreted less effectively, so patients are prone to volume overload.
7. Nerve conduction velocity decreases. Pain sensation in the elderly is diminished.
8. Thirst diminishes with age. The elderly frequently do not have adequate fluid intake and often are chronically dehydrated.
9. The brain decreases in size relative to the cranial cavity. Onset of signs and symptoms of subdural hematoma may be delayed.
10. Detection of shock may be more difficult. By blocking the beta effects of sympathetic stimulation, beta-blockers mask early signs and symptoms of shock.
11. The spinal canal tends to narrow, and degeneration tends to occur in the vertebral bodies. The risk of cervical spine fracture and of spinal cord injury increases.
12. Hepatic blood flow and ability to metabolize drugs decrease. Doses of most drugs must be decreased to compensate.

Chapter 44

Abuse and Assault

INTRODUCTION

Abuse (which can be physical, psychological, or both) and assault (physical violence toward another person) are overwhelmingly serious and common problems. These are complex situations for paramedics to handle because the provider must address physical and psychological issues of medical care and provide appropriate management from the perspective of law enforcement. It can be very difficult to support a distraught patient, perform an adequate assessment and medical intervention, and obtain evidence for possible legal action. In some cases, providers must also remain aware that the patient's safety, and perhaps their own, is not secure. This chapter discusses incidence rates and categories of abuse, as well as profiles of perpetrators and persons at risk for abuse. It details medical aspects of care and a provider's legal responsibilities, as well as lists the resources that a provider may be able to access to assist patients who are victims of abuse and assault.

TOTAL TEACHING TIME: 4.25 HOURS
The total teaching time is only a guideline based on the didactic and practical lab averages in the National Standard Curriculum. Instructors should take into consideration such factors as the pace at which students learn, the size of the class, and breaks. The actual time devoted to teaching objectives is the responsibility of the instructor.

CHAPTER OBJECTIVES

After reading this chapter, you should be able to:

1. Discuss the incidence of abuse and assault. (p. 1716)
2. Describe the categories of abuse. (pp. 1716–1725)
3. Discuss examples of spouse, elder, child, and sexual abuse. (pp. 1716–1725)
4. Describe the characteristics associated with the profile of a typical spouse, elder, or child abuser and the typical assailant of sexual abuse. (pp. 1717, 1719–1720, 1720–1721, 1725)
5. Identify the profile of the "at-risk" spouse, elder, and child. (pp. 1717–1718, 1719, 1721, 1724–1725)
6. Discuss the assessment and management of the abused patient. (pp. 1717, 1718, 1719, 1721–1723, 1726)
7. Discuss the legal aspects associated with abuse situations. (pp. 1718, 1723, 1726–1727)
8. Identify community resources that are able to assist victims of abuse and assault. (pp. 1718, 1723, 1726–1727)
9. Discuss the documentation necessary when caring for abused and assaulted patients. (pp. 1723, 1726–1727)

FRAMING THE LESSON

Begin by reviewing the important points from Chapter 43, "Geriatric Emergencies." Discuss any points that the class does not completely understand. Then move on to Chapter 44. Ask the students to name types of abuse and the typical victims associated with abuse and assault. Encourage all students to participate and stretch themselves on points of age, gender, or type of partner relationship. Persons of any age may be victims of abuse, as can males or females. Partner relationships can include heterosexual ones (with either the male or female as victim) or homosexual ones (again, including male or female victims). If you have time, encourage students who wish to mention a case with which they are personally familiar to discuss these instances; doing so will make personal the complex and sad situations that they will encounter as paramedics in the field. (Be prepared that one or more students may confide in you that they have been abused or are in an abusive relationship.) After this exercise is complete, students will have a better understanding of the scope of the problems of abuse and assault as well as its seriousness as a medical and legal emergency.

TEACHING STRATEGIES

People learn in a variety of ways. Some do better with the spoken word, whereas others prefer the written. Some prefer to work alone, whereas others profit from working in groups. Recognizing these different ways of acquiring knowledge, the authors of this *Instructor's Resource Manual* have provided a variety of teaching strategies for the different types of learners. These strategies are intended to foster higher-level cognitive skills and encourage creative learning and problem solving. For greatest effectiveness, incorporate these strategies into your class lecture. Symbols in the Lecture Outline indicate the points at which various exercises might be most appropriate. Other strategies can be used to preview the lesson or to summarize it.

The following strategies are keyed to specific sections of the lesson:

1. ***Understanding Victims of Abuse.*** It is important for students to learn that the victims of abuse are often regular people, not so different from themselves. To do this, they must spend time with people who have suffered abuse and assaults. Have the class create a volunteer project, fundraiser, or social event for a local shelter or survivor program. The gift of their time will be much appreciated, but the cooperation shared between your students and these people in need will go a long way the next time one cares for a victim of abuse or assault.

2. ***Creating a Reporting System for Identifying Abuse.*** Suggest to students that they create a reporting structure for victims that begins in the field and transfers to the hospital. For example, Rural/Metro of Syracuse, New York, has a simple half sheet of colored paper that can be removed from the run report that includes the facts surrounding suspicion of abuse or assault. Whenever the ED staff sees the report on this special colored paper, the patient gets a consult with social services, a division of the hospital better equipped to deal with the issues of abuse than a busy ED. Additionally, when a file is pulled for a patient, multiple reports on this special colored paper are an easy visual cue that previous providers have suspected abuse. Share great examples like this of EMS making a difference to inspire creative problem solving in your students.

3. ***Researching Community Agencies That Aid the Abused.*** Have students research the agencies in their communities equipped to handle victims of abuse.

They should include shelters, hospitals, clinics, and counseling programs. Require them to create a pocket card so that this information is at the ready should they need to refer a patient or abuser in the future.

4. Psychologist-Led Workshop on Communicating with Victims of Abuse. Ask a counselor or psychologist with expertise in victims of abuse to help you conduct a workshop on interviewing and communicating with these patients. Be sure it is not just a lecture but a real chance to practice the techniques taught by this professional during role playing or scenarios. This is a difficult skill that often includes sensitive and embarrassing subject matter. The student will be woefully inept unless these skills are developed first in the classroom.

5. Improving the Index of Suspicion. Improve your students' index of suspicion for abuse by brainstorming physical and emotional findings that might suggest abuse. Ask students to give examples of contexts in which the finding would or would not be indicative of abuse. Being alert to the possibilities will increase the likelihood that students will assess for and report potential abuse.

6. Newspaper Articles and Case Studies of Abuse. Gather newspaper clippings and case studies of abuse and neglect for reading in class during this unit. Often providers cannot identify with the trauma of abuse until they meet a victim and realize that the people are just like themselves or their family members. Gathering clippings lends realism to the topic.

The following strategies can be used at various points throughout the lesson or to help summarize and demonstrate what students have learned.

Learning Local Protocol for Reporting Abuse. Be sure students understand the reporting policy in your locale. EMS professionals are not mandatory reporters in every state. If the policy exists in your area, supply students with phone numbers, contact names, and timelines for reporting. This information is probably available from your Department of Health Services.

Guest Speakers. This strategy will help students see the faces behind the profiles. If you have appropriate contacts with a battered women's shelter, sexual assault nurse examiner (SANE), police officer, or public prosecutor, consider getting someone with extensive firsthand experience to speak to the students. Another possibility is someone who has recovered from a background of abuse or assault, preferably someone who had contact with EMS at some point in their background and could address what EMTs did in their case or did not do.

Role Playing Abuse Scenarios. If your students feel comfortable doing so, ask them to take roles in different scenarios. One scenario might have parents involved in child abuse, the child, and an EMS provider; another may have an abused elder, an adult child caregiver who is abusive or neglectful, and an EMS provider.

Ask the students who watch each role play to take notes of things the participants say or do (such as body posture, not making eye contact with provider) that give them insight into the situation and the provider's response to the medical, social, and legal aspects of the case.

Distinguishing Abuse from Medical Problems. Invite your students to brainstorm about situations (for partner, elder, child, and sexual abuse) that might be mistaken for abuse but are not. Then have them act out the roles and get feedback from participants and viewers about their feelings for the people suspected of abuse and the provider who feels there is real suspicion of an abuse situation in this case.

Practice in the Field. If possible, talk with the appropriate liaison individuals and consider sending students (one at a time or in pairs) to any of the following types of sites or groups:

- the sexual assault unit of the local police force or district attorney's office
- a correctional institute or community group for persons convicted of abuse or assault or undergoing therapy for anger management or abuse
- a meeting of sexual assault nurse examiners (SANEs)
- a facility caring for children who have been abused
- a home that takes in elders who have been abused or provides day care for at-risk elders whose adult children work outside the home

Cultural Considerations, Legal Notes, and Patho Pearls. The Student CD-ROM contains this series of informative features to enhance the student's understanding of the material covered in this chapter.

TEACHING OUTLINE

Chapter 44 is the fourth lesson in Division 5, *Special Considerations/Operations*. Distribute Handout 44-1 so that students can familiarize themselves with the learning goals for this chapter. If students have any questions about the objectives, answer them at this time.

Then present the chapter. One possible lecture outline follows. In the outline, the parenthetical references in regular type are references to text pages; those in bold type are references to figures, tables, or procedures.

I. Introduction. Millions of children, adults, and elderly persons are abused and assaulted each year in the United States, and the EMS system is involved with many cases of abuse. It is crucial that EMS providers be prepared for all aspects of care involved in handling these patients. (p. 1716)

- **A.** Magnitude of the problem (p. 1716)
    1. Nearly 3 million children are abused each year, with more than 1,000 deaths.
    2. Between 2 and 4 million women are battered each year by their partners.
    3. Between 700,000 and 1.1 million elders are abused each year.
- **B.** Scope of the problem (p. 1716)
    1. Abuse situations transcend gender, race, age, and socioeconomic status.
    2. Effects are serious and long-lasting and may form a cycle in which a victim of abuse later becomes an abuser.
- **C.** Ramifications for EMS providers (p. 1716)
    1. Cooperate with law enforcement when they are present.
    2. Identify victims and initiate responsive action when law enforcement is not present.

II. Partner abuse (pp. 1716–1718)

- **A.** May occur in any type of domestic partnership (p. 1716)
- **B.** Both men and women may be victim or abuser. (p. 1716)
- **C.** Abuse of women by men most widespread form of partner abuse (p. 1716)
- **D.** Characterizations of this form of abuse extend generally to most battery situations. (p. 1716)
- **E.** Categories of abuse (p. 1716)
    1. Physical
        a. Application of force

  b. Causes direct personal injury
  c. May exacerbate existing medical conditions
   i. Hypertension
   ii. Diabetes
   iii. Asthma
 2. Verbal
  a. Words chosen to control or harm
  b. Damages self-esteem
  c. May exacerbate existing medical conditions
  d. Can lead to self-destructive behavior
   i. Depression
   ii. Substance abuse
   iii. Suicidal behavior
 3. Sexual
  a. Forced sexual contact
  b. Form of physical abuse
  c. Includes marital or date rape

F. Reasons for not reporting abuse (pp. 1716–1717)
 1. Fear of reprisal
 2. Fear of humiliation
 3. Denial
 4. Lack of knowledge
 5. Lack of financial resources

G. Identification of partner abuse (10 generic risk factors) (p. 1717)
 1. Male is unemployed.
 2. Male uses illegal drugs at least once a year.
 3. Partners have different religious backgrounds.
 4. Family income is below the poverty level.
 5. Partners are unmarried.
 6. Either partner is violent toward children at home.
 7. Male did not graduate from high school.
 8. Male is unemployed or has a blue-collar job.
 9. Male is between 18 and 30 years old.
 10. Male saw his father hit his mother.

H. Characteristics of partner abusers (p. 1717)
 1. History of family violence
 2. Two partners who do not know how to back down from conflict
 3. Overly aggressive personality in abusers
 4. Use of alcohol or drugs by abuser
 5. Cycle of feeling out of control then remorseful, then repetition of cycle by abuser

I. Characteristics of abused partners (pp. 1717–1718)
 1. Pregnancy
  a. 45 percent of abused women suffer some form of battery while pregnant
 2. Substance abuse to seek a numbing effect
 3. Emotional disorders such as depression, anxiety, or suicidal behavior
 4. Tendency to protect attacker

J. Approaching the battered patient (p. 1718)
 1. Use direct questioning techniques.
 2. Avoid judgmental comments and questions.
 3. Listen carefully, assuring patient of your respect and attention.
 4. Encourage victims to regain control of their lives.
 5. Advise patient to take all precautions.
  a. Be knowledgeable about local resources for assistance.

TEACHING STRATEGY 2
Creating a Reporting System for Identifying Abuse

READING/REFERENCE
Criss, E. "EMS—Resource for Battered Women," *JEMS*, July 2000.

TEACHING STRATEGY 3
Researching Community Agencies That Aid the Abused

TEACHING STRATEGY 4
Psychologist-Led Workshop on Communicating with Victims of Abuse

POWERPOINT PRESENTATION
Chapter 44 PowerPoint slides 13–16

III. Elder abuse (pp. 1718–1720)
  A. Contributing factors (see also Chapter 43) (p. 1718)
    1. Increased life expectancy
    2. Increased dependency on others as a result of longevity
    3. Decreased productivity in later years
    4. Physical and mental impairments, especially among the very old
    5. Limited resources for long-term care of elderly
    6. Economic factors
    7. Stress on middle-aged caretakers responsible for two generations
  B. Identification of elder abuse (p. 1719)
    1. Domestic
      a. Elder in home-based setting
    2. Institutional
      a. Elder being cared for by a person paid to provide care
    3. Acts of commission
      a. Physical
      b. Sexual
      c. Emotional violence
    4. Acts of omission
      a. Neglect
  C. Theories about causes of domestic elder abuse (p. 1719)
    1. Stressed and overburdened caregivers
    2. Physical or mental impairment in elderly victim
    3. Family history of violence
    4. Personal problems for caregiver
  D. Characteristics of abused elders (p. 1719)
    1. If abuse
      a. Likely that elder is dependent upon another
    2. If neglect
      a. Likely elder lives alone and is afraid to ask for help
  E. Characteristics of elder abusers (pp. 1719–1720) (**Table 44-1, p. 1719**)

POWERPOINT PRESENTATION
Chapter 44 PowerPoint slides 17–28

IV. Child abuse (pp. 1720–1722)
  A. One of most difficult situations paramedic will face (p. 1720)
  B. Cases may range from neglect to violence resulting in emotional or physical impairment. (p. 1720)
  C. Occurs among children of all ages (birth to 18 years) (p. 1720)
  D. Can be inflicted by any caregiver, including a sibling or other child (p. 1720)
  E. May be physical, emotional, or sexual (p. 1720) (**Fig. 44-1, p. 1720**)
  F. Characteristics of child abusers (pp. 1720–1721)
    1. Any one or combination of the following should raise index of suspicion
      a. Family history of abuse
      b. Use or abuse of drugs and/or alcohol
      c. Immaturity and preoccupation with self
      d. Lack of obvious feeling for the child, rarely looking at or touching the child
      e. Seemingly unconcerned about the child's injury, treatment, or prognosis
      f. Openly critical of the child, with little indication of guilt or remorse for involvement in the child's condition
      g. Little identification with the child's pain, whether it be physical or emotional
  G. Characteristics of abused children (p. 1721)
    1. Any one or combination of the following should raise index of suspicion
      a. Crying (often hopelessly) during treatment or not crying at all

TEACHING STRATEGY 5
Improving the Index of Suspicion

- b. Avoiding parents or showing little concern for their absence
- c. Unusually wary or fearful of physical contact
- d. Apprehensive and/or constantly on the alert for danger
- e. Prone to sudden behavioral changes
- f. Absence of nearly all emotions
- g. Neediness, constantly requesting favors, food, or things

H. Identification of the abused child (pp. 1721–1723)
   1. Assessment
      a. Discrepancies in history
      b. Evidence of physical or emotional abuse
      c. Environmental clues of neglect
      d. Conditions commonly mistaken for abuse
         i. Car seat burns
         ii. Staphylococcal scalded skin syndrome
         iii. Chickenpox (cigarette burns)
         iv. Hematological disorders associated with easy bruising
   2. Indicators of abuse on physical exam often relate to soft-tissue injury. (Table 44-2, p. 1722) (Fig. 44-2, p. 1722)
      a. Burns and scalds
         i. Especially those indicating the implement or source
         ii. Common locations
            a) Soles of the feet
            b) Palms of the hands
            c) Back
            d) Buttocks
      b. Fractures sites
         i. Skull
         ii. Nose
         iii. Facial features
         iv. Upper extremities
      c. Head injuries
         i. Account for most mortality and long-term morbidity
         ii. Scalp wounds
         iii. Skull fractures
         iv. Subdural hematomas
         v. Repeated contusions
         vi. Note head injuries
      d. Shaken baby syndrome
         i. Signs of brain damage
         ii. Neck and/or spine injury
         iii. Retinal hemorrhages
      e. Abdominal injuries
         i. Infrequent but can be very serious with trauma to liver, spleen, or mesentery due to blunt force
   3. Signs of neglect
      a. Malnutrition
         i. Sometimes as severely underweight as up to 30 percent
      b. Severe diaper rash
      c. Diarrhea and/or dehydration
      d. Hair loss
      e. Untreated medical conditions
      f. Inappropriate, dirty, or torn clothing
      g. Tired and listless attitude
      h. Nearly constant demands for physical contact or attention
   4. Signs of emotional abuse
      a. Caregiver ignoring child and showing indifference
      b. Caregiver rejecting, humiliating, or criticizing child

> **TEACHING STRATEGY 6**
> Newspaper Articles and Case Studies of Abuse

           c. Isolation of child with deprivation of normal human nurturing
           d. Terrorizing child with verbal bullying
           e. Caregiver encouraging destructive or antisocial behavior
           f. Overpressuring child with unrealistic expectations of success
    I. Recording and reporting child abuse (p. 1723)
        1. You have a responsibility to report suspected cases of child abuse.
        2. Pay attention to requests for help or other signals from the abuser.
        3. Conduct examinations in suspected or known cases with a colleague present, if at all possible.
        4. Final documentation should be objective, legible, and written with the knowledge that it may be used in legal action.

> **POWERPOINT PRESENTATION**
> Chapter 44 PowerPoint slides 28–48

V. Sexual assault (pp. 1724–1727)

    A. Sexual assault (p. 1724)
        1. Unwanted oral, genital, rectal, or manual sexual contact
    B. Rape (p. 1724)
        1. Penile penetration of genitalia or rectum without victim's consent
    C. Legal definition of rape varies from state to state. (p. 1724)
    D. Characteristics of victims of sexual assault/rape (p. 1724)
        1. Patterns
           a. Victim most likely to be a female adolescent under age 18
           b. Incidence most likely
               i. Between 6 P.M. and 6 A.M.
               ii. At victim's home or home of friend, relative, or acquaintance
           c. Assailant more likely to be someone known by victim
        2. Symptoms of sexual abuse (molestation)
           a. Nightmares
           b. Restlessness
           c. Withdrawal tendencies
           d. Hostility
           e. Phobias related to the offender
           f. Regressive behavior such as bed-wetting
           g. Truancy
           h. Promiscuity in older children and teens
           i. Drug and alcohol abuse
    E. Characteristics of sexual assailants (p. 1725)
        1. Assailants come from every background.
        2. Victimizers of children are more likely to have been abused themselves as children.
        3. Many, especially adolescents and abusive adults, believe domination is part of any relationship.
        4. Assaults often occur when assailant is under influence of alcohol or other drugs.
        5. Nearly 30 percent of rapists use weapons.
        6. Assailants may use date rape drugs.
    F. Date rape drugs (predator drugs) (p. 1725)
        1. Occurring with increasing frequency
        2. Actions
           a. Render a person unresponsive
           b. Weaken them to a point where they are unable to resist an attacker
           c. Some of these medications cause amnesia, thus eliminating or distorting the victim's recall of the assault
        3. Rohypnol
           a. Characteristics
               i. Potent benzodiazepine
               ii. Colorless

   iii. Odorless
   iv. Tasteless
   v. Can be dissolved in a drink without being detected
   vi. Alcohol intensifies its effects.
  b. Body responses
   i. Sedative effect
   ii. Amnesia
   iii. Muscle relaxation
   iv. Slowing of the psychomotor response
  c. Street names
   i. Roofies
   ii. Rope
   iii. Ruffies
   iv. R2
   v. Ruffles
   vi. Roche
   vii. Forget-Pill
   viii. Mexican Valium
4. Gamma-hydroxybutyrate (GHB)
  a. Characteristics
   i. Liquid
   ii. Odorless
   iii. Colorless
   iv. Depressant with anesthetic-type qualities
   v. Used as an amino acid supplement by body builders
  b. Body responses
   i. Relaxation
   ii. Tranquility
   iii. Sensuality
   iv. Loss of inhibitions
  c. Street names
   i. Liquid Ecstasy
   ii. Liquid X
   iii. Scoop
   iv. Easy Lay
   v. Grievous Bodily Harm
5. Ketamine
  a. Characteristics
   i. Potent anesthetic agent
   ii. Widely used in veterinary practice
   iii. Used in human anesthesia
   iv. Chemically similar to the hallucinogenic LSD
  b. Body responses
   i. Hallucinations
   ii. Amnesia
   iii. Dissociation
  c. Street names
   i. K
   ii. Special K
   iii. Vitamin K
   iv. Jet
   v. Super Acid
6. MDMA
  a. Characteristics
   i. Most commonly known as Ecstasy
  b. Body responses
   i. Psychological difficulties

                    a) Confusion
                    b) Depression
                    c) Sleep problems
                    d) Drug craving
                    e) Severe anxiety
                    f) Paranoia
                        1) During and sometimes weeks after taking the drug
                ii. Physical symptoms
                    a) Muscle tension
                    b) Involuntary teeth clenching
                    c) Nausea
                    d) Blurred vision
                    e) Rapid eye movement
                    f) Faintness
                    g) Chills or sweating
            c. Street names for MDMA
                i. Ecstasy
                ii. Beans
                iii. Adam
                iv. XTC
                v. Roll
                vi. E
                vii. M
        7. Precautions
            a. Persons attending parties and other events should be cautious in regard to predator drugs.
            b. It is best not to drink from a punch bowl or a bottle passed around.
            c. Notice the behavior of others at the party.
            d. If a person seems more intoxicated than the amount of alcohol consumed would warrant, then consider the possibility of predator drugs.
            e. If a rape victim thinks she has been drugged, a drug screen should be requested upon arrival at the emergency department.
            f. EMS personnel should note any suspicions or observations that may point to the use of a predator drug.
    G. EMS responsibilities (p. 1726)
        1. Ensure own and patient's safety foremost.
        2. Never enter a scene if you feel your safety is compromised; leave if you feel unsafe.
        3. Provide safety and privacy during patient care.
        4. Consider care by a same-sex provider.
        5. Give patient some feelings of control by offering choices wherever possible.
    H. Legal considerations (pp. 1726–1727)
        1. Responsibility to report cases to appropriate law enforcement officials
        2. Obligation to know about available victim and witness protection programs
        3. Responsibility to know about specialized resources
            a. Shelters
            b. State agencies
            c. Nurses trained as sexual assault nurse examiners (SANEs)
        4. Evidence
            a. Rules on obtaining possible evidence of crime
            b. Understanding of concept of chain of evidence
        5. Familiarity with local protocols for abuse and assault

VI. Chapter summary (p. 1727). The incidence of abuse is widespread today, and you will encounter many cases during your paramedic career. You should learn the hallmarks of partner abuse, elder abuse, child abuse, and sexual assaults. You should also learn to recognize significant physical and emotional assessment findings as well as characteristics of the victims and assailants. Proper treatment of victims of abuse and assault includes knowing the legal requirements of your area, protecting evidence, and properly documenting your findings and actions.

POWERPOINT PRESENTATION
Chapter 44 PowerPoint slide 49

SKILLS DEMONSTRATION AND PRACTICE

Students can practice skills discussed in the chapter in the following role play:

Form groups of students and have each write a role play scenario for partner, child, or elder abuse or for sexual assault. Have each writing group come up with a list of items that are present in the script (or should be present in the acting) that are historical, environmental, or behavioral clues to the type of abuse or assault being presented. They may wish to do this before or after writing the script itself.

Have another group present the scenario, and then have the class as a whole discuss what they have seen. See if class members find all of the clues that the writing group listed or if they come up with different or additional clues.

If you have had speakers come to the group or had students make field visits, have the students with firsthand experience compare and contrast their actual experience with what they saw in the scenario and heard in the group discussion.

ADVANCED LIFE SUPPORT SKILLS
Larmon & Davis. *Advanced Life Support Skills.*

ADVANCED LIFE SKILLS REVIEW
Larmon & Davis. *Advanced Life Skills Review.*

BRADY SKILLS SERIES: ALS
Larmon & Davis. *Brady Skills Series: ALS.*

WORKBOOK
Chapter 44 Activities

ASSIGNMENTS

Assign students to complete Chapter 44, "Abuse and Assault," of the workbook. Also assign them to read Chapter 45, "The Challenged Patient," before the next class.

READING/REFERENCE
Textbook, pp. 1729–1745

HANDOUT 44-2
Chapter 44 Quiz

EVALUATION

Chapter Quiz and Scenario   Distribute copies of the Chapter Quiz provided in Handout 44-2 to evaluate student understanding of this chapter. Make sure each student reads the scenario to reinforce critical thinking on the scene. Remind students not to use their notes or textbooks while taking the quiz.

Student CD   Quizzes for every chapter are contained on the dynamic and highly visual in-text student CD.

Companion Website   Additional quizzes for every chapter are contained on this exciting website.

TestGen   You may wish to create a custom-tailored test using *Prentice Hall TestGen for Essentials of Paramedic Care,* 2nd Edition to evaluate student understanding of this chapter.

On-line Test Preparation (for students and instructors)   Additional test preparation is available through Brady's new on-line product, *EMT Achieve: Paramedic Test Preparation* at *http://www.prenhall.com/emtachieve/.* Instructors can also monitor student mastery on-line.

HANDOUT 44-3
Chapter 44 Scenario

PARAMEDIC STUDENT CD
Student Activities

COMPANION WEBSITE
http://www.prenhall.com/bledsoe

TESTGEN
Chapter 44

EMT ACHIEVE: PARAMEDIC TEST PREPARATION
Mistovich & Beasley. *EMT Achieve: Paramedic Test Preparation.*
www.prenhall.com/emtachieve/

©2007 Pearson Education, Inc.
Essentials of Paramedic Care, 2nd ed.

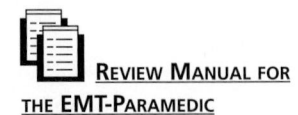

Review Manual for the EMT-Paramedic This comprehensive exam review contains hundreds of test questions and rationales, including scenarios, along with two 180-question practice tests on CD.

REVIEW MANUAL FOR THE EMT-PARAMEDIC
Cherry & Mistovich. *Review Manual for the EMT-Paramedic*, 3rd edition.

REINFORCEMENT

HANDOUTS 44-4 AND 44-5
Reinforcement Activities

Handouts If classroom discussion or performance on the quiz indicates that some students have not fully mastered the chapter content, you may wish to assign some or all of the Reinforcement Handouts for this chapter.

PARAMEDIC STUDENT CD
Student Activities

Student CD (for students) A wide variety of material on this CD-ROM will reinforce and also expand student knowledge and skills.

POWERPOINT PRESENTATION
Chapter 44

PowerPoint Presentation (for instructors) The PowerPoint material developed for this chapter offers useful reinforcement of chapter content.

COMPANION WEBSITE
http://www.prenhall.com/bledsoe

Companion Website (for students) Additional review quizzes and links to EMS resources will contribute to further reinforcement of the chapter.

ONEKEY
Chapter 44

OneKey On-line support is offered for this course on one of three platforms: CourseCompass, Blackboard, or Web CT. Includes the IRM, PowerPoints, TestGen, and Companion Website for instruction. Ask your local sales representative for more information.

ADVANCED LIFE SUPPORT SKILLS
Larmon & Davis. *Advanced Life Support Skills.*

Brady Skills Series: Advanced Life Skills (Video or CD) Have your students watch the skills come to life on VHS or CD-ROM, or they can purchase the highly visual, full-color text with step-by-step procedures and rationales.

ADVANCED LIFE SKILLS REVIEW
Larmon & Davis. *Advanced Life Skills Review.*

BRADY SKILLS SERIES: ALS
Larmon & Davis. *Brady Skills Series: ALS.*

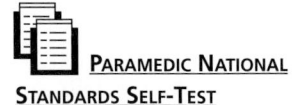

PARAMEDIC NATIONAL STANDARDS SELF-TEST
Miller. *Paramedic National Standards Self-Test*, 4th edition.

HANDOUT 44-1

Student's Name _____

CHAPTER 44 OBJECTIVES CHECKLIST

Knowledge	Date Mastered
1. Discuss the incidence of abuse and assault.	
2. Describe the categories of abuse.	
3. Discuss examples of spouse, elder, child, and sexual abuse.	
4. Describe the characteristics associated with the profile of a typical spouse, elder, or child abuser and the typical assailant of sexual abuse.	
5. Identify the profile of the "at-risk" spouse, elder, and child.	
6. Discuss the assessment and management of the abused patient.	
7. Discuss the legal aspects associated with abuse situations.	
8. Identify community resources that are able to assist victims of abuse and assault.	
9. Discuss the documentation necessary when caring for abused and assaulted patients.	

Handout 44-2

Student's Name _____

CHAPTER 44 QUIZ

Write the letter of the best answer in the space provided.

_____ 1. Which of the following is NOT one of the several common reasons why a domestic partner does not report that he or she is being abused?
   A. fear of reprisal by the abusing partner
   B. lack of knowledge of how to report abuse or seek help
   C. fear that he or she will not be believed
   D. denial that their situation is one of abuse

_____ 2. Characteristics of abused partners include all of the following EXCEPT:
   A. pregnancy in a female partner.
   B. chronic physical condition.
   C. substance abuse.
   D. emotional disorders.

_____ 3. Elder abusers are often all EXCEPT which of the following individuals?
   A. a grandchild
   B. an adult child
   C. a spouse
   D. a different kind of familial relative

_____ 4. All of the following injuries in a child should give you a high level of suspicion that child abuse is involved EXCEPT:
   A. burns on the soles of the feet, palms of the hands, back, or buttocks.
   B. head injuries.
   C. fractures of the skull, nose, or ribs.
   D. burns in a "splash" pattern.

_____ 5. All of the following are common clues that a child is being neglected EXCEPT:
   A. severe diaper rash.
   B. malnutrition and underweight condition.
   C. a child patient ignoring and avoiding physical contact with EMS provider.
   D. untreated medical conditions.

_____ 6. Common characteristics of victims of sexual assault include all of the following EXCEPT:
   A. celibacy and denial of own sexuality.
   B. phobias related to the offender.
   C. regressive behavior such as bed-wetting.
   D. withdrawal tendencies.

_____ 7. Which of the following medical conditions is NOT easily mistaken for a sign of abuse?
   A. chickenpox
   B. car seat burns
   C. blood disorders that cause easy bruising
   D. measles

_____ 8. All of the following are correct correlations between the age of a bruise and its skin appearance EXCEPT:
   A. 0–2 days and a reddened, swollen, tender appearance.
   B. 10 or more days and a yellow color.
   C. 0–5 days and blue or purple color.
   D. 5–7 days and a green color.

_____ 9. Which of the following is NOT one of the common characteristics of a child abuser?
   A. history of having been abused themselves
   B. overly concerned with child's welfare and severity of any injury during interview
   C. pattern over time of becoming more frequently and more severely abusive
   D. immaturity and preoccupation with self

HANDOUT 44-2 Continued

_____ 10. All of the following are common characteristics of abused children EXCEPT:
   A. constant crying or no crying during treatment.
   B. absence of emotion or constant neediness for attention from the EMS provider.
   C. avoiding parents or constantly asking for parents' attention.
   D. sudden behavioral changes during interview and treatment.

_____ 11. All of the following are characteristic of abusers of women EXCEPT:
   A. unemployment.
   B. use of illegal drugs at least once a year.
   C. family income over $95,000 a year.
   D. different religious background from the woman.

_____ 12. In cases of neglect, the elders most commonly:
   A. have incomes less than $75,000 a year.
   B. live alone.
   C. live with grandchildren.
   D. have a chronic medical condition requiring medication.

_____ 13. The physical or emotional violence or neglect that is carried out when an elder is being cared for by a person paid to provide care is:
   A. professional elder abuse.   C. common elder abuse.
   B. institutional elder abuse.   D. mercenary elder abuse.

_____ 14. The number of states that require health care workers to report suspected cases of child abuse is:
   A. 35.   C. 45.
   B. 40.   D. 50.

_____ 15. Your primary responsibility at a call to a scene of suspected abuse is:
   A. preserving the chain of evidence.
   B. discovering the identity of the abuser.
   C. your safety and that of the patient.
   D. psychological support.

Handout 44-3

Student's Name _____

CHAPTER 44 SCENARIO

Review the following real-life situation. Then answer the questions that follow.

A team is called to a neighborhood nursing home to check "an elderly woman who fell." On arrival, the team waits in the lobby until an aide comes for them.

They walk down the hall and find an elderly lady sitting up in bed, clutching the side rails with both hands. Her hair is uncombed, and she looks vacantly out before her. The aide says she is busy and cannot stay, and then leaves them with the patient.

They introduce themselves, and the lady says her name is Lillian Good and that she is 84 years old. Kerry starts to ask her whether she fell when a nurse comes into the room and answers the question by saying, "Lillian knew she shouldn't get out of bed without help, but she tried anyway." Lillian is quiet. Kerry says she needs to examine the patient, but then has to squeeze past the nurse to get to the bedside. Kerry asks Mrs. Good about the fall as she gently takes a hand to check a pulse and looks closely at the patient.

Kerry notes that the lady looks and smells as if she has not bathed recently, and there is a clear odor of urine. The bottom sheet is crisp and white in contrast to the top sheet, which has a variety of food stains on it. As Kerry gently asks her question about the fall again, the nurse interrupts to say that Mrs. Good falls often and a new aide called the paramedics. "It was really a mistake," she says. "We don't need your help. If you just want to check her vital signs, you can leave."

1. Based on initial impressions, what, if any, problems do you suspect in addition to your need to work up the alleged fall?

2. Does the nurse's behavior arouse your index of suspicion? Why or why not?

3. Based on this impression, are there any signs you should look for while conducting a physical examination of the patient?

4. If your physical is within normal limits, the patient does not supply any information, and there is no evidence of injury from the (alleged) fall, is there anything more you should do before discussing the case with medical direction?

HANDOUT 44-4

Student's Name _____

CHAPTER 44 REVIEW

Write the word or words that best complete each sentence in the space(s) provided.

1. The pattern of abuse and assault forms a(n) _____ that is difficult to break.

2. Victims of partner abuse hesitate or fail to report the problem because of fear of _____, fear of humiliation, denial, lack of knowledge, and lack of _____ _____.

3. Partner abuse may be categorized as _____ abuse, the most obvious form, _____ abuse, which damages self-esteem, and _____ abuse, a form of physical abuse.

4. A history of _____ _____ makes a person more likely to repeat the pattern of partner abuse as an adult.

5. The three characteristics of abused partners are _____ (45 percent of abused women), _____ _____, and emotional disorders such as _____, evasiveness, anxiety, and suicidal behavior.

6. When speaking with an abused partner, be prepared to share your knowledge of _____ _____.

7. _____ _____ _____ takes place when an elder is being cared for in a home situation; _____ elder abuse occurs when an elder is being cared for by a person who is paid for such care.

8. One of the four main theories about the causes of elder abuse is that caregivers feel _____ or _____.

9. Elder abuse can be either acts of _____ (physical, sexual, or emotional violence) or acts of _____ (neglect).

10. _____ _____ make up the largest group of perpetrators of domestic elder abuse.

11. Most _____ _____ were physically or emotionally abused as children.

12. In cases of reported physical child abuse, perpetrators tend to be _____.

13. Abused children may be unusually wary and fearful of _____ _____.

14. Abused children under 6 usually appear excessively _____, while those over age 6 appear _____.

15. Frequent behavioral traits of child abusers include immaturity and preoccupation with _____, seeming _____ about a child's injury, treatment, or prognosis, and little indication of _____ or _____ for involvement in the child's condition.

16. A green bruise on a child who has been abused is _____ to _____ days old.

17. The paramedic can frequently recognize the source of intentional burns to children by their _____ and/or _____.

18. _____ _____ _____ may occur when a parent or caregiver becomes frustrated with a crying child.

19. Neglected children are frequently _____, causing them to be underweight, sometimes by up to 30 percent.

20. Neglected children may also exhibit _____ or _____ attitudes or make near constant demands for _____ _____.

REINFORCEMENT

©2007 Pearson Education, Inc.
Essentials of Paramedic Care, 2nd ed.

HANDOUT 44-4 Continued

21. _____ _____ is unwanted sexual contact, while _____ is generally defined as penile penetration of the genitalia or rectum.

22. The group most likely to be the victims of sexual assault/rape are _____ younger than age _____.

23. Government figures show that approximately one third of all juvenile victims of assault/rape are younger than _____ years of age.

24. In cases of date rape, the assailant may have drugged the victim with _____, known by the street names of roofie, roche, rib, and rope.

25. As well as physical care, the paramedic is responsible for providing proper _____ care for the victims of assault and rape.

ABUSE AND ASSAULT TRUE OR FALSE

Indicate whether the following statements are true or false by writing T or F in the space provided.

_____ 1. Abuse and assault in the United States involves persons of each gender and of every race, age, and socioeconomic status.

_____ 2. Partner abuse can involve heterosexual couples or same-sex couples, but men are the abusers in relationships that involve a man.

_____ 3. You may find that an abuse victim who is a patient of yours has both direct injury and indirect injury, with the latter represented by aggravation of an existing medical condition such as asthma or diabetes.

_____ 4. When you are talking with a patient who has been physically battered, you will find that direct, nonjudgmental questioning generally works best.

_____ 5. Elder abuse commonly takes place in homes, but not in institutional settings such as a nursing home.

_____ 6. Approximately 1 million women in the United States are battered by their spouses each year.

_____ 7. Nearly 3 million children in the United States suffer abuse each year.

_____ 8. Battery is not a problem between same-sex couples.

_____ 9. Forty-five percent of women suffer some form of battery during pregnancy.

_____ 10. One of the most common theories holds that caregivers in cases of elder abuse feel stressed and overburdened.

_____ 11. A child's behavior is one of the most important indicators of abuse.

_____ 12. Because rib fractures are common in children, they are not a good indicator of abuse.

_____ 13. When confronted with a case of child abuse, try to conduct the examination with another colleague present.

_____ 14. One in two U.S. rape victims is under age 18.

_____ 15. In case of rape, allow the victim to urinate or defecate if it will calm her.

Chapter 44 Answer Key

Handout 44-2: Chapter 44 Quiz

1. C	5. C	9. B	13. B
2. B	6. A	10. C	14. D
3. A	7. D	11. C	15. C
4. D	8. B	12. B	

Handout 44-3: Chapter 44 Scenario

1. There should be a high level of suspicion of institutional elder neglect or abuse. There are signs that the patient's personal hygiene has not been adequately addressed (uncombed hair, indications that she hasn't bathed or been bathed), her environment has not been adequately cared for (top sheet with old and new food stains, indicating it hasn't been changed), and that she hasn't had needed care (the clear smell of urine and signs that the bottom sheet has just been changed).
2. The nurse is excluding the patient from conversation with the paramedics and is dismissive of the incident. She clearly wants the team to leave as soon as possible.
3. There may be signs of direct abuse or further evidence of neglect. Signs of abuse might include bruises of various ages. Signs of neglect might include bedsores on the buttocks, heels, or elbows or evidence of urine or fecal material on the bedding, clothing, or patient. Other potential signs of abuse or neglect would include any indications of dehydration or malnutrition.
4. You must organize the reasons for your suspicion of elder abuse or neglect for yourselves, as well as document them thoroughly. You must further evaluate your impressions of the nurse as well as any other staff you encounter while on-scene and appraise medical direction of any concerns you may have for the patient's safety if she is not transported to a facility for evaluation. You should also ask (if it is not clear per local protocol) whether the nurse or another member of the nursing home staff can refuse transport of the patient.

Handout 44-4: Chapter 44 Review

1. cycle
2. reprisal, financial resources
3. physical, verbal, sexual
4. family abuse
5. pregnancy, substance abuse, depression
6. community resources
7. Domestic elder abuse, institutional
8. stressed, overburdened
9. commission, omission
10. Adult children
11. child abusers
12. men
13. physical contact
14. passive, aggressive
15. self, unconcerned, guilt, remorse
16. 5, 7
17. shape, pattern
18. Shaken Baby Syndrome
19. malnourished
20. tired, listless, physical contact
21. Sexual assault, rape
22. females, 18
23. 6
24. flunitrazepam (Rohypnol)
25. psychosocial

Handout 44-5: Abuse and Assault True or False

1. T	5. F	9. T	13. T
2. F	6. F	10. T	14. T
3. T	7. T	11. T	15. F
4. T	8. F	12. F	

Chapter 45

The Challenged Patient

INTRODUCTION

Throughout your students' careers, they will encounter patients who live with a challenge, who may present special needs. The challenges that these patients face may be obvious to the EMS provider (such as complete blindness, cerebral palsy, or paraplegia). In other cases, they may be so subtle that they are not identified readily in initial conversation with the patient (such as slight mental retardation or some degree of traumatic brain injury, some degree of hearing impairment, some forms of mental illness). In still other cases, the challenges are not medical at all—the patient might speak a different language than the provider's, live in a community culture with very different expectations for health care, or be a foreign citizen in the United States. In all these and in many other cases, it is important for the provider to realize that individuals with challenges—"challenged patients"—exist and may require some level of accommodation for proper patient care to be given.

TOTAL TEACHING TIME:
5.09 HOURS
The total teaching time is only a guideline based on the didactic and practical lab averages in the National Standard Curriculum. Instructors should take into consideration such factors as the pace at which students learn, the size of the class, and breaks. The actual time devoted to teaching objectives is the responsibility of the instructor.

CHAPTER OBJECTIVES

After reading this chapter, you should be able to:

1. Describe the various etiologies and types of hearing impairments. (p. 1731)
2. Recognize the patient with a hearing impairment. (p. 1732)
3. Anticipate accommodations that may be needed in order to properly manage the patient with a hearing impairment. (p. 1732)
4. Describe the various etiologies and types, recognize patients with, and anticipate accommodations that may be needed in order to properly manage each of the following conditions:

    - Visual impairments (pp. 1732–1733)
    - Speech impairments (pp. 1733–1734)
    - Obesity (pp. 1734–1736)
    - Paraplegia/quadriplegia (p. 1736)
    - Mental illness (p. 1736)
    - Developmentally disabled (pp. 1736–1737)
    - Down syndrome (pp. 1737–1738)
    - Emotional impairment (p. 1736)
    - Emotional/mental impairment (p. 1736)

©2007 Pearson Education, Inc.
Essentials of Paramedic Care, 2nd ed.

5. Describe, identify possible presenting signs of, and anticipate accommodations for the following diseases/illnesses:

   - Arthritis (pp. 1738–1739)
   - Cancer (pp. 1739–1740)
   - Cerebral palsy (p. 1740)
   - Cystic fibrosis (p. 1741)
   - Multiple sclerosis (p. 1741)
   - Muscular dystrophy (pp. 1741–1742)
   - Myasthenia gravis (p. 1743)
   - Poliomyelitis (p. 1742)
   - Spina bifida (pp. 1742–1743)
   - Patients with a previous head injury (p. 1742)

6. Define, recognize, and anticipate accommodations needed to properly manage patients who:

   - Are culturally diverse (pp. 1743–1744)
   - Are terminally ill (p. 1744)
   - Have a communicable disease (p. 1744)
   - Have a financial impairment (p. 1744)

7. Given several challenged patients, provide the appropriate assessment, management, and transportation. (pp. 1730–1744)

FRAMING THE LESSON

Begin by reviewing the important points from Chapter 44, "Abuse and Assault." Discuss any points that the class does not completely understand. Then move on to Chapter 45. Start by splitting students into groups and assigning each group to a general type of challenge: Ask them to name as many examples as they can think of. For instance, types might include congenital conditions, changes due to aging, permanent disabilities, short-term disabilities, chronic conditions, or nonmedical challenges. As the students develop their list, have them think about the way in which a patient would manifest or try to hide each example and how they, as providers, might recognize and respond to that challenge.

For instance, a patient might be a foreign citizen in the United States. A tourist might be concerned about her ability to express herself in the English language or be unclear about the structure and funding of American health care. If the EMS provider raised the concern and asked if the person or her family had any questions, a constructive conversation might follow. However, if the patient were an unregistered alien living in the United States, her ability to voice her concerns might be much less and the provider might not realize the level of the patient's anxiety over getting caught up in the EMS system.

- Congenital conditions might involve sensory impairment (blindness or deafness), motor and speech ability (cerebral palsy), appearance (cleft lip or palate, hare lip, birthmarks) or even immune function (in a child born with immune deficiency due to HIV/AIDS or a genetic immune deficiency syndrome).
- Changes due to aging might be as subtle as poor flexibility and balance while on steps or uneven ground or as obvious as nearly total sensory loss. Severe osteoarthritis or osteoporosis may cause chronic pain or disfigurement. Macular degeneration may cause partial or total loss of vision.
- Permanent disabilities include motor loss (paraplegia, quadriplegia, amputation of a limb), sensory loss, and visible scarring from a burn or

other injury. One type of long-term disability that requires accommodation is immune compromise due to either therapy for cancer or diseases such as AIDS.
- Short-term disabilities might include pregnancy, anxiety over health in someone who had a recent MI or other major medical condition, impaired mobility in someone who had recent major surgery, or even the confusion and fatigue of someone with a high fever due to the flu or other infectious illness. One common instance providers might see is a patient with vomiting or diarrhea who feels uncomfortable saying "excuse me" and running to the bathroom.
- Chronic conditions are numerous and include impairment secondary to stroke or head injury, asthma, COPD, heart failure, diabetes, epilepsy, inflammatory bowel disease, and different forms of anemia.
- Nonmedical challenges other than the citizenship example already given include poor finances, difficulties with English as a communication language, and membership in a community culture with possible differences in expectations about health care and interaction between men and women (for instance, Asian health beliefs, or membership in Hasidic Judaism or Amish culture).

TEACHING STRATEGIES

People learn in a variety of ways. Some do better with the spoken word, whereas others prefer the written. Some prefer to work alone, whereas others profit from working in groups. Recognizing these different ways of acquiring knowledge, the authors of this *Instructor's Resource Manual* have provided a variety of teaching strategies for the different types of learners. These strategies are intended to foster higher-level cognitive skills and encourage creative learning and problem solving. For greatest effectiveness, incorporate these strategies into your class lecture. Symbols in the Lecture Outline indicate the points at which various exercises might be most appropriate. Other strategies can be used to preview the lesson or to summarize it.

The following strategies are keyed to specific sections of the lesson.

1. Creating a Device to Improve Communication. Have students work in groups to create a device or implement to improve communication with a challenged patient. This could be hearing or visually impaired, wheelchair bound, and so on. Give them plenty of time, then have them present their ideas to the group. Some might be good enough to install in your local emergency vehicles. This activity is kinesthetic and improves problem-solving skills.

2. Simulated Deafness. Simulate deafness in your classroom for an entire session by having everyone wear disposable earplugs. Be sure the students attend lectures, ask questions, and socialize, all while wearing their earplugs. At the end of the day, note how much longer it took to accomplish the same amount of material you normally cover. Ask students to record their feelings about the challenge by writing a paragraph at the end of the day. This empathy exercise is an affective domain activity.

3. Learning to Communicate through an Interpreter. Assessment and treatment of a patient using an interpreter is extremely challenging. Set up scenarios in your class that require the use of an interpreter or other means of communication. Consider using family members of students, community members, members of cultural groups, or foreign language students to act as your patients and interpreters. Emphasize that a paramedic cannot give up on the assessment or fail to communicate altogether simply because of a language barrier.

4. Teacher's Aide Assignment. Many students with special challenges are being mainstreamed into regular schools and classrooms. Assign students to assist the teachers and caregivers in these classrooms in order to better understand the physical and mental abilities and limitations of these students. Additionally, the often overworked teachers will appreciate the extra set of hands.

5. Speaker from Arthritis Foundation. A speaker from the Arthritis Foundation is probably available in your area. He or she can teach students about the disease, including current pharmacology, special challenges for arthritis patients, and accommodations that health care providers could make to improve the care provided to arthritis patients. Most of us could modify our handling and positioning of patients to make emergency procedures less painful and improve cooperation of patients suffering from this disease.

6. Diversity Exercise. To help students appreciate their differences and discover how easily one can be labeled "different," have them write on a Post-it one thing that makes them different, insecure, or afraid. Then, have the class guess who belongs to each of the differences. Discuss how it feels to be vulnerable. Emphasize the importance of tolerance and impartiality in health care providers.

The following strategies can be used at various points throughout the lesson or to help summarize and demonstrate what students have learned.

Understanding Both Sides of the Problem. For one or more medical challenges (hearing impairment, visual impairment, obesity, requirement for a wheelchair), split students into small groups. Ask one student to simulate a patient with that challenge (through placement of earplugs, use of blindfold, wearing multiple jackets and pants, being confined to a wheelchair) while the others act as the EMS team. Afterward, have the students discuss their experiences: What discomforts did the patients feel? What actions by the EMS team eased or worsened the experience for them? For the EMS providers, what actions by the patients or themselves did they feel improved the quality of communication or the ease of patient care?

Repeat this exercise after the chapter is completed to reinforce the chapter content regarding approach to the challenged patient.

Listening to Firsthand Experience. Ask individuals with a variety of challenges who have had experience with EMS to talk to the students about their interactions with EMS providers and what recommendations they have for the students.

In the Field. Take the students to an EMS unit that is off-duty and have them ask the team what equipment/procedural accommodations they can readily make for patients with a variety of challenges (blind or deaf, wheelchair-bound, obese, spastic limbs, etc.).

Cultural Considerations, Legal Notes, and Patho Pearls. The Student CD-ROM contains this series of informative features to enhance the student's understanding of the material covered in this chapter.

HANDOUT 45-1
Chapter 45 Objectives Checklist

TEACHING OUTLINE

Chapter 45 is the fifth lesson in Division 5, *Special Considerations/Operations*. Distribute Handout 45-1 so that students can familiarize themselves with the learning goals for this chapter. If students have any questions about the objectives, answer them at this time.

Then present the chapter. One possible lecture outline follows. In the outline, the parenthetical references in regular type are references to text pages; those in bold type are references to figures, tables, or procedures.

I. Introduction. A wide variety of challenges and impairments may be present in the patients paramedics encounter. Thus, they will need to understand and recognize these special conditions and make accommodations needed for proper patient care. (p. 1730)

II. Physical challenges (pp. 1730–1736)

A. Hearing impairments (pp. 1730–1732)
  1. Decrease in or loss of ability to hear or distinguish sounds, especially speech
  2. Conductive deafness
     a. Blockage of sound wave transmission through external ear canal to middle or inner ear
     b. May be treated or cured
     c. In children, rule out congenital deafness and consider otitis media.
     d. In all, consider impacted cerumen, water, or another irritant.
     e. In trauma cases, consider trauma-related causes such as hematoma.
  3. Sensorineural deafness
     a. Inability of nerve impulses to reach auditory center in brain because of nerve damage to either inner ear or the brain
     b. Is usually permanent
     c. At-risk infants and children include
        i. Preterm infants
        ii. Those treated with ototoxic drugs
        iii. Those exposed *in utero* to rubella or cytomegalovirus (CMV)
     d. Impairment may be secondary to infection
        i. Bacterial meningitis or viruses
     e. Impairment may be temporary
        i. Aspirin toxicity
           a) Manifested as ringing in the ears, tinnitus
     f. Among elderly, presbycusis (progressive age-related impairment) becomes significant in persons over age 65 years.
  4. Recognition of deafness
     a. Typical behaviors that may be mistaken for evidence of head injury
        i. Asking questions repeatedly
        ii. Misunderstanding questions or answers to their questions
        iii. Responding inappropriately to questions or requests
     b. Clues that may aid recognition
        i. Presence of hearing aid
        ii. Use of sign language
        iii. Continual positioning to be squarely in front of your face (so patient can lip read)
  5. Accommodations for deaf patients
     a. Address patient face-to-face and make sure patient understands each question or request.
     b. Speak slowly and in low-pitched voice; do not yell or overtly gesture as these may be perceived as threatening.
     c. Reduce background noise to a minimum.
     d. On night calls, consider the following:
        i. Looking for hearing aid
        ii. Placing stethoscope on patient and speaking into it
        iii. Using pen and paper

POWERPOINT PRESENTATION
Chapter 45 PowerPoint slides 4–19

TEACHING STRATEGY 1
Creating a Device to Improve Communication

TEACHING STRATEGY 2
Simulated Deafness

READING/REFERENCE
Deschamp, C., and R. C. Sneed. "EMS for Children with Special Healthcare Needs." *EMS*, Nov. 1999.

TEACHING STRATEGY 3
Learning to Communicate through an Interpreter

POINT TO EMPHASIZE
Address deaf patients face-to-face to give them the opportunity to read lips and interpret expressions.

- **iv.** Trying to find an American Sign Language (ASL) interpreter
  - **a)** Call ahead if one will be needed at hospital.
- **B.** Visual impairments (pp. 1732–1733)
  1. Etiologies
     - **a.** Injury
       - **i.** Previous injury usually includes eye and tissue around orbit.
       - **ii.** Penetrating injury often results in enucleation, removal of the eyeball.
       - **iii.** Permanent blindness may be caused by chemical and thermal burns.
       - **iv.** Causes of temporary impairment includes
         - **a)** Deployment of an airbag
         - **b)** Corneal abrasion
     - **b.** Disease
       - **i.** Glaucoma
       - **ii.** Diabetic retinopathy
     - **c.** Congenital conditions
       - **i.** Cerebral palsy
       - **ii.** Premature birth
     - **d.** Infection
       - **i.** Cytomegalovirus (CMV) infection in AIDS patients can lead to blindness via retinitis.
     - **e.** Degeneration of retina, optic nerve, or nerve pathways
  2. Recognizing and accommodating visual impairments (**Fig. 45-1, p. 1733**)
     - **a.** Identify yourself on approach.
     - **b.** Describe everything you do before/as you do it.
     - **c.** Do not touch or disturb a guide dog without patient's permission.
     - **d.** Refer to local protocol regarding transportation of a guide dog.
     - **e.** If there is no guide dog, ask if there are any tools (such as a white cane) that the patient wants to have transported with him/her.
     - **f.** Allow patient to take your arm rather than taking patient's arm if you are guiding him/her.
- **C.** Speech impairments (pp. 1733–1734)
  1. Language disorders
     - **a.** Impaired ability to understand spoken or written word
     - **b.** Aphasia
       - **i.** Loss of ability to communicate in speech, writing, or signs
     - **c.** Sensory aphasia
       - **i.** Patient cannot understand the spoken word, what you are saying.
     - **d.** Motor aphasia (expressive aphasia)
       - **i.** Patient understands what is said but cannot speak.
     - **e.** Global aphasia
       - **i.** Patient has both sensory and motor aphasia.
       - **ii.** Brain tumor in Broca's region is one cause.
  2. Articulation disorders (dysarthria)
     - **a.** Occur when sounds are produced or put together incorrectly in a way that makes it difficult for the listener to understand
     - **b.** Can occur in children or adults
  3. Voice production disorders
     - **a.** Affect the quality of the person's voice
     - **b.** Patients will show
       - **i.** Hoarseness
       - **ii.** Harshness
       - **iii.** Inappropriate pitch
       - **iv.** Abnormal nasal resonance

- c. Causes
    - i. Trauma to the vocal cords
    - ii. Infection to the vocal cords
    - iii. Cancer of the larynx is a cause in adults.
- 4. Fluency disorders
    - a. Present as a form of stuttering
    - b. More common in males than females
- 5. Accommodations for speech impairments (Fig. 45-2, p. 1735)
    - a. Listen to what is said, not how it's said.
    - b. Listen carefully and wait for complete responses.
    - c. Never assume that patient's intelligence is affected.
        - i. Use normal phrasing of questions.
    - d. Do not rush patient or finish responses.
    - e. Use question phrasing that invites short, direct answers.
    - f. Be prepared that the interview may take longer than usual.
    - g. Look directly at patient when asking questions.
    - h. Ask for a repeated response if you didn't understand the first time.
    - i. Never pretend to understand when you do not.
    - j. Be prepared to offer pen/paper or alternative means of communication.

POINT TO EMPHASIZE
When speaking to a patient with a speech impairment, try to form questions that require short, direct answers.

D. Obesity (pp. 1734–1736)
1. Over 40 percent of Americans are obese.
2. Complicates EMS care
    - a. Directly
        - i. Making lifting and moving more difficult
    - b. Indirectly
        - i. Aggravating medical conditions
            - a) Hypertension
            - b) Heart disease
            - c) Stroke
            - d) Diabetes
            - e) Musculoskeletal problems
3. Etiologies
    - a. Defined as 20 to 30 percent or more over ideal weight
    - b. Causes
        - i. Improper diet
        - ii. Lack of exercise
        - iii. Genetic factors or medical conditions that lower metabolism
            - a) Usually hypothyroidism
4. Accommodations for obese patients
    - a. Obtain a complete history.
    - b. Don't allow patient to dismiss a complaint (such as shortness of breath) as related to their obesity.
    - c. Make necessary accommodations during assessment.
        - i. ECG electrode placement on the arms and thighs if chest is unavailable
        - ii. Lung auscultation on anterior surface if patient cannot lean forward for you
    - d. Before transporting, ensure that your equipment is rated for the patient's weight.
    - e. Call for transportation assistance if necessary from another EMS crew or the fire department.
    - f. Be sure to let receiving facility know the patient's weight.
    - g. Try not to bring unneeded attention to patient to protect his or her dignity.

> **POINT TO EMPHASIZE**
> If a person has halo traction, be sure to stabilize the traction before transport.

> **TEACHING STRATEGY 4**
> Teacher's Aide Assignment

> **POWERPOINT PRESENTATION**
> Chapter 45 PowerPoint slides 20–23

> **POINT TO EMPHASIZE**
> Patients with Down syndrome are often loving and trusting. Be sure to treat them with respect and patience.

E. Paralysis (p. 1736)
  1. Ventilators
     a. If patient requires a ventilator, be sure you maintain airway (suction may be needed) and keep ventilator functioning.
     b. If ventilator isn't easily portable, use a BVM device while transporting patient to ambulance.
     c. When possible, use onboard ventilator to minimize strain on patient's battery-powered unit.
     d. Reassure patient before making any changes in life-support system.
  2. Halo traction
     a. Stabilize traction before transport.
     b. Ask patient, and check with physician, if there is any question.
  3. Colostomy
     a. Be sure not to disturb external bag or stoma site.
  4. Assistance devices
     a. Be sure to ask patient what devices (e.g., canes, walkers, wheelchairs) should be transported to give patient some autonomy after arrival at receiving facility.

III. **Mental challenges and emotional impairments** (p. 1736)

  A. Wide range, from psychotic states and mood disorders to emotional responses to a recent or ongoing traumatic experience (p. 1736)
  B. Review Chapter 38 for details on assessment, management, and treatment of patients with these types of disorders. (p. 1736)

IV. **Developmental disabilities** (pp. 1736–1738)

  A. Impaired or insufficient brain development that causes learning disabilities (p. 1736)
  B. Accommodations for developmental disabilities (p. 1737)
     1. Many will be fully competent on interview, and no accommodation is required.
     2. Some may require help in history and physical from a familiar caregiver. (Fig. 45-3, p. 1737)
     3. Remember that patients will recognize your body language and verbal tone, so it is especially important that they see your respect for them.
     4. Establish trust and explain what you need from the patient during interview, physical, or treatment and keep in mind that patients may be confused or anxious, especially the severely impaired.
     5. It may be necessary to keep the primary caregiver with patient at all times, depending on age and degree of disability.
     6. Be sure to assess the level of impairment of the individual patient before establishing plan.
  C. Down syndrome (pp. 1737–1738)
     1. Typical physical features
        a. Eyes sloped upward at outer corners
        b. Folds of skin on either side of the nose that cover the inner corner of the eye
        c. Small face and features
        d. Large and protruding tongue
        e. Flattening on back of head
        f. Short, broad hands
     2. Medical associations
        a. Heart or intestinal defects and chronic lung problems
        b. At high risk for development of cataracts and early-onset Alzheimer's disease

D. Fetal alcohol syndrome (p. 1738)
  1. May physically resemble Down syndrome but is due to excessive alcohol consumption during pregnancy
  2. Typical physical features
     a. Small head with multiple facial abnormalities
     b. Small eyes with short slits
     c. Wide, flat nose bridge
     d. Lack of a groove between nose and upper lip
     e. Small jaw
  3. Developmental associations
     a. Delayed physical growth
     b. Mental disabilities
     c. Hyperactivity

V. Pathological challenges (pp. 1738–1743)

A. Arthritis (pp. 1738–1739)
  1. Three most common types
     a. Juvenile rheumatoid arthritis (JRA)
        i. Connective tissue disorder that presents before age 16 years
     b. Rheumatoid arthritis
        i. Autoimmune disorder
     c. Osteoarthritis
        i. Degenerative joint disease that is the most common arthritis seen in elderly patients
  2. Common characteristics
     a. Painful swelling and irritation of joints
     b. Joint stiffness
     c. Limited range of motion
     d. Sometimes deformity of smaller joints of hands and feet (**Fig. 45-4, p. 1739**)
     e. Children with JRA may have liver or spleen complications.
  3. Treatment
     a. Includes use of aspirin and nonsteroidal antiinflammatory drugs (NSAIDs), and/or corticosteroids
     b. Side effects of these drugs to distinguish symptoms from those of a disease:
        i. NSAIDs
           a) Can cause stomach upset and vomiting, with or without blood emesis.
        ii. Corticosteroids
           a) Can cause hyperglycemia, bloody emesis, and decreased immune function.
  4. Management
     a. Be sure you get complete list of medications to avoid inadvertently giving something that will interact with a medication.
     b. Keep the physical discomfort of patient in mind when examining and transporting; special padding may be required.

B. Cancer (pp. 1739–1740)
  1. All cancers are caused by abnormal growth of cells.
  2. Type of cancer determined by site of origin of malignant cells.
     a. Carcinomas arise in epithelial tissue.
     b. Sarcomas arise in connective tissue.
  3. Sometimes most obvious sign is not of disease but rather of treatment.
     a. Anorexia and weight loss
     b. Hair loss (alopecia)

POWERPOINT PRESENTATION
Chapter 45 PowerPoint slides 24–27

TEACHING STRATEGY 5
Speaker from Arthritis Foundation

> **POINT TO EMPHASIZE**
> If a patient has been undergoing chemotherapy, assume he or she is neutropenic and keep a mask on the patient to reduce risk of infection.

    c. Skin markings to show radiation therapy portals
    d. Evidence of surgery such as mastectomy
  4. Effects of cancer treatment on EMS care
    a. Poor immune function and high vulnerability to infection secondary to chemotherapy-induced neutropenia
     i. Loss of neutrophilic white blood cells
     ii. Keep a mask on patient during transport and in emergency department. (Fig. 45-5, p. 1740)
    b. Poor veins for establishing IV access
     i. Look for possible implanted infusion port, but do NOT use such a port unless you have the specific training to do so.
     ii. If patient requests that you not start a peripheral IV, consider whether you can do so (is IV a life-saving necessity or not?).
     iii. If patient has a peripheral access device such as a Groshong or Hickman catheter, consider using it if IV access is needed.
  5. Remember, whenever possible, to involve patient in decision making and defer to his/her requests.
 C. Cerebral palsy (p. 1740)
  1. Group of disorders caused by cerebral damage in utero or during birth
  2. Causes include:
    a. Prenatal rubella exposure
    b. Hypoxia during birth
    c. Postnatal infections or trauma
  3. General characteristics
    a. Difficulty with motor control
     i. Spasticity of single limb or full body
    b. About two thirds of persons affected have below-normal intellectual capacity.
    c. About half of persons affected have seizures.
  4. Types
    a. Spastic paralysis
     i. Most common
     ii. Forces muscles into state of permanent contracture
    b. Athetosis
     i. Involuntary writhing movement
     ii. Usually affecting upper and lower extremities
     iii. If face affected, drooling or grimacing common
    c. Ataxia
     i. Least common
     ii. Causes uncoordinated gait and balance
  5. Management
    a. Don't assume below-normal intelligence
     i. Many people with cerebral palsy are highly intelligent and can communicate if special devices allow them to do so.
    b. Be sure to recognize, use, and transport all necessary communication and mobility special devices.
    c. Make accommodations for transport to prevent further injury
     i. Pillows and extra blankets to pad extremities that are not in proper alignment
     ii. Ready suction if drool is a concern.
    d. If there is a caregiver, get his or her help during assessment.
    e. If the patient uses sign language, call ahead for an interpreter if one will be needed at the receiving facility.
 D. Cystic fibrosis (CF or mucoviscidosis) (p. 1741)
  1. Genetic disease that involves mucus glands, primarily in the lungs and digestive system

2. Pathology
      a. Thick, abnormal mucus causes bronchial obstruction and atelectasis in the lungs
      b. Blockages in the exocrine ducts of the pancreas lead to decrease in pancreatic enzymes and malnutrition.
   3. Complete medical history important in detecting CF
      a. "Sweat test" detects high chloride concentration in sweat.
      b. Disease present from birth with typical prognosis of death by early adulthood
         i. With late outliers extending life span into the thirties
   4. Medical characteristics
      a. High chloride concentration in sweat
      b. Frequent lung infections
      c. Clay-colored stool
      d. Clubbing of fingers and toes
   5. Management
      a. Transport issues may be difficult for both patient and family because most patients you will see are children or adolescents who do not want another trip to the hospital.
      b. Be prepared to give oxygen therapy to all CF patients, either by mask or as blow-by oxygen with patient or family member holding source if patient won't tolerate mask.
      c. Be prepared to suction airway secretions.
      d. Be sure to get list of medications (antibiotics and Mucomyst are typical) and bring all along to the hospital.
E. Multiple sclerosis (MS) (p. 1741)
   1. Disorder of the CNS
   2. Perhaps autoimmune in origin
   3. Pathology
      a. Centers on inflammation and damage to myelin sheaths of neurons
      b. Causes formation of scar tissue that blocks impulses to affected area
   4. Most often affects persons ages 20–40, women more than men.
   5. Symptoms and progression
      a. Typical onset is slow, with slight strength change in muscle associated with numbness or tingling.
      b. Disease may progress till gait unsteady or wheelchair is necessary.
      c. Speech may slur.
      d. Double vision or eye pain is common.
      e. Symptoms often have a come-and-go pattern and become more frequent, more severe, and longer lasting over time.
      f. Patients may eventually be bedridden and lose bladder control.
      g. Death is often due to infection.
   6. Management
      a. Know that, as with other patients with chronic illness, persons may experience mood swings and sometimes seek medical care for their feelings.
      b. Transport may require oxygen therapy and other supportive care.
      c. Position for comfort and safety and do not expect patient to walk to ambulance.
      d. Be sure to transport all assistive devices (e.g., wheelchair or cane) with patient. **(Fig. 45-6, p. 1741)**
F. Muscular dystrophy (MD) (pp. 1741–1742)
   1. Group of genetic diseases characterized by progressive weakness and wasting of muscle tissue

POINT TO EMPHASIZE
CF patients may have been chronically ill all their lives. The last thing they want is another trip to the hospital.

2. Multiple forms, most classified by age of onset, muscles affected, and history
3. Most common type is Duchenne MD
   a. Typically develops in boys ages 3–6 and leads to progressive muscle weakness, paralysis, and death by age 12 or so.
4. Death is often due to involvement of respiratory muscles and/or heart.
5. Management
   a. Be sure to get full family history, if possible.
   b. Be sure to note which muscles are affected and any muscle groups that the patient cannot move.
   c. Because most of the patients you will see are children, use age-appropriate language.
   d. Supportive therapy, particularly oxygen, may be needed, especially late in course of disease.

G. Poliomyelitis (polio) (p. 1742)
   1. Viral communicable disease that affects brain gray matter and the spinal cord
   2. Now rare in developed nations due to immunization
   3. Although polio is now rare in United States there are many people born before 1950s who are affected by the disease (recall case study at opening of chapter).
   4. Pathology
      a. Initial attack centers on virus entering body through GI tract, entering bloodstream, and then traveling to CNS where the virus enters nerve cells and alters them.
   5. Paralytic polio
      a. Patients experience asymmetrical muscle weakness that leads to permanent paralysis.
   6. Most patients recover from initial attack, but are left with permanent paralysis in affected muscles.
      a. Look for assistive devices, muscle atrophy of affected limb, or even ventilator if respiratory muscles are involved.
   7. Post-polio syndrome
      a. Affects persons who suffered severely more than 30 years ago and who currently have syndrome constellation of easy fatiguing, especially after exercise, and develop cold intolerance in extremities.
   8. Management
      a. Make appropriate accommodations for patients on long-term ventilator assistance who may have tracheotomies.
      b. Know that because many patients pride themselves on their independence, transport may be frustrating.
      c. Transport patient with all assistive devices.
      d. Encourage them not to get fatigued by walking to ambulance.
      e. Try to alleviate patient's anxiety as much as possible.

H. Previous head injury (p. 1742)
   1. Wide range of presentations, depending on site and severity of brain injury
   2. Patients may have stroke-like symptoms
      a. Aphasia
      b. Slurred speech
      c. Loss of vision or hearing
      d. Learning disabled
      e. Affected by frequent seizures
   3. A complete history of preexisting deficits is crucial to assessment, but some patients may not remember or be able to give historical information.
   4. Where possible, document symptoms known to be new or recurrent.

5. Conduct physical slowly and look carefully for signs of trauma or responses typical of pain, especially if patient cannot talk.
6. Transport depends on current complaint.
7. Regardless of complaint, give as much information as possible to receiving facility about the previous head injury.

I. Spina bifida (pp. 1742–1743)
  1. Congenital anomaly within the group called neural tube defects in which the spinal canal and spinal column did not close properly (p. 00)
  2. Types
     a. Spina bifida occulta
        i. Condition may be nearly invisible and asymptomatic.
        ii. Bone underneath skin did not close properly.
     b. Spina bifida cystica
        i. Either bone of vertebra(e), the bone and meninges surrounding the spinal cord, or all three types of tissue protrude from the back with obvious deformity
  3. Symptoms
     a. Depend on degree of tissue protrusion and vertebral level of deformity
     b. Paralysis of lower extremities and lack of bowel or bladder control common
     c. Hydrocephalus, accumulated fluid within brain, common in children born with spina bifida cystica
        i. Requires surgical implantation of a shunt
  4. Management
     a. Because a significant proportion of affected children and adolescents have latex allergy, assume that all spina bifida patients have the allergy.
     b. Be sure to transport all assistive devices with patient.
     c. Should transport infant in car seat unless contraindicated.

J. Myasthenia gravis (p. 1743)
  1. Autoimmune disease characterized by chronic weakness of voluntary muscles and progressive fatigue
  2. Develops most frequently in women between ages 20 and 50
  3. Pathology centers on blockage of neural impulse from nerve cell to nerve cell.
  4. Symptoms commonly include
     a. Double vision
     b. Complete lack of energy
        i. Especially in evening
        ii. Often involving facial muscles
           a) Drooping eyelid
           b) Difficulty in chewing or swallowing.
  5. In severe cases, respiratory muscles may be affected, leading to respiratory arrest, and these patients may require assisted ventilation en route to receiving facility.
  6. Other accommodations are specific to the individual patient's needs.

VI. **Other challenges** (pp. 1743–1744)
A. Culturally diverse patients (pp. 1743–1744) (Fig. 45-7, p. 1743)
  1. It is your ethical responsibility to treat all patients in the same manner.
  2. Respect the folk medicine beliefs of ethnic groups.
  3. Respect a patient's right to refuse treatment even after you fully explain the need and possible consequences.
  4. Always make sure you obtain a signed refusal of treatment and transportation form for your records.

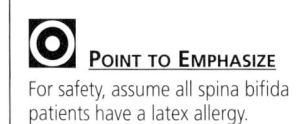

POINT TO EMPHASIZE
For safety, assume all spina bifida patients have a latex allergy.

POWERPOINT PRESENTATION
Chapter 45 PowerPoint slides 28–32

TEACHING STRATEGY 6
Diversity Exercise

POINT TO EMPHASIZE
Treat the patient, not the patient's financial condition.

POWERPOINT PRESENTATION
Chapter 45 PowerPoint slide 33

WORKBOOK
Chapter 45 Activities

READING/REFERENCE
Textbook, pp. 1746–1777

HANDOUT 45-2
Chapter 45 Quiz

HANDOUT 45-3
Chapter 45 Scenario

PARAMEDIC STUDENT CD
Student Activities

COMPANION WEBSITE
http://www.prenhall.com/bledsoe

TESTGEN
Chapter 45

   5. Be familiar with any foreign language spoken by a significant number of residents in your area and look for translation help from family or through use of a translator device or telephone language line.
      a. Always let receiving facility know if they will need a translator.
  B. Terminally ill patients (p. 1744)
   1. Paramedic may be called when a patient has decided to die at home but the family gets to a crisis point in management and calls an ambulance or when a new medical condition has developed that (in the patient's or family's view) merits EMS evaluation.
   2. Review Chapter 46 of text for guidelines on caring for the terminally ill patient either at home or in a hospice setting.
  C. Patients with communicable diseases (p. 1744)
   1. Take all appropriate BSI precautions while refraining from any judgments and keeping the patient's sensitivities in mind.
   2. Explain that BSI measures are specific to the disease, not the patient; all patients with a similar disease are treated similarly.
   3. Refer to Chapter 37 for details on communicable diseases.
  D. Patients with financial challenges (p. 1744)
   1. Always treat the patient, not his or her financial condition.
   2. Become familiar with public hospitals and clinics that provide services to patients who do not have adequate funds or insurance
   3. Calm the patient while discussing this information. (**Fig. 45-8, p. 1744**)

VII. Chapter summary (p. 1744). It is important to be aware of the pathophysiology of diseases that you may encounter throughout your career. You should also know the characteristics of impairments that are commonly found in the medical setting. They may be the primary reason that your patient seeks help, or they may not be the reason your patient called at all. Whatever the circumstances, it is important to learn the various etiologies of these impairments and illnesses in order to treat your patients with the knowledge and respect that each one deserves.

ASSIGNMENTS

Assign students to complete Chapter 45, "The Challenged Patient," of the workbook. Also assign them to read Chapter 46, "Acute Interventions for the Chronic-Care Patient," before the next class.

EVALUATION

Chapter Quiz and Scenario   Distribute copies of the Chapter Quiz provided in Handout 45-2 to evaluate student understanding of this chapter. Make sure each student reads the scenario to reinforce critical thinking on the scene. Remind students not to use their notes or textbooks while taking the quiz.

Student CD   Quizzes for every chapter are contained on the dynamic and highly visual in-text student CD.

Companion Website   Additional quizzes for every chapter are contained on this exciting website.

TestGen You may wish to create a custom-tailored test using *Prentice Hall TestGen for Essentials of Paramedic Care,* 2nd Edition to evaluate student understanding of this chapter.

On-line Test Preparation (for students and instructors) Additional test preparation is available through Brady's new on-line product, *EMT Achieve: Paramedic Test Preparation* at *http://www.prenhall.com/emtachieve/*. Instructors can also monitor student mastery on-line.

Review Manual for the EMT-Paramedic This comprehensive exam review contains hundreds of test questions and rationales, including scenarios, along with two 180-question practice tests on CD.

REINFORCEMENT

Handouts If classroom discussion or performance on the quiz indicates that some students have not fully mastered the chapter content, you may wish to assign some or all of the Reinforcement Handouts for this chapter.

Student CD (for students) A wide variety of material on this CD-ROM will reinforce and also expand student knowledge and skills.

PowerPoint Presentation (for instructors) The PowerPoint material developed for this chapter offers useful reinforcement of chapter content.

Companion Website (for students) Additional review quizzes and links to EMS resources will contribute to further reinforcement of the chapter.

OneKey On-line support is offered for this course on one of three platforms: CourseCompass, Blackboard, or Web CT. Includes the IRM, PowerPoints, TestGen, and Companion Website for instruction. Ask your local sales representative for more information.

Brady Skills Series: Advanced Life Skills (Video or CD) Have your students watch the skills come to life on VHS or CD-ROM, or they can purchase the highly visual, full-color text with step-by-step procedures and rationales.

EMT ACHIEVE: PARAMEDIC TEST PREPARATION
Mistovich & Beasley. *EMT Achieve: Paramedic Test Preparation.*
www.prenhall.com/emtachieve/

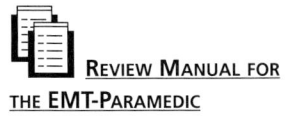

REVIEW MANUAL FOR THE EMT-PARAMEDIC
Cherry & Mistovich. *Review Manual for the EMT-Paramedic,* 3rd edition.

HANDOUTS 45-4 AND 45-5
Reinforcement Activities

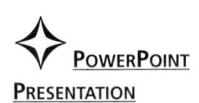

PARAMEDIC STUDENT CD
Student Activities

POWERPOINT PRESENTATION
Chapter 45

COMPANION WEBSITE
http://www.prenhall.com/bledsoe

ONEKEY
Chapter 45

ADVANCED LIFE SUPPORT SKILLS
Larmon & Davis. *Advanced Life Support Skills.*

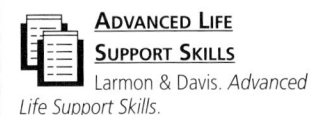

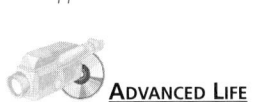

ADVANCED LIFE SKILLS REVIEW
Larmon & Davis. *Advanced Life Skills Review.*

BRADY SKILLS SERIES: ALS
Larmon & Davis. *Brady Skills Series: ALS.*

PARAMEDIC NATIONAL STANDARDS SELF-TEST
Miller. *Paramedic National Standards Self-Test,* 4th edition.

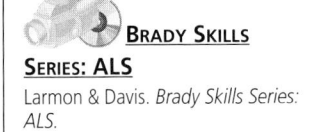

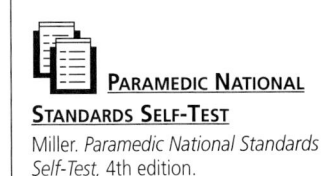

Handout 45-1

Student's Name _____

CHAPTER 45 OBJECTIVES CHECKLIST

Knowledge	Date Mastered
1. Describe the various etiologies and types of hearing impairments.	
2. Recognize the patient with a hearing impairment.	
3. Anticipate accommodations that may be needed in order to properly manage the patient with a hearing impairment.	
4. Describe the various etiologies and types, recognize patients with, and anticipate accommodations that may be needed in order to properly manage each of the following conditions: • Visual impairments • Speech impairments • Obesity • Paraplegia/quadriplegia • Mental illness • Developmentally disabled • Down syndrome • Emotional impairment • Emotional/mental impairment	
5. Describe, identify possible presenting signs of, and anticipate accommodations for the following diseases/illnesses: • Arthritis • Cancer • Cerebral palsy • Cystic fibrosis • Multiple sclerosis • Muscular dystrophy • Myasthenia gravis • Poliomyelitis • Spina bifida • Patients with a previous head injury	
6. Define, recognize, and anticipate accommodations needed to properly manage patients who: • Are culturally diverse • Are terminally ill • Have a communicable disease • Have a financial impairment	
7. Given several challenged patients, provide the appropriate assessment, management, and transportation.	

HANDOUT 45-2

Student's Name _____

CHAPTER 45 QUIZ

Write the letter of the best answer in the space provided.

_____ 1. Persons with impaired maturation of the brain who are unable to learn at the usual rate are considered to have what type of challenge?
   A. physical challenge
   B. developmental challenge
   C. mental challenge
   D. pathological challenge

_____ 2. Which one of the following is NOT a cause of conductive hearing impairment?
   A. neonatal asphyxia
   B. childhood otitis media
   C. impacted cerumen
   D. trauma to the mandible or ear

_____ 3. The types of speech impairments are called:
   A. articulation disorders.
   B. language disorders.
   C. fluency disorders.
   D. aphasia disorders.

_____ 4. Patients with _____ have been ill for their entire lives, and you need to remember that the last thing they want is another exposure to the medical system or another hospitalization.
   A. multiple sclerosis
   B. cystic fibrosis
   C. muscular dystrophy
   D. spina bifida

_____ 5. Always assume that patients with this condition have a latex allergy.
   A. cerebral palsy
   B. cancer
   C. cystic fibrosis
   D. spina bifida

_____ 6. Clues that a person may have cancer include all of the following EXCEPT:
   A. alopecia (hair loss).
   B. significant weight loss.
   C. thirstiness and frequent urination.
   D. implanted infusion port.

_____ 7. Assume that a person who has recently undergone chemotherapy as a form of cancer therapy is neutropenic and thus vulnerable to:
   A. infection.
   B. hypoglycemia.
   C. bradycardia.
   D. tachypnea.

_____ 8. Common accommodations you should make for persons with severe hearing impairment do NOT include which of the following?
   A. Make initial connection with the patient via movement or by gently touching them.
   B. Maintain a face-to-face position.
   C. Exaggerate facial and body language to make points more clear.
   D. Reduce background noise to lowest possible level.

_____ 9. One cause of temporary vision loss is:
   A. injury.
   B. infection.
   C. deployment of vehicle airbag.
   D. disease.

_____ 10. Individuals who may need to be transported with the patient for medical reasons include all of the following EXCEPT a(n):
   A. home nurse.
   B. interpreter (either sign language or spoken language).
   C. caregiver for the severely mentally impaired.
   D. assistance dog.

_____ 11. A large proportion of persons with cerebral palsy are:
   A. developmentally challenged.
   B. highly intelligent.
   C. unable to communicate in any way.
   D. mentally challenged.

HANDOUT 45-2 Continued

_____ 12. Persons who may have difficulty walking to the ambulance when ill do NOT include patients with:
   A. myasthenia gravis.
   B. multiple sclerosis.
   C. post-polio syndrome.
   D. spina bifida.

_____ 13. Whenever possible when dealing with a culturally diverse patient, you should:
   A. maintain face-to-face positioning.
   B. remember that some folk remedies may interact with medical therapies.
   C. work through an interpreter.
   D. document the fact that the patient is culturally diverse.

_____ 14. It is particularly important to explain all BSI precautionary procedures as they arise with patients who:
   A. have a communicable disease.
   B. have had recent chemotherapy.
   C. have cystic fibrosis.
   D. are terminally ill.

_____ 15. Causes of permanent vision loss include all of the following EXCEPT:
   A. glaucoma.
   B. diabetic retinopathy.
   C. CMV infection.
   D. corneal abrasion.

HANDOUT 45-3

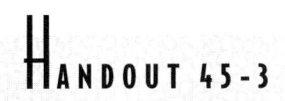

Student's Name _____

CHAPTER 45 SCENARIO

Review the following situation, and then answer the questions that follow.

You and your partner are called out shortly after 1:00 A.M. to the site of a single-vehicle accident. When you arrive at the scene, you see a fair amount of debris in the right lane that looks like cardboard or paneling and an apparently undamaged car on the shoulder. A police officer is talking with an older man who appears to be physically unhurt. As you walk toward them, you see an older woman standing quietly on the far side of the car.

The two men explain that the couple, Mr. and Mrs. Barrett, had been awakened by a phone call that their daughter had gone into labor with her first child. The couple dressed quickly and set out for the hospital. Unfortunately, Mr. Barrett did not see the debris in his lane until too late, and the car went over some of the cardboard as he tried to swerve away into another lane. Mr. Barrett tells you that both he and his wife were wearing their seat belts, and he thinks they were "just a bit shaken up."

Your partner, who is standing near Mrs. Barrett, gestures, and you walk over to them. He tells you in a quiet voice that she only shook her head in response to his questions, and, although he can't see any blood or bruises in the darkness, he is worried about head injury.

You touch Mrs. Barrett gently on her arm, and she looks up, almost surprised to see you. She doesn't say anything when you ask her if she has any discomfort anywhere, but she continues to watch your face. Suddenly, you get an idea, and you tell her you'd like to walk over to the ambulance and talk there. As you take her arm gently, she says "all right" and willingly walks with you toward the lights of the ambulance. As you glance at her, you see no sign of injury.

1. What clues, if any, suggest that Mrs. Barrett may have a type of challenge rather than head trauma? What type of challenge do you suspect?

2. When you reach the relatively well-lit area beside the ambulance, what accommodations should you make, on the assumption Mrs. Barrett may be hearing impaired, as you try to begin an interview with her?

3. When you ask Mrs. Barrett whether she can hear you all right, she reaches up to touch her ears and says "Oh, my. I forgot to put my hearing aids in." What question should you ask next?

EVALUATION

©2007 Pearson Education, Inc.
Essentials of Paramedic Care, 2nd ed.

CHAPTER 45 *The Challenged Patient* **1101**

HANDOUT 45-4

Student's Name _____

CHAPTER 45 REVIEW

Write the word or words that best complete each sentence in the space(s) provided.

1. Physical challenges include sensory impairments such as visual or hearing loss, as well as speech impairments and physical states such as _____ or _____.

2. When obesity complicates positioning of ECG electrodes, remember that you can place electrodes on the _____ and _____ instead of on the chest.

3. A person with _____ aphasia cannot understand the spoken word, whereas a person with _____ aphasia cannot clearly articulate a response to what you say.

4. When speaking with a person who has a speech impairment, try to phrase questions so that they can be answered with _____, direct responses.

5. An individual with paralysis due to an injury among the cervical vertebrae may have compromise of _____ muscles and require use of a home _____.

6. Be sure to have _____ ready when you treat quadriplegic patients in case there are excess secretions in the airway.

7. If a patient is wearing a halo device, be sure to _____ _____ before transport.

8. It may be necessary to spend extra time on the physical examination of an adult with a(n) _____ disability if they do not have sufficient cognitive or communicative skills to give you history information.

9. Remember that individuals with Down syndrome may have other physical conditions involving one or more of these three organs: _____, _____, and _____.

10. _____ _____ syndrome is sometimes confused with Down syndrome because of similar facial characteristics, even though it is due to a form of toxic injury during pregnancy.

11. Because _____ distress is highly probable in patients with cystic fibrosis, be prepared to give oxygen therapy.

12. If you use an interpreter for any reason, be sure to document the _____ _____ and the _____ _____ _____.

13. Remember that every patient who has decision-making ability has the right to _____ _____; if this occurs, be sure it is documented properly.

14. One axiom about caring for patients with monetary challenges is to care for the _____, not the _____ _____.

15. Signs of myasthenia gravis that are readily observed in the face are _____ _____ and difficulty with _____ or _____.

REINFORCEMENT

1102 ESSENTIALS OF PARAMEDIC CARE

©2007 Pearson Education, Inc.
Essentials of Paramedic Care, 2nd ed.

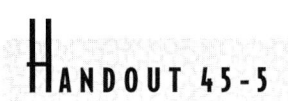

THE MANY TYPES OF CHALLENGED PATIENTS

Fill in the blanks to complete the information on different types of challenged patients.

1. Examples of physical challenges:
   a. _____ impairment with _____ deafness and _____ deafness
   b. _____ impairment
   c. _____ impairment with _____ aphasia, _____ aphasia, and _____ aphasia
   d. _____
   e. _____ with possible paraplegia or quadriplegia

2. _____ challenges and _____ impairment (including the psychoses, mood disorders, personality disorders, and responses to a traumatic experience)

3. _____ disabilities (including patients with Down syndrome, fetal alcohol syndrome, and disabilities of many other origins)

4. Examples of _____ challenges (chronic conditions):
   a. Arthritis
   b. _____
   c. _____ palsy
   d. _____ _____ (mucoviscidosis)
   e. _____ _____ (MS)
   f. _____ _____ (MD)
   g. _____ and post- _____ syndrome
   h. Previous _____ _____
   i. _____ _____ with _____ _____ occulta or _____ _____ cystica
   j. _____ gravis

5. Other challenges include:
   a. _____ _____ patients
   b. _____ _____ patients
   c. Patients with _____ diseases
   d. Patients with _____ challenges

Chapter 45 Answer Key

Handout 45-2: Chapter 45 Quiz

1. B	6. C	11. B
2. A	7. A	12. D
3. D	8. C	13. B
4. B	9. B	14. A
5. D	10. A	15. D

Handout 45-3: Chapter 45 Scenario

1. The undamaged appearance of the car, the uninjured appearance and settled voice of Mr. Barrett, as well as the information that the couple were both wearing seat belts, by no means rules out head injury in Mrs. Barrett, but they do not raise your level of concern, either.

   Her surprise when you walk close to her and her fixing on your face in the darkness are clues that she might be hearing impaired. It is difficult to assess her status in the darkness. You realize that the poor light—if she has a hearing impairment—is making it harder for her, especially after the news of her daughter's labor and the minor car accident, to focus on and respond to what you say.

   The fact that she said "all right" clearly when you asked her to walk over to the ambulance does not rule out a speech impairment, but it does make it somewhat less likely than hearing impairment.

2. You should assume a directly face-to-face position. Speak clearly in a low-pitched voice and without exaggeration. Look for a hearing aid. Ask her directly if she can hear you properly because you need to ask her a few questions about how she feels. Reduce background noise as much as possible. (For instance, make sure radio is turned down or partner sits in ambulance to listen to any incoming calls. Stand at the side farther from the highway to muffle any road noise.)

3. Any question that directly calls for a response on whether she can hear you well enough to answer a few questions is proper. If she can't hear well enough, ask her husband to stand with her and ask them questions jointly to ascertain whether either has been injured sufficiently to require intervention. Be matter-of-fact. Hearing impairment is a complication to patient interview but not a problem itself.

Handout 45-4: Chapter 45 Review

1. obesity, paralysis
2. arms, thighs
3. sensory, motor (expressive)
4. short
5. respiratory, ventilator
6. suction
7. stabilize traction
8. developmental
9. heart, intestines, lungs
10. Fetal alcohol
11. respiratory
12. person's name, information they provided
13. refuse treatment
14. patient, financial condition
15. drooping eyelid, swallowing, chewing

Handout 45-5: The Many Types of Challenged Patients

1. a. Hearing, conductive, sensorineural
   b. Visual
   c. Speech, sensory, motor (expressive), global
   d. Obesity
   e. Paralysis
2. Mental, emotional
3. Developmental
4. pathological
   a. *Arthritis*
   b. Cancer
   c. Cerebral
   d. Cystic fibrosis
   e. Multiple sclerosis
   f. Muscular dystrophy
   g. Poliomyelitis, *post*-polio
   h. head injury
   i. Spina bifida, spina bifida, spina bifida
   j. Myasthenia
5. a. Culturally diverse
   b. Terminally ill
   c. communicable
   d. financial

Chapter 46
Acute Interventions for the Chronic-Care Patient

INTRODUCTION

Because of the movement toward early hospital discharge followed by home care, there has been a huge increase in home health care needs and services over the past 30 to 40 years. Currently, more than 665,000 caregivers—nurses, home health aides, physical therapists, occupational therapists, and other health care professionals—support patients who receive home care. Experts expect this trend to continue. Thus, an increasingly large number of patients will receive treatment, even for terminal illness, in an out-of-hospital setting. Your students will receive calls to assess and treat patients with chronic conditions who are receiving care at home. This chapter will teach them how to assess whether the EMS call is for an acute problem unrelated to the chronic condition, reflects an exacerbation of the chronic condition, is related to home care equipment, or is due to another reason. This chapter covers the epidemiology of home care, reasons for ALS intervention in home care cases, as well as pertinent general system pathophysiology, assessment, and management.

TOTAL TEACHING TIME: 5.69 HOURS
The total teaching time is only a guideline based on the didactic and practical lab averages in the National Standard Curriculum. Instructors should take into consideration such factors as the pace at which students learn, the size of the class, and breaks. The actual time devoted to teaching objectives is the responsibility of the instructor.

CHAPTER OBJECTIVES

After reading this chapter, you should be able to:

1. Compare and contrast the primary objectives of the paramedic and the home care provider. (pp. 1748, 1752)
2. Identify the importance of home health care medicine as it relates to emergency medical services. (pp. 1747–1748)
3. Differentiate between the role of the paramedic and the role of the home care provider. (pp. 1748, 1752)
4. Compare and contrast the primary objectives of acute care, home care, and hospice care. (pp. 1747–1748, 1752, 1774–1775)
5. Discuss aspects of home care that enhance the quality of patient care and aspects that have the potential to become detrimental. (pp. 1747–1748)
6. List pathologies and complications in home care patients that commonly result in ALS intervention. (pp. 1748–1753, 1757–1776)

7. Compare the cost, mortality, and quality of care for a given patient in the hospital versus the home care setting. (pp. 1747–1748)
8. Discuss the significance of palliative care programs as related to a patient in a home health care or hospice setting. (pp. 1752, 1774–1775)
9. Define hospice care, comfort care, and DNR/DNAR as they relate to local practice, law, and policy. (pp. 1758–1759, 1774–1776)
10. List and describe the characteristics of typical home care devices related to airway maintenance, artificial and alveolar ventilation, vascular access, drug administration, and the GI/GU tract. (pp. 1748–1749, 1750, 1752, 1757, 1761–1772)
11. Discuss the complications of assessing each of the devices described above. (pp. 1761–1762)
12. Describe indications, contraindications, and techniques for urinary catheter insertion in the male and female patient in an out-of-hospital setting. (pp. 1769–1770)
13. Identify failure of GI/GU, ventilatory, vascular access, and drain devices found in the home care setting. (pp. 1761–1772)
14. Discuss the relationship between local home care treatment protocols/SOPs and local EMS protocols/SOPs. (p. 1752)
15. Discuss differences in the ability of individuals to accept and cope with their own impending death. (p. 1776)
16. List the stages of the grief process and relate them to an individual in hospice care. (p. 1776)
17. Discuss the rights of the terminally ill patient. (pp. 1774–1776)
18. Summarize the types of home health care available in your area and the services provided. (pp. 1747–1753)
19. Given a series of home care scenarios, determine which patients should receive follow-up home care and which should be transported to an emergency care facility. (pp. 1753–1757)
20. Given a series of scenarios, demonstrate interaction and support with the family members/support persons for a patient who has died. (pp. 1774–1776)

FRAMING THE LESSON

Begin by reviewing the important points from Chapter 45, "The Challenged Patient." Discuss any points that the class does not completely understand. Then move on to Chapter 46. Break students into groups to brainstorm examples of patients who receive home care. You may wish to use categories based on age or health condition. For instance, a group asked to think about age-related reasons for home care might think of these examples:

- A premature infant who needs follow-up care after hospital discharge
- A small child with a serious, chronic disorder requiring special respiratory, GI, or other care
- Elderly individuals who require monitoring of blood sugar, blood pressure, or another variable or who require in-home care because of physical disability, dementia, or another medical problem

A group challenged to think of short-term or temporary conditions requiring home care might come up with examples such as these:

- A new mother who had significant delivery complications and needs follow-up home care

- A patient returning home from a rehab center who requires in-home personal care and support with exercises and other rehabilitation measures
- A patient who has had transplant surgery and requires at-home health care to recuperate from surgery and learn how to handle the medications and other needs associated with post-transplantation living
- A patient who is terminally ill and has come home to die

Students asked to think of long-term examples of home care will probably focus on the major chronic conditions that affect North Americans, especially elderly persons:

- A patient with diabetes and complications such as diabetic retinopathy and/or extremity amputation who requires medical monitoring and personal care
- A person with a developmental disability and a chronic condition such as inflammatory bowel disease who needs personal and medical support
- A patient with paraplegia or quadriplegia who requires intensive medical support on a constant basis
- A patient with severe atherosclerosis who has had previous MIs and amputation because of vascular insufficiency

TEACHING STRATEGIES

People learn in a variety of ways. Some do better with the spoken word, whereas others prefer the written. Some prefer to work alone, whereas others profit from working in groups. Recognizing these different ways of acquiring knowledge, the authors of this *Instructor's Resource Manual* have provided a variety of teaching strategies for the different types of learners. These strategies are intended to foster higher-level cognitive skills and encourage creative learning and problem solving. For greatest effectiveness, incorporate these strategies into your class lecture. Symbols in the Lecture Outline indicate the points at which various exercises might be most appropriate. Other strategies can be used to preview the lesson or to summarize it.

The following strategies are keyed to specific sections of the lesson.

1. A Day with a Home Health Care Provider. Arrange for students to spend a day of clinical time with a home health care provider. It could be enlightening for students to witness the depth and scope of home health care. Additionally, students should gain an appreciation for the challenges of caring for terminal and chronic care patients. Often the conditions of a patient's home are far more difficult to work within than in the hospital. Home health providers are excellent creative problem solvers and can teach students a great deal about their role, chronic care patients, and the advanced care devices in homes today.

2. Home Health Care Device In-Service. Conduct an in-service with students on the advanced technology of home care devices so they are more likely to know how to use this equipment when they encounter it in the field. Have a representative from the manufacturer, a medical equipment representative, or home care nurse bring the equipment and manuals to class. Also, emphasize to students that patients and family members are often good resources for use of the equipment. Be sure the representative provides students with a contact number to call should they encounter an equipment problem in the field.

3. Hospital Clinical Time with Wounds and Ostomies. Consider clinical time for students on the hospital floor that deals with wounds and ostomies, or with a wound care clinic. The paramedic's knowledge of wound care is often limited to direct pressure and elevation. Intensive time spent learning to recognize the early signs of local and systemic infection will be helpful in their careers. Additionally, caring for wounds, managing dressing changes, and cleaning ostomies will likely be part of the expected practice of the paramedic in the near future.

4. Simulating Bodily Functions. Students are often taken aback by the products of bodily functions encountered on calls because classroom simulations lack this type of realism. When appropriate, simulate an incontinent patient by using Depends and chocolate cake frosting, fill an ostomy bag with mushroom soup, or attach (tape) a seemingly full Foley to the patient. These additions seem small but can derail an assessment and treatment plan when encountered on an actual call.

5. Questioning Techniques. Emphasize to students how to respect a person's intelligence by directing questions *first* to the patient. It is appropriate to interview the family or caregiver in lieu of the patient *only after* the patient has been determined by you to be incapable of providing an accurate history. Too many providers insult and alienate patients by *assuming* they are incompetent to answer questions.

6. Practicing Ostomy Care on Ostomy and Stoma Mannequins. Ostomy and stoma mannequins are available from all of the major mannequins manufacturers. If your budget does not allow a purchase, consider borrowing one from your nursing education department or home health care company. Create skills sheets for ostomy care much the way you would for other emergency procedures such as intubation or patient assessment. By practicing and testing these procedures and skills in class, you place importance on these competencies. This is an important message for students about caring for all patients equally well, regardless of level of acuity of the call.

The following strategies can be used at various points throughout the lesson or to help summarize and demonstrate what students have learned.

The Nature of EMS Calls for Chronic-Care Patients. Have students break into groups to discuss the patients listed for each category in the exercise for Framing the Lesson. This time, have your students think of possible reasons for EMS calls to these patients. Encourage them to think about the kinds of chief complaints these patients might have, as well as any kind of equipment or procedural difficulty that might result in an EMS call.

Cultural Considerations, Legal Notes, and Patho Pearls. The Student CD-ROM contains this series of informative features to enhance the student's understanding of the material covered in this chapter.

TEACHING OUTLINE

Chapter 46 is the sixth lesson in Division 5, *Special Considerations/Operations*. Distribute Handout 46-1 so that students can familiarize themselves with the learning goals for this chapter. If students have any questions about the objectives, answer them at this time.

Then present the chapter. One possible lecture outline follows. In the outline, the parenthetical references in regular type are references to text pages; those in bold type are references to figures, tables, or procedures.

I. Introduction. The movement in the United States toward early hospital discharge (or no hospital admission) and establishment of home care has resulted in large numbers of people cared for at home. Note that this number will probably only increase with time. The primary driving force in home health care is cost containment. (p. 1747)

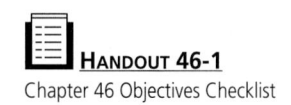

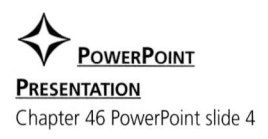

II. Epidemiology of home care (pp. 1747–1753)
- **A.** Factors that promoted the growth of home health care in recent years (pp. 1747–1748)
    1. Enactment of Medicare in 1965
    2. Advent of health maintenance organizations (HMOs)
    3. Improved medical technology
    4. Changes in attitudes of doctors and patients toward hospital care
- **B.** Arguments in favor of home health care (pp. 1747–1748)
    1. Recovery often faster in familiar environment
    2. Speeds dismissal from hospitals and nursing homes
    3. Costs less
- **C.** Patients receiving home care (pp. 1747–1748)
    1. In 1992, almost 75 percent of home care patients were 65 years or older.
    2. In 1992, of elderly home care patients, almost two thirds (66 percent) were women.
    3. Today some 8 million patients—both acute and chronic—receive formal health care treatment from paid providers.
    4. Patients require home care for various reasons.
- **D.** ALS response to home care patients (p. 1748) (**Fig. 46-1, p. 1748**)
    1. Common reasons for ALS intervention
        - a. Equipment failure
        - b. Unexpected complications
        - c. Absence of a caregiver
        - d. Need for transport
        - e. Inability to operate a device
    2. Primary role of the paramedic is to identify and treat any life-threatening problems.
- **E.** Typical responses (pp. 1748–1752)
    1. Chief complaints are similar to those in other populations, but the home care patient is fragile and more likely to decompensate and go into crisis more quickly than general population.
    2. Airway complications
    3. Respiratory failure
        - a. Emphysema
        - b. Bronchitis
        - c. Asthma
        - d. Cystic fibrosis
        - e. Congestive heart failure
        - f. Pulmonary embolus
        - g. Sleep apnea
        - h. Guillain-Barré syndrome
        - i. Myasthenia gravis
    4. Cardiac decompensation
        - a. Congestive heart failure
        - b. Acute MI
            - i. Home care patients are at higher risk
        - c. Cardiac hypertrophy
        - d. Calcification or degeneration of the heart's conductive system
        - e. Heart transplant
        - f. Sepsis
    5. Alterations in peripheral circulation
    6. Altered mental status
        - a. Common reason for EMS calls
        - b. Causes
            - i. Hypoxia
            - ii. Hypotension

POWERPOINT PRESENTATION
Chapter 46 PowerPoint slides 5–13

TEACHING STRATEGY 1
A Day with a Home Health Care Provider

TEACHING STRATEGY 2
Home Health Care Device In-Service

TEACHING STRATEGY 3
Hospital Clinical Time with Wounds and Ostomies

POINT TO EMPHASIZE
Remember that cardiac decompensation is a true medical emergency that can lead to life-threatening shock.

                    iii. Sepsis
                    iv. Altered electrolytes or blood chemistries
                    v. Hypoglycemia
                    vi. Alzheimer's disease
                    vii. Cancerous tumor or brain lesions
                    viii. Overdose
                    ix. Stroke (brain attack)
            7. GI/GU crises (gastrointestinal/genitourinary)
            8. Infections and septic complications
                a. Be alert to infections in the home care patient with any of the following.
                    i. Indwelling devices
                        a) Gastrostomy tubes
                        b) PICC lines
                        c) Foley catheters
                        d) Colostomies
                    ii. Limited lung function and tracheotomies
                    iii. Patients with decreased sensorium
                    iv. Surgically implanted drains
                    v. Decubitus wounds (bedsores) (**Fig. 46-2, p. 1751**)
                b. Signs of infection
                    i. Redness and/or swelling, especially at insertion site of indwelling device
                    ii. Purulent discharge at the insertion site
                    iii. Warm skin at the insertion site
                    iv. Fever
                c. Signs and symptoms of sepsis
                    i. Redness at an insertion site
                    ii. Fever
                    iii. Altered mental status
                    iv. Poor skin color and turgor
                    v. Signs of shock
                    vi. Vomiting
                    vii. Diarrhea
            9. Equipment malfunction
                a. Home ventilators
                b. Oxygen delivery systems
                c. Apnea monitors
                d. Home dialysis machines
            10. Other medical disorders and home care patients
                a. Brain or spinal trauma
                b. Arthritis
                c. Psychological disorders
                d. Cancer
                e. Hepatitis
                f. AIDS
                g. Transplants (including patients awaiting transplantation)
    F. Commonly found medical devices (p. 1752)
        1. Glucometers
        2. IV infusions and indwelling IV sites
        3. Nebulized and aerosolized medication administrators
        4. Shunts, fistulas, and venous grafts
        5. Oxygen concentrators, oxygen tanks, and liquid oxygen systems
        6. Oxygen masks and nebulizers
        7. Tracheotomies and home ventilators
        8. G-tubes, colostomies, and urostomies
        9. Surgical drains

POINT TO EMPHASIZE
You will be foolish and endanger the patient if you pretend to understand a device, but don't.

  10. Apnea monitors, cardiac monitors, and pulse oximeters
  11. Wheelchairs, canes, and walkers
 G. Intervention by a home health care practitioner or physician (p. 1752)
  1. Most cases require acute intervention.
  2. In some cases the paramedic's role is supportive.
   a. Chemotherapy
   b. Pain management
   c. Hospice care
 H. Injury control and prevention (pp. 1752–1753)
  1. Prevent the creation of the hazard to begin with.
  2. Reduce the amount of the hazard brought into existence.
  3. Prevent the release of the hazard that already exists.
  4. Modify the rate of distribution of the hazard from the source.
  5. Separate the hazard and that which is to be protected in both time and space.
  6. Separate the hazard and that which is to be protected by a barrier.
  7. Modify the basic qualities of the hazard.
  8. Make that which is to be protected more resistant to the hazard.
  9. Counter the damage already done by the hazard.
  10. Stabilize, repair, and rehabilitate the object of the damage.

III. General system pathophysiology, assessment, and management (pp. 1753–1757)

 A. Assessment (pp. 1753–1755)
  1. Scene size-up: safety
   a. Any patient with limited movement may be contaminated with urine, feces, or emesis.
   b. Any bed-bound patient may have weeping wounds, bleeding, or decubitus ulcers.
   c. Sharps may be present.
   d. Collection bags for urine or feces sometimes leak.
   e. Tracheostomy patients clear mucus by coughing, which can spray.
   f. Any electrical machine has the potential for electric shock.
   g. A hospital bed, wheelchair, or walker could be contaminated with body fluid.
   h. Contaminated medical devices, such as a nebulizer, may be left around unprotected.
   i. Oxygen in the presence of flame has the potential for fire or explosion.
   j. Equipment may be in the way and cause you to fall, or it may be unstable and fall on you.
   k. Medical wastes may not be properly contained or discarded.
  2. Scene size-up: patient milieu
   a. Evaluate patient's environment.
   b. Assess quality of home care received by patient.
   c. Note any signs of abuse of neglect.
   d. Note condition of medical devices.
   e. Remember: The paramedic not only has a responsibility to treat the patient but also to act as an advocate.
 B. Initial assessment, focused history, physical exam (pp. 1755–1757)
  1. Initial assessment
   a. Try to establish a baseline presentation for patient.
   b. Assess for changes from the norm.
   c. If unable to stabilize a patient, complete the rapid assessment and transport immediately.

POINT TO EMPHASIZE
On any call involving a home care patient, be sure to ask whether another health care professional has been called.

TEACHING STRATEGY 4
Simulating Bodily Functions

POWERPOINT PRESENTATION
Chapter 46 PowerPoint slides 14–16

POINT TO EMPHASIZE
Be sure to remove any medical waste you generate so that the patient does not return to an unsafe environment.

Teaching Strategy 5
Questioning Techniques

  d. In noncritical patients, compare vital signs to bedside records if they are kept.
  e. Focus your exam on the chief complaint and how it might relate to the patient's chronic condition.
  f. Be sure to check for decubiti, as they pose a significant danger to the patient through infection.
  g. Be meticulous.
 2. Mental status (**Fig. 46-3, p. 1756**)
  a. If patient has preexisting altered mental status, have a good understanding of patient's normal mentation before transport.
  b. Follow same general procedures as with other patients.
  c. If patient unable to answer questions, rely on family members or caregivers.
  d. Remember that home care patients, particularly older or terminal patients, may fear being moved from the home.
 3. Other considerations
  a. Take into account the condition that led to home care and the events that led to the current crisis.
  b. Talk to the health care provider and the patient.
  c. Before beginning any life-saving measures ascertain whether or not the patient has DNR or DNAR orders.
 C. Transport and management treatment plan (p. 1757)
  1. Paramedic may have to replace home treatment modalities with ALS modalities.
  2. Paramedic may have to transport patient's home devices.

Point to Emphasize
Home care patients often have a high dosing regimen, which may make them less responsive to medications.

PowerPoint Presentation
Chapter 46 PowerPoint slides 17–38

IV. **Specific acute home health situations** (pp. 1757–1776)
 A. Respiratory disorders (pp. 1757–1767)
  1. Common home respiratory equipment
   a. Oxygen equipment
   b. Portable suctioning machines
   c. Aerosol equipment and nebulizers
   d. Incentive spirometers
   e. Home ventilators
   f. Tracheostomy tubes and collars
  2. Chronic diseases requiring home respiratory support
   a. COPD (**Fig. 46-4, p. 1758**)
    i. Bronchitis
    ii. Emphysema
    iii. Asthma
   b. Congestive heart failure (CHF)
   c. Cystic fibrosis (CF)
   d. Bronchopulmonary dysplasia (BPD)
   e. Neuromuscular degenerative diseases
    i. Muscular dystrophy
    ii. Poliomyelitis
    iii. Guillain-Barré syndrome
    iv. Myasthenia gravis
   f. Sleep apnea
   g. Patients awaiting lung transplants
  3. Medical therapy found in the home setting
   a. Home oxygen therapy
   b. Artificial airways/tracheostomies
    i. Common complications
    ii. Management (**Fig. 46-5, p. 1764**)

Teaching Strategy 6
Practicing Ostomy Care on Ostomy and Stoma Mannequins

- **c.** Home ventilation
  - **i.** Positive-pressure ventilators
  - **ii.** Negative-pressure ventilators
  - **iii.** PEEP, CPAP, and BIPAP (**Fig. 46-6, p. 1766**)
- **d.** General assessment considerations
- **e.** General management considerations

B. Vascular access devices (pp. 1767–1768)
  1. Types of VADs
     - **a.** Hickman, Broviac, and Groshong catheters
     - **b.** Peripherally inserted central catheters (PICC)
     - **c.** Surgically implanted medication delivery systems
     - **d.** Dialysis shunts (**Fig. 46-7, p. 1767**)
  2. Anticoagulant therapy
  3. VAD complications
     - **a.** Various types of obstructions cause most common complications.
       - **i.** Thrombus at catheter site
       - **ii.** Air embolus at catheter site
       - **iii.** Catheter kinking
       - **iv.** Catheter tip embolus
     - **b.** Signs and symptoms of an air embolus
       - **i.** Headache
       - **ii.** Shortness of breath with clear lungs
       - **iii.** Hypoxia
       - **iv.** Chest pain
       - **v.** Other indications of myocardial ischemia
       - **vi.** Altered mental status

C. Cardiac conditions (pp. 1768–1769)
  1. Post-MI recovery
  2. Post–cardiac surgery
  3. Heart transplant
  4. CHF
  5. Hypertension
  6. Implanted pacemaker
  7. Atherosclerosis
  8. Congenital malformation (pediatric)

D. GI/GU crisis (pp. 1769–1772)
  1. Urinary tract devices (**Figs. 46-8 and 46-9, p. 1769**)
  2. Urinary device complications
  3. Gastrointestinal tract devices (**Fig. 46-10, p. 1770; Fig. 46-11, p. 1771; Fig. 46-12, p. 1772**)
  4. Gastrointestinal tract complications
  5. Psychosocial implications

E. Acute infections (pp. 1772–1773)

F. Maternal and newborn care (pp. 1773–1774)
  1. Common maternal complications
     - **a.** Massage of uterus, if not already contracted
     - **b.** Administration of fluids to correct hypotension
     - **c.** Administration of certain medications, such as Pitocin, if ordered
     - **d.** Rapid transport to hospital, if necessary
  2. Common infant/child complications
     - **a.** Cyanosis
     - **b.** Bradycardia (<100 b/m)
     - **c.** Crackles
     - **d.** Respiratory distress

G. Hospice and comfort care (pp. 1774–1776) (**Table 46-1, p. 1775**)
  1. ALS intervention (**Fig. 46-13, p. 1776**)
  2. Common diseases at hospice

POINT TO EMPHASIZE
The goal of hospice care is to provide palliative or comfort care rather than curative care.

     a. Congestive heart failure
     b. Cystic fibrosis
     c. COPD
     d. AIDS
     e. Alzheimer's
     f. Cancer
  3. Stages of death and grief
     a. Denial
     b. Anger
     c. Depression
     d. Bargaining
     e. Acceptance

V. Chapter summary (p. 1776). The shift toward home health care is one of the most important trends of the 2000s and will have a great impact on the ALS profession. You can expect in your career to provide acute intervention for a growing number of chronic care patients of all ages and in all stages of the disease process. These calls will challenge you to use all of your assessment skills in developing an effective management plan, which in many cases will be based on input from an extended team of home health care workers.

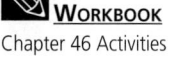

ASSIGNMENTS

Assign students to complete Chapter 46, "Acute Interventions for the Chronic-Care Patient," of the workbook. Also assign them to read Chapter 47, "Assessment-Based Management," before the next class.

EVALUATION

Chapter Quiz and Scenario   Distribute copies of the Chapter Quiz provided in Handout 46-2 to evaluate student understanding of this chapter. Make sure each student reads the scenario to reinforce critical thinking on the scene. Remind students not to use their notes or textbooks while taking the quiz.

Student CD   Quizzes for every chapter are contained on the dynamic and highly visual in-text student CD.

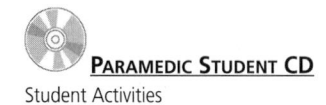

Companion Website   Additional quizzes for every chapter are contained on this exciting website.

TestGen   You may wish to create a custom-tailored test using *Prentice Hall TestGen for Essentials of Paramedic Care*, 2nd Edition to evaluate student understanding of this chapter.

On-line Test Preparation (for students and instructors)   Additional test preparation is available through Brady's new on-line product, *EMT Achieve: Paramedic Test Preparation* at *http://www.prenhall.com/emtachieve/*. Instructors can also monitor student mastery on-line.

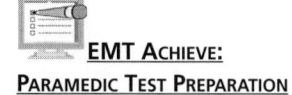

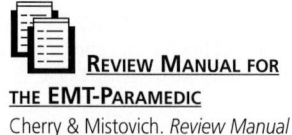

Review Manual for the EMT-Paramedic   This comprehensive exam review contains hundreds of test questions and rationales, including scenarios, along with two 180-question practice tests on CD.

REINFORCEMENT

Handouts If classroom discussion or performance on the quiz indicates that some students have not fully mastered the chapter content, you may wish to assign some or all of the Reinforcement Handouts for this chapter.

Student CD (for students) A wide variety of material on this CD-ROM will reinforce and also expand student knowledge and skills.

PowerPoint Presentation (for instructors) The PowerPoint material developed for this chapter offers useful reinforcement of chapter content.

Companion Website (for students) Additional review quizzes and links to EMS resources will contribute to further reinforcement of the chapter.

OneKey On-line support is offered for this course on one of three platforms: CourseCompass, Blackboard, or Web CT. Includes the IRM, PowerPoints, TestGen, and Companion Website for instruction. Ask your local sales representative for more information.

Brady Skills Series: Advanced Life Skills (Video or CD) Have your students watch the skills come to life on VHS or CD-ROM, or they can purchase the highly visual, full-color text with step-by-step procedures and rationales.

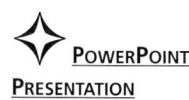

HANDOUTS 46-4 TO 46-7
Reinforcement Activities

PARAMEDIC STUDENT CD
Student Activities

POWERPOINT PRESENTATION
Chapter 46

COMPANION WEBSITE
http://www.prenhall.com/bledsoe

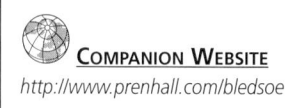

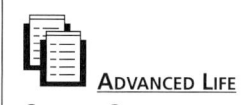

ONEKEY
Chapter 46

ADVANCED LIFE SUPPORT SKILLS
Larmon & Davis. *Advanced Life Support Skills.*

ADVANCED LIFE SKILLS REVIEW
Larmon & Davis. *Advanced Life Skills Review.*

BRADY SKILLS SERIES: ALS
Larmon & Davis. *Brady Skills Series: ALS.*

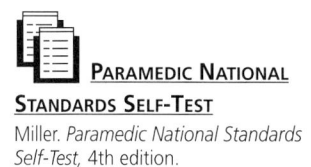

PARAMEDIC NATIONAL STANDARDS SELF-TEST
Miller. *Paramedic National Standards Self-Test,* 4th edition.

Handout 46-1

Student's Name _____

CHAPTER 46 OBJECTIVES CHECKLIST

Knowledge	Date Mastered
1. Compare and contrast the primary objectives of the paramedic and the home care provider.	
2. Identify the importance of home health care medicine as it relates to emergency medical services.	
3. Differentiate between the role of the paramedic and the role of the home care provider.	
4. Compare and contrast the primary objectives of acute care, home care, and hospice care.	
5. Discuss aspects of home care that enhance the quality of patient care and aspects that have the potential to become detrimental.	
6. List pathologies and complications in home care patients that commonly result in ALS intervention.	
7. Compare the cost, mortality, and quality of care for a given patient in the hospital versus the home care setting.	
8. Discuss the significance of palliative care programs as related to a patient in a home health care or hospice setting.	
9. Define hospice care, comfort care, and DNR/DNAR as they relate to local practice, law, and policy.	
10. List and describe the characteristics of typical home care devices related to airway maintenance, artificial and alveolar ventilation, vascular access, drug administration, and the GI/GU tract.	
11. Discuss the complications of assessing each of the devices described above.	
12. Describe indications, contraindications, and techniques for urinary catheter insertion in the male and female patient in an out-of-hospital setting.	
13. Identify failure of GI/GU, ventilatory, vascular access, and drain devices found in the home care setting.	
14. Discuss the relationship between local home care treatment protocols/SOPs and local EMS Protocols/SOPs.	
15. Discuss differences in the ability of individuals to accept and cope with their own impending death.	

OBJECTIVES

1116 ESSENTIALS OF PARAMEDIC CARE

©2007 Pearson Education, Inc.
Essentials of Paramedic Care, 2nd ed.

HANDOUT 46-1 Continued

Knowledge	Date Mastered
16. List the stages of the grief process and relate them to an individual in hospice care.	
17. Discuss the rights of the terminally ill patient.	
18. Summarize the types of home health care available in your area and the services provided.	
19. Given a series of home care scenarios, determine which patients should receive follow-up home care and which should be transported to an emergency care facility.	
20. Given a series of scenarios, demonstrate interaction and support with the family members/support persons for a patient who has died.	

HANDOUT 46-2

Student's Name _____

CHAPTER 46 QUIZ

Write the letter of the best answer in the space provided.

_____ 1. Common reasons for ALS intervention in home care settings include all of the following EXCEPT:
   A. equipment failure.
   B. absence of a caregiver.
   C. unexpected complications.
   D. arguments between caregiver and patient.

_____ 2. Patients with which disease are at high risk for unhealed wounds or ulcers, particularly on the feet?
   A. Atherosclerosis
   B. Diabetes mellitus
   C. Coronary heart disease
   D. Deep vein thrombophlebitis (DVT)

_____ 3. Pressure sores are classified:
   A. by the depth of tissue destruction.
   B. as diabetes-related and nondiabetes-related.
   C. by the location on the body.
   D. as gravity-dependent or nongravity-dependent.

_____ 4. Settings in which the scope of treatment is beyond your training include all of the following EXCEPT:
   A. chemotherapy.
   B. pain management.
   C. hospice care.
   D. home dialysis.

_____ 5. Bronchopulmonary dysplasia (BPD) primarily affects:
   A. older persons, especially heavy smokers.
   B. children with cystic fibrosis.
   C. infants of low birth weight.
   D. older persons with hypertension.

_____ 6. Chronic dilation of a bronchus or bronchi with secondary infection is termed:
   A. atelectasis.
   B. bronchiectasis.
   C. chronic bronchitis.
   D. bronchopneumonia.

_____ 7. What form of ventilation is the recommended support for acute respiratory disorders?
   A. positive-pressure ventilation (PPV)
   B. negative-pressure ventilation (NPV)
   C. positive end-expiratory pressure (PEEP)
   D. bilevel positive airway pressure (BIPAP)

_____ 8. Types of vascular access devices used in the home setting include all of the following EXCEPT:
   A. heparin lock.
   B. Hickman or Broviac catheter.
   C. peripherally inserted central catheter.
   D. dialysis shunt.

_____ 9. Signs and symptoms of an air embolus include all of the following EXCEPT:
   A. shortness of breath with clear lung sounds.
   B. chest pain.
   C. back pain.
   D. headache.

HANDOUT 46-2 Continued

_____ 10. Signs of postpartum depression are found in what proportion of mothers?
   A. 10–20 percent
   B. 30–35 percent (roughly one third)
   C. 45–55 percent (roughly one half)
   D. 70–80 percent (roughly three quarters)

_____ 11. Signs and symptoms of cardiac or respiratory insufficiency in newborns include all of the following EXCEPT:
   A. hypotension.
   B. cyanosis.
   C. bradycardia.
   D. lung crackles.

_____ 12. Common diseases you will see in a hospice setting include all of the following EXCEPT:
   A. congestive heart failure (CHF).
   B. chronic obstructive pulmonary disease (COPD).
   C. cerebral palsy.
   D. Alzheimer's disease.

_____ 13. A surgical diversion of the urinary tract to a stoma, or hole, in the abdominal wall is called:
   A. ureterostomy.
   B. urostomy.
   C. cytostomy.
   D. nephrostomy.

_____ 14. Signs and symptoms of respiratory distress include all of the following EXCEPT:
   A. tachypnea.
   B. use of accessory muscles.
   C. upright posturing.
   D. wheezing or crackles on auscultation.

_____ 15. Common causes for calls from patients with cystic fibrosis include all of the following EXCEPT:
   A. pneumothorax.
   B. hemoptysis.
   C. cor pulmonale.
   D. hematemesis.

HANDOUT 46-3

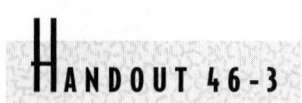

Student's Name _____

CHAPTER 46 SCENARIO

Review the following situation, and then answer the questions that follow.

The dispatcher calls you to investigate a "hysterical" call about a "man who is coughing blood." As you pull up to the house, a young woman runs down the lawn toward your unit, and you recognize her as the wife of a previous patient of yours, a man in his early 30s with advanced cystic fibrosis. He had a DNR order in place when you transported him to the hospital last month for diarrhea and dehydration.

Her husband is sitting on the floor of the living room with his back against a couch. He is breathing rapidly, shallowly, and with great effort; the muscles in his neck stand out as he leans forward. He is staring blankly at the blood that is on his hands and the front of his sweatshirt. His nasal cannula hangs loosely from his neck. As your partner goes to his side, the woman tells you that he "has had bronchitis" but had been "doing so well" on antibiotics. She says she heard coughing and came into the living room in time to see him start "coughing up all that blood" and slump from the couch to the floor.

Your partner rapidly replaces the nasal cannula, dials up the oxygen, and suctions the patient's airway. He no longer sounds as if he is choking, but he begins to cough again. He doesn't seem to be responding to your partner's presence. She shakes her head at you and reaches out to take his pulse and grab her stethoscope.

1. List two pieces of information that you need to know right away in order to provide the appropriate level and type of intervention for the patient.

She says she didn't call the cystic fibrosis clinic because "they're so negative. He needs help!" In response to your request to see current orders and plans, she reluctantly gives you information that states he has been accepted into hospice care and gives contact information for the service. The DNR order stipulates that the patient may receive oxygen and airway protection (e.g., suctioning), but intubation and ventilatory assistance are precluded. You note the patient's signature on the form, as well as his doctor's.

The patient is still in a semi-seated position on the floor with your partner kneeling behind him. She says he has a very rapid (about 180 bpm), weak pulse and that she can't yet hear any clear areas in his lung fields. As he coughs, more blood comes out of his mouth. She suctions. The wife leans against the wall and begins to cry helplessly.

2. What is the immediate medical need? What is the immediate need in terms of coordinating your care with the established plan?

A large amount of blood comes from the man's mouth, and he falls forward so that he is lying across your partner's lap. She continues to suction, and the blood continues to come. She leans over him closely, then looks up and says, "He isn't breathing, and he's nonresponsive." She places her hand over his carotid and says, "Pulse is weakening, too."

As his wife clings to you, crying and trembling, you look over again, and your partner shakes her head once. Then she gently lays the man's body out on the floor and begins to wipe the blood off his face. Without looking, she extends her arm backward to turn off the oxygen.

3. What is your immediate medical responsibility to the patient? To his wife?

EVALUATION

1120 ESSENTIALS OF PARAMEDIC CARE

©2007 Pearson Education, Inc.
Essentials of Paramedic Care, 2nd ed.

HANDOUT 46-4

Student's Name _____

CHAPTER 46 REVIEW

Write the word or words that best complete each sentence in the space(s) provided.

1. Total health care expenditures are expected to rise by _____ percent in the first decade of the 2000s.

2. Almost _____ percent of home care patients are 65 or older.

3. The primary goal of the ALS provider in home care situations is to identify and treat any _____-_____ problems.

4. The disease that is characterized by episodic muscle weakness triggered by an autoimmune attack on the acetylcholine receptors is _____ _____.

5. A program of palliative care and support services that addresses the physical, social, economic, and spiritual needs of terminally ill patients and their families is _____.

6. The one thing home care calls have in common is their _____.

7. When making a home care call, try to ascertain from the primary care provider (if present) a(n) _____ presentation for the patient.

8. _____ habits, _____ intake, and minor _____ or _____ can have a dramatic effect on the seriously ill home-bound patient.

9. Many home care patients suffer from COPD, which is a triad of diseases including _____, _____ _____, and _____.

10. Common home treatments for respiratory illnesses include oxygen, _____ or _____ medications, and possibly a ventilator utilizing _____, _____, or _____.

11. The most common problems faced by tracheostomy patients include _____ of the airway by _____ and a dislodged _____.

12. _____ _____ _____ are used to provide any parenteral treatment on a long-term basis.

13. The most common complications seen in patients with VADs result from _____ of various types.

14. Most complications related to urinary support devices result from _____ or _____ _____.

15. For the mother who has recently given birth, the most common complications are _____ _____ and _____.

Handout 46-5

Student's Name _____

ACUTE INTERVENTIONS TRUE OR FALSE

Indicate whether each statement is true or false by writing T or F in the space provided.

_____ 1. Almost 75 percent of home care patients are age 65 or older, and about 75 percent are female.

_____ 2. A home care patient is more likely to decompensate and go into crisis more quickly than a patient in the general population.

_____ 3. Cardiac decompensation is considered a true medical emergency in patients with preexisting cardiac or pulmonary compromise.

_____ 4. A high risk of infection is not seen in all patients with decreased immune response.

_____ 5. A Stage 2 pressure sore involves the epidermis, whereas a Stage 3 sore involves the full thickness of the skin, exposing subcutaneous tissue.

_____ 6. On any call involving a home care patient, ask whether another health care professional, in addition to EMS, has been called.

_____ 7. Many home care patients have a baseline lung capacity that only minimally meets their normal requirements.

_____ 8. Home care patients usually have a high dosing regimen, which may make them more responsive to additional medication.

_____ 9. When treating a patient with cystic fibrosis, always inquire about the stage of the disease and about any standing orders.

_____ 10. Pulmonary congestion or frank pulmonary edema may develop in infants with bronchopulmonary dysplasia when excessive amounts of fluid have been given.

_____ 11. Tracheostomy patients who have had a laryngectomy do not have any remaining air connection with the nasopharynx, so it is not necessary to block nose and mouth when ventilating the patient.

_____ 12. Tracheostomy stomas close slowly when the tube is not replaced.

_____ 13. Some common reasons patients use a home ventilator include decreased respiratory drive, weakness of respiratory muscles, obstructive pulmonary disorders, and sleep apnea.

_____ 15. Do not obtain vascular access or blood pressure readings in an extremity with a shunt.

_____ 16. Have a high index of suspicion for infection in the wounds of home care patients.

HANDOUT 46-6

Student's Name _____

ACUTE INTERVENTIONS ABBREVIATIONS

Interpret the following Chapter 46 abbreviations by writing out their meanings in the spaces provided.

1. DNR _____
2. DNAR _____
3. GI/GU _____
4. PEG _____
5. G-tube _____
6. COPD _____
7. VAD _____
8. PEEP _____
9. CPAP _____
10. BIPAP _____
11. CNS _____
12. CHF _____
13. CF _____
14. BPD _____
15. IMV _____
16. TPN _____
17. ARDS _____
18. PPV _____
19. NPV _____
20. PICC _____

Handout 46-7   Student's Name _____

HOME CARE SAFETY GUIDELINES

In responding to any home care situation, keep in mind the following guidelines about scene safety:

1. Any patient with limited movement may be contaminated with feces, urine, or emesis.
2. Any bed-bound patient may have weeping wounds, bleeding, or decubitus ulcers (bedsores).
3. Sharps may be present.
4. Collection bags for urine or feces sometimes leak.
5. Tracheostomy patients clear mucus by coughing, which can spray.
6. Any electrical machine has the potential for electric shock.
7. A hospital bed, wheelchair, or walker could be contaminated with body fluid.
8. Contaminated medical devices, such as a nebulizer, may be left around unprotected.
9. Oxygen in the presence of flame has the potential for fire or explosion.
10. Equipment may be in the way and cause you to fall, or it may be unstable and fall on you.
11. Medical wastes may not be properly contained or discarded.

Be sure that the following safety tips on home use of oxygen are followed.

1. Alert the local fire department to the presence of oxygen in the home.
2. Keep a fire extinguisher on hand.
3. If a fire does start, turn off the oxygen immediately and leave the house.
4. Don't smoke—and do not allow others to smoke—near the oxygen system. (No open flames or smoking within 10 feet of oxygen.)
5. Do not use electrical equipment near oxygen administration.
6. Store the oxygen tank in an approved, upright position.
7. Keep a tank or reservoir away from direct sunlight or heat.
8. Ground all oxygen cylinders.

Additional guidelines on oxygen use that you should know include the following:

1. Ensure the ability of the patient/home care provider to administer oxygen.
2. Make sure the patient knows what to do in case of a power failure.
3. Evaluate sterile conditions, especially disinfection of reusable equipment.
4. As with any patient with chronic respiratory problems, remain alert to signs and symptoms of hypoxemia.

Chapter 46 Answer Key

Handout 46-2: Chapter 46 Quiz

1. D	5. C	9. C	13. B
2. B	6. B	10. D	14. C
3. A	7. A	11. A	15. D
4. D	8. A	12. C	

Handout 46-3: Chapter 46 Scenario

1. You need to ask the wife whether she called the patient's physician or other telephone contact and, if so, what instructions were given. Secondly, exactly what DNR or other orders are currently in place?
2. Medically, you and your partner need to support airway, breathing, and circulation to the extent you can do so within the DNR order. You need to ask the wife once again whether she has called anyone—doctor at the clinic, hospice service, or other family—and what, if anything, she was told.
3. You and your partner need to confirm lack of heartbeat and respiration and notify medical control of the patient's death. After an initial cleanup of the patient's body, one of you needs to assist his wife in sitting with and grieving him. The other needs to call hospice to see what support they will get in place for his wife before you leave. Finally, you need to attend to whatever responsibilities are yours in the situation of a home death from natural causes.

Handout 46-4: Chapter 46 Review

1. 7.5
2. 75
3. life-threatening
4. myasthenia gravis
5. hospice
6. diversity
7. baseline
8. Eating, fluid, illnesses, injuries
9. emphysema, chronic bronchitis, asthma
10. nebulized, aerosol, PEEP, CPAP, BIPAP
11. blockage, mucus, cannula
12. Vascular access devices
13. obstructions
14. infection, device malfunctions
15. postpartum bleeding, embolus

Handout 46-5: Acute Interventions True or False

1. F	5. T	9. T	13. T
2. T	6. T	10. T	14. T
3. F	7. T	11. F	15. T
4. F	8. F	12. F	16. T

Handout 46-6: Acute Interventions Abbreviations

1. Do not resuscitate
2. Do not attempt resuscitation
3. Gastrointestinal/genitourinary
4. Percutaneous endoscopic gastrostomy (tube)
5. Gastrostomy tube
6. Chronic obstructive pulmonary disease
7. Vascular access device
8. Positive end-expiratory pressure
9. Continuous positive airway pressure
10. Bilevel positive airway pressure
11. Central nervous system
12. Congestive heart failure
13. Cystic fibrosis
14. Bronchopulmonary dysplasia
15. Intermittent mandatory ventilation
16. Total parenteral nutrition
17. Acute respiratory distress syndrome
18. Positive-pressure ventilation
19. Negative-pressure ventilation
20. Peripherally inserted central catheter

Chapter 47
Assessment-Based Management

INTRODUCTION

You need to think before you act as a paramedic in a manner similar to that for many other roles in life. This chapter addresses the focal role of thoughtful assessment in decision making regarding patient care and in ongoing evaluation and reassessment of the patient's condition. The chapter opens with presentation of the core concept of inverted pyramid thinking, clinical decision making. Then it addresses the components of effective assessment and presentation of patient information, as well as factors that may hinder either or both elements of patient care. After working through this chapter, students should be able to synthesize a large amount of material they have already encountered into a working model of a paramedic in action.

TOTAL TEACHING TIME:
14.40 HOURS
The total teaching time is only a guideline based on the didactic and practical lab averages in the National Standard Curriculum. Instructors should take into consideration such factors as the pace at which students learn, the size of the class, and breaks. The actual time devoted to teaching objectives is the responsibility of the instructor.

CHAPTER OBJECTIVES

After reading this chapter, you should be able to:

1. Explain how effective assessment is critical to clinical decision making. (pp. 1779–1781)
2. Explain how the paramedic's attitude and uncooperative patients affect assessment and decision making. (pp. 1781–1782)
3. Explain strategies to prevent labeling, tunnel vision, and decrease environmental distractions. (pp. 1780–1784)
4. Describe how personnel considerations and staffing configurations affect assessment and decision making. (pp. 1782–1784)
5. Synthesize and apply concepts of scene management and choreography to simulated emergency calls. (pp. 1783–1784)
6. Explain the roles of the team leader and the patient care person. (pp. 1783–1784)
7. List and explain the rationale for bringing the essential care items to the patient. (pp. 1784–1785)
8. When given a simulated call, list the appropriate equipment to be taken to the patient. (pp. 1784–1785)
9. Explain the general approach to the emergency patient. (pp. 1785–1788)

10. Explain the general approach, patient assessment differentials, and management priorities for patients with various types of emergencies that may be experienced in prehospital care. (pp. 1779–1788)
11. Describe how to effectively communicate patient information face to face, over the telephone, by radio, and in writing. (pp. 1788–1790)
12. Given various preprogrammed and moulaged patients, provide the appropriate scene size-up, initial assessment, focused assessment, and detailed assessment, then provide the appropriate care, ongoing assessments, and patient transport. (pp. 1779–1791)

FRAMING THE LESSON

Begin by reviewing the important points from Chapter 46, "Acute Interventions for the Chronic-Care Patient." Discuss any points that the class does not completely understand. Then move on to Chapter 47. You might begin the lesson by demonstrating use of the inverted pyramid of clinical thinking to your students through interaction with a paramedic on an actual case. Ask a paramedic to bring in blinded records of a medical or injury case that he/she feels is a good example of the importance of critical thinking/clinical decision-making skills. Have the paramedic read the dispatcher's comments and then have the class (or the group working with her/him) brainstorm about questions that occur to them. Have them work through the case to the point at which the patient is transferred to the receiving team. Have one student write down the major time points (dispatcher call, arrival on-scene, scene size-up, initial assessment, focused history and physical exam, ongoing assessment, and detailed physical exam) and the questions/thoughts that are on the paramedic's mind.

After the exercise is complete, review the questions to demonstrate the inverted pyramid of broad/multiple questions narrowing down toward more focused and fewer questions as patient care progresses. As a last step, ask students to name factors that helped or hindered their thinking. (If you have a radio playing softly in the background, someone may think of background noise or other environmental factors. If you have a large group of students rather than a small group, someone may think that too many providers present makes proceeding more difficult. Use the list of factors given in the chapter for other suggestions.)

Make sure students understand—before you proceed with the chapter—that this chapter should help them synthesize a lot of material they have already encountered, from differential diagnoses for various organ systems to the basic steps of an encounter. It is a capstone to previous work, not simply a repetition of earlier material.

TEACHING STRATEGIES

People learn in a variety of ways. Some do better with the spoken word, whereas others prefer the written. Some prefer to work alone, whereas others profit from working in groups. Recognizing these different ways of acquiring knowledge, the authors of this *Instructor's Resource Manual* have provided a variety of teaching strategies for the different types of learners. These strategies are intended to foster higher-level cognitive skills and encourage creative learning and problem solving. For greatest effectiveness, incorporate these strategies into

your class lecture. Symbols in the Lecture Outline indicate the points at which various exercises might be most appropriate. Other strategies can be used to preview the lesson or to summarize it.

The following strategies are keyed to specific sections of the lesson.

1. 20 Questions. Use a variation of "20 questions" to get students to see how they start with broad questions and work down to more focused ones. Place students in small groups. Have one student in each group think of an illness or injury they have had. Then have the others ask questions about the chief complaint, history, or expected findings and guess the diagnosis or diagnoses that would need further testing to confirm.

2. Making a Diagnosis. Assign common chief complaints to small groups of students. Have them create a list of differential diagnoses as a group, then complete the narrowing process with the class, finally arriving at a field diagnosis by asking for additional information as needed. This cooperative learning exercise prevents tunnel vision while working toward a field diagnosis. Additionally, it builds oral presentation skills.

3. Thinking about Diagnoses. Get in the habit of asking students to present a list of differentials and a field diagnosis during simulations and patient assessment labs. This encourages the inverted pyramid format of critical thinking and will help you identify the students who are unsure of their assessment skills. This early identification of students needing patient assessment or pathophysiology remediation will save you and the students much anxiety later in the field internship.

4. Stressing Patient History. Be sure to share with students the fact that diagnoses are made with as much as 80 percent of the decision coming from the history. This fact adds justification to the reason paramedics should ask so many questions in the field. Too often paramedics feel that a comprehensive history is the job of the hospital staff or doctor and take shortcuts with patients. This is inappropriate and could lead to a mistake or oversight. Encourage students to obtain a full history on every patient.

5. Thinking about Biases. To help students identify the biases they may harbor, ask students to describe different types of patients that they encounter. Give them categories according to dispatch information such as "drunk," "homeless person," "domestic violence," or "nursing home patient." Allow them to free-form ideas without regard for being polite or politically correct. Then, help them work through the negative connotations and stereotypes with facts and information that clearly debunk their "theories." This activity helps students to identify biases and replace opinions based on feelings with those based in reality.

The following strategies can be used at various points throughout the lesson or to help summarize and demonstrate what students have learned.

Clipping File. Gather newspaper clippings and case law rulings about EMS providers who have failed to treat legitimate medical conditions because the provider assumed the patient to be faking or not worthy of care. Many of these cases have harsh consequences for the providers, including fines, loss of income, suspensions, and job loss. This lends reality to the discussion of why we always treat every patient with the same level of respect and professionalism. Oftentimes, those not motivated by morals can be motivated to do the right thing by fear of the consequences.

HANDOUT 47-1
Chapter 47 Objectives Checklist

TEACHING STRATEGY 1
20 Questions

POINT TO EMPHASIZE
The decisions you make as a paramedic will be only as good as the information you gather.

TEACHING STRATEGY 2
Making a Diagnosis

TEACHING STRATEGY 3
Thinking about Diagnoses

TEACHING STRATEGY 4
Stressing Patient History

POWERPOINT PRESENTATION
Chapter 47 PowerPoint slides 4–6

POWERPOINT PRESENTATION
Chapter 47 PowerPoint slides 7–17

TEACHING STRATEGY 5
Thinking about Biases

POINT TO EMPHASIZE
A large number of rescuers moving around can be as distracting as a large number of bystanders.

READING/REFERENCE
Stein, L., and D. M. Meade. "Follow the Signs." *EMS*, Nov. 1997.
Werfel, P. "20 Tips to Perfect Your Assessment Skills." *JEMS*, Jan. 2000.

POWERPOINT PRESENTATION
Chapter 47 PowerPoint slide 17

Role Play. If you don't do the group exercise as a start for the lesson, use group role play to teach and reinforce the main points of the lesson. Have one group of students write a scenario, including dispatch call, scene size-up, initial assessment, pertinent history, physical exam, vitals, and so on. Then give the scenario to one student in a second group. He plays patient with the information given to him while the others act as EMS providers. Get everyone's perspective—those who wrote the scenario and watch the role play, the patient, and the providers. Show students how much "thinking" really goes on during a provider-patient interaction.

Cultural Considerations, Legal Notes, and Patho Pearls. The Student CD-ROM contains this series of informative features to enhance the student's understanding of the material covered in this chapter.

TEACHING OUTLINE

Chapter 47 is the seventh lesson in Division 5, *Special Considerations/Operations*. Distribute Handout 47-1 so that students can familiarize themselves with the learning goals for this chapter. If students have any questions about the objectives, answer them at this time. Then present the chapter. One possible lecture outline follows. In the outline, the parenthetical references in regular type are references to text pages; those in bold type are reference to figures, tables, or procedures.

I. Introduction. Much of patient assessment is based on concepts of inverted pyramid reasoning (called clinical decision making or critical thinking) and differential diagnosis. (p. 1779) (**Fig. 47-1, p. 1779**)

II. Effective assessment. Proper assessment is the foundation for patient care. (pp. 1779–1784)

  A. Importance of accurate information. (pp. 1780–1781)
     1. Decisions are only as good as the information collected.
     2. The history (**Fig. 47-2, p. 1780**)
     3. The physical exam
     4. Pattern recognition
     5. Assessment/field diagnosis
     6. BLS/ALS protocols

  B. Factors affecting assessment and decision making (pp. 1781–1783)
     1. Personal attitudes
     2. Uncooperative patients (**Fig. 47-3, p. 1782**)
     3. Patient compliance
     4. Distracting injuries
     5. Environmental and personnel considerations

  C. Assessment/management choreography (pp. 1783–1784) (**Fig. 47-4, p. 1783**)
     1. Team leader
     2. Patient care provider

III. The right equipment. The paramedic should learn to think of equipment as essential items carried in a backpack. (pp. 1784–1785)

  A. Infection control supplies (p. 1784)
  B. Airway control items (p. 1784)
     1. Airways (oral and nasal)
     2. Suction
     3. Catheters
     4. Laryngoscopes and blades
     5. ET tubes and equipment

C. Breathing (p. 1784)
1. Pocket mask
2. BVM
3. Variously sized masks
4. Oxygen tank and regulator
5. Oxygen masks and cannulas
6. Occlusive dressings
7. IV catheter for decompression

D. Circulation (p. 1784)
1. Dressings
2. Bandages
3. Tape
4. Sphygmomanometer
5. Stethoscope
6. Notebook and pen/pencil

E. Disability (p. 1784)
1. Rigid collars
2. Flashlight

F. Dysrhythmia (p. 1785)
1. Cardiac monitor/defibrillator

G. Exposure and protection (p. 1785)
1. Scissors
2. Space blankets

IV. General approach to the patient. Use an ordered approach when confronting a patient. Use the basic elements of the assessment process. (pp. 1785–1788)

A. Scene size-up (p. 1785)
B. Initial assessment (p. 1786)
1. Resuscitative approach
2. Contemplative approach
3. Immediate evacuation (**Fig. 47-5, p. 1787**)

C. Focused history and physical exam: four categories of patients (pp. 1786–1787)
1. Trauma patient with a significant mechanism of injury or altered mental status
2. Trauma patient with an isolated injury
3. Medical patient who is responsive
4. Medical patient who is unresponsive

D. Ongoing assessment and the detailed physical exam (pp. 1787–1788)
E. Identification of life-threatening problems (p. 1788)

V. Presenting the patient. Learning to communicate effectively is key to transferring patient information. (pp. 1788–1790)

A. Establishing trust and credibility is best done through use of the SOAP (Subjective findings, Objective findings, Assessment, Plan) format. (pp. 1788–1789) (**Fig. 47-6, p. 1789**)

B. Developing effective presentation skills (pp. 1789–1790)
1. Guidelines for effective presentation
   a. Lasts less than 1 minute
   b. Is very concise and clear
   c. Avoids extensive use of medical jargon
   d. Follows a basic format, usually the SOAP format or variation
   e. Includes both pertinent findings and pertinent negatives (findings that might be expected, given the patient's complaint or condition, but are absent or denied by the patient)

POINT OF INTEREST

Although the tasks assigned to the team leader and patient care provider are great, be aware that many systems have variations of these roles and responsibilities. For instance, the Los Angeles County Fire Department makes the team leader responsible for scene management, history, documentation, and radio communication, while the patient care provider actually does the physical assessment, vitals, and rescue skills such as bandaging, IV, and medication administration. Be sure to make students aware if services in your area differ from that of the model in the text.

POWERPOINT PRESENTATION
Chapter 47 PowerPoint slides 18–21

POINT TO EMPHASIZE
Be aware of your body language and the messages it sends.

POWERPOINT PRESENTATION
Chapter 47 PowerPoint slides 22–23

POINT TO EMPHASIZE
Plan ahead. Know what particular areas of information will be asked for or expected so that you can be ready with that information.

          f. Concludes with specific actions, requests, or questions related to the plan
     2. Information in ideal presentation
          a. Patient identification
          b. Chief complaint
          c. Present illness/injury
          d. Past medical history
          e. Physical signs
          f. Assessment
          g. Plan

VI. Review of common complaints (pp. 1790–1791)

  A. Practice sessions (p. 1790)
  B. Laboratory-based simulations (p. 1791)
  C. Self-motivation (p. 1791)

VII. Chapter summary (p. 1791). Assessment forms the basis of patient care. To make correct decisions, you must gather information and then evaluate and synthesize it. A variety of factors may affect assessment and the decision-making process itself. Some of these factors include paramedic attitude; uncooperative patients; obvious, but distracting injuries; narrow, or tunnel, vision; the environment; patient compliance; and personnel considerations.

    It is important to have the right equipment readily available to treat immediately life-threatening conditions. Effective communication and transfer of patient information—whether done face to face, over the telephone or radio, or in writing—is crucial to presenting the patient and ensuring continuation of effective care.

    Remember, the best way to develop good assessment skills is to practice until you become comfortable with a wide range of patient complaints.

SKILLS DEMONSTRATION AND PRACTICE

Assessment Practice You can distribute Handouts 47-5 through 47-21 to students at any point during the lesson. Use the handouts in the same manner as the ones in the text were used. Encourage students to put themselves one step ahead of the paramedics in the scenarios. If the paramedics in the scenarios take actions, see if the students arrive at reasons for the actions similar to those given in the handout. What would they have done differently? Or for different reasons? Have class discussions about each of the scenarios.

ASSIGNMENTS

Assign students to complete Chapter 47, "Assessment-Based Management," of the workbook. Also assign them to read Chapter 48, "Operations," before the next class.

EVALUATION

Chapter Quiz and Scenario Distribute copies of the Chapter Quiz provided in Handout 47-2 to evaluate student understanding of this chapter. Make sure each student reads the scenario to reinforce critical thinking on the scene. Remind students not to use their notes or textbooks while taking the quiz.

POWERPOINT PRESENTATION
Chapter 47 PowerPoint slide 24

HANDOUTS 47-7 THROUGH 47-21
Case Scenarios

ADVANCED LIFE SUPPORT SKILLS
Larmon & Davis. *Advanced Life Support Skills.*

ADVANCED LIFE SKILLS REVIEW
Larmon & Davis. *Advanced Life Skills Review.*

BRADY SKILLS SERIES: ALS
Larmon & Davis. *Brady Skills Series: ALS.*

WORKBOOK
Chapter 47 Activities

READING/REFERENCE
Textbook, pp. 1793–1889

HANDOUT 47-2
Chapter 47 Quiz

HANDOUTS 47-3 AND 47-5 TO 47-21
Chapter 47 Scenarios

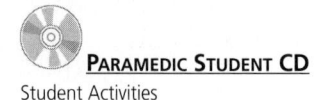

PARAMEDIC STUDENT CD
Student Activities

Student CD Quizzes for every chapter are contained on the dynamic and highly visual in-text student CD.

Companion Website Additional quizzes for every chapter are contained on this exciting website.

TestGen You may wish to create a custom-tailored test using *Prentice Hall TestGen for Essentials of Paramedic Care,* 2nd Edition to evaluate student understanding of this chapter.

On-line Test Preparation (for students and instructors) Additional test preparation is available through Brady's new on-line product, *EMT Achieve: Paramedic Test Preparation* at *http://www.prenhall.com/emtachieve/.* Instructors can also monitor student mastery on-line.

Review Manual for the EMT-Paramedic This comprehensive exam review contains hundreds of test questions and rationales, including scenarios, along with two 180-question practice tests on CD.

REINFORCEMENT

Handouts If classroom discussion or performance on the quiz indicates that some students have not fully mastered the chapter content, you may wish to assign the Reinforcement Handout for this chapter.

Student CD (for students) A wide variety of material on this CD-ROM will reinforce and also expand student knowledge and skills.

PowerPoint Presentation (for instructors) The PowerPoint material developed for this chapter offers useful reinforcement of chapter content.

Companion Website (for students) Additional review quizzes and links to EMS resources will contribute to further reinforcement of the chapter.

OneKey On-line support is offered for this course on one of three platforms: CourseCompass, Blackboard, or Web CT. Includes the IRM, PowerPoints, TestGen, and Companion Website for instruction. Ask your local sales representative for more information.

Brady Skills Series: Advanced Life Skills (Video or CD) Have your students watch the skills come to life on VHS or CD-ROM, or they can purchase the highly visual, full-color text with step-by-step procedures and rationales.

COMPANION WEBSITE
http://www.prenhall.com/bledsoe

TESTGEN
Chapter 47

EMT ACHIEVE: PARAMEDIC TEST PREPARATION
Mistovich & Beasley. *EMT Achieve: Paramedic Test Preparation.*
www.prenhall.com/emtachieve/

REVIEW MANUAL FOR THE EMT-PARAMEDIC
Cherry & Mistovich. *Review Manual for the EMT-Paramedic,* 3rd edition.

HANDOUT 47-5
Reinforcement Activities

PARAMEDIC STUDENT CD
Student Activities

POWERPOINT PRESENTATION
Chapter 47

COMPANION WEBSITE
http://www.prenhall.com/bledsoe

ONEKEY
Chapter 47

ADVANCED LIFE SUPPORT SKILLS
Larmon & Davis. *Advanced Life Support Skills.*

ADVANCED LIFE SKILLS REVIEW
Larmon & Davis. *Advanced Life Skills Review.*

BRADY SKILLS SERIES: ALS
Larmon & Davis. *Brady Skills Series: ALS.*

PARAMEDIC NATIONAL STANDARDS SELF-TEST
Miller. *Paramedic National Standards Self-Test,* 4th edition.

Handout 47-1

Student's Name _____

CHAPTER 47 OBJECTIVES CHECKLIST

Knowledge	Date Mastered
1. Explain how effective assessment is critical to clinical decision making.	
2. Explain how the paramedic's attitude and uncooperative patients affect assessment and decision making.	
3. Explain strategies to prevent labeling, tunnel vision, and decrease environmental distractions.	
4. Describe how personnel considerations and staffing configurations affect assessment and decision making.	
5. Synthesize and apply concepts of scene management and choreography to simulated emergency calls.	
6. Explain the roles of the team leader and the patient care person.	
7. List and explain the rationale for bringing the essential care items to the patient.	
8. When given a simulated call, list the appropriate equipment to be taken to the patient.	
9. Explain the general approach to the emergency patient.	
10. Explain the general approach, patient assessment differentials, and management priorities for patients with various types of emergencies that may be experienced in prehospital care.	
11. Describe how to effectively communicate patient information face to face, over the telephone, by radio, and in writing.	
12. Given various preprogrammed and moulaged patients, provide the appropriate scene size-up, initial assessment, focused assessment, and detailed assessment, then provide the appropriate care, ongoing assessments, and patient transport.	

OBJECTIVES

HANDOUT 47-2

Student's Name _____

CHAPTER 47 QUIZ

Write the letter of the best answer in the space provided.

_____ 1. When the patient has a medical (nontrauma) complaint, as much as _____ of the diagnosis will be made based upon the history.
   A. 30 percent
   B. 50 percent
   C. 66 percent
   D. 80 percent

_____ 2. Your ability to recognize patterns in the history and physical findings depends on your knowledge base and:
   A. the patient's ability to provide a full history.
   B. your experience.
   C. the quality of your medical direction.
   D. the quality of your local protocols.

_____ 3. Medical causes of patient restlessness and lack of cooperation with the paramedic include all of the following EXCEPT:
   A. emotional response to poor previous EMS experiences.
   B. hypoxia.
   C. intoxication with alcohol or other drugs.
   D. hypoglycemia.

_____ 4. Factors that can affect assessment and decision making negatively include all of the following EXCEPT:
   A. patients who are not compliant.
   B. environmental considerations such as scene chaos and dangerous situations.
   C. having only one paramedic for assessment.
   D. presence of distracting injuries.

_____ 5. In multiple casualty situations, who acts as the triage group leader?
   A. most experienced provider present
   B. patient care provider
   C. team leader
   D. equipment manager

_____ 6. The list of essential equipment for all calls includes all of the following EXCEPT:
   A. a long spine board.
   B. cardiac monitor/defibrillator.
   C. oral and nasal airways.
   D. oxygen tank and regulator.

_____ 7. If you may need additional equipment or support, call for it during the:
   A. initial assessment.
   B. focused history and physical exam.
   C. scene size-up.
   D. detailed physical exam.

_____ 8. Whenever you suspect a life-threatening problem, use the:
   A. contemplative approach.
   B. immediate evacuation approach.
   C. ABC approach.
   D. resuscitative approach.

_____ 9. A patient who hit a tree while sledding and appears to have broken an ankle but seems fine otherwise without positive finding would probably fit into what category after the focused history and physical exam is done?
   A. trauma patient with a significant mechanism of injury or altered mental status
   B. trauma patient with an isolated injury
   C. medical patient who is responsive
   D. medical patient who is unresponsive

©2007 Pearson Education, Inc.
Essentials of Paramedic Care, 2nd ed.

CHAPTER 47 *Assessment-Based Management* 1135

EVALUATION

HANDOUT 47-2 Continued

_____ 10. A patient in great distress who is complaining of angina-like pain that hasn't subsided with nitroglycerin would probably fit into what category after the focused history and physical exam is done?
   A. trauma patient with a significant mechanism of injury or altered mental status
   B. trauma patient with an isolated injury
   C. medical patient who is responsive
   D. medical patient who is unresponsive

_____ 11. Ongoing assessments should be done at which interval if the patient is stable and at which interval if unstable?
   A. 10 minutes, 2 minutes   C. 15 minutes, 2 minutes
   B. 10 minutes, 5 minutes   D. 15 minutes, 5 minutes

_____ 12. For trauma patients, if time and patient condition permit you should perform a:
   A. focused physical exam.   C. rapid trauma assessment.
   B. detailed physical exam.   D. thorough trauma assessment.

_____ 13. The resuscitative approach would be taken with all of the following conditions EXCEPT:
   A. respiratory distress or failure.   C. all spinal injuries.
   B. altered mental status.   D. status epilepticus.

_____ 14. The ongoing assessment includes all of the following EXCEPT the:
   A. transport priority consideration. C. mental status.
   B. rapid head-to-toe exam.   D. vital signs.

_____ 15. The most effective oral presentations of patients include all of the following characteristics EXCEPT:
   A. avoiding extensive use of medical jargon.
   B. following a basic format, usually SOAP or a variation.
   C. lasting less than 5 minutes.
   D. concluding with actions, requests, or questions related to the plan.

HANDOUT 47-3

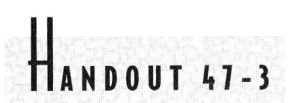

Student's Name _____

CHAPTER 47 SCENARIO

Review the following real-life situation. Then answer the questions that follow.

Dispatch sends you to a local park for "a child hurt while sledding." While your partner drives, you wish you knew the approximate age of the child and what kind of trauma is suggested by the word "hurt."

1. What other thoughts might go through your head while en route to the scene?

On arrival at the park, you and your partner head toward a large group of people near a stand of tall pine trees. As you approach, you see a child of perhaps age 7 or 8 years lying still on the ground. You don't see any blood on the snow.

2. What thoughts run through your head now?

You are told that the little girl was playing happily. Then she took "one last" afternoon ride down the hill, went straight into a tree, and fell off the sled. She seemed to be dazed, then complained of a headache and laid down. She hasn't spoken since, but moans intermittently.

Your partner notes that the child is lying on her back with limbs in seemingly proper alignment, no bleeding, and abrasions on one side of face. She focuses on his face as he kneels by her side but doesn't move.

3. What thoughts are probably running through the partner's head as he gets an immediate impression of the patient?

As your partner talks to the little girl, he learns her name is Emily, she is 7 years old, and she feels sick. When asked for specifics, she says her head hurts and she feels very dizzy if she moves at all. She is not sure what happened, but does know she is at the park near her grandmother's house and that she had gone sledding with friends. She can feel all four extremities but doesn't want to move because that makes her feel as if she might vomit.

The only additional historical information is that the child might have been unconscious briefly after the accident, but mostly she "just seemed out of it." No adults or children have any impression of whether her level of consciousness or mental status have changed since the accident.

4. What are your thoughts on the nature of injury and how to proceed?

EVALUATION

©2007 Pearson Education, Inc.
Essentials of Paramedic Care, 2nd ed.

CHAPTER 47 *Assessment-Based Management* 1137

HANDOUT 47-3 Continued

Your partner places a cervical collar on the little girl. As you position the spine board to move her onto it, she sits up suddenly and leans against your partner. Head examination reveals a large swelling on the patient's forehead, mostly behind the hairline. There is only slight oozing from surface abrasions. The child's pupils are equal and reactive to light. There is no evidence of any foreign matter in either eye. The rest of the rapid exam is notable only for tachycardia. There is no tenderness or swelling around the collarbones or on any of her extremities. She has no chest or abdominal discomfort.

At this point, the child becomes increasingly aware of the people staring at her and she begins to cry. An adult tells you that someone has gone to her grandmother's house and her parents are on the way and should be here within 5 minutes.

5. What do you do next? Is your next action affected by the fact the patient is a child and not an adult?

The patient is moved to the ambulance. Medical direction suggests immediate transport, with the parents to meet the ambulance at the hospital, which is about 15 minutes away by car.

6. What elements should be emphasized during the ongoing assessment of this child?

The parents arrive at the hospital shortly after Emily is transferred to the care of the emergency department staff. Her vitals remained stable during transport and her mental status improved somewhat, with greater ability to show orientation to day, place, nature of her situation ("I'm riding in the ambulance with you"), and the names of her paramedics.

She is eventually diagnosed with a concussion, from which she recovers without sequelae.

Handout 47-4

Student's Name _____

CHAPTER 47 REVIEW

Write the word or words that best complete each sentence in the space(s) provided.

1. The three elements of the inverted pyramid are _____ _____, _____ _____, and _____ _____.
2. _____ forms the foundation for patient care.
3. You must be as nonjudgmental as possible to avoid "short circuiting" data collection and pattern recognition by _____ conclusions before _____ a thorough assessment.
4. The roles of the team leader include the following:

5. The roles of the patient care provider include the following:

6. Be aware of your _____ _____ and the messages it sends, either intentionally or unintentionally.
7. The scene size-up has four components, which are:

8. The initial assessment has six components, which are:

HANDOUT 47-4 Continued

9. After the focused history and physical exam are complete, patients can be classified into one of four groups:
   _____
   _____
   _____
   _____

10. The seven components of the ongoing assessment are:
    _____
    _____
    _____
    _____
    _____
    _____
    _____

11. At all stages of the assessment, you must actively and continuously look for and manage any _____-_____ _____.

12. The underlying principle of assessment-based management is to rapidly and accurately assess the patient and then to treat for the _____-_____ _____.

13. SOAP stands for S _____ _____, O _____ _____, A _____, P _____.

14. The ability to _____ _____ is the key to transferring patient information.

15. The most effective oral presentations usually last less than _____ _____.

1140 ESSENTIALS OF PARAMEDIC CARE

Handout 47-5   Student's Name _____

CHECKLIST OF ESSENTIAL EQUIPMENT

- Infection Control
  - infection control supplies, namely gloves and eye shields
- Airway Control
  - oral airways
  - nasal airways
  - suction (electric or manual)
  - rigid tonsil-tip and flexible suction catheters
  - laryngoscope and blades
  - endotracheal tubes, stylettes, syringes, tape
- Breathing
  - pocket mask
  - manual ventilation bag-valve mask
  - spare masks in various sizes
  - oxygen tank and regulator
  - oxygen masks, cannulas, and extension tubing
  - occlusive dressings
  - large-bore IV catheter for thoracic decompression
- Circulation
  - dressings
  - bandages and tape
  - sphygmomanometer, stethoscope
  - note pad and pen or pencil
- Disability
  - rigid collars
  - flashlight
- Dysrhythmia
  - cardiac monitor/defibrillator
- Exposure and Protection
  - scissors
  - space blankets or something to cover the patient

(NOTE: See text page 1785 for discussion on how to determine additional "take in" equipment.)

Handout 47-6   Student's Name _____

CHECKLIST FOR ELEMENTS IN PATIENT PRESENTATION

✔ Patient identification, age, sex, and degree of distress
✔ Chief complaint (why EMS call was made)
✔ Present illness/injury
  —Pertinent details about present problem
  —Pertinent negatives
✔ Past medical history
  —Allergies
  —Medications
  —Pertinent medical history
✔ Physical signs
  —Vital signs
  —Pertinent positive findings
  —Pertinent negative findings
✔ Assessment
  —Paramedic impression
✔ Plan
  —What has been done
  —Orders requested

Handout 47-7

Student's Name _____

CHEST PAIN SCENARIO

ACTIONS	REASONING
DISPATCH	
I am working overtime at Medic 3 when we get dispatched to a 63-year-old male with chest pain. My partner, John, and I head to the ambulance and sign on en route to the call 2 minutes later.	I recognize the street that we are going to and realize I have 4 to 5 minutes to think about the situation on the way to the call. Chest pain in a 63-year-old male can be any one of a number of things, from a heart attack to an aneurysm to musculoskeletal chest pain. I have to be prepared for anything, so when we arrive on-scene, I grab the O_2 and the monitor while John grabs the drug bag. We throw it all onto the stretcher and head into the house.
SCENE SIZE-UP	
We arrive on-scene and find a one-story ranch house with only two steps up to the front door. I am grateful that I don't have to carry my stretcher up a flight of stairs. The house looks clean and well kept.	I have always been concerned about a back injury working this job. Easy access to the patient decreases my chances of that happening. The walkway to the house is clear of any obstacles, and the porch appears to be in good repair.
INITIAL ASSESSMENT	
We get into the living room to find a gentleman sitting straight up in his recliner. He is pale, short of breath, and holding his chest. I notice a walker beside the chair. John places our pulse oximeter on the patient's finger for a room air reading as he prepares to place the patient on high-flow O_2. He will place the patient on the monitor after the oxygen.	I am concerned because the patient is pale and appears to be in significant pain. I immediately wonder if he is having an MI due to his chest pain. Although he is pale, he does not appear diaphoretic, so I can't rule out several other possibilities as well. His pulse ox reads 88 percent on room air, which has me wondering why he is not oxygenating well. Does he have a history of COPD? I would like to see what his ECG strip shows, to help me narrow down what is going on.

©2007 Pearson Education, Inc.
Essentials of Paramedic Care, 2nd ed.

CHAPTER 47 *Assessment-Based Management*

HANDOUT 47-7 *Continued*

ACTIONS	REASONING
HISTORY	
Our patient introduces himself as Steven Willis. He tells us that he was sitting in the recliner, and as he sat up to get himself something to drink he had a sudden onset of sharp left-sided chest pain that took his breath away. He has been feeling short of breath ever since. He tried to rest for several minutes, hoping it was just a pulled muscle, but the pain hasn't gotten any better so he called 911.	As Mr. Willis is telling us that he is short of breath, I notice that his breathing is slightly labored, although he can speak in complete sentences. I have approached him, and as he is talking I check a radial pulse and find a rapid, regular pulse rate. I count the rate in the 120s, which rules out SVT as the cause of his chest pain. The oxygen that he has been getting seems to be helping a little, and his breathing is starting to slow down.
John now has Mr. Willis on the monitor, and Mr. Willis appears to be in a sinus tachycardia.	I am relieved to see that he is not in v-tach or having any other rhythm disturbances such as PVCs. His rate could be fast due to the fact that he is having pain, or it could also be related to his chest pain.
John has rechecked Mr. Willis's pulse ox, and it is now at 94 percent. He takes a blood pressure reading and reports 132/88.	I am happy to see that he is oxygenating better, but I am concerned about what caused the decreased oxygen saturation to begin with. The fact that Mr. Willis is able to sit up without complaining of lightheadedness or diaphoresis, plus the fact that he has a strong radial pulse, leads me to believe that he has a good blood pressure. Mr. Willis described his pain as "sharp" and not as "ripping" or "tearing." This, along with the fact that he is normotensive, leads me to rule out a dissecting thoracic aneurysm.
When asked, Mr. Willis describes the pain as sharp. His shortness of breath is somewhat relieved with the oxygen. He denies nausea, vomiting, and diaphoresis. The pain started as soon as he sat up, and until then he had been pain-free at rest.	I know from experience that patients having an MI describe their pain as "pressure" or "tightness in the chest," not usually as sharp, so I am thinking that this is probably not an MI. The fact that the pain started with movement and not at rest also leads me to think that this is not unstable angina, although I would like to know what his medical history is.
Mr. Willis tells us that he has a history of non-insulin dependent diabetes, hypertension, and has recently been discharged from a rehabilitation unit for a hip fracture he suffered 3 weeks ago. He had surgery on the hip 2½ weeks ago.	With this last piece of medical history, I think I can narrow down Mr. Willis's chest pain and shortness of breath to a pulmonary embolism. He is post-op from a recent hip fracture and has been sedentary for 3 weeks. A pulmonary embolism would explain his decreased oxygenation level, due to an occluded vessel in his lung. I would like to finish a physical exam, though, before I make a final decision.

SCENARIOS

1144 ESSENTIALS OF PARAMEDIC CARE

HANDOUT 47-7 Continued

ACTIONS	REASONING
PHYSICAL EXAM	
I ask Mr. Willis to lean forward so I can listen to his lung sounds. He has decreased breath sounds with scattered wheezes bilaterally. At this point he admits to being a two-pack-a-day smoker.	My last thought was that perhaps Mr. Willis had a spontaneous pneumothorax, but since I can hear breath sounds in all lung fields, I can rule this out as a cause of his chest pain and shortness of breath.
We place Mr. Willis on the stretcher carefully, due to his recent fractured hip. I take this opportunity to palpate femoral pulses bilaterally, which he indeed does have.	If Mr. Willis had a dissecting aneurysm, I would not be able to palpate femoral pulses due to the aorta leaking blood into the retroperitoneal cavity. This helps to confirm my thought that Mr. Willis is suffering from a pulmonary embolism.
INTERVENTIONS	
We move Mr. Willis to the ambulance, where we place him on onboard oxygen, which continues through a nonrebreather mask at 15 L/min. I start an IV as John starts to drive to the hospital with lights and sirens. Unfortunately, there isn't much more for me to do for Mr. Willis besides supportive care and frequent vital sign checks.	I would like to get Mr. Willis to the hospital quickly so they can get him to V/Q scan or CT for a final diagnosis. If he is having a pulmonary embolism, they need to start him on heparin as soon as possible.
ONGOING ASSESSMENT	
During the short trip to the hospital, Mr. Willis states he is starting to feel increased relief from his shortness of breath with the oxygen, but the sharp chest pain remains.	I note his pulse ox is up to 95 percent, so I know he is oxygenating better, but this just doesn't seem to be helping his pain.
COMMUNICATIONS AND WRITTEN REPORT	
I called ahead to the ED to let them know we were coming. As it turned out, they were having a quiet shift and had already called ahead for the V/Q scan. We settle him on an ED stretcher and give a final report with a final set of vital signs.	I had started filling out my run sheet in the back of the ambulance, so I just need to finish the narrative section. I grab a cup of coffee and head to the EMS room to finish my chart so I can leave it with his nurse before I go.
FOLLOW-UP	
I called the ED the next day to see what happened with Mr. Willis. The V/Q scan did indeed show a PE, and they heparinized him pretty quickly.	Well, at least I got that one right! I just wish there was more we could do for these patients in the field.

Handout 47-8

Student's Name _____

CARDIAC ARREST—PULSELESS ELECTRICAL ACTIVITY SCENARIO

ACTIONS	REASONING
DISPATCH	
My partner, Sue, and I are hanging out in the dispatch center after dropping off a box of donuts when a 911 call comes in for a woman down on the street about three blocks away. Because we aren't doing anything, we volunteer to take the call. We are already in the ambulance and heading to the call when we are officially dispatched.	"Woman down on the street." I'm thinking, in this city, this could be anything. Is she awake, dead, drunk? I tell Sue that I'll grab the monitor and the drug box if she grabs the airway kit and the O_2. We arrive on the scene in about 2 minutes.
SCENE SIZE-UP	
By the time we get there, a large crowd has gathered around our patient, so we really can't see her. There is a police officer there trying to clear an area with easy access to the patient for us to park. I can see that there are a couple of people, one of whom is another police officer, kneeling on the ground near the patient. When the crowd sees us get out of our ambulance they clear an area for us.	I am relieved to see the scene is safe. It adds to my comfort level on this job to see the police arrive ahead of me. A job outside like this attracts a crowd, and you never know when the scene can get hostile. The crowd seems concerned about the woman and allows us through easily.
INITIAL ASSESSMENT	
We find the woman in the supine position, with a man doing chest compressions and the police officer holding a nonrebreather mask over the patient's face. She is cyanotic. I get down next to her and ask the man to hold compressions while I check for a carotid pulse. There isn't one. I ask him to continue compressions.	"Oh great!" Sue says to me as she looks at the patient's oxygen mask. She goes to the woman's head and proceeds to take out the airway equipment. I am trying to figure out what is going on here. Was this woman walking down the street when she suddenly collapsed? Could this have been a traumatic event? I start to look around for any evidence of trauma.

HANDOUT 47-8 Continued

ACTIONS	REASONING
HISTORY	
"Can anyone around here tell me what happened?" I yell to the crowd as I start to get out the drug box and the IV kit. A man tells me that he saw the woman walking down the street when two men gave her a shove, grabbed her bag, and then ran down the street. She staggered a bit after being pushed, started to run after them while yelling, and then fell to the ground.	This is interesting. While trying to figure out the cause of the cardiac arrest, several things go through my head. How hard did they shove her? Could they have caused some kind of blunt trauma, like a tension pneumothorax or a cardiac tamponade? Does she have a cardiac history, and the exertion of what has happened to her put too much strain on her heart?
I ask the man doing compressions if he is doing OK and if he needs relief. He says he is fine, that he took a CPR class at the gym, and he doesn't mind continuing. I take advantage of this and get out some epinephrine for Sue to put down her ET tube once she gets that in. As I start to take out the monitor, a woman comes running through the crowd. She is crying and tells us that the woman is her mother and she had just left her apartment down the street. Her elevator is broken, and she had just run down six flights of stairs after a neighbor told her what had happened to her mother. Just then our supervisor shows up as well. He puts the patient on the monitor for me.	I am glad we have someone here who could tell us something about our patient. We still don't know what has caused this woman to go into cardiac arrest.
When asked, she tells us her mother has a history of heart disease and has recently been told she needed to have a cardiac catheterization and possible angioplasty. She has high blood pressure and her cholesterol level has been high.	This may help narrow things down, but I don't want to rule out trauma as the cause of this event yet. After all, who knows how hard she got pushed and if that could have caused any problems.
PHYSICAL EXAM	
Sue gets the ET tube in, and I watch for equal rise and fall of her chest. I listen for breath sounds over the epigastrium, which I don't hear, and then I listen for breath sounds bilaterally.	She has clear and equal breath sounds bilaterally, with equal rise and fall of her chest. Sue hyperventilates her, and I do not note any tracheal deviation. I can now rule out a tension pneumothorax as a cause for this cardiac arrest.
Sue dumps around 2 times the normal dose of epi down the tube, followed by 20 cc of saline.	Looking around, I don't see any other cause for blunt trauma. There is nothing she could have been pushed into to cause electrocution. It is pretty warm out, so I can safely say she wasn't hypothermic, and she obviously didn't drown.

HANDOUT 47-8 Continued

ACTIONS	REASONING
INTERVENTIONS	
I ask the man to hold compressions so I can see if there is any activity on the monitor. I note a coarse v-fib and get ready to shock her. I make sure everyone is clear and shock at 200 joules.	I know she's got a cardiac history, so I'm thinking that she just had too much stress put on her heart as she was mugged and then tried to run down the street.
I note that she is still in v-fib, so I shock again. I have to shock her a third time, which converts her to bradycardia with a rate of 46. I ask the man to hold compressions so I can check for a pulse. She still does not have a pulse. I give Sue an atropine to give down the tube.	Now I note that she is in PEA. I go through all of the causes for PEA in my head. I've already decided that she isn't hypothermic, she doesn't have a tension pneumothorax, and there is no reason to think she has suffered from a drug overdose, and I didn't get anything from her history that would lead me to believe she had a pulmonary embolism. I need to get an IV started, so I can give her a fluid bolus in case she is bleeding out from trauma from the fall and she needs drugs.
We continue compressions as I get the IV started. I run normal saline wide open as I secure the IV. Sue has been hyperventilating the patient after the epi. Just then I hear someone in the crowd telling the patient's daughter what happened. I hear him say that right before she fell, he saw her clutch her chest and take a few deep breaths; then she fell.	Why couldn't he have told me this? I'm thinking. It appears as if she might have suffered an MI from the activity. I go back to thinking about the PEA and what I can do next to convert her to a perfusing rhythm. If the PEA is being caused by hypoxia, then the hyperventilation should have helped. The atropine hasn't increased her rate.
I give the patient another epi via the IV.	Still no pulse. Maybe she is acidotic. If she doesn't convert soon, I'll consider giving her some bicarb.
It is time to get her loaded into the ambulance. As we load her up, I profusely thank the man for doing compressions.	
ONGOING ASSESSMENT	
We head to the hospital with lights and sirens. Our supervisor is driving, so we can work on the patient in the back. Sue continues to bag the patient as I do compressions. We continue to give epi and atropine IV, but her rhythm never changes.	Once again I consider pericardial tamponade, but it appears that this event occurred before the woman fell to the ground, so I have ruled out trauma as the cause for the arrest. If she is in PEA from hypokalemia, a round of sodium bicarb may help now.
I give her sodium bicarbonate 1 mEq/kg via IV	I know this can work if the patient is hypokalemic or acidotic, two more causes of PEA. I hope something works.
We hold compressions and check again for a pulse. There is still no pulse, so we continue CPR.	

HANDOUT 47-8 Continued

ACTIONS	REASONING
COMMUNICATIONS AND WRITTEN REPORT	
My supervisor called ahead, so the hospital knew we were coming. They had the code room ready for us. I give a report as someone takes over compressions for me. We hang back and watch as they continue working on her. She soon goes from PEA to asystole, and they call the code.	The only thing left that they could have done was a pericardiocentesis, but the ED staff decided that they didn't want to do this once she converted to asystole.
FOLLOW-UP	
It turns out that the cops grabbed the kids that did this just a few blocks away. They had stolen a few bags that day but didn't think anything like this would happen.	I love being a paramedic, but sometimes the job is a little distressing. I can't help but feel bad for this woman and her daughter.

Handout 47-9

Student's Name _____

ACUTE ABDOMINAL PAIN SCENARIO

ACTIONS	REASONING
DISPATCH	
It's 2:00 in the afternoon and Chris and I have had a pretty slow day when we get dispatched for a 78-year-old female with abdominal pain. It's my turn to work up the patient, so Chris hops in the driver's seat as I jump in the front seat next to him. I know the address, and I know that we have about a 5-minute response time.	I've been doing this job for a long time, so I realize that although this is probably just a routine call, it could turn out to be more than that. The patient could have a long-standing history of abdominal problems, such as colitis or diverticulitis, but there is also a chance that this could be an acute problem, such as an aortic aneurysm. That's what I like about this job; you just never know.
SCENE SIZE-UP	
We arrive on scene to find two cars in the driveway, so we park on the road in front of the house. This makes it difficult for us to get our stretcher to the door, because we now have to take it up the front yard. Then I notice five steps leading up to the front door. This does not make me happy.	I am always concerned about a back injury working this job. We try to minimize the amount of lifting we need to do. Hopefully there will be someone in the house who can move the car blocking the driveway. If we have to, we can call for lifting assistance.
INITIAL ASSESSMENT	
We've made it into the house with the stretcher, our jump kit, oxygen, and the monitor. There is a middle-aged woman, who is not our patient, waiting at the door, telling us that her mother is in the bedroom on the first floor (thank goodness for the small things!). I get to the bedroom and find the patient lying in bed in her nightclothes, pale but dry, sitting up in the bed. There is a bedside commode at the side of the bed and several pill bottles on the bedside table.	For several reasons, I am guessing that my patient has chronic medical problems. The bedside commode makes me wonder if she is bedridden, and the number of pill bottles leads me to think that she has a significant medical history. I need to start asking her some questions to find out what is going on.

SCENARIOS

1150 ESSENTIALS OF PARAMEDIC CARE

©2007 Pearson Education, Inc.
Essentials of Paramedic Care, 2nd ed.

HANDOUT 47-9 Continued

ACTIONS	REASONING
HISTORY	
I introduce myself and my partner, and the patient tells me her name is Nancy. She hasn't been feeling well for several days, and over the last 2 days she has been having abdominal pain which is getting worse. She says she has also been short of breath, which has been getting worse as well.	Well, so far this doesn't really help me narrow down what is going on. I need to find out where exactly the pain is. If she is having pain that she describes as indigestion and shortness of breath, this may not be an abdominal problem but could be an MI. I ask her to show me exactly where her pain is.
Nancy uses her hands to cover her entire abdomen and says she cannot pinpoint exactly where the pain is. When asked, she denies feeling indigestion or heartburn.	Well, this at least rules out a cardiac problem. And if she were having renal colic, she would be complaining more of back pain and not generalized abdominal pain, so I don't think that is what is going on, either. I still need more information. This could still be something quite serious, like a dissecting abdominal aortic aneurysm (AAA).
She tells me that she has been having small, frequent episodes of diarrhea for about 2 days and started vomiting this morning. She points to a bowl sitting on her bedside table.	Although patients may experience vomiting from a dissecting AAA, they usually don't have several days of diarrhea prior to it. This could still be appendicitis, but I think that by now her pain would have localized to the right lower quadrant. I also don't think that this is cholecystitis, since she doesn't have epigastric pain that is radiating to her back between her shoulder blades.
I ask Nancy what her medical history is as Chris starts getting a set of vital signs. Nancy's daughter starts handing me the pill bottles. I see that she is on blood pressure medication, an antidepressant, an antiinflammatory, and a narcotic. I am told that Nancy has recently been having pain in her left knee after a fall and that she has been taking the narcotic on a regular basis. She denies any heart disease. She tells me her last normal bowel movement was 3 days ago.	Well, now we are getting somewhere. The fact that she has recently been placed on narcotics helps me. I know that narcotics can cause constipation, especially if the patient is not mobile, and Nancy apparently isn't mobile due to knee pain. In a patient Nancy's age, constipation can easily lead to a bowel obstruction.

HANDOUT 47-9 Continued

ACTIONS	REASONING
PHYSICAL EXAM	
Chris tells me that Nancy's blood pressure is 92/70 and her heart rate is 102. On physical exam, I find Nancy's abdomen to be firm and distended. I try not to press too hard, but even with slight palpation she complains of pain. I have her lean forward so I can listen to her breath sounds, which are clear and equal throughout all lung fields. Her skin is cool and dry. I look over to the bowl at the side of her bed and find a small amount of dark brown emesis.	I am pretty certain that Nancy is suffering from a bowel obstruction. Her abdomen is distended and she has pain with palpation. She hasn't had a normal bowel movement for 3 days. I am also concerned, due to her vital signs, that she is bordering on shock. This could be caused by necrosis within an organ, in this case her intestines.
INTERVENTIONS	
Nancy needs an IV so we can give her a fluid bolus. Chris takes out the oxygen and puts her on a nonrebreather at 15 lpm as I start her IV. We assist her to the stretcher, and, although her blood pressure is a little low, she tells me she is more comfortable sitting at a 45-degree angle. We move her down the hall, and together are able to carry her down the stairs and into the ambulance.	She is not experiencing all of the signs of hypovolemic shock, and she is tolerating her vital signs well. I am not going to aggressively treat her for shock but will just give supportive care. I do want to see if a 500-cc fluid bolus will help her.
ONGOING ASSESSMENT	
En route to the hospital, I place Nancy on the monitor and notice a sinus tach of 104. Her pulse ox is 100 percent on the nonrebreather mask. Her blood pressure hasn't changed. Nancy continues to complain of nausea, so I've given her an emesis basin.	Since I just started the fluid bolus I don't really expect to see any immediate changes. I will check again in a few minutes.
Five minutes later, I note her heart rate is now in the 90s and her BP is 100/72. It seems that the fluid bolus is doing her some good. She still feels cool and remains pale.	I give her another blanket to help warm her up. We are almost at the hospital now.

HANDOUT 47-9 Continued

ACTIONS	REASONING
COMMUNICATIONS AND WRITTEN REPORT	
I call ahead to let the ED know that they are receiving a 79-year-old female with a probable bowel obstruction. They say that they will give me a room assignment upon arrival.	Since it is a quick trip to the hospital, I haven't got much charting done. I can get that finished after I've given my patient report.
FOLLOW-UP	
Before we leave the ED, I check on Nancy one last time. Her vitals signs have stabilized, although she isn't feeling any better. They are doing blood work and X-rays and have already consulted with a surgeon. It looks like she does, indeed, have a bowel obstruction.	Chris and I say goodbye to Nancy as we head out. I hope she does well, because she apparently has a long road ahead of her.

GI BLEEDING SCENARIO

ACTIONS	REASONING
DISPATCH	
"Medic 210, respond to 5891 Cedar Lane, Apartment 3, for a 56-year-old male vomiting blood." Robin and I had just sat down to eat lunch when our radio sounded. "Great, another day without a meal," Robin says as we head to the ambulance.	"Vomiting blood. This is not going to be pleasant," I'm thinking as we head to the call. Especially on an empty stomach.
SCENE SIZE-UP	
The apartment complex is large, and we are having a little trouble finding the right apartment. This isn't in a great part of town, so the police respond to calls here with us, and the officer in front of us has finally found the right one. Lucky for us, this is a first-floor apartment. The officer gets to the door first and finds it unlocked, so he heads in the door in front of us. We find our patient on the floor of the bathroom, sitting up against the wall near the toilet.	It eases my mind to have the police on the scene with us. We don't always get this lucky, but when I am concerned about my safety on a call, it is a relief to have them there. After looking around the apartment, I don't see any reason to feel unsafe here.
INITIAL ASSESSMENT	
The patient is pale and sitting straight up against the wall. When we come in, he tries to get up, but winces as if in pain, so he goes right back to the same position he was in. We introduce ourselves, and I go over to the patient, whose name is John.	John is probably pale due to blood loss from his vomiting. I don't have any information from him yet, but I am guessing he may have lost a significant amount of blood. He also seems hesitant to move, probably from extreme abdominal pain. I quickly try to find out what is going on.
HISTORY	
John tells us that he hasn't been able to work the last couple of days due to abdominal pain. At first, he thought it was indigestion, so he went out and bought some antacids, hoping they would help, which they did for a few hours.	I'm wondering if John has any history of peptic ulcer disease. I'm guessing that he doesn't because he didn't recognize the signs of it and tried medicating himself. I know this is common prior to patients complaining of upper GI bleeds.

HANDOUT 47-10 Continued

ACTIONS	REASONING
HISTORY (*Continued*)	
Yesterday the pain got worse, and he just lay in his bed. This morning he woke up nauseous and had several episodes of vomiting blood along with one episode of soft stool. He tells us he was barely able to get up and call 911 when he had to come back into the bathroom to vomit again.	Bleeding in the GI tract can be very irritating to the stomach and intestines. I ask him to describe the bleeding for me before I jump to any conclusions about what is going on.
John says that he has been vomiting bright red blood, but he noted that his stool was black and tarry.	John is having an upper GI bleed. This has been going on long enough for older blood to pass through his lower GI tract. If this were a lower GI bleed, the blood in his stool would be a brighter color and he would probably be vomiting blood that looked like coffee grounds, if he were vomiting at all.
PHYSICAL EXAM	
We need to get a quick set of vital signs and then get some treatment started. Robin gets out the BP cuff as I get ready to do a physical assessment. I would like to do this quickly so we can get him comfortable on the stretcher.	His blood pressure is 104/72, and his heart rate is 98. He is still hemodynamically stable, but I know this can change quickly so I still want to get two large-bore IVs started.
On physical exam, John is very tender on palpation of the right upper quadrant. I also note bulging in the RUQ.	We assist John onto the stretcher and place him supine on it. I would like to perform a tilt test to see if there are any changes in his blood pressure or his pulse. When we stand him up, I am going to get another set of vital signs.
Robin and I help John to his feet. He complains of severe pain with movement, but I explain why I am getting another set of vital signs before he sits on the stretcher. He agrees to let us do this, so Robin helps hold him up while I check his blood pressure and pulse.	His blood pressure is now 88/52, and his pulse rate has gone to 118. This means that he has failed his tilt test and will need aggressive fluid resuscitation.

HANDOUT 47-10 Continued

ACTIONS	REASONING
INTERVENTIONS	
Once John is on the stretcher, I start one of the two IVs that he will need. I figure I can get a fluid bolus going while we load him into the ambulance and then start another IV en route to the hospital. We also put him on oxygen. I am concerned about his positioning on the stretcher. I know that he continues to vomit and, because he has a decreasing level of consciousness, there is risk for aspiration. However, with his vital signs, I don't want to sit him up straight on the stretcher. I place John in the left lateral recumbent position, which should help avoid aspiration.	John needs the fluid resuscitation because he is beginning to go into hypovolemic shock. I don't want him to decompensate any more than he already has. Although he has been awake, alert, and oriented times 3 up until this point, I still want to make sure I do everything for him I can to prevent aspiration.
ONGOING ASSESSMENT	
I've got two IVs started, and I've drawn some blood off the second IV. His bolus continues, and he hasn't vomited since we've been in the ambulance. I continue to check his vital signs every 5 minutes until we get to the hospital.	I need to continue to monitor John for signs of worsening shock. His vitals remain stable, and he has maintained his level of consciousness. He reports no change in his pain.
COMMUNICATIONS AND WRITTEN REPORT	
I alert the ED that we are en route with an active upper GI bleed. They tell us to report to their trauma room, where they can easily do fluid resuscitation and give blood if necessary.	Once in the ED, I report to the waiting nurse. I've labeled my bloods, and they get sent to the lab quickly for a CBC and type and crossmatch in case John needs a blood transfusion.
FOLLOW-UP	
I follow up with the nursing staff later in the day. John's first set of blood work came back within normal limits, but the second set, done a couple of hours later, showed a significant blood loss, and he wound up needing to get a couple of units of blood.	I'm glad John called when he did. If he had continued to decompensate while alone in his apartment, his outcome could have been a lot worse.

SCENARIOS

HANDOUT 47-11

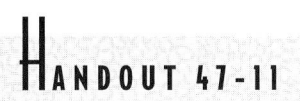

Student's Name _____

ALTERED MENTAL STATUS SCENARIO

ACTIONS	REASONING
DISPATCH	
What a day! Matt and I are both on overtime at Medic 3, which is usually a quiet station, but we haven't stopped all day. We just sit down to put our feet up for 5 minutes when we get dispatched. "Medic 3, respond to 176 West 59th Street, Apartment 5J, for an unconscious male." When we sign on that we are responding, dispatch tells us that we have an unconscious male in his early-to-mid-30s, and the caller has no idea what is going on.	Matt hops in the driver's seat and hits the lights and sirens as I get in the passenger's seat. We start discussing what is going on here, and he starts testing me. "OK," he says, "let's review our AEIOU-TIPS," as he tests my memory. "I'll buy lunch if you can remember them all." This time I can outsmart him, and I know I'll be saving $5 on lunch today. AEIOU-TIPS is a mnemonic that helps us remember some of the common causes for altered mental status. I tell him I know them all. A is acidosis, E is epilepsy, I is infection, O is an overdose, U is uremia, or kidney failure, T can be trauma, tumor, or a toxin, I is for insulin, or diabetic emergency, P is for psychosis or poisoning, and S is for stroke or seizure. "I'm in the mood for Italian today," I tell him as we arrive on scene.
SCENE SIZE-UP	
We pull up to a pretty old apartment building with a several-step walk up to the front door. There is a doorway to get into the building, which I am assuming is locked, then a vestibule, and then another doorway. I only hope this building has a working elevator. There is no one around this afternoon, and this is usually a pretty safe neighborhood, but I always look around to see who is hanging around and who can mess with the ambulance while we're inside. Matt locks up the front as I grab the stretcher from the back. We grab all of our equipment and he finishes locking up.	We have to stay on our toes with regard to our safety, as far as lifting and moving and environmental factors as well. We both know how to lift and move stretchers and patients up and down stairs without getting hurt, but you can never be too cautious. And scene safety is important no matter where you work, whether it's in the heart of the city or in the quietest suburb.

©2007 Pearson Education, Inc.
Essentials of Paramedic Care, 2nd ed.

CHAPTER 47 *Assessment-Based Management* 1157

SCENARIOS

HANDOUT 47-11 Continued

ACTIONS	REASONING
INITIAL ASSESSMENT	
The elevator is working and we head up to 5J. We get off the elevator to find a man waiting at the door of one of the apartments. He yells down to us when he sees us.	
We get inside to find a male, mid 30s, in the bed, profusely sweaty, pale, bordering on unconscious. He is in gym clothes, and there is a gym bag at the side of the bed. His friend tells us he doesn't know anything about the patient's medical history; he came to pick him up for lunch and found him like this.	Matt starts getting out the monitor and IV equipment while I start assessing the patient. He is cool to the touch and very sweaty. I start getting a blood pressure. I look around to see if there are any pill bottles or alcohol around; perhaps this was an overdose, or maybe he had a seizure. I am glad we reviewed the mnemonic on the way here, because I am now going through them all again in my head.
HISTORY	
Our patient's friend, John, tells us that he called Larry, our patient, this morning to see if he wanted to go to lunch. Larry was off from work today, so they made plans for John to pick Larry up at 12:00. John didn't show up until 12:45, and Larry didn't answer the buzzer downstairs. Someone let him into the building, and luckily Larry didn't lock his door, so John let himself in and found Larry like this. There is also vomitus in the bathroom.	I ask John to start looking around the apartment for any medications his friend may take or to find anything that may give us a clue as to what's going on.

I don't see any alcohol bottles nearby, and I don't smell it on Larry's breath, and with the story that John has told us, I don't think Larry is drunk. He breath doesn't smell fruity, so I don't think this is acidosis. He could have had a seizure, and if he takes seizure meds, hopefully John will find them. I think I can also rule out an infectious process, as he was willing to go to lunch up to the last minute, so he must have been feeling well. I guess this could be a drug overdose, but again, if there are any bottles, hopefully John will find them. I get to "T" for trauma, and I think, maybe this is a head injury—he could have really suffered a head injury, didn't feel well afterwards, and decided to lie down and that's how he got to the bed. So far, I'm not really getting anywhere here. Now I'm at "I" for insulin. There is a good chance that Larry could be hypoglycemic, since he hadn't eaten lunch yet. When Matt gets the IV started, we'll have to check his dex stick. I guess Larry could have a psych history or could have been poisoned in some way. We'll find out about the psych history if John can find any meds. I think it is unlikely that Larry had a stroke, based on his initial presentation of diaphoresis and vomiting. |

HANDOUT 47-11 Continued

ACTIONS	REASONING
PHYSICAL EXAM	
Matt keeps calling Larry's name, and Larry is looking at him but isn't speaking. Matt has him on the monitor, which shows a sinus tach. Matt reports a weak, rapid pulse. Larry can move all extremities and even tries to fight Matt as Matt takes his arm to start the IV.	I yell out to John, who is looking through Larry's medicine cabinet, to see if he has found anything yet. When he says he hasn't, I tell him to look in the kitchen and to make sure he checks the refrigerator. If Larry is diabetic, there should be insulin in there.
Matt is having trouble with the IV because Larry is really fighting now. He has strong movements of his extremities, so I go to hold him down.	I tell Matt that I don't think Larry had a stroke, due to the strong, equal movements of his extremities. Since it appears that he just came back from the gym, I don't think this is an intentional overdose or alcohol-related, but we can't rule that out just yet.
We get the IV started, and Matt draws blood and gets a dex stick, which I throw in the glucometer. Just then John comes into the room with two bottles of insulin, NPH and regular, and a box of syringes.	Larry's glucose reading is 23. He is diabetic and is hypoglycemic.
INTERVENTIONS	
I grab the drug kit and throw Matt an ampule of 50 percent dextrose. He is pushing it as fast as he can, but the dextrose is thick and it takes some time.	While we are waiting for Larry to become more alert, we are trying to piece together what happened. We are guessing that Larry had been exercising prior to lunch. Regular exercise can actually lead to a decrease in the amount of insulin a patient needs to take. He may have then taken his regular insulin, expecting to eat lunch at a certain time, but then John was late and Larry probably didn't eat. All this could have led to Larry becoming severely hypoglycemic.
ONGOING ASSESSMENT	
A few minutes later Larry starts to wake up and looks around. He manages to sit up in the bed, and his skin is becoming dry. He begins to regain color in his face.	The D_{50} is working and Larry's blood sugar is coming up. He is alert and oriented and can tell us what is going on. Basically, we got the story right. He tells us he usually wears a medical ID bracelet, but one of the links broke and he hadn't replaced it yet.

HANDOUT 47-11 Continued

ACTIONS	REASONING
ONGOING ASSESSMENT (*Continued*)	
This episode has scared Larry because this is the first time that this has happened to him. He agrees to go the hospital with us, and transport is uneventful. His heart rate is coming down, and his skin is warm and dry.	Many diabetics, once they wake up, refuse transport to the hospital. In order to avoid medical liability for not transporting a patient for whom we have begun treatment, we call a supervisor who reviews with the patient the procedure for refusal of medical transport, and then has the patient sign a refusal form. In this case, Larry realizes that his insulin needs to be adjusted because he has been working out regularly and wants to be seen in the ED.
COMMUNICATIONS AND WRITTEN REPORT	
We call ahead to the ED and let them know we are coming. They give us a room assignment as we head in without an emergency.	This is a nonemergent transport because Larry has regained his normal mental status and he is no longer hypoglycemic. I write my report en route to the hospital.
FOLLOW-UP	
The ED runs Larry's pre-glucose blood for a glucose level, which shows 23. His dextrose stick is now 69, so they give him some orange juice and lunch to eat, because they would like to see it a little higher.	We say goodbye and head to lunch ourselves. After all, it's time for Matt to pay off his bet.

Handout 47-12

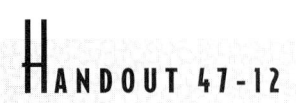

Student's Name _____

DYSPNEA SCENARIO

ACTIONS	REASONING
DISPATCH	
It is 4:30 in the afternoon, and we've just had one of the slowest days I can remember for a long time. I'm telling my partner, Maria, that I am almost bored when we are dispatched for a 26-year-old male in a local park complaining of shortness of breath. I am actually relieved to have some work to do.	The park that we are dispatched to has several different areas. We are directed to go to the basketball courts when we get there. The park is very busy this time of year, with lots of ball players coming around in the afternoon for pickup games, but there is also a crowd that is into the drug scene, and you can usually find one or two drug dealers there. The occasional crack overdose or drug bust is never a surprise here, so we don't know what we are getting into when we head to the park.
SCENE SIZE-UP	
We pull into the parking lot at the basketball courts to find a crowd of people standing around in a circle. There are two cop cars already there, and I can see at least three police officers in the crowd. One car has its trunk open, and I see an officer heading toward the crowd with an oxygen tank.	The fact that there are several police officers there is not surprising. The city is pretty good about making sure that EMS is not alone in areas that have a reputation for drugs and crime, even in the middle of the day. Maria and I grab our monitor, airway kit, and stretcher and head toward the basketball courts.
INITIAL ASSESSMENT	
A young man is sitting up against a basketball pole with labored respirations, sternal retractions, and diaphoresis. He is complaining of chest pain.	En route to the scene, I had been thinking that this could be drug-related due to the location. Perhaps the patient had been smoking crack or inhaling fumes as some kids have become fond of doing, but it appears that the patient had been playing ball. He is working hard to breathe, but I don't hear any stridor, so I can rule out a foreign body obstruction. Although it is hard to say right now, the fact that he was playing ball leads me to think he is in good health, so I don't think there is anything infectious like pneumonia. He may be a smoker, but he is too young to have any chronic breathing problems from it, like emphysema or acute bronchitis. He is tall and thin, so I can't rule out a spontaneous pneumothorax or even a pneumothorax from trauma, if he was hit in the chest by another player. He is breathing fast and his respirations are obviously labored, so he is clearly not hyperventilating. I need to get a little medical history and do a respiratory assessment to rule out heart failure, MI, and pulmonary embolism.

HANDOUT 47-12 Continued

ACTIONS	REASONING
HISTORY	
Our patient, Jason, cannot speak in complete sentences due to his shortness of breath. Another player tells us that they had been playing ball for about an hour when Jason started to slow down and walk toward the bench. Then he couldn't walk anymore. He sat down against the pole because he was able to breathe a little better sitting straight up, but he didn't have the strength to hold himself up.	Since Jason cannot speak, I ask him only to answer yes or no to my questions. When asked, he denies any cardiac history. He does tell me that he has a history of asthma. I ask him if he uses medicine for his asthma every day, and he shakes his head no and points to his bag. I give it to him and he pulls out an albuterol inhaler. He manages to get out that he only uses it when he becomes short of breath with exercise. I shake it, and it feels empty. He tells me he can't remember when he used it last.
PHYSICAL EXAM	
As we are getting Jason's medical history, Maria puts the pulse ox on Jason's finger. He is already on 15 L/min of oxygen via a nonrebreather mask that one of the police officers put on him. His pulse ox reading is 90 percent.	He isn't oxygenating well, which means he must be pretty tight, meaning that his bronchioles are pretty closed up.
I ask Jason to lean forward so I can listen to his lungs. He has high-pitched inspiratory and expiratory wheezing throughout all lung fields.	He doesn't have unilateral wheezing, so I can rule out an aspirated foreign body and a pneumothorax. The wheezing is clearly related to his asthma, so I am no longer concerned that his shortness of breath and chest pain are from a pulmonary embolism.
INTERVENTIONS	
Maria puts Jason on the albuterol treatment and assists him to our stretcher. I place him on the monitor and note sinus tachycardia in the 110s. His respiratory rate is 36.	Shortness of breath can lead to tachypnea and tachycardia. I want to monitor his vital signs regularly to watch for any changes.
ONGOING ASSESSMENT	
En route to the ED, I start an IV in case the physician wants to give steroids when Jason gets to the ED. When the first albuterol treatment is over, I start a second. I note that his heart rate is now in the 120s, but his respiratory rate is now 28. I reassess his breath sounds, and the wheezing is becoming a little coarser.	Steroids are important to relieve the inflammation in the bronchioles. Albuterol is a beta-agonist, and one of its side effects is tachycardia. As Jason's airway starts to open, the wheezing should become less high-pitched, like whistling, and become coarser. This means that he is having more air movement. He is still breathing fast, although it is good to see his respiratory rate come down a little.

HANDOUT 47-12 Continued

ACTIONS	REASONING
COMMUNICATIONS AND WRITTEN REPORT	
We call ahead to the ED to let them know we are coming. It is a quick trip, so I don't have time to get my chart written in the back of the ambulance.	I give the report and sit down in the EMS room to get my chart done while Maria restocks the respiratory equipment.
FOLLOW-UP	
Jason has finished his third treatment by the time I am done with my chart. He is still on oxygen, but they've put him on a nasal cannula and his pulse ox is now 95 percent. He is speaking in complete sentences and thanks us for our help.	I remind him that he needs to keep a new inhaler in his bag if he is going to play ball. Even if he had gotten to the one he had with him, it wouldn't have done him any good.

Handout 47-13

Student's Name _____

SYNCOPE SCENARIO

ACTIONS	REASONING
DISPATCH	
Miguel and I have just spent the day cleaning the ambulance. It is 4:30 P.M. and we are looking forward to resting for the rest of the shift when we get dispatched for a 59-year-old female with a syncopal episode. We clear the buckets and mop out of the way so we can get the ambulance out and sign on en route to the scene.	Well, so much for getting some rest this afternoon. I ask the dispatcher if they have any more information for us, since syncope is kind of vague—at least let us know if the patient is conscious. We find out that the caller is the patient's daughter, who was a bit hysterical on the phone and didn't give much information. We do know that the patient is now awake. That's a start.
SCENE SIZE-UP	
We arrive on scene 6 minutes later. We are in a typical suburban neighborhood and there are bikes and toys in the driveway, so we park in the street. We usually don't have police on the scene with us, unless there is reason to believe the scene is unsafe, so we are the only ones to arrive. A young woman comes running out of the house, telling us to hurry up.	We look at each other and move a little quicker. Perhaps something has changed and her mother is no longer awake.
INITIAL ASSESSMENT	
We are shown to the living room, where a middle-aged woman is lying on the couch with her feet up on some pillows. She looks pale and clammy. She is awake, alert, and oriented times 3. Her respirations are easy and nonlabored. When she sees us, she begins to sit up, but we encourage her to lie back down.	At least someone knew to lie her down and elevate her feet to help the blood flow back to her head. I wonder if she was here in the living room when she experienced the syncope or if she was helped here after she woke up.

SCENARIOS

1164   ESSENTIALS OF PARAMEDIC CARE

©2007 Pearson Education, Inc.
Essentials of Paramedic Care, 2nd ed.

HANDOUT 47-13 Continued

ACTIONS	REASONING
HISTORY	
Mrs. Dunn, our patient, tells us that she was standing at the sink, washing dishes, when she felt lightheaded and became sweaty. As she was reaching the table to sit down, she fell to the floor, and that is where her daughter found her. Her daughter, Lynn, tells us through her tears that her mother "was out" for a long time but woke up and was able to walk to the couch.	I can see we are going to have trouble getting information from the daughter, but Mrs. Dunn seems to be doing pretty well. She was standing at the sink when she became lightheaded. I wonder if she became orthostatic due to a fluid volume problem or if she had a vasovagal episode. Her respirations are easy and nonlabored, so her syncope does not appear to be caused by hyperventilation. She may have a sugar problem or a cardiac problem that we don't know about yet. I saw her move all extremities equally when she sat up, so I don't think she had a stroke, although she may have had a TIA. Her daughter did not describe any seizure activity, so I am ruling that out as a cause for her syncope.
When asked, Mrs. Dunn denies any chest pain or shortness of breath prior to her syncopal episode, nor is she experiencing either one now.	This can still be cardiac-related, such as an arrhythmia. Since she denies chest pain, I don't think this is an MI.
PHYSICAL EXAM	
Miguel gets out the monitor as I start my physical assessment. Mrs. Dunn is cool and clammy to the touch. She has clear lung sounds bilaterally and no pedal edema. I've checked her pulse and it feels pretty slow. I'd like to see what her rhythm looks like.	With a quick pulse check, I can rule out SVT and v-tach as a cause for the syncope. Her rate is pretty slow, so I am thinking that her bradycardia could be the problem. I'd like to know more about that.
Miguel reports a sinus bradycardia on the monitor with no ectopy. Mrs. Dunn's blood pressure is 180/110. Her daughter reminds her to tell us about her blood pressure problem.	I wonder what this blood pressure problem is all about? She may have been hypotensive due to a fluid volume problem, although with a BP of 180/110 I doubt that is what happened.
Mrs. Dunn has recently been diagnosed with hypertension. Her daughter comes back with the pill bottle and I see that Mrs. Dunn is taking atenolol. She just started the medication this past week.	Atenolol is a beta-blocker that is used for hypertension. It can also cause bradycardia. Mrs. Dunn just couldn't compensate for her low heart rate while standing up washing dishes, and that is what caused her syncopal episode.
INTERVENTIONS	
Miguel starts an IV and draws blood. He starts a line of normal saline at a KVO rate.	If Mrs. Dunn remains symptomatic from the bradycardia, we may need to give her atropine or possibly even use our pacer. We need to have an IV started to be prepared for either.

HANDOUT 47-13 Continued

ACTIONS	REASONING
ONGOING ASSESSMENT	
We get Mrs. Dunn loaded into the ambulance, and I recheck her vital signs. Her blood pressure is 176/112, and her heart rate is 42.	Mrs. Dunn is tolerating her vital signs well, but I realize that this could easily change. I've taken out an amp of atropine just to be on the safe side. I also have my pacer pads ready, in case I need to take them out quickly. If she were still feeling lightheaded, I may even consider putting the pads on her in case I needed to use the pacer quickly, but I don't think it is necessary at this time.
COMMUNICATIONS AND WRITTEN REPORT	
I let the ED know that we need a monitored bed for a syncopal episode related to bradycardia. They give me a room assignment as I finish my report. We now have about a 10-minute transport, so Mrs. Dunn and I talk in the back of the ambulance as I finish my run sheet.	The trip to the ED was uneventful. Mrs. Dunn remained asymptomatic, with no change in her vital signs. I give the report to the ED nurse and hand her my run sheet. Now maybe we can head back to the station to put our feet up.
FOLLOW-UP	
Mrs. Dunn was admitted to the hospital for monitoring. She shouldn't be there for more than a day or two. Her physician will also be changing her blood pressure medication.	There are many other drugs out there that will keep Mrs. Dunn's blood pressure under control but will not cause the bradycardia and syncope that she experienced today.

HANDOUT 47-14

Student's Name _____

SEIZURE SCENARIO

ACTIONS	REASONING
DISPATCH	
The call comes in the middle of the night. "Medic 206, respond to 218 Treebrooke Road for a seizure." Kayla and I throw our boots on and head out the door. I knew it was too much to expect to be able to sleep through the night on a Friday. Things were just going too well.	Kayla is driving as I am looking up the street on the map. Treebrooke is in one of the little subdivisions in our district—it is just a matter of finding the right one.
SCENE SIZE-UP	
We arrive in a quiet little neighborhood to find the house well lit. This is always a relief in the middle of the night. There is one step up to the front door. We head up the driveway with our stretcher and equipment.	I am always concerned about going out to someone's house in the middle of the night. If they don't turn lights on, we never know what we may find the hard way. I have tripped over children's toys and fallen off porches. Thankfully, none of this ever led to an injury.
INITIAL ASSESSMENT	
We get into the house, and a woman named Pat meets us at the door and quickly directs us upstairs. We carry up our equipment and leave the stretcher downstairs. We are led into the bathroom of the master bedroom to find a man in his mid-40s on the bathroom floor, with jerking motions noted in his arms and legs. He has vomited on the floor.	The patient appears to still be seizing. I grab suction equipment as Kayla grabs the oxygen and a bag-valve mask. While I start to suction, Pat tells us the seizure is getting better and that he isn't jerking as much. Kayla passes me the BVM, and I start to bag our patient, Bobby, as Kayla gets out the IV kit and prepares to start an IV.
HISTORY	
As I am bagging Bobby, his jerking continues. I yell out a bunch of questions to Pat: Does Bobby have any medical problems we need to know about? Does he have a history of seizures? Can she tell us what happened prior to Bobby having the seizure? I ask specifically about medical history. Has he been complaining of not feeling well recently, specifically asking if he's been complaining of a headache? She tells me that Bobby does not have any medical problems at all.	Bobby does not have a history of seizures. Pat now starts getting upset, so I have to start asking more specific questions. I want to know exactly what is causing this seizure, but Pat is becoming less helpful the more upset she is getting. By asking about any recent headaches, I can rule out more than one cause of the seizure. I am concerned that he may have an infectious process going on, such as meningitis. Pat denies any recent headaches. The fact that she denies any medical history doesn't mean that this isn't caused by something like a brain tumor or a neurovascular disease. He may have either one, and this could be the initial presentation.

©2007 Pearson Education, Inc.
Essentials of Paramedic Care, 2nd ed.

CHAPTER 47 *Assessment-Based Management* 1167

HANDOUT 47-14 Continued

ACTIONS	REASONING
HISTORY (*Continued*)	
Has Bobby recently experienced any trauma or head injury?	A head injury, even several days ago, could have led to a cerebral bleed or contusion, which could result in a seizure several days later. Pat is unaware of any head injury.
I tell her I have to ask some sensitive questions. I ask if Bobby takes drugs or drinks alcohol on a regular basis. She starts to cry and tells me that he usually drinks at least 2 six-packs over the course of the day, but lately they have been arguing about it. Two days ago he told her he could prove that he wasn't an alcoholic by going "cold turkey" and not drinking anymore. Tonight he was shaking and sweating and complaining of nausea before going to bed.	It appears that Bobby is going through alcohol withdrawal. Pat describes the symptoms of detoxification, and patients going through withdrawal frequently have seizures.
PHYSICAL EXAM	
Bobby continues to have jerking motions in his arms and his legs. He has urinated in his pajama pants. I take the bag-valve mask off his face to look in his mouth to see if he has bitten his tongue.	Incontinence and a bitten tongue are both signs of a generalized tonic-clonic, or grand mal, seizure.
INTERVENTIONS	
Since Bobby hasn't stopped jerking yet, we are concerned that he may have another seizure. Kayla calls medical direction for an order for Valium so we can get this seizure activity stopped.	Due to local protocols, we need to call the hospital for medical direction before we give any narcotics. We get an order for 10 mg of Valium, which I give via slow IV push through the normal saline IV that Kayla started. We start a normal saline IV on seizure patients due to the fact that if the physician wants to give the patient IV Dilantin, it is compatible only with normal saline.
As we are waiting for the fire department to show up, we have time to put Bobby on the monitor. He is now breathing on his own, so I switch him to a nonrebreather mask.	I also call for lifting assistance, because I am concerned that Kayla and I will not be able to safely carry this patient down the stairs by ourselves, especially if he starts to seize again.
ONGOING ASSESSMENT	
We get Bobby loaded into the ambulance. His seizure activity has stopped, and he is postictal. He is taking slow deep breaths, so I check his respiratory rate, which is 12. His pulse ox is 99 percent on the nonrebreather mask. His blood pressure is 132/78, and his heart rate is 92.	I need to closely monitor his vital signs. Valium is a CNS depressant, which means he could stop breathing due to the medication. It can also lower his blood pressure, so I need to make sure that his BP stays within normal limits.

HANDOUT 47-14 Continued

ACTIONS	REASONING
COMMUNICATIONS AND WRITTEN REPORT	
We notify the ED that we are coming, and we are told that we will get a room assignment on arrival.	I wait until I get to the ED to write my report. I want to monitor Bobby closely in case he seizes again or has any change in his vital signs.
FOLLOW-UP	
Bobby is starting to come around as we are getting ready to leave the ED. Pat has arrived at the hospital and thanks us for helping her husband.	If there were any doubts that Bobby has an alcohol problem, this incident should settle it. Bobby has a long road ahead of him.

Handout 47-15

Student's Name _____

HYPOTHERMIA SCENARIO

ACTIONS	REASONING
DISPATCH	
"Medic 112, respond to 357 South East Drive for an elderly male, unresponsive." Our radio alerts us of a call, and Lucas and I head out to the rig.	While en route, I call dispatch to see if there is any other information I can get. I know the address—it's one of the many nursing homes in our district. Many times they call us and the chief complaint isn't even close to what's going on when we get there, so we like to have a little more information prior to our arrival. We find out that the patient had been missing for several hours and was found outside in nightclothes.
SCENE SIZE-UP	
We arrive on scene to find several police cars and fire trucks already on location. We are directed to the ambulance entrance by a police officer, who escorts us into the building and fills us in on what is going on. The police had been called several hours ago because one of the Alzheimer's patients was missing. The police and fire department searched for 3 hours and found the patient in the woods behind the nursing home. It is close to winter and the temperatures dropped into the low 40s last night. They wrapped the patient in some blankets, carried him back to the nursing home on a Reeves stretcher, and called us.	I do not have any concerns regarding my safety or the safety of my partner on this call. However, I wonder how this patient was able to just leave during the night without anybody noticing. But this is not my problem. I just need to make sure I do the best I can for this patient.
INITIAL ASSESSMENT	
We arrive in the patient's room to find him wrapped in several blankets. He is unresponsive and lying very still, and his muscles are stiff and rigid. He has shallow respirations and a weak pulse. He is not on any oxygen or monitoring equipment. I ask what the patient's temperature is and no one seems to know.	This patient is exhibiting signs of severe hypothermia. He is not shivering, which means his body temperature must be pretty low. I am concerned about his shallow respirations, because this may indicate an impending respiratory or cardiac arrest.

SCENARIOS

ESSENTIALS OF PARAMEDIC CARE

©2007 Pearson Education, Inc.
Essentials of Paramedic Care, 2nd ed.

HANDOUT 47-15 Continued

ACTIONS	REASONING
HISTORY	
The head nurse comes in to give us a report, but doesn't add much more to what we already know. The patient has been a resident for several months and has a history of wandering the halls, but has never tried to leave the building before. He has a medical history of hypertension and coronary artery disease. She also tells us that he has a Do Not Resuscitate order on his chart and that his daughter is on her way.	This medical history doesn't really change anything that we are going to do for the patient right now. However, I am concerned about cardiac and respiratory arrest, and the fact that he is a DNR can completely change the way we care for this patient.
PHYSICAL EXAM	
Lucas starts to get out the monitor and IV equipment as I start a physical assessment. I unwrap the blankets the patient is in and find that he is still in the wet nightclothes that he was found in. A nursing assistant takes a quick rectal temperature and reports 30°C (86°F).	I immediately take out my shears and start cutting off the wet clothes. I ask for some new blankets, and a nursing assistant runs to get some. His body temperature indicates that he is in need of active internal rewarming, which should not be attempted in the field unless we have more than a 15-minute response time to the hospital.
We place the patient on the monitor and find he is in atrial fibrillation. I ask the head nurse if he has a history of a-fib, which she denies. I attempt to get a blood pressure, but I cannot hear one.	A-fib is the most common presenting dysrhythmia seen in hypothermia and can be seen in those patients with a body temperature of less than 30°C. This concerns me, because if he gets any cooler, the patient can easily go into ventricular fibrillation.
INTERVENTIONS	
The patient is still lying in the Reeves stretcher, and I would like to get it out from under him because it is also cold and a little damp. I ask for some moving assistance from the firefighters who are still there.	I know it is important to limit handling of the patient and to move him carefully, since rough handling can lead to ventricular fibrillation. However, I want to do everything I can to get whatever is cold and wet away from the patient. We can move him to our stretcher on a sheet when the time comes.
The nursing assistant hands me some heat packs, which she wants me to place under his arms and in his groin. I say thanks but no thanks and continue doing what I am doing.	Applying external heat to this patient can result in rewarming shock by causing reflex peripheral vasodilation. This causes the return of cool blood and acids from the extremities to the core. This may cause a paradoxical "afterdrop" core temperature decrease and further worsen core hypothermia.

HANDOUT 47-15 *Continued*

ACTIONS	REASONING
INTERVENTIONS *(Continued)*	
I want to get this patient to the hospital quickly, because there is nothing more that I can do for him here. I quickly get him covered up in dry blankets after we start an IV. We slowly and carefully move him over to our stretcher and load him carefully into the back of the ambulance. We keep warm IV fluids in an IV warmer in the ambulance, so I grab a bag and hang it on the patient en route to the hospital.	Active internal rewarming requires warm IV fluids, warm, humidified oxygen, peritoneal lavage, and extracorporeal rewarming. I know that the warmed IV fluids that I have will contribute little to the rewarming effort, but their use may prevent further heat loss and can prevent the onset of rewarming shock. We have less than a 15-minute response time to the hospital, so even if I had the means of further active rewarming, I wouldn't attempt it in the field.
ONGOING ASSESSMENT	
We transport the patient to the hospital slightly inclined with his head down. Although Lucas is using his lights and sirens, he is driving slowly to avoid any rough handling of the patient. The patient remains in a-fib.	I am still concerned about the possibility of v-fib, so we do our best to keep the patient still. Although we have the heat blasting in the back of the truck and we are hanging warm IV fluids, nothing is going to help this patient until we get him to the hospital.
COMMUNICATIONS AND WRITTEN REPORT	
I call the ED and let them know we have a 7-minute ETA with a severely hypothermic patient. They tell me to report to the trauma room, where they keep all of their equipment for active rewarming.	We head to the trauma room and I quickly give the report and hand them the patient's DNR order, along with the rest of the copies of his chart. The DNR order will become very important, should the patient convert to v-fib. This is going to be a long report to write, so I grab a cup of coffee and head to the EMS room.
FOLLOW-UP	
We head out about 25 minutes later. The ED staff has started the active rewarming process and his core temperature is now 32°C. His daughter has arrived and would like to know what happened, so we take a few minutes to fill her in a little on what we know took place prior to our arrival.	It's a shame that this patient was able to get out of the nursing home as easily as he was. They need to review how they care for Alzheimer's patients, because it is all too common for them to wander off as this man did.

Handout 47-16

Student's Name _____

HAZARDOUS MATERIALS/TOXICOLOGY SCENARIO

ACTIONS	REASONING
DISPATCH	
I am working an overtime night shift at Station 3 with Mary. It's the middle of the night, and we get called out for a 36-year-old male in respiratory arrest. Lucky for him, the call is right down the street.	I throw my boots on and head out the door. I offer to drive, but because Mary is used to working nights and I'm not, she says she would prefer to drive. It's fine with me because it gives me a minute or two to shake the sleep out of my head. I tell her that I'll grab the oxygen, monitor, and airway kit if she takes the jump box. We'll just throw it all on the stretcher as we head inside.
SCENE SIZE-UP	
We arrive on the scene to find a dark, rundown apartment building. I can't believe anyone even lives here. The neighborhood is known for the drug dealers and addicts who hang around, and it is protocol to dispatch police along with the ambulance on any calls here. Just as I am getting ready to ask if the police are on the way, I hear their siren in the background. We follow protocol and wait in the ambulance until the cops arrive.	This is a frustrating part of the job. I remember learning the very first day of EMT class that I always have to make sure the scene is safe for me and my crew. This scene is definitely not safe, and, although I am told that the patient is in respiratory arrest, I am not going to take any chances with my own safety.
INITIAL ASSESSMENT	
We are escorted up the stairs and find ourselves in an abandoned apartment. Several people run out the door when they see the police arrive. A woman stands in the doorway to another room and motions for us to come in there. We find a man in his mid 30s leaning up against a wall, breathing at about 4 times a minute. I look around him before I get down next to him to make sure I don't get stuck with any needles. As I kneel down, I feel for a pulse, which is slow.	I am assuming that this is a heroin overdose, based on what I know about the area and the fact that this patient is experiencing severe respiratory depression and bradycardia.

©2007 Pearson Education, Inc.
Essentials of Paramedic Care, 2nd ed.

CHAPTER 47 *Assessment-Based Management* 1173

SCENARIOS

HANDOUT 47-16 Continued

ACTIONS	REASONING
HISTORY	
We ask the woman what happened, but she looks at the cops and says she doesn't know; she just found him like this.	She obviously isn't going to tell us the truth, especially with the cops around.
I ask if she knows if he has any medical problems, and she says she has no idea and that she hasn't known him for very long.	Although I am assuming that this is a heroin overdose, I cannot rule out the possibility of a medical problem. However, as my husband always says, "When you hear hoofbeats, think horses and not zebras," so we are going to treat the obvious first.
PHYSICAL EXAM	
We lay him down and Mary gets out the oxygen and bag-valve mask. I do a quick pupil check with my flashlight while she is doing this and find constricted pupils.	Constricted pupils are another sign of a heroin overdose.
INTERVENTIONS	
I then start bagging the patient with 100 percent oxygen.	The patient is basically in a coma and isn't fighting the BVM at all. Mary puts the pulse ox on his finger, and his oxygen saturation goes from 79 to 98 percent after a short time. This gives Mary a little more time to get an IV started, as I am not having any difficulty managing his airway.
Because I am not having any problems managing the patient's airway with a bag-valve mask, Mary attempts an IV rather than intubation. We both know that this patient needs naloxone as soon as possible.	I don't want to bag him for too long, due to increased gastric distention and the risk of aspiration from vomiting. However, we both know that the opiate antagonist naloxone can reverse a heroin overdose quickly, thereby reversing the respiratory depression quickly. Many times these patients wake up intubated and proceed to pull out their tubes, which can cause trauma to the airway.
Mary gets lucky and finds a good vein in the patient's thumb and is able to start an IV on the second attempt.	Frequently, IV drug abusers are very difficult IV sticks. They have been abusing their veins for a long time and therefore don't have any usable veins left. If this were to happen, we would give the naloxone as an intramuscular injection. Although it takes longer to work this way, the advantage of IM naloxone is that it lasts longer as well.
Mary gives the patient naloxone 2 mg slow IV push.	We have both had the experience of giving this drug too rapidly, causing vomiting.

HANDOUT 47-16 Continued

ACTIONS	REASONING
INTERVENTIONS *(Continued)*	
The patient starts to breathe on his own and starts to become combative, pushing the BVM off his face. Mary had just finished securing the IV.	Many times these patients wake up combative. I have also had the experience of the patient getting very angry because we have taken away his high. They don't realize that we have saved their lives, as they weren't breathing and would have died.
The police jump in and secure him until he has had a chance to calm down. He becomes quiet and cooperative once he realizes what is going on. We convince him to go to the hospital with us and load him up on the stretcher.	Naloxone reverses the symptoms of a narcotic overdose, but has a shorter half-life than the drug that the patient overdosed on. It is important to get the patient to the hospital in case the drug wears off before the heroin does.
ONGOING ASSESSMENT	
En route to the hospital, I get a full set of vital signs, which are now all within normal limits. He is breathing 20 times a minute, and he is in a normal sinus rhythm at 88. His blood pressure is 118/62. I recheck his vital signs every 5 minutes.	I want to do frequent vital sign checks in case the naloxone wears off and he starts to experience signs of overdose again.
COMMUNICATIONS AND WRITTEN REPORT	
Mary calls in a report from the front of the ambulance as I ride in the back with the patient. We have a short trip to the hospital, and transport is uneventful.	I give the report to the nurse in charge and sit at the desk to finish the run sheet while Mary restocks the equipment we used.
FOLLOW-UP	
While in the ED, the patient starts to exhibit signs of the overdose again, so they give him another dose of naloxone. Although he wants to leave, he isn't going anywhere for a while.	The patient won't be discharged until the physician is convinced that the patient won't go into respiratory arrest when he leaves. We head back to the station to hopefully finish out our shift quietly.

Handout 47-17

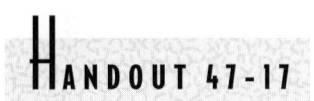

Student's Name _____

BLUNT TRAUMA SCENARIO

ACTIONS	REASONING
DISPATCH	
My partner, Antonio, and I are just cleaning up at the hospital after bringing in a bad MI when dispatch calls us on the radio to see if we are available to take a call. The last thing we want to do is run another call right now, but we have just finished cleaning up so we agree to do it. The call is for a pedestrian struck at the corner of Howard and Mills, which is just a few blocks from the hospital.	Great, we go from taking care of a huge MI to a trauma. I call dispatch to find out if this is a child or an adult, since this type of trauma affects these types of patients differently. I am told that this is a male patient in his mid-to-late 20s.
SCENE SIZE-UP	
We reach Howard pretty quickly, but traffic is backed up, presumably because of the accident. Antonio maneuvers around the cars that are trying to get out of our way. We get to the intersection to find a car in the middle of it, with a man lying in the road about 12 feet away. There are a few people around the man, including a police officer. I get out of the ambulance and note that the engine of the car is turned off. I don't see any fluids leaking from the car.	I want to make sure the scene is safe. The car is safely turned off, and I don't need to worry about any leaking fluids causing a problem.
INITIAL ASSESSMENT	
We approach the patient and find him lying on his stomach. He appears to be unconscious and is not moving. There is a moderate amount of blood by his head, but I can't see where it is coming from. I can see that he is breathing, but I am not certain about airway compromise.	Right away I am concerned about a head injury, due to the mechanisms of injury and the bleeding from his head. We also need to protect his c-spine, in case he has a cervical-spine injury.
HISTORY	
The driver of the car is clearly upset, stating that he didn't see the patient walk in front of the car. Witnesses say that the patient was trying to run across the street against the light when he got hit. They saw him roll onto the hood of the car and slide into the windshield, then get thrown to the ground as the car stopped suddenly. Another witness says that she didn't think the car was going very fast when it hit the victim.	From this story I am figuring that he got hit on the side, possibly causing a lower leg injury on the side that was hit. Hitting the hood could have caused a femur or chest injury. Hitting the windshield could have caused head, neck, or shoulder trauma. He could have suffered additional trauma from being thrown to the ground.

HANDOUT 47-17 Continued

ACTIONS	REASONING
PHYSICAL EXAM AND INTERVENTIONS	
Antonio immediately measures the patient for a cervical immobilization collar, while at the same time he assesses the patient's airway, breathing, and circulation. The patient is breathing on his own but has blood coming from his mouth. He has a radial pulse, which means he has a blood pressure of at least 60 systolic. I help Antonio put the c-collar on, and, with the assistance of the police officer, we gently logroll the patient onto his back.	The blood in the patient's mouth concerns me. If the patient cannot protect his airway, then he can aspirate on the blood or any teeth that may have been loosened.
I use the portable suction to suction his mouth and find out where the bleeding is coming from. This starts to wake the patient up. I don't see any loose teeth or other objects, and I see that he has a cut on his tongue, probably from biting it. Once I finish suctioning, I see the cut isn't bleeding anymore. I start the patient on 100 percent oxygen via a nonrebreather mask.	Suctioning is important to clear the airway and to visualize the mouth for trauma even though the patient has a patent airway.
Now that he is on his back and his airway is clear, I can evaluate for a flail chest or other chest injury such as pneumothorax or hemothorax. I note equal expansion of the chest cavity and as I listen to his breath sounds I note clear and equal breath sounds bilaterally.	The type of blunt trauma that this patient suffered can lead to internal chest injuries. If he were having any compromise in his breathing, this could lead to respiratory arrest.
The patient starts to moan and starts moving his arms to grab at his c-collar. He opens his eyes after I ask him to several times. He is trying to speak, but I don't understand what he is saying, and he is withdrawing from pain. I figure his Glasgow Coma Score at 10.	The Glasgow Coma Score is a moderately good predictor of head injury severity. A score between 9 and 12 indicates moderate injury. I had been considering intubating him to protect his airway, especially with the blood in his mouth, but I think I can hold off on that for now.
I instruct the patient to lie still and not to move his head or neck and to stop grabbing at his collar. I explain that if he has a neck injury, all the movement can make the injury worse. I do a quick neuro assessment and ask him to squeeze my hands and to push down and then pull up with his feet. I find he moves all extremities equally.	The fact that he is moving his arms and legs is a good sign that he hasn't suffered an obvious c-spine injury. This certainly is not a guarantee, however, and if he has any broken bones in his neck, I want to keep him from moving them to prevent further injury.
I already know that the patient has a strong radial pulse. I check capillary refill, and it is less than 2 seconds. I do a quick look to see if there is evident bleeding from additional injuries, and right now I don't see any.	A capillary refill of more than 3 seconds can be caused by hypovolemia, although I also realized that if he were a smoker or taking certain meds, those things could also cause a delayed capillary refill. It is important to detect any signs of early shock.

©2007 Pearson Education, Inc.
Essentials of Paramedic Care, 2nd ed.

HANDOUT 47-17 Continued

ACTIONS	REASONING
PHYSICAL EXAM AND INTERVENTIONS (*Continued*)	
Due to the mechanism of injury, I decide that this patient needs a rapid trauma assessment. I have already done a quick evaluation of the patient's head, neck, and chest during my initial assessment. I need to now evaluate his abdomen, pelvis, and extremities.	I focus on these areas first because they are where serious life threats are most likely to occur.
Because we are concerned about hypothermia, we don't want to leave him lying on the ground, especially since we'll have to cut off his clothes to perform our exam, further lowering his body temperature. Since the ambulance is right here, we decide to quickly get him loaded in the back before going any further. We know he has a decent blood pressure and pulse from our initial assessment, so we take a few minutes to put him in the ambulance now.	We want to keep the patient as warm as possible to prevent hypothermia.
We are now in the back of the ambulance. The patient has become more alert and is starting to ask questions. As a matter of fact, he has asked the same questions several times. I do a quick pupil check and find his pupils are equal and reactive.	The repetitive questioning convinces me that the patient has a concussion, as exhibited by the memory loss. He is not suffering any herniation in his brain from swelling or bleeding, at least not yet, which I note since his pupils are equal and reactive.
Antonio checks the patient's vital signs and gets the following: blood pressure 102/68, pulse 104, with sinus tachycardia on the monitor, and respirations 22.	His vital signs are good but bordering on possible shock. We need to check them frequently and do what we can to prevent the patient from going into shock. If he is bleeding, I need to find out from where.
I try to get the patient to tell me if he is having any pain anywhere, but he isn't answering my questions. I try to get him to pay attention, but I'm not getting anywhere. Antonio gets ready to start his IVs as I go on with my assessment. I start cutting his clothes off so I can do a visual inspection, but I cover him up with blankets so I can keep him warm.	My physical evaluation of the patient is going to be very important, because he is not answering my questions due to his head injury.
I inspect his abdomen for any asymmetry or apparent pulsing masses. I palpate each quadrant to see if this elicits any pain response from the patient, which it does not.	I carefully palpate all four quadrants of his abdomen, and I watch his face for any evidence of pain, but this does not seem to bother him. He denies pain on palpation when I ask him.
Next, I evaluate his pelvis. I place firm pressure on the iliac crests directed medially and on the pubic bone directed downward. Everything feels fine, and again the patient denies pain in the area.	I am checking for crepitus and/or any instability of the pelvis. A patient can bleed heavily from a pelvic fracture.

SCENARIOS

1178 ESSENTIALS OF PARAMEDIC CARE

HANDOUT 47-17 Continued

ACTIONS	REASONING
PHYSICAL EXAM AND INTERVENTIONS (*Continued*)	
I carefully examine each extremity for muscle tone, distal pulse, temperature, color, and capillary refill time. I also check for motor response, sensory response, and limb strength. I do not see any evidence of injury.	When a patient has a major area of injury, such as a head injury, he may not complain about pain from a broken bone in an extremity because he is focused on the major injury.
Antonio and I now need to logroll the patient to check his back for injury. I examine the total surface of the back and palpate the spinal column from top to bottom. Again, the patient has no complaints of pain, although I still find his answers unreliable.	Careful examination for slight deformities, minor reddening, and very subtle pain or tenderness may reveal the only signs or symptoms of a spinal cord injury.
Antonio takes one more set of vitals before heading up front to drive. The patient's blood pressure remains stable at 108/70, pulse rate is 107, still in sinus tach, and his respirations are still 22.	His vital signs are stable, and there really isn't much more to do for this patient except transport him to the hospital.
ONGOING ASSESSMENT	
I recheck vital signs every 5 minutes en route to the hospital. I also do a repeat neuro exam and check the patient's pupils for any changes. He is responding to my questions better, although he is still asking repetitive questions. I'm glad it's a short ride to the hospital!	With any major trauma, a patient can compensate for a while and then decompensate quickly. This is why I am checking vital signs and neuro status frequently.
COMMUNICATIONS AND WRITTEN REPORT	
Our dispatcher has called the ED for us to let them know they are getting a trauma. The trauma team is waiting for us in the trauma bay. The leader of the trauma team takes my report and takes over from here.	A trauma chart is a hard one to write. I have to make sure I have documented every assessment that I have done. This chart is going to take a while to complete.
FOLLOW-UP	
By the time we clean up the ambulance and finish charting, the patient is back from a CT scan. Miraculously for the patient, it is negative. So far, all X-rays have been negative as well. It seems that he is going to walk away from this with just a bad concussion.	I realize that not everyone is this lucky, and I'm glad he is going to have a good outcome.

Handout 47-18

Student's Name _____

ALLERGIC REACTION SCENARIO

ACTIONS	REASONING
DISPATCH	
It's a warm Sunday afternoon, and I'm sitting around the station feeling sorry for myself. It's too nice to be working today! My partner, Luz, is taking a nap and I'm watching the Yankees game when the tones go off. We are dispatched for an allergic reaction. Why are we getting this call? The closer unit must already be out.	En route to the call we are told that our patient is a 42-year-old male who was stung by several bees while mowing the lawn. The caller's wife states that the patient is in the back yard, too weak to go into the house.
SCENE SIZE-UP	
We arrive in 9 minutes and pull up to the house. I am concerned about the fact that if the patient is still in the back, then the bees are, too. The patient's son meets us at the ambulance and tells us that his father is "passed out." We ask about the bees, and he says that his father was able to move away from the hive before he got sick.	We don't normally think of insects when we think of scene safety, but I was concerned about what we would find when we got there. The last thing I would want to do is have to approach a patient who is still surrounded by angry bees.
INITIAL ASSESSMENT	
We get to the yard to find our patient, Mr. Mann, sitting in a deck chair, with his upper body lying across the picnic table. His skin is red, and I can see hives on his exposed skin. His breathing is labored. He sees us coming and weakly lifts up his head.	Without even talking to the patient I can see he is in anaphylaxis, a severe allergic reaction. Although his condition appears to be bad, we want to make sure he isn't in shock and then prevent that from happening.
HISTORY	
His wife tells us that he was mowing the lawn, and suddenly she heard him screaming. She ran outside and found him running from the bees after being stung several times. When asked, she says that he has been stung by a bee twice before. The first time he was fine; the second time the area where he was stung became red and swollen, but he never got this bad.	Before a patient has an allergic reaction, he needs to have an initial exposure to the antigen, known as sensitization. A subsequent exposure induces a much stronger secondary response, such as the localized reaction that Mr. Mann had with the second bee sting. Hypersensitivity is an unexpected and exaggerated reaction to a particular antigen, such as the multiple bee stings that Mr. Mann experienced.

SCENARIOS

1180 ESSENTIALS OF PARAMEDIC CARE

©2007 Pearson Education, Inc.
Essentials of Paramedic Care, 2nd ed.

HANDOUT 47-18 Continued

ACTIONS	REASONING
PHYSICAL EXAM	
We get a quick set of vital signs and find the following: BP 90/60, pulse 110, respirations 28. Mr. Mann has wheezing throughout all lung fields. He is complaining of dizziness and abdominal pain.	Mr. Mann is experiencing many of the symptoms of anaphylactic shock. We need to get him treated immediately.
INTERVENTIONS	
Luz gets out a nonrebreather mask and starts Mr. Mann on high-flow oxygen.	Oxygen is the first drug to administer in anaphylactic shock.
Mr. Mann needs an IV, but first I am going to give him epinephrine 1:10,000 subcutaneously.	Epinephrine is a sympathetic agonist, the primary drug used in anaphylaxis. It causes increased cardiac contractility and peripheral vasodilation and can also reverse some of the bronchospasm that Mr. Mann is having.
Luz starts Mr. Mann on an albuterol treatment as I start his IV.	As a beta-agonist, albuterol will help reverse some of the bronchospasm and laryngeal edema associated with anaphylaxis. Mr. Mann needs an IV so that we can administer additional medication, and for a fluid bolus.
Mr. Mann's IV is started, and I give him 50 mg of IV diphenhydramine. I also start a 500-cc fluid bolus.	Antihistamines are the second-line drugs used in anaphylaxis. Antihistamines block the effects of histamine, which is the principal chemical mediator in allergic reactions. I give him a fluid bolus in order to correct the hypotension.
ONGOING ASSESSMENT	
Treating Mr. Mann takes several minutes. Once we have completed the initial round of drugs and fluid, I recheck his vital signs. His BP is 100/62, pulse is 122, and respirations are 24.	We are starting to see some improvement. His blood pressure is coming up, and he is breathing a little slower. I am not surprised that his pulse rate is higher, because the epinephrine and the albuterol can both raise a patient's heart rate.
I reassess Mr. Mann's breath sounds, and the wheezing is getting coarser.	His airway is opening, so he is getting more airflow through his bronchioles.
Mr. Mann is still in the deck chair, but we have brought the stretcher over to him and assist him onto it. He says his dizziness is getting better and he wants to sit up a little bit.	Since his blood pressure is coming up, I assist Mr. Mann in sitting up to a semi-Fowler position. This helps with his breathing, but he is still wheezing.
En route to the ED, I take another set of vital signs, which remain stable.	I could have given another dose of epinephrine 3–5 minutes after the first dose, but Mr. Mann didn't need it.

HANDOUT 47-18 Continued

ACTIONS	REASONING
COMMUNICATIONS AND WRITTEN REPORT	
We load Mr. Mann into the ambulance and head to the ED. We call to let them know we are coming. They will give additional medication, such as corticosteroids.	Corticosteroids do not help in the initial stages of anaphylaxis, but they help suppress the inflammatory response later on.
We arrive at the hospital and give a report. The first albuterol treatment is done, but Mr. Mann is still wheezing, so the ED staff starts another one as soon as he is transferred to the stretcher.	I sit down to write up the run report. This call went very quickly, so this shouldn't take me very long.
FOLLOW-UP	
I stick my head in Mr. Mann's room to see how he is doing before I go. I ask him if anyone has told him that he could give himself epinephrine if he should get stung again, and he laughs and tells me that three different people have already told him this. He won't be leaving without a prescription.	Patients who experience severe allergic reactions can give self-administered epinephrine. Hopefully, this will help Mr. Mann avoid any more incidents like this in the future.

Handout 47-19

Student's Name _____

BEHAVIORAL DEPRESSION SCENARIO

ACTIONS	REASONING
DISPATCH	
It's 3:34 in the morning, and Brandon and I get dispatched for a patient requesting transport due to suicidal thoughts. We have just gotten back from another call, and I am tired. "Hopefully, this won't take very long," I think as I am getting in the ambulance.	This could turn out to be a simple transport to the hospital, or it could be much more difficult than that, especially if the patient has already made an attempt to end his life. If that's the case, he may not want to go willingly with us. We'll have to see when we get there.
SCENE SIZE-UP	
We arrive on scene and find we are the first ones here. It is departmental policy that we do not enter the scene of the call until we have a police escort, so we wait a few minutes until they show up.	Although I know that most patients experiencing behavioral emergencies are not violent, if this patient is in crisis his behavior is unpredictable. We approach these patients cautiously, in order to protect ourselves from potential injury.
INITIAL ASSESSMENT	
The police officer goes in the house and comes to get us after a couple of minutes. We go into the house and find the patient sitting at the kitchen table with three pill bottles in front of him. He is fully dressed and speaks quietly. His affect is flat, and he doesn't look at me.	As soon as I see the bottles I am concerned that he may have taken an overdose of the medication. We need to find out what is going on as quickly as possible, but I don't want to proceed too fast and cause the patient any extra anxiety.
HISTORY	
I approach the patient, who is named Sam, quietly and sit down next to him. Brandon keeps his distance, along with the police officer. I ask him if he has taken any of the pills in the bottles, and he says he hasn't. I look at them and note two antidepressants and an antianxiety medication. I see they were just filled the day before. I ask him if Brandon can count them, and he tells us to go ahead.	Brandon takes the bottles to count the pills and make sure that they are all accounted for. Unfortunately, we cannot believe a patient when he says he hasn't taken an overdose. By counting out the pills, Brandon can confirm that he hasn't. All of the pills, except for his daily dose, are accounted for.

©2007 Pearson Education, Inc.
Essentials of Paramedic Care, 2nd ed.

CHAPTER 47 *Assessment-Based Management* 1183

SCENARIOS

HANDOUT 47-19 Continued

ACTIONS	REASONING
HISTORY	
I ask Sam what is going on. He tells me that over the last couple of weeks he has been feeling worthless and depressed and that he went to see his doctor for it yesterday. He can barely get himself up in the morning to go to work, and he didn't make it in at all the last 2 days. He hasn't been able to sleep and hasn't been eating much. Tonight he sat up thinking that everything would be much better if he just took all of his pills and "got it over with." That scared him, so he called us.	Sam is experiencing five of the symptoms that must be present in a 2-week period in order to be diagnosed with major depressive disorder.
He denies any recent events that could have caused him to feel this way, such as a recent death of a family member. He also denies drug and alcohol abuse. When asked, he states he doesn't have any medical history.	Before a patient can be diagnosed with depression, other causes of these symptoms need to be ruled out. Bereavement can cause symptoms similar to depression, as can drug and alcohol abuse. A medical condition, such as hypothyroidism, can also cause such symptoms.
PHYSICAL EXAM	
I take a quick set of vital signs and find them to be within normal limits. We then walk him out to the ambulance and seat him in the captain's chair in the back with his seat belt on.	We need to remove the patient from the crisis area, so we decide to head to the hospital. I can get the rest of the information I need en route to the ED.
INTERVENTIONS	
I talk to Sam in a quiet, nonthreatening tone. I start to ask some open-ended questions about what has been going on over the last 2 weeks. I do not interrupt him while he is speaking.	There isn't much I can do for Sam except to make him feel nonthreatened and cared for. By listening and paying attention, I show that I am not ignoring his problems.
ONGOING ASSESSMENT	
Sam starts to open up and tells me that he has a history of depression, but this is the first time he has seen a doctor for it or has taken medication. He also tells me that he has never attempted suicide, although he has thought about it before. It scared him, because he has never come this close to actually trying to kill himself.	Since he has opened up and started talking to me, I don't want to interrupt him by taking another set of vital signs, although I normally would get a set en route to the hospital.

SCENARIOS

1184 ESSENTIALS OF PARAMEDIC CARE

©2007 Pearson Education, Inc.
Essentials of Paramedic Care, 2nd ed.

HANDOUT 47-19 Continued

ACTIONS	REASONING
COMMUNICATIONS AND WRITTEN REPORT	
Brandon is driving to the hospital and notifies them that we are en route with a quiet and cooperative patient who is feeling suicidal. He is instructed to take the patient to one of the three behavioral emergency rooms when we get there.	Many hospitals have BE rooms for psych patients. If a patient becomes violent or cannot be controlled, there isn't anything in the room that can cause harm to the patient or a staff member.
Upon arrival we walk Sam to BE 3 and give a report to the nurse and the social worker.	The social worker will talk with Sam and will determine the safest plan for him, whether that is admission to a psychiatric hospital or sending him home.
FOLLOW-UP	
I follow up the next day and find out that Sam was admitted to the psychiatric hospital for depression and suicidal thoughts.	I hope they get his medication under control and he starts to feel better. He is a nice man, and I hope everything works out well for him.

Handout 47-20

Student's Name _____

VAGINAL BLEEDING SCENARIO

ACTIONS	REASONING
DISPATCH	
"Medic 12, respond to 5234 North Main Street, 5th floor, for an obstetrical emergency." It's 2:00 in the afternoon, and we just finished watching our daily soap when Trevor and I got dispatched to one of the office buildings downtown.	We sign on that we are en route to the scene, and dispatch tells us that we are responding to a 27-year-old who is having vaginal bleeding in her first trimester. This is good to know. We know we don't have an impending delivery, which, although it can be exciting, can also be very dangerous for the mother and the baby.
SCENE SIZE-UP	
We pull up to the door and security is waiting for us, keeping the elevator clear. We get to the 5th floor and we are directed to the ladies' restroom, where several women are standing in the doorway. They clear out of the way, and we find the patient sitting on the bathroom counter, crying softly.	The scene is safe and well controlled. We have no difficulty getting upstairs or finding the patient.
INITIAL ASSESSMENT	
I approach the patient and introduce Trevor and myself. I do a quick pulse check and find it to be within normal limits. Her skin is warm and dry, and her color is good.	If she were having heavy vaginal bleeding, she would be in danger of going into hypovolemic shock. So far, she does not display any symptoms of shock.
HISTORY	
As Trevor takes her blood pressure, I try to find out more about what is going on. She tells me she is 6 weeks pregnant after trying to get pregnant for a year. She woke up with mild cramping this morning, which has gotten worse throughout the day. She came into the bathroom this afternoon and noted "a lot" of bleeding. The cramping has been continuing to get worse, and now she is starting to have a backache.	What our patient is describing are all signs and symptoms of spontaneous abortion, or miscarriage. If she has passed the fetus and placenta, this would have been considered a complete abortion.

HANDOUT 47-20 Continued

ACTIONS	REASONING
HISTORY (*Continued*)	
I ask her if she has noticed any clots or tissue, and she said she was too upset to notice.	If she hasn't passed tissue or only partially passed tissue, then this may be considered a threatened abortion, which in some cases, the fetus can actually be saved. Or it could be an incomplete abortion, which may need surgery. Vaginal bleeding and cramping can also be signs of an ectopic pregnancy, in which the fertilized egg is implanted in the fallopian tube instead of the uterus. This is an obstetrical emergency and may require emergency surgery if the patient suffers a ruptured tube and is bleeding excessively.
PHYSICAL EXAM	
We assist the patient to the stretcher and place her in a position of comfort. I ask her if her pain feels like it is more on one side than the other, which she denies. I palpate her abdomen to see if I can localize the pain, but again she denies any sharp pain in the right or left lower quadrant.	Ectopic pregnancies most often present as abdominal pain, which then localizes in the affected lower quadrant of the abdomen. Syncope, vaginal bleeding, and shock can accompany the pain. Although she would need an ultrasound to rule it out, I am willing to bet that this is not an ectopic pregnancy.
We do a set of orthostatic vital signs to note changes in order to determine impending shock.	Her orthostatic vital signs remain within normal limits.
INTERVENTIONS	
We head downstairs and place the patient in the ambulance. Trevor jumps up front to drive, and I get in the back. En route to the hospital I start an IV of normal saline at a KVO rate after drawing a set of blood samples.	The ED staff is going to run a set of basic blood work, and, because I started an IV, I drew the blood in order to avoid a second needle stick for the patient. I prefer to have the IV line in case the patient starts to bleed heavily and goes into shock.
ONGOING ASSESSMENT	
I repeat a set of vital signs every few minutes to monitor for blood loss. The patient does not report any changes in pain or bleeding.	Everything remains within normal limits en route to the ED. Transport remains uneventful.
The patient continues to cry softly and tells me how excited she was to be having a baby.	A miscarriage is a very sad occurrence for a patient to go through and requires emotional support during transport.

©2007 Pearson Education, Inc.
Essentials of Paramedic Care, 2nd ed.

HANDOUT 47-20 Continued

ACTIONS	REASONING
COMMUNICATIONS AND WRITTEN REPORT	
We alert the ED that we are coming and are told that Room 8, the pelvic room, is empty. We give our report to the nurse taking the patient and head to the EMS room to write the report.	This was a quick run and shouldn't require much time to write the report.
FOLLOW-UP	
The ED doctor hasn't even seen the patient yet by the time we leave. She thanks us for our help, and we say goodbye.	I think about our patient later in the day and hope everything turned out all right for her.

Handout 47-21

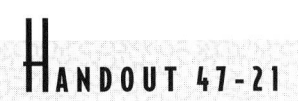

Student's Name _____

PEDIATRIC SCENARIO

ACTIONS	REASONING
DISPATCH	
At 1:13 A.M., my partner, Jim, and I are sleeping when our radio tones go off. "Medic 206, respond to Tree Top Trailer Park, Lot #3, for a pediatric respiratory arrest." I don't think either of us has ever moved any quicker to the ambulance as we sign on en route. I know this trailer park, which is right up the street.	A pediatric patient always gets my blood flowing, but a pediatric respiratory arrest is even worse. We ask the dispatcher if they have any more information for us, but we are told that the caller doesn't have a telephone and had gone to the end of the road to use a pay phone to call us.
SCENE SIZE-UP	
We pull into the trailer park and find #3 in the front. There is a gentleman waiting for us, waving his arms up and down so we can see him. As we get out, we hear him telling us to hurry up, his baby isn't breathing. I grab our pediatric emergency bag as Jim grabs the oxygen and monitor. We leave the stretcher in the back for now.	The father is obviously frantic but does not appear to be any danger to us. The scene is not well lit, and we have to carefully watch where we are going so we don't fall.
INITIAL ASSESSMENT	
We get inside to find an approximately 10-month-old baby in his mother's arms, pinking and breathing on his own. Mom is crying and rocking the baby.	Immediately I can see that the baby is no longer in respiratory arrest. He has spontaneous respirations and good color.
HISTORY	
I try to calm the parents down so we can get some information. I ask what happened, and Dad tells me that they heard a funny noise coming from the crib and went in and found the baby blue, with his arms and legs jerking. He was making a "funny, gagging sound" and wasn't breathing.	It sounds like the parents are describing a seizure. When a patient has a seizure, he is unable to breathe, and babies tend to become cyanotic quickly. The "funny, gagging sound" could have been the baby's tongue causing an airway obstruction during the seizure.

HANDOUT 47-21 Continued

ACTIONS	REASONING
PHYSICAL EXAM	
I ask Mom to unwrap the baby so I can do a patient assessment. She tells me that she would prefer to keep him wrapped up because he feels very warm and is afraid he has a fever.	This is making more sense now. Febrile seizures are those seizures that occur as a result of a sudden increase in body temperature. They occur most commonly between the ages of 6 months and 6 years.
I explain to the mother that it is really important that I take a good look at the baby. She unwraps him, and this wakes him up. He starts to cry a little and sounds irritable. I do a quick head-to-toe assessment. He has rhonchi throughout all lung fields.	I ask Mom if the baby has been sick, and she says he has had a cold for about 2 days. He started coughing before bedtime tonight. The irritable cry could be because he is postictal, or it could mean that he has a CNS infection.
INTERVENTIONS	
I explain to the parents that even though the baby is breathing now and appears to have had a febrile seizure, it is important to take him to the hospital to make sure there isn't anything else going on.	The parents agree that the baby needs to be seen. Mom asks to come with us, and Dad says he'll follow us in the car.
Before we leave for the ED, I ask Jim to give me a hand in the back starting an IV.	I need to have IV access in case the patient has another seizure and needs medication. I would also like to check a glucose level to make sure we aren't missing hypoglycemia.
I call medical direction and ask for an order to give Valium in case the patient has another seizure. I am told I can give 0.2 mg/kg every 2 to 5 minutes if the patient should seize again.	I don't want to have to take the time to call should the baby start to have another seizure.
I start some blow-by oxygen, as the patient still appears postictal.	
I take a set of vital signs on the patient and get a pulse rate of 180 and a respiratory rate of 66. We do not have a thermometer on the ambulance, but he is hot to the touch and his vital signs, plus his medical history, indicate that he has a fever.	I convince Mom to unwrap the baby, because keeping him wrapped up in the blanket does not allow him to cool off.
ONGOING ASSESSMENT	
I monitor the patient's airway and color, which remain good.	The airway obstruction that his parents described may have been from his tongue during the seizure, but he also could have had a lot of mucus in his airway, as his lungs sound infected. I want to make sure he doesn't choke again.

HANDOUT 47-21 Continued

ACTIONS	REASONING
COMMUNICATIONS AND WRITTEN REPORT	
I had already notified the ED that we were coming when I called medical direction. They are waiting for us when we get there. We give a report and Mom walks toward an exam room with the nurse.	We sit down at the desk, and I start to write up the run sheet.
FOLLOW-UP	
It turns out the baby had a fever of 104.2°. He was doing much better after a little ibuprofen and was actually playful by the time we left the ED.	His fever got very high, quickly, which is what caused the seizure. He was like a new child after the fever reducer.

Chapter 47 Answer Key

Handout 47-2: Chapter 47 Quiz

1. D	6. A	11. D
2. B	7. C	12. B
3. A	8. D	13. C
4. C	9. B	14. B
5. B	10. C	15. C

Handout 47-3: Chapter 47 Scenario

1. The questions should be broad and without preconception. Possible questions include the following:
   - Parents/guardians there or not?
   - Trauma to head, chest, abdomen, limbs?
   - Neurologic deficits, need for spinal immobilization?
   - Fractured ribs or extremity(ies)?
   - Internal bleeding?
   - Abrasions or other surface injuries?
   - Any significant underlying medical problems?

2. These impressions may overlap with those already given, but many will be more specific to the case of possibly severe trauma in a child:
   - Is airway open, and is patient breathing?
   - Has patient had loss of consciousness or altered mental status?
   - Possible head or spinal injury?
   - Possible chest or abdominal trauma?
   - Fracture or serious trauma to limbs?
   - Signs of internal or external hemorrhage?

3. There are no obvious signs of major trauma and the child is conscious and responding to his presence. Thoughts might include the following:
   - Did anyone talk to her after the accident, and has her apparent mental status changed since then?
   - Can she respond to basic questions I might ask, such as her name and whether anything hurts her?

4. Thoughts on the nature of injury and how to proceed:
   - Head injury is definitely possible. Should we immobilize her neck and possibly put her on a spine board before further examination?
   - Should we do a quick check for other signs of head injury, such as state of pupils or swelling or bruising of the head, or should we proceed with rapid assessment of the rest of her body?
   - When proper protective steps have been taken, should we position her or take other measures to protect the airway, especially if there is threat of vomiting?

5. Because of the cold environmental conditions and the child's anxiety, it is definitely time to move her to the ambulance and call medical direction to see whether she should be transported immediately or it is acceptable to wait 5 minutes to see if the parents arrive.

6. Components of ongoing assessment should include the following:
   - Ongoing assessment of airway, breathing, circulation. Look at least once for signs of cold injury to feet and hands.
   - Otherwise focus on vital signs and neurological reassessment for mental status, other evidence of head injury.
   - If patient is able to talk without additional distress, ask for historical information on medications, allergies, chronic problems, or recent illness or accident.

Handout 47-4: Chapter 47 Review

1. differential diagnosis, narrowing process, field diagnosis
2. Assessment
3. reaching, completing (or synonyms)
4. obtains history, performs physical exam, presents patient, handles documentation, acts as EMS commander
5. provides scene cover, gathers scene information, talks to relatives/bystanders, obtains vital signs, performs interventions, acts as triage group leader
6. body language
7. body substance isolation, scene safety, location of all patients, determination of mechanism of injury or nature of illness
8. forming a general impression, mental status assessment (AVPU), airway assessment, breathing assessment, circulation assessment, determining patient's priority for further on-scene care or immediate transport
9. trauma patient with a significant mechanism of injury or altered mental status, trauma patient with an isolated injury, medical patient who is responsive, medical patient who is unresponsive
10. mental status, airway/breathing/circulation, transport priorities, vital signs, focused assessment of any problem areas or conditions, effectiveness of interventions, management plans
11. life-threatening problems
12. worst-case scenario
13. subjective findings, objective findings, assessment, plan
14. communicate effectively
15. one minute

Chapter 48
Operations

INTRODUCTION

Operations forms a crucial part of a paramedic's career. Although students are already familiar with many aspects of EMS operations, they must repeatedly reinforce operational procedures to ensure the safety of EMS providers, patients, and bystanders. The time to review these procedures is not during high-stress emergency situations; instead the procedures must come as second nature. Chapter 48, "Operations," has been divided into five parts: Part 1: Ambulance Operations; Part 2: Medical Incident Management; Part 3: Rescue Awareness and Operations; Part 4: Hazardous Materials Incidents; and Part 5: Crime Scene Awareness.

PART 1: AMBULANCE OPERATIONS

Most students readily identify medical knowledge and procedural skills as types of content to be mastered before they become proficient as paramedics. Far fewer think of knowledge about standards for ambulances and medical equipment or skills necessary to methodically check and restock an ambulance's equipment and supplies. Yet the ability of a paramedic to function safely and effectively in the field depends on proper ambulance operation. This chapter covers five related topics: ambulance standards, maintenance of ambulance equipment and supplies, ambulance stationing, safe ambulance operations, and utilization of air medical transport.

TOTAL TEACHING TIME
There is no specific time requirement for this topic in the National Standard Curriculum for paramedic. Instructors should take into consideration such factors as the pace at which students learn, the size of the class, and breaks. The actual time devoted to teaching objectives is the responsibility of the instructor.

PART 2: MEDICAL INCIDENT MANAGEMENT

In almost all of the material your students have read so far, the emphasis has been on the relationship between one or two EMS providers and a single patient. This chapter deals with incidents that involve multiple patients. Situations that your students may see frequently range from multiple-vehicle accidents to home fires to scenes of domestic or other violence. Less frequent incidents such as chain-reaction vehicular accidents, bus or train accidents, and natural disasters can be much more complicated and involve many more patients. Efficient responses in cases involving multiple patients depend on the skills and discipline your students will learn from this chapter and other training materials and exercises. Because EMS providers almost always interact in the larger situations with police and firefighters, and possibly even disaster officials, this chapter introduces them to the logistics of working with other types of emergency personnel.

TOTAL TEACHING TIME:
8.17 HOURS
The total teaching time is only a guideline based on the didactic and practical lab averages in the National Standard Curriculum. Instructors should take into consideration such factors as the pace at which students learn, the size of the class, and breaks. The actual time devoted to teaching objectives is the responsibility of the instructor.

©2007 Pearson Education, Inc.
Essentials of Paramedic Care, 2nd ed.

TOTAL TEACHING TIME:
35.99 HOURS
The total teaching time is only a guideline based on the didactic and practical lab averages in the National Standard Curriculum. Instructors should take into consideration such factors as the pace at which students learn, the size of the class, and breaks. The actual time devoted to teaching objectives is the responsibility of the instructor.

TOTAL TEACHING TIME:
12.50 HOURS
The total teaching time is only a guideline based on the didactic and practical lab averages in the National Standard Curriculum. Instructors should take into consideration such factors as the pace at which students learn, the size of the class, and breaks. The actual time devoted to teaching objectives is the responsibility of the instructor.

TOTAL TEACHING TIME:
5.39 HOURS
The total teaching time is only a guideline based on the didactic and practical lab averages in the National Standard Curriculum. Instructors should take into consideration such factors as the pace at which students learn, the size of the class, and breaks. The actual time devoted to teaching objectives is the responsibility of the instructor.

PART 3: RESCUE AWARENESS AND OPERATIONS

In almost all of the material your students have encountered so far in their course work, physical access to the patient has not been an issue. The concept of rescue—that some victims need to be extricated before they can become patients who can be treated—was raised in Chapter 47 and is discussed in detail in this chapter. The goal of Chapter 48 is to give your students an "awareness level" of knowledge about rescues in different settings (namely, surface water, hazardous atmospheres, highway operations, and hazardous terrains) so that they can collaborate comfortably and efficiently with other personnel during a wide range of rescue operations.

PART 4: HAZARDOUS MATERIALS INCIDENTS

Students were introduced to the concept of EMS calls related to toxicological emergencies in Chapter 34 and environmental emergencies in Chapter 36. This chapter expands on that base to discuss incidents in which hazardous materials are spilled or released as a result of an accident, equipment failure, human error, or intentional actions designed to skirt regulations regarding such compounds. Students will learn about the role of the paramedic in such hazardous materials (hazmat) incidents as well as specifics about medical care for patients contaminated with a hazardous material.

PART 5: CRIME SCENE AWARENESS

Students were introduced to the concepts of scene danger and criminal activity relates to abuse and neglect in Chapter 44 and incident management system in Chapter 48. This chapter discusses the possibility of danger in every setting, on every call, and it teaches safety strategies that your students can use throughout their working lives. In addition, the chapter explains basic guidelines for collaboration with law enforcement when EMS providers need to provide medical care at a crime scene. After reading this chapter, your students will understand the principles of evidence preservation and documentation.

CHAPTER OBJECTIVES

Part 1: Ambulance Operations (pp. 1798–1809)

After reading Part 1 of this chapter, you should be able to:

1. Identify current local and state standards that influence ambulance design, equipment requirements, and staffing of ambulances. (pp. 1798–1800)
2. Discuss the importance of completing an ambulance equipment/supply checklist. (pp. 1800–1801)
3. Discuss factors used to determine ambulance stationing and staffing within a community. (pp. 1801–1802)
4. Describe the advantages and disadvantages of air medical transport and identify conditions/situations in which air medical transport should be considered. (pp. 1806–1809)

Part 2: Medical Incident Management (pp. 1809–1830)

After reading Part 2 of this chapter, you should be able to:

1. Explain the need for the incident management system (IMS)/Incident command system (ICS) in managing emergency medical services incidents. (pp. 1809–1810)
2. Describe the functional components (command, finance, logistics, operations, and planning) of the incident management system. (pp. 1810–1811, 1816–1819, 1823)
3. Differentiate between singular and unified command and identify when each is most applicable. (pp. 1813–1814)
4. Describe the role of command, the need for command transfer, and procedures for transferring it. (pp. 1811–1816)
5. List and describe the functions of the following groups and leaders in the ICS as they pertain to EMS incidents:
   - Safety (pp. 1812, 1816–1817)
   - Logistics (p. 1818)
   - Rehabilitation (rehab) (p. 1826)
   - Staging (p. 1825)
   - Treatment (pp. 1824–1825)
   - Triage (pp. 1820–1824)
   - Transportation (pp. 1825–1826)
   - Extrication/rescue (p. 1826)
   - Disposition of deceased (morgue) (p. 1824)
   - Communications (pp. 1814, 1826–1827)
6. Describe the methods and rationale for identifying specific functions and leaders for the functions in the ICS. (pp. 1810–1811, 1814)
7. Describe essential elements of the scene size-up when arriving at a potential MCI. (pp. 1812–1813)
8. Define the terms *multiple-casualty incident (MCI)*, *disaster management*, *open or uncontained incident*, and *closed or contained incident*. (pp. 1809, 1812, 1813, 1827)
9. Describe the role of the paramedics and EMS system in planning for MCIs and disasters. (pp. 1819, 1827–1828, 1829)
10. Explain the local/regional threshold for establishing command and implementation of the incident management system including MCI declaration. (pp. 1809, 1811–1812)
11. Describe the role of both command posts and emergency operations centers in MCI and disaster management. (pp. 1811–1816)
12. Describe the role of the on-scene physician at multiple-casualty incidents. (p. 1825)
13. Define triage and describe the principles of triage. (pp. 1820–1824)
14. Describe the START (simple triage and rapid transport) method of initial triage. (pp. 1821–1822)
15. Given color-coded tags and numerical priorities, assign the following terms to each (pp. 1821–1822):
    - Immediate
    - Delayed
    - Minimal
    - Expectant
16. Define primary, secondary, and ongoing triage and their implementation techniques. (p. 1821)

17. Describe techniques used to allocate patients to hospitals and track them. (pp. 1825–1826)
18. Describe the techniques used in tracking patients during multiple-casualty incidents and the need for such techniques. (pp. 1822–1826)
19. Describe modifications of telecommunications procedures during multiple-casualty incidents. (pp. 1814, 1826–1827)
20. List and describe the essential equipment to provide logistical support to MCI operations to include (pp. 1818, 1824–1825):

    - Airway, respiratory, and hemorrhage control
    - Burn management
    - Patient packaging/immobilization

21. Describe the role of mental health support in MCIs. (pp. 1817–1818, 1826, 1829–1830)
22. Describe the role of the following exercises in preparation for MCIs (p. 1829):

    - Tabletop exercises
    - Small and large MCI drills

23. Given several incident scenarios with preprogrammed patients, provide the appropriate triage, treatment, and transport options for MCI operations based on local resources and protocols. (pp. 1809–1830)

Part 3: Rescue Awareness and Operations (pp. 1830–1856)

After reading Part 3 of this chapter, you should be able to:

1. Define the term *rescue*, and explain the medical and mechanical aspects of rescue operations. (pp. 1830–1831)
2. Describe the phases of a rescue operation, and the role of the paramedic at each phase. (pp. 1835–1838)
3. List and describe the personal protective equipment needed to safely operate in the rescue environment to include: head, eye, and hand protection; personal flotation devices; thermal protection/layering systems; high visibility clothing. (pp. 1831–1833)
4. Explain the risks and complications associated with rescues involving moving water, low head dams, flat water, trenches, motor vehicles, and confined spaces. (pp. 1838–1845, 1846–1851)
5. Explain the effects of immersion hypothermia on the ability to survive sudden immersion and self-rescue. (pp. 1839–1840)
6. Explain the benefits and disadvantages of water-entry or "go techniques" versus the reach-throw-row-go approach to water rescue. (pp. 1840–1841)
7. Explain the self-rescue position if unexpectedly immersed in moving water. (pp. 1840, 1843)
8. Describe the use of apparatus placement, headlights and emergency vehicle lighting, cone and flare placement, and reflective and high visibility clothing to reduce scene risk at highway incidents. (pp. 1846–1847)
9. List and describe the design element hazards and associated protective actions associated with autos and trucks, including energy-absorbing bumpers, air bag/supplemental restraint systems, catalytic converters, and conventional and nonconventional fuel systems. (pp. 1848–1849)
10. Given a diagram of a passenger auto, identify the A, B, C, and D posts, firewall, and unibody versus frame construction. (pp. 1849–1850)
11. Explain the difference between tempered and safety glass, identify its locations on a vehicle, and describe how to break it. (p. 1850)

12. Explain typical door anatomy and methods to access through stuck doors. (p. 1850)
13. Describe methods for emergency stabilization using rope, cribbing, jacks, spare tires, and come-a-longs for vehicles found in various positions. (pp. 1849, 1850–1851)
14. Describe electrical and other hazards commonly found at highway incidents (above and below the ground). (pp. 1848–1849)
15. Define low-angle rescue, high-angle rescue, belay, rappel, scrambling, and hasty rope slide. (pp. 1851–1852)
16. Describe the procedure for Stokes litter packaging for low-angle evacuations. (pp. 1852–1854)
17. Explain anchoring, litter/rope attachment, and lowering and raising procedures as they apply to low-angle litter evacuation. (pp. 1852, 1854)
18. Explain techniques used in nontechnical litter carries over rough terrain. (p. 1854)
19. Explain nontechnical high-angle rescue procedures using aerial apparatus. (p. 1854)
20. Explain assessment and care modifications (including pain medication, temperature control, and hydration) necessary for attending to entrapped patients. (pp. 1855–1856)
21. List the equipment necessary for an "off road" medical pack. (pp. 1833, 1856)
22. Explain the different types of "Stokes" or basket stretchers and the advantages and disadvantages associated with each. (pp. 1852–1854)
23. Given a list of rescue scenarios, provide the victim survivability profile and identify which are rescue versus body recovery situations. (pp. 1830–1856)
24. Given a series of pictures, identify those considered "confined spaces" and potentially oxygen deficient. (pp. 1845–1846)

Part 4: Hazardous Materials Incidents (pp. 1857–1872)

After reading Part 4 of this chapter, you should be able to:

1. Explain the role of the paramedic/EMS responder at the hazardous material incident. (pp. 1857–1858)
2. Identify resources for substance identification, decontamination, and treatment information. (pp. 1862–1863)
3. Identify primary and secondary decontamination risk. (p. 1865)
4. Describe topical, respiratory, gastrointestinal, and parenteral routes of exposure. (pp. 1865–1866)
5. Explain acute and delayed toxicity, local versus systemic effects, dose response, and synergistic effects. (p. 1866)
6. Explain how the substance and route of contamination alters triage and decontamination methods. (pp. 1868–1869)
7. Explain the employment and limitations of field decontamination procedures. (pp. 1870–1871)
8. Explain the use and limitations of personal protective equipment (PPE) in hazardous material situations. (p. 1871)
9. List and explain the common signs, symptoms, and treatment of exposures to corrosives, pulmonary irritants, pesticides, chemical asphyxiants, and hydrocarbon solvents. (pp. 1866–1868)
10. Describe the characteristics of hazardous materials and explain their importance to the risk assessment process. (pp. 1857, 1858–1863, 1869–1870)

11. Describe the hazards and protection strategies for alpha, beta, and gamma radiation. (pp. 1864–1865)
12. Define the toxicologic terms and their use in the risk assessment process. (p. 1865)
13. Given a specific hazardous material, research the appropriate information about its physical and chemical properties and hazards, suggest the appropriate medical response, and determine the risk of secondary contamination. (pp. 1862–1863)
14. Identify the factors that determine where and when to treat a hazardous material incident patient. (pp. 1863, 1869–1870)
15. Determine the appropriate level of PPE for various hazardous material incidents. (p. 1871)
16. Explain decontamination procedures including critical patient rapid two-step decontamination and noncritical patient eight-step decontamination. (p. 1870)
17. Identify the four most common solutions used for decontamination. (p. 1870)
18. Identify the body areas that are difficult to decontaminate. (p. 1870)
19. Explain the medical monitoring procedures for hazardous material team members. (p. 1872)
20. Explain the factors that influence the heat stress of hazardous material team personnel. (p. 1872)
21. Explain the documentation necessary for hazmat medical monitoring and rehabilitation operations. (p. 1872)
22. Given a stimulated hazardous substance, use reference material to determine the appropriate actions. (pp. 1862–1863)
23. Integrate the principles and practices of hazardous materials response in an effective manner to prevent and limit contamination, morbidity, and mortality. (pp. 1857–1872)
24. Size up a hazardous material (hazmat) incident and determine: potential hazards to the rescuers, public, and environment and potential risk of primary contamination to patients and secondary contamination to rescuers. (pp. 1858–1863, 1865–1871)
25. Given a contaminated patient, determine the necessary level of decontamination, level of rescuer PPE, decontamination methods, treatment, and transportation and patient isolation techniques. (pp. 1866–1871)
26. Determine the hazards present to the patient and paramedic given an incident involving a hazardous material. (pp. 1857–1872)

Part 5: Crime Scene Awareness (pp. 1872–1885)

After reading Part 5 of this chapter, you should be able to:

1. Explain how EMS providers are often mistaken for the police. (pp. 1873–1878)
2. Explain specific techniques for risk reduction when approaching highway encounters, violent street incidents, residences, and "dark houses." (pp. 1873–1879)
3. Describe the warning signs of potentially violent situations. (pp. 1873–1877)
4. Explain emergency evasive techniques for potentially violent situations, including threats of physical violence, firearms encounters, and edged weapons encounters. (pp. 1873–1883)

5. Explain EMS considerations for the following types of violent or potentially violent situations: gangs and gang violence, hostages/sniper situations, clandestine drug labs, domestic violence, and emotionally disturbed people. (pp. 1873–1879)
6. Explain the following techniques: field "contact and cover" procedures during assessment and care, evasive tactics, and concealment techniques. (pp. 1879–1883)
7. Describe police evidence considerations and techniques to assist in evidence preservation. (pp. 1883–1885)
8. Given several crime scene scenarios, identify potential hazards and determine if the scene is safe to enter, then provide care, preserving the crime scene as appropriate. (pp. 1872–1885)

FRAMING THE LESSON

Begin by reviewing the important points from Chapter 47, "Assessment-Based Management." Discuss any points that the class does not completely understand. Then move on to Chapter 48.

PART 1: AMBULANCE OPERATIONS

You can use the following exercise to get students to recognize for themselves the critical importance of sound ambulance operation: Lay out a scenario for your students, perhaps a call for a middle-aged man with a suspected acute MI or a two-vehicle car accident. Have them brainstorm about the thought and action steps they take after they receive the call (this also reinforces the concepts they learned in the preceding lesson, Chapter 47). When someone makes initial mention of a piece of equipment (such as a cardiac monitor/defibrillator) or supplies (such as those necessary for body substance isolation procedures, or BSI) say, "Oh, that isn't working correctly" or "the only gloves are much too large for your hands" and view their reactions.

PART 2: MEDICAL INCIDENT MANAGEMENT

Select a variety of photos of multiple-casualty incidents and disasters. If possible, have at least some of them represent local events. Have the students look at the photos, consider the cases (such as chain-reaction vehicular accidents, fire in a hospital or school, an earthquake, tornado, or even mass shooting or bombing) and think about the following issues that are critical to medical incident command:

- The complexities of responding as EMS providers to situations where there are many patients scattered over the scene and patients range from the slightly physically injured to the dying or deceased
- The need to collaborate efficiently with firefighters, police, or other officials
- The problems that operating in an unsafe or hazardous environment may present

PART 3: RESCUE AWARENESS AND OPERATIONS

Explore the variety of settings that require rescue. Have your students brainstorm about situations that might require victim rescue. Some examples, such as motor vehicle accidents, will come readily. Others, such as home occupants affected by carbon monoxide poisoning, children caught in a dry well or other confined space, or persons who fall through ice, may come only with prompting.

Try to get students to think of examples that fit the major categories discussed in the chapter: surface water (flat and moving water), hazardous atmospheres (trenches, hazmat incidents), highway operations (unstable vehicles, hazardous cargo, volatile fuel), and hazardous terrain (high-angle cliffs, off-road wilderness areas). Then get them to name the four major categories for themselves. Emphasize any categories of rescue that are particularly common in your area.

PART 4: HAZARDOUS MATERIALS INCIDENTS

Where do you find hazardous materials? Ask students to list situations in which an EMS responder might find hazardous materials. Get students to list examples of the three major settings: residential, industrial, transportation, and then have them work to identify specific local sites that might be considered at high risk for a hazmat incident if an accident or terrorist act occurred there. Examples might include home fires, gas explosion, or gasoline vapor inhalation from a ruptured container, industrial manufacturing settings (as well as industries that use chemicals, which range from photo development sites to dry cleaners to hair parlors), buried pipelines, bombings or fires, and highway accidents and train derailments.

PART 5: CRIME SCENE AWARENESS

What makes up a dangerous situation? Have students recollect case studies from previous chapters of this book, as well as previous discussions in class, that focus on personal and scene safety. Students should recollect the chapter on abuse and neglect, as well as mention personal safety in the setting of major multiple-casualty incidents and in settings of violence (such as hostage/sniper incidents and terrorist acts). Some students may bring up environmental hazards such as highway accidents and physically unstable scenes and other rescue (or potential rescue) settings.

Get your students to see that potential dangers exist in almost every call and that it becomes crucial to have safety strategies in mind each time dispatch sends out their unit. Teach them that good safety skills may avert violence or save them from it and that the same types of awareness and tactical skills will help them to collaborate effectively with police when they need to give medical care at a crime scene.

TEACHING STRATEGIES

People learn in a variety of ways. Some do better with the spoken word, whereas others prefer the written. Some prefer to work alone, whereas others profit from working in groups. Recognizing these different ways of acquiring knowledge, the authors of this *Instructor's Resource Manual* have provided a variety of teaching strategies for the different types of learners. These strategies are intended to foster higher-level cognitive skills and encourage creative learning and problem solving. For greatest effectiveness, incorporate these strategies into your class lecture. Symbols in the Lecture Outline indicate the points at which various exercises might be most appropriate. Other strategies can be used to preview the lesson or to summarize it.

PART 1: AMBULANCE OPERATIONS

The following strategies are keyed to specific sections of the lesson.

1. Recognizing State Codes. Because the book explains that the "State EMS Code" dictates the standards for most ambulances, obtain a copy of this code, or one provided by your county health department, for students to read. There is no better reinforcement to learning than real-world examples, especially when the text refers to one of these examples.

2. Designing an Ambulance. As a class, design a new ambulance. Include all the "wish list" items such as TV and VCR but also help students create solutions to current vehicle problems such as inability to stand up inside the vehicle or sharps containers located in the wrong places. When you have the "ultimate" vehicle, have a draftsperson draw you one or make a model and keep it in the classroom as evidence of student creativity and ingenuity. This cooperative learning exercise builds teamwork and employs problem solving.

3. Thinking about Maintenance. To emphasize the importance of equipment maintenance and calibration, challenge students to implement a system for these activities in their service or your school. Be sure they obtain the manufacturers' recommendations for each piece of equipment to be included. This activity brings the classroom to the workplace and lends realism to your lecture.

4. Staff Planning. Arm students with the description of a community and vital call volume statistics. Have each small group create a system status and staffing plan for their community using a tabletop town or actual city map. Ask them to indicate how many ambulances should be on duty at any given time, create a shift schedule, establish acceptable response times, and post their units to accomplish this goal. This activity is kinesthetic and requires actual problem-solving skills. Additionally, it may lend some empathy for their dispatch and staffing personnel.

5. Thinking about Safety. Few things are as frightening to providers as the thought of causing an injury ourselves. To emphasize the importance of meticulous care when driving, obtain a dispatch audio of an accident involving an ambulance that caused injury to another human being. The reality of this mistake will leave a powerful impression for many years to come.

The following strategies can be used at various points throughout the lesson or to help summarize and demonstrate what students have learned.

Building Air Medical Awareness. Ask any of your local air medical rescue crews to land at or near your school for a helicopter safety drill. This is a special situation that cannot be fully realized with lecture alone. Several factors make helicopter evacuations unique, including the loud noise, flying debris, danger of rotors, limited cargo space, expertise of staff, and so on. The students will remember this information much better by actually seeing the helicopter land and hearing the crew cover safety information.

Cultural Considerations, Legal Notes, and Patho Pearls. The Student CD-ROM contains this series of informative features to enhance the student's understanding of the material covered in this chapter.

PART 2: MEDICAL INCIDENT MANAGEMENT

The following strategies are keyed to specific sections of the lesson.

6. Fire Service Guest Speaker. Most classes would be served well by inviting a fire official to teach the concept of incident command. The fire department has been using this system of incident management on every call for many years, while EMS has really just begun using incident command. Often, inviting an expert in a subject attracts the students' attention for a subject they might otherwise see as boring.

7. Reviewing Command Structures. To emphasize the difference between unified and singular command, have students report on a notable incident of each type cited in the media or from your local area. Ask them to compare and contrast the types of incident and the manner in which they were handled. This activity reinforces research and oral presentation skills while clarifying these concepts.

8. Recognizing Roles in MCIs. Describe different activities involved in an MCI and have students identify which officer would be responsible for handling each task. If possible, identify titles ahead of time and have students role play the situation so that they actually have a chance to act in the assigned role. This kinesthetic activity helps students perform behaviors required of the assigned role, improving the likelihood of responding correctly in the future.

9. Triage Practice. Create packages of paper-doll patients to be triaged by students. If possible, color in the injuries on one side of the doll and describe their situation on the back. For the less artistically inclined, make the doll a silhouette of color construction paper and describe the patient's condition on the back. Have students triage their victims using the START triage system.

10. Recognizing Disaster Management Factors. Place the names of several potential disasters on strips of paper and place them in a hat. Have small groups of students draw a disaster and identify mitigating factors for their chosen disaster. If these factors do not exist in your community, brainstorm solutions and share important ideas with folks who can make a difference in the form of a letter to your councilperson, fire chief, city planner, and so on. This activity lends realism to the disaster management concepts and promotes community activism.

The following strategies can be used at various points throughout the lesson or to help summarize and demonstrate what students have learned.

Reviewing MCIs. Retrieve records of MCIs handled locally or regionally or create one or more scenarios. Discuss them with the students after you teach the lesson, asking them about their roles as paramedics as well as the overall roles of other emergency personnel at the scene. Get them to synthesize the material taught in the chapter as they discuss triage and rescue, treatment and transport, and so on. Make sure they know the proper names of the different roles involved, as they will need to know them in the case of an actual MCI emergency.

Field Trips. If an MCI occurred locally and the scene conveys some sense of what the incident was like (perhaps a local stretch of highway where a chain reaction occurred in blizzard conditions), visit the scene. Discuss how EMS and other types of personnel would have covered the scene, negotiated any hazards, and fulfilled their roles as part of the overall incident team.

Participating in MCI Drills. Nearly every health department in the United States requires at least annual mass casualty drills. Obtain the schedule and have your class included. When possible, have them integrated into the responding unit crews. If it is not possible for students to play patient care roles, be sure they are included as victims. Even observing a large-scale drill will be educational. Asking to participate in an already scheduled drill will save you the enormous effort required to stage a drill of your own. Additionally, students will have an opportunity to work side by side with professionals in their chosen field during the drill.

Cultural Considerations, Legal Notes, and Patho Pearls. The Student CD-ROM contains this series of informative features to enhance the student's understanding of the material covered in this chapter.

PART 3: RESCUE AWARENESS AND OPERATIONS
The following strategies are keyed to specific sections of the lesson.

11. Thinking about Rescue Equipment. Hold a "Protective Equipment Fashion Show." Among members of your class will be many who own or have access to specialized personal protective equipment for various rescue situations. Have them model the gear in class. An announcer can read from the script about the type of clothing, its protective function, and its availability. This activity involves all of the senses and learning domains and is great fun!

12. More on Rescue Equipment. Create a "treasure chest" of specialized clothing and equipment for your class to use. Be sure to include helmets, gloves, eye protection, BSI gear, turnout gear, body armor, and so on. When lab session scenarios present a hazardous situation, students can return to their vehicle (or your treasure chest) to don the appropriate gear. Remember, students will play like they practice, so it is your responsibility to instill good safety habits in the classroom.

13. Researching Rescue Situations. As an exercise in preplanning, have students research the training and gear required for various rescue situations. Be sure they learn the extent and technicality of the training, where to get this training, continuing education requirements, and the cost associated with the training. Ask that they identify an individual who has this training to interview for their experiences. Photos or brochures would be an added plus. This activity emphasizes research skills taught earlier in the program. Additionally, verbal communication skills are enhanced through the interview and report. Last, this activity lends realism to adult learners by connecting with a professional or role model already trained in their topic area.

The following strategies can be used at various points throughout the lesson or to help summarize and demonstrate what students have learned.

Wilderness Rescue. Two fantastic programs in Colorado exist as information sources and role models for a variety of wilderness medical topic areas. The Wilderness Medical Institute in Pitkin, Colorado, provides Wilderness EMT training and adventures. Colorado Mountain College in Breckenridge, Colorado, offers one of only three Wilderness Paramedic programs in the country. These programs teach the core EMT or Paramedic curricula along with special emphasis on backcountry survival, swiftwater rescue, avalanche rescue, rock climbing and rappelling, and decision making in the absence of communication with medical control.

River Rafting. A river rafting trip is a great way to teach the principles of swiftwater rescue in a fun environment. Most states have day river trips for $20 to $50 per person. Make special arrangements so that the guide will allow stops to practice rescue techniques. You will likely be surprised at how much water safety the guide covers in the normal introduction. Whenever possible, bring students out of the classroom into the real world. Involvement of the senses engages the right brain and facilitates the learning of new ideas, concepts, and techniques.

Water Rescue. In most areas of the country, water rescue is a real possibility. Not every community is equipped with lifeguards for its pools, lakes, rivers, and oceans. Therefore, your students may be called upon to apply ground rescue techniques to the water. They will need practice in order to do this safely and effectively. Rent or borrow space at your local pool to practice spinal immobilization, wound care, airway management, and more in this new, wet, and relatively unstable environment.

Cultural Considerations, Legal Notes, and Patho Pearls. The Student CD-ROM contains this series of informative features to enhance the student's understanding of the material covered in this chapter.

PART 4: HAZARDOUS MATERIALS INCIDENTS

The following strategies are keyed to specific sections of the lesson.

14. Using Guidebooks. Be sure to have a library of guidebooks available for student reference because most will be used too infrequently to warrant a purchase by the students. The library should include the following guidebooks: *Hazardous Waste Operations and Emergency Response Standard*, *NFPA 473: Standard for Competencies for EMS Personnel Responding to Hazardous Materials Incidents*, and the *North American Emergency Response Guidebook*. Encourage students to establish their own reference library as well as use your school's professional library. This demonstrates a commitment to lifelong learning that is important in prehospital care.

15. Reviewing the Curriculum. If they aren't already, be sure the hazmat awareness competencies are included in your core curriculum. Not only are they the standard for all emergency personnel, the information is imperative to your students' future personal safety.

16. Hazmat Simulator. Large or well-endowed fire departments possess simulators for hazmat operations much the way EMS does for rhythm generation and ACLS. Borrow or buy time with one of these simulators to give students a more realistic vision of the types of hazmat incidents they may encounter. The simulators use a mix of video and computer graphics to show the scene, victims, and even smoke, fumes, and fire. When using the simulator or other scenarios, be sure to focus on the paramedics' approach to the incident. Emphasize the difference in tactics used when the EMS responder is responsible for patient care versus hazmat operations in which the responder might be acting with the fire department.

17. Tabletop Scenarios. Use your tabletop town for hazmat scenarios. Use toy or cardboard buildings and small cars to simulate hazmat incidents involving tanker trucks, school buses, farm equipment, and cargo trains. When you use your imagination, your students will too, improving their creative problem-solving skills.

18. Thinking about Hazards. Map out the block on which your school sits. Have students identify, either by educated guess or by actual investigation, the hazardous materials that exist in each building or space. Whether you are on a college campus, in a hospital, or on a block with a hair salon, you are likely to have numerous hazardous materials lurking around your building. Facilitate a discussion about how those materials would need to be handled if an incident occurred at one of those facilities. You might even use your *Emergency Response Guidebook* to identify the proper decontamination and secure handling required in the event of an incident.

19. Assigned Reading. *Vector* by Robin Cook is a novel based in reality and research that addresses the use and danger of biological weapons. Invite students to read the book and report on the themes. Or buy several paperback copies and use them as prizes when playing review games in class. Robin Cook has written many books that address particular medical topics, such as foodborne illness, cancer treatments, and female reproductive issues.

20. Hazmat Placards. Make your class a set of "placard flashcards" with colored cardstock. The symbols and numbers can be changed by affixing Velcro to them. When doing hazmat simulations or scenarios, use your placards. Similarly, drill the recall of the colors and numbers by using your placard flashcards for review.

The following strategies can be used at various points throughout the lesson or to help summarize and demonstrate what students have learned.

Field Trip. If a hazmat incident occurred in your area, consider a field trip to the site, preferably in the company of an EMS provider who served there. Discuss relevant details on the nature of the hazardous substance; the degree of contamination of persons, equipment, and environment; and the medical care provided on site and during transportation (including decontamination on site and precautions taken against secondary contamination during packaging and transport). If there is no appropriate local site, consider use of photos as a case study aid.

Cultural Considerations, Legal Notes, and Patho Pearls. The Student CD-ROM contains this series of informative features to enhance the student's understanding of the material covered in this chapter.

PART 5: CRIME SCENE AWARENESS

The following strategies are keyed to specific sections of the lesson.

21. Developing Checklists. As you look at a typical call in your local area from time of dispatch to time of return, get students to develop a checklist of physical and mental actions they should take at every step. The list should cover each time point from dispatch (full information on call/caller, location of call) to scene arrival (inconspicuous arrival, initial scene size-up before leaving ambulance) to patient transport (watching family and bystanders for signs of incipient violence or threat, requesting backup if necessary).

22. Verbal Judo. "Verbal Judo" is a program that specializes in using verbal and body language to mitigate the potential for violent behavior in emergency situations. There is a full course offered by certified professionals in this program, as well as a book by the same name and a website at *www.verbaljudo.com*.

23. Gang Awareness. Most law enforcement agencies have a division or officer who specializes in gang intelligence. If you live in a small or rural area, call upon the services of your nearest urban law enforcement agency for this expertise. They will be able to share with students critical information about gang identification, behavior, and danger. Do not underestimate the penetration of gangs into your area, no matter how small or rural your community. Additionally, many students may go on to practice in cities beyond the immediate community. If this information is omitted from your curriculum, your students will be ill-prepared in potentially dangerous situations.

24. Identifying Hazards. Many reality crime and law enforcement shows exist on television today. Select a few clips to show in class so that students can identify possible hazards and mitigation or safety approaches to the situation. This visual activity can be done as a cooperative learning exercise. Students will be amazed at how poor their memory is and how many details they miss. You may have to replay the tape several times before all hazards can be identified. Be sure to discuss the consequences of careless scene safety practices specific to the clips you are showing.

25. Preserving Evidence. Invite a crime scene technician or medical examiner to speak to your class about the preservation of evidence. Many students will be impressed by the type of evidence that can solve a case or lead to a conviction. Most will have a new respect for the consideration of evidence when treating persons involved in a crime. Few things will make as strong an impression as a trip to the morgue to watch a medical examiner gather the forensic evidence. Try arranging this with your ME office.

The following strategies can be used at various points throughout the lesson or to help summarize and demonstrate what students have learned.

Tactical Training. Borrow a tactical training area to run simulations for a day. A CONTOMS, TEMS, SWAT, or other law enforcement academy will likely have a mock city area in which to practice scenarios that mimic crime scenes. Your students will benefit from getting out of the classroom where they can actually approach an area from the side yard, peer through windows, and find areas of cover; all concepts you have taught in this chapter. This change of environment will definitely prepare students better than the standard classroom scenario situations.

Self-Defense. Offer a personal safety or self-defense course to your students after class or on a weekend. Though this type of skill is not necessarily a psychomotor objective of the curriculum, many of the principles of personal safety are applicable.

Most of these programs are low cost and can be contracted through a health club, gym, or law enforcement agency.

Cultural Considerations, Legal Notes, and Patho Pearls. The Student CD-ROM contains this series of informative features to enhance the student's understanding of the material covered in this chapter.

TEACHING OUTLINE

Chapter 48 is the eighth lesson in Division 5, *Special Considerations/Operations*. Distribute Handouts 48-1, 48-9, 48-16, 48-22, and 48-27 so that students can familiarize themselves with the learning goals for this chapter. If students have any questions about the objectives, answer them at this time.

Then present the chapter. One possible lecture outline follows. In the outline, the parenthetical references in regular type are references to text pages; those in bold type are references to figures, tables, or procedures.

PART 1: AMBULANCE OPERATIONS

I. Introduction. Ambulance standards, maintenance of ambulance equipment and supplies, ambulance stationing, safe ambulance operations, and utilization of air medical transport are all core concepts for effective ambulance maintenance and operation. (p. 1798)

II. Ambulance standards (pp. 1798–1800)
  A. Levels of oversight (pp. 1798–1799)
    1. Federal (DOT)
    2. State
    3. Local
  B. Ambulance design (pp. 1799–1800) (**Fig. 48-1, p. 1799**)
    1. Type I
      a. Conventional truck cab-chassis with a modular ambulance body
    2. Type II
      a. Standard van, forward control integral cab-body
    3. Type III
      a. Specialty van, forward control integral cab-body ambulance
  C. Medical equipment standards (p. 1800)
    1. OSHA
    2. NIOSH
    3. NFPA
  D. Additional guidelines (p. 1800)
    1. Commission on Accreditation of Ambulance Services (CAAS)

III. Checking and maintaining ambulances (pp. 1800–1801)
  A. Vehicle checklists (p. 1800)
  B. Equipment checklists (pp. 1800–1801)

IV. Ambulance deployment and staffing (pp. 1801–1802)
  A. Deployment factors (p. 1801)
    1. Demographics
    2. Primary area of responsibility
  B. Traffic congestion (pp. 1801–1802)
    1. System status management
    2. Tiered response system
  C. Operational staffing (p. 1802)

V. Safe ambulance operations (pp. 1802–1806)

  A. Educating providers (pp. 1802–1803)
  B. Reducing ambulance collisions (p. 1803)
  C. Standard operating procedures (pp. 1803–1804) (**Fig. 48-2, p. 1804**)
  D. The due regard standard (p. 1804)
  E. Lights and siren: a false sense of security (pp. 1804–1805)
  F. Escorts and multivehicle responses (p. 1805)
  G. Parking and loading the ambulance (pp. 1805–1806)
  H. The deadly intersection (p. 1806)

VI. Utilizing air medical transport (pp. 1806–1809)

  A. Fixed-wing aircraft (p. 1806)
  B. Rotorcraft (pp. 1806–1807) (**Fig. 48-3, p. 1807**)
  C. Advantages and disadvantages of air transport (p. 1807)
  D. Activation (p. 1807)
  E. Indications for patient use (pp. 1807–1808)
      1. Clinical criteria (**Table 48-1, p. 1808**)
      2. Mechanism of injury
      3. Difficult assessment situations
      4. Time/distance factors
  F. Patient preparation and transfer (pp. 1808–1809)
  G. Scene safety and the landing zone (p. 1809)

PART 2: MEDICAL INCIDENT MANAGEMENT

I. Introduction. As a paramedic, you will be involved in a wide variety of responses including the single-patient incidents, such as a cardiac patient or simple trauma patient; the small-scale multiple-patient incidents, such as motor vehicle crashes, house fires, or gang activity; and the large-scale multiple-casualty incidents (MCIs), such as airplane crashes and natural disasters. (p. 1809)

II. Origins of emergency incident management (pp. 1810–1811)

  A. Incident Command System (ICS) (p. 1810)
  B. Incident Management System (IMS) (p. 1810)
  C. National Incident Management System (NIMS) (p. 1810)
  D. Regulations and standards (p. 1810)
  E. Emergency Operations Center (EOC) (p. 1810)
  F. A uniform, flexible system (C-FLOP) (pp. 1810–1811)
      1. C — command
      2. F — finance/administration
      3. L — logistics
      4. O — operations
      5. P — planning

III. Command (pp. 1811–1816)

  A. Concept of command as most important functional area (p. 1811)
      1. Incident commander (IC)
      2. Span of control
  B. Establishing command (pp. 1811–1812) (**Fig. 48-4, p. 1812**)
  C. Incident size-up (pp. 1812–1813)
      1. Life safety
      2. Incident stabilization
          a. Open incident
          b. Closed incident
      3. Property conservation

POWERPOINT PRESENTATION
Chapter 48 PowerPoint slides 14–23 (Part 1)

TEACHING STRATEGY 5
Thinking about Safety

HANDOUT 48-8
Lights, Sirens, and Intersections

POWERPOINT PRESENTATION
Chapter 48 PowerPoint slides 24–37 (Part 1)

POINT TO EMPHASIZE
As a general rule, do not rely solely on lights and siren to alert other motorists to your approach.

POINT TO EMPHASIZE
Exercise extreme caution whenever you approach an intersection.

POINT TO EMPHASIZE
Stable patients who are accessible to ground vehicles are best transported by ground vehicles.

POWERPOINT PRESENTATION
Chapter 48 PowerPoint slide 4 (Part 2)

POWERPOINT PRESENTATION
Chapter 48 PowerPoint slides 5–9 (Part 2)

HANDOUT 48-9
Chapter 48, Part 2 Objectives Checklist

TEACHING STRATEGY 6
Fire Service Guest Speaker

POWERPOINT PRESENTATION
Chapter 48 PowerPoint slides 10–24 (Part 2)

TEACHING STRATEGY 7
Reviewing Command Structures

POINT TO EMPHASIZE
The ultimate authority for decision making rests with the incident commander.

PowerPoint Presentation
Chapter 48 PowerPoint slides 25–33 (Part 2)

Teaching Strategy 8
Recognizing Roles in MCIs

PowerPoint Presentation
Chapter 48 PowerPoint slides 34–38 (Part 2)

PowerPoint Presentation
Chapter 48 PowerPoint slides 39–52 (Part 2)

Teaching Strategy 9
Triage Practice

Point to Emphasize
All personnel should be trained in triage techniques, and all response units should carry triage equipment.

Point to Emphasize
The routing of patients to hospitals is as important as getting them into an ambulance.

Teaching Strategy 10
Recognizing Disaster Management Factors

D. Singular versus unified command (pp. 1813–1814)
   1. Incident command post (CP)
E. Identifying a staging area (p. 1814)
F. Incident communications (p. 1814)
G. Resource utilization (p. 1815)
H. Command procedures (pp. 1815–1816) (**Fig. 48-5, p. 1815**)
I. Termination of command (p. 1816)

IV. **Support of incident command** (pp. 1816–1819) (**Fig. 48-6, p. 1817**)
   A. Command staff (pp. 1816–1818)
      1. Safety officer (SO)
      2. Liaison officer (LO)
      3. Information officer (IO)
      4. Mental health support
         a. Small incidents
         b. Major incidents/disasters
   B. Finance/Administration (p. 1818)
   C. Logistics (p. 1818)
   D. Operations (pp. 1818–1819)
   E. Planning (p. 1819)

V. **Division of operation functions** (pp. 1819–1820) (**Fig. 48-7, p. 1820**)
   A. Branches (p. 1819)
   B. Groups and divisions (p. 1819)
   C. Units (p. 1819)
   D. Sectors (p. 1819)

VI. **Functional groups within an EMS branch** (pp. 1820–1827)
   A. Triage (pp. 1820–1824)
      1. Primary triage
      2. Secondary triage
      3. The START system (**Fig. 48-8, p. 1822**)
         a. Ability to walk
         b. Respiratory effort
         c. Pulse/perfusion
         d. Neurological status
      4. Triage tagging/labeling (**Fig. 48-9, p. 1823**)
      5. The need for speed
   B. Morgue (p. 1824)
   C. Treatment (pp. 1824–1825)
      1. Red treatment unit
      2. Yellow treatment unit
      3. Green treatment unit
      4. Supervision of treatment units
   D. On-scene physicians (p. 1825)
   E. Staging (p. 1825)
   F. Transport unit (pp. 1825–1826)
   G. Extrication/rescue unit (p. 1826)
   H. Rehabilitation unit (p. 1826)
   I. Communications (pp. 1826–1827)
      1. EMS communications officer
      2. Alternative means of communication

VII. Disaster management (pp. 1827–1828)

A. Mitigation (p. 1827)
B. Planning (pp. 1827–1828)
C. Response (p. 1828)
D. Recovery (p. 1828)

VIII. Meeting the challenge of multiple-casualty incidents (pp. 1828–1830)

A. Common problems (pp. 1828–1829)
B. Preplanning, drills, and critiques (p. 1829)
C. Disaster mental health services (pp. 1829–1830)
   1. Psychological first aid to meet providers' emotional needs
   2. Screening of rescuers and victims for abnormal signs and symptoms of traumatic stress

PART 3: RESCUE AWARENESS AND OPERATIONS

I. Introduction. Rescue is the concept/definition of extrication and/or disentangling the victims who will become your patients after rescue is complete. (p. 1830)

II. Role of the paramedic (pp. 1830–1831)

A. The paramedic must have proficiency up to at least the "awareness level" for rescues involving (pp. 1830–1831)
   1. Surface water
   2. Hazardous atmospheres
   3. Highway operations
   4. Hazardous terrains (**Fig. 48-10, p. 1830**)

III. Protective equipment (pp. 1831–1833)

A. Rescuer protection (pp. 1831–1833) (**Fig. 48-11, p. 1832**)
   1. Helmets
   2. Eye protection
   3. Hearing protection
   4. Respiratory protection
   5. Gloves
   6. Foot protection
   7. Flame/flash protection
   8. Personal flotation devices
   9. Lighting
   10. Hazmat suits or SCBA (self-contained breathing apparatus)
   11. Extended, remote, or wilderness protection
B. Patient protection (p. 1833)
   1. Helmets
   2. Eye protection
   3. Hearing and respiratory protection
   4. Protective blankets
   5. Protective shielding

IV. Safety procedures (pp. 1833–1834)

A. Rescue SOPs (p. 1833)
B. Crew assignments (p. 1834) (**Fig. 48-12, p. 1834**)
C. Preplanning (p. 1834)

POWERPOINT PRESENTATION
Chapter 48 PowerPoint slide 53 (Part 2)

POINT TO EMPHASIZE
Never say "It will never happen here."

POWERPOINT PRESENTATION
Chapter 48 PowerPoint slides 54–58 (Part 2)

HANDOUT 48-16
Chapter 48, Part 3 Objectives Checklist

POWERPOINT PRESENTATION
Chapter 48 PowerPoint slide 4 (Part 3)

TEACHING STRATEGY 11
Thinking about Rescue Equipment

POWERPOINT PRESENTATION
Chapter 48 PowerPoint slides 5–6 (Part 3)

POINT TO EMPHASIZE
The application of safety equipment—both to rescuers and patients—is paramount in any rescue situation.

POWERPOINT PRESENTATION
Chapter 48 PowerPoint slides 7–9 (Part 3)

HANDOUT 48-21
Rescuer Protective Equipment

TEACHING STRATEGY 12
More on Rescue Equipment

POINT TO EMPHASIZE
Always be sure to avoid covering the victim's mouth and nose during rescue operations.

TEACHING STRATEGY 13
Researching Rescue Situations

POWERPOINT PRESENTATION
Chapter 48 PowerPoint slides 10–11 (Part 3)

POINT TO EMPHASIZE
Rescue operations should only be attempted by personnel with special training and experience in these areas.

POWERPOINT PRESENTATION
Chapter 48 PowerPoint slides 12–21 (Part 3)

POINT TO EMPHASIZE
It is paramount that the rescuer knows how to properly package the patient to prevent further injury.

POWERPOINT PRESENTATION
Chapter 48 PowerPoint slides 22–30 (Part 3)

POINT TO EMPHASIZE
Water entry is a last resort—and is an action best left to specialized water rescuers.

V. Rescue operations (pp. 1835–1838)
   A. Phase 1: Arrival and size-up (p. 1835)
   B. Phase 2: Hazard control (p. 1835)
   C. Phase 3: Patient access (pp. 1835–1836)
   D. Phase 4: Medical treatment (pp. 1836–1837) (**Fig. 48-13, p. 1836**)
      1. Basic responsibilities
         a. Initiate patient assessment.
         b. Maintain patient care procedures.
         c. Accompany patient during removal and transport.
      2. Basic care steps
         a. Initial assessment of MS-ABCs
         b. Management of life-threatening ABC problems
         c. Spinal immobilization
         d. Splinting of major fractures
         e. Appropriate patient packaging
         f. Ongoing reassessment
   E. Phase 5: Disentanglement (pp. 1837–1838) (**Fig. 48-14, p. 1838**)
      1. Basic responsibilities
         a. Skills to function in active rescue zone
         b. Readiness to provide prolonged patient care
         c. Ability to call for and use special rescue resources
   F. Phase 6: Patient packaging (p. 1838) (**Fig. 48-15, p. 1839**)
   G. Phase 7: Removal/Transport (p. 1838)

VI. Surface water rescues (pp. 1838–1845)
   A. General background (pp. 1839–1841)
      1. Rescuers should know how to swim.
      2. Use PFDs.
      3. Water temperature
         a. Hypothermia
         b. HELP
         c. HUDDLE
      4. Basic rescue techniques (**Fig. 48-16, p. 1840**)
   B. Moving water (pp. 1841–1843)
      1. Recirculating currents (**Fig. 48-17, p. 1842**)
      2. Strainers (**Fig. 48-18, p. 1842**)
      3. Foot/extremity pins
      4. Dams/hydroelectric intakes
      5. Self-rescue techniques
         a. Cover mouth and nose during entry.
         b. Protect the head; keep face out of water.
         c. Do not attempt to stand in moving water.
         d. Float on back, feet downstream.
         e. Steer with feet.
         f. Remember that water moves faster around outside of a bend.
         g. Watch out for rocks and strainers.
         h. Watch for eddies.
         i. Be careful not to fall in the first place.
   C. Flat water (pp. 1843–1845)
      1. Factors affecting survival
         a. Personal flotation devices
         b. Cold protective response
      2. Location of submerged victims
      3. Rescue versus body recovery
      4. In-water patient immobilization
         a. Phase one: In-water spinal immobilization

      b. Phase two: Rigid cervical collar application
      c. Phase three: Back boarding and extrication from the water

VII. Hazardous atmosphere rescues (pp. 1845–1847) (**Fig. 48-19, p. 1845**)
  A. Confined-space hazards (p. 1846)
    1. Oxygen-deficient atmospheres
    2. Toxic or explosive chemicals (**Fig. 48-20, p. 1846**)
    3. Engulfment
    4. Machinery entrapment
    5. Electricity
    6. Structural concerns
  B. Confined-space protections in the workplace (p. 1846)
  C. Cave-ins and structural collapses (p. 1847)
    1. Reasons for collapses/cave-ins
      a. Poor construction techniques
      b. Lip of trench caves in
      c. Wall shears away in entirety
      d. "Spoil pile" too close to edge of hole
      e. Water seepage, ground vibrations, intersecting trenches, disturbed soil
    2. Rescue from trenches/cave-ins

VIII. Highway operations and vehicle rescues (pp. 1847–1851)
  A. Hazards in highway operations (pp. 1847–1849)
    1. Traffic hazards
      a. Staging
      b. Positioning of apparatus
      c. Emergency lighting
      d. Redirection of traffic
      e. High visibility
    2. Other hazards
      a. Fire and fuel
      b. Alternative fuel systems
      c. Sharp objects
      d. Electric power (**Fig. 48-21, p. 1849**)
      e. Energy-absorbing bumpers
      f. Supplemental restraint systems (SRSs)/airbags
      g. Hazardous cargoes
      h. Rolling vehicles
      i. Unstable vehicles
  B. Auto anatomy (pp. 1849–1850)
    1. Basic constructions
    2. Firewall and engine compartment
    3. Glass
    4. Doors
  C. Rescue strategies (pp. 1850–1851)
    1. Initial scene size-up
    2. Control hazards.
    3. Assess the degree of entrapment and fastest means of extrication. (**Fig. 48-22, p. 1850**)
    4. Establish circles of operation.
    5. Treatment, packaging, removal
  D. Rescue skills practice (p. 1851)

POWERPOINT PRESENTATION
Chapter 48 PowerPoint slides 38–42 (Part 3)

READING/REFERENCE
Sargent, C. "Close Encounters: EMS at Confined Space Operations." *JEMS,* July 1999.

POWERPOINT PRESENTATION
Chapter 48 PowerPoint slides 00–00

POINT TO EMPHASIZE
Suspect hazmat at any scene involving commercial vehicles.

POWERPOINT PRESENTATION
Chapter 48 PowerPoint slides 43–50 (Part 3)

IX. Hazardous terrain rescues (pp. 1851–1856)
  A. Types of hazardous terrain (pp. 1851–1852)
  B. Patient access in hazardous terrain (p. 1852)
    1. High-angle rescues (**Figs. 48-23a and 23b, p. 1853**)
    2. Low-angle rescues
    3. Flat terrain with obstructions
  C. Patient packaging for rough terrain (pp. 1852–1854) (**Figs. 48-24a and 24b, p. 1853**)
  D. Patient removal from hazardous terrain (pp. 1854–1855)
    1. Flat rough terrain
    2. Low-angle/high-angle evacuation
    3. Use of helicopters
    4. Packaging/evacuation practice
  E. Extended care assessment and environmental issues (pp. 1855–1856)
    1. Need for protocols to address patient-related concerns and topics
      a. Long-term rehydration management
      b. Cleansing and care of wounds
      c. Removal of impaled objects
      d. Nonpharmacological pain management
      e. Pharmacological pain management
      f. Assessment/care of head and spine injuries
      g. Management of hypo- or hyperthermia
      h. Termination of CPR
      i. Treatment of crush injury/compartment syndrome
    2. Environmental issues that can affect assessment
      a. Weather/temperature
      b. Limited patient access
      c. Difficulty transporting equipment
      d. Cumbersome PPE
      e. Patient exposure
      f. Use of ALS skills
      g. Patient monitoring
      h. Improvisation

HANDOUT 48-22
Chapter 48, Part 4 Objectives Checklist

TEACHING STRATEGY 14
Using Guidebooks

POWERPOINT PRESENTATION
Chapter 48 PowerPoint slides 4–5 (Part 4)

TEACHING STRATEGY 15
Reviewing the Curriculum

POWERPOINT PRESENTATION
Chapter 48 PowerPoint slides 6–8 (Part 4)

TEACHING STRATEGY 16
Hazmat Simulator

TEACHING STRATEGY 17
Tabletop Scenarios

PART 4: HAZARDOUS MATERIALS INCIDENTS

I. Introduction. Hazardous materials (hazmat) are very common in all regions and in all settings. Definition per DOT is "any substance which may pose an unreasonable risk to health and safety of operating or emergency personnel, the public, and/or the environment if not properly controlled during handling, storage, manufacture, processing, packaging, use, disposal, or transportation." (p. 1857) (**Fig. 48-25, p. 1857**)

II. Role of the paramedic (pp. 1857–1858)
  A. If first responders, roles include (p. 1857)
    1. Scene size-up
    2. Assessment of toxicological risk
    3. Activation of IMS
    4. Establishment of command
  B. Requirements and standards (p. 1857)
    1. OSHA
    2. EPA
    3. NFPA
  C. Levels of training (p. 1858)
    1. Awareness level
    2. EMS Level 1
    3. EMS Level 2

III. Incident size-up (pp. 1858–1863)

A. IMS and hazmat emergencies (p. 1858)
B. Incident awareness (pp. 1858–1860)
  1. Transportation (**Fig. 48-26, p. 1859**)
  2. Fixed facilities (**Fig. 48-27, p. 1859**)
  3. Terrorism
C. Recognition of hazards (pp. 1860–1861)
  1. Placard classifications (**Fig. 48-28, p. 1861**)
  2. NFPA 704 system (**Figs. 48-29a and 48-29b, p. 1861**)
D. Identification of substances (pp. 1862–1863)
  1. *Emergency Response Guidebook* (ERG)
  2. Shipping papers
  3. Material safety data sheets (MSDS)
  4. Monitors and testing
  5. Other sources of information
     a. CAMEO
     b. CHEMTREC
     c. CHEMTEL
E. Hazardous materials zones (p. 1863) (**Fig. 48-30, p. 1864**)
  1. Hot (exlusionary or red) zone
  2. Warm (contamination reduction or yellow) zone
  3. Cold (safe or green) zone

IV. Specialized terminology (pp. 1863–1865)

A. Terms for medical hazmat operations (pp. 1863–1865)
  1. Boiling point
  2. Flammable/explosive limits
  3. Flash point
  4. Ignition temperature
  5. Specific gravity
  6. Vapor density
  7. Vapor pressure
  8. Water solubility
  9. Alpha radiation
  10. Beta radiation
  11. Gamma radiation
B. Toxicological terms (p. 1865)
  1. Threshold limit value/time weighted average (TLV/TWA)
  2. Threshold limit value/short-term exposure limit (TLV/STEL)
  3. Threshold limit value/ceiling level (TLV/CL)
  4. Lethal concentration/lethal dose (LCt/LD)
  5. Parts per million/parts per billion (ppm/ppb)
  6. Immediately dangerous to life and health (IDLH)

V. Contamination and toxicology review (pp. 1865–1868)

A. Types of contamination (p. 1865)
  1. Primary
     a. Direct exposure to a hazardous substance
  2. Secondary
     a. Transfer of a hazardous substance to a noncontaminated person via contact with someone or something already contaminated
B. Routes of exposure (pp. 1865–1866)
  1. Respiratory
  2. Topical

POWERPOINT PRESENTATION
Chapter 48 PowerPoint slides 9–31 (Part 4)

TEACHING STRATEGY 18
Thinking about Hazards

TEACHING STRATEGY 19
Assigned Reading

POINT TO EMPHASIZE
Placards may only provide minimal information about a hazardous substance. Some materials, when shipped in smaller quantities, may not require a placard at all.

TEACHING STRATEGY 20
Hazmat Placards

POWERPOINT PRESENTATION
Chapter 48 PowerPoint slides 32–36 (Part 4)

POINT TO EMPHASIZE
At a hazmat incident, keep a bad situation from becoming worse by evacuating uncontaminated people from the area around the incident.

POWERPOINT PRESENTATION
Chapter 48 PowerPoint slides 37–51 (Part 4)

3. Parenteral
4. Gastrointestinal
C. Cycles and actions of poisons (p. 1866)
   1. Acute effects
      a. Signs and symptoms displayed rapidly on exposure to a substance
   2. Delayed effects
      a. Signs and symptoms that develop well after exposure
   3. Local effects
      a. Effects involving the area around the immediate site of exposure
   4. Systemic effects
      a. Effects that occur throughout the body after exposure to a toxic substance
D. Treatment of common exposures (pp. 1866–1868)
   1. Corrosives
   2. Pulmonary irritants
   3. Pesticides
   4. Chemical asphyxiants
   5. Hydrocarbon solvents

VI. **Approaches to decontamination** (pp. 1868–1871)
   A. Methods of decontamination (pp. 1868–1869)
      1. Dilution
      2. Absorption
      3. Neutralization
      4. Isolation/disposal
   B. Decontamination decision making (pp. 1869–1870)
      1. Modes of operation
         a. Fast-break decision making
         b. Long-term decision making
   C. Field decontamination (pp. 1870–1871)
      1. Two-step process
         a. Removal of clothing and personal effects
         b. Gross decontamination (two times)
      2. Eight-step process
         a. Step 1: Workers enter decon area and mechanically remove contaminants from victims
         b. Step 2: Drop equipment in tool-drop area; remove outer gloves
         c. Step 3: Decon personnel showers for victims and rescuers
         d. Step 4: Removal and isolation of SCBA
         e. Step 5: Removal of all protective clothing
         f. Step 6: Removal of personal clothing from victims and rescuers
         g. Step 7: Full-body wash for rescuers and victims
         h. Step 8: Assessment and transport of victims; monitoring of rescuers
      3. Transportation considerations

VII. **Hazmat protection equipment** (p. 1871)
   A. Level A (p. 1871)
      1. Highest-level respiratory and splash protection
      2. Sealed, impenetrable, fully encapsulating hazmat suits
   B. Level B (p. 1871)
      1. Full respiratory protection
      2. Nonencapsulating but chemical resistant
   C. Level C (p. 1871)
      1. Nonpermeable suit with air-purifying respirator

POWERPOINT PRESENTATION
Chapter 48 PowerPoint slides 52–60 (Part 4)

POINT TO EMPHASIZE
If life threat exists, the patients come first, environmental considerations last.

POWERPOINT PRESENTATION
Chapter 48 PowerPoint slides 61–67 (Part 4)

D. Level D (p. 1871)
  1. Turnout gear

VIII. Medical monitoring and rehabilitation (p. 1872)

A. Entry readiness (p. 1872)
B. Postexit "rehab" (p. 1872)
C. Heat stress factors (p. 1872)

IX. Importance of practice (p. 1872)

A. Potential incident scene activities (p. 1872)
  1. Establish command
  2. Make the first incident decisions
  3. Help protect all on-scene personnel
B. To achieve proficiency, paramedics must become actively involved in drills and exercises to prepare for a hazardous materials incident (p. 1872)
C. Become involved with local emergency operations planning (p. 1872)

PART 5: CRIME SCENE AWARENESS

I. Introduction. Violence is widespread, and you may be caught up in it during EMS calls. Learn safety tactics, know your local area, and familiarize yourself with protocols for handling dangerous situations and interacting with police. (pp. 1872–1873)

II. Approach to the scene. Begin consideration of safety strategies at the time of dispatch (pp. 1873–1875) (**Fig. 48-31, p. 1874**)

A. Possible scenarios (pp. 1873–1875)
  1. Advised of danger en route
  2. Observing danger on arrival (**Fig. 48-32, p. 1874; Fig. 48-33, p. 1875; Fig. 48-34, p. 1876**)
  3. Eruption of danger during care or transport

III. Specific dangerous scenes (pp. 1875–1879)

A. Highway encounters (pp. 1876–1877)
B. Violent street incidents (pp. 1877–1878)
  1. Murder, assault, robbery
  2. Dangerous crowds and bystanders
     a. Signs of danger
        i. Shouts or loud voices
        ii. Pushing or shoving
        iii. Hostilities toward anyone on scene
        iv. Rapid increase in crowd size
        v. Inability of law officers to control crowd
  3. Street gangs
     a. Appearance
     b. Graffiti
     c. Tattoos
     d. Hand signals/language
C. Drug-related crimes (pp. 1878–1879)
  1. Signs of drug involvement
     a. Prior history of drugs in neighborhood of call
     b. Clinical evidence that patient used drugs
     c. Drug-related comments by bystanders
     d. Drug paraphernalia at scene

POWERPOINT PRESENTATION
Chapter 48 PowerPoint slides 68–71 (Part 4)

POWERPOINT PRESENTATION
Chapter 48 PowerPoint slide 72 (Part 4)

POINT TO EMPHASIZE
If you observe anything abnormal during preentry medical monitoring, do not allow the hazmat team member to attempt a rescue.

HANDOUT 48-27
Chapter 48, Part 5 Objectives Checklist

POWERPOINT PRESENTATION
Chapter 48 PowerPoint slides 4–9 (Part 5)

POWERPOINT PRESENTATION
Chapter 48 PowerPoint slides 10–16 (Part 5)

TEACHING STRATEGY 21
Developing Checklists

POINT TO EMPHASIZE
There is no such thing as a dead hero!

POINT TO EMPHASIZE
In most cases, you can legally leave behind a patient when there is a documented danger.

TEACHING STRATEGY 22
Verbal Judo

TEACHING STRATEGY 23
Gang Awareness

PowerPoint Presentation
Chapter 48 PowerPoint slides 17–27 (Part 5)

Teaching Strategy 24
Identifying Hazards

Point to Emphasize
Nothing in the ambulance is worth your life. Retreat by foot or whatever means possible to avoid violence that threatens your life.

Point to Emphasize
If you must touch or move an item, remember to tell police.

PowerPoint Presentation
Chapter 48 PowerPoint slides 28–31 (Part 5)

Teaching Strategy 25
Preserving Evidence

PowerPoint Presentation
Chapter 48 PowerPoint slides 38 (Part 1), 59 (Part 2), 51 (Part 3), 73 (Part 4), 32 (Part 5)

D. Clandestine drug laboratories (p. 1879)
 1. Actions to take on discovering a clandestine drug lab
  a. Leave area immediately.
  b. Do not touch anything.
  c. Do not stop chemical reactions in process.
  d. Do not smoke or bring a source of flame into lab.
  e. Notify police.
  f. Initiate ICS and hazmat procedures.
  g. Consider evacuation.
E. Domestic violence (p. 1879)

IV. **Tactical considerations** (pp. 1879–1883)
 A. Safety tactics (pp. 1880–1882)
  1. Retreat
  2. Cover and concealment (**Figs. 48-35a and 48-35b, p. 1880**)
  3. Distraction and evasion
  4. Contact and cover (**Table 48-2, p. 1881**)
  5. Warning signals and communication
 B. Tactical patient care (pp. 1882–1883)
  1. Body armor
  2. Tactical EMS
   a. Members and organizations
    i. TEMS
    ii. SWAT-Medics
    iii. EMT-Tacticals
    iv. CONTOMS
    v. NTOA
   b. Possible scenarios
    i. Raids on clandestine drug labs
    ii. EMS in barricade situations
    iii. Wounding by weapons or booby traps
     a) Special gear for tactical operations
    iv. Use of CS, OC, or other gas
    v. Blank-firing weapons
    vi. Helicopter operations
    vii. Pyrotechnics
    viii. Extreme conditions
    ix. Firefighting and hazmat operations

V. **EMS at crime scenes** (pp. 1883–1885)
 A. EMS and police operations (pp. 1883–1884)
 B. Preserving evidence (pp. 1884–1885)
  1. Types of evidence
   a. Prints
   b. Blood and body fluids
   c. Particulate evidence
   d. On-scene observations
  2. Documenting evidence

VI. **Chapter summary** (pp. 1885–1886). As a paramedic, you should be familiar with standards that influence ambulance design, equipment requirements, and staffing. You should also regularly complete all checklists regarding on-board equipment and essential supplies. Be aware of items that require routine maintenance or calibration as well as the expiration dates on all drugs. Keep in mind OSHA safety requirements and know how to report equipment problems or failures. Be familiar with the profile of a typical ambulance collision and develop strategies for preventing it from occurring. Also be aware of the issues and policies surrounding the staging and staffing of ambulances. Appreciate the conditions or situations that merit air medical transport and the safety issues involved in packaging the patient, selecting a landing site, and approaching the aircraft.

Every paramedic should be thoroughly familiar with the procedures used in a typical incident management system. You should be able to follow these procedures at every multiple-patient, multiple-unit response—from the smallest incident to the largest. Expect to respond to several MCIs during your EMS career. A good preplan, regular use of the IMS, and MCI training will allow you to handle each event calmly and professionally.

Whenever you function in any phase of a rescue, you must be properly outfitted with protective equipment. You must also have training specific to the type of rescue. During the operational phases of a rescue, you must provide direct patient care and work with technical teams to assure optimal patient management. Any paramedic assigned to rescue duties should have training in the care of patients who may require prolonged management.

Every member of an EMS team should be prepared to face the challenges of the hazmat incident. As with any EMS operation, the primary consideration is your own safety. You become useless at a hazmat incident if you become contaminated yourself. Similarly, your first priority at any crime scene is your own safety. To protect your life and the lives of others, you need to develop a "crime scene awareness." Do not needlessly expose yourself to dangers better left to professional emergency medical personnel such as SWAT-Medics or EMT-Ts. When you do treat the victim(s) at a crime scene, keep in mind that police and EMS personnel must work together to preserve the evidence. Touch only those items or objects that pertain directly to patient care.

ASSIGNMENTS

Assign students to complete Chapter 48, "Operations," of the workbook. Also assign them to read Chapter 49, "Responding to Terrorist Acts," before the next class.

EVALUATION

Chapter Quizzes and Scenarios Distribute copies of the Chapter Quizzes provided in Handouts 48-2, 48-10, 48-17, 48-23, and 48-28; and the Chapter Scenarios provided in Handouts 48-3, 48-11, 48-18, 48-24, and 48-29 to evaluate student understanding of this chapter. Make sure each student reads the scenarios to reinforce critical thinking on the scene. Remind students not to use their notes or textbooks while taking the quiz.

Student CD Quizzes for every chapter are contained on the dynamic and highly visual in-text student CD.

Companion Website Additional quizzes for every chapter are contained on this exciting website.

TestGen You may wish to create a custom-tailored test using *Prentice Hall TestGen for Essentials of Paramedic Care*, 2nd Edition to evaluate student understanding of this chapter.

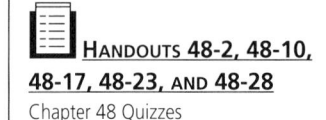

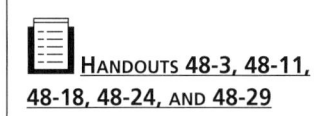

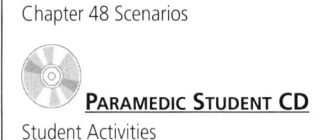

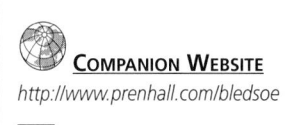

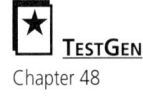

WORKBOOK
Chapter 48 Activities

READING/REFERENCE
Textbook, pp.1890–1904

HANDOUTS 48-2, 48-10, 48-17, 48-23, AND 48-28
Chapter 48 Quizzes

HANDOUTS 48-3, 48-11, 48-18, 48-24, AND 48-29
Chapter 48 Scenarios

PARAMEDIC STUDENT CD
Student Activities

COMPANION WEBSITE
http://www.prenhall.com/bledsoe

TESTGEN
Chapter 48

EMT ACHIEVE: PARAMEDIC TEST PREPARATION
Mistovich & Beasley. *EMT Achieve: Paramedic Test Preparation.* www.prenhall.com/emtachieve/

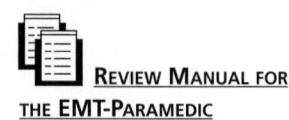

REVIEW MANUAL FOR THE EMT-PARAMEDIC
Cherry & Mistovich. *Review Manual for the EMT-Paramedic*, 3rd edition.

HANDOUTS 48-4 TO 48-8; 48-12 TO 48-15; 48-19 TO 48-21; 48-25 AND 48-26; 48-30 TO 48-32
Reinforcement Activities

PARAMEDIC STUDENT CD
Student Activities

POWERPOINT PRESENTATION
Chapter 48

COMPANION WEBSITE
http://www.prenhall.com/bledsoe

ONEKEY
Chapter 48

ADVANCED LIFE SUPPORT SKILLS
Larmon & Davis. *Advanced Life Support Skills.*

ADVANCED LIFE SKILLS REVIEW
Larmon & Davis. *Advanced Life Skills Review.*

BRADY SKILLS SERIES: ALS
Larmon & Davis. *Brady Skills Series: ALS.*

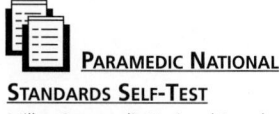

PARAMEDIC NATIONAL STANDARDS SELF-TEST
Miller. *Paramedic National Standards Self-Test,* 4th edition.

On-line Test Preparation (for students and instructors) Additional test preparation is available through Brady's new on-line product, *EMT Achieve: Paramedic Test Preparation* at *http://www.prenhall.com/emtachieve/*. Instructors can also monitor student mastery on-line.

Review Manual for the EMT-Paramedic This comprehensive exam review contains hundreds of test questions and rationales, including scenarios, along with two 180-question practice tests on CD.

REINFORCEMENT

Handouts If classroom discussion or performance on the quiz indicates that some students have not fully mastered the chapter content, you may wish to assign some or all of the Reinforcement Handouts for this chapter.

Student CD (for students) A wide variety of material on this CD-ROM will reinforce and also expand student knowledge and skills.

PowerPoint Presentation (for instructors) The PowerPoint material developed for this chapter offers useful reinforcement of chapter content.

Companion Website (for students) Additional review quizzes and links to EMS resources will contribute to further reinforcement of the chapter.

OneKey On-line support is offered for this course on one of three platforms: CourseCompass, Blackboard, or Web CT. Includes the IRM, PowerPoints, TestGen, and Companion Website for instruction. Ask your local sales representative for more information.

Brady Skills Series: Advanced Life Skills (Video or CD) Have your students watch the skills come to life on VHS or CD-ROM, or they can purchase the highly visual, full-color text with step-by-step procedures and rationales.

HANDOUT 48-1

Student's Name _____

CHAPTER 48 OBJECTIVES CHECKLIST

PART 1: AMBULANCE OPERATIONS

Knowledge	Date Mastered
1. Identify current local and state standards that influence ambulance design, equipment requirements, and staffing of ambulances.	
2. Discuss the importance of completing an ambulance equipment/supply checklist.	
3. Discuss factors used to determine ambulance stationing and staffing within a community.	
4. Describe the advantages and disadvantages of air medical transport and identify conditions/situations in which air medical transport should be considered.	

CHAPTER 48 QUIZ

PART 1: AMBULANCE OPERATIONS

Write the letter of the best answer in the space provided.

_____ 1. The plan used by an EMS agency to maneuver its ambulances and crews in an effort to reduce response times is called:
   A. use strategy.
   B. operational strategy.
   C. deployment strategy.
   D. staffing/stationing strategy.

_____ 2. Oversight for EMS services is usually handled at which level?
   A. federal government
   B. state government
   C. regional level
   D. local level

_____ 3. The agency charged with worker safety is abbreviated as:
   A. OSHA.
   B. NIOSH.
   C. NFPA.
   D. CAAS.

_____ 4. Deployment factors commonly considered by an EMS agency include all of the following EXCEPT:
   A. location of hospitals.
   B. location of possible facilities to house ambulances.
   C. safety of neighborhood with possible housing facility.
   D. local geographic and traffic considerations.

_____ 5. Analysis of accident data indicates that almost three quarters of ambulance collisions take place:
   A. at dusk or after dark.
   B. in inclement weather.
   C. during daylight hours.
   D. at intersections.

_____ 6. Steps to reduce ambulance collisions commonly include all of the following EXCEPT:
   A. hands-on driver training with experienced field officers.
   B. ordering paramedics to report all personal citations or accidents.
   C. use of slow-speed vehicle operations course.
   D. demonstrated knowledge of primary and backup routes to hospitals.

_____ 7. Ambulances are rarely, if ever, legally exempted from:
   A. operating during night hours with lights and siren.
   B. highway speed limits.
   C. following posted directions of travel.
   D. passing a school bus with flashing lights.

_____ 8. Common guidelines for siren use include all of the following EXCEPT:
   A. using the siren as a standard warning device during daylight hours.
   B. assuming that some motorists will hear the siren but ignore it.
   C. being prepared for erratic maneuvers from some drivers who hear the siren.
   D. never assuming all motorists will hear the siren.

_____ 9. Fixed-wing aircraft are generally employed:
   A. in areas with regional airports and landing sites.
   B. in weather conditions that make helicopter flight unsafe.
   C. whenever helicopters are unavailable.
   D. when transport distances exceed 100 miles.

HANDOUT 48-2 Continued

_____ 10. Indications for patient transport by helicopter include all of the following EXCEPT:
  A. certain clinical criteria relating to trauma score, crush injury, major burns, and so on.
  B. trauma team preference for the receiving facility.
  C. situations that are difficult for ground transportation.
  D. transport time to a trauma center greater than 15 minutes by a ground ambulance.

_____ 11. When you are first to arrive at the scene of a motor vehicle collision, park the ambulance, if possible, upwind and uphill from the wreckage by:
  A. 50 feet.   C. 200 feet.
  B. 100 feet.   D. 250 feet.

_____ 12. If the scene of a motor vehicle crash has been secured when you arrive, you should park the ambulance:
  A. next to the wreckage.   C. in front of the wreckage.
  B. behind the wreckage.   D. behind a police vehicle.

_____ 13. An organization that allows multiple vehicles to arrive at an EMS call at different times, often providing different levels of care or transport, is:
  A. system status management. C. PAR.
  B. reserve capacity.   D. a tiered response system.

_____ 14. A situation likely to require patient transport by helicopter is a:
  A. multivehicle crash.   C. wilderness rescue.
  B. hazardous materials incident. D. multialarm fire.

_____ 15. The landing zone for a helicopter should be:
  A. 25 by 25 feet.   C. 75 by 75 feet.
  B. 50 by 50 feet.   D. 100 by 100 feet.

HANDOUT 48-3

Student's Name _____

CHAPTER 48 SCENARIO

PART 1: AMBULANCE OPERATIONS

Review the following real-life situation. Then answer the questions that follow.

Your unit has been based for a number of years at a fire station in a residential section of the city. Because recent development has significantly increased the number of homes in your area and has expanded the residential neighborhood into the adjacent foothills, your area of responsibility has grown much larger. This winter has been hard, with frequent snow that has accumulated on the shoulders of roads and made some of the outlying, previously country roads very difficult to negotiate, particularly those running to a recreational area at the edge of your area. Your unit is a Type II van ambulance.

You have an in-service meeting coming up with your city administrator, and you and the other ambulance crews that staff your unit would like to present your concerns regarding the difficulty of using your ambulance on the outlying roads and your concerns about the large geographic area you cover.

1. What, if any, suggestions might you make regarding the matching of ambulance type with the roads of your expanded area of operation?

2. You have heard that the EMS administration is considering a review of deployment over the city as a whole based on growth in city size and population over the last decade. In order to make your input as useful as possible, what should you consider about the peak loads in your sector and how that might affect citywide deployment plans?

HANDOUT 48-4

Student's Name _____

CHAPTER 48 REVIEW

PART 1: AMBULANCE OPERATIONS

Write the word or words that best complete each sentence in the space(s) provided.

1. Most state regulations set _____ standards rather than a(n) _____ standard for operation.
2. _____ is an organization that makes the work environment safer by ensuring mechanical maintenance and the availability of personal protection equipment.
3. _____ _____ on medications should be checked each shift, and the older, in-date drugs marked appropriately so they are used first.
4. Ideal deployment decisions take into account two sets of data: past _____ _____ and projected _____ _____.
5. The highest volume of calls, or _____ _____, should be expressed in terms of day or week and time of day.
6. When vehicles are positioned for calls in specific high-volume areas, the crew's location is known as their _____ _____ of _____ (_____).
7. In _____ _____ management, a computerized personnel and ambulance deployment system enables the EMS service to meet service demands with fewer resources and still ensure appropriate response time and vehicle location.
8. Communities that have several levels of response, from designated first responders to backup ALS units, are said to have a(n) _____ _____ system.
9. A number of backup accidents could be avoided by use of a(n) _____.
10. The situation in which it is most likely that a police escort is appropriate for an ambulance is when the ambulance is operating in _____ _____ and needs to be guided to the scene or the hospital.
11. If your ambulance is the first vehicle on the scene, park _____ _____ _____ the wreckage so your warning lights alert approaching motorists.
12. Exercise _____ _____ whenever you approach an intersection.
13. In order for a helicopter program to be effective, the frontline first responders must consider _____ as early as possible.
14. A standard van with a forward control integral cab-body is called a(n) _____ _____ ambulance.
15. Flight crews suggest that EMS crews mark the landing zone with a single _____ in the _____ position.

REINFORCEMENT

©2007 Pearson Education, Inc.
Essentials of Paramedic Care, 2nd ed.

CHAPTER 48 *Operations* 1223

HANDOUT 48-5

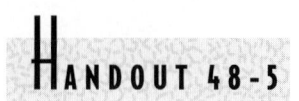

Student's Name _____

AMBULANCE OPERATIONS TRUE OR FALSE

PART 1: AMBULANCE OPERATIONS

Indicate whether the following statements are true or false by writing T or F in the space provided.

_____ 1. The days of "blowing through" intersections at high speed with lights and sirens engaged have passed.

_____ 2. Routine, detailed shift checks of ambulances are insufficient to minimize issues associated with risk management.

_____ 3. OSHA has helped to ensure there are equipment lists calling for disinfecting agents, sharps containers, red bags, HEPA masks, and personal protective equipment.

_____ 4. In general, ambulance staffing takes into account ample coverage for peak load times as well as the need for reserve capacity.

_____ 5. The New York State data on ambulance collisions included reportable collisions and crashes occurring while the ambulance was backing up.

_____ 6. The legal standard for drivers of ambulances is based on the concept of due regard.

_____ 7. As a general rule, do not rely solely on lights and siren to alert other motorists to your approach.

_____ 8. Recent data have indicated that lights/siren use shaves roughly a minute from response time, but significantly increases the possibility of injury to the responding crew.

_____ 9. The most important point in ambulance lighting is visibility: The ambulance must be clearly visible from 360 degrees to all other motorists as well as pedestrians.

_____ 10. Stable patients who are accessible to ground vehicles are best transported by ground vehicles.

_____ 11. You should consider air medical transport for any patient who has a Glasgow Coma Scale score of less than 12.

_____ 12. Most EMS agencies no longer suggest the use of a police escort for ambulances.

_____ 13. If your ambulance is the first vehicle on the emergency scene of a motor vehicle collision, make sure that you park in back of the wreckage.

_____ 14. Always go around cars stopped at an intersection on their left (driver's) side.

_____ 15. In general, a helicopter requires a landing zone of 75 by 75 feet.

Handout 48-6

Student's Name _____

AMBULANCE OPERATIONS ABBREVIATIONS

PART 1: AMBULANCE OPERATIONS

Fill in the words for each abbreviation used in the chapter.

1. DOT _____
2. FCC _____
3. OSHA _____
4. NIOSH _____
5. NFPA _____
6. CAAS _____
7. ACS _____
8. SOPs _____
9. AED _____
10. SSM _____
11. CAAMS _____
12. LZ _____
13. PAR _____
14. FAA _____

Handout 48-7

Student's Name _____

TYPICAL UNIT CHECKLISTS

PART 1: AMBULANCE OPERATIONS

The components of a typical vehicle/equipment checklist include the following:

- Patient infection control, comfort, and protection supplies
- Initial and focused assessment equipment
- Equipment for the transfer of the patient
- Equipment for airway maintenance, ventilation, and resuscitation
- Oxygen therapy and suction equipment
- Equipment for assisting with cardiac resuscitation
- Supplies and equipment for immobilization of suspected bone injuries
- Supplies for wound care and treatment of shock
- Supplies for childbirth
- Supplies, equipment, and medications for the treatment of acute poisonings, snakebites, chemical burns, and diabetic emergencies
- Advanced life support equipment, medications, and supplies
- Safety and miscellaneous equipment
- Information on the operation and inspection of the ambulance itself

Equipment items that should be checked regularly include the following:

- Automated external defibrillator (AED)
- Glucometer
- Cardiac monitor
- Oxygen systems
- Automated transport ventilator (ATV)
- Pulse oximeter
- Suction units
- Laryngoscope blades
- Lighted stylets
- Penlights
- Any other battery-operated equipment

Handout 48-8

Student's Name _____

LIGHTS, SIRENS, AND INTERSECTIONS

PART 1: AMBULANCE OPERATIONS

Guidelines on Use of Lights and Siren

Consider the following before turning on the siren:

- Motorists are less inclined to yield to an ambulance when the siren is continually sounded.
- Many motorists feel that the right-of-way privileges given to ambulances are abused when sirens are sounded.
- Inexperienced motorists tend to increase their driving speeds by 10 to 15 miles per hour when a siren is sounded.
- The continuous sound of a siren can possibly worsen sick or injured patients by increasing their anxiety.
- Ambulance operators may also develop anxiety from sirens used on long runs, not to mention the possibility of hearing problems.

Some useful guidelines on use of sirens include the following:

- Use the siren sparingly and only when you must.
- Never assume all motorists hear your siren.
- Assume that some motorists will hear your siren, but choose to ignore it.
- Be prepared for panic and erratic maneuvers when drivers do hear your siren.
- Never use the siren to scare someone.

Intersections

Helpful tips for negotiating an intersection include the following:

- Stop at all red lights and stop signs and then proceed with caution.
- Always proceed through an intersection slowly.
- Make eye contact with other motorists to ensure they understand your intentions.
- If you are using any of the exemptions offered to you as an emergency vehicle, such as passing through a red light or a stop sign, make sure you warn motorists by appropriately flashing your lights and sounding the siren.
- Remember that lights and siren only "ask" the public to yield the right of way. If the public does not yield, it may be because they misunderstand your intentions, cannot hear the siren due to noise in their own vehicles, or cannot see your lights. Never assume that other motorists have a clue as to what you plan on doing at the intersection.
- Always go around cars stopped at the intersection on their left (driver's) side. In some instances, this may involve passing into the oncoming lane, which should be done slowly and very cautiously. You invite trouble when you use a clear right lane to sneak past a group of cars at an intersection. If motorists are doing what they should do under motor vehicle laws, they may pull into the right lane just as you attempt to pass.

©2007 Pearson Education, Inc.
Essentials of Paramedic Care, 2nd ed.

HANDOUT 48-8 Continued

- Know how long it takes for your ambulance to cross an intersection. This will help you judge whether you have enough time to pass through safely.

- Watch pedestrians at an intersection carefully. If they all seem to be staring in another direction, rather than at your ambulance, they may well be looking at the fire truck headed your way.

- Remember that there is no such thing as a rolling stop in an ambulance weighing over 10,000 pounds or a medium-duty vehicle weighing some 24,000 pounds. Even at speeds as slow as 30 miles per hour, these vehicles will not stop on a dime. When negotiating an intersection, consider "covering the brake" to shorten the stopping distance.

Chapter 48 Answer Key

Part 1: Ambulance Operations

Handout 48-2: Chapter 48 Quiz

1. C
2. B
3. A
4. C
5. D
6. B
7. D
8. A
9. D
10. B
11. B
12. C
13. D
14. C
15. D

Handout 48-3: Chapter 48 Scenario

1. Your unit is not built for rough roads. If a significant proportion of your current area is in the foothills and supplied by rough roads, perhaps a medium-duty ambulance or other vehicle type would be a better match for this sector.
2. Your operations area is almost entirely residential, which means you have a lower volume of people in that area during working hours on weekdays. Because people are home evenings and on weekends and your area abuts a recreational area, your peak times are weekday evenings and weekends. If deployment plans are being reviewed, that information may be helpful to the administrators. They can actually look at the records of number of calls in your area to confirm peak times and compare your peak times with those for sections of the city that are primarily business or industrial. If necessary, the administration could consider shifting your primary area of responsibility during business hours on weekdays to include some business/industrial areas. Another possibility might be to collaborate with the agency that covers the recreational area itself to see if a heavier-duty ambulance might cover the most difficult roads, at least in winter.

Handout 48-4: Chapter 48 Review

1. minimum, gold
2. OSHA (Occupational Safety and Health Administration)
3. Expiration dates
4. community responses, demographic changes
5. peak load
6. primary area of responsibility (PAR)
7. system status
8. tiered response
9. spotter
10. unfamiliar territory
11. in front of
12. extreme caution
13. medevac
14. Type II
15. flare, upwind

Handout 48-5: Ambulance Operations True or False

1. T
2. F
3. T
4. T
5. F
6. T
7. T
8. F
9. T
10. T
11. F
12. T
13. F
14. T
15. F

Handout 48-6: Ambulance Operations Abbreviations

1. Department of Transportation
2. Federal Communications Commission
3. Occupational Safety and Health Administration
4. National Institute for Occupational Safety and Health
5. National Fire Protection Association
6. Commission on Accreditation of Ambulance Services
7. American College of Surgeons
8. standard operating procedures
9. automated external defibrillator
10. system status management
11. Commission on Accreditation of Air Medical Services
12. landing zone
13. primary area of responsibility
14. Federal Aviation Agency

Handout 48-9

Student's Name _____

CHAPTER 48 OBJECTIVES CHECKLIST

PART 2: MEDICAL INCIDENT MANAGEMENT

Knowledge	Date Mastered
1. Explain the need for the incident management system (IMS)/Incident Command System (ICS) in managing emergency medical services incidents.	
2. Describe the functional components (command, finance, logistics, operations, and planning) of the incident management system.	
3. Differentiate between singular and unified command and identify when each is most applicable.	
4. Describe the role of command, the need for command transfer, and procedures for transferring it.	
5. List and describe the functions of the following groups and leaders in the ICS as they pertain to EMS incidents: • Safety • Logistics • Rehabilitation (rehab) • Staging • Treatment • Triage • Transportation • Extrication/rescue • Disposition of deceased (morgue) • Communications	
6. Describe the methods and rationale for identifying specific functions and leaders for the functions in the ICS.	
7. Describe essential elements of the scene size-up when arriving at a potential MCI.	
8. Define the terms *multiple-casualty incident (MCI)*, *disaster management*, *open or uncontained incident*, and *closed or contained incident*.	
9. Describe the role of the paramedics and EMS system in planning for MCIs and disasters.	
10. Explain the local/regional threshold for establishing command and implementation of the incident management system including MCI declaration.	
11. Describe the role of both command posts and emergency operations centers in MCI and disaster management.	

1230 ESSENTIALS OF PARAMEDIC CARE

©2007 Pearson Education, Inc.
Essentials of Paramedic Care, 2nd ed.

HANDOUT 48-9 Continued

Knowledge	Date Mastered
12. Describe the role of the on-scene physician at multiple-casualty incidents.	
13. Define triage and describe the principles of triage.	
14. Describe the START (simple triage and rapid transport) method of initial triage.	
15. Given color-coded tags and numerical priorities, assign the following terms to each: • Immediate • Delayed • Minimal • Expectant	
16. Define primary, secondary, and ongoing triage and their implementation techniques.	
17. Describe techniques used to allocate patients to hospitals and track them.	
18. Describe the techniques used in tracking patients during multiple-casualty incidents and the need for such techniques.	
19. Describe modifications of telecommunications procedures during multiple-casualty incidents.	
20. List and describe the essential equipment to provide logistical support to MCI operations to include: • Airway, respiratory, and hemorrhage control • Burn management • Patient packaging/immobilization	
21. Describe the role of mental health support in MCIs.	
22. Describe the role of the following exercises in preparation for MCIs: • Tabletop exercises • Small and large MCI drills	
23. Given several incident scenarios with preprogrammed patients, provide the appropriate triage, treatment, and transport options for MCI operations based on local resources and protocols.	

Handout 48-10

Student's Name _____

CHAPTER 48 QUIZ

PART 2: MEDICAL INCIDENT MANAGEMENT

Write the letter of the best answer in the space provided.

_____ 1. The individual who runs the management of a multiple-casualty incident (MCI) and has ultimate authority for decision making is called the:
  A. incident senior official.
  B. incident commander.
  C. incident coordinator.
  D. incident manager.

_____ 2. Incident priorities during scene size-up include all of the following EXCEPT:
  A. life safety.
  B. incident stabilization.
  C. incident containment.
  D. property conservation.

_____ 3. In all cases of a(n) _____, it is better to request more resources than are needed rather than to request an insufficient amount.
  A. multiple casualty incident
  B. closed incident
  C. open incident
  D. unified incident

_____ 4. Incident commanders should radio a brief progress report roughly every _____ minutes until the incident has been stabilized.
  A. 5
  B. 10
  C. 15
  D. 20

_____ 5. The use of _____ by the incident commander and other senior officers makes identification easier for incoming personnel.
  A. special reflective vests
  B. special reflective hats
  C. special reflective jackets
  D. special reflective tags on CP positions

_____ 6. At an MCI, the _____ monitors all actions to ensure no potentially harmful conditions are created.
  A. scene officer
  B. hazards officer
  C. size-up officer
  D. safety officer

_____ 7. The functions of the EMS branch of operations include all of the following EXCEPT:
  A. triage.
  B. treatment.
  C. staging.
  D. transport.

_____ 8. In triage, the highest priority is given to patients tagged with the color:
  A. black.
  B. yellow.
  C. green.
  D. red.

_____ 9. Under the START triage system, the first distinction among patients is based on their:
  A. ability to tell you their name.
  B. ability to walk.
  C. ability to follow a simple command.
  D. ability to breathe spontaneously at a rate of 30 breaths per minute or less.

_____ 10. In triage, the best way to assess perfusion is:
  A. capillary refill.
  B. carotid pulse.
  C. radial pulse.
  D. assessment of mental status.

HANDOUT 48-10 Continued

_____ 11. The signs in START include all of the following EXCEPT:
  A. an open airway.
  B. respirations over 30 breaths per minute.
  C. the ability to follow commands.
  D. visible hemorrhage.

_____ 12. Use of triage tags provides quick recognition of:
  A. who did the triage.
  B. priority of patient treatment.
  C. the patient's name.
  D. the facility to which the patient should be sent.

_____ 13. Medical materials that should be carried by the triage officer include all of the following EXCEPT:
  A. a bag-valve-mask (BVM) device.   C. oral airways.
  B. infection control supplies.   D. trauma dressings.

_____ 14. Ideally, it should take _____ to triage each patient.
  A. less than 20 seconds   C. roughly 30–45 seconds
  B. less than 30 seconds   D. roughly 45–60 seconds

_____ 15. Patients who are deceased are triaged as:
  A. red.   C. yellow.
  B. white.   D. black.

Handout 48-11

Student's Name _____

CHAPTER 48 SCENARIO

PART 2: MEDICAL INCIDENT MANAGEMENT

Review the following real-life situation. Then answer the questions that follow.

You and your partner are called out at 9:07 P.M. for a motor vehicle collision involving two cars, injuries unknown. The night is foggy, and you have to drive fairly slow. Fortunately, the scene is only minutes away from your station and the two cars are clearly visible in the right lane and shoulder of the highway. You park in front of the cars and set your lights to bright flashers so the scene will be as visible as possible to oncoming traffic. No other responders are on the scene yet, and there are no bystanders.

A quick survey of the two cars reveals that one rear-ended the other, sending the first car into the sign for an exit ramp. The driver of the second car is sitting, apparently stunned, in his seat. You note that he looks up as you approach, that there is no visible blood, and that he is wearing his seat belt. The car, which is an older model, does not have an airbag. The driver's side door appears to be intact.

The first car is significantly more damaged, with rear-end damage from the collision and a broken windshield from the impact with the exit sign. The driver is sitting in her seat, contained between an airbag and the seat back. She is not moving and does not respond to your presence. She is clearly breathing. A young woman in the front passenger seat is also contained by an airbag. She is yelling "Help!" and trying to wipe blood and loose hair from her face. A toddler in the backseat is half in, half out of a car seat that has swung across the rear seat, and you can see bruising and abrasions on the side of her face that hit the side window. She is crying. The driver's side door appears to be intact, but the front passenger door has caved inward somewhat and the highway sign has been bent over the front bumper; it hangs over the windshield and the forward part of the passenger door. The rear doors appear to be intact. As you check the rear doors of the car, you realize that there is a faint smell of gasoline.

1. Does this appear to be a multiple-casualty incident (MCI)? If so, what type?

2. What roles should the EMS responders assume, and what should they do next?

3. Should they call in more resources as they size up the scene? If so, what resources?

4. A police cruiser pulls up while the incident commander is on the radio. What, if any, briefing and instructions should the commander give the officers?

1234 ESSENTIALS OF PARAMEDIC CARE

©2007 Pearson Education, Inc.
Essentials of Paramedic Care, 2nd ed.

HANDOUT 48-12

Student's Name _____

CHAPTER 48 REVIEW

PART 2: MEDICAL INCIDENT MANAGEMENT

Write the word or words that best complete each sentence in the space(s) provided.

1. Whenever _____ or more units respond to an emergency, it is a sound idea to implement IMS.

2. The standardized, national structure used to handle large-scale emergencies is called the _____ _____ _____ (_____), and it covers coordination of response elements such as triage, treatment, transport, and staging.

3. Check if your state has passed specific legislation called a _____-_____ law to specify who has ultimate authority at a multiple-casualty incident.

4. The major elements of IMS can be remembered with the mnemonic C-FLOP: C for _____, F for _____ / _____, L for _____, O for _____, and P for _____.

5. In _____ _____, one individual is responsible for coordinating response to an incident, whereas managers from different jurisdictions such as law enforcement, fire, and EMS coordinate activity in the process of _____ _____.

6. Never forget the importance of assigning _____ early in the incident.

7. _____ forms the cornerstone of the incident management system (IMS).

8. Command is only transferred _____-_____-_____, with a short but complete briefing on incident status.

9. At an MCI, the _____ _____ coordinates all operations that involve outside agencies.

10. The operations section at an MCI may have many _____, each of which represents one functional level based on role or geographic location.

11. _____ _____ takes place after patients have been moved to a treatment area and is done to determine any changes in status.

12. The four components of START are the signs/symptoms of _____ _____ _____, _____ _____, _____ / _____, and _____ _____.

13. Any triage tags you use should meet these two criteria: easy to _____ and provide rapid visual identification of _____.

14. The routing of patients to _____ is as important as getting them to an ambulance.

15. The _____ area at an MCI is the location established to support on-scene rescuers, and the _____ _____ _____ is the ambulance crew dedicated to standing by to treat any ill or injured rescuers.

©2007 Pearson Education, Inc.
Essentials of Paramedic Care, 2nd ed.

Handout 48-13

Student's Name _____

MEDICAL INCIDENT MANAGEMENT ABBREVIATIONS

PART 2: MEDICAL INCIDENT MANAGEMENT

Write the words represented by the following abbreviations in the spaces provided.

1. MCI _____
2. MVC _____
3. IMS _____
4. ICS _____
5. IC _____
6. CP _____
7. IO _____
8. CISM _____
9. START _____
10. NIMS _____

HANDOUT 48-14

Student's Name _____

STRUCTURES OF THE INCIDENT MANAGEMENT SYSTEM

PART 2: MEDICAL INCIDENT MANAGEMENT

Each of the following diagrams represents a figure from the text that highlights key information about IMS. Fill in each box with the missing labels.

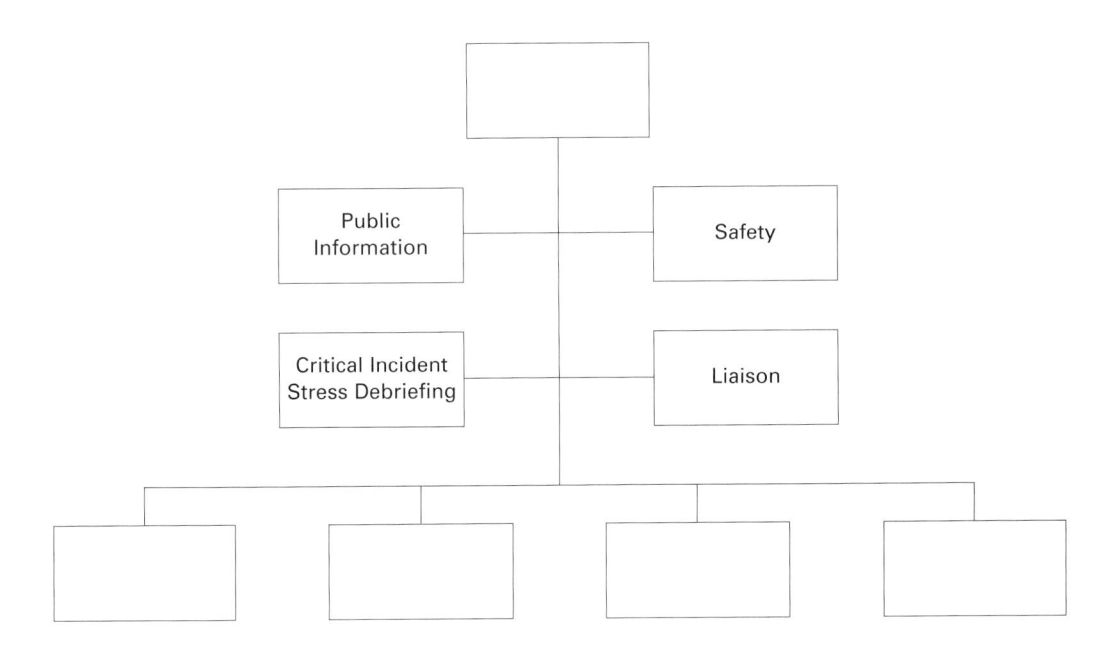

Basic Elements of the Incident Management System

HANDOUT 48-14 Continued

```
                    ┌─────────┐
                    │         │
                    └────┬────┘
                         │
                    ┌────┴────┐
                    │         │
                    └────┬────┘
                         │
                    ┌────┴────┐
                    │         │
                    └────┬────┘
         ┌───────────┬───┴───────┬───────────┐
    ┌────┴────┐ ┌────┴────┐ ┌────┴────┐ ┌────┴────┐
    │         │ │         │ │         │ │         │
    └────┬────┘ └────┬────┘ └────┬────┘ └────┬────┘
         │           │           │           │
```

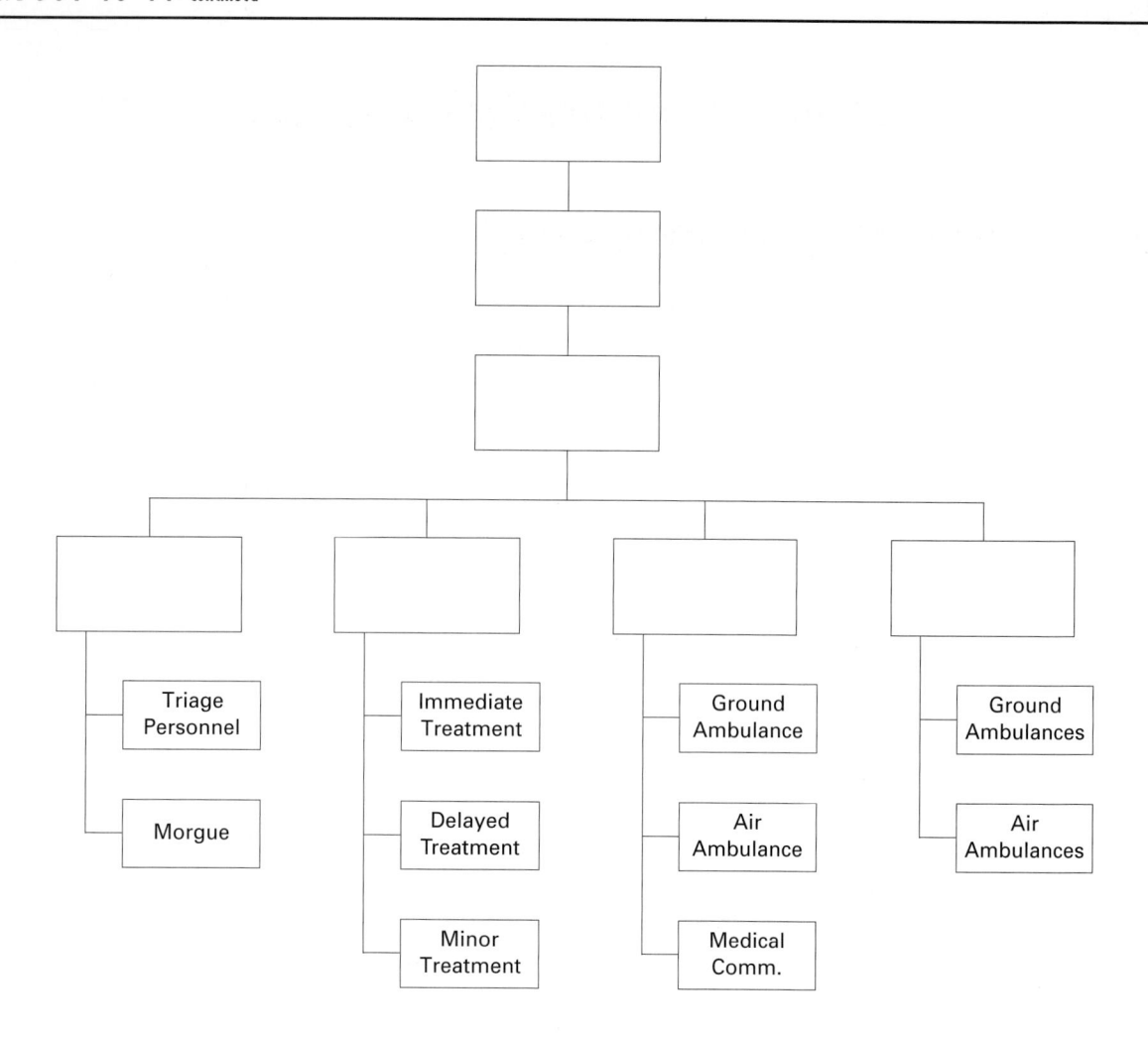

Triage Personnel	Immediate Treatment	Ground Ambulance	Ground Ambulances
Morgue	Delayed Treatment	Air Ambulance	Air Ambulances
	Minor Treatment	Medical Comm.	

IMS EMS Branch

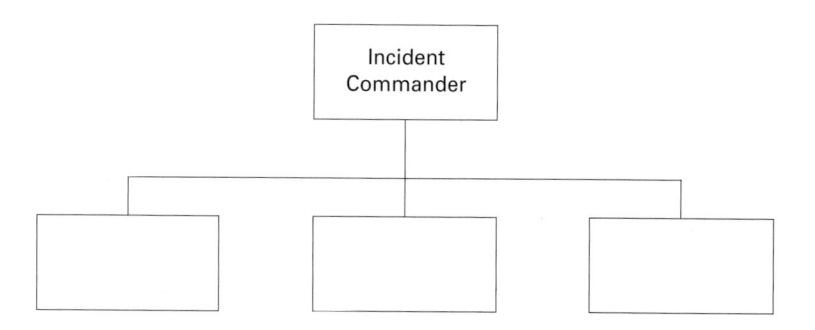

```
              ┌──────────────┐
              │   Incident   │
              │  Commander   │
              └──────┬───────┘
         ┌───────────┼───────────┐
    ┌────┴───┐  ┌────┴───┐  ┌────┴───┐
    │        │  │        │  │        │
    └────────┘  └────────┘  └────────┘
```

**Basic IMS Organization
EMS Operations**

Handout 48-15

Student's Name _____

THE START TRIAGE SYSTEM

PART 2: MEDICAL INCIDENT MANAGEMENT

The following diagram represents the operation of the START triage system. Fill in each missing label to complete the flow chart.

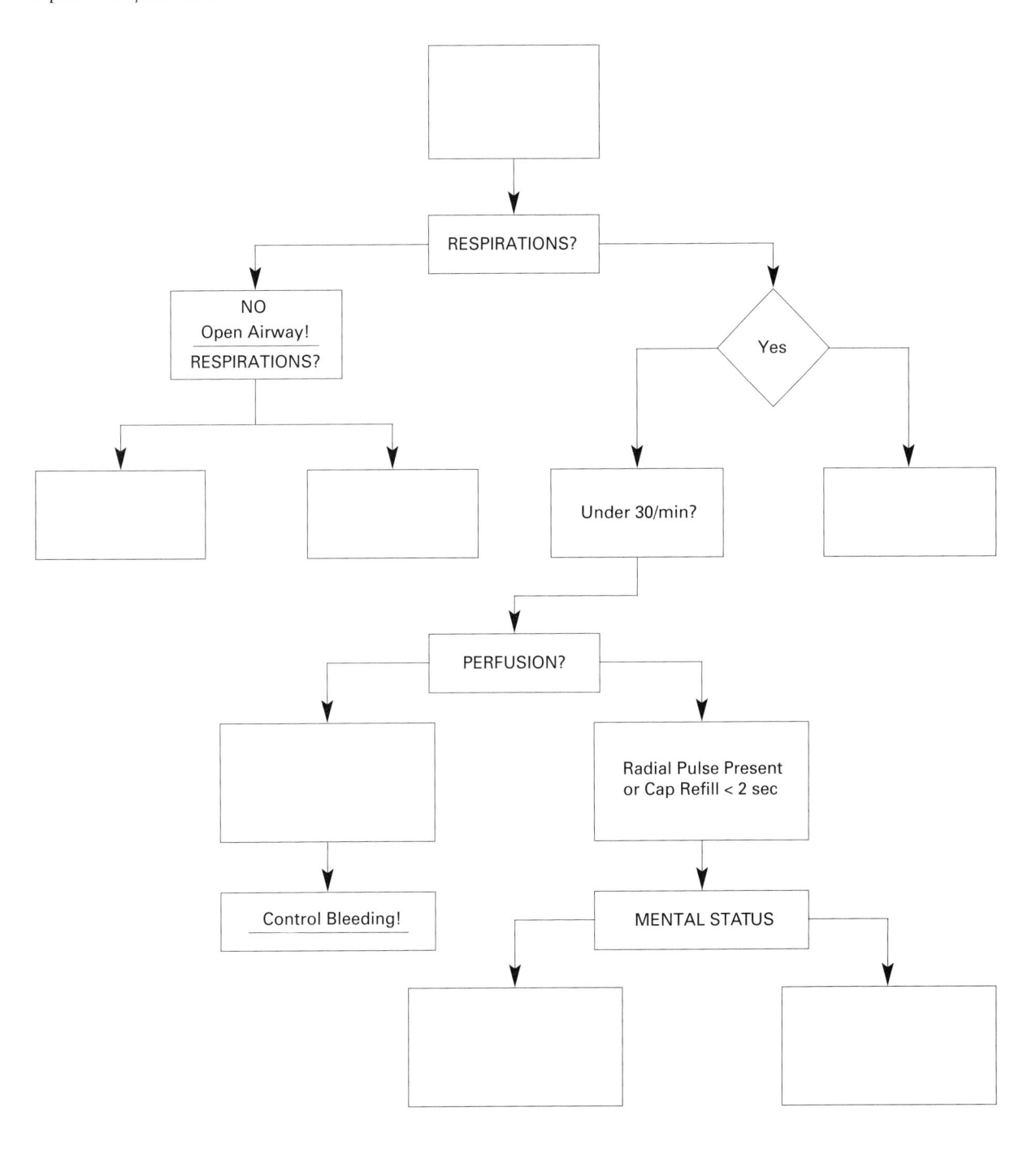

©2007 Pearson Education, Inc.
Essentials of Paramedic Care, 2nd ed.

CHAPTER 48   Operations   1239

Chapter 48 Answer Key

Part 2: Medical Incident Management

Handout 48-10: Chapter 48 Quiz

1. B	5. A	9. B	13. A
2. C	6. D	10. C	14. B
3. C	7. C	11. D	15. D
4. B	8. D	12. B	

Handout 48-11: Chapter 48 Scenario

1. This is a multiple-casualty incident with four known victims. It is an uncontained (or open) incident because there is traffic on the highway, visibility is very poor, and, thus, there is real potential for additional collisions near or with the involved vehicles. IMS (incident management system) should be implemented because of the number of victims and the potential for more injuries from additional collisions or gasoline-related fire or explosion.
2. One provider should act as incident commander and size up the scene with three priorities:
   1. Life safety. Is there a visible gasoline spill, and what is the fire or explosion risk? What needs to be done to secure rescuer safety? Are there additional victims (perhaps from the second car) who are not in a car but are nearby and in need of help?
   2. Incident stabilization. The ambulance has already been parked in position to alert oncoming motorists to the accident. However, the second vehicle is still in the right travel lane.
   3. Property conservation. Not a primary issue during scene size-up on the highway.

   The other provider conducts triage of the four victims.
3. The incident commander needs to call dispatch and initiate IMS. At least one additional ambulance unit will be needed, dependent on the findings of the triage officer and the presence of any additional victims outside of the cars. Police will need to be on scene to handle traffic and any bystanders who arrive, as well as to document any legal aspects of the collision. Fire will need to be called because of the possible gasoline leak, and there are also questions about possible need for extrication of at least one passenger (the young woman in the front passenger seat) from the first car.
4. The incident commander holds singular command unless the situation changes. He should direct the police to help stabilize the incident (by putting out flares and taking any other measures necessary to block off and protect the accident scene, making their own assessment of gasoline risk, and making a second check for other possible victims) and to make their initial report to their base command.

Handout 48-12: Chapter 48 Review

1. two
2. incident management system (IMS)
3. scene-authority
4. Command, Finance/administration, Logistics, Operations, Planning
5. singular command, unified command
6. command
7. Communications
8. face-to-face
9. liaison officer
10. branches
11. Secondary triage
12. ability to walk, respiratory effort, pulses/perfusion, neurological status
13. use, priorities
14. hospitals
15. rehabilitation, rapid intervention team

Handout 48-13: Medical Incident Management Abbreviations

1. multiple-casualty incident
2. motor vehicle collision
3. incident management system
4. incident command system
5. incident commander
6. command post
7. information officer
8. critical incident stress management
9. simple triage and rapid transport
10. National Incident Management System

Handout 48-14: Structures of the Incident Management System

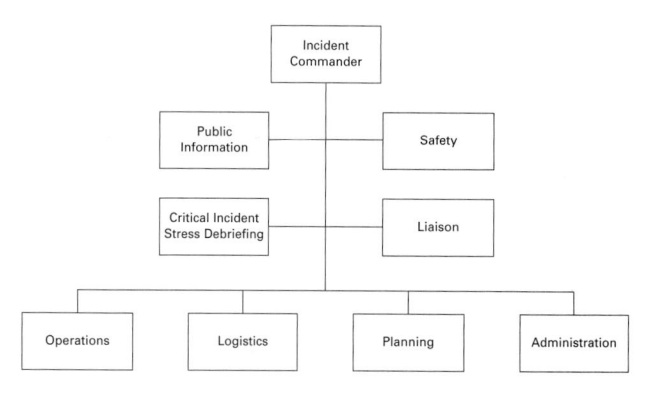

```
                Incident
              Commander
                   |
      +------------+------------+
      |                         |
   Public                     Safety
   Information
      |                         |
   Critical Incident         Liaison
   Stress Debriefing
      |
  +---------+---------+---------+
  |         |         |         |
Operations Logistics Planning Administration
```

Basic Elements of the Incident Management System

1240 ESSENTIALS OF PARAMEDIC CARE

Handout 48-14: Structures of the Incident Management System (Continued)

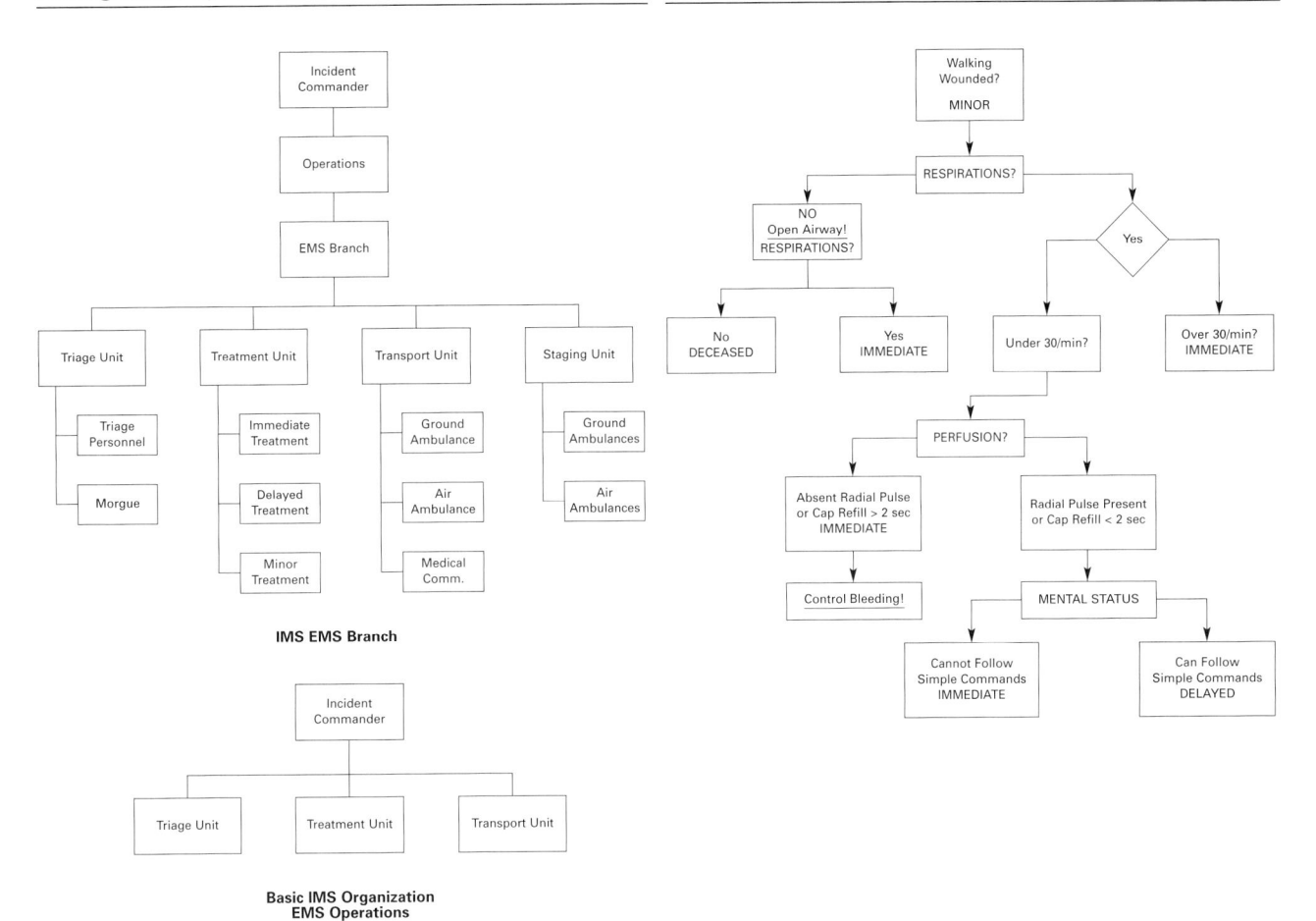

IMS EMS Branch

- Incident Commander
  - Operations
    - EMS Branch
      - Triage Unit
        - Triage Personnel
        - Morgue
      - Treatment Unit
        - Immediate Treatment
        - Delayed Treatment
        - Minor Treatment
      - Transport Unit
        - Ground Ambulance
        - Air Ambulance
        - Medical Comm.
      - Staging Unit
        - Ground Ambulances
        - Air Ambulances

Basic IMS Organization EMS Operations

- Incident Commander
  - Triage Unit
  - Treatment Unit
  - Transport Unit

Handout 48-15: The Start Triage System

- Walking Wounded? → MINOR
- RESPIRATIONS?
  - NO → Open Airway! RESPIRATIONS?
    - No → DECEASED
    - Yes → IMMEDIATE
  - Yes
    - Under 30/min?
      - PERFUSION?
        - Absent Radial Pulse or Cap Refill > 2 sec → IMMEDIATE → Control Bleeding!
        - Radial Pulse Present or Cap Refill < 2 sec → MENTAL STATUS
          - Cannot Follow Simple Commands → IMMEDIATE
          - Can Follow Simple Commands → DELAYED
    - Over 30/min? → IMMEDIATE

Handout 48-16

Student's Name _____

CHAPTER 48 OBJECTIVES CHECKLIST

PART 3: RESCUE AWARENESS AND OPERATIONS

Knowledge	Date Mastered
1. Define the term *rescue*, and explain the medical and mechanical aspects of rescue operations.	
2. Describe the phases of a rescue operation, and the role of the paramedic at each phase.	
3. List and describe the personal protective equipment needed to safely operate in the rescue environment to include: head, eye, and hand protection; personal flotation devices; thermal protection/layering systems; high visibility clothing.	
4. Explain the risks and complications associated with rescues involving moving water, low head dams, flat water, trenches, motor vehicles, and confined spaces.	
5. Explain the effects of immersion hypothermia on the ability to survive sudden immersion and self-rescue.	
6. Explain the benefits and disadvantages of water-entry or "go techniques" versus the reach-throw-row-go approach to water rescue.	
7. Explain the self-rescue position if unexpectedly immersed in moving water.	
8. Describe the use of apparatus placement, headlights and emergency vehicle lighting, cone and flare placement, and reflective and high visibility clothing to reduce scene risk at highway incidents.	
9. List and describe the design element hazards and associated protective actions associated with autos and trucks, including energy-absorbing bumpers, air bag/supplemental restraint systems, catalytic converters, and conventional and nonconventional fuel systems.	
10. Given a diagram of a passenger auto, identify the A, B, C, and D posts, firewall, and unibody versus frame construction.	
11. Explain the difference between tempered and safety glass, identify its locations on a vehicle, and describe how to break it.	
12. Explain typical door anatomy and methods to access through stuck doors.	
13. Describe methods for emergency stabilization using rope, cribbing, jacks, spare tires, and come-a-longs for vehicles found in various positions.	

HANDOUT 48-16 Continued

Knowledge	Date Mastered
14. Describe electrical and other hazards commonly found at highway incidents (above and below the ground).	
15. Define low-angle rescue, high-angle rescue, belay, rappel, scrambling, and hasty rope slide.	
16. Describe the procedure for Stokes litter packaging for low-angle evacuations.	
17. Explain anchoring, litter/rope attachment, and lowering and raising procedures as they apply to low-angle litter evacuation.	
18. Explain techniques used in nontechnical litter carries over rough terrain.	
19. Explain nontechnical high-angle rescue procedures using aerial apparatus.	
20. Explain assessment and care modifications (including pain medication, temperature control, and hydration) necessary for attending to entrapped patients.	
21. List the equipment necessary for an "off road" medical pack.	
22. Explain the different types of "Stokes" or basket stretchers and the advantages and disadvantages associated with each.	
23. Given a list of rescue scenarios, provide the victim survivability profile and identify which are rescue versus body recovery situations.	
24. Given a series of pictures, identify those considered "confined spaces" and potentially oxygen deficient.	

©2007 Pearson Education, Inc.
Essentials of Paramedic Care, 2nd ed.

CHAPTER 48 *Operations* 1243

OBJECTIVES

HANDOUT 48-17

Student's Name _____

CHAPTER 48 QUIZ

PART 3: RESCUE AWARENESS AND OPERATIONS

Write the letter of the best answer in the space provided.

_____ 1. The use of _____ is paramount in any rescue situation.
   A. appropriately skilled personnel
   B. safety equipment
   C. appropriate time-saving measures
   D. portable medical equipment and supplies

_____ 2. Vital rescuer protective equipment includes all of the following EXCEPT:
   A. protective shielding.   C. hearing protection.
   B. respiratory protection.   D. a helmet.

_____ 3. The presence of electrical wires at the rescue scene indicates a possible threat of:
   A. fire.   C. shock.
   B. explosion.   D. both A and C

_____ 4. Hazards that may not be visible during scene size-up include all of the following EXCEPT the presence of:
   A. infected material.
   B. poisonous substances.
   C. potential sources of violence or emotional trauma.
   D. a potentially unstable environment.

_____ 5. The goals of rescue assessment include all of the following EXCEPT:
   A. identification and care for existing patient problems.
   B. anticipation of changes in patient condition.
   C. anticipation of changes in physical environment.
   D. advance determination of needed assistance and equipment.

_____ 6. Because of the possibility of extended time in the field, for rescue patients you must be prepared to provide:
   A. ongoing assessment.   C. treatment protocols.
   B. stabilization techniques.   D. psychological support.

_____ 7. The use of force to free a patient from entrapment is called:
   A. extrication.   C. release.
   B. disentrapment.   D. removal.

_____ 8. Methods used to disentangle the patient must constantly be analyzed:
   A. to look for the shortest method of release.
   B. on a risk-to-benefits basis.
   C. to look for the technique that allows greatest paramedic access.
   D. to look for the methods safest for rescuers and the patient.

_____ 9. It is paramount that the rescuer know how to prevent further patient injury by adapting techniques of:
   A. disentanglement.   C. packaging.
   B. removal.   D. transport.

EVALUATION

1244 ESSENTIALS OF PARAMEDIC CARE

HANDOUT 48-17 Continued

___ 10. While en route to the hospital, you should perform ongoing assessments at these intervals if the patient is stable/unstable.
  A. 3 minutes/5 minutes
  B. 5 minutes/10 minutes
  C. 5 minutes/15 minutes
  D. 5–7 minutes/17–20 minutes

___ 11. HELP (Heat Escape Lessening Position) is an in-water position designed to reduce heat loss by as much as:
  A. 40 percent.
  B. 60 percent.
  C. 75 percent.
  D. 90 percent.

___ 12. Factors contributing to the death of a hypothermic patient include all of the following EXCEPT:
  A. inability to grasp a line or flotation device.
  B. inability to follow simple directions.
  C. bronchospasm, which increases risk of drowning.
  D. laryngospasm, which increases risk of drowning.

___ 13. Recirculating currents, strainers, foot/extremity pins, and dams/hydroelectric intakes are examples of what type of scenario?
  A. fresh-water
  B. swift-water
  C. water obstacle
  D. hazardous water

___ 14. General factors in a person's survivability profile for a water accident include all of the following EXCEPT:
  A. age.
  B. lung volume.
  C. water temperature.
  D. use of alcohol and/or other drugs.

___ 15. One of the MOST serious threats in a confined-space rescue is:
  A. physical instability.
  B. presence of toxic or caustic substances.
  C. oxygen deficiency.
  D. the presence of sharp or otherwise hazardous objects.

EVALUATION

Handout 48-18

Student's Name _____

CHAPTER 48 SCENARIO

PART 3: RESCUE AWARENESS AND OPERATIONS

Review the following real-life situation. Then answer the questions that follow.

It is 10:40 P.M., and you and your partner are about to finish your shift on this pleasantly cool summer night. Then dispatch calls and sends you to a nearby residential neighborhood for "a woman who fell in a swimming pool."

You and your partner grab your personal flotation jackets as you leave the ambulance. When you arrive at the pool area, you find a middle-aged man standing by lawn chairs. When you look in the water, you see a woman on the far side of the pool crying and struggling to hold onto a ladder. She repeatedly tries to climb up the ladder but appears unable to coordinate her movements enough to get out of the pool.

Your partner jogs to the far side of the pool toward the woman while you turn toward the man. You notice he is dressed in light summer clothing, not swimwear, and there is a distinct odor of alcohol. He quickly tells you the woman is his wife and she fell in the swimming pool while they were walking to the house from the garage. "Got home from a party," he says. "She just lost her balance. Stupid, really."

He sits in a pool chair while you join your partner. A quick scan of the scene shows no flotation devices or other floatable object for you to throw or hand to the woman. The area around the pool is dry and level. There is nothing visible in the pool except the woman, who you notice is struggling to hold the ladder with one hand and pull up a skirt with the other. Your partner, who has knelt beside her, tells you her name is Frances and she is unable to say what happened except that she feels sick and can't pull herself up and out of the pool. She has blood dripping from the left temple and what appears to be the beginning of a black eye on the same side. You don't see any other obvious injuries, but the lighting is poor. She is spitting out some water but appears to be breathing relatively easily.

1. Is this a rescue situation? Do you see any potential hazards during your scene size-up?

2. Do you need any additional resources, and, if so, what?

3. What should be done to care for the patient while you wait for additional help (if you decide to wait)?

4. What steps will you need to take to remove the woman safely from the pool when the proper time comes?

Handout 48-19

Student's Name _____

CHAPTER 48 REVIEW

PART 3: RESCUE AWARENESS AND OPERATIONS

Write the word or words that best complete each sentence in the space(s) provided.

1. The checklist for backcountry work includes protective equipment for _____ _____, provisions for personal _____ _____, snacks, temporary _____, _____ lighter, and redundant _____.

2. Most rescue calls have at least seven defined phases: _____ and size-up, _____ control, _____ access, _____ _____, _____, patient _____, and _____ and transport.

3. _____ triggers the technical beginning of the rescue.

4. During the fourth rescue phase, medical treatment, the paramedic has three responsibilities: initiation or _____ _____, maintenance of _____ _____ procedures during disentanglement, and accompaniment of the patient during _____ and _____.

5. The area in which special rescue teams operate is known as the _____ _____ _____.

6. Actions to delay hypothermia include use of _____ _____ _____ (_____), use of _____ _____ _____ _____ (_____), and _____ _____.

7. The water rescue model is called _____ - _____ - _____ - _____.

8. _____ plays a role in many water accidents, including nearly 50 percent of fatal boating accidents.

9. Always put on a(n) _____ whenever you approach water.

10. Water rescue patients are never dead until they are _____ and _____.

11. The three phases of in-water patient immobilization are in-water _____ _____, _____ _____ application, and _____ _____ and extrication from the water.

12. It only takes one spark to trigger an explosion: Always be careful of all potential sources of _____.

13. If a collapsed trench or cave-in has caused a burial, a _____ _____ is likely.

14. _____ _____ is the largest single hazard associated with EMS highway operations.

15. Do not _____ a vehicle until you have ruled out all electrical hazards.

16. For rescuer safety, suspect _____ _____ at any scene involving commercial vehicles.

17. _____ glass can produce glass dust or fracture into long shards, whereas _____ glass fractures into many small beads of glass.

18. Three types of hazardous terrain are _____ - _____ terrain, _____ - _____ terrain, and _____ _____ with obstructions.

19. Be aware of the _____ in mission, crew training, and capabilities of helicopters that do air medical care and those of helicopters that do rescue.

20. Good _____ skills are mandatory in hazardous terrains, but limit _____ skills to those that are really needed: Do not complicate any already complicated operation.

HANDOUT 48-20

Student's Name _____

RESCUE AWARENESS TRUE OR FALSE

PART 3: RESCUE AWARENESS AND OPERATIONS

Indicate whether the following statements are true or false by writing T or F in the space provided.

_____ 1. Failure to train paramedics in rescue awareness will eventually end in the injury or death of EMS personnel, patients, or both.

_____ 2. In general, all paramedics should have the training and personal protective equipment to allow them to access and assess the patient and establish incident command.

_____ 3. Personal flotation devices only need to be worn if you operate in water.

_____ 4. Personnel screening for rescue unit training should include physical and psychological testing.

_____ 5. Practice exercises with clear protocols and simulated patients will give you and your unit ample opportunity to train and to utilize IMS in rescue situations.

_____ 6. If you are the first unit on scene, be careful not to underestimate your ability to handle a rescue situation: Remember not to stretch resources farther than necessary.

_____ 7. During the access phase, key medical, technical, and other personnel should confer with the incident commander on the safest strategy to accomplish the rescue.

_____ 8. Disentanglement may be the most technical and time-consuming portion of the rescue.

_____ 9. Nearly all incidents in and around water are preventable.

_____ 10. Water causes heat loss 10 times faster than air.

_____ 11. Water entry is a last-resort measure.

_____ 12. It is always unsafe to walk in fast-moving water over mid-calf depth because of the danger of entrapping a foot or extremity.

_____ 13. The mammalian diving reflex is more pronounced in adults than in children.

_____ 14. Confined space is defined as any space with limited access/egress that is not designed for human occupation.

_____ 15. Over half of all fatalities associated with confined spaces are rescuers, not the original victim(s).

HANDOUT 48-21

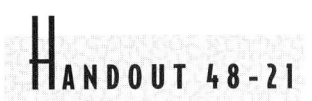

Student's Name _____

RESCUER PROTECTIVE EQUIPMENT

PART 3: RESCUE AWARENESS AND OPERATIONS

- **Helmets:** The best helmets have a four-point, nonelastic suspension system. Avoid helmets with nonremovable "duck bills" in back because they can compromise your ability to wear the helmet in tight spaces. A compact firefighting helmet that meets NFPA standards is adequate for most vehicle and structural applications.

- **Eye protection:** Two essential pieces of eye gear include goggles (vented to prevent fogging) and industrial safety glasses. These should be ANSI approved. Do not rely on the face shields found in fire helmets. They usually provide inadequate eye protection.

- **Hearing protection:** High-quality earmuff styles provide the best hearing protection. However, you must take into account other factors such as practicality, convenience, availability, and environmental considerations. In high-noise areas, for example, you might use the multibaffled rubber earplugs used by the military or sponge-like disposable earplugs.

- **Respiratory protection:** Surgical masks or commercial dust masks prove adequate for most occasions. These should be routinely carried on all EMS units.

- **Gloves:** Leather gloves usually protect against cuts and punctures. They allow for free movement of the fingers and ample dexterity. As a rule, heavy, gauntlet-style gloves are too awkward for most rescue work.

- **Foot protection:** As a rule, the best general boots for EMS work are high-top, steel-toed and/or shank boots with a coarse lug sole to provide traction and prevent slipping. For rescue operations, lace-up boots offer greater stability and better ankle support by limiting the range of motion. They also don't come off as easily as pull-on boots when walking through deep mud.

- **Flame/flash protection:** Whenever there is the potential for fire, turnout gear, coveralls, and jumpsuits all offer some arm and leg protection and help prevent damage to your uniform. They also have the added advantage of quick and easy application. For protection against the sharp, jagged metal or glass found at many motor vehicle accidents or structural collapses, turnout gear generally works best.

- **Personal flotation devices (PFDs):** If your service includes areas where water emergencies can result, your unit should carry PFDs that meet the U.S. Coast Guard standards for flotation. They should be worn whenever operating in or around water. You should also attach a knife, strobe light, and whistle to the PFD so that they are easily accessible.

- **Lighting:** Depending upon the type and location of the rescue, you might also consider portable lighting. Many rescuers carry at least a flashlight or, better yet, a headlamp that can be attached to a helmet for hands-free operation.

- **Hazmat suits or SCBA (self-contained breathing apparatus):** These items should only be made available to the personnel trained to use them.

- **Extended, remote, or wilderness protection:** If your unit provides service to a remote or wilderness area, you would be advised to have a backcountry survival pack as part of your gear. This backpack should be loaded with PPE for inclement weather, provisions for personal drinking water (iodine tablets/water filter), snacks for a few hours, temporary shelter, butane lighter, and some redundancy in lighting in case of light source failure.

Chapter 48 Answer Key

Part 3: Rescue Awareness and Operations

Handout 48-17: Chapter 48 Quiz

1. B	5. C	9. C	13. B
2. A	6. D	10. C	14. D
3. D	7. A	11. B	15. C
4. D	8. B	12. C	

Handout 48-18: Chapter 48 Scenario

1. This is a rescue situation because the woman is unable to get herself out of the pool and she has traumatic injury, although you can't yet determine the specifics. The presence of an early black eye and bleeding from the left temple suggests the possibility of a head injury.

    You should examine the rest of the pool perimeter for potential safety hazards, as well as for evidence of where she fell into the pool (perhaps the presence of blood at the edge of the pool, if she hit her head while falling into the pool).

    There is already evidence of potential hazard at the scene: The man is under the influence of alcohol and shows no concern about his wife. Not only has he not been helpful, he is a potential risk to you and your partner. The situation also has some suggestions of possible domestic violence, which further complicates matters for you and your partner and suggests the woman may have injuries unrelated to her exposure in the pool.

2. You should call for immediate police backup and consider a second EMS unit to help you evaluate the woman's condition in the pool and assist in her rescue.

3. While you wait for the scene to be secured, your partner should continue to talk with her to get any historical information about the incident or admission of complicating factors (namely, she didn't fall into the pool on her own) and as part of an ongoing assessment of mental status. You also need to monitor for any signs of hypothermia or other change in condition that would override a delay in removal until the scene is clearly secured and sufficient help is on hand.

4. When the scene has been secured for your safety, you will need to perform in-water spinal immobilization, apply a rigid cervical collar, and apply a spine board before removing the patient from the water.

Handout 48-19: Chapter 48 Review

1. inclement weather, drinking water, shelter, butane, lighting
2. arrival, hazard, patient, medical treatment, disentanglement, packaging, removal
3. Access
4. patient assessment, patient care, removal, transport
5. active rescue zone
6. personal flotation devices (PFDs), Heat Escape Lessening Position (HELP), huddling together
7. reach-throw-row-go
8. Alcohol
9. PFD
10. warm, dead
11. spinal immobilization, rigid cervical collar, back boarding
12. electricity
13. secondary collapse
14. Traffic flow
15. touch
16. hazardous materials
17. Safety, tempered
18. low-angle, high-angle, flat terrain
19. differences
20. BLS, ALS

Handout 48-20: Rescue Awareness True or False

1. T	5. F	9. T	13. F
2. F	6. F	10. F	14. T
3. F	7. F	11. T	15. T
4. T	8. T	12. F	

HANDOUT 48-22

Student's Name _____

CHAPTER 48 OBJECTIVES CHECKLIST

PART 4: HAZARDOUS MATERIALS INCIDENTS

Knowledge	Date Mastered
1. Explain the role of the paramedic/EMS responder at the hazardous material incident.	
2. Identify resources for substance identification, decontamination, and treatment information.	
3. Identify primary and secondary decontamination risk.	
4. Describe topical, respiratory, gastrointestinal, and parenteral routes of exposure.	
5. Explain acute and delayed toxicity, local versus systemic effects, dose response, and synergistic effects.	
6. Explain how the substance and route of contamination alters triage and decontamination methods.	
7. Explain the employment and limitations of field decontamination procedures.	
8. Explain the use and limitations of personal protective equipment (PPE) in hazardous material situations.	
9. List and explain the common signs, symptoms, and treatment of exposures to corrosives, pulmonary irritants, pesticides, chemical asphyxiants, and hydrocarbon solvents.	
10. Describe the characteristics of hazardous materials and explain their importance to the risk assessment process.	
11. Describe the hazards and protection strategies for alpha, beta, and gamma radiation.	
12. Define the toxicologic terms and their use in the risk assessment process.	
13. Given a specific hazardous material, research the appropriate information about its physical and chemical properties and hazards, suggest the appropriate medical response, and determine the risk of secondary contamination.	
14. Identify the factors that determine where and when to treat a hazardous material incident patient.	

HANDOUT 48-22 Continued

Knowledge	Date Mastered
15. Determine the appropriate level of PPE for various hazardous material incidents.	
16. Explain decontamination procedures including critical patient rapid two-step decontamination and noncritical patient eight-step decontamination.	
17. Identify the four most common solutions used for decontamination.	
18. Identify the body areas that are difficult to decontaminate.	
19. Explain the medical monitoring procedures for hazardous material team members.	
20. Explain the factors that influence the heat stress of hazardous material team personnel.	
21. Explain the documentation necessary for hazmat medical monitoring and rehabilitation operations.	
22. Given a stimulated hazardous substance, use reference material to determine the appropriate actions.	
23. Integrate the principles and practices of hazardous materials response in an effective manner to prevent and limit contamination, morbidity, and mortality.	
24. Size up a hazardous material (hazmat) incident and determine: potential hazards to the rescuers, public, and environment and potential risk of primary contamination to patients and secondary contamination to rescuers.	
25. Given a contaminated patient, determine the necessary level of decontamination, level of rescuer PPE, decontamination methods, treatment, and transportation and patient isolation techniques.	
26. Determine the hazards present to the patient and paramedic given an incident involving a hazardous material.	

HANDOUT 48-23

Student's Name _____

CHAPTER 48 QUIZ

PART 4: HAZARDOUS MATERIALS INCIDENTS

Write the letter of the best answer in the space provided.

_____ 1. Roles of EMS providers who are the first responders to a hazmat incident include all of the following EXCEPT:
   A. assessment of toxicological risk.
   B. activation of IMS.
   C. initial containment procedures.
   D. establishment of incident command.

_____ 2. The three levels of training that an EMS provider may acquire include all of the following EXCEPT:
   A. awareness level.   C. operations level.
   B. supervisory level.   D. technician level.

_____ 3. The transportation warning placard for a flammable gas will have:
   A. red or green color and a flame symbol.
   B. red or green color and a ball-on-fire symbol.
   C. orange color and a flame symbol.
   D. yellow color and a ball-on-fire symbol.

_____ 4. At fixed facilities, the diamond segments of the hazmat placard give information on all of the following EXCEPT:
   A. health hazards.   C. fire hazards.
   B. explosion hazards.   D. reactivity.

_____ 5. CHEMTREC is an example of a:
   A. telephone hotline.   C. printed reference book.
   B. computerized database.   D. poison control center.

_____ 6. At a fixed facility, suggested emergency first-aid treatment may be found:
   A. at a central safety office. C. on the container label.
   B. on the NFPA placard.   D. on a material safety data sheet.

_____ 7. Colorimetric tubes are used to:
   A. measure approximate pH of a liquid.
   B. measure approximate concentration of a given gas in the air.
   C. search air for specific chemicals.
   D. measure approximate concentration of oxygen in air.

_____ 8. Early in scene size-up of a hazmat incident, make sure to:
   A. evacuate all people from the scene of the incident.
   B. evacuate uncontaminated people from the region around the incident.
   C. rescue uncontaminated people from the scene of the incident.
   D. triage contaminated people at the scene of the incident.

_____ 9. The lowest temperature at which a liquid will give off enough vapors to ignite is called the:
   A. lower ignition limit.   C. ignition temperature.
   B. flash point.   D. vapor density temperature.

EVALUATION

HANDOUT 48-23 Continued

_____ 10. The most hazardous type of radiation is called:
   A. alpha radiation.
   B. beta radiation.
   C. delta radiation.
   D. gamma radiation.

_____ 11. The toxicological term used to express the level of exposure safe for someone with full-time occupational exposure is abbreviated as:
   A. LD.
   B. TLV/CL.
   C. TLV/TWA.
   D. IDLH.

_____ 12. Secondary contamination is quite likely with:
   A. liquids and particulates.
   B. gases and liquids.
   C. gases, liquids, and particulates.
   D. liquids only.

_____ 13. In hazmat incidents, the least common route of exposure is:
   A. respiratory inhalation.
   B. topical absorption.
   C. gastrointestinal ingestion.
   D. parenteral injection.

_____ 14. Decontamination for pesticide exposure features:
   A. topical administration of water and green soap.
   B. oral administration of water.
   C. inhalation administration with high-flow oxygen.
   D. IV administration of sodium nitrite.

_____ 15. Among the general methods of decontamination, the one almost never used by EMS personnel is:
   A. dilution.
   B. absorption.
   C. isolation/disposal.
   D. neutralization.

HANDOUT 48-24

Student's Name _____

CHAPTER 48 SCENARIO

PART 4: HAZARDOUS MATERIALS INCIDENTS

Review the following real-life situation. Then answer the questions that follow.

You and your partner are called to an area near the railroad tracks that is frequented by homeless adults. The dispatcher tells you a small fire has been reported and there may be casualties.

When you arrive, you and your partner walk through a dumping area to reach a sheltered area near a bridge. Firefighters have already doused the fire, which burned down a makeshift tent made of cardboard and plastic sheeting. Two adults are sitting on a pile of tires near the fire scene: Each has visibly labored breathing, leaning forward and straining to breathe. One man looks as if he is barely conscious. A firefighter runs up to tell you that the two men stayed in the shelter after it started to burn because it was so cold outside. He moved them to their current position. He is concerned about smoke inhalation injury and possible hypothermia.

1. During initial scene size-up, what, if any, clues are present that might indicate a hazmat incident?

2. What needs to be done to confirm scene and personal safety?

3. Assume there is no evidence of hazardous substances other than those to which the men were exposed while they were in the burning shelter. What decontamination and treatment steps do you take?

HANDOUT 48-25

Student's Name _____

CHAPTER 48 REVIEW

PART 4: HAZARDOUS MATERIALS INCIDENTS

Write the word or words that best complete each statement in the space(s) provided.

1. Even a small-scale hazmat incident may turn into a multijurisdictional event, triggering use of the _____ _____ _____ (_____).

2. The federal agencies that have published the most important requirements and standards are _____ and _____.

3. Never compromise _____ _____ during the early phase of a hazmat operation or you risk becoming a patient yourself.

4. Basic IMS structure at a hazmat incident includes a(n) _____ _____, a(n) _____ _____, and a(n) _____ _____. Be sure you establish backup plans in case wind conditions or other environmental factors change quickly.

5. Hazardous materials may be present in any setting: residential, business, or highway. If you suspect hazmat, use _____ to inspect the scene from a distance.

6. When hazardous materials are transported in _____ _____, the use of a placard may not be required.

7. With the NFPA system, the scale of 0–4 represents _____ _____ on one end of the scale and _____ _____ on the other end.

8. After you have determined that one or more hazardous materials is present at a scene, you need to find _____ or more concurring reference sources regarding identification before taking any specific actions.

9. Two limitations of the *North American Emergency Response Guidebook* (ERG) are the presence of only _____ information on medical treatment and the fact that more than one _____ may have the same UN number.

10. The three control zones at a hazmat incident are coded as red (hot, exclusionary) zone, _____ (_____, _____ _____) zone, and _____ (_____, _____) zone.

11. Unless you or your crew have appropriate training, support, and equipment, you should remain inside the _____ zone.

12. Specific gravity compares a chemical with _____, whereas vapor density compares a chemical with _____.

13. Two sets of terms used to describe the action of a poison are _____ or _____ effects and _____ or _____ effects.

14. Primary respiratory exposure cannot be decontaminated; however, you should _____ _____ _____ and _____ _____ to release any trapped gas.

15. Assess patients with smoke inhalation for these two byproducts of combustion: _____ _____ and _____.

16. The four general methods of decontamination are _____, _____, _____, and _____/_____.

17. The first rule of EMS in hazmat situations is DO NOT _____ _____ _____!

1256 ESSENTIALS OF PARAMEDIC CARE

HANDOUT 48-25 Continued

18. Fast-break decision making is often employed at incidents with _____ injured patients and unknown or life-threatening materials.

19. When possible, use _____ - _____ decision making because of its many advantages.

20. The two measures in two-step decontamination are removal of _____ and _____ _____ and _____ _____.

21. The four most common decontamination solvents are _____, _____ _____, _____ _____, and _____ _____.

22. Another term for a field-decontaminated patient is a _____ - _____ patient.

23. A hazmat suit that offers full respiratory protection and chemically resistant material that is nonencapsulating is termed _____ _____.

24. For a hazmat incident, always remember that some level of protection is better than none: Use _____ gloves and wear _____ boots.

25. Be sure to document seven variables for each member of the hazmat team at preentry and at postexit: _____ _____, _____, _____ rate, _____, _____ _____, _____, and _____/_____ status.

Handout 48-26

Student's Name _____

HAZMAT ABBREVIATIONS

PART 4: HAZARDOUS MATERIALS INCIDENTS

Write out the term represented by each of the abbreviations used in Chapter 48.

1. DOT _____
2. IMS _____
3. OSHA _____
4. EPA _____
5. NFPA _____
6. MVC _____
7. WMD _____
8. UN _____
9. NA _____
10. ERG _____
11. CAMEO _____
12. CHEMTREC _____
13. CHEMTEL _____
14. MSDS _____
15. LEL _____
16. UEL _____
17. TLV/TWA _____
18. PEL _____
19. TLV/STEL _____
20. TLV/CL _____
21. LCt _____
22. LD _____
23. ppm _____
24. ppb _____
25. IDLH _____
26. SLUDGE _____
27. SCBA _____
28. APR _____

Chapter 48 Answer Key

Part 4: Hazardous Materials Incidents

Handout 48-23: Chapter 48 Quiz

1. C	5. A	9. B	13. C
2. B	6. D	10. D	14. A
3. A	7. C	11. C	15. D
4. B	8. B	12. A	

Handout 48-24: Chapter 48 Scenario

1. Fire always produces byproducts, among them carbon monoxide and cyanides. Every patient with smoke inhalation has a possible exposure to one or both compounds. In addition, this fire involved burning plastic (a chemical compound) and may have involved one or more of the dumped items in the area. Thus, there is the potential for other hazardous substances to be present.
2. You should check with the firefighters to see what, if any, steps they took to identify possible hazards and remove them from the fire scene. Either you or your partner should make a quick scene check for possible hazardous substances while the other evaluates the two patients for possible surface contamination and then for medical needs. Both you and your partner should have donned personal protective gear including rubber boots and other protection (Level C or D gear, depending upon local protocol).
3. Both patients show respiratory distress or respiratory failure. Decontamination for carbon monoxide and cyanides would include immediate removal of clothing and personal effects. (Watch for signs of hypothermia as you help them change into clean clothing.) Field medical treatment for carbon monoxide is oxygenation. Cyanide exposure is treated with use of a cyanide kit, which contains amyl nitrite, sodium nitrite, and sodium thiosulfate. Medical care still includes support of the ABCs, prevention or treatment of hypothermia, and any other needs suggested by patient assessment.

Handout 48-25: Chapter 48 Review

1. incident management system (IMS)
2. OSHA, EPA
3. scene safety
4. command post, staging area, decontamination corridor
5. binoculars
6. small quantities
7. no hazard, extreme hazard
8. two
9. general, chemical
10. yellow (warm, contamination reduction), green (cold, safe)
11. green
12. water, air
13. acute, delayed, local, systemic
14. remove all clothing, personal effects
15. carbon monoxide, cyanides
16. dilution, absorption, neutralization, isolation/disposal
17. become a patient
18. critically
19. long-term
20. clothing, personal effects, gross decontamination
21. water, green soap, isopropyl alcohol, vegetable oil
22. semi-decontaminated
23. Level B
24. nitrile, rubber
25. blood pressure, pulse, respiratory, temperature, body weight, ECG, mental/neurologic

Handout 48-26: Hazmat Abbreviations

1. Department of Transportation
2. incident management system
3. Occupational Safety and Health Administration
4. Environmental Protection Agency
5. National Fire Protection Association
6. motor vehicle collision
7. weapons of mass destruction
8. United Nations
9. North America(n)
10. *Emergency Response Guidebook*
11. Computer-Aided Management of Emergency Operations
12. Chemical Transportation Emergency Center
13. Chemical Telephone, Inc.
14. material safety data sheets
15. lower explosive limit
16. upper explosive limit
17. threshold limit value/time weighted average
18. permissible exposure limit
19. threshold limit value/short-term exposure limit
20. threshold limit value/ceiling limit
21. lethal concentration
22. lethal dose
23. parts per million
24. parts per billion
25. immediately dangerous to life and health
26. salivation, lacrimation, urination, diarrhea, gastrointestinal distress, emesis
27. self-contained breathing apparatus
28. air-purifying respirator

Handout 48-27

Student's Name _____

CHAPTER 48 OBJECTIVES CHECKLIST

PART 5: CRIME SCENE AWARENESS

Knowledge	Date Mastered
1. Explain how EMS providers are often mistaken for the police.	
2. Explain specific techniques for risk reduction when approaching highway encounters, violent street incidents, residences, and "dark houses."	
3. Describe the warning signs of potentially violent situations.	
4. Explain emergency evasive techniques for potentially violent situations, including threats of physical violence, firearms encounters, and edged weapons encounters.	
5. Explain EMS considerations for the following types of violent or potentially violent situations: gangs and gang violence, hostages/sniper situations, clandestine drug labs, domestic violence, and emotionally disturbed people.	
6. Explain the following techniques: field "contact and cover" procedures during assessment and care, evasive tactics, and concealment techniques.	
7. Describe police evidence considerations and techniques to assist in evidence preservation.	
8. Given several crime scene scenarios, identify potential hazards and determine if the scene is safe to enter, then provide care, preserving the crime scene as appropriate.	

HANDOUT 48-28

Student's Name _____

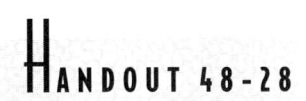

CHAPTER 48 QUIZ

PART 5: CRIME SCENE AWARENESS

Write the letter of the best answer in the space provided.

_____ 1. Arrest rates for violent crime have risen most in which age group?
  A. 10–20 years old
  B. 17–25 years old
  C. 15–34 years old
  D. 35–50 years old

_____ 2. Safety information about a location for an upcoming call commonly comes from all of the following EXCEPT:
  A. information from CAD on the location.
  B. information from law enforcement officers on the location.
  C. your familiarity with the neighborhood.
  D. your experience (or lack of it) at that address.

_____ 3. Signs of impending danger in the setting of a crowd include all of the following EXCEPT:
  A. hostilities toward anyone on the scene.
  B. increasingly loud voices.
  C. inability of police to control bystanders.
  D. rapid decrease in crowd size.

_____ 4. The difference between cover and concealment relates to the degree to which you:
  A. can rapidly exit if needed.
  B. are protected from bullets.
  C. can be seen by others.
  D. can be identified by law enforcement.

_____ 5. Common safety tactics include all of the following EXCEPT:
  A. contact and cover.
  B. retreat.
  C. distraction and evasion.
  D. persuasion and retreat.

_____ 6. Your physical well-being is key to which tactic?
  A. distraction and evasion
  B. retreat
  C. contact and cover
  D. cover and concealment

_____ 7. With the use of contact and cover, the contact provider is responsible for all of the following EXCEPT:
  A. initiating direct patient care.
  B. providing limited function such as handling equipment.
  C. performing patient assessment.
  D. handling most interpersonal contacts at the scene.

_____ 8. Differences in care offered by a TEMS unit and a standard EMS unit include all of the following EXCEPT:
  A. the major priority of patient extraction from the hot zone.
  B. the fact that trauma patients are more frequently encountered than medical patients.
  C. the use of metal clipboards and chemical agents.
  D. consultation with incident commander regarding treatment and transport.

HANDOUT 48-28 Continued

_____ 9. The best material in which to collect potential evidence is:
  A. a plastic bag.
  B. a brown paper bag.
  C. any airtight container.
  D. a glass container.

_____ 10. Evidence that you may be asked to provide includes all of the following EXCEPT:
  A. clothing or other personal effects you removed from the patient.
  B. your scene size-up regarding possible safety threats.
  C. your on-scene observations of setting and persons present.
  D. precautions you took to preserve blood evidence.

HANDOUT 48-29

Student's Name _____

CHAPTER 48 SCENARIO

PART 5: CRIME SCENE AWARENESS

Review the following real-life situation. Then answer the questions that follow.

Dispatch calls at 10:43 P.M. on a hot summer night with a call for "person down in the street" in an area of the city you know well during daylight hours: a neighborhood with two hospitals, medical offices, and other businesses. The dispatcher has no additional information on the call because the caller hung up before she could ask any questions.

As your partner drives down a main street in the neighborhood, you notice how few people are walking by. There isn't much vehicular traffic, either. When your partner turns into the street given in the call, you don't see any cars or pedestrians and almost all of the buildings are completely dark.

Partway down the block, a young man runs into the street and starts waving his arms. You decide to get out and approach the man by walking up the opposite sidewalk. Your partner agrees to park on that side of the street near the corner. He will radio for police backup and come out to cover you from the street if you signal him. If you feel the scene is insecure, you are to retreat toward him and he'll drive forward to pick you up.

The young man looks frightened and is waving his arms frantically. "Hurry up, man. He's bleeding. You've got to help him." He points to a figure slumped on the sidewalk in the shadow of an office building.

You turn toward your partner and use your agreed-upon signal that he should call for police backup, move the ambulance somewhat closer, and then get out to cover you. The young man says "Thanks, man," touches your shoulder gently, and moves toward the figure, who you see is another young man in similar clothes. The second man looks up, sees you, and says, "Please help me. He stuck me with a knife. I'm bleeding."

1. List the information given in the case study that would raise your suspicion of the possibility of danger at the scene or the possibility that the call involves violent crime.

2. The paramedic crew chose to use contact and cover as a safety tactic. Do you agree or disagree with their choice? Explain.

3. Is there any additional information that might have been available to the paramedics that might have influenced their choice of tactic?

CHAPTER 48 REVIEW

PART 5: CRIME SCENE AWARENESS

Write the word or words that best complete each sentence in the space(s) provided.

1. Your most important safety tactic is an ability to identify _____ _____ _____ as soon as possible.
2. A(n) _____ _____ (_____) unit is designed and staffed to handle on-site medical support to law enforcement.
3. Never follow a(n) _____ _____ to the scene of a call: Use lights and siren _____.
4. Two factors that might lead bystanders to confuse EMS providers with police officers are use of _____ and _____ on a vehicle and similarity in _____ or _____.
5. Potentially dangerous scenes include _____, _____, _____, and _____, to name a few.
6. _____ _____ should be well thought out in advance of the response to a hate crime.
7. Remember that EMS and law enforcement officials are on the same side: Be sure to have good _____ _____ with law enforcement.
8. Types of evidence include _____, _____, and _____.
9. Record only the _____ at the scene of a crime, and record them accurately.
10. If you must _____ or _____ an item at a crime scene, remember to tell the police.

HANDOUT 48-31

Student's Name _____

CRIME SCENE AWARENESS TRUE OR FALSE

PART 5: CRIME SCENE AWARENESS

Indicate whether each statement is true or false by writing T or F in the space provided.

_____ 1. Because a significant number of people do not report violent crime to the police, an EMS provider may be the only contact a victim has with a professional who can intervene to prevent further harm.

_____ 2. On arrival at a scene, you should rule out all immediate hazards before you knock on a door for entrance.

_____ 3. Remember that there are only a few cases in which you can legally and ethically retreat without taking the patient with you.

_____ 4. If you have to limit assessment and proceed with rapid transport of a patient because of on-scene danger, be sure to document your reasons for acting quickly.

_____ 5. Retreat signals the end of the call: Thorough documentation will reduce liability and refute charges of abandonment.

_____ 6. The effectiveness of body armor is largely unaffected by wetness or temperature, although it can get uncomfortably warm when worn in hot conditions.

_____ 7. Never jeopardize patient care for the sake of evidence, but do treat every object that may be important as potential evidence in your handling and documentation.

_____ 8. Remember that everything that you and your EMS colleagues see or hear can become evidence in a criminal case.

_____ 9. If you have to move a gun, do not handle it on the grips or handles because you will destroy potentially valuable fingerprints.

_____ 10. Most current body armor will prevent many types of penetration and severe cavitation.

Handout 48-32

Student's Name _____

CRIME SCENE AWARENESS REFERENCE SHEET

PART 5: CRIME SCENE AWARENESS

Some potential warning signs of danger include:

- Violent or abusive behavior
- An altered mental state
- Grabbing or hiding items from inside the vehicle
- Arguing or fighting among passengers
- Lack of activity where activity is expected
- Physical signs of alcohol or drug abuse—namely, liquor bottles, beer cans, or syringes
- Open or unlatched trunks—a potential hiding spot for people or weapons
- Differences among stories told by occupants

To make a safe approach to a vehicle at a roadside emergency, follow these steps:

- Park the ambulance in a position that provides safety from traffic.
- Notify dispatch of the situation, location, the vehicle make and model, and the state and number of the license plate.
- Use a one-person approach. The driver should remain in the ambulance, which is elevated and provides greater visibility.
- The driver should remain prepared to radio for immediate help and to back or drive away rapidly once the other medic returns.
- At nighttime, use the ambulance lights to illuminate the vehicle. However, do not walk between the ambulance and the other vehicle. You will be backlit, forming an easy target.
- Because police approach vehicles from the driver's side, you should approach from the passenger's side—an unexpected route.
- Use the A, B, and C door posts for cover.
- Observe the rear seat. Do not move forward of the C post unless you are sure there are no threats in the rear seat or foot wells.
- Retreat to the ambulance (or another strategic position of cover) at the first sign of danger.
- Make sure you have mapped out your intended retreat and escape with the ambulance driver.

In responding to the scene of any violent crime, keep these precautions in mind:

- Dangerous weapons may have been used in the crime.
- Perpetrators may still be on scene or could return to the scene.
- Patients may sometimes exhibit violence toward EMS, particularly if they risk criminal penalties as a result of the original incident.

HANDOUT 48-32 Continued

Whenever a crowd is present, look for these warning signs of impending danger:

- Shouts or increasingly loud voices
- Pushing or shoving
- Hostilities toward anyone on scene, including the perpetrator of a crime, the victim, the police, and so on
- Rapid increase in crowd size
- Inability of law enforcement officials to control bystanders

Commonly observed gang characteristics include the following:

- Appearance—Gang members frequently wear unique clothing specific to the group. Because the clothing is often a particular color, even a bandana can signify gang membership. Within the gang itself, members sometimes wear different articles to signify rank.
- Graffiti—Gangs have definite territories, or "turfs." Members often mark their turf with graffiti broadcasting the gang's logo, warning away intruders, bragging about crimes, insulting rival gangs, or taunting police.
- Tattoos—Many gang members wear tattoos or other body markings to identify their gang affiliations. Some gangs even require these tattoos. The tattoos will be in the gang's colors and often contain the gang's motto or logo.
- Hand signals/language—Gangs commonly create their own methods of communication. They give gang-related meanings to everyday words or create codes. Hand signals provide quick identification among gang members, warn of approaching law enforcement, or show disrespect to other gangs. Gang members often perform signals so quickly that an uninformed outsider may not spot them, much less understand them.

There are a number of signs that can alert you to the involvement of drugs at an EMS call. These include the following:

- Prior history of drugs in the neighborhood of the call
- Clinical evidence that the patient has used drugs of some kind
- Drug-related comments by bystanders
- Drug paraphernalia visible at the scene such as
  - tiny zip-top bags or vials
  - sandwich bags with the corners torn off (indicating drug packaging) or untied corners of sandwich bags (indicating drug use)
  - syringes or needles
  - glass tubes, pipes, or homemade devices for smoking drugs
  - chemical odors or residues

If you ever come upon a clandestine laboratory, take these actions:

- Leave the area immediately.
- Do not touch anything.
- Never stop any chemical reactions already in progress.
- Do not smoke or bring any source of flame near the lab.
- Notify the police.
- Initiate IMS and hazmat procedures.
- Consider evacuation of the area.

Chapter 48 Answer Key

Part 5: Crime Scene Awareness

Handout 48-28: Chapter 48 Quiz

1. C	4. B	7. B	10. B
2. B	5. D	8. C	
3. D	6. A	9. B	

Handout 48-29: Chapter 48 Scenario

1. Answers include the following:
   - The call to 911 itself is suspicious: It comes long after dark and notes only that a person is down in a nonresidential area. The dispatcher cannot elicit any details because the caller hangs up right away.
   - In addition, there may be an element of concern at time of dispatch that any possible crime would involve drugs, given that the area has hospitals and doctors' offices.
   - While driving to the scene, you note there are few vehicles or pedestrians, which means you are more isolated.
   - In addition, the street location itself has no vehicles or pedestrians and is deserted and dark.
   - At the scene, you see only one person, a young man (in the age group [15–34 years] most likely to commit violent crime) who is visibly distraught.
   - The apparent patient, described only as "bleeding," is in a poorly lit, isolated spot.
   - The patient is another young man wearing clothes similar to the distraught man's, which might signal possible gang involvement.
   - The patient says he was stabbed, which makes it a crime scene.

2. There is no one way to handle an incident, and often wisdom comes only with hindsight. In the scenario, the contact provider decided that the scene was sufficiently safe to initiate patient contact with appropriate cover given by his partner (and with the knowledge that police had been notified). He may have noted that the man in the street seemed genuinely frightened and concerned for the patient and showed no hostility or fear toward the paramedic. In fact, he seemed grateful for help. A more conservative option would have been to call for police backup and wait for its arrival before exiting the ambulance. The unit would then have been capable of quickest retreat. This option could have been justified on the basis of the following:
   - The isolated nature of the scene
   - The lack of bystanders
   - The darkness of the scene (which could have been concealing individuals intent on harming the paramedics or stealing drugs from the ambulance)
   - The possibility of street crime or gang involvement
   - The presence of a number of doctors' offices, any of which could have been robbed for drugs or medical equipment

3. Answers might include any of the following:
   - Information from the dispatcher (or personal knowledge) about whether there had been incidents of attacks/thefts from ambulance crews in the city, particularly in that neighborhood
   - Information from the dispatcher (or personal knowledge) about whether the area had a high incidence of street crime, gang-related violence, or drug-related violence
   - Information from the dispatcher (or personal knowledge) of average time for police backup to arrive in that area at that time of night

Handout 48-30: Chapter 48 Review

1. potentially violent situations
2. tactical EMS (TEMS)
3. police car, cautiously (if at all)
4. lights, siren, uniforms, badges
5. Any four of the following are acceptable: highway encounters, violent street incidents, murders/assaults/robberies, dangerous crowds, street gangs, drug-related crimes, clandestine drug labs, domestic violence
6. Crew assignments
7. ongoing communication
8. Any three of the following are acceptable: prints (fingerprints, footprints, tire prints, etc.), blood and blood splatter, body fluids, particulate evidence, on-scene EMS observations
9. facts
10. touch, move

Handout 48-31: Crime Scene Awareness True or False

1. T	4. T	7. T	10. F
2. F	5. F	8. T	
3. F	6. F	9. F	

Chapter 49

Responding To Terrorist Acts

INTRODUCTION

The events of September 11, 2001, have greatly impacted our society and our sensitivity to the threat of terrorist acts. This new awareness forces the EMS community to prepare itself to respond to acts of terrorism. Though the weapon of choice used by terrorist groups worldwide is the conventional explosive, it is clear that the twenty-first century will bring new terrorism threats using more unconventional means, such as commercial aircraft to bring down structures and weapons of mass destruction including nuclear, biological, and chemical weapons.

CHAPTER OBJECTIVES

After reading this chapter, you should be able to:

*1. Identify the typical weapons of mass destruction likely to be used by terrorists. (pp. 1891–1902)

*2. Explain the mechanisms of injury associated with conventional and nuclear weapons of mass destruction. (pp. 1892–1895)

*3. Identify and describe the major subclassifications of chemical and biological weapons of mass destruction. (pp. 1895–1902)

*4. List the scene evidence that might alert the EMS provider to a terrorist attack that involves a weapon of mass destruction. (pp. 1902–1903)

*5. Describe the special safety precautions and safety equipment appropriate for an incident involving nuclear, biological, or chemical weapons. (pp. 1902–1903)

*6. Identify the assessment and management concerns for victims of conventional, nuclear, biological, and chemical weapons. (pp. 1892–1902)

*7. Given a narrative description of a conventional, nuclear, biological, or chemical terrorist attack, identify the elements of scene size-up that suggest terrorism and identify the likely injuries and any special patient management considerations necessary. (pp. 1891–1903)

*NOTE: The objectives for this chapter are not included in the DOT Paramedic curriculum.

TOTAL TEACHING TIME

There is no specific time requirement for this topic in the National Standard Curriculum for Paramedic. Instructors should take into consideration such factors as the pace at which students learn, the size of the class, and breaks. The actual time devoted to teaching objectives is the responsibility of the instructor.

©2007 Pearson Education, Inc.
Essentials of Paramedic Care, 2nd ed.

FRAMING THE LESSON

Begin by reviewing the important points from Chapter 48, "Operations." Discuss any points that the class does not completely understand. Then move on to Chapter 49. Briefly highlight recent incidents of WMD, including the London subway bombing (2005); the Madrid train bombing (2004); anthrax-laced letters (2001); destruction of the World Trade Center Towers (2001); sarin gas release in the Tokyo Subway System (1996); Oklahoma City federal building bombing (1995); and first World Trade Center bombing (1993). Discuss that terrorism is a worldwide problem. During their career in EMS, it is possible students will be called upon to respond to some type of terrorist act or mass casualty incident (MCI).

TEACHING STRATEGIES

People learn in a variety of ways. Some do better with the spoken word, whereas others prefer the written. Some prefer to work alone, whereas others profit from working in groups. Recognizing these different ways of acquiring knowledge, the authors of this *Instructor's Resource Manual* have provided a variety of teaching strategies for the different types of learners. These strategies are intended to foster higher-level cognitive skills and encourage creative learning and problem solving. For greatest effectiveness, incorporate these strategies into your class lecture. Symbols in the Lecture Outline indicate the points at which various exercises might be most appropriate. Other strategies can be used to preview the lesson or to summarize it.

The following strategies are keyed to specific sections of the lesson.

1. Thinking about Associated Dangers. Have students consider the effects of an explosive agent in their own communities. Map out a section of the community in which your school stands. If possible, include both commercial and residential areas. Have students identify, either by educated guess or by actual investigation, the potential hazards that exist in each building or space. Facilitate a discussion about how those materials would need to be handled if a terrorist incident occurred at one of those buildings.

2. Assigned Reading. *Vector* by Robin Cook is one novel among many that addresses the use and danger of biological weapons. Encourage students to read one such book and report on the themes. Or buy several paperback copies and use them as prizes when playing review games in class.

3. Assigned Viewing. *Outbreak* (1995) by Warner Brothers is a movie that addresses the spread of an ebola outbreak from its African origins to a small California community. Encourage students to view this video and report on the themes.

4. Guest Speaker: ESDA/OEM Official. Consider inviting a representative from your area ESDA/OEM office to discuss response preparedness and the role of EMS.

5. Table-Top Exercise. Use a community layout and Matchbox-type vehicles to role play management of a terrorist act on "Anywhere, USA." Students should utilize the incident command system (ICM) to manage the situation.

The following strategies can be used at various points throughout the lesson or to help summarize and demonstrate what students have learned.

Field Trip. If an explosive hazmat incident occurred in your area, consider a field trip to the site, preferably in the company of an EMS provider who served there. Discuss relevant details on the nature of the hazardous materials involved and the extent of contamination. Also consider the equipment and the medical care provided on site and during transportation, including decontamination efforts and precautions taken against secondary contamination during packaging and transport.

Recognizing Disaster Management Factors. Write the names of several potential disasters on strips of paper and place them in a hat. Have small groups of students draw a disaster and identify mitigating factors. If these factors do not exist in your community, brainstorm solutions and share important ideas with folks who can make a difference, such as by way of a letter to your council representative, fire chief, city planner, and so on. This activity lends realism to disaster management concepts and promotes community activism.

Participating in MCI Drills. Nearly every health department in the nation has annual mass-casualty drills. Obtain the schedule and have your class included. When possible, have them integrated into the responding unit crews. If it is not possible for students to play patient care roles, be sure they are included as patients. Even observing a large-scale drill will be educational. Asking to participate in an already scheduled drill will save you the enormous effort required to stage one of your own.

Cultural Considerations, Legal Notes, and Patho Pearls. The Student CD-ROM contains this series of informative features to enhance the student's understanding of the material covered in this chapter.

TEACHING OUTLINE

Chapter 49 is the ninth lesson in Division 5, *Special Considerations/Operations*. Distribute Handout 49-1. If students have any questions about the objectives, answer them at this time.

Then present the chapter. One possible lecture outline follows. In the outline, the parenthetical references in regular type are references to text pages; those in bold type are references to figures, tables, or procedures.

I. Introduction. Terrorism threats may involve weapons of mass destruction (WMD) including nuclear, biological, and chemical (NBC) weapons. (p. 1891) (**Fig. 49-1, p. 1891**)

II. Explosive agents (p. 1892) (**Fig. 49-2, p. 1902**)

  A. Explosives (p. 1892)
      1. Most likely method by which terrorists will strike
      2. Compression/decompression injuries
      3. Secondary explosions
  B. Incendiary agents (p. 1892)
      1. Less explosive power and greater heat and burn potential
  C. Incorporating other agents with explosives (p. 1892)

III. Nuclear detonation (pp. 1893–1895) (**Figs. 49-3, p. 1893**)

  A. Release of energy that is generated when heavy nuclei split (fission) or light nuclei combine (fusion) to form new elements (p. 1893)
  B. Nuclear radiation cannot be felt, seen, or otherwise detected by any of our senses (p. 1893)

HANDOUT 49-1
Chapter 49 Objectives Checklist

READING/REFERENCES
Erich, J. "The Expert Take: Assessing the Terrorism Issues Facing EMS," *Emergency Medical Services*, Jan. 2002.

POWERPOINT PRESENTATION
Chapter 49 PowerPoint slides 4–5

POWERPOINT PRESENTATION
Chapter 49 PowerPoint slides 6–7

READING/REFERENCES
Sachs, E. M. "The Bubonic Man: Lessons from a Bioterrorism Incident," *Emergency Medical Services*, Aug. 2000.

POWERPOINT PRESENTATION
Chapter 49 PowerPoint slide 8

C. Mechanisms of injury (pp. 1893–1894)
  1. Initial detonation
  2. Fallout
D. Nuclear incident response (p. 1894)
  1. First hour spent moving patients to safety
  2. Evacuation of fallout area
  3. Geiger counter
  4. Dosimeter
  5. Sodium iodine tablets
E. Radioactive contamination (pp. 1894–1895)
  1. Results in an explosion site, with radioactive material contaminating the immediate vicinity

IV. Chemical agents (pp. 1895–1900)
A. Volatility (p. 1895)
B. Specific gravity (p. 1895)
C. Nerve agents (pp. 1895–1896)
  1. Agents generally inhibit the degradation of a neurotransmitter (acetylcholine) and quickly cause a nervous system overload.
  2. SLUDGE signs and symptoms
     a. Salivation
     b. Lacrimation
     c. Urination
     d. Defecation
     e. Gastric Emptying (also may see this as *Gastric distress and Emesis* in some sources)
  3. Treatment includes the administration of atropine and then pralidoxime chloride (Mark I kit)
D. Vesicants (blistering agents) (p. 1896)
  1. agents that damage exposed tissue, frequently causing vesicles (blisters)
E. Pulmonary agents (p. 1896)
F. Biotoxins (p. 1897)
G. Incapacitating agents (pp. 1897–1898)
H. Other hazardous chemicals (p. 1898)
I. Recognition of a chemical agent release (p. 1898)
J. Management of a chemical agent release (pp. 1898–1900) (**Fig. 49-4, p. 1899**)

V. Biologic agents (pp. 1900–1902) (**Table 49-1, p. 1900**)
A. Pneumonia-like agents (p. 1901)
B. Encephalitis-like agents (p. 1901)
C. Other agents (p. 1901)
D. Protection against biologic agent transmission (pp. 1901–1902) (**Fig. 49-5, p. 1901**)

VI. General considerations regarding terrorist attacks (pp. 1902–1903)
A. Scene safety (p. 1902)
B. Recognizing a terrorist attack (pp. 1902–1903)
C. Responding to a terrorist attack (p. 1903)

VII. Chapter summary (p. 1903). Many of the mechanisms of injury used by terrorists subtly induce their damage (toxic gases, radiation contamination, or biological agents) so that there is little scene evidence. Your responsibility is to maintain an enhanced lookout for any signs of NBC release or exposure and limit the contact you, the general population, and your patients have to such an agent. In general, it is not the role of EMS to deal with NBC agents. Your role as a paramedic is likely to be providing supportive care after patient decontamination.

ASSIGNMENTS

Assign students to complete Chapter 49, "Responding to Terrorist Acts," of the workbook.

EVALUATION

Chapter Quiz and Scenario   Distribute copies of the Chapter Quiz provided in Handout 49-2 to evaluate student understanding of this chapter. Make sure each student reads the scenario to reinforce critical thinking on the scene. Remind students not to use their notes or textbooks while taking the quiz.

Student CD   Quizzes for every chapter are contained on the dynamic and highly visual in-text student CD.

Companion Website   Additional quizzes for every chapter are contained on this exciting website.

TestGen   You may wish to create a custom-tailored test using *Prentice Hall TestGen for Essentials of Paramedic Care*, 2nd Edition to evaluate student understanding of this chapter.

On-line Test Preparation   (for students and instructors). Additional test preparation is available through Brady's new on-line product, *EMT Achieve: Paramedic Test Preparation* at *http://www.prenhall.com/emtachieve/*. Instructors can also monitor student mastery on-line.

Review Manual for the EMT-Paramedic   This comprehensive exam review contains hundreds of test questions and rationales, including scenarios, along with two 180-question practice tests on CD.

REINFORCEMENT

Handouts   If classroom discussion or performance on the quiz indicates that some students have not fully mastered the chapter content, you may wish to assign some or all of the Reinforcement Handouts for this chapter.

Student CD (for students)   A wide variety of material on this CD-ROM will reinforce and also expand student knowledge and skills.

PowerPoint Presentation (for instructors)   The PowerPoint material developed for this chapter offers useful reinforcement of chapter content.

Companion Website (for students)   Additional review quizzes and links to EMS resources will contribute to further reinforcement of the chapter.

OneKey   On-line support is offered for this course on one of three platforms: CourseCompass, Blackboard, or Web CT. Includes the IRM, PowerPoints, TestGen, and Companion Website for instruction. Ask your local sales representative for more information.

Brady Skills Series: Advanced Life Skills (Video or CD)   Have your students watch the skills come to life on VHS or CD-ROM, or they can purchase the highly visual, full-color text with step-by-step procedures with rationales.

TESTGEN
Chapter 49

EMT ACHIEVE: PARAMEDIC TEST PREPARATION
Mistovich & Beasley. *EMT Achieve: Paramedic Test Preparation,* www.prenhall.com/emtachieve/

REVIEW MANUAL FOR THE EMT-PARAMEDIC
Cherry & Mistovich. *Review Manual for the EMT-Paramedic,* 3rd edition.

HANDOUT 49-4
Reinforcement Activity

PARAMEDIC STUDENT CD
Student Activities

POWERPOINT PRESENTATION
Chapter 49

COMPANION WEBSITE
http://www.prenhall.com/bledsoe

ONEKEY
Chapter 49

ADVANCED LIFE SUPPORT SKILLS
Larmon & Davis. *Advanced Life Support Skills.*

ADVANCED LIFE SKILLS REVIEW
Larmon & Davis. *Advanced Life Skills Review.*

BRADY SKILLS SERIES: ALS
Larmon & Davis. *Brady Skills Series: ALS.*

PARAMEDIC NATIONAL STANDARDS SELF-TEST
Miller. *Paramedic National Standards Self-Test,* 4th edition.

HANDOUT 49-1

Student's Name _____

CHAPTER 49 OBJECTIVES CHECKLIST

Knowledge	Date Mastered
1. Identify the typical weapons of mass destruction likely to be used by terrorists.	
2. Explain the mechanisms of injury associated with conventional and nuclear weapons of mass destruction.	
3. Identify and describe the major subclassifications of chemical and biological weapons of mass destruction.	
4. List the scene evidence that might alert the EMS provider to a terrorist attack that involves a weapon of mass destruction.	
5. Describe the special safety precautions and safety equipment appropriate for an incident involving nuclear, biological, or chemical weapons.	
6. Identify the assessment and management concerns for victims of conventional, nuclear, biological, and chemical weapons.	
7. Given a narrative description of a conventional, nuclear, biological, or chemical terrorist attack, identify the elements of scene size-up that suggest terrorism and identify the likely injuries and any special patient management considerations necessary.	

HANDOUT 49-2

Student's Name _____

CHAPTER 49 QUIZ

Write the letter of the best answer in the space provided.

_____ 1. Which of the following is considered a weapon of mass destruction?
   A. nuclear bomb
   B. chemical weapon
   C. biological agent
   D. all of the these

_____ 2. Which one of the following injuries is NOT expected from a conventional explosive blast?
   A. blunt trauma
   B. penetrating trauma
   C. severe and extensive burns
   D. compression/decompression injury

_____ 3. Which one of the following is considered an incendiary agent?
   A. tularemia
   B. napalm
   C. sarin
   D. ebola

_____ 4. The danger that separates the conventional from the nuclear detonation is:
   A. radiation.
   B. strength of the explosion.
   C. high incidence of burn injury.
   D. all of the these

_____ 5. The site of a nuclear detonation is generally radiation free from moments after the blast until _____ hour(s) post ignition.
   A. 1
   B. 6
   C. 12
   D. 48

_____ 6. In addition to an explosive agent, the "dirty bomb" contains which one of the following?
   A. chemical agent
   B. radioactive material
   C. biological agent only
   D. both chemical and biological agents

_____ 7. A volatile chemical agent does which one of the following?
   A. gathers in low spots like a subway
   B. converts quickly to a gas from a liquid
   C. causes blistering and respiratory injury
   D. interrupts the transmission of central nervous system impulses

_____ 8. The chemical agent that produces the SLUDGE signs is a:
   A. vesicant.
   B. biotoxin.
   C. nerve agent.
   D. pulmonary agent.

_____ 9. One of the most deadly toxic agents known is a:
   A. vesicant.
   B. biotoxin.
   C. nerve agent.
   D. pulmonary agent.

_____ 10. Which one of the following agents is most likely to produce blistering?
   A. vesicant
   B. biotoxin
   C. nerve agent
   D. pulmonary agent

_____ 11. Which one of the following is the most likely and most dependable clue to the release of a chemical agent?
   A. strange smell
   B. cloud of vapor
   C. multiple patients with similar signs and symptoms
   D. large numbers of dead insects found crushed on your windshield

HANDOUT 49-2 Continued

_____ 12. Which one of the following statements about the time of release of a biological agent is CORRECT?
   A. The patient's breath usually has a strange odor.
   B. You can see a cloud of vapor above storage containers.
   C. Multiple patients immediately complain of similar symptoms.
   D. There may be no indication of an agent being released at all.

_____ 13. Who most likely will recognize a biological agent release?
   A. emergency department personnel
   B. hazardous materials team
   C. EMT-Intermediates
   D. first responders

_____ 14. Which one of the following is the recommended and most effective form of protection against an infectious biological agent?
   A. body substance isolation precautions
   B. self-contained breathing apparatus
   C. 10 percent hypochlorite solution
   D. Mark I kit

_____ 15. The victim of a chemical or nuclear attack needs which one of the following before you begin care?
   A. iodine tablets
   B. proper decontamination
   C. application of a HEPA respirator
   D. administration of the Mark I Kit contents

HANDOUT 49-3

Student's Name _____

CHAPTER 49 SCENARIO

Review the following real-life situation. Then answer the question that follows.

It is a warm, summer weekend and your community's annual street festival is in full swing. Officials report that this is the largest turnout in the festival's history. You are dispatched to the main grandstand area where a large crowd has gathered to hear a highly publicized band performance. Tony and Hilda are on duty and dispatched to the festival's first aid station for a burn patient. Upon arriving at the first aid station, you are advised there are additional patients, all presenting with similar signs and symptoms. After calling for additional assistance, you begin to evaluate and triage the patients. Common signs and symptoms include burns to exposed arms and legs, some blistering; rhinorrhea, cough and dyspnea; and nausea and vomiting.

1. Given your initial assessment of the scene and patients, what is the probable mechanism of injury?

2. How should additional ambulances respond to the scene? How should the other spectators be managed?

3. What treatment should be provided to these patients?

Handout 49-4

Student's Name _____

CHAPTER 49 REVIEW

Write the word or words that best complete each sentence in the space(s) provided.

1. Called ____ ____ ____ ____, the chemical, biological, and nuclear weapons used by terrorists are meant to create a maximum number of casualties.

2. The use of violence to provoke fear and influence behavior for political, social, religious, or ethnic goals is called a ____ act.

3. A special subset of explosives, ____ ____ have less explosive power but greater heat and burn potential.

4. Radioactive dust and particles that threaten the lives of people far from the epicenter of a nuclear detonation are called ____.

5. A(n) ____ ____ is an instrument used to detect and measure the radiation given off by an object or area.

6. A(n) ____ is an instrument that measures the cumulative amount of radiation absorbed.

7. A conventional explosive device that distributes radioactive material over a large area is called a(n) ____ ____.

8. The term ____ refers to the ease by which a chemical changes from a liquid to a gas.

9. ____ ____ refers to the density or weight of a vapor or gas as compared to air.

10. The term ____ ____ refers to chemicals that restrict the degradation of neurotransmitters such as acetylcholine and quickly facilitate a nervous system overload.

11. The ____ ____ ____ is a two-part auto-injector set that the military uses as treatment for nerve-agent exposure.

12. A(n) ____ is an agent that damages exposed skin, frequently causing vesicles (blisters).

13. ____ agents are chemicals that primarily cause injury to the lungs.

14. A(n) ____ is a poison that is produced by living organisms but is itself not alive.

15. A(n) ____ agent is either a living organism or a toxin produced by a living organism that is deliberately distributed to cause disease and death.